Thoracolumbar Spine Fractures

Thoracolumbar Spine Fractures

Editors

Yizhar Floman, M.D.
*Professor of Orthopaedic Surgery
Department of Orthopaedic Surgery
Spine Surgery Unit
Hebrew University—Hadassah Medical School
Hadassah University Hospital
Jerusalem, Israel*

Jean-Pierre C. Farcy, M.D.
*Associate Clinical Professor of Orthopaedics
Columbia University College of
Physicians and Surgeons
Associate Attending Orthopaedic Surgeon
Columbia-Presbyterian Medical Center
New York, New York*

Claude Argenson, M.D.
*Professor of Orthopaedic Surgery
University of Nice
Chief of Service
Department of Orthopaedic Surgery
St. Roch University Hospital
Nice, France*

Raven Press 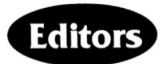 New York

Raven Press, Ltd., 1185 Avenue of the Americas, New York, New York 10036

© 1993 Raven Press, Ltd. All rights reserved. This book is protected by copyright. No part of it may be reproduced, stored in a retrieval system, or transmitted, in any form or by any means, electronic, mechanical, photocopying, or recording, or otherwise, without the written permission of the publisher.

Made in the United States of America

Library of Congress Cataloging-in-Publication Data

Thoracolumbar spine fractures / editors, Yizhar Floman, Jean-Pierre C.
  Farcy, Claude Argenson.
      p. cm.
    Includes bibliographical references and index.
    ISBN 0-7817-0049-3
    1. Thoracic vertebrae—Fractures. 2. Lumbar vertebrae—Fractures.
  3. Spinal cord—Wounds and injuries. I. Floman, Yizhar.
  II. Farcy, Jean-Pierre C. III. Argenson, Claude.
    [DNLM: 1. Lumbar Vertebrae—injuries. 2. Spinal Cord Injuries.
  3. Spinal Fractures. 4. Thoracic Vertebrae—injuries. WE 725
  T4875 1993]
  RD768.T47 1993
  617.15'1—dc20
  DNLM/DLC
  for Library of Congress   92-48559

The material contained in this volume was submitted as previously unpublished material, except in the instances in which credit has been given to the source from which some of the illustrative material was derived.

Great care has been taken to maintain the accuracy of the information contained in the volume. However, neither Raven Press nor the editors can be held responsible for errors or for any consequences arising from the use of the information contained herein.

Materials appearing in this book prepared by individuals as part of their official duties as U.S. Government employees are not covered by the above-mentioned copyright.

9 8 7 6 5 4 3 2 1

Dedication

To all patients who have suffered a thoracolumbar spine fracture, and especially to those who still fight a subsequent disability.

Thoracolumbar spine fractures and the resultant complications may be devastating and result in lifetime problems for patients who were, most often, young and active.

Any effort to better comprehend, analyze, and treat the consequences of spine disruption and the damaged neural structures is a remarkable endeavor.

Each contributor to this book is committed to improving the treatment of thoracolumbar spine fractures. It is hoped their contributions will help to improve the prognosis for these injuries.

Y.F.
J-P.C.F.
C.A.

and

To Efrat, Roni, Yonathan, Omri, and Ori, with love.

Y.F.

To my family, with admiration and love.

J.-P.C.F.

*To my wife, Any
and my children, Jean-Noël, and Christopher
for their love and support.*

C.A.

Contents

Contributors xi

Acknowledgments xv

Preface xvii

Section I. Basic Sciences

1. Organogenesis and Development of the Thoracic, Lumbar, and Sacral Spine 1
   Fernand de Peretti and Claude Argenson

2. Anatomy of the Thoracolumbar and Sacral Spine with Special Consideration for Implant Insertion 11
   Fernand de Peretti and Claude Argenson

3. Physiology and Pathophysiology of the Neural Elements 35
   Jean-Pierre C. Farcy and Bernard A. Rawlins

4. Biomechanics of the Normal Thoracolumbar Spine and Their Applications to Fractures 45
   Alain Tanguy

5. Epidemiology of Traumatic Spinal Column and Cord Injuries ... 59
   Milka Donchin

6. Descriptive Epidemiology of Traumatic Spinal Cord Injury in New York State 65
   John H. Relethford

Section II. Imaging and Diagnostic Modalities

7. Imaging of Thoracic and Lumbar Vertebral Fractures 69
   Richard H. Daffner

8. Electrophysiology of the Normal and Diseased Spine 99
   Jörg Herdmann and Jiří Dvořák

9. Intraoperative Ultrasonography in Spinal Trauma 123
   Nathan H. Lebwohl and Parley W. Madsen

Section III: Classification and Management

10. Classification of Thoracolumbar Spine Fractures 131
Claude Argenson and Pascal Boileau

11. Neurologic Injuries: Syndromes, Diagnosis, and Prognosis 157
E. Shannon Stauffer

12. Intensive Care of the Spinal Cord Injured Patient 167
Reuven Pizov, Leonid Eidelman, and Yizhar Floman

13. Early Management of Spinal Cord Injury 173
Paul C. McCormick and Bennett M. Stein

14. Orthopaedic Principles of Surgical Management 179
Claude Argenson

15. Specific Injuries and Management 195
Claude Argenson and Pascal Boileau

16. Conservative Management of Burst Fractures 215
Joseph E. Mumford and James N. Weinstein

17. Low Lumbar (L3-L4-L5) Burst Fractures 223
Keith H. Bridwell

18. Considerations in Management of Facet Joint Injuries 235
Mark Weidenbaum and Jean-Pierre C. Farcy

19. Sacral Fractures: Diagnosis and Management 245
Francis Denis

Section IV: Techniques and Spinal Instrumentation

20. Anterior Techniques of Decompression and Fixation 251
James C. Bayley, Hansen A. Yuan, and Bruce E. Fredrickson

21. Anterior Decompression and Instrumentation in the Management of Thoracolumbar Injuries, with Special Reference to Burst Fractures 267
Yizhar Floman

22. Posterior Instrumentation in the Management of Thoracolumbar Injuries 279
Yizhar Floman

Section V: Specific Problems Related to Age and Etiology

23. Thoracic and Lumbar Spine Injuries in Children 307
Gerard Bollini

24. Spinal Deformities Secondary to Traumatic Lesions Involving the Spine and Spinal Cord in Children 327
Jean Dubousset

25. Thoracolumbar Fractures in Osteoporosis 339
Felicia Cosman and Robert Lindsay

26. Surgical Management of Primary and Secondary Bone Tumors of the Thoracolumbar Spine 359
Joseph Y. Margulies, Yizhar Floman, and Michael G. Neuwirth

27. Fractures of the Spine in Ankylosing Spondylitis 385
Edward H. Simmons and Avi J. Bernstein

Section VI: Management of Complications and Rehabilitation

28. Systemic Complications of Spinal Cord Injuries 409
Avital Fast

29. Post-Traumatic Syringomyelia: A General Review 421
Jafar J. Jafar, Ramesh Babu, Bernard Sigel, and Junju Machi

30. Post-Traumatic Syringomyelia: Surgical Management and Case Reports .. 429
Bernard Williams

31. Late Deformities 449
Steven D. Glassman and Jean-Pierre C. Farcy

32. Rehabilitation Principles in the Management of Thoracolumbar Spine Fractures 463
Kristjan T. Ragnarsson

Subject Index 485

Contributors

Claude Argenson, M.D. *Professor of Orthopaedic Surgery, Chief of Service, Service de Chirurgie Orthopedique et Traumatologique, Centre Hospitalier Regional et Universitaire de Nice, St. Roch University Hospital, Pierre Devoluy Street 5, 06000 Nice, France*

Ramesh Babu, M.D. *Department of Neurosurgery, New York University, 530 First Avenue, New York, New York 10016*

James C. Bayley, M.D. *Assistant Professor, Department of Orthopaedic Surgery, Harvard Medical School, and Beth Israel Hospital, 330 Brookline Avenue, Boston, Massachusetts 02215*

Avi J. Bernstein, M.D. *Clinical Instructor, Department of Orthopaedic Surgery, University of Chicago, The Pritzker School of Medicine, and the Lutheran General Hospital, 1875 Dempster Street, Suite 425, Park Ridge, Illinois 60068-1145*

Pascal Boileau, M.D. *Chief of Clinic, Department of Orthopaedic Surgery, St. Roch University Hospital, Pierre Devoluy Street 5, 06031 Nice, France*

Gerard Bollini, M.D. *Chief of Service, Professor of Orthopaedic Surgery, Hôpital Timone Enfants, Bd Jean Moulin, 13385 Marseille Cedex 5, France*

Keith H. Bridwell, M.D. *Associate Professor, Division of Orthopedic Surgery, Washington University School of Medicine, Suite 11300, West Pavilion, One Barnes Hospital Plaza, St. Louis, Missouri 63110*

Felicia Cosman, M.D. *Assistant Professor of Clinical Medicine, Department of Medicine, Columbia University College of Physicians and Surgeons, New York, New York, and Regional Bone Center, Helen Hayes Hospital, Route 9-W, West Haverstraw, New York 10993*

Richard H. Daffner, M.D., F.A.C.R. *Professor of Radiologic Sciences, Department of Diagnostic Radiology, The Medical College of Pennsylvania, Allegheny Campus, and Allegheny General Hospital, 320 East North Avenue, Pittsburgh, Pennsylvania 15212-9986*

Francis Denis, M.D. *Clinical Assistant Professor of Orthopaedic Surgery, University of Minnesota, and Minnesota Spine Center, 606 24th Avenue South, Suite 602, Minneapolis, Minnesota 55454*

Milka Donchin, M.D., M.P.H. *Department of Social Medicine, Hebrew University Hadassah School of Public Health and Community Medicine, and Hadassah Medical Organization, P.O. Box 12000, Jerusalem 91120, Israel*

Jean Dubousset, M.D. *Professor, University of René Descartes, Department of Pediatric Orthopaedic Surgery, St. Vincent de Paul Hospital, 82 Av Denfert Rochereau, 75014 Paris Cedex 14, France*

Jiří Dvořák, M.D. *PD Dr. med., Department of Neurology, Spine Unit, W. Schulthess Hospitals, Neumünsterallee 3, 8008 Zürich, Switzerland*

Leonid Eidelman, M.D. *Lecturer, Departments of Anesthesiology and Critical Care Medicine, Hadassah University Hospital, Kiryat Hadassah, P.O. Box 12000, Jerusalem 91120, Israel*

Jean-Pierre C. Farcy, M.D. *Associate Clinical Professor of Orthopaedics, Columbia University College of Physicians and Surgeons, and Associate Attending Orthopaedic Surgeon, Columbia-Presbyterian Medical Center, 161 Fort Washington Avenue, New York, New York 10032*

Avital Fast, M.D. *Chairman, Department of Rehabilitation Medicine, St. Vincent's Hospital & Medical Center of New York, 153 West 11th Street, New York, New York 10011, and Associate Professor of Rehabilitation Medicine, New York Medical College, New York, New York*

Yizhar Floman, M.D. *Professor of Orthopaedic Surgery, Department of Orthopaedic Surgery and Spine Surgery Unit, Hebrew University—Hadassah Medical School, Hadassah University Hospital, P.O. Box 12000, Jerusalem 91120, Israel*

Bruce E. Fredrickson, M.D. *Professor, Department of Orthopaedic Surgery, State University of New York, Health Science Center at Syracuse, 550 Harrison Street, Suite 100, Syracuse, New York 13202-3072*

Steven D. Glassman, M.D. *Instructor, Department of Orthopaedic Surgery, University of Louisville, School of Medicine, Louisville, Kentucky 40292*

Jörg Herdmann, M.D. *Dr. med., Department of Neurosurgery, Heinrich-Heine-University of Düsseldorf, Moorenstrasse 5, 4000 Düsseldorf 1, Germany*

Jafar J. Jafar, M.D. *Associate Professor, Department of Neurosurgery, New York University Medical Center, 560 First Avenue, New York, New York 10016*

Nathan H. Lebwohl, M.D. *Assistant Professor, Department of Orthopaedics and Rehabilitation, University of Miami/Jackson Memorial Medical Center, Rehabilitation Center Room 303, 1611 N.W. 12th Avenue, Miami, Florida 33101*

Robert Lindsay, M.B.Ch.B., Ph.D., F.R.C.P. *Professor of Clinical Medicine, Department of Medicine, Columbia University College of Physicians and Surgeons, New York, New York, and Regional Bone Center, Helen Hayes Hospital, Route 9-W, West Haverstrew, New York 10993*

Junju Machi, M.D., Ph.D. *Research Assistant Professor, Surgical Research Division, Department of Surgery, Medical College of Pennsylvania, 3300 Henry Avenue, Philadelphia, Pennsylvania 19129*

Parley W. Madsen, M.D., Ph.D. *Assistant Professor, Department of Neurological Surgery, University of Miami School of Medicine, Miami, Florida 33101*

Joseph Y. Margulies, M.D., Ph.D. *Orthopaedic Department/Spine Service, Hospital for Joint Disease/Orthopaedic Institute, 301 East 17th Street, New York, New York 10003*

Paul C. McCormick, M.D. *Assistant Professor of Neurological Surgery, Columbia-Presbyterian Medical Center, NI2-204, 710 West 168 Street, New York, New York 10032*

Joseph E. Mumford, M.D. *Orthopedic Associates, P.A., 909 Mulvane Avenue, Topeka, Kansas 66606*

Michael G. Neuwirth, M.D. *Chief of Spine Service, Hospital for Joint Disease/Orthopaedic Institute, 301 East 17th Street, New York, New York 10003*

Fernand de Peretti, M.D. *Associate Professor of Anatomy, Department of Orthopaedic Surgery, St. Roch University Hospital, Pierre Devoluy Street 5, 06030 Nice, France*

Reuven Pizov, M.D. *Intensive Care Unit, Department of Anesthesiology, Hadassah University Hospital, P.O.B. 12000, Jerusalem 91120, Israel*

Kristjan T. Ragnarsson, M.D. *Dr. Lucy G. Moses Professor and Chairman, Department of Rehabilitation Medicine, Mount Sinai School of Medicine, Box 1240, New York, New York 10029*

Bernard A. Rawlins, M.D., M.S. *Chief Resident, Department of Orthopaedic Surgery, Columbia-Presbyterian Medical Center, 161 Fort Washington Avenue, New York, New York 10032*

John H. Relethford, Ph.D. *Associate Professor and Chair, Department of Anthropology, State University of New York College at Oneonta, Oneonta, New York 13820-4015*

Bernard Sigel, M.D. *Professor of Surgery, and Director, Surgical Research Division, Department of Surgery, Medical College of Pennsylvania, 3300 Henry Avenue, Philadelphia, Pennsylvania 19129*

Edward H. Simmons, M.D., F.R.C.S.(C.), M.S.(T.O.R.), F.A.C.S. *Professor, Department of Orthopaedic Surgery, State University of New York at Buffalo, 50 High Street, Suite 805, Buffalo, New York 14203, and Director of University Orthopaedic Spine Service, Head, Orthopaedic Department, Buffalo General Hospital, Buffalo, New York*

E. Shannon Stauffer, M.D. *Department of Orthopaedic Surgery, Southern Illinois School of Medicine, P.O. Box 19230, Springfield, Illinois 62794*

Bennett M. Stein, M.D. *Chairman, Department of Neurological Surgery, Columbia-Presbyterian Medical Center, NI-4, 710 West 168th Street, New York, New York 10032*

Alain Tanguy, M.D. *Professor of Pediatric Orthopaedics, Service Chirurgie Infantile, Hotel-Dieu, BP69, 63000 Clermont-Ferrand, France*

Mark Weidenbaum, M.D. *Assistant Professor, Department of Orthopaedic Surgery, College of Physicians and Surgeons, Columbia-Presbyterian Medical Center, 622 West 168th Street, New York, New York 10032*

James N. Weinstein, M.S., D.O. *Professor, Department of Orthopaedic Surgery, Director, Spine Diagnostic & Treatment Center, University of Iowa Hospitals and Clinics, 200 Hawkins Drive, #1201-1 RCP, Iowa City, Iowa 52242-1088*

Bernard Williams, M.D., Ch.M., F.R.C.S. *Midland Centre for Neurosurgery and Neurology, Warley, Birmingham B67 7JX, United Kingdom*

Hansen A. Yuan, M.D. *Professor, Department of Orthopaedic and Neurological Surgery, State University of New York, Health Science Center at Syracuse, 550 Harrison Street, Suite 100, Syracuse, New York 13202-3072*

Acknowledgments

We wish to thank the illustrators, E. Hovorka and P. M. Cambas (for Dr. Argenson's chapters) and Dr. G. Chaimsky (for Dr. Floman's chapters), for their excellent art work.

A special word of thanks to Dr. Jean-Pierre C. Farcy for his help in the English translation of several chapters.

The completion of this book could not have been accomplished without the enormous dedication, competence, and humor of Mary Bennett.

Grateful acknowledgment is extended to Hana Reis and Sarah Mazar for their excellent assistance in the preparation of the manuscripts.

Preface

The management of fractures of the thoracic and lumbar spine, with or without neurologic impairment, is a challenging task that requires a team approach. Management of acute spinal injuries has undergone significant progress in the last decade; nevertheless, many issues of surgical management remain controversial. The increasing sophistication of the various diagnostic, medical, surgical and rehabilitation techniques mandates not only the sharing of this knowledge among the various specialties managing these patients, but also the exchange of knowledge and comprehension among international experts. *Thoracolumbar Spine Fractures* compiles this knowledge and closes the gaps of information among specialists.

The goal of this work is to delineate the methods of diagnosis, treatment, and rehabilitation of thoracolumbar injuries. The book is a collective effort of anatomists, biomechanicists, epidemiologists, neuroradiologists, neurophysiologists, spine surgeons from both orthopaedic surgery and neurosurgery, and experts from the fields of medicine, anesthesia, physical medicine, and rehabilitation. In addition, this volume represents the experience gained in North America and Europe, especially France. Indeed, the immense contributions of French spine surgeons have revolutionized spine surgery in the last decade.

This volume presents not only personal philosophies in managing the most challenging injuries, but also provides critical analysis of advantages and disadvantages of the various techniques. It identifies specific injury patterns and presents the most effective techniques of management. The book summarizes the latest knowledge in management of these devastating injuries and contains a wealth of information that will enhance the work of health care professionals managing spine injuries. Traumatic as well as non-traumatic spine fractures are discussed, including osteoporotic fractures and fractures due to primary and secondary vertebral tumors.

Embryology of the axial skeleton as well as the anatomy of the thoracic, lumbar, and sacral spine are discussed in depth, and various anatomical peculiarities pertinent to diagnosis and modern surgical treatment are examined. The anatomy, physiology and pathophysiology of the spinal cord are described and discussed. Clinical biomechanics of the normal spine and spine fractures are provided. The scope of these injuries and their epidemiological importance are delineated. The various diagnostic techniques such as imaging (plain radiographs, computerized tomography, and magnetic resonance imaging scans), neurophysiologic diagnostic and monitoring techniques, and sonography are emphasized and illustrated. A new comprehensive classification of thoracic and lumbar spine fractures is presented along with the older more traditional classifications. In addition, a classification of sacral fractures and a thorough discussion of its various types is presented. The various clinical neurologic syndromes caused by spinal cord injuries are described and illustrated. Early intensive care management of patients with thoracic spinal cord injuries is delineated. The principles of conservative and surgical management are outlined, both from the orthopaedic and neurosurgical points of view. In addition, specific thoracic, lumbar, and sacral injuries are recapitulated with detailed in-depth descriptions of their surgical management. Specific injuries in uncommon anatomical locations are also described and illustrated. The pros and cons of surgical approaches to the thoracic and lumbar spine and spinal instrumentation techniques, both anterior and posterior, are described, illustrated, and discussed in depth. In addition, the specific features of pediatric spine injuries, including the principles of reconstruction of late pediatric deformities, are outlined and discussed. Other spine fractures such as those due to osteoporosis, ankylosing spondylitis, and spine tumors are described in detail, and their specific management is outlined.

The management of various late sequelae of spinal fractures and spinal cord injuries such as chronic complications of paraplegia, post-traumatic syringomyelia and surgical reconstruction of late spinal deformities are discussed. Finally, rehabilitation of spinal cord injuries is outlined and discussed.

The book is aimed at orthopaedic surgeons, spine surgeons, neurosurgeons, physiatrists, and medical students.

Yizhar Floman
Jean-Pierre C. Farcy
Claude Argenson

Thoracolumbar Spine Fractures

Organogenesis and Development of the Thoracic, Lumbar, and Sacral Spine

Fernand de Peretti and Claude Argenson

ORGANOGENESIS AND OSSIFICATION

The spine is somitic, or mesodermic, in origin (1,8,11,12,18). Organogenesis of the spine takes place around the spinal cord (medulla spinalis), which is the most caudal section of the neural tube (tubus neuralis). Therefore it is useful to outline the origin of the neural tube and the somite (somitus) before studying the organogenesis of the spine.

Formation of the Trilaminar Embryonic Disc

The primitive line (linea primitiva) appears on the surface of the epiblast at the end of the second week. At the cranial extremity of the primitive line, the primitive node (nodus primitivus) appears. Soon after the appearance of the primitive node, a narrow tract develops. The tract is directed caudocranially and opens toward the primitive, or Hensen's node (original orifice) (Fig. 1). On the 16th day, the epiblast cells migrate toward the primitive line, invaginate into the primitive line, and migrate laterally between the ectoblast (ectoderm) and the endoblast (endoderm) to form the mesoblast (mesoderm), or middle layer.

Formation of the Notochordal Process (Processus Notochordalis)

Around the 16th day, ectoblast cells migrate from the primitive node toward the cranial pole and form a cord, the notochordal process along the midline (Fig. 1A). The notochordal process develops between the ectoblast and the endoblast and proceeds cranially to-

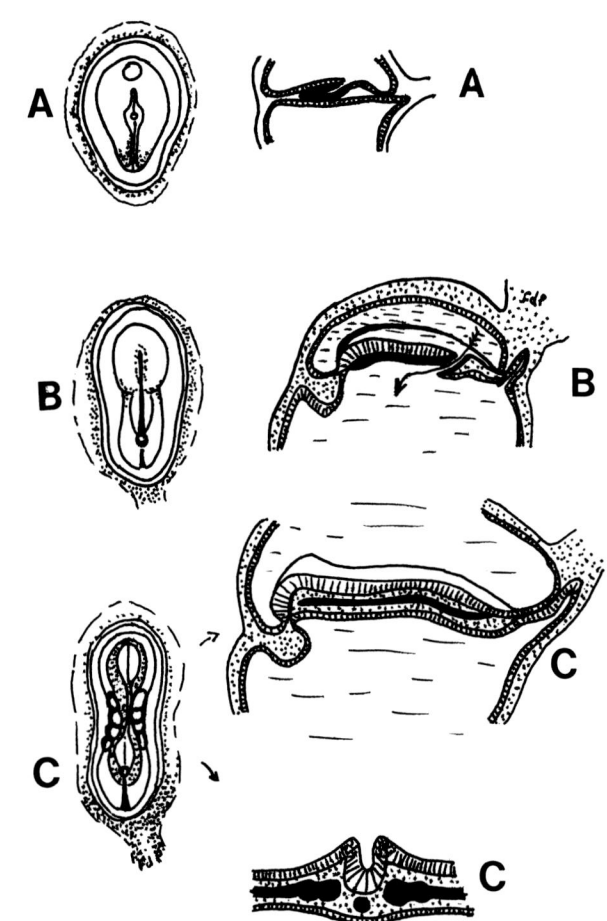

FIG. 1. Development of the notochord. **A:** Note the primitive line and Hansen's node (nodus primitivus). The notochord extends cranially from Hansen's node between the ectoderm and the endoderm. **B:** The neurenteric canal is a temporary phenomenon. **C:** Emergence of the somite and formation of the sulcus neuralis. The notochord lies in its final location between the neural tube and the endoderm.

F. de Peretti: Department of Orthopaedic Surgery, St. Roch University Hospital, 06000 Nice, France.
C. Argenson: Department of Orthopaedic Surgery, Service de Chirurgie Orthopedique et Traumatologique, Centre Hospitalier Regional et Universitaire de Nice, St. Roch University Hospital, 06000 Nice, France.

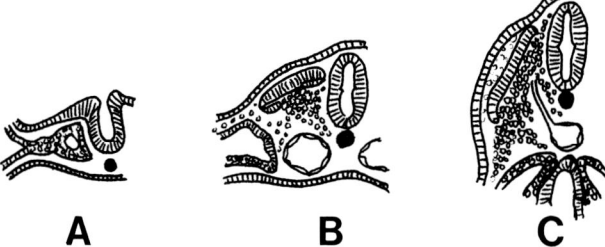

FIG. 2. Development of the somite. **A:** Horizontal cross section showing the position of a somite. **B:** Formation of the sclerotome and incipient migration. **C:** Development of an intersegmental arteria.

ward the prechordal lamina (lamina prechordalis). Thus the mesoblast is organized around a central axis, the notochordal process, that stretches from the primitive node to the prechordal lamina; the prechordal lamina is derived from a fusion of the epiblast and the endoblast.

On the 19th day, the floor of the notochordal canal disappears, after the merger of orifices that appear in the floor (Fig. 1B). Caudally, the orifice of the neurocentral canal (canalis neurentericus) allows temporary communication between the amniotic cavity and the vitellin sac. This is the prechordal stage, characterized by a cellular plate situated between the ectoblast and the vitellin sac.

Around the 20th day, the notochordal process forms a plate that folds back on itself to form the notochord, which is then situated between the ectoblast and the endoblast (Fig. 1C). The somite becomes organized laterally along this primitive axis, and along the neural tube dorsally.

Development of the Neural Tube

The embryonic ectoblast facing the notochord thickens and forms the lamina neuralis on the 18th day (Fig. 2A). The lamina neuralis develops into a groove and then closes dorsally to form the neural tube. The tube temporarily remains open at the neuroporus cranialis (closure on day 26) and at the neuroporus caudalis (closure around day 28). Proliferation of nervous tissue causes plication of the embryo along the longitudinal axis. The cranial section of the neural tube retains the three primitive cerebral vesicles. This lumen communicates with the lumen in the caudal section of the neural tube, which ultimately becomes the spinal cord.

At the third month, the spinal cord occupies the entire length of the embryo, and the spinal nerves (nervi spinales) cross the future intervertebral foramina at their point of origin.

From the fourth month, the length of the spinal column (columna vertebralis) and the dura mater increases more rapidly than the neural tube. This causes the caudal portion of the spinal cord to move gradually to a higher location (Fig. 3).

At birth, the caudal end of the spinal cord is located at L3. After birth, the vertebral column will grow

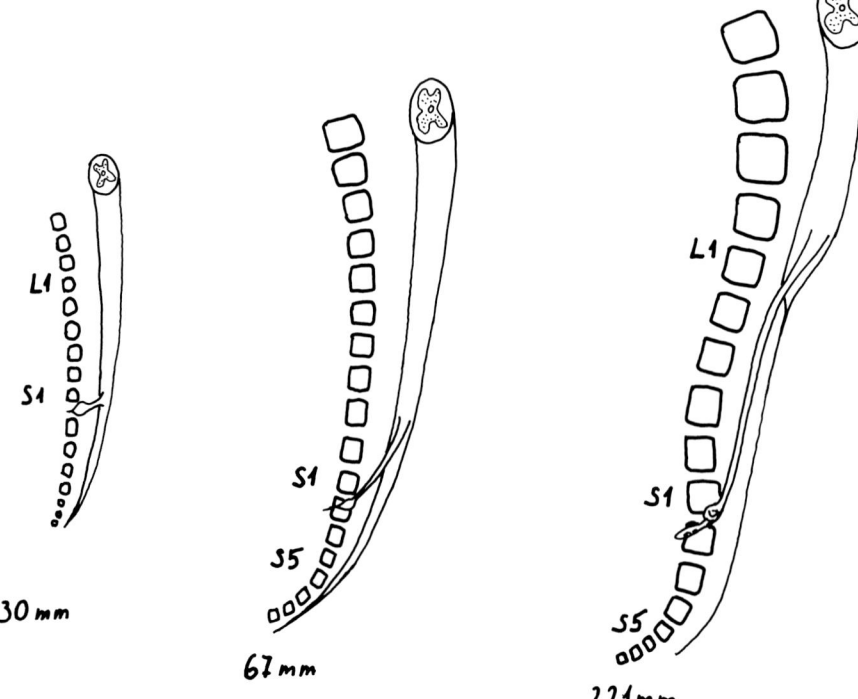

FIG. 3. Unequal growth patterns of the spine and spinal cord.

around the spinal cord. The caudal extremity of the spinal cord will be at the level of L1 on a fully grown adolescent.

Because of this unequal growth rate, the spinal nerve roots (radici nervi spinalis) travel obliquely from the spinal cord segment of origin toward the corresponding vertebral level. The dura mater remains attached to the bony column down to the sacrum.

ORGANOGENESIS OF THE SPINE

Formation of the Somite

During formation of the notochord and the neural tube, the embryonic mesoblast (mesoderma embryonicum) forms longitudinal columns on both sides. The paraxial mesoblast is elongated laterally by the lateral mesoblast.

Around the 20th day, the paraxial mesoblast divides into segments that give rise to the somite (Fig. 2). These provide the bulk of the axial skeleton, the associated muscles, and the skin. Initially, they take the form of a pluripotential tissue, the mesenchyma. Roughly 38 pairs of somites are formed; they constitute superficial elevations. Each somite develops a variable cavity, the myocele (Fig. 2A,B). The dorsal wall of the myocele forms the dermamyotome at the origin of the dermatome, which forms the subcutaneous tissue, and of the myotome, which provides the muscles. The ventral wall of the myocele forms the sclerotome (sclerotomus), which forms the spine.

Migration of the Sclerotome

During the fourth week, the sclerotome cells migrate toward the midline and surround the spinal cord and the notochord (Fig. 2C).

Ossification of the Spine

The ossification of the spine is an endochondral ossification (ossification endochondralis).

Precartilaginous Stage

The cells of the sclerotome migrate in three directions.

1. *Dorsally*. The mesenchyma of the sclerotome covers the neural tube and forms the vertebral arch (arcus vertebrae). It also participates in the formation of the transverse process (processus transversus) of the thoracic vertebrae (vertebrae thoracicae).
2. *Ventrolaterally*. The mesenchyma of the sclerotome forms the costal process (processus costarius) and the ribs of the thorax. The costal process participates entirely in the formation of the transverse process of the lumbar vertebrae (vertebrae lumbales), but only partially in the formation of the sacral ala (ala ossis sacri) (Fig. 3).
3. *Ventromedially*. The migration phenomenon is most complex in the ventromedial direction (Fig. 4). The cells of each sclerotome migrate ventromedially to take up a position between the spinal cord and the aorta (arteria aortica) (Fig. 4A,B), thereby surrounding the notochord.

Initially, the spinal nerve of each somite is located at the same level as the sclerotome (Fig. 4A,B). The parietal arteries emerge from the aorta and are initially located between the sclerotomes (Fig. 4A).

At a second stage, each sclerotome divides into two parts, the cranial and the caudal. The caudal part of each sclerotome, which faces the spinal nerve, will give rise to the intervertebral disc (discus intervertebralis) (Fig. 4C) to produce the vertebral body (corpus vertebrae).

Thus the vertebral body presents as an intersegmental formation. The intervertebral disc is derived from the most cranial part of each caudal section of sclerotome and thereby locates between two vertebral bodies. The vertebral arch and the costal process also retain their segmental origin. After formation of the vertebral body, the spinal nerve is initially situated at the sclerotome and provides its nerve supply. The spinal nerve will be located at the intervertebral foramen (foramen intervertebrale).

The notochord disappears completely at the level of the vertebral body but persists as the nucleus pulposus of the intervertebral disc. The notochord induces the formation of the vertebral body, and the neural tube induces the formation of the vertebral arch.

Chondrification Stage

During the sixth week, the chondrification centers make their appearance. There are two chondrification centers within each vertebral body. At the end of the embryonic period, the centers fuse to form the cartilaginous center of the vertebral body. Two other chondrification centers appear in the vertebral arch; they also fuse with one another and with the body center. Further developments of the neural tube give rise to the spinous process (processus spinosus) and the transverse process (processus transversus). The vertebral arch gradually closes posteriorly, beginning in the thoracic region (regio thoracius) and terminating in the cervical and lumbar regions (regiones cervicalis and lumbalis). Posterior spina bifida is more frequent in the cervical and low lumbar spines.

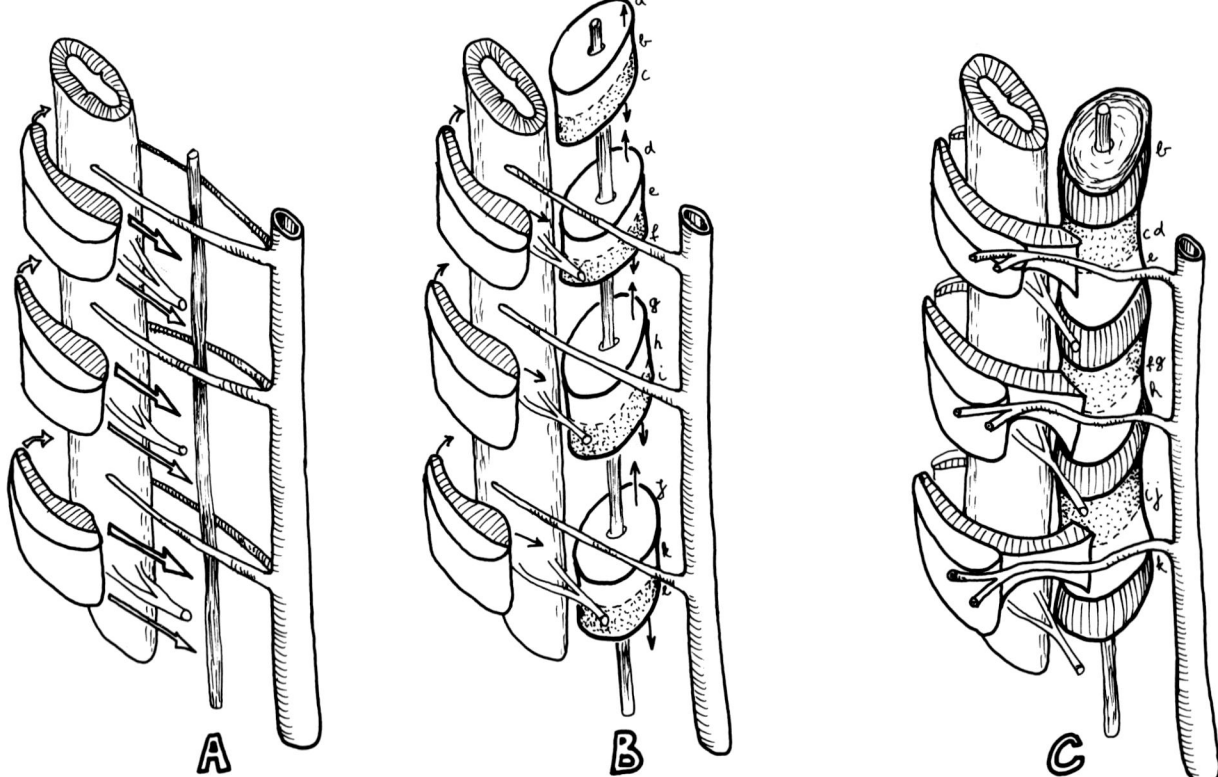

FIG. 4. Organogenesis of the spine (schematic diagram). **A:** Position of the somite lateral to the neural tube. The notochord lies ventral to the neural tube. Note the spinal nerves and the intersegmental arteries. The sclerotome is shown by the *shaded area* inside each somite. *Arrows* indicate the direction of sclerotome migration. **B:** Sclerotome surrounds the notochord, forming the vertebral bodies to be. Each sclerotome possesses a cranial and caudal mass. *Arrows* show the direction of future migration. The arteries still lie in an intersegmental position. The spinal nerves are still found at the same level as the sclerotomes. **C:** Formation of the definitive vertebral bodies. The vertebral disc stems from the cranial zone of the caudal section of each sclerotome. The intersegmental arteries are now situated opposite the vertebral bodies. The spinal nerves now emerge through the vertebral foramen. The vertebral arch develops from the sclerotome and preserves its segmental origin.

The Ossification Stage

This stage begins during the embryonic period and terminates approximately at age 25 (3,4,12). During the prenatal period, three growing osteogenic nuclei (gemmae osteogeneticae primariae) are visible (Fig. 5). One is ventral in the vertebral body, and one is dorsal in each one-half of the vertebral notch.

At birth, the vertebra is composed of three primary ossification centers (centra primaria ossificationis), connected by cartilaginous bridges (Fig. 5). The cartilage between the arch and the body is called the neurocentral cartilage.

The postnatal period is marked by (a) the fusion of the two halves of the vertebral arch during the first year; (b) the fusion of the arch with the vertebral body between the third and sixth years of age; and (c) the appearance of the secondary ossification centers (centra secundaria ossificationis).

After the onset of puberty, five ossification centers (15,16) appear (Fig. 5): one for the dorsal extremity of the spinous process (processus spinosus), one for the lateral extremity of each transverse process, and two that, with each other, form an annular ossification center on the upper and lower surfaces of the vertebral body. All the secondary ossification centers merge with the rest of the vertebrae between the ages of 16 and 25. However, although the vertebral body is mostly formed by the ventral primary ossification center, some elements of the vertebral arch and the lower and upper rib facets (foveae costales) also contribute to its formation.

The radiological appearance of infantile vertebrae varies with the onset and development of the ossification centers (3,10,12,13) (Figs. 6–10).

Until age 6 or 7, the vertebral body resembles the head of a tortoise (Fig. 6). It is oval in shape and becomes roughly rectangular with rounded corners. The

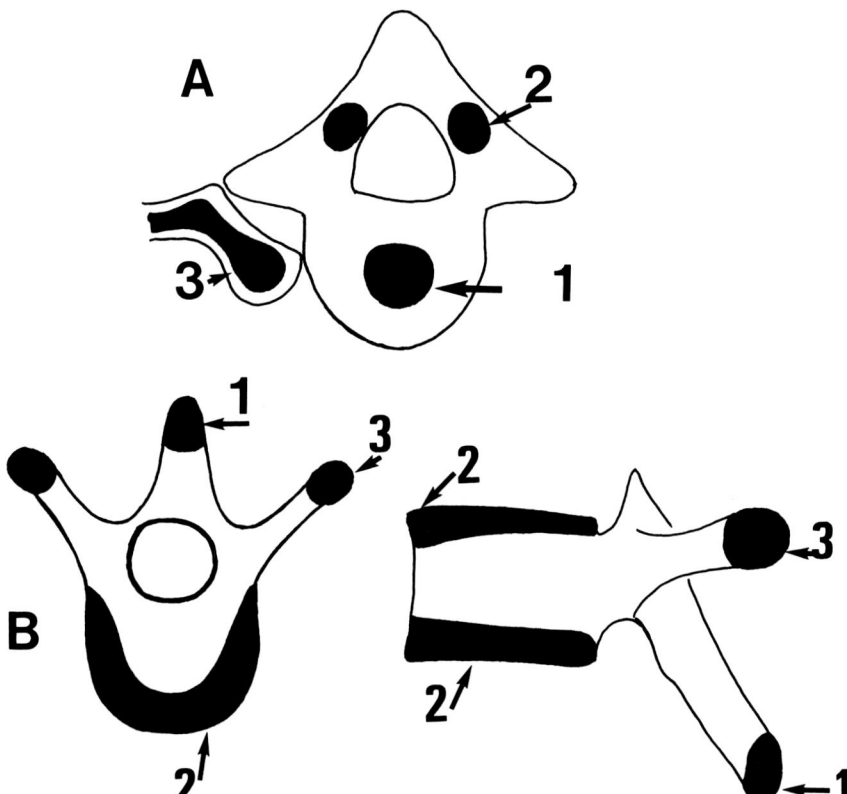

FIG. 5. Ossification of the vertebra. **A:** The three primary ossification centers. *1*, The primary body center; *2*, the two primary centers of the vertebral arches; and *3*, the center of the rib. **B:** The five secondary ossification centers. *1*, Centers of the spinous processes; *2*, the two annular cranial and caudal centers of the vertebral body; and *3*, centers of the transverse processes.

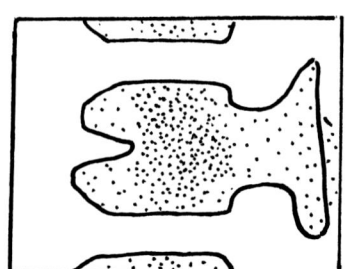

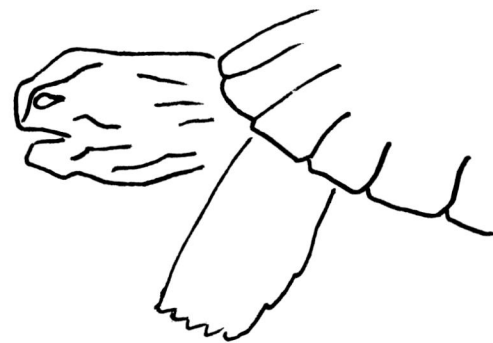

FIG. 6. Radiological view of the vertebral body before age 6. Note the tortoise-head shape.

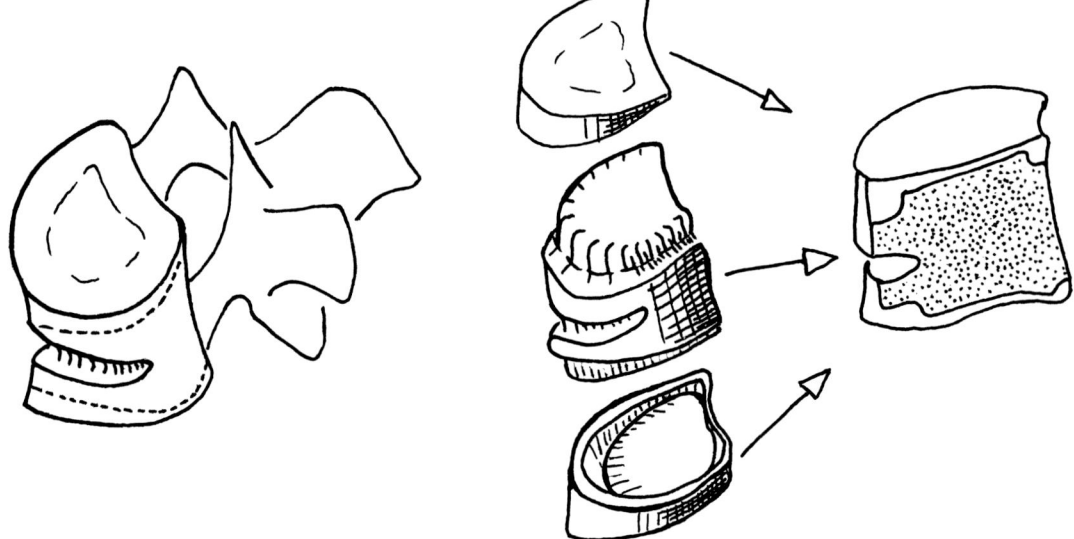

FIG. 7. Development of the ossification centers of the vertebral body and of the anterior vascular groove at <8 to 9 years. The cranial and caudal cartilaginous caps give rise to a marginal rim.

anterior part of the ossification center is hollowed by a horizontal slit that is reminiscent of a tortoise's mouth. This slit corresponds to the vascular orifices.

Between 6 and 9 years of age, the anterosuperior and anteroinferior angles take the shape of a flight of steps (Figs. 7 and 8). Cartilaginous plates cover the vertebral body, rather like the lid of a tin can. At the periphery, in the "flight of stairs," the cartilaginous plates form the marginal cartilaginous rim.

Toward age 9 or 10, sometimes a little earlier, particularly in girls, the secondary ossification center, which initially consists of tiny calcifications, appears in the marginal rim (Fig. 8). By the age of 11 to 12 in girls and age 12 to 13 in boys, the marginal bony rim is completely formed. It takes the shape of a bony anterolateral crescent that is thicker anteriorly than posteriorly, both in reality and in radiographs. In lateral radiographs, the hollows in the "steps" are occupied by these ossification centers (Fig. 9). Normally, the radiographic image is discrete and shows no anterior or lateral overlap. Any exuberant "wildcat" growth may raise the question of a spinal growth dystrophy.

Between ages 13 and 14 in girls and ages 14 and 15 in boys, the bony marginal rim begins to fuse with the vertebral body (Fig. 10).

The vertebral fusion of the bony rim occurs very late, although earlier at the thoracic than the lumbar level.

This development is visible on a radiograph and provides evidence of enchondral ossification. Thorough examination is necessary to distinguish it from a pathological process.

Organogenesis and ossification of the sacrum (4) (Fig. 11), although more complex, are similar to those observed in other vertebrae. The fusion of the sacral vertebrae occurs early, although fibrocartilaginous differentiation of the mesenchyma can persist in the form of fragments of disc included (discus inclusus) between two sacral vertebrae, particularly at S1 and S2. The sacral ala has two origins: the anterior and lateral section emanate from the S1 costal process, and the posterior third branches from the vertebral arch.

Apart from the vertebral bodies and the sacral ala, ossification is produced by a mosaic of more than 30 ossification centers.

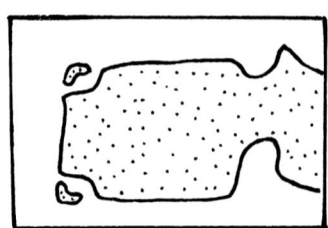

FIG. 8. Radiological view before age 10. Girls, 8 to 10 years; boys 9 to 10 years.

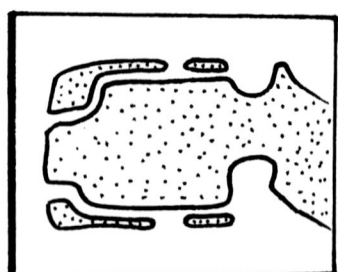

FIG. 9. Radiological view between 11 and 13 years of age. Girls, 11 to 12 years; boys 12 to 13 years.

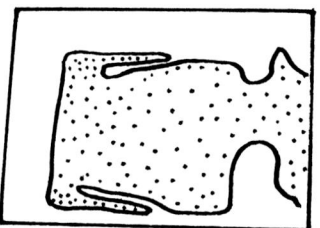

FIG. 10. Radiological view between 13 and 15 years of age. Girls, 13 to 14 years; boys, 14 to 15 years.

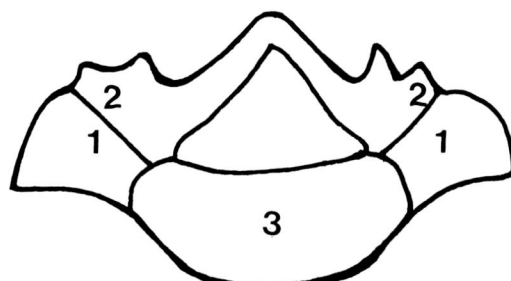

FIG. 11. Ossification of the sacrum. *1*, The lateral part stemming from the S1 costal process. *2*, Dorsal section of the sacral wing stemming from the vertebral arch. *3*, The body of the sacral corpus stemming from the primary centers of the body.

ORGANOGENETIC DEFECTS

Combined Neurological and Bone Anomalies (9,15)

The most common defect is spina bifida (Fig. 12). It is caused either by the nonclosure of the neural tube or, more frequently, by the nonclosure of the neuroporus caudalis when the spina bifida is situated in the lumbosacral region. In its classic form, spina bifida occurs when the vertebral arch does not fuse dorsally. This is spina bifida occulta, the most common form, and is discovered radiologically in 15% to 20% of the population. If more than one or two vertebrae are affected, the meninges protrude through the orifice to form a skin covered sac. This condition is termed meningocele. If it is fairly large, the sac may also contain spinal cord and spinal nerves. This is termed myelomeningocele. The sac is covered by a thin, fragile membrane. Neurologic deficits are part of this entity or syndrome.

If there is a complete posterior failure to close, the spinal cord and the roots are superficially exposed to the surface. In this case, it is called myelocele.

This type of malformation is often associated with caudal displacement of the spinal bulb (medulla oblongata) and the cerebellum into the vertebral canal. Hydrocephaly with Arnold–Chiari malformation is frequently observed, as well.

Diastematomyelia is a rare defect that is characterized by localized splitting of the spinal cord associated with a cartilaginous or osseous defect (septum median and spina bifida), the genesis of which is unknown. Reference is sometimes made to defects in the closure of the neural tube, splitting of the notochord, persistence of the neurenteric canal (canalis neurentericus), and disturbances in the hydrodynamic equilibrium. Clinically, a patch of hair with modified skin color can be found at the level of the lumbosacral spine.

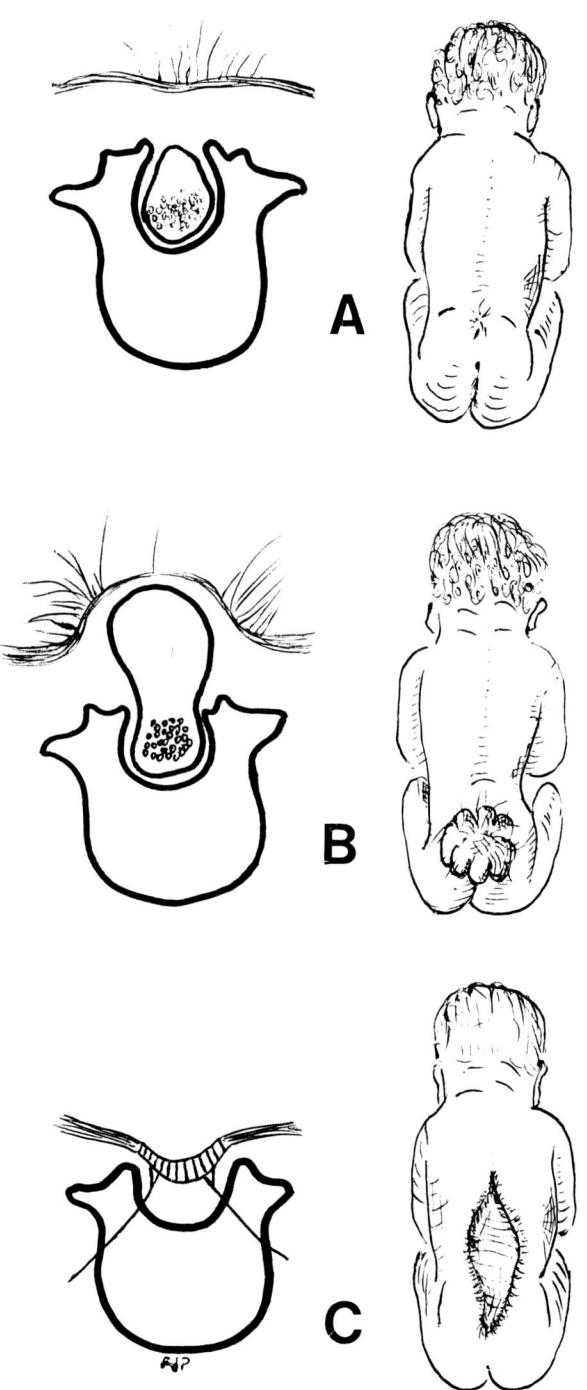

FIG. 12. Closure defects of the neuroporus caudalis. **A:** Spina bifida occulta. **B:** Spina bifida with meningocele. **C:** Myelocelia with rachischisis.

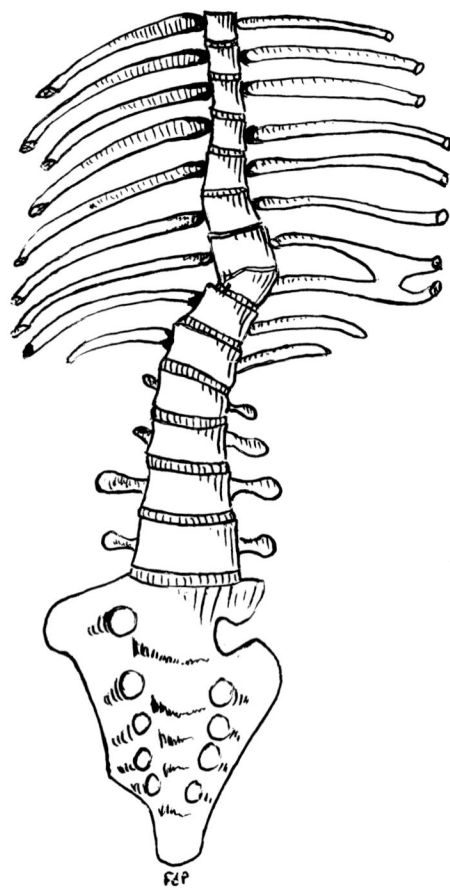

FIG. 13. Hemivertebra with formation of scoliosis.

BONE-RELATED ANOMALIES

Some bone-related anomalies are merely frequent transitional variations, found in the lumbosacral region. Many have no clinical significance, as in the lumbarization of S1 or the sacralization of L5. Defects can be complete, partial, or unilateral and are often asymptomatic.

Other anomalies result from complete, symmetrical vertebral fusions that trap parts of the disc. This is undetectable on a radiograph. They are asymptomatic, often located between C1 and C7.

The most serious defects involve incomplete and asymmetrical vertebral fusions with the development of hemivertebra due to the presence either of a missing vertebra or vertebrae in excess. If the malformation is in the thoracic spine, the hemivertebra is associated with the presence of a rib on the same side. This is due to the complexity of the formation and rearrangement of the sclerotome during development and migration. This malformation may be responsible for asymmetric growth accompanied by scoliosis (Fig. 13). It is occasionally associated with diastematomyelia.

Development of Spinal Curvature

The embryo, as does a child who has not started to walk, exhibits pronounced curvature with ventral concavity (Fig. 14). Cervical curvature appears only

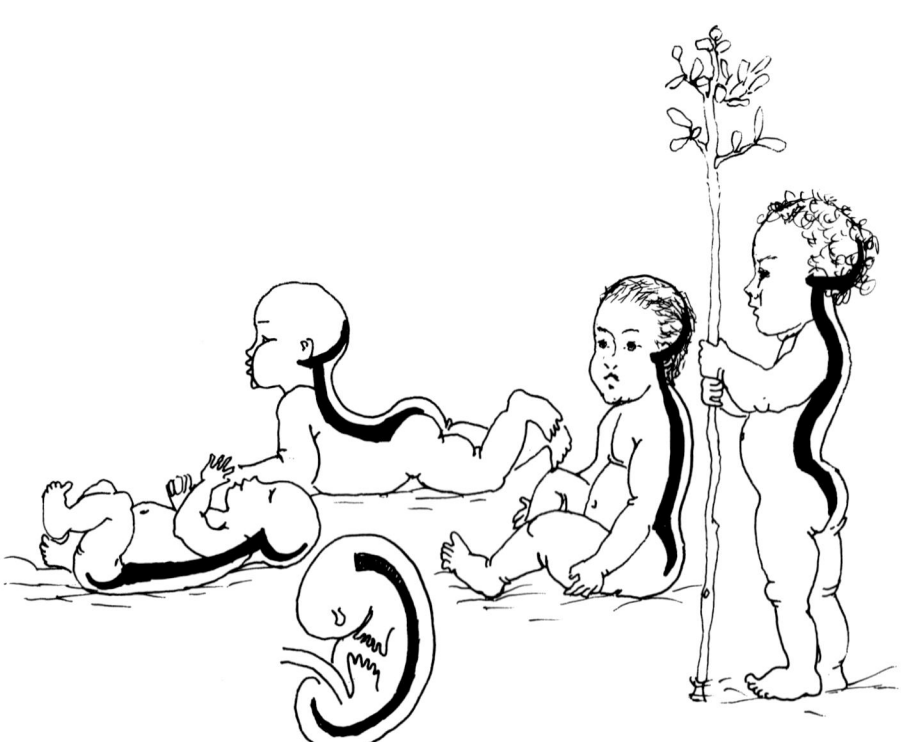

FIG. 14. Development of sagittal curves of the spine.

with the advent of the sitting position (Fig. 14). Lumbar curvature begins when the upright position, specific to humans, is adopted.

GROWTH OF THE SPINE

Analytic Study

The spine is the product of enchondral bone formation. Each vertebral body includes an ossification center and an upper and lower epiphyseal cartilage (17) (cartilago epiphysialis). The ossification center behaves as a metaphysis. The junction between the vertebral body and the vertebral arch is composed of cartilage with a dual potential action. The anterior aspect contributes to the development of 30% of the vertebral body, and the posterior aspect contributes to the formation of the vertebral arch. Growth is due to four main cartilages. In addition, the secondary ossification centers impart morphological identity to each vertebra.

Synthetical Study

The length of the spine triples between the time of birth and adulthood (Fig. 15), increasing from 24 to 70 cm in men and to 60 cm in women. The lengthening of the spine follows a growth pattern that parallels the height of the child in a sitting position (4).

The thoracic spine measures 11 cm at birth; at the end of the growth period, it measures approximately 28 cm in boys and 26 cm in girls. It represents 30% of the sitting height and 40% of the spine. The intervertebral discs account for 18% of the length of the thoracic spine (2).

The lumbar spine measures 7 cm at birth, and 16 cm in boys and 15.5 cm in girls at the end of the growth period. It represents 18% of the sitting height and 23% of the vertebral column; the intervertebral discs represent 35% of the length of the lumbar spine. The sacrum measures 14% of the sitting height and 18% of the spine.

The spine as a whole, like the rest of the body, does not experience regular growth (5–7) (Fig. 15). The first growth peak occurs during the first year, when the child doubles his/her size. The growth rate then slows gradually to a plateau-like curve at approximately age 7. The second growth peak starts with the onset of puberty, and gradually levels off 2 or 3 years later. Nevertheless, the spine continues to mature and is considered to be complete only when the ossification center of the iliac crest (crista iliaca) has fused totally with the iliac wing (ala ossis ilii) (14).

The growth pattern resembles a volumetric explosion. While the vertebral length triples or quadruples during growth, the volume of the spine can multiply by a factor of over 20.

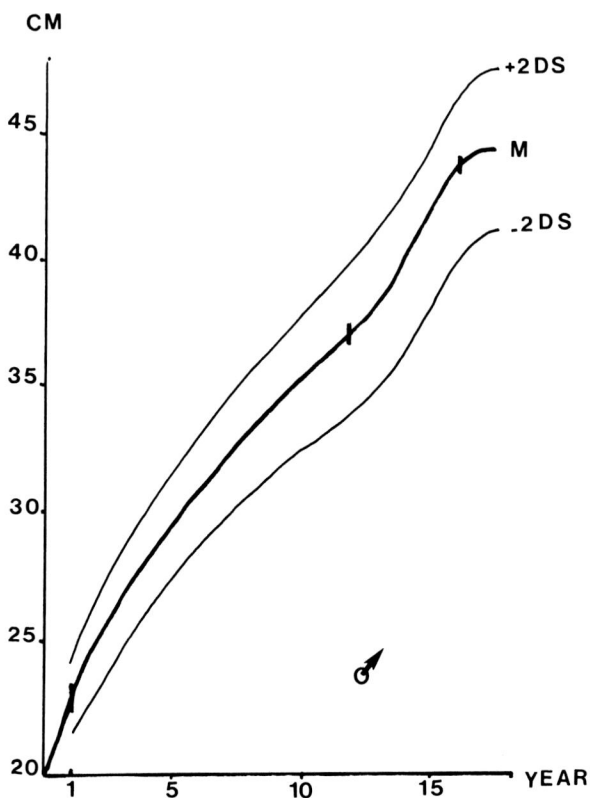

FIG. 15. Thoracic and lumbar spinal growth curve showing growth peak at 1 year of age and at puberty. DS, standard deviation.

CONCLUSION

The spine undergoes enchondral bone formation. The maturing process is completed by the onset of adulthood. Initially, the development of the notochord and the neural tube is closely associated with that of the vertebral body and the vertebral arch.

The vertebral body has an inter- and bi-metameric origin. The vertebral arch has a purely metameric origin. During the entire growth period, the spine is vulnerable to all forms of insult, which traditionally injure growth cartilages.

REFERENCES

1. Ben Pansky P. *Review of medical embryology*. New York: Macmillan, 1982.
2. Brandner ME. Normal values of the vertebral body and intervertebral disc index during growth. *AJR* 1970;110:618.
3. Castaing J, Santini JJ. *Anatomie fonctionnelle de l'appareil locomoteur: le rachis*. Paris: Medicorama, Epri, 1976.
4. DiMeglio A, Bonnel F. *Le rachis en croissance*. Paris: Springer Verlag, 1990.

5. Duval-Beaupere G, Sayet A. Contribution respective des segments superieur et inferieur a la croissance des garcons. *Arch Fr Pediatr* 1979;36:369–378.
6. Duval-Beaupere G, Barthel T. La croissance des scoliotiques. *Rev Chir Orthop* 1983;69:201–206.
7. Duval-Beaupere G, Lamireau T. Scoliosis at less than 30°. Properties of the evolutivity (Risk of progression). *Spine* 1985;10:421–424.
8. Falkner F, Tanner JM. *Human growth*. London: Baillere Tindall, 1976.
9. Goto S, Uhthoff HK. Notochord and spinal malformations. *Acta Orthop Scand* 1986;57:149–153.
10. Greulich WW, Pyle SY. *Radiographic atlas of skeletal development of the hand and wrist*. Stanford, CA: Stanford University Press, 1959.
11. Langman J. *Medical embryology*. Baltimore: Williams & Wilkins, 1981.
12. O'Rahilly R, Benson D. The development of the vertebral column. In Bradford DS, Hensinger RN, eds. *The pediatric spine*. New York: Thieme, 1985;3–17.
13. Petersson H, Daneman A, Hardwood-Nash DC. *Computed tomography in pediatric orthopedic radiology*. Ekelund: Boijsen, 1983;26–48.
14. Risser JC. The iliac apophysis: an invaluable sign in the management of scoliosis. *Clin Orthop* 1958;11:111–119.
15. Schmorl G. *The human spine in health and disease*, 2nd ed. New York: Grune & Stratton, 1971.
16. Schwytzer FX. Study of the growth of the vertebral bodies in adolescents. *Acta Anat* 1977;98:52–61.
17. Taylor JP. Growth of human intervertebral disks and vertebral bodies. *J Anat* 1975;120:49–68.
18. Tuchman-Duplessis H, David G, Haegel P. *Illustrated human embryology. Embryogenesis*, vol 1. New York: Springer-Verlag, 1972.

2

Anatomy of the Thoracolumbar and Sacral Spine with Special Consideration for Implant Insertion

Fernand de Peretti and Claude Argenson

The anatomic nomenclature used in this chapter is the internationally adopted "Nomina Anatomica" (Sixth International Congress of Anatomists held in Paris in 1955).

This chapter includes analytic studies of the following:

1. The vertebrae.
2. The intervertebral joints.
3. The global view of the entire spine.
4. The nerve connections and the principles governing laminectomies and corporectomies.
5. The anatomic principles of pedicular targeting and sacral screw insertion.

ANALYTIC STUDY OF THE VERTEBRAE

The External Configuration of Standard Vertebra

The standard vertebra (28) is composed of two features: the anterior vertebral body (corpus vertebrae) and the posterior vertebral arch (arcus vertebrae). The body and the arch enclose the intervertebral foramen (foramen vertebrale). Posteriorly, the vertebral body presents an abraded, concave surface that constitutes the anterior aspect of the medullary spinal canal, and two smooth cartilage-encrusted surfaces that are the upper and lower vertebral endplates.

From anterior to posterior and on both sides, the vertebral arch is composed of the following:

1. The pedicle (pediculus), situated laterally on the posterior surface of the corpus vertebrae.
2. The pars interarticularis, or vertebral isthmus, which connects the superior and inferior articular processes (processus articularis superior and inferior) to the transverse processes (processus transversus) laterally. Irrespective of the vertebra, the pedicle (pediculus) is always situated below the superior articular process (processus articularis superior), at the level of the transverse process. This serves as a landmark for introduction of pedicle screws. Full, comprehensive knowledge of this pars interarticularis anatomy at each level makes possible the selection of the most desirable entry point and to gain proper orientation in order to perform pedicular anchorage with vertebral screws.
3. The lamina of the vertebral arch (lamina arcus vertebrae), always directed caudally and posteriorly, joins its contralateral equivalent on the implantation site of the spinous process (processus spinosus). This results in its alignment with the middle or lower two-thirds of the vertebral body that bears the same designation. It reaches as far as the upper quarter of the next underlying vertebral body. Thus, there is a discrepancy between vertebral body and lamina at any given level. This must be remembered while undertaking decompressive laminectomy: the lamina that is removed belongs to the vertebral body that is a level above, and the

---

F. de Peretti: Department of Orthopaedic Surgery, St. Roch University Hospital, 06000 Nice, France.
C. Argenson: Department of Orthopaedic Surgery, Service de Chirurgie Orthopedique et Traumatologique, Centre Hospitalier Regional et Universitaire de Nice, St. Roch University Hospital, 06000 Nice, France.

disc space exposed is always under the laminectomized vertebra.

Structure

The vertebral body (2) consists of a sheath of cortical bone (substantia compacta) that encloses the cancellous bone (substantia spongiosa) (Fig. 1). Several networks of lamellae, layers of cancellous bone, can be distinguished within the body. The vertical lamellae reach from one vertebral endplate to the other. These lamellae are particularly closely packed at the posterior part of the vertebral body. The oblique lamellae originate from the endplates, concentrate at the level of the pedicles, and terminate in the articular processes. They are organized into interlacing arches at the level of the upper one-half of the posterior vertebral body. Thus one can describe a triangle of weakness with an anterior base anterior to the vertebral body, the base of which corresponds to the anterior part of the vertebral body. It is within this triangle, with its low density cancellous bone, that compression fractures occur.

In addition to the above-mentioned lamellae, there are also horizontal lamellae that stretch from one side to the other.

In the posterior aspect of the vertebral body, the cancellous bone is very dense and forms the posterior vertebral wall, which constitutes the feature most resistant to compression (9,30).

The pedicle consists of a sleeve of cortical bone, inside of which there is extremely dense cancellous bone. This allows for excellent anchorage of pedicular screws. The cancellous oblique lamellae inside the pedicle open anteriorly into the articular process (processus articularis) and the pars interarticularis, or isthmus.

The less dense parts, containing the least cancellous lamellae, are the lamina and the transverse and spinous processes (processus transversus and spinosus). This explains the failure of internal fixation techniques, such as Wilson or Crawford plates, which were screwed into the spinous processes.

CHARACTERISTICS OF THE DIFFERENT VERTEBRAL LEVELS

The Thoracic Vertebrae

The thoracic vertebrae (Fig. 2) are smaller than the lumbar vertebrae. The vertebral body presents an anteroposterior diameter that is slightly larger than the transverse diameter. The vertebral foramen is oval or circular in shape. The pedicle is narrow, flattens in the transverse plane, and is laterally implanted on the upper one-half or two-thirds of the vertebral body.

The articular processes are smooth and lie in a frontal plane. During a posterior surgical approach, the superior articular facet is masked by the inferior articular process of the vertebra immediately above it. The transverse processes project markedly both laterally and posteriorly. They are on the same posterior plane as the spinous processes.

The processus spinosus has a marked caudal and posterior orientation that extends downward to the lower edge of the underlying vertebra; the lamina extends as far as the pedicle of the underlying vertebra. As a result, there is no posterior space between the two thoracic vertebrae that can be penetrated by a needle inserted posteriorly; the vertebral canal cannot be punctured at the thoracic level. In the thoracic spine, the lamina and the spinous process overlap like shingles on a roof.

The Lumbar Vertebrae (Vertebrae Lumbalis)

These vertebrae (Fig. 3) are extremely large. The transverse diameter of the vertebral body is greater

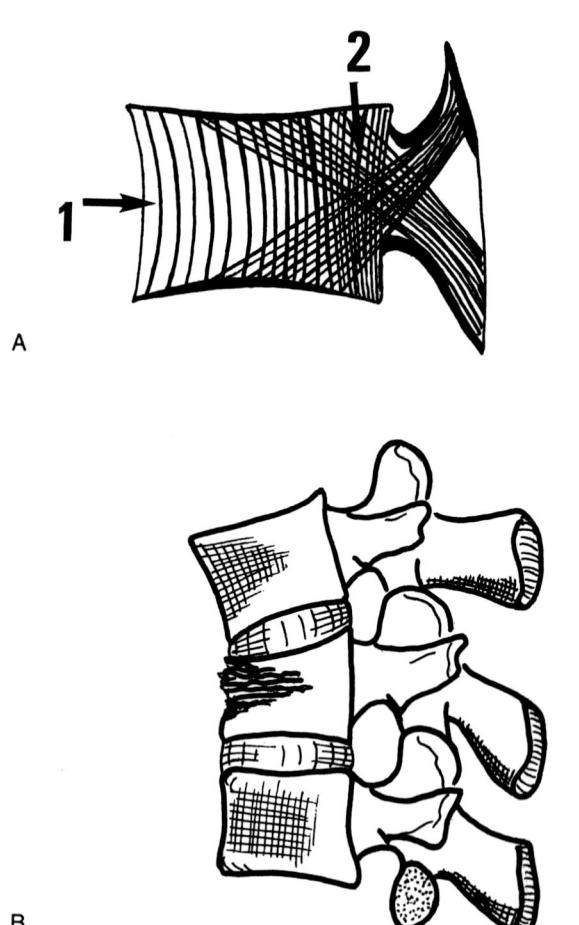

FIG. 1. A: The cancellous bone of the vertebra showing (*1*) the triangle of anterior weakness of the vertebral body and (*2*) the posterior wall. **B:** Wedge fracture.

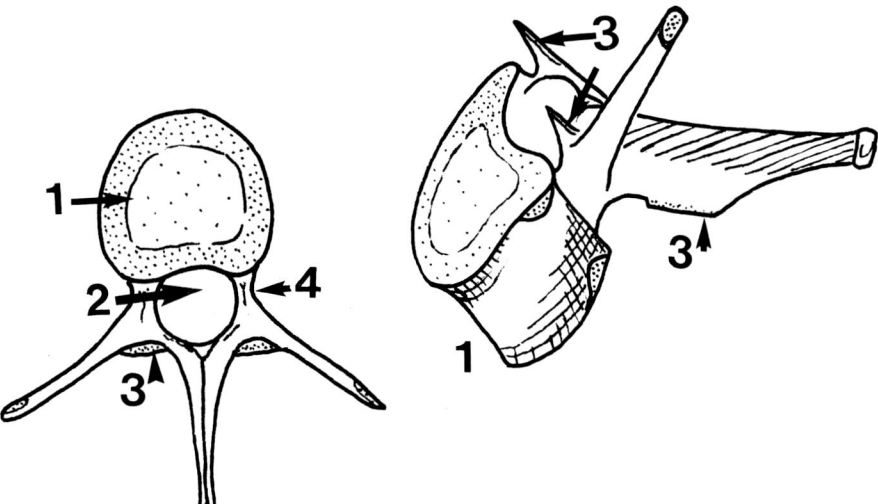

FIG. 2. The thoracic vertebra: *1*, corpus; *2*, circular or oval-shaped vertebral foramen; *3*, articular process in the frontal plane; and *4*, extremely narrow pedicle.

than the anteroposterior diameter. The vertebral foramen is triangular with an anterior base.

The pedicle is very solid and implants laterally at the upper one-third. It is beveled caudally and medially to accommodate the spinal root (radix spinalis).

The superior articular process is shaped like a fragment of a hollow cylinder and faces posteriorly and medially. The inferior articular process is shaped like a fragment of a solid cylinder, facing anteriorly and externally. However, the joint cavity (cavum articularis) develops in a sagittal plane in such a way that, in a posterior approach, the surgeon, in using a rongeur or gouge at the joint capsule, will uncover zygapophyseal joints (see Fig. 20).

The transverse processes are somewhat obliquely inclined in the anterior plane. They are called the costal processes (processus costali) because they share the same origin as the ribs. They are quite long; the longest is L3.

The lamina is shorter caudally than at the level of the thoracic vertebrae and thus allows a posterior opening between two laminae. Between L3 and L4, L4 and L5, and L5 and S1, this window allows ample room for a lumbar puncture through the ligamentum flavum.

The spinous process flattens transversely and is rectangular and sturdy. On a patient in the anatomical reference position, their posterior development is greater as one progresses caudally. Two tubercles need to be given special mention. The first is the mammillary process (processus mammilaris), a posterior and lateral continuation of the superior articular process. During a posterior approach, it masks the apophyseal joint cavity. The second tubercle is the accessory process (processus accessorius), which is situated at the lower edge of the implantation of the costal process. This can serve as a surgical landmark during insertion of pedicular screws.

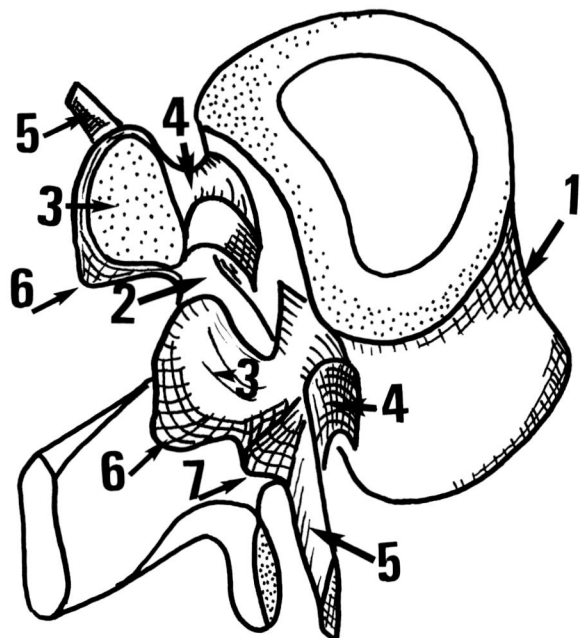

FIG. 3. The lumbar vertebra: *1*, vertebral body presenting a transverse diameter larger than the anteroposterior diameter; *2*, triangular vertebral foramen; *3*, articular process in the sagittal plane; *4*, large pedicle; *5*, costal process; *6*, mammillary process; and *7*, accessory process.

The Thoracolumbar Transitional Vertebrae (1,6,16,25)

In the majority of cases, thoracolumbar transition is achieved at T12. The superior articular processes are situated in the frontal plane; the inferior articular processes are located in the sagittal plane.

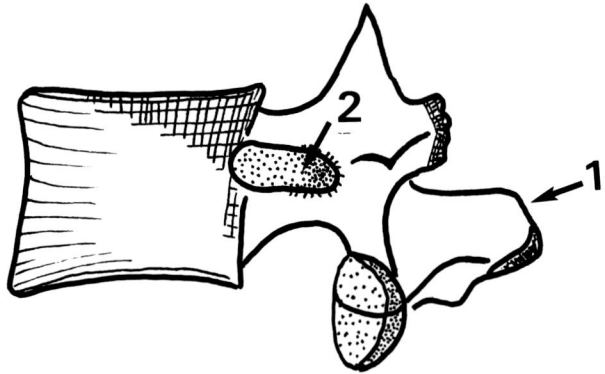

FIG. 4. T12: *1*, spinous process; *2*, costovertebral joint (12 ribs). Note the absence of transverse process.

Three other features of T12 deserve to be mentioned (Fig. 4). The T12 spinous process is the smallest in size. The thoracic and lumbar spinous processes converge on it, a phenomenon referred to as anticlinal (Fig. 5). The head of the rib articulates with a cartilaginous facet in pedicular position. There is not transverse process.

The T11 vertebra also presents a costal joint in the pedicular location, with identical surgical consequences. The transverse process is visible, but its dimensions are small.

Occasionally (28), all the characteristics of thoracolumbar transition can be found at T11. In these cases, T12 presents as a lumbar vertebra.

In exceptional circumstances, thoracolumbar transition characteristics will be found at L1. They may be shared by two vertebrae, and asymmetry may be found in the ribs. The surgeon should not rely on the external appearance of the vertebra to locate landmarks but should use radiographic means to verify the location.

The First Two Sacral Vertebrae (Vertebrae Sacrales)

The first two sacral vertebrae share a characteristic anomaly, all features of which should be familiar to the surgeon (11,12). The superior articular process of S1 does not lie in the sagittal plane as it does in the lumbar vertebrae. Its orientation can vary considerably from one individual to another, and even from one side to

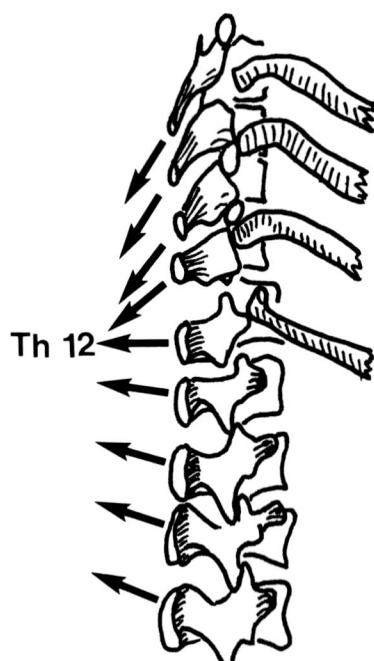

FIG. 5. Anticlinal phenomenon. Note the convergence of the thoracic and lumbar spinous processes near T12. (T = Th)

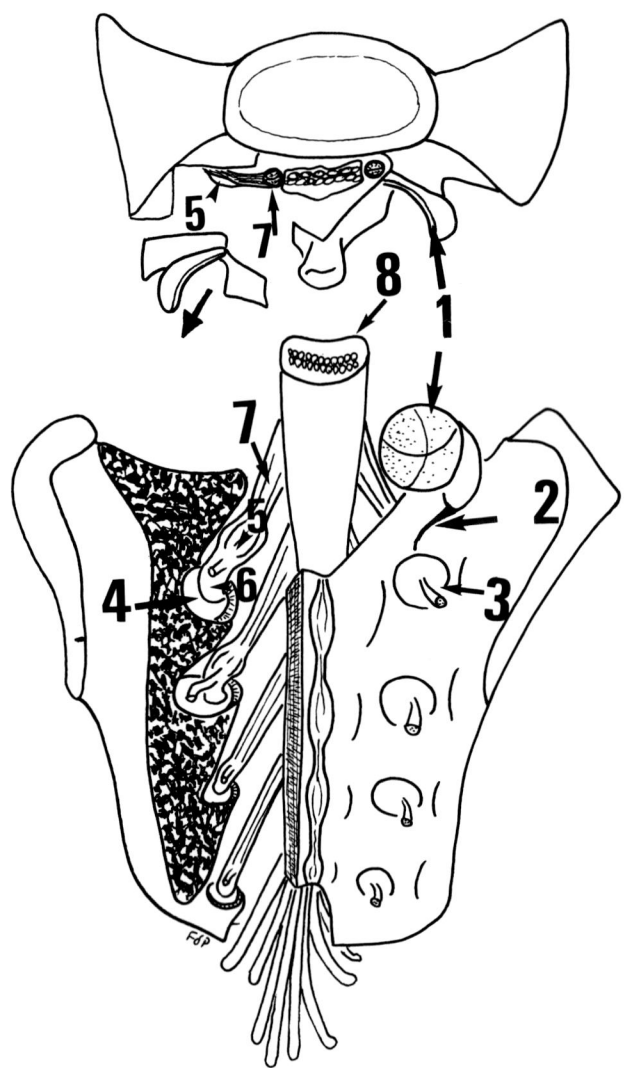

FIG. 6. Posterior and superior views of the sacrum. Left hemilaminectomy was performed to reveal the pathways of the sacral roots. *1*, Articular process, which generally lies in a more frontal plane than that of the lumbar vertebra; *2*, caudal extension of the articular process along a bone crest; *3*, sacral foramen with extremely small dorsal ramus; *4*, pelvic sacral foramen; *5*, spinal ganglion; *6*, ventral branch of the spinal nerve (ramus ventralis of the nervus spinalis); *7*, S1 sacral root; and *8*, dura mater.

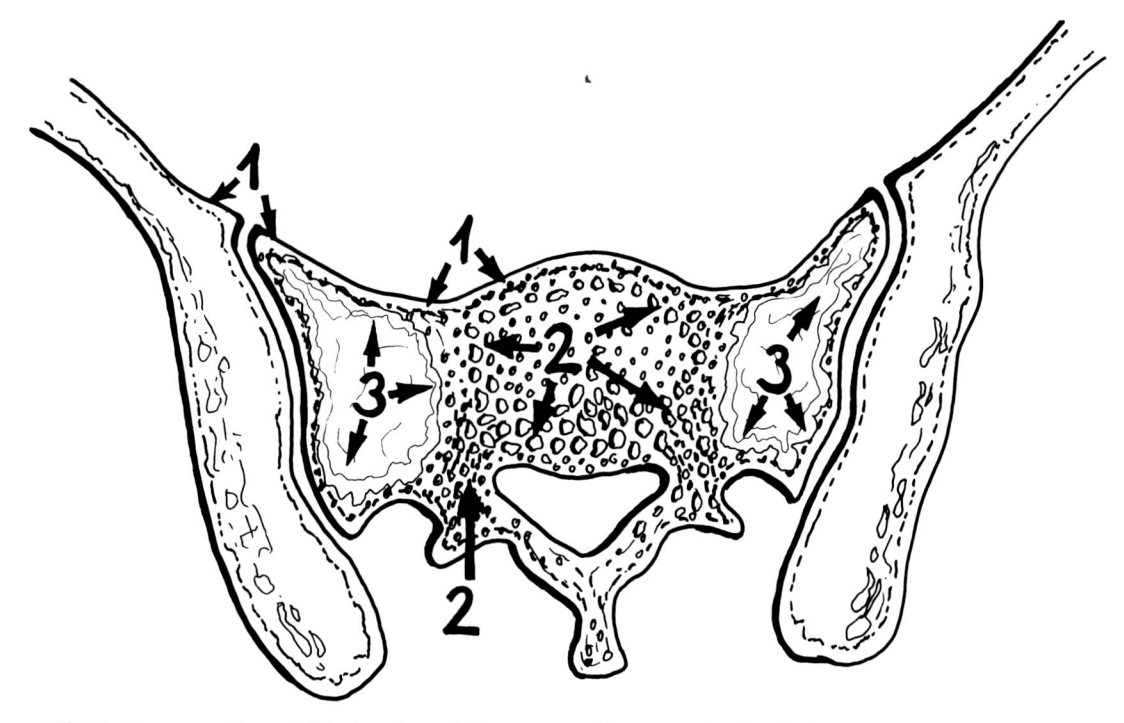

FIG. 7. Cross section of S1 showing: *1*, the compact bone at the level of the promontory (promentorium) and the sacroiliac joint; *2*, the cancellous bone at the level of the vertebral body and the pedicle; and *3*, the ball of fatty tissue at the lateral mass.

the other. It faces posteriorly and medially, at an angle of 0° to 60° on the frontal plane; the average angle is 30°. During a posterior surgical approach, the S1 articular process is totally masked by the articular process of the L5 vertebra. Resection of the L5 inferior articular process is required in order to see the S1 articular processes and their cartilaginous surfaces (Figs. 6 and 7).

The sacral canal is triangular in shape and very flat in the frontal plane. It opens laterally into the anterior and posterior sacral foramina (foramina sacralio pelvina and dorsalia). The bodies of S1 and S2 and the pedicle contain dense cancellous bone. In contrast, the lateral sacral mass (pars lateralis ossis sacri) contains more fatty tissue (11,12). Anatomic dissection of 20 cadaveric sacrums from laboratory specimens were studied in the anatomy laboratory in Nice. The results were compared to those of 20 healthy subjects who were younger than 55 years of age who were studied using computerized axial tomography with three-dimensional reconstruction (11,12).

The compact bone (substantia corticalis) is dense only in the region of the S1 endplate, particularly in the region of the promontory (promontorium), the arcuate line of the pelvis (linea terminalis), and the sacroiliac joint (junctura sacroiliaca). Hence the medial architecture of the sacrum is a bone that acts as a keystone, transmitting loads between the spine and the pelvis.

Finally, the sacrum presents a marked anterior concavity and tapers caudally. Thus S2 is decidedly smaller than S1. This can be seen clearly in horizontal cross sections.

The S1 and S2 pedicles (pediculi) are oriented medially. In a recent study of 20 dry spines (11,12), we found an anteromedial orientation for the S1 pedicle. The average angle was 23° from the sagittal plane, with variations at the extremes from 18° to 30°. Measurements were made on the medial margin of the pedicle at the upper orifice of the sacral canal.

Like the lumbar vertebrae, the sacral pedicles present a medial face and are beveled medially. The root and the spinal ganglion (ganglion spinale) have direct contact with this surface (Fig. 6).

THE VERTEBRAL JOINTS (JUNCTURAE COLUMNAE VERTEBRALIS)

The vertebral joints include three distinct features: the intervertebral disc (juncturae intercorporealis), the zygapophyseal joints (juncturae zygapophyseales), and the ligaments (ligamenta).

The Junctura Intercorporealis

This is a symphysis, a joint with no articular cavity but with a fibrocartilage situated between the two cartilage-encrusted surfaces. This fibrocartilage is called the intervertebral disc (discus intervertebralis).

The Intervertebral Disc (Discus Intervertebralis)

The intervertebral disc consists of two components, the annulus fibrosus and the nucleus pulposus (29). The annulus fibrosus consists of almost complete fibrocartilaginous concentric rings, which are extended below the vertebral endplates. The nucleus pulposus is enclosed in the annulus, although there is no clear definition between the two structures, which are avascular and therefore have poor healing potential.

With age (5), the disc tends to creep and subsequently tear. Posterior tears may permit the posterior ejection of the contents of the disc, that is, nucleus pulposus. This can readily be seen on a sagittal section of the spine of an elderly subject. Over the age of 60, in the lower lumbar spine, the annulus extends beyond the physiologic boundaries of the vertebral body and bulges mildly into the vertebral foramen and spinal canal.

The Ligaments

The intervertebral disc is strengthened by an articular capsule. The capsule is strengthened anteriorly by the anterior longitudinal ligament (ligamentum longitudinale anterius), posteriorly by the posterior longitudinal ligament (ligamentum longitudinale posterius), and laterally by the extensions of these two ligaments (Fig. 8).

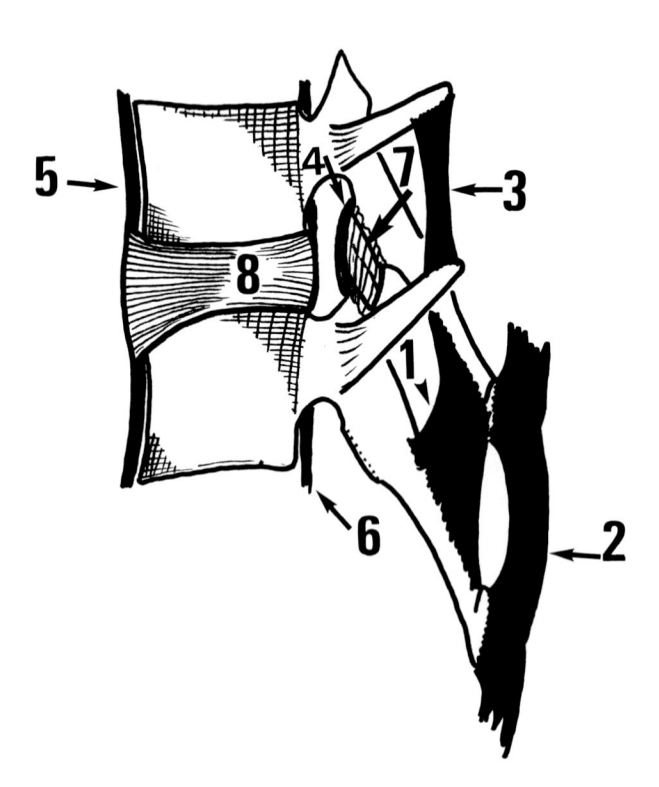

The Posterior Joints (Juncturae Zygapophyseales)

The posterior joints are synovial joints (juncturae synoviales). Their articular surfaces have been detailed. The joint capsule is thicker in the lumbar spine than in the thoracic region. The posterior joints are reinforced by the following remote ligaments: interspinous ligament (ligamentum interspinale), supraspinous ligament (ligamentum supraspinale), intertransverse ligament (ligamentum intertransversarium), and flaval ligament (ligamentum flavum).

The ligamentum flavum, or yellow ligament, derives its name from its color. It extends from the lower margin of a posterior arch to the upper rim of the underlying vertebral arch. The ligament is very narrow in the thoracic region but is much thicker at the lumbar vertebrae, where it measures up to 2 to 3 mm in lateral width and 3 to 4 mm in thickness in its central part. Along its medial line, sometimes there is a slit through which a freer can be inserted. This slit separates the right side from the left side of the ligamentum flavum. In the lumbar vertebrae, it inserts cranially in a notch that faces caudally and anteriorly in the lower edge of the lamina. It attaches caudally in a notch that faces cranially and posteriorly; this notch is cut into the upper edge of the lamina of the underlying vertebra. As a result, the vertebral laminae (laminae arcus vertebrae) and the ligamentum flavum cover one another like shingles on a roof. Laterally, the ligamentum flavum extends to the anteromedial face of the articular capsule.

The ligamentum flavum forms a frontal "screen" that closes the interlaminar space posteriorly (Fig. 9).

FIG. 8. The ligaments of the vertebral column: *1*, interspinous ligament; *2*, Supraspinous ligament; *3*, intertransverse ligament; *4*, ligamentum flavum; *5*, anterior longitudinal ligament; *6*, posterior longitudinal ligament; *7*, articular capsule; and *8*, intervertebral disc.

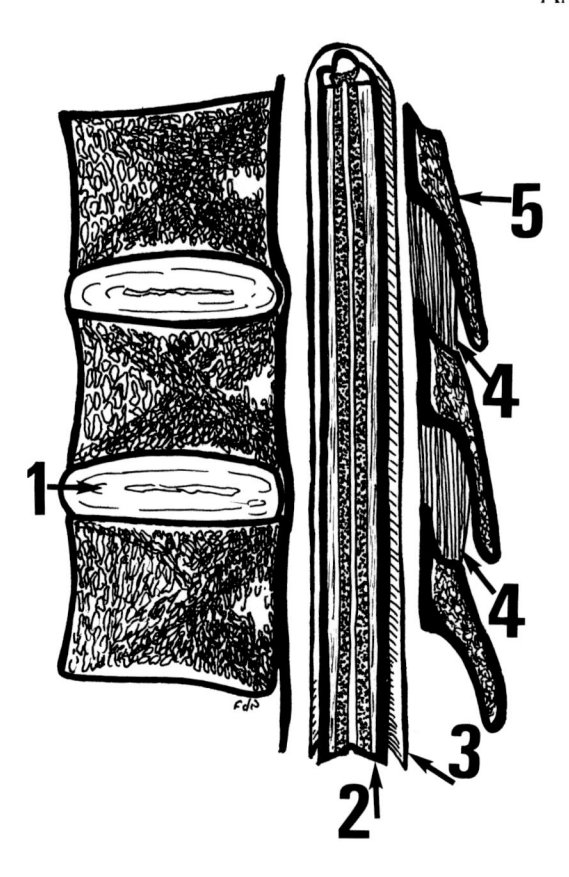

FIG. 9. Paramedian sagittal section of the thoracic spine: *1*, disc; *2*, spinal cord; *3*, dura mater; *4*, ligamentum flavum; and *5*, vertebral lamina projecting two-thirds of the way down the vertebral body and at the level of the underlying intervertebral disc.

At the lamina, and particularly at the implantation of the spinous process, it lines the ventral face of these structures, thus forming an open anterior angle. The top of this angle is situated at the medial fissure of the ligamentum flavum.

These structural characteristics have anatomic and surgical consequences. The posterior aspect of the vertebral canal is formed by the superimposition of the laminae and the ligamentum flavum. The latter bulges into the vertebral canal, particularly when the spine is extended. When the ligamentum flavum is resected, the midline vertical fissure that divides the ligament into two parts can be found; after partial resection of the spinous process of the vertebra above, this vertical fissure is more clearly visible. Because of its bony insertion, the ligamentum flavum needs to be detached with a special curette. Cranially, the curette must be inserted anterior to the caudal border of the lamina. Caudally, the cutting edge of the elevator or a scalpel blade must pass posterior to the cranial border of the lamina.

OVERVIEW OF THE ENTIRE SPINE

The vertebral column (columna vertebralis) has three curvatures in the sagittal plane—the cervical lordosis, the thoracic kyphosis, and the lumbar lordosis—below which lies the anterior sacral concavity (21,36,37).

The thoracic kyphosis extends caudally to T10. It is essentially discal in origin and is caused by the posterior opening of the intervertebral disc. Most frequently, the horizontal vertebra corresponds to T7, which is thus located at the highest point of the curvature.

The thoracolumbar junction is situated between T11 and L1. It is essentially discal in origin, resulting from the posterior widening of the intervertebral discs. It also has a secondary bone-related origin, since the vertebral bodies are slightly higher at the posterior aspect than at the anterior.

The lumbar lordosis extends from L1 to L5. It is discal in origin and results from the anterior widening of the discs. The horizontal vertebra is most often L3, which therefore marks the top point of the curvature.

The lumbosacral junction starts at L4. It involves both the anterior opening of the intervertebral disc and the asymmetric features in the vertebral body, which is higher in the anterior plane than in the posterior.

There are great variations of spinal curvature from one individual to another. Table 1 shows the respective angles between the various vertebrae (27,36,37).

It is crucial to know the vertebral endplates' angle of obliquity from the horizontal plane, as well as the obliquity of the endplates relative to each other. The

TABLE 1. Respective angles of the

	S	L5	L4	L3	L2	L1
S	0(0)0					
L5	−35(−21)−10	−27(−8)5				
L4	−53(−36)−18	−42(23)−10	−10(−1)8			
L3	−64(−47)−26	−54(−33)−16	−26(−12)0	−7(1)10		
L2	−74(−54)−28	−62(−40)−19	−36(−19)−6	−17(−6)7	−5(3)11	
L1	−79(−56)−33	−69(−42)−18	−44(−21)−2	−23(−8)11	−13(0)13	−3(5)12
T12	−82(−55)−32	−72(−41)−19	−43(−20)1	−27(−7)13	−16(1)20	−7(5)17
T11	−83(−53)−28	−70(−39)−17	−46(−18)3	−30(−5)15	−21(3)23	−11(7)20
T10	−81(−51)−24	−68(−37)−14	−43(−16)9	−28(−3)21	−22(5)29	−14(9)25
T9	−80(−48)−23	−70(−35)−10	−42(−13)11	−29(0)23	−23(8)33	−15(12)30
T8	−81(−44)−20	−71(−31)−6	−36(−9)14	−28(4)26	−22(12)40	−14(16)37
T7	−68(−39)−13	−58(−25)−2	−32(−4)19	−23(9)27	−17(17)37	−9(21)44
T6	−62(−33)−8	−51(−20)2	−27(2)27	−18(15)35	−12(23)45	−4(27)51
T5	−61(−28)−3	−51(−14)10	−29(7)32	−21(20)41	−15(28)51	−6(32)56
T4	−51(−23)4	−38(−10)17	−20(12)36	−5(25)47	1(33)57	9(37)61

From ref. 37. Statistical study involving 100 adults. Negative values are assigned to angles opening anteriorly (lordosis). In each box, the left-hand figure represents the minimum value. The right-hand figure shows the maximum value. The figure in parentheses represents the mean value.

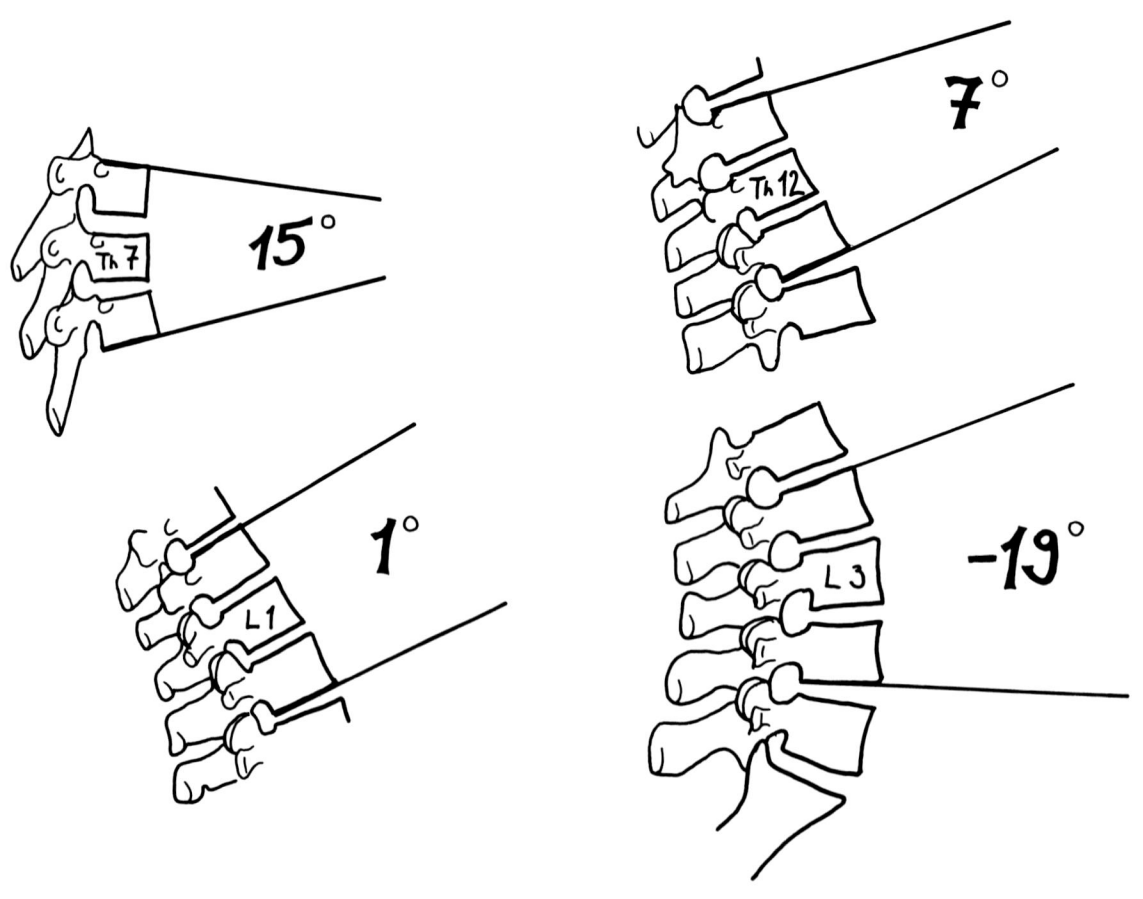

FIG. 10. The most frequently calculated angles in traumatology.

vertebral bodies from T4 and S1

T12	T11	T10	T9	T8	T7	T6	T5	T4
−5(5)14								
−7(7)17	−3(5)12							
−12(9)22	−5(6)17	−5(3)11						
−12(11)29	−5(9)27	−6(6)24	−4(4)22					
−11(15)36	−4(13)36	−6(10)37	−5(8)36	−9(4)14				
−6(21)44	1(18)47	1(15)44	4(13)35	0(10)22	−6(5)20			
−2(26)52	5(24)55	5(21)51	6(19)44	4(15)29	1(11)22	−6(4)14		
−4(32)56	3(29)60	4(26)56	7(24)52	6(21)36	6(16)31	−2(10)23	−6(4)19	
12(36)60	12(34)63	7(31)61	7(29)60	8(25)42	6(21)38	1(14)26	−2(9)17	−8(4)11

term "regional kyphosis" is improperly used to describe the angle formed by the cranial vertebral endplate of the upper vertebra and the caudal vertebral endplate of the lower vertebra of a given region. All these features need to be calculated in the event of spine trauma. Figure 10 shows the angles most frequently encountered. The sagittal index is calculated at each level and is measured as one disc and one vertebral body.

NERVE CONNECTIONS IN THORACIC AND LUMBAR VERTEBRAE

Some basic principles must be reviewed here. The spinal cord (medulla spinalis) most often ends at L2; in exceptional cases, it ends at a lower level (21). Below L2, the roots form the cauda equina. The dura mater generally ends at S2. The surgeon needs to be particularly aware of a number of specific features: the vascularization of the medulla and roots, the surface area and occupancy rates of the vertebral canal, and the basic features of decompressive surgery.

Medullar Vascularization: The Arteries of the Thoracic and Lumbar Spinal Cord (Medulla Thoracica and Lumbalis)

The main artery is the anterior spinal artery (arteria spinalis anterior), which basically acts as a central blood supply for the gray matter (substantia grisea). Ancillary arteries include the left and right posterior spinal arteries (arteria spinalis posterior). Between the posterior arteries and the anterior spinal artery (arteria spinalis anterior), there is an anastomotic pia mater network that distributes peripherally toward the funicles of the spinal cord (funiculi medullae spinalis). The anterior and posterior arteries anastomose at the conus medullaris to form an anastomotic loop.

The supply vessels branch from the radicular arteries (arteriae radiculares medullarae) of the spinal cord (4,8,13,20). The thoracic cord is principally vascularized by a small artery that originates in the spinal branches of the fourth and fifth intercostal arteries. The lumbar intumescentia is chiefly vascularized by a single radicular anterior artery stemming from the spinal branch. This, in turn, originates from an intercostal artery between T8 and T12, or from a lumbar artery at L1 or L2, most often on the left side. The

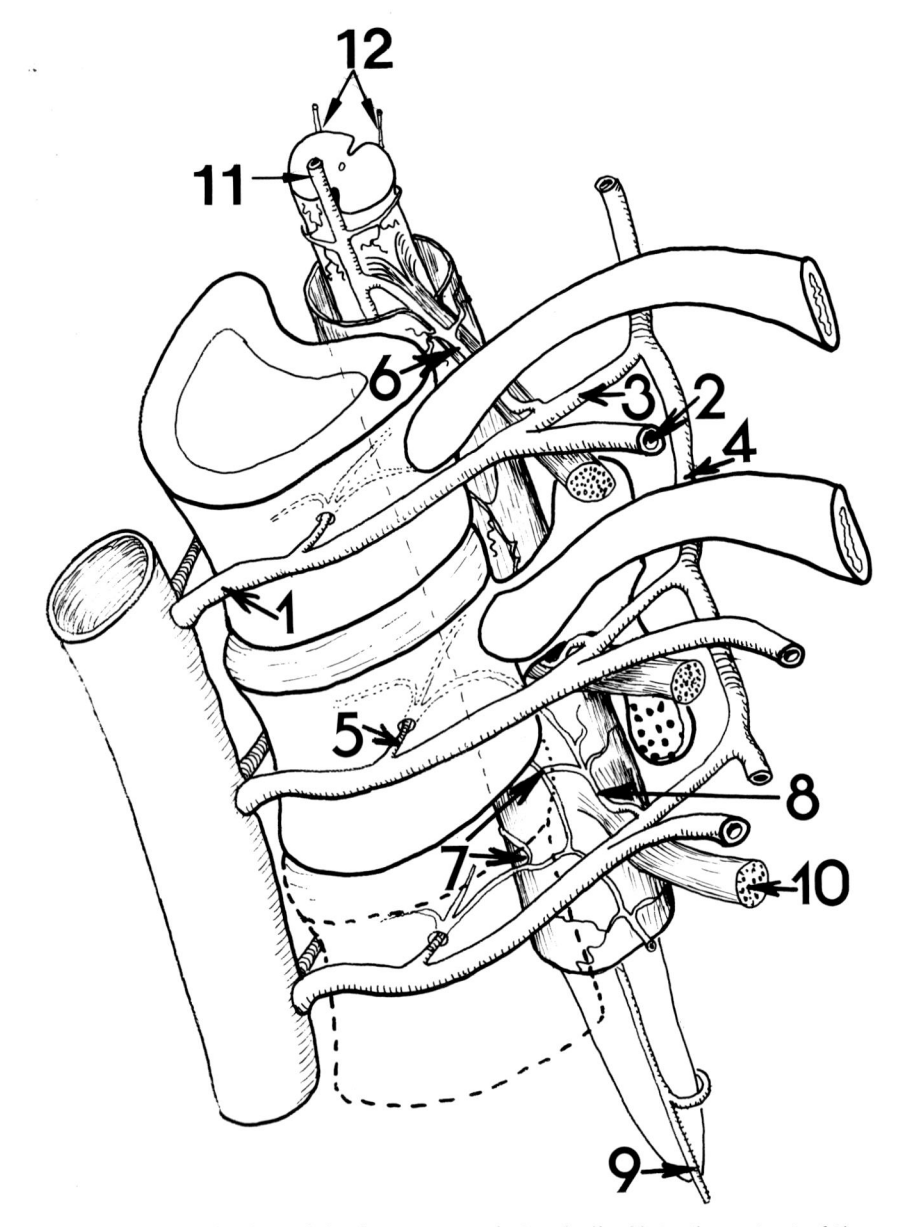

FIG. 11. Arterial vascularization of the intumescentia lumbalis. Note the extent of the anastomoses around the intervertebral foramen. *1*, Parietal artery; *2*, ventral branch; *3*, dorsal branch; *4*, posterior intramuscular anastomoses; *5*, vertebral anastomoses; *6*, radiculomedullary artery of the intumescentia lumbalis; *7*, intraspinal anastomoses; *8*, radicular artery; *9*, anastomotic loop of the conus medullaris; *10*, spinal nerve; *11*, anterior spinal artery; and *12*, dorsal spinal artery.

lumbar intumescentia and the conus medullaris receive secondary vascularization from the posterior radicular arteries, which follow the roots of the cauda equina.

There are several anastomotic levels (Fig. 11); three are of particular interest to the surgeon. The first, at the level of the pia mater, is narrow and no doubt provides only a complementary metameric supply. In general, it is not damaged by surgery.

The second level is spinal via the arteries that vascularize the vertebral column. The third level is extraspinal, involving anterior and posterior anastomoses. Posteriorly, they are situated between the dorsal branches of the intercostal arteries and the lumbar arteries. These anastomoses travel along the vertebral grooves. Anteriorly, they pass between the anterior and posterior intercostal arteries and, in the lumbar region (regio lumbalis), between the abdominal branches of the lumbar arteries. Hence the isolated sectioning of an intercostal or lumbar artery during corporectomy generally has no effect on medullar vascularization. In contrast, however, an anterior spinal approach with ligation of the intercostal or lumbar artery in association with a posterior approach involving destruction of the posterior anastomotic network can give rise to cord ischemia. In such cases, some authors (4,32) advocate a preliminary arteriogram of the spine.

Venous Drainage

Venous drainage connects the veins in the dura mater to their termination in the internal vertebral venous plexus (plexus venosus vertebralis internus) in the anterior epidural cavity and, secondarily, in the posterior epidural cavity of the lumbar and sacral spines. This plexus anastomoses abundantly with the intervertebral veins (venae intertebrales) and the anterior and posterior external vertebral plexus (plexus venosus vertebralis externus). These large veins form anastomoses between the lower and the upper vena cava systems. They also can act as a portocaval derivation via the sacral veins, which are closely connected to the medial rectal veins (venae rectales mediae) and therefore to the superior rectal vein (vena rectalis superior). Occasionally, they are responsible for catastrophic hemorrhages during corporectomies performed on patients who have had recent fractures. For these reasons, the patient necessarily must be positioned in a way that leaves the abdomen "clear," with no external pressure so venous drainage can be as efficient as possible.

The Spinal Roots

The nerve roots (radices spinales) in the thoracic spine are positioned horizontally and their direction is slightly anterior. They are covered by the dura mater and cross through the center of the vertebral foramen equidistant from the pedicles. The nerve roots are embedded in fatty tissue and are surrounded by the intervertebral veins (venae intertebrales). In the lateral part of the foramen, the roots are connected to the bony structure by fibrous expansions. Thoracic roots are vulnerable to the penetration of a pedicular screw into the intervertebral foramen.

In the lumbar and sacral vertebrae, the roots are anterior. Their axes are increasingly vertical as the roots progress caudally (Fig. 12).

In the lumbar vertebrae, the roots cross the dura mater and pass at the level of the intervertebral disc before passing into the lateral recess (recessus lateralis) and the intervertebral foramen. The root is highly vulnerable at each of these three segments.

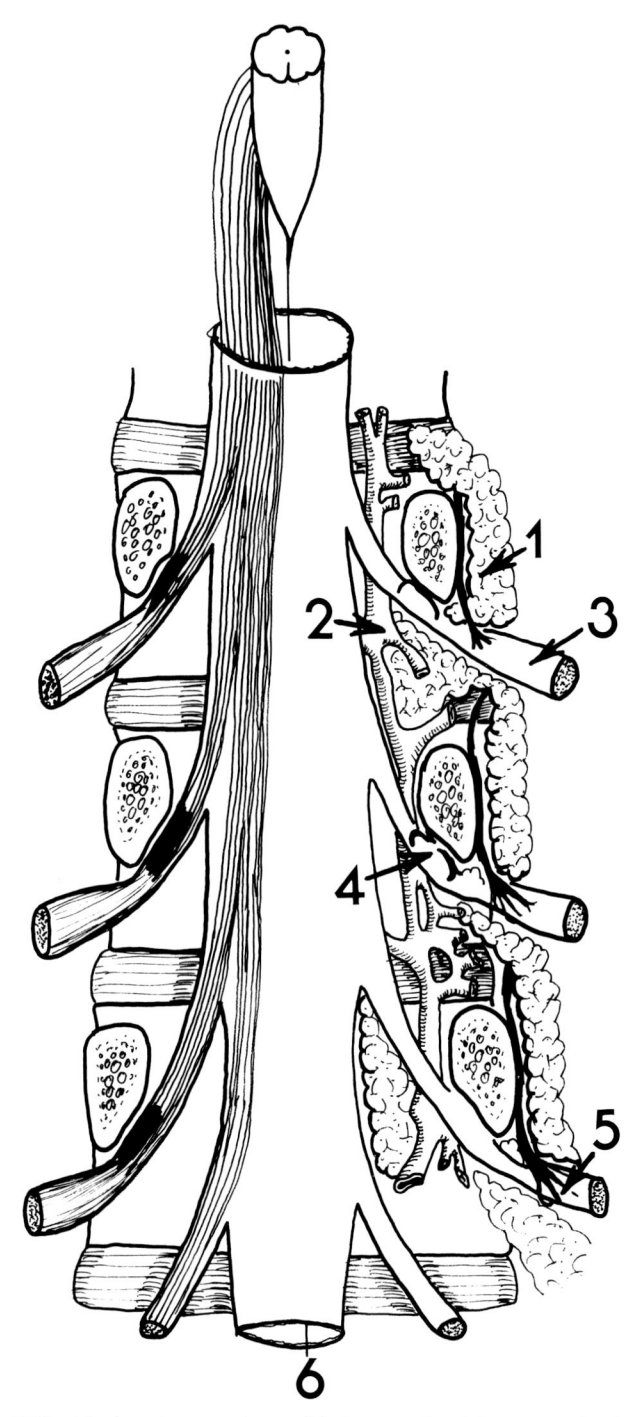

FIG. 12. Lumbar roots and intervertebral foramen (radices lumbales and foramen intervertebrale): *1*, fatty tissue; *2*, venous plexus; *3*, spinal nerve; *4*, spinal ganglion immediately under the pedicle; *5*, ligamentous bridge between the spinal nerve and the bony frame of the intervertebral foramen; and *6*, terminal filaments (filum terminale). There is no ligamentous bridge between the ganglion and the pedicle. The root can be moved with little difficulty within the spinal canal.

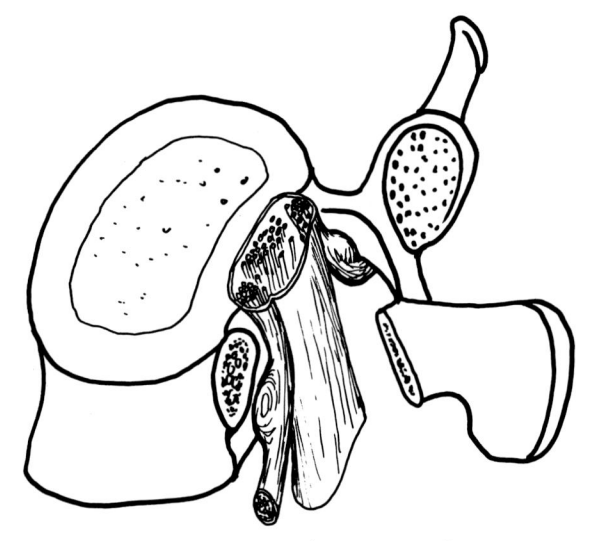

FIG. 13. The lateral recess is a narrow, bony groove.

TABLE 2. *Sagittal and transverse diameters of the vertebral foramen*

Level	Sagittal diameters (mm)		Transversal diameters (mm)	
	Mean values	Extremes	Mean values	Extremes
T1	12.4	10–14	18.3	15–20
T2	13.2	11–16	16.6	14–20
T3	14.2	11–17	14.6	12–18
T4	11.8	11–17	14.6	12–17
T5	13.5	11–17	14.4	13–17
T6	13.6	10–18	14.4	13–18
T7	13.4	10–18	14.4	13–18
T8	13.3	12–17	14.7	13–20
T9	13	10–17	14.5	13–20
T10	12.8	11–16	14.5	12–17
T11	12.9	11–16	16.7	13–20
T12	13.5	12–17	18.1	15–20
L1	13.3	11–17	18.9	16–21
L2	12.2	10–16	19	17–21
L3	9.9	10–15	19.5	17–21
L4	11.3	9–12	20.4	17–24
L5	11.3	9–15	22.5	20–25

The lateral recess (recessus lateralis) (Fig. 13) is a narrow channel enclosed ventrally by the posterior surface of the vertebral body, by the pedicle at the lateral aspect, and by the zygapophyseal joints dorsally. In the lumbar vertebrae, these joints are covered anteriorly by the extremely thick ligamentum flavum.

In the intervertebral foramen, the root passes directly under the pedicle, which is beveled caudally and medially. The spinal ganglion is located directly under this edge, into which it sometimes imprints its shape (10). At the lateral edge of the intervertebral foramen, the spinal nerve develops numerous extensions, which anchor it to the bony frame (10).

Some authors (14,17,35) have described the ligaments that attach the root to the vertebra on the root's intraspinal part. We believe the root is embedded in the internal vertebral venous plexus and the fatty tissue (corpus adiposum) of the epidural cavity. The venous plexus and fatty tissue act as a kind of shock absorber, allowing some measure of mobility. More specifically, they allow mobility for the root.

Connections in the sacral region are similar. The pedicles are beveled caudally and medially, while the ganglion is situated under the pedicle. The spinal nerve originates in the canalis sacralis and immediately divides into its two branches, which emerge through the pelvic and thoracic sacral foramina (Fig. 6).

Occupancy Rates of the Vertebral Canal

The vertebral canal is formed by the superimposition of the vertebral foramina. At T1 and T2, the vertebral foramen is oval in shape and flattens at the posterior axis. From T3 to T8, it is circular in shape before again becoming oval from T9 to L1. Downward from L2, it is triangular, with an anterior base, and becomes progressively flatter in the posterior axis.

Table 2 shows the sagittal and transverse diameters of the vertebral foramina. These dimensions were obtained from millimetric measurements on 20 dry spines in the Nice anatomy laboratory.

The anterior aspect of the vertebral canal is formed by the superimposition of the vertebral bodies and the vertebral discs. Laterally, it is formed by the superimposition of the pedicles and intervertebral foramina. Dorsally, the vertebral canal is formed by the superimposition of the laminae and ligamentum flavum. The anterior surface of the ligamentum flavum bulges into the vertebral canal. The bulge increases when the spine is extended.

Caudally and posteriorly, the inclination of the laminae is oblique. The ligamentum flavum occupies the space created by this oblique angulation. Computerized axial tomography can provide high quality horizontal sections of the spine. However, evaluation of the real anteroposterior diameter of the vertebral canal depends on identification of the ligamentum flavum (Fig. 14). Failure to do this means the anteroposterior diameter will be overestimated. The same is true for measurement of the surface of the vertebral canal.

Magnetic resonance imaging provides excellent visualization of the ligamentum flavum and precludes errors of this kind.

Current imaging techniques allow evaluation of the degree of traumatic stenosis in the vertebral canal by indicating the extent of posterior wall retropulsion and the occupancy rate of the vertebral canal.

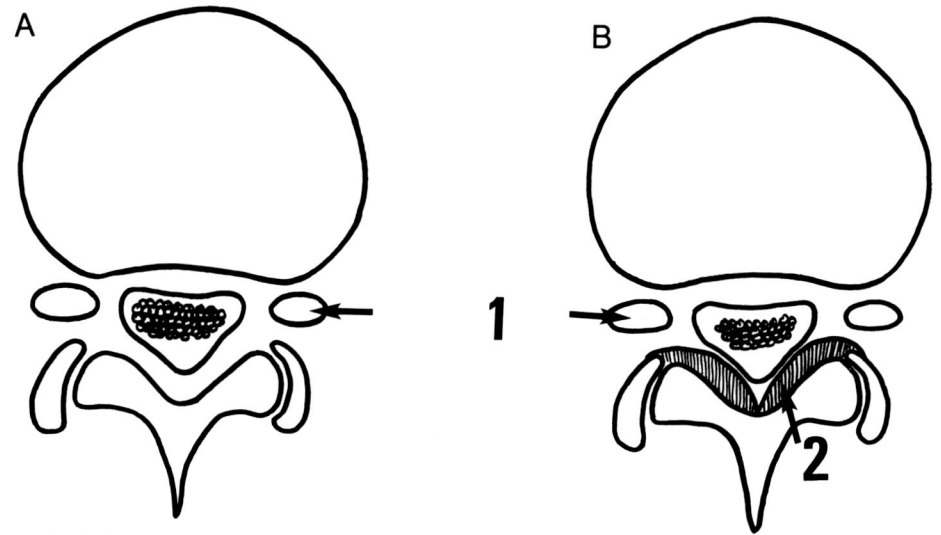

FIG. 14. **A:** Schematic horizontal section as shown by CT scan. **B:** The same cross section showing the ligamentum flavum. Note the thickness of this ligament.

Rene Louis (21) observed that the thoracic spinal cord (medulla spinale thoracica) occupies two-thirds of the sagittal diameter of the vertebral canal and five-eighths of the transverse diameter.

Our analysis (Table 3) of the sections confirmed these figures and showed that the sheath formed by the dura mater of the spinal cord is situated 3 mm from the pedicle and 1 or 2 mm from the posterior surface of the vertebral body. However, the sheath of the dura mater, covering the lumbar roots, is in direct contact with the pedicles. In the region of the thoracic and lumbar vertebrae, the dura mater does not adhere to the vertebral body.

The spinal cord is situated 2 to 4 mm from the posterior face of the vertebral body, depending on the position of the spine. It is located an average of 4 mm from the pedicle.

We undertook five deep-frozen horizontal cross sections on five laboratory subjects. The cross sections were photographed and enlarged, and the surfaces of the various features were measured on graph paper and expressed in percentages of the total surface of the vertebral canal. It should be stressed that the surface of the vertebral canal is measured inside the boundaries imposed by the ligamentum flavum. If the surface area were measured exclusively within the lamina of the vertebral arch, without taking into consideration the thickness of the ligamentum flavum, higher values would be obtained with caudal progression within a given vertebra, since the lamina is obliquely oriented in the caudal and posterior axes (Fig. 9).

The mean values obtained are given in Table 3. We observed considerable variations at the thoracolumbar junction due to variations in the length of the spinal cord.

It should be noted that the cross section of the spinal cord does not exceed 30% of the surface area of the vertebral canal. This explains why, in some cases, a 60% narrowing has no clinical symptoms.

TABLE 3. *Vertebral canal surface occupation rates (in percentages) of the spinal cord, the roots, the fatty tissue, the vessels, the dura mater, and the cerebrospinal fluid*

Level	Medulla	Radices	Corpus adiposum	Arteriae and venae	Dura mater and liquor cerebrospinalis
T1	30%			44%	26%
T4	30%			50%	20%
T12	20%			40%	40%
L1	2%	28%	15%	15%	40%
L3		17%	20%	25%	36%
S1		8%	45%	15%	32%

The study was undertaken using five adult cadavers.

THE ANATOMIC RUDIMENTS OF DECOMPRESSIVE SURGERY

The thoracic portion of the spinal cord (pars thoracica medullae) is attached anteriorly to the vertebral bodies by the roots, which have a lateral and slightly anterior orientation. The thoracic spinal cord can be compared to a man clinging to a column with his upper limbs. This renders the thoracic spinal cord very vulnerable to anterior compression and displacement.

Figure 15 shows the action of the classic posterosuperior fragment observed in burst fractures (3). After reduction of the deformity, surgical decompression can be undertaken using an anterior or posterior approach. Whether an anterior or posterior approach is used, the surgeon must verify abdominal *freedom* in order to reduce venous bleeding. Corporectomy allows in situ decompression and has no detrimental effect on arterial vascularization if an anterior approach is used exclusively.

In the thoracic vertebral column, posterior laminectomy is effective only if it removes the lower section of the upper lamina as well as the lamina of the fractured vertebra. In the region of the lumbar spine, the ligamentum flavum situated posterior to the lesion should be removed. Laminectomy can be extended to the pedicle (3), thus removing the vertebral arch, which allows a posterolateral approach to the vertebral body. During excision of the pedicle, the lumbar root can be damaged in the lateral recess (recessus lateralis). The thoracic spinal root (radix spinalis thoracica) is situated farther from the pedicle, which is narrower than in the lumbar vertebrae. All these procedures are associated with considerable bleeding.

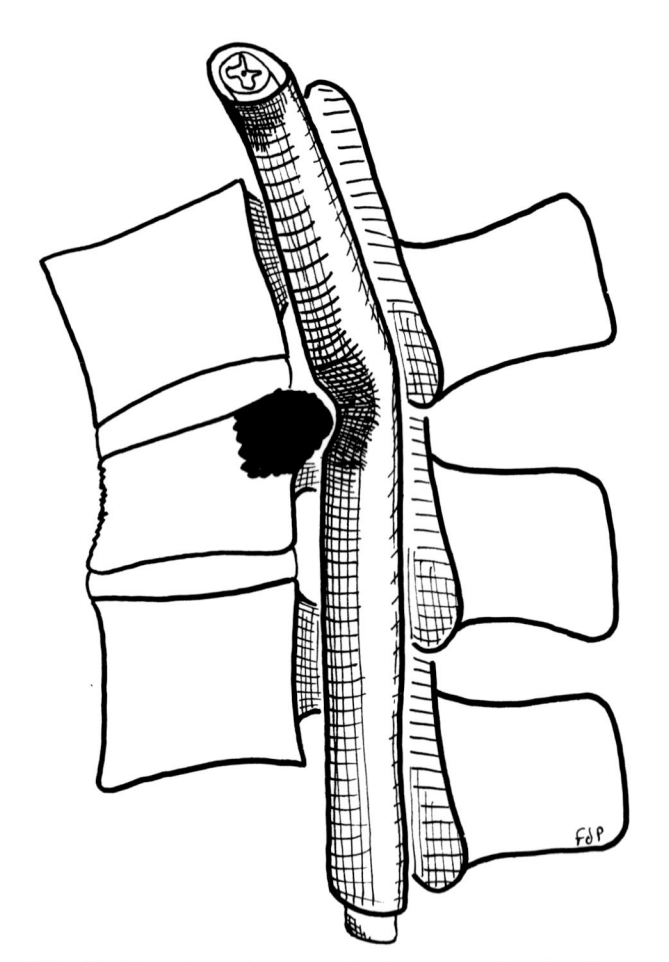

FIG. 15. Classic posterosuperior fragment showing its effect on the dura mater. Laminectomy of the affected vertebra involves no posterior decompression because the lamina juts out, covering the lower two-thirds of the vertebral body. Partial laminectomy of the overlying vertebra should be performed concurrently.

ANATOMIC RUDIMENTS OF PEDICULAR AND SACRAL SCREW INSERTION

Pedicular screw insertion by posterior approach presupposes awareness of both the anatomy of the pedicles and their various landmarks.

Anatomy of the Pedicle

Using 20 dry spines, we measured the height, thickness, and orientation of the pedicles in the horizontal plane (Fig. 16). The results are given in Table 4. Our results are the same as those of other authors (19,24,32,39,40).

The following can be concluded:

1. The T1 and T2 pedicles can accommodate a screw with a diameter of 5 mm or less.
2. The thoracic pedicles from T3 to T10 are narrow. A 4-mm screw may perforate the pedicle, since some pedicles are less than 3 mm in width.
3. The pedicle size of T11 and the vertebrae below it allows the use of screws with a diameter of 5 or 6 mm. This can be assessed by preoperative CT scan.
4. In the lower lumbar vertebrae, it may be possible to use 7-mm screws.
5. During insertion of the screw, the surgeon must be aware of the pedicle convergence angle. The T1 and T2 pedicles are the most convergent pedicles in the anterior and internal planes. They describe open anterior and medial angles and lie from 10° to 40° from the sagittal plane. From T3 to T10, the pedicles are oriented a few degrees medially. From T11 to L1, the pedicles are oriented in the sagittal

TABLE 4. Variations of width and orientation of pedicles

Level	Width (mm)		Height (mm)		Orientation	
	Mean	Extremes	Mean	Extremes	Mean	Extremes
T1	7	5–10	8	6–11	28°	20–40°
T2	5.25	4–7	10.25	8–11	20°	10–30°
T3	4.5	3–7	9.6	7–11	14°	5–20°
T4	3.62	3–5	10.37	8–12	9°	5–15°
T5	3.75	3–5	10	7–12	9°	5–15°
T6	4.25	3–6	10	7–12	6°	0–10°
T7	4.25	3–6	9.87	8–12	5°	0–10°
T8	4.25	3–6	11	8–12	5°	0–10°
T9	4.75	3–7	11.62	9–16	4°	0–5°
T10	6.12	4–10	13.75	9–18	3°	0–5°
T11	7.37	5–10	15.5	12–20	1°	−5 to +5°
T12	7.25	5–11	14.5	12–18	−2°	−5 to +5°
L1	6	3–9	11.5	8–15	1°	0–5°
L2	6.75	4–12	13.75	11–17	4°	0–10°
L3	7.62	5–12	13.75	11–17	7°	5–10°
L4	10.37	7–18	13.12	10–15	9°	5–15°
L5	15.71	13–18	12	10–15	16°	5–20°

Study was undertaken using 20 dry spines.

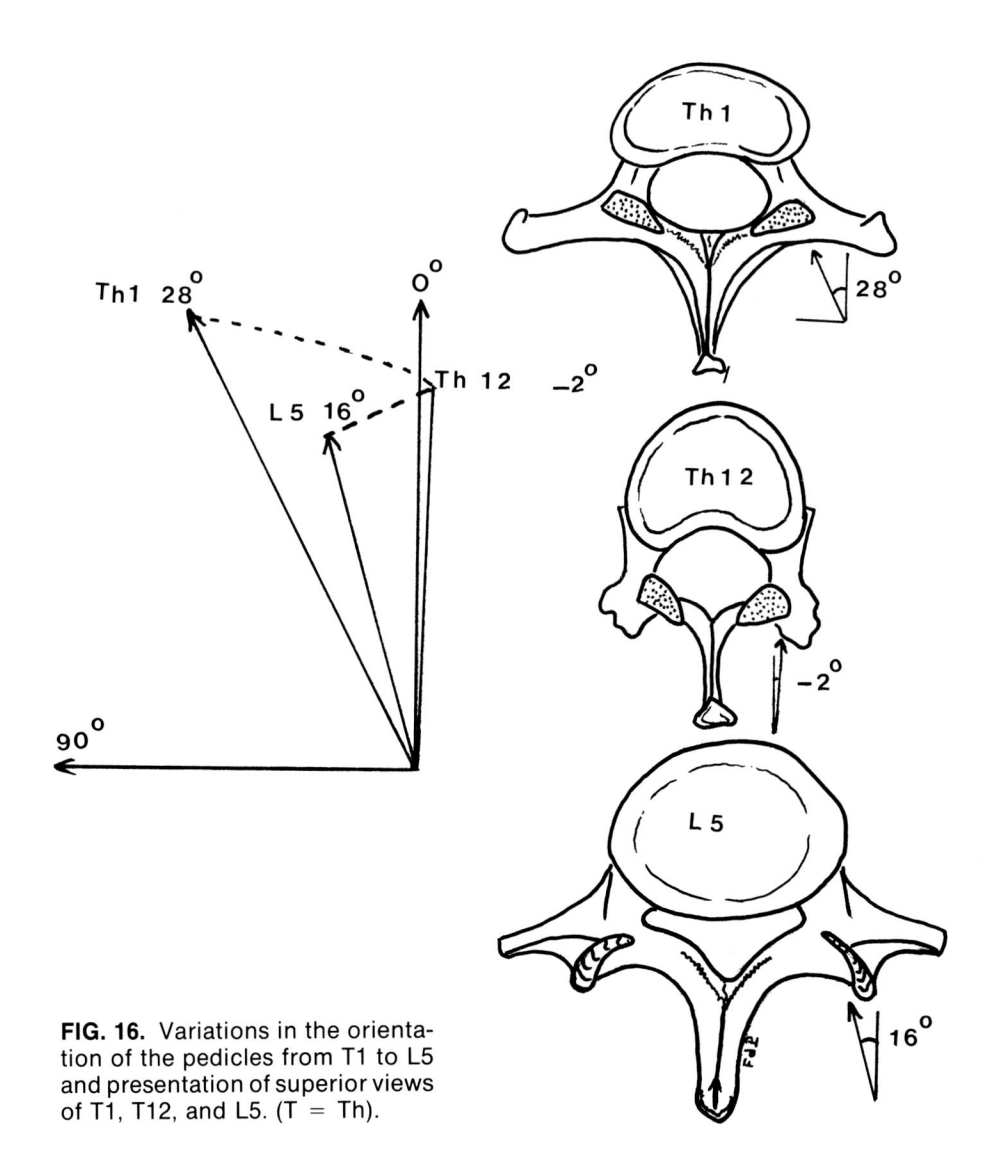

FIG. 16. Variations in the orientation of the pedicles from T1 to L5 and presentation of superior views of T1, T12, and L5. (T = Th).

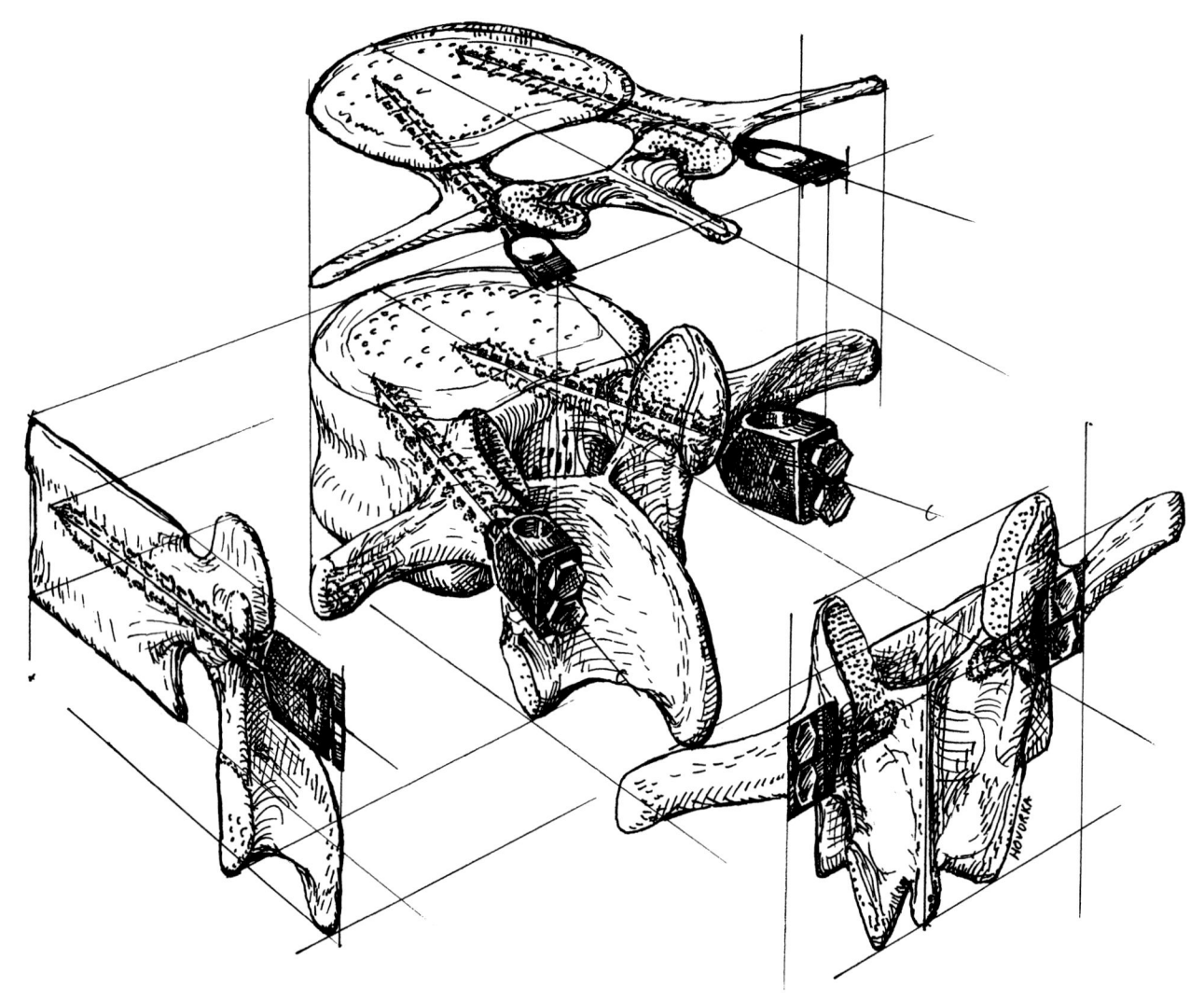

FIG. 17. Insertion of a pedicular screw [Cotrel–Dubousset (7–15)] along the axis of the pedicle. The insertion point is located in the center of the base of the transverse process.

plane, slightly medially and ventrally. Below L1, the pedicles are increasingly medially oriented and describe an open ventral and medial angle of 4° to the sagittal plane at L2. This angle is 16° at L5.

Using these data, the surgeon can drill "straight forward" as described by Raymond Roy-Camille et al. (31,32,34), inserting a pedicular screw in the sagittal plane, or a pedicular screw can be inserted along the axis of the pedicle (Fig. 17). If a large diameter screw (7,38) is required, the surgeon could adopt the "axis" technique. In the strictly sagittal screw insertion, the screw often *re-emerges* if the size of the screw is *approximately the same* as that of the pedicle (Fig. 18). Finally, sagittal screws are prone to reemerge ventrally at the circumferential surface of the vertebra. Thus, since there are two types of pedicle screw techniques, the "straight ahead" and "axis" methods, there are two pedicular targeting techniques (Fig. 19).

The "Straight Ahead" ("Droit Devant") Technique

The "straight ahead" technique (31,32,34) is subject to a hard and fast rule: the center of the pediculus is located below the lower margin of the superior articular process. Targeting is undertaken differently for the thoracic and lumbar vertebrae.

Targeting the Thoracic Vertebrae

The articular processes are situated in a frontal plane, and the center of the pedicle projects below the middle of the superior articular process (Fig. 20). As a result, it is essential to use scalpel and curette to incise and resect the articular capsule. The articular cavity becomes visible after resection of the fatty margins of the synovial folds (plicae synovialis). The lateral and medial extremity of the articular cavity must be per-

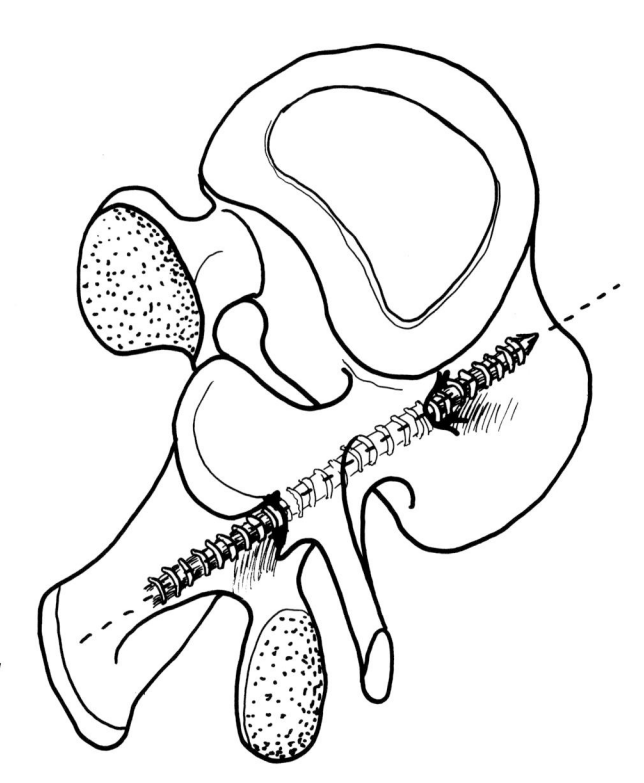

FIG. 18. Schematic diagram of a strictly sagittal screw emerging from the vertebra.

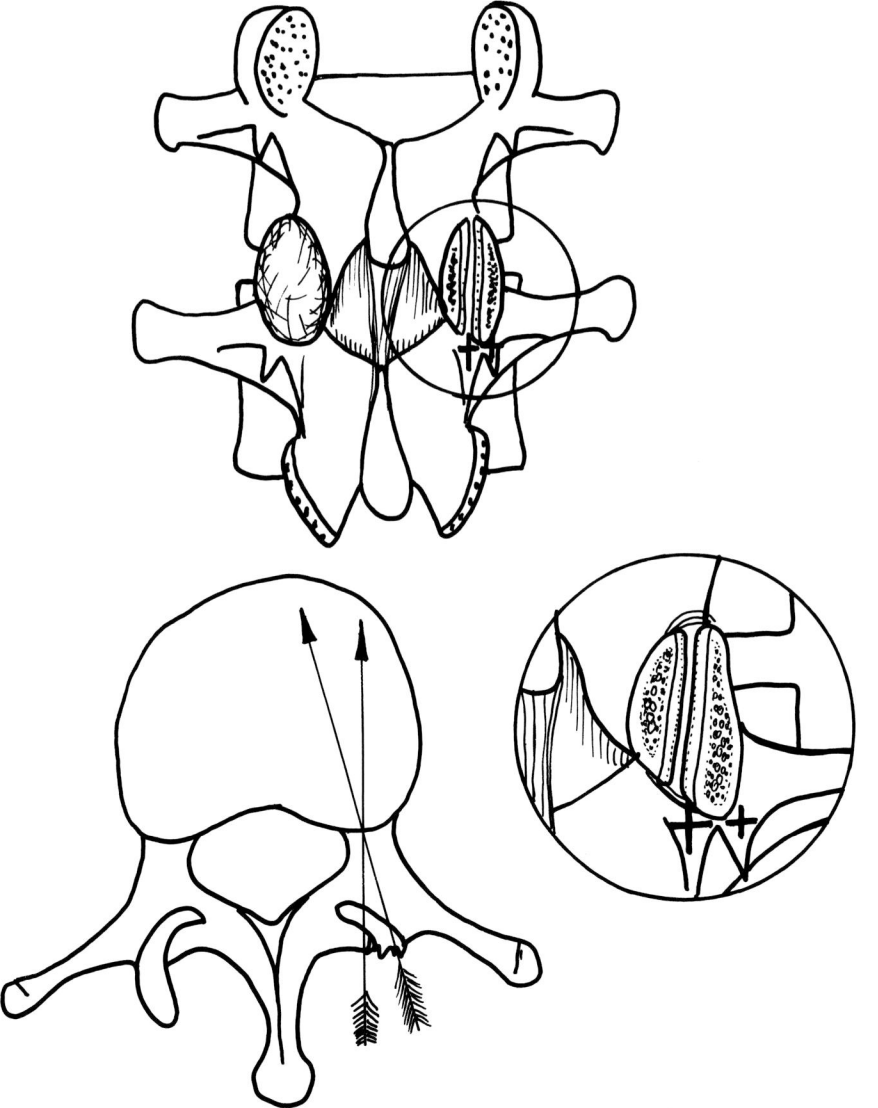

FIG. 19. The two types of pedicular screw insertion techniques at the lumbar level. The **inset** shows the articular cavity after resection of the zygapophyseal joint. The two *crosses* indicate possible screw insertion points: below the articular cavity in the "straight ahead" technique; and outside the articular cavity at the base of the transverse process for medial and frontal screw insertion along the axis of the pedicle.

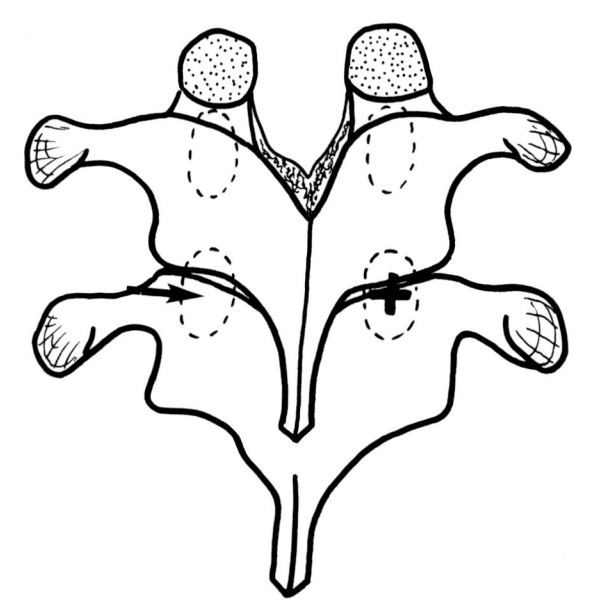

FIG. 20. Posterior view of two thoracic vertebrae showing the insertion point of the pedicular screw in the "straight ahead" technique.

fectly exposed. This is a delicate maneuver medially, since the surgeon must guard against penetrating the vertebral canal. The surgeon can mobilize the articular cavity by grasping the spinous processes with a Kocher clamp. The center of the articular cavity must be located and the hole drilled 1 mm below the lower margin of the superior articular process of the vertebra. At this level, a bony hump corresponding to the upper rim of the lamina is observed. To prevent the drill from slipping, the hump must be flattened with a rongeur, or the hole is countersunk with a square point.

Targeting the Lumbar Vertebrae

The articular cavity is located in the sagittal plane. It is essential to resect the posterior projection of the zygapophyseal joints with a large rongeur. Then, the articular cavity can be seen as a vertical line, which can easily be visualized by moving the vertebrae together. The surgeon can follow this vertical line and countersink a hole 1 mm below the articular cavity. In this region, a bony crest corresponding to the cranial part of the pars interarticularis is noted. This crest must be smoothed with a small gouge or rongeur before countersinking the screw hole (Fig. 17).

Screw Insertion Along the Pedicular Axis

First, the articular cavity of the posterior intervertebral joints must be located, using the same procedure as for the "straight ahead" technique. This allows the instruments to make contact with the spine.

The second stage involves preparing the entry point by breaking through the compact bone that forms the posterior part of the base of the transverse process. In the lumbar vertebrae, there is a clear distinction between the transverse process and the vertebral lamina. The line between the two structures is marked (Figs. 3, 17, and 19) by the accessory process, which must be resected using a small rongeur to prepare the hole for insertion of the screw.

In the thoracic vertebrae, the transverse process slopes gently into the vertebral lamina, and the base of the transverse process can be located on the line that connects the lateral edges (Fig. 21) of the superior and inferior articular processes. At T1 and T2, the entry

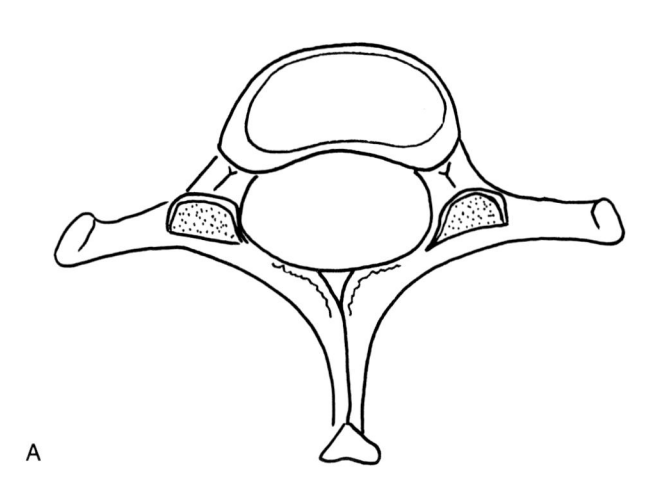

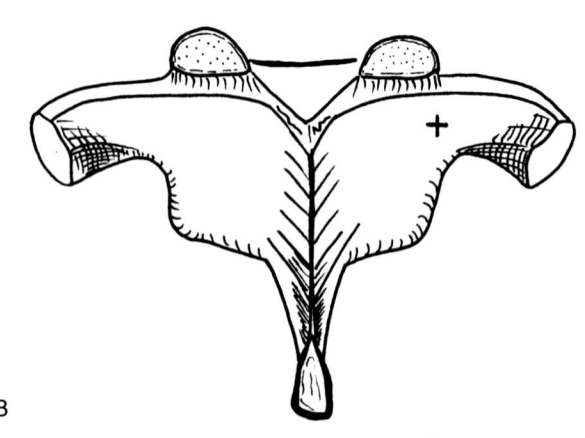

FIG. 21. Vertebra T1. **A:** Superior view of T1 showing the marked medial and frontal orientation of the pedicle. **B:** Posterior view. The *cross* marks the entry point of the screw, which has been inserted along the pedicular axis.

point will appear to be located in a very lateral position, much more so than in the underlying vertebrae. This is because the vertebral foramen flattens considerably in the transverse plane at T1 and T2. After the cortex has been penetrated, the screw insertion path can be prepared.

The third stage involves preparing the path for screw insertion using a bit or a square-point punch, bearing in mind the mean orientation values of the pedicle (see section on pedicular anatomy). A safer procedure involves starting the screw hole with a fine curette, which is rotated on its axis and guided through the dense sheath of compact bone to penetrate the cancellous bone. During one of our training courses, we asked 30 surgeons to use this method to insert a 6-mm diameter screw into two low lumbar pedicles on anatomical specimens, which were then radiographed and autopsied. Only two screws reemerged from the pedicles. Surgeons are advised to place a reference mark and to obtain perioperative radiographs before proceeding with final screw insertion.

Anatomic Features for Sacral Vertebrae Screw Insertion

The articular cavity of the zygoapophyseal joints of the lumbosacral junction is located in neither the frontal nor sagittal plane. The location varies from individual to individual, and even from one side to the other. It is oriented in a posteromedial plane and describes an open external angle with the frontal plane, varying from 0° to 60° and averaging approximately 30°. The articular cavity is prolonged caudally by a bony crest, similar to the lumbar vertebrae (Figs. 6 and 22).

The lateral part of the sacrum ala is filled with fat (Fig. 7). The surgeon must bear in mind that the base of the sacrum (basis ossis sacri) faces cranially and ventrally and describes an average angle of 42° to the horizontal plane in a subject in the anatomic reference position. This is important for screw placement. A perioperative radiograph is crucial to check the orientation of the sacrum on the subject in the prone position (Fig. 23).

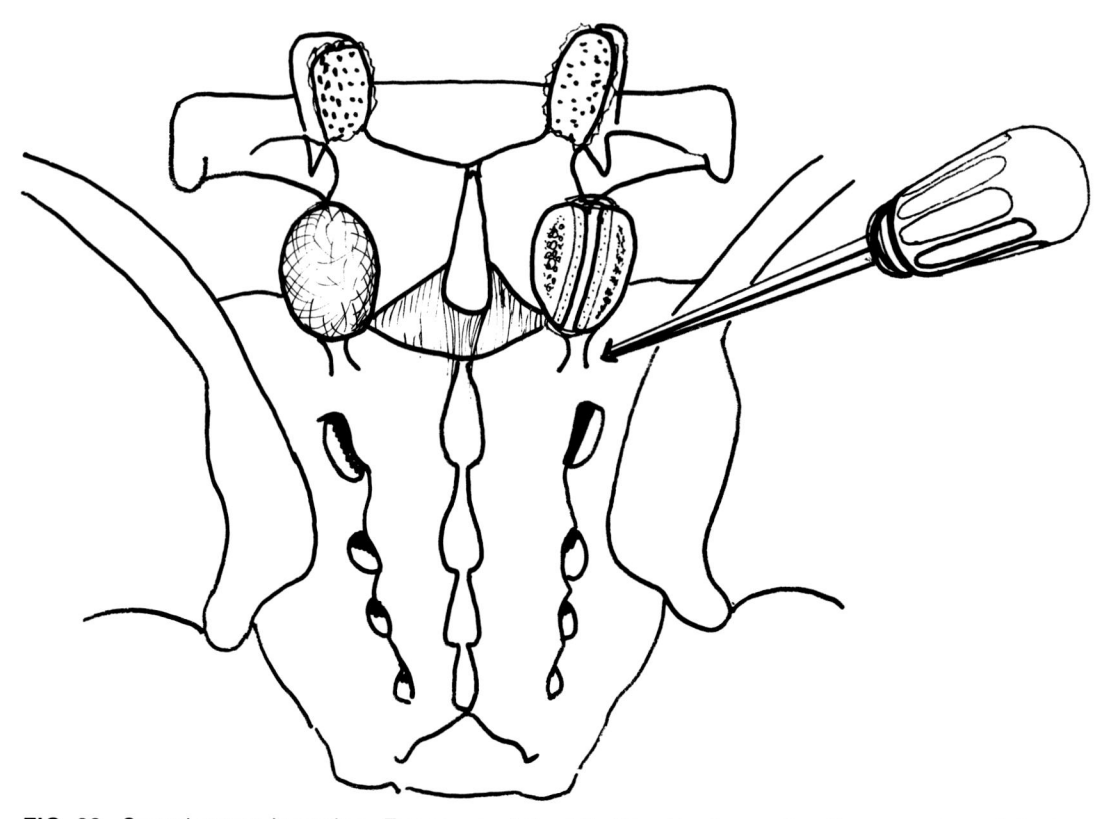

FIG. 22. Sacral screw insertion. Exposure of the L5–S1 articular cavity after resection of the L5 inferior articular process. The square-tipped point is inserted in order to prepare the pathway of an S1 corporeo pedicular screw. It is oriented as medially and frontally as the posterior projection of the iliac crest allows.

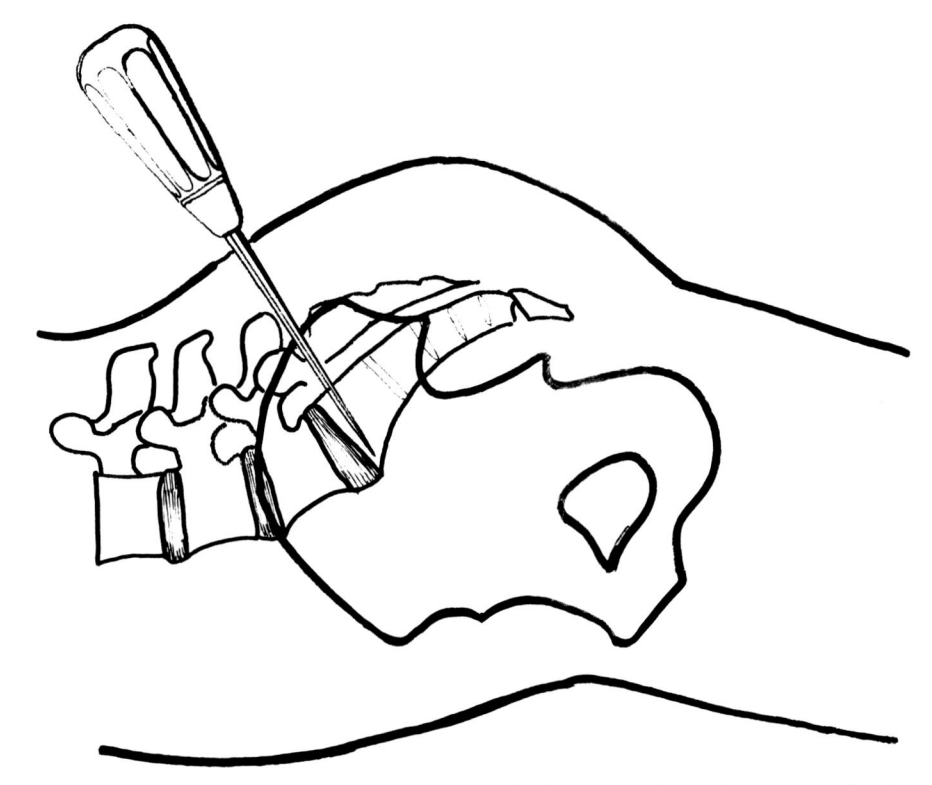

FIG. 23. Diagram of perioperative radiograph control of a square-tipped point inserted to prepare the path of a sacral screw.

At S1, three different screw insertion orientations are advocated. Raymond Roy-Camille et al. (33) advises the "straight ahead" orientation, parallel to the S1 endplate (Fig. 24). Rene Louis (22,23) suggests an oblique, anterior, external, caudal orientation that describes an angle of 30° to 45° to the horizontal and sagittal planes (Fig. 24).

Following experimental work (11,12), we suggest "corporeo pedicular" screw insertion close to the S1 endplate (Fig. 25) or, even better, perforating this endplate to obtain a more solid anchorage in bone.

Whatever technique is adopted, the first stage involves exposing the S1 articular processes by resecting the lower facet of L5. A bony crest is below the S1 articular facet. The drill hole for the "corporeo pedicular" technique is 3 mm lower and external to the S1 articular facet or, in other words, 3 mm external to the above-mentioned bony crest and oriented from lateral to medial.

At the S2 level, the landmarks are easily determined between the first and second dorsal sacral foramina (foramina sacralia dorsalia). However, two possible

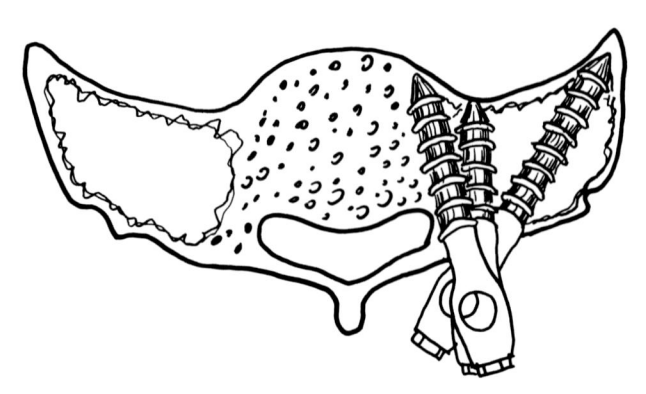

FIG. 24. Insertion of a corporeo pedicular screw at S1. See the three types of screws in S1. See also Fig. 7.

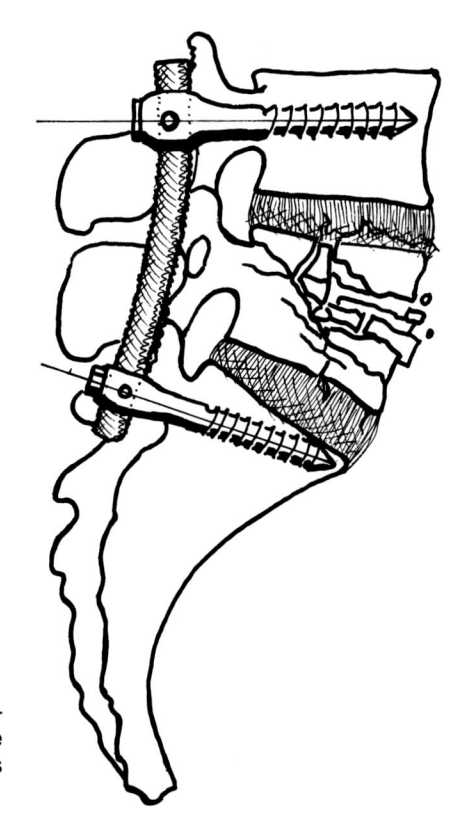

FIG. 25. Diagram of a Cotrel–Dubousset (7,15) lumbo-sacral fixture using the authors' method. The sacral screw lies flush with the S1 sacral endplate.

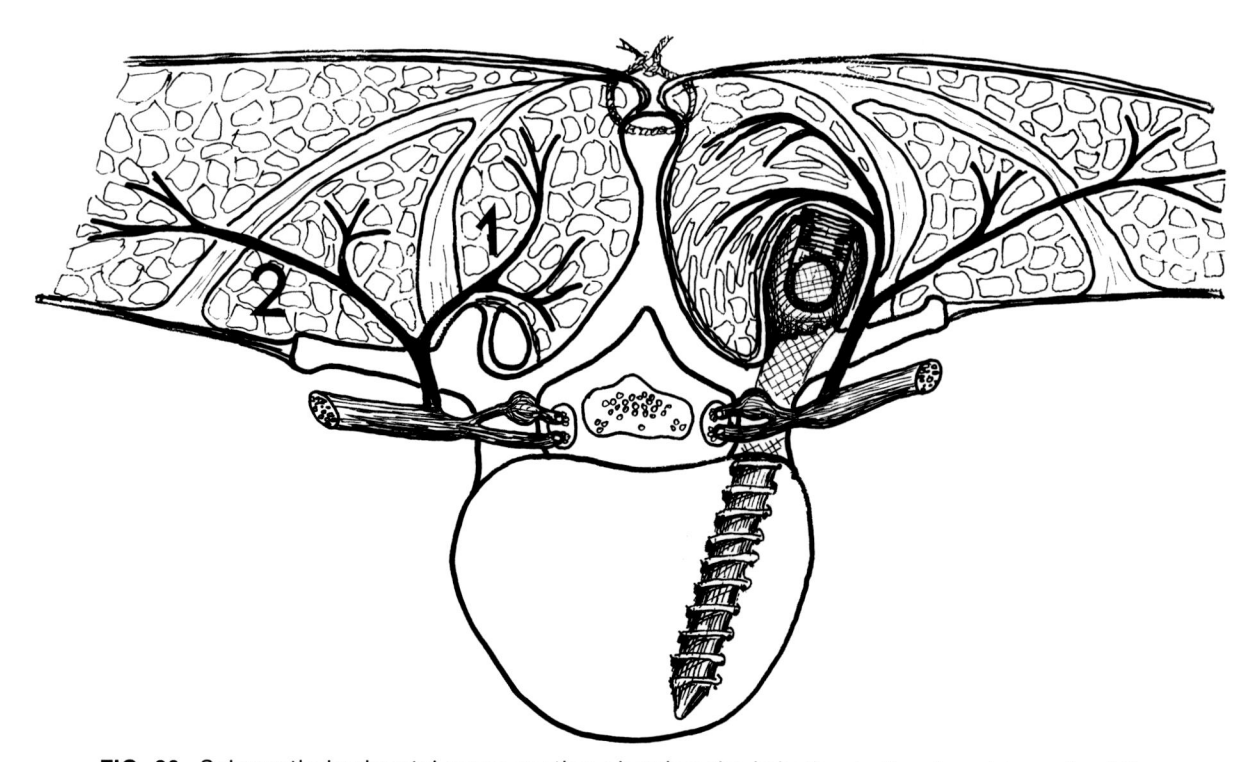

FIG. 26. Schematic horizontal cross section showing the irritation in the dorsal branch of the spinal nerve caused by fixtures (a screw head shown here) used in extreme lateral osteosynthesis. *1*, Medial branch of the dorsal branch; and *2*, lateral branch of the dorsal branch.

orientations can be adopted, either "straight ahead" or anterior and external, into the lateral mass of the sacrum. The "corporeo pedicular" orientation (i.e., ventral and medial) is impossible because of the posterior and internal projections of the posterior superior iliac spine (spina iliaca posterior superior), which protrudes exactly between the first and second sacral dorsal foramina.

Hazards Related to Pedicular Screws

The hazards inherent in the use of pedicular screws are essentially related to the nerves. Investigations of the nervous connections in the spine have shown us that the dura mater sheath of the spinal cord is situated at least 2 mm from the pedicle; the spinal cord is located at least 4 mm from the pedicle. This explains why it is possible to have encroachment of the screw without incurring neurologic damage (18).

In the thoracic vertebrae, the roots are horizontal and emerge from the center of the intervertebral foramen, therefore some distance from the upper and lower pedicles.

In the lumbar and sacral vertebrae, the nerve roots descend almost vertically. They pass into the lateral recesses (recessus lateralis) and directly under the pedicle of the vertebra of the same name, and the spinal ganglion is situated directly beneath the pedicle. Thus the sacral and lumbar nerve roots, especially the ganglion, are directly vulnerable to the medial or caudal projection of a pedicular screw. Suprapedicular projection involves no danger for the nerves.

Figure 26 illustrates the danger of compression of the dorsal branch (ramus dorsalis) of the spinal nerve due to extreme lateral screw insertion when pedicular screws were placed along the axis of the pedicle. Likewise, an extensive approach to the transverse process can cause damage to the dorsal branch.

Pedicular screws also constitute a hazard to the vascular system when screws project too far. Although there is little need to insist on the presence of the aorta, the inferior vena cava, and the intercostal and lumbar arteries, it should be noted that the median sacral artery (arteria sacralis mediana) is located anterior to the sacrum, and that the internal iliac artery (arteria iliaca interna) and its branches are anterior to the sacroiliac joint.

REFERENCES

1. Aman-Jean F. *La region thoraco-lombaire.* These de Paris, No. 450. Paris: Gaston Doin et Cie, 1928.
2. Amstutz HC, Sissons HA. The structure of the vertebral spongiosa. *J Bone Joint Surg* 1969;51B:540.
3. Argenson C. Traitement des fractures du rachis dorso-lombaire chez l'adulte. In: *Conferences d'Enseignement.* Paris: Expansion Scientifique Francaise, 1984;5–27.
4. Argenson C. Cals vicieux et pseudarthroses du rachis thoracolombaire. In: *Cahiers d'Enseignement de la SOFCOT, Conferences d'Enseignement.* Paris: Expansion Scientifique Fransaise, 1990;205–234.
5. Boden S, McCowin P, Davis D, Dina T, Mark A, Weisel S. Abnormal magnetic resonance scans of the cervical spine in asymptomatic subjects. *J Bone Joint Surg* 1990;72A:1178–1184.
6. Branchereau A, et al. Abord de la charniere dorso-lombaire par voie sous pleuro-peritoneale. *Nouv Presse Med* 1975;4–9: 649–651.
7. Cotrel Y, Dubousset J. Nouvelle technique d'osteosynthese rachidienne segmentaire par voie posterieure. *Rev Chir Orthop* 1984;70:489–494.
8. Crock HV, Yoshizawa H. *The blood supply of the vertebral column and spinal cord in man.* New York: Springer-Verlag, 1977.
9. Decoulx P, Rienau G. Les fractures du rachis dorso-lombaire sans troubles nerveux. *Rev Chir Orthop* 1958;44(4):254–328.
10. de Peretti F, Micalef JP, Bourgeon A, Argenson C, Rabischong P. Biomechanics of the lumbar spinal nerve roots and the first sacral root within the intervertebral foramina. *Surg Radiol Anat* 1989;11:221–225.
11. de Peretti F, et al. Bases anatomiques du traitement chirurgical par le materiel Cotrel–Dubousset des fractures du rachis thoracique et lombaire. *Acta Orthop Belg* 1991;57:126–136.
12. de Peretti F, Argenson C, Bourgeon A, Eude P, Aboulker C. Bases anatomiques et experimentales de la mise en place d'une vis d'osteosynthese au niveau de la premiere vertebre sacree. *Surg Radiol Anat* 1991;13:133–137.
13. Dommisse GF. The blood supply of the spinal cord. *J Bone Joint Surg* 1974;56B(2):225–235.
14. Falconer MA, McGeorge M, Begg A. Observations on the cause and mechanism of symptom-production in sciatica and low back pain. *J Neurol Neurosurg Psychiatry* 1948;11:13J.
15. Farcy JPC, Weidenbaum M, Hoeltzel DA, Athanasiou KA. A comparative biomechanical study of spine fixation using Cotrel–Dubousset instrumentation. *Spine* 1987;12(9):877–881.
16. Fey B. L'abord du rein par voie thoraco-abdominale. *Arch Urol* 1925;159(5):169–178.
17. Forestier J. Le trou de conjugaison vertebral et l'espace epidural. Etude anatomique et clinique. These de Paris, 1922.
18. Gertzbein S, Robbins S. Accuracy of pedicular screw placement in vivo. *Spine* 1990;15(1):11–14.
19. Gonon GP, Rousson B, Fischer LP, DeMourgues G. Interet chirurgical de la connaissance anatomique des directions pediculaires au niveau du rachis dorso-lombaire. *Lyon Chirurgical* 1974;70(6):408–410.
20. Lazorthes G, Gouaze A, Zadeh J, Santini JJ, Lazorthes Y. Arterial vascularization of the spinal cord. *J Neurosurg* 1991;35: 253–262.
21. Louis R. *Chirurgie du rachis: anatomie chirurgicale et voies d'abord.* Berlin: Springer-Verlag, 1982.
22. Louis R. Fusion of the lumbar and sacral spine by internal fixation with screw plates. *Clin Orthop* 1986;203:18–33.
23. Louis R. Reconstruction isthmique des spondylolyses par plaque vissee et greffes sans arthrodeses. A propos de 78 cas. *Rev Chir Orthop* 1988;74(6):549–557.
24. Marchesi D, Schneider E, Glauser P, Aebi M. Morphometric analysis of the thoracolumbar and lumbar pedicles, anatomoradiologic study. *Surg Radiol Anat* 1988;10:317–322.
25. Mitchell M, Mirbaha MD. Anterior approach to the thoracolumbar junction of the spine by a retroperitoneal extrapleural technique. *Clin Orthop* 1973;91:41–47.
26. Mitchell M, Mirbaha MD. Exposure of the vertebral bodies of the proximal lumbar segments: some anatomic points. *Spine* 1978;3–4:329–335.
27. Niedermann E. *Normwerte der sagittalen Krummung von Brust und Lendenwirbelsaule Erwchsener, Ergebnisse einer Reihenuntersuchung.* Verlag Zurich, Germany: Juris Druck, 1968.
28. Paturet G. *Traite d'anatomie humaine,* vols I, II, and IV. Paris: Masson et Cie, 1951.

29. Rabischong P, Louis R, Vignaud J, Massare G. Le disque intervertebral. *Anat Clin* 1978;1:55–64.
30. Rieunau G. Etude biomecanique des forces de rupture des corps vertebraux dorso-lombaires. *Bordeaux Chir* 1970;41(2):133–135.
31. Roy-Camille R, Saillant G, Berteauu D, Salago V. Osteosynthesis of thoraco-lumbar spine fractures with metal plates screwed through the vertebral pedicles. *Reconstr Surg Traumatol* 1976;15:2.
32. Roy-Camille R, et al. *Rachis dorso-lombaire traumatique non neurologique*. Deuxiemes Journees d'Orthopedie de la Pitie. Paris: Masson, 1980;1–152.
33. Roy-Camille R, et al. *Spondylolisthesis L4 L5 et L5 S1*. 3emes Journees d'Orthopedie de la Pitie. Paris: Masson, 1983;91–144.
34. Roy-Camille R, Saillant G, Mazel C. Internal fixation of the lumbar spine with pedicle screw plating. *Clin Orthop* 1988;203:7–17.
35. Spencer D, Irwin G, Miller J. Anatomy and significance of fixation of the lumbosacral nerve roots in sciatica. *Spine* 1983;8(6):672–679.
36. Stagnara P, DeMauroy JC, Dran G, Gonon GP, Costanzo G, Dimnet J, Pasquet A. Reciprocal angulation of vertebral bodies in a sagittal plane: approach to references for the evaluation of kyphosis and lordosis. *Spine* 1982;7(4):335–342.
37. Stagnara P. *Les deformations du rachis*. Paris: Masson, 1985.
38. Steffee A, Biscup R, Sitkowski D. Segmental spine plates with pedicle screw fixation: a new internal fixation device for disorders of the lumbar and thoracic spine. *Clin Orthop* 1986;203:45.
39. Zindrick M, Wiltse L, Widell E, Thomas J, Holland W, Field B, Spencer C. A biomechanical study of intrapeduncular screw fixation in the lumbosacral spine. *Clin Orthop* 1986;203:99–112.
40. Zindrick M, Wiltse L, Dornick A, et al. Analysis of the morphometric characteristics of the thoracic and lumbar pedicles. *Spine* 1987;12:160–166.

Physiology and Pathophysiology of the Neural Elements

Jean-Pierre C. Farcy and Bernard A. Rawlins

The cord is the most important part of the neural axis with regard to its development and evolution as well as its functional importance. All neural elements above the cord are the result of progressive improvement and additions that developed as the species climbed the scale of animal sophistication.

Looking at worms and arthropods, it is possible to conceive an individual composed of segments, all alike and stacked one on top of the other. Each segment would have muscles, skeleton, vessels, viscera, and nervous systems to provide a theoretical autonomy. This segment, foreseen by the succession of somites in the gastrula, is called a metamere. The cord, along with the vertebral column, carries this metameric constitution in an obvious manner, by the segmental outgrowth of the nerve roots. However, each theoretically independent segment functionally depends on the connection between each other segment, and their functional solidarity.

Systematic understanding requires a description of the spinal cord as a metameric organ. This description is segmental; after this, a synthesis of the connected segments in a multimetameric organ. It would appear along the lines that this multimetameric organ falls under the control of a suprastructure to which it is connected and which provides the ultimate regulation.

EMBRYOLOGY

On the seventh day of gestation, modified ectodermal cells invaginate and migrate between the ectodermal and endodermal layers to form the neural plate, the lateral margin of which shifts up while the midline caves in, forming the neural tube. Caudal to the fourth somite, the neural tube gives rise to the future spinal cord, while cranially it will give rise to the upper neural elements of the brain. Rapid differentiation takes place at the end of the first month of fetal life, and the cells of the neural ectoderm are organized in three layers: the inner layer surrounds the ependymal canal; the middle layer forms neuroblasts, the future gray matter of the cord; and the outer layer, which will become the white matter of the spinal cord (41).

The spinal cord, which occupies the full length of the spinal canal at the third month of fetal life, will grow less rapidly than the spine. The result is an apparent ascension of the spinal cord inside the spinal canal, and thus the caudal end of the cord lies at L4 by the ninth week of gestation; it will be at the level of the lower endplate of L2 at birth (9).

The spinal cord is therefore bound to the spinal canal at both ends, caudally and cranially. The filum terminale represents, terminally, a vestigial inner layer attached caudally at the coccyx. The shape of the cord is cylindrical from T1 to a zone of enlargement that is always found above the conus, which ends as a narrow tip.

MENINGES

The spinal cord is enclosed in three membranes, called meninges. The meninges are formed from the inside-out by the pia mater, the arachnoid, and the dura mater. They are separated from each other by the sub-

---

J.-P. C. Farcy and B. A. Rawlins: Department of Orthopaedics, Columbia University College of Physicians and Surgeons, and Columbia–Presbyterian Medical Center, New York, NY 10032.

arachnoid space and the subdural space, respectively. While the subdural space is merely potential space, the subarachnoid space is filled by cerebrospinal fluid.

The meninges serve as a support to the nervous system, especially in association with the buoyant effect of the fluid. As connective tissues, the meninges provide an access route for vessels of the nervous system.

The spinal pia mater is thicker, firmer, and less vascular than the cerebral pia mater, and it consists of an outer epipia and an inner intima pia that is in direct contact with the nervous tissues. The spinal pia mater covers the spinal cord and is intimately adherent to the cord. The ligamentum denticulum, situated on each side of the cord, presents, on its lateral border, triangular and tooth-like processes fixed at regular intervals to the dura.

The spinal portion of the arachnoid is a delicate membrane around the spinal cord, surrounding the cauda equina, and ending at the level of the lower border of S2. The subarachnoid space between the arachnoid and the pia mater contains the cerebrospinal fluid and a network of thin, trabeculated, connective tissues that connect the arachnoid to the pia mater. The denticulate ligament is an extension of the pia mater and is triangular in configuration within the coronal plane and has points of fixation to the dura along the spinal canal. Changes in the form and position of the denticulate ligament during spinal movement were demonstrated by Epstein (24) with use of cineradiographic techniques in 1966. This showed the actual participation of the denticulate ligament in stabilization of the cord within the spinal canal during motion.

The dura mater is a fibrous structure made of collagen and elastic fibers. The spinal dura mater is attached to the posterior longitudinal ligament of the vertebrae, especially near the lower end of the vertebral canal. The dura mater has trabecular prolongations along the roots of the spinal nerves as they pass through the intervertebral foramina. An extradural space exists between the dura and the periosteum of the inner aspect of the vertebral canal. This space is called the epidural space and is filled by loose fat and connective tissues.

CORD MORPHOLOGY

The cord and nerve roots are defined as the neuraxis or the neural elements and are protected by the vertebral canal. We have already seen the intimate relationship between the neural elements, envelopes, and the bony elements of the vertebral canal. Any disruption of the bony elements of the vertebral canal could potentially injure the neural elements, which they protect. The cord itself is cylindrical, and its diameter varies according to the emergence of the nerves of the upper and lower extremities. These two parts present a larger diameter and an oblong shape. The cord is potentially damaged by any injury, including surgical intervention. A discrepancy between the length of the vertebral column and the length of the cord results in a variation in the length and direction of the nerve roots. The nerve roots are almost horizontal in the cervical spine. They are more oblique and longer in the thoracic spine. The roots are almost vertical and much longer at the level of the lumbar spine, where they occupy the vertebral canal caudally to the conus, forming the cauda equina. The average length of the cord is 45 cm, with filum terminale extending the length of the cord an additional 25 cm.

The cord may be anatomically separated into the gray and white matter each containing tracts, described as zones, which contain neural elements of specialized function. The gray matter contains a somatosensory zone in the dorsal gray horn and a somatomotor zone in the ventral gray horn. A third, intermediate zone is present in autonomic visceral centers, posterior to the sulcus limitans, and in autonomic visceral centers, which are anterior to the sulcus limitans. The sympathetic and parasympathetic centers are found between the somatomotor and somatosensory zones. The center for the simple arc reflex is also found within the gray matter.

The dorsal gray horn carries sensitivity through fasciculi, or tracks, including Lissauer's track, Waldeyer's nucleus, Foland's substantia gelatinosa, Crosby's dorsal funicular nucleus, and Clark's column, which occupies the neck.

The ventral gray horn is the central column for the phrenic nucleus, C3 to C7, and lumbosacral nucleus, L2 to S2. The lateral nuclei control the upper girdle, pelvic girdle, and muscles of the limbs. The median nuclei control flexion and extension of the muscles of the head and trunk.

The intermediate zone is composed of the base of both horns and the lateral gray column. This zone contains the visceral sensory nuclei dorsali and the visceral motor nuclei ventrali.

There are also two centers for somatic reflexes. This is the simplest arc reflex generated between one sensitive neuron and one motor neuron. The same arc reflex is also generated between three or more neurons, including one or more associative neurons. An abnormal reflex on clinical examination means an impairment of the corresponding cord myelomere.

The parasympathetic centers are located in the brain stem and sacral spinal cord. The sympathetic centers are located in the thoracolumbar cord from C8 to L4. Sympathetic centers located along the cord may be identified with specific somatic functions. Budge's ciliospinal center is located at C8 to T3 and is involved in iridodilation. The cardioaccelerator center is found at the level of T1 to T4. Pilomotor, sudorific, and vasomotor centers located at C8 to L2 are involved in thermoregulation. The bronchopulmonary center located at T3 to T5 affects the caliber and secretion of the bronchi. The abdominal splanchnic center between T6 and L2 acts on the supramesocolic viscera, colon, and small bowel. The center of anorectal and bladder continence is located at L2 to L4. The ejaculation center is located at L1 to L3.

Parasympathetic centers include the center of anorectal expulsion at S1 to S2, the center of bladder expulsion or micturition at S3 to S4, and the erection center located at S2 (41).

The white matter contains three types of fibers differentiated by their function. Two types of fibers are involved in the most elementary function. The simple arc reflex utilizes fibers that constitute part of the nerve root and peripheral nerves. Reflex units are connected by longitudinal association fibers grouped in tracts. Sensitivity and motricity follow different pathways and as described by Sherrington they are ascending fibers for sensitivity and descending fibers for motricity. Each group of fibers is specialized and follows a specific tract.

There are three types of ascending fibers that are specialized in carrying exteroceptive, proprioceptive, and combined complex sensitive information.

Exteroceptive sensitivity comprises tactile sharp pain, dull pain, and thermal sensitivity. Sharp pain is transmitted on the side of its spinal ganglia where it originates and follows the Goll and Burdack tract on the ipsilateral side of the cord to the brain. Thermal sensitivity, dull pain, and tactile sensation are transmitted across the cord to the contralateral side and ascend in the lateral and anterior spinothalamic tracts that form the Dejerine arcuate tract. The fact that one connective neuron crosses the center of the gray matter to carry thermic information to the opposite side explains the loss of thermic sensitivity in cases of central cord syndrome or necrosis and syringomyelia. The proprioceptive sensibility uses two ascending pathways, either the anterior ventral spinocerebellar tract, marked with decussation, or the posterior spinocerebellar tract, which is without decussation. The third type of ascending fibers are more complex and follow the spinotectalis track localized within the arcuate Dejerine track.

The descending fibers progress from the cortex to the spine, where connection is provided by an arc synapse in the gray matter of the anterior horn that transmits motricity to muscles. There are two types of descending fibers for specialized motor commands, the pyramidal and extrapyramidal tracts. The face, larynx, and tongue muscles follow the pyramidal tract. There is a direct pyramidal tract without decussation and a lateral pyramidal tract with decussation. The extrapyramidal motricity commands autonomic and voluntary movements. All motor tracts decussate and terminate in the ventral horn of the spinal gray matter, which is the "final common pathway."

VASCULARIZATION OF THE SPINE

Vascularization of the cord has been better understood since the works of Lazorthes (39) and Adamkiewicz (1–3). This resulted in a somewhat frightening concept of a barely unique blood supply to the spinal cord that could easily be jeopardized while performing spinal surgery. In 1969, Louis (40) contributed a description of the origin of spine vascularization.

In 1978, Louis performed more thorough research that gave a more realistic view of the real blood supply to the cord, confirming the work of Crock and Yoshizawa (18). They suggested that a metameric radiculomedullary spinal artery accompanied each spinal nerve. These arteries anastomose in ladder fashion, arising from the posterior intercostalis and traveling in the foramina, along the epidural surface. They penetrate the subarachnoid space where it divides into two branches. Two pairs of arteries anastomose with the opposite side and constitute the posterior spinal arteries. The rest of the cord, the anterior white matter and anterior horn, receives blood from the branch of the anterior spinal artery.

Therefore, in spinal surgery, it is dangerous to use cautery in the vertebral foramina and its vicinity while performing cautery hemostasis, especially when the surgery is performed on both sides of the spine.

The venous return system drains the blood to the cava system and, under physiologic conditions such as coughing or sneezing, the venous pressure increases in the spinal venous system. Compression of the jugular veins and the abdomen by Valsalva maneuver increases the venous pressure and therefore the cerebrospinal fluid (CSF) pressure. This maneuver is useful for recognition of CSF obstruction in the subarachnoid space and was described by Quiqenstead.

NEUROMENINGEAL DYNAMICS

The spinal vertebrae are linked together by ligaments and discs, constituting a flexible structure that protects the neural elements during motion. The neural elements are located between the posterior and middle column of the spine. Since the vertebral canal is in flexion, the soft tissues, such as the posterior longitudinal ligament, the discs, and the ligamentum flavum bind the bony elements and allow motion.

In flexion, the length of the posterior and middle columns increases, but the middle column increases to a lesser extent. The total lengthening of the vertebral canal can be calculated by summation of the individual lengths of the ligamentous structures at each spinal level in flexion as described by Bradford and Spurling (14).

This variation in length of the canal is due to the elastic behavior of the ligamentous tissues and discs and varies with age. The average increase in length is 7.5 cm in adults. Under normal physiologic range of motion, the increased length in flexion in a child's spine averages 12 cm. The spinal structures must accommodate these modifications of length at each step through normal range of motion.

Most of the lengthening takes place where the spine is the most mobile (16). Therefore the cervical and lumbar elements reflect the largest changes when amplitude is measured. This discrepancy in length between the spinal canal and the spinal cord can be responsible for "spinal cord injury without radiographic abnormalities," an injury that happens in children who sustain rapid hyperflexion. The cord is stretched to rupture inside the spinal canal, the length of which has increased abruptly.

To the contrary, the shortening that takes place during the course of extension is, by far, less important than the lengthening in flexion. At most, in hyperextension, the overall shortening does not exceed 9 to 10 cm.

The dural envelope is the structure that accommodates this variation in length. In flexion, the diameter of the dural sac decreases as the dura mater stretches and slides inside the canal, where the epidural space offers the potential to improve this ability to slide. Most of these variations in length take place in the cervical and lumbar parts of the spinal canal. The accommodation of the neural elements is more dramatic and therefore simpler to measure at these two levels. In the thoracic segment, the motion is of reduced amplitude, and only a few modifications of length take place during range of motion.

The cord inside the dural sac is maintained in equilibrium by the denticulate ligament, which provides cranial attachment and suspension to the conus. Below the conus, the cauda equina, made up of the lumbosacral nerve roots, offers more possibilities to accommodate the most dramatic changes in length during hyperflexion (41).

There are two parts in the nerve roots that were measured by Rene Louis. One part, after emergence from the cord or conus, goes to the point where it traverses the dura mater. This is the subarachnoid part of the nerve root; the second part is a subdural section of the root that goes from the point at which the roots perforate the dura to the point where they fuse into a nerve, distal from the spinal ganglia.

It appears that, below L3, the length of the roots accommodates the largest flexion radius; distally each root must stretch to accommodate the same range of flexion. S1 will stretch far more than L3.

Charnley showed that nerve roots glide freely through the intervertebral foramina. Lassegue described pain elicited by stretching the sciatic nerve by slowly evaluating the stretched leg of a patient in a supine position.

The pain elicited in performing such a maneuver can be similar in location and distribution to the pain to which the patient is accustomed. The pain can be excruciating if the elevation of the stretched leg is not done gently and gradually. This maneuver corresponds to pulling on the nerve with a 3-kg load.

At the level of the foraminal canal, the subdural part of the roots glides. This results in a pull-out of 12 mm at the level of the L5 root (36).

In flexion, extension, and lateral bending, the angulation at which the roots exit varies from the cervical to the lumbar spine, and between extension and flexion. Louis obtained data that showed a great deal of mobility between the two extreme positions in flexion and extension. These variations in angulation offer the possibility for gliding without undergoing distension.

THE ACUTE SPINAL CORD INJURY

The acute spinal cord injury is a devastating injury that carries a high level of mortality when it affects the upper spine, resulting in permanent nerve damage distal to the injury site.

In this book, which addresses only thoracolumbar and sacral fractures, the cord injuries are localized at the levels of the thoracic cord, conus medullaris, cauda equina, and nerve roots.

The sequence of events necessary to create cord injury are: first, a mechanical insult to the neural tissues; and second, changes in spinal cord blood flow (SCBF), which are very interdependent with biochemical changes.

These events must be controlled, as must the consequences of their insufficiency. It has been demonstrated that any of these events can play a role in the vicious circle that creates such a devastating outcome to the acute spine injury.

The Mechanical Insult

The displacement of bony elements and loss of stability with disruption of the elements of the spine by high velocity energy result from a direct blow to the cord.

Any type of injury can be described from the transection or the complete strangulation due to injuries that range in severity from large displacement fracture-dislocation to simple stretching from a minimal blow. Any perforating agent, from a sharp bone splinter resulting from a local, comminuted fracture to the high velocity gun projectile, can lacerate meninges and cord with greater or lesser destruction.

In an attempt to better understand the mechanism of the mechanical insult, models were designed to evaluate experimental spinal cord injury. A morphometric study was conducted after contusion of the cat thoracic spine by Blight (10).

This study indicated that tissue extrusion into the neural elements is a major determinant of axon disruption and the pattern of central necrosis. Flexion, extension, longitudinal distraction, and compression as well as rotation and shear, or any combination of these, result in a similar type of damage that is classified as tissue extrusion.

This mechanical insult results in neuron damage but, surprisingly enough, the human's highly specialized neural cord can tolerate gray matter loss better than white matter loss. This apparent contradiction is explained by the fact that, at a given level, a loss of gray matter corresponds to a limited loss of neurons, which can be supplied by a level above or a level below. But a loss of white matter means a loss of connection between all the gray matter levels of the cord to the brain, which can jeopardize more dramatically the function of such a sophisticated system. To a lesser extent, cord concussion can happen like a brain concussion and appears to be a reversible dysfunction. This transitory situation seems related to short lasting, low energy tissue deformities with definite, minimal anatomic lesions.

Among the other types of mechanical insults, there are two different aspects of secondary injury. One is due to an unstable bony lesion that is responsible for ongoing cord damage. When the spinal canal is unstable, there is a repetition of injuries that maintains the vicious cycle (21).

Physical movements at the site of a spinal cord injury have a detrimental effect on the clinical course and accentuate pathology, as demonstrated by Ducker. Stabilization helps to maintain the integrity of the fibers, tracts, and neurons that have survived.

In the last few years, the awareness and progressive understanding of spine stability have made continuous progress. However, it remains as controversial to define spine instability as it is to attain it. The consensus is the pursuit for ideal stabilization and therefore stability. A less controversial issue is compression and its corollary, decompression.

Compression can be the result of focal impingement of bone, soft tissue, or foreign body on the neural tissues. Impingement results in a mechanical distortion of the blood vessels, which can be occluded by extrinsic compression. The occlusion of blood vessels is responsible for ischemia and a subsequent, vicious cycle of edema, microhemorrhage, more ischemia, and necrosis. This reality was described in 1975 by Griffiths (29).

When a traumatic event leads to spinal cord injury by a disruption in the protection afforded by the vertebral column, the initial event results in disruption of axons at the level of injury. This initial event is the primary injury. However, a cascade of events seen on a cellular level results in progressive pathologic changes. These changes result in the further destruction of axons that were not disrupted at the time of initial injury. The process that leads to further disruption of additional axons is described as secondary injury (53,55).

An enormous effort has been made to obtain data that will help to demonstrate the pathophysiologic mechanism that takes place during secondary injury. With information on the pathophysiologic mechanism of injury, the clinician and researcher can attempt to reverse or halt the events that cause secondary injury, thereby preventing damage to additional axons.

With the extensive research data generated for the different types of mechanisms of canal injury, a critical review of the mechanisms is required. Certain mechanisms that are thought to be responsible for secondary injury could be a response to initial injury and necrotic changes.

In 1960, Davison (20) already had made a report of examination with the naked eye of the spinal cord after compression. He described the cord as "oedematory, soft, mush, sometimes grayish-red and constricted." Under microscopic vision the vessels are collapsed and have undergone hyalinization. There is fragmentation of the myelin sheets and axon cylinders, demonstrating different types of demyelinization, which results in decreased axoplasmic flow.

It appears that the neural dysfunction correlated with compression is a physical injury to the neural membrane, regardless of hemodynamic changes (33,38).

Magnetic resonance imaging (MRI) gives a direct assessment of neural tissue compression and offers an accurate evaluation of the materials responsible for focal compression. The most appropriate decompression must be performed, bearing in mind the long-term spine stability.

This task can be surgically performed and achieved at the level of the nerve roots. Rydevik et al. (46) demonstrated that compression is responsible for changes in nerve root microcirculation, leading to ischemia, intraneural edema, and, ultimately, demyelinization. Olmarker et al. (44) also demonstrated that edema formation was more pronounced after rapid onset than progressive onset of compression. These studies confirm the intuitive notion that high velocity, rapid onset of compression mechanically created a wave of damage that went far beyond the damage caused by slow progressive compression.

Another important reality is the direct relationship between the duration of the compression applied to the nerve and the degree of nerve injury (19). This work on nerves by Rydevik and his associates demonstrates the general reaction of myelinized fibers to long-term compression. Other, more recent work demonstrates the long-held, intuitive feeling that decompression gives the best possible environment for the nervous fibers to regenerate. Recovery of conduction in demyelinated axons may permit recovery of function and can be mediated by several mechanisms, including remyelination by oligodendrocytes or Schwann cells (54).

All these recent works open a door on hope for the future; if we consider that it has been demonstrated that 10% of the total number of axons can support acceptable recovery, the work done with the assistance of Sir George Bedbrook in Australia shows a continuity of CNS tissue at the level of the lesion. Even with complete paraplegia, some continuity across the injured segment was found. As found on a group of rats that recovered somatosensory evoked potentials (SSEP) 4 months after injury, ultrastructural investigations testified to the existence of reparative processes of the nervous system (27). In summary, the mechanical insult creates direct damage (i.e., progressive or acute compression), results in microvascular changes, microscopic hemorrhages, and a thrombosis followed by edema, anoxia, and necrosis. This vicious cycle will be addressed in the following paragraphs.

Hemodynamic Changes

A succession of changes occur in the blood supply at the level of the spinal cord surface, as observed in the microvessels, where a sludging phenomenon that precedes stasis is described as a first manifestation of blood flow impairment (8). The result is ischemia, which is responsible for many unsalvageable lesions of the neural tissues. The role of ischemia in spinal cord injury is obvious (5).

Necrosis can result from hemorrhage and is described as a constant pattern of injury (35). The vessels dilate progressively, and flame-shaped hemorrhages are visible. In other tissues, the partial pressure of carbon dioxide in arterial blood increases locally and results in local vasodilation and increases blood flow. This response is impaired in cases of spinal cord injury; the only increase of blood flow is in the capillaries and venules.

The end result is a combination of central ischemia and peripheral hyperemia that can be demonstrated by blood flow studies (37,49). The change in SCBF can be analyzed in different steps. (a) There is a short, favorable delay before the SCBF decreases to dangerous, ischemic levels. This period of time, even when short, constitutes a time window in which pharmaceutical agents can be efficient. (b) SCBF reduction is dominant in the central gray matter of the cord and less dominant in the peripheral white matter. (c) The loss of vasomotor responsiveness and autoregulation has a dramatic effect on the pathologic development of lesions. (d) Blood pressure impairment dramatically affects the outcome of the lesion. (e) Parallel changes in partial oxygen pressure in tissues will ultimately affect cord metabolic functions.

All possible means of multifaceted treatment must be activated to take the best advantage of this very short, favorable delay to prevent SCBF impairment. In 1969, this was described from a pharmacological point of view: a statistically significant improvement and recovery of neurologic function were associated with dexamethasone in experimental canine studies of incomplete cord injury (22). At the end of this chapter, we will see how new studies have confirmed this first research and how protocol has been designed to indicate steroid use in patients affected with acute spinal cord injury.

BIOCHEMICAL DERANGEMENT

The safety system, the blood–brain barrier, allows only oxygen, sugar, and a few selected amino acids to cross over into the central nervous system. The acute injury to the spinal cord is responsible for a phenomenon similar to an impairment of the blood–brain barrier (52). Accumulation of catecholamines, perhaps lactates, and other ischemic products maintains a permanent chemical insult to neural tissue (34).

Reduced blood flow at the lesion site has been implicated by a number of investigators as one of the causes of secondary injury (48). Monitoring of injured spinal cords with evoked potentials has demonstrated a loss in response immediately following contusion. The response is regained for a short period of time and then lost hours or days later. Products to explain these deteriorating events have been sought by investigators.

A number of mechanisms and substances have been identified in an effort to explain the neurophysiologic changes. The release of vasoactive and neurotoxic substances (45), edema, the change in the ionic environment with entry of calcium ions into cells (56), the breakdown of lysosomes, and release of free radicals (25) are all implicated in this secondary injury event.

In the normal mammalian neuron, an ionic gradient is maintained through the sodium–potassium-activated adenosine triphosphatase transport system, referred to as an electrogenic pump. This electrogenic pump is found as a protein within the cell membranes. Tissue concentrations of Na^+ and K^+ are maintained at 15.0 mM and 150.0 mM, respectively, while extracellular concentrations are maintained at 150.0 mM and 5.5 mM, respectively. Spine contusion and resulting disruption of the membrane's integrity lead to increased extracellular K^+ concentration and decreased extracellular Na^+ concentration. This shift in ions profoundly affects the membrane potentials, which are dependent on the Na^+ and K^+ transmembrane gradients. A disruption of the transmembrane gradients will then block action potential conduction in axons. Animal studies have shown that extracellular K^+ increases from a normal of 4 mM to a mean of 54 mM within seconds after injury (56,59). Similarly, extracellular Na^+ concentrate falls from 150 mM to less than 70 mM. Shifts in sodium from the extracellular space to the intracellular space result in an osmotic gradient with shift of water from the extracellular space to the tissue, and this results in tissue edema. The increased pressure developed may be the result of decreasing the blood flow to 50% in the white and gray matter (48).

Also noted with more pronounced effect is the extracellular reduction in calcium concentration with membrane damage as calcium accumulates in cells at the time of injury (58). Calcium can serve as a messenger in numerous intracellular processes including metabolism and control of membrane ionic permeability. Calcium ions bind to the mitochondria and interrupt the production of phosphorylated metabolic substrates. Calcium ions activate phospholipase, which breaks down membrane phospholipids and releases free fatty acids (15). The free fatty acids are converted to prostaglandins.

Cytochrome oxidase activity occurs in the center of the traumatic site. Cytochrome oxidase is the rate limiting enzyme of electron transport and is located on the inner membrane of the mitochondria. Calcium ions, in blocking electron transport in mitochondria, generate free radicals, which break down membranes, worsening the influx of calcium into cells and generating lipid peroxides (31). The combination of lipid peroxides and fatty acids is a potent vasoactive agent and edema producing compounds (17).

Interest in lipid peroxides is enhanced by the presence of drugs that could reduce the lipid peroxides in tissues. Superoxide dismutase converts free radicals to hydrogen peroxide. Drugs that can interrupt the effects of free radicals include methylprednisolone and vitamin E (6,7). Certain catalysts in the formation of prostaglandins can also be blocked, and lipid peroxides have shown it to be suppressed by methylprednisolone in animal studies (30,31).

In addition to focusing on prevention of secondary injury through pharmacologic agents, there has been an attempt to look at the regeneration of damaged tissue. Recent studies have shown that GM_1 gangliosides enhance the neurologic recovery of patients and are considered safe in treating spinal cord injury. Nonetheless, this study looked at a sample population of 34 patients; a larger patient population study is required (28).

The use of pharmacologic agents in the routine treatment of patients with spinal cord injuries remains controversial. There has been a reported high incidence of gastrointestinal bleeding, in particular with head trauma and spinal injury patients compared to other types of trauma (51). The influence of steroids in development of gastrointestinal bleeding remains controversial. Given the lack of studies that demonstrate the efficacy of these pharmacologic agents in reducing the effects of secondary injury, their use in routine treatment was not recommended in the past (43).

It has been observed that a succession of events following spinal cord injury, including destruction, hemorrhage, anoxia, edema, and necrosis, resulted in axoplasmic transport inhibition within 2 hr after injury. Complete inhibition of function occurs within 6 hr following a severe crush injury (4).

More recent studies have demonstrated that use of glucocorticosteroids soon after injury, and certainly within 6 to 8 hr, does help to improve motor scores (12,13,53). The initial dose of methylprednisolone is high, 30 mg/kg, followed by 5.2 mg/kg/hr for the subsequent 23-hr period. No additional glucocorticosteroids are recommended after this 24-hr period (23).

NEUROLOGIC ASSESSMENT OF CORD INJURY

Spinal shock is a dysfunction in the nervous tissue due to physiologic processes and is said to have resolved when reflex arcs below the level of the injury return. Neurogenic shock is defined as hypotension and bradycardia following spinal injury.

Initial assessment of a patient with spinal cord injury should distinguish between complete or incomplete neurologic deficit. Complete neurologic deficit exists when there is no sensory or motor function caudal to the injury level. Classification is not possible in the initial evaluation if there is no bulbocavernosus reflex. The return of the bulbocavernosus or anoanal reflex signifies the end of spinal shock, and this usually occurs within 24 hr in 99% of patients. A complete lesion is generally classified as paraplegic or quadriplegic.

An incomplete neurologic lesion has some function below the level of injury, and a detailed physical examination of all muscle groups is required (Table 1). In general, the more function the patient has below the lesion, the better the prognosis.

Incomplete neurologic lesions can be classified in syndromes. The syndromes implicate the area of the spinal cord damaged by the injury. In a posterior cord syndrome, the posterior aspect of the cord is damaged,

TABLE 1. *Innervation of lower limb muscles affected with thoracic lumber lesions*

Level	Muscles
L1	Iliopsoas, hip flexors
L2	Sartorius
L3	Quadriceps, adductor longus, adductor brevis
L4	Tibialis anterior
L5	Extensor hallucis longus, gluteus medius and minimus
S1	Gastrocnemius
S2	Flexor hallucis longus and brevis
S3	Foot intrinsics

TABLE 3. *Motor index score*

Muscle	Right	Left
Diaphragm		2
Deltoid	5	5
Biceps	5	5
Triceps	5	5
Flexor digitorum superficialis	5	5
Abductor digiti minimi	5	5
Intercostals		2
Upper abdominals		2
Lower abdominals		2
Iliopsoas	5	5
Quadriceps	5	5
Extensor digiti minimi	5	5
Gastrocnemius	5	5
Anal		2
Total (= 100)	45	10	45

and the anterior spinothalamic tracts are spared, maintaining crude touch sensation clinically. In the anterior cord syndrome, the anterior cord is damaged while the posterior cord is spared. Clinically, patients demonstrate motor paraplegia and a sensory level with intact position sense, vibratory sensation, and proprioception due to an intact posterior column. In a central cord syndrome, there is damage to central gray and white matter at the level of injury. Clinically, this is expressed as loss in motor function at the level of injury, with sparing of function below this level. When the lesion occurs at the cervical region, it might present as loss in motor function in the arms and hands, with sparing of the lower extremities. At the thoracolumbar level, this might present as inability to lift the legs off the table while maintaining motor function at the feet. A descriptive classification of spine injuries, while helpful in delineating the pathophysiology, is not helpful with quantifying the injury or useful in predicting or evaluating treatment protocols. A useful and popular method of classification of an incomplete lesion is the Frankel classification system (26) (Table 2).

The motor classification of patients with spinal cord injury first described by Lucas and Ducker is a further step to quantify the results of cord injury (11,42). A standard motor function scale is used: 0, no neurologic function; 1, trace; 2, poor; 3, fair; 4, good; 5, normal. A standard motor examination, which incorporated 14 different muscle groups, was used in their initial study. Muscles such as the diaphragm, abdominals, and the anal sphincter that could be assessed only as strong, abnormal, or paralyzed were graded from 0 to 2. By selection of certain muscle groups, a 100-point grading system is developed (Table 3). This can be used to evaluate recovery rate based on the patient's initial and follow-up examinations. The American Spinal Injury Association motor score uses a 100-point grading system developed from motor tests of 20 specific muscles.

TABLE 2. *Frankel classification*

A. Absent motor and sensory function below a given level
B. Sensation present, complete motor paralysis
C. Sensation present, motor function not useful (Grade 2–3/5)
D. Sensation present, motor function weak but useful (Grade 4/5)
E. Neurologically intact

SUMMARY

Cord injuries and subsequent paraplegia rarely are due to a complete cord transsection. Rather, they are due to a crushed cord with incomplete primary lesions.

From the instant of injury through the following hours, all the stages of inflammation develop. Microhemorrhage, edema, and ischemia are part of a vicious cycle that causes nerve cells to be anoxic and therefore to die.

In the following hours and days, fibrous degeneration is responsible for multiple interactions in the connective neuron cell network, and paralysis becomes spastic and irreversible. Reversing this process has been one of the neurophysiologist's major concerns in decreasing the inflammatory reaction through the use of systemic drugs.

The immediate post-traumatic use of steroids is still in the process of being documented as efficient. The other concern is to protect and to facilitate neural cells and axon regeneration. In that respect, a high concentration of gangliosides may facilitate regeneration and therefore interconnections of neurons.

REFERENCES

1. Adamkiewicz AA. Ueber die mikroskopischeen Gefässe des Menschlichen Rückenmarkes. Trans 7th Session, Int Med Congress 1881;1:155–157.
2. Adamkiewicz AA. Die Blutgefässe des Menschlichen Ruckenmarkes I: Die Gefässe der Ruckenmarkssubstanz. Situngs bdk. Akad d Wissensch, Math-naturw Cl 1881;84:469.
3. Adamkiewicz AA. Die Blutgefässe des Menschlichen Rucken-

markes II: Die Gefässe der Rückenmarksoberflache. Situngs bdk. Adad d Wissensch, Math-naturw, Cl 1882;85:101–130.
4. Albin MS, White RJ. Epidemiology, physiopathology, and experimental therapeutics of acute spinal cord injury. *Crit Care Clin* 1987;3:441.
5. Allen AR. Remarks on histopathological changes in spinal cord due to impact: an experimental study. *J Nerv Ment Dis* 1914;41:141–147.
6. Anderson DK, Means ED, Waters TR, Green ES. Microvascular perfusion and metabolism in injured spinal cord after methylprednisolone treatment. *J Neurosurg* 1982;56:106–113.
7. Anderson DK, Saunders RD, Demedick P, Dugan LL, Braughler JM, Hall ED, Means ED, Horrocks LA. Lipid hydrolysis and peroxidation in injured spinal cord: partial protection with methylprednisolone or vitamin E and selenium. *CNS Trauma* 1985;2:257–267.
8. Assenmacher DR, Ducker TB. Experimental traumatic paraplegia: the vascular and pathologic changes seen in reversible and irreversible spinal cord lesions. *J Bone Joint Surg* 1971;53:617–680.
9. Barson AT. The vertebral level of termination of the spinal cord during normal and abnormal development. *J Anat* 1970;106(3):489.
10. Blight A. Mechanical factors in experimental spinal cord injury. *J Am Paraplegia Soc* 1988;2:6–34.
11. Bohlman HH, Ducker TB, Lucas JT. Spine and spinal cord injuries. In: Rothman RH, Simeone FA, eds. *The spine*, 2nd ed. Philadelphia: Saunders, 1982;661–756.
12. Bracken MB, Collins WF, Freeman DF, et al. Efficiency of methylprednisolone in acute spinal cord injury. *JAMA* 1984;251:45–52.
13. Bracken MB, Shepard MJ, Colins WF, et al. A randomized controlled trial of methylprednisolone or naloxone in the treatment of acute spinal cord injury: results of the Second National Acute Spinal Cord Injury Study. *N Engl J Med* 1990;322:1405–1411.
14. Bradford FK, Spurling RG, eds. *The intervertebral disc*. Springfield IL: Charles C Thomas, 1945.
15. Braughler JM, Duncan LA, Goodman T. Calcium enhances in vitro free radical induced damage to brain synaptosomes, mitochondria, and cultured spinal cord neurones. *J Neurochem* 1985;45:1288–1293.
16. Breig A. *Biomechanics of the central nervous system*. Chicago: Year Book Medical Publishers, 1960.
17. Chan PH, Schmidley JW, Fishman RA, Langor SM. Brain injury edema and vascular permeability changes induced by oxygen-derived free radicals. *Neurology* 1984;34:315–320.
18. Crock HW, Yoshizawa H. *The blood supply of the vertebral column and spinal cord in man*. New York: Springer-Verlag, 1977.
19. Dahlin LB, Danielsen N, Ehira T, Lundborg G, Rydevik B. Mechanical effects of compression of peripheral nerves. *J Biomech Eng* 1986;108(2):120–122.
20. Davison C. General pathological considerations in injuries of the spinal cord. In: Brook S, ed. *Injuries of the brain and the spinal cord and their covering*. New York: Springer, 1960;515–517.
21. Ducker TB. In: Cowley RA, Trump BE, eds. *Pathophysiology of shock*. Baltimore: Williams & Wilkins, 1982.
22. Ducker TB, Harriet HF. Experimental treatments of acute spinal cord injury. *J Neurosurg* 1969;30:693–697.
23. Ducker TB, Spengler DM. Commentary: spinal cord injury and glucocortical steroid therapy: good news and bad. *J Spinal Disord* 1990;3(4):433–435.
24. Epstein BNS. An anatomic, myelographic, and cinemyelographic study of the dentate ligament. *AJR* 1966;98:704–712.
25. Flamm ES, Demopoulous HB, Seligman ML, et al. Free radicals in cerebral ischemia. *Stroke* 1978;9:445.
26. Frankel HL, Hancock DO, Hyslop G, Melzak J, Michaelis LS, Ungar GH, Vernon JD, Walsh JJ. The value of postural reduction in the initial management of closed injuries of the spine with paraplegia and tetraplegia: Part I. *Paraplegia* 1969;7:179–192.
27. Frascarelli M, Oppido PA, Ricchi L, Delfini R, D'Orazi G. Chronic damage after spinal trauma in rat(s): neurophysiological and ultrastructural investigations. *J Neurosurg Sci* 1990;34(1):1–6.
28. Geisler FH, Dorsey FC, Coleman WP. Recovery of motor function after spinal-cord injury—a randomized, placebo-controlled trial with GM-1 ganglioside. *N Engl J Med* 1991;324(26):1829–1838.
29. Griffiths JR. Vasogenic edema following acute and chronic spinal cord compression in the dog. *J Neurosurg* 1975;42:155–165.
30. Hall ED, Wolf DL. A pharmacological analysis of the pathophysiological mechanisms of posttraumatic spinal cord ischemia. *J Neurosurg* 1986;64:951–961.
31. Hall ED, Wolf DL, Braughler JM. Effects of a single large dose of methylprednisolone sodium succinate on experimental posttraumatic spinal cord ischemia: dose–response and time–action analysis. *J Neurosurg* 1984;61:124–130.
32. Hsu CY, Haleshka PV, Hogan EL, Banik NL, Lee WA, Perot PC. Alterations of thromboxanes and prostacylin levels in experimental spinal cord injury. *Neurology* 1985;35:1003–1009.
33. Hukuda S, Wilson CB. Experimental cervical myelopathy: effects of compression and ischemia on the canine cervical cord. *J Neurosurg* 1972;37:631–652.
34. Ito T, Allen M, Yashon D. A mitochondrial lesion in experimental spinal cord trauma. *J Neurosurg* 1987;48:434–442.
35. Kakulas BA, Bedbrook GM. Pathology of injuries of the vertebral spinal cord with emphasis on the microscopic aspects. In: Vinken PJ, Bruyn GW, eds. *Handbook of clinical neurology, Volume 25. Injuries of the spine and spinal cord*. Amsterdam: North-Holland, 1976;27–42.
36. Kapandji IA. *Physiology of the joints*, vol 3. New York: Churchill Livingstone, 1974.
37. Kobrine AI, Doyle TF, Rizzoli HV. Spinal cord blood flow as affected by changes in systemic arterial blood pressure. *J Neurosurg* 1976;44:12–15.
38. Kobrine AI, Evans DE, Rizzoli HV. Experimental acute balloon compression of the spinal cord. *J Neurosurg* 1979;51:841–845.
39. Lazorthes G, Poulhes J, Bastide G, Roulleau J, Chancholle AR: Recherches sur la vascularisation artérielle de la moelle. Application à lá pathologie médullaire. *Bull Acad Natl Med* (Paris) 1957;41:464.
40. Louis R: Topographie vertébromédullaire. *Bull Assoc Anat* (Nancy) 1969;54:272.
41. Louis R. *Surgery of the spine*. Berlin: Springer-Verlag, 1983.
42. Lucas JT, Ducker TB. Motor classification of spinal cord injuries with mobility, morbidity and recovery indices. *Am Surg* 1979;945:151–158.
43. Montesano PX, Benson DR. Fracture and dislocation of the spine, Part II: The thoracolumbar spine. In: Rockwood CA Jr, Green DP, Bucholz RW, eds. *Rockwood and Green's fractures in adults*, 3rd ed. Philadelphia: Lippincott, 1991;1358–1397.
44. Olmarker K, Rydevik B, Holm S. Edema formation in spinal nerve roots induced by experimental, graded compression: an experimental study on the pig cauda equina with special reference to differences in effects between rapid and slow onset of compression. *Spine* 1989;14:569–673.
45. Osterholm JL. The pathophysiological response in spinal cord injury. *J Neurosurg* 1974;40:5–33.
46. Rydevik B, Brown MD, Lundborg G. Pathoanatomy and pathophysiology of nerve root compression. *Spine* 1984;9:7–15.
47. Rydevik BL, Myers RR, Powell HC. Pressure increase in the dorsal root ganglion following mechanical compression. *Spine* 1989;14:574–576.
48. Sandler AN, Tator CH. Review of the effect of spinal cord trauma on the vessels and blood flow in the spinal cord. *J Neurosurg* 1976;45:638–645.
49. Schmith AJ, McCrary DB, Bloedel JR. Hyperemia, CO_2 responsiveness and autoregulation in the white matter following experimental spinal cord injury. *J Neurosurg* 1978;48:239–251.
50. Soderstrom CA, Ducker TB. Increased susceptibility of patients with cervical cord lesion to peptic GI complications. *J Trauma* 1983;23:1061–1065.
51. Stauffer ES. Diagnosis and prognosis of the acute cervical cord injury. *Clin Orthop* 1975;112:9–15.
52. Vise WM, Yashon D, Hunt WE. Mechanisms of norepinephrine accumulation within site of spinal cord injuries. *J Neurosurg* 1984;40:76–82.

53. Walker MD. Acute spinal-cord injury. *N Engl J Med* 1991; 324(26):1885–1887.
54. Waxman SG. Demyelination in spinal cord injury. *J Neurol Sci* 1989;1(2):1–14.
55. Young W. Pharmacologic therapy of acute spinal cord injury. In: Errico TJ, Bauer RD, Waugh T, eds. *Spinal trauma*. Philadelphia: Lippincott, 1991;415–433.
56. Young W, Koreh I. Potassium and calcium changes in injured spinal cords. *Brain Res* 1986;365:42–53.
57. Young W, Ransohoff J. Injuries to the cervical cord. In: Sherk H, ed. *The cervical spine*, 2nd ed. Philadelphia: Lippincott, 1989;464–495.
58. Young W, Yen V, Blight A. Extracellular calcium ionic activity in experimental spinal cord contusion. *Brain Res* 1982;253: 105–113.
59. Young W, Koreh I, Yen V, Lindsay A. Effect of sympathectomy on extracellular potassium ionic activity and blood flow in experimental spinal cord contusion. *Brain Res* 1982;253:115–124.

4

Biomechanics of the Normal Thoracolumbar Spine and Their Application to Fractures

Alain Tanguy

The thoracolumbar spine is frequently involved in spinal injuries, with more than 50% of all vertebral body fractures occurring between the 12th thoracic vertebra and the second lumbar vertebra. Specific mechanical conditions exist at this level that may explain its vulnerability under certain trauma conditions. Under normal conditions of daily life, however, the strength and stability of the thoracolumbar spine prevent mechanical failure, thereby protecting the spinal cord while allowing mobility with movement in various planes.

THE POTENTIAL VULNERABILITY OF THE THORACOLUMBAR SPINE

The thoracolumbar spine is a transition area (Fig. 1) between rigid and flexible segments, so that stress concentration arises at this level. The thoracic spine is rigid because there is less deformable disc material than in the lumbar spine. The ratio of disc height to vertebral height is 1:6 at the thoracic level compared to 1:3 at the lumbar level (42). Movements of the thoracic spine also are restricted by the rib cage and costovertebral ligaments. Thoracic intervertebral sagittal mobility is 2° to 6°, compared to 10° to 24° at the lumbar level.

The thoracolumbar spine also is a transition area in degrees of freedom of movement. In the thoracic spine, the ribs restrict flexion, extension, and lateral bending. Their parallel orientation offers comparatively little restriction of torsion, but the rib cage as a whole has a rigidifying effect. Extension is limited further by the length and obliquity of the spinous processes. At the

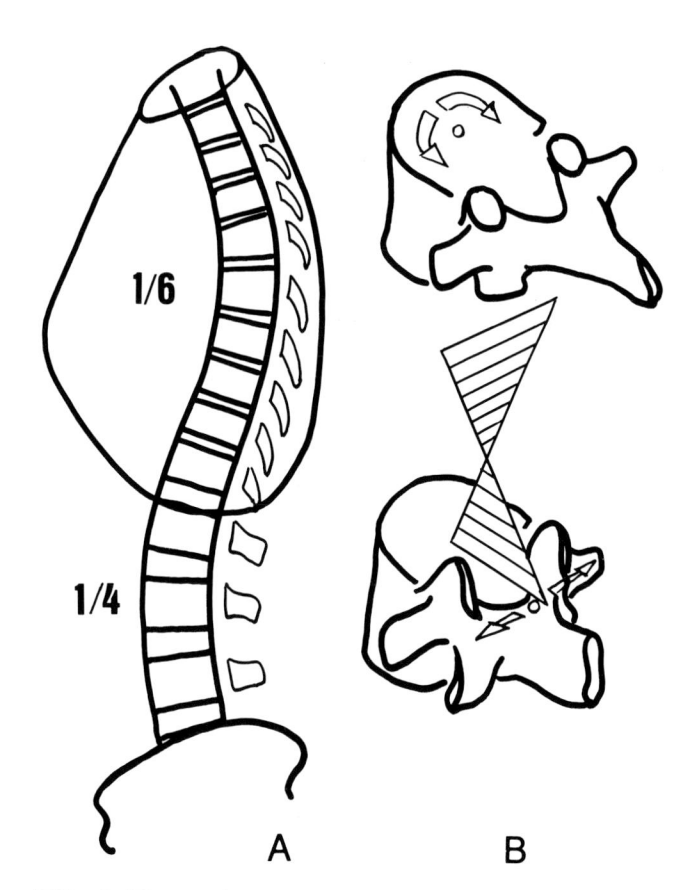

FIG. 1. Thoracolumbar transition. **A:** Rigid rib cage, oblique spinous processes, and disc material, which is less deformable at the thoracic level. **B:** Modification in the orientation of articular facets and the location of the axis of horizontal rotation.

A. Tanguy: Department of Pediatric Orthopaedics, Service Chirurgie Infantile, Hotel-Dieu, 63000 Clermont-Ferrand, France.

T11 and T12 levels, the ribs are completely independent from the rib cage so there is no more restriction of movement. Below this junction, the lumbar region is mainly devoted to flexion–extension, and the anteroposterior diameter of the vertebral body is smaller than the transverse diameter. There is progressive sagittal orientation of the articular facet joints. Lateral bending is allowed to a lesser degree, while rotation is strongly limited (11) by the facets because the center of their arc of rotation is far posterior to the center of the intervertebral disc (25). The thoracolumbar junction has neither the restriction of movement of the thoracic elements nor the facet geometry of the lumbar level. Therefore it is particularly at risk for torsion injuries, since tensile stresses can be resisted only by the capsule and ligaments.

Finally, the thoracolumbar spine is an area of transition between the anterior concavity of the thoracic spine (kyphosis) and the posterior concavity of the lumbar spine (lordosis). Stagnara et al. (36) measured the reciprocal angulation of the vertebral bodies in the sagittal plane and found the transitional vertebra to vary between T9 and L3. The most frequent was L1 (33%), followed by T12 (22%) and L2 (21%). At these levels, more load is carried along the longitudinal axis and there is a decrease in the obliquity of intervertebral disc spaces.

BIOMECHANICS OF THE PROTECTION OF THE THORACOLUMBAR SPINE FROM MECHANICAL FAILURE

The vulnerability of the thoracolumbar spine only appears under certain conditions. Otherwise, it can safely meet the requirements of strength, mobility, and stability without irreversible damage through the ability of its components to adapt to various loads and its inclusion in an efficiently organized spine.

THE ACCOMMODATION OF SPINAL COMPONENTS TO LOAD

Compression

Axial compression loads are carried mainly through the vertebral body, the endplate, and the disc; each component resists the load differently.

The Intervertebral Disc

When a motion segment (two vertebrae with the intervening disc and connecting soft tissues) is compressed vertically, it is readily apparent that there is more deformation in the disc than in the vertebra, leading to the simple concept of the disc as a shock absorber. It is possible to relate deformation to the load: as would be expected, the higher the load, the higher the deformation. In fact, this relationship is not maintained. Above a given load, there is little further deformation; the disc becomes stiffer (5), to the point where other structures fail (27), allowing penetration of nuclear material into the vertebral body. Thus the intervertebral disc is very deformable for small loads but highly rigid for large loads, so that it is impossible to produce experimentally an annular injury under pure compressive loads because other structures fail first. Stiffening of the disc can be induced by a compressive preload. Janevic et al. (18) determined that through this mechanism, a compressive preload of 2200 N resulted in 2.6, 4.5, and 6.1 times decreased flexibility in bending, axial torsion, and shear, respectively, resulting in considerable modification in spine mobility. This mechanism is useful to adjust the stability of the spine, to attenuate the transition between the rigid thoracic spine and the mobile lumbar spine, and to limit motion within physiological range. Preliminary computer simulations suggest that the preload stiffening effect can reduce some trunk muscle stresses by as much as 30% from those predicted in the absence of this effect.

Time is a very important factor because the disc exhibits viscoelastic properties. Load rate is an essential parameter, since the faster the disc is loaded, the stiffer it becomes, resulting in decreased shock absorbing capacity. Also, maintaining a suddenly applied load allows deformation to increase with time: this is the creep behavior of the disc. In the same way, if a given deformity is maintained constant, the deforming forces tend to decrease with time: this is the load relaxation phenomenon.

The fact that these characteristics of compressive stiffness, creep, and load relaxation are maintained after complete removal of the nucleus (24) demonstrates the major role played by the annulus in the management of compression loads. With its high water content, the nucleus has hydrostatic properties and provides radial transmission of forces, which are resisted through the fiber arrangement of the annulus as tensile stresses. Thus the compressive load applied axially to the disc is transmitted radially by the nucleus and distributed transversely within the annulus, which yields centrally and resists strongly at the periphery, decreasing the risk of mechanical failure (Fig. 2A).

Endplate

Along with radial transmission of load by the nucleus, there is an axial endplate bulge that corresponds in magnitude to the linear compression of the motion segment (4). This is a useful mechanism to reduce the

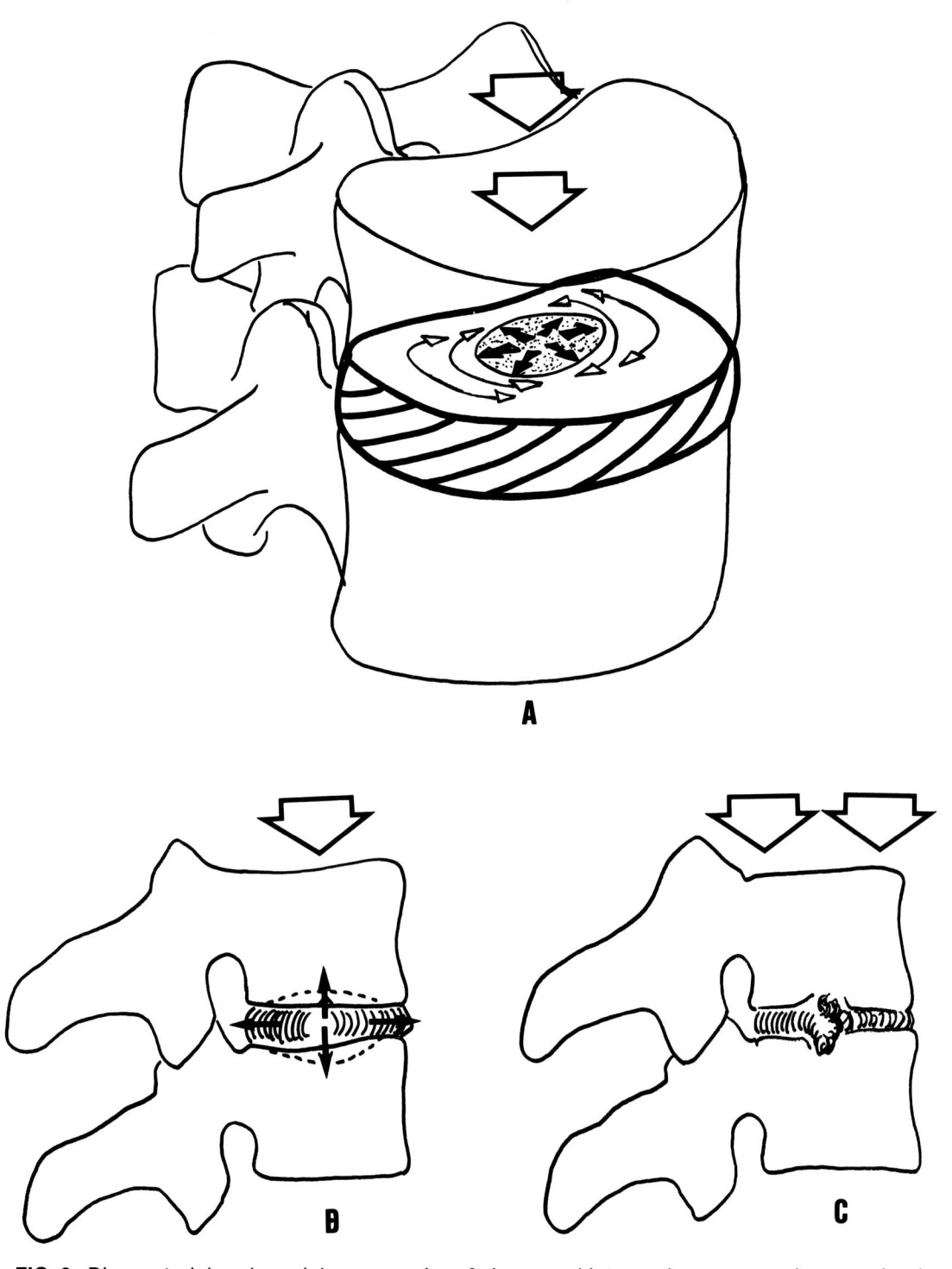

FIG. 2. Disc material under axial compression. **A:** Increased intranuclear pressure is transmitted to the annulus fibers as tensile stresses. **B:** Axial endplate bulging. **C:** With increasing loads, disc material penetrates through endplate fissures.

strain on the annulus fibers (Fig. 2B). With axial overload, the endplate is one of the first structures to fail, as proved by static and dynamic tests conducted by Perey (27). Such failures are associated with penetration of nuclear material through endplate fissures into the vertebral body (Schmorl's nodes) (Fig. 2C).

Vertebral Body

It should be remembered that vertebral body strength is related to osseous tissue content. A 25% decrease in bone content (which occurs normally through aging) results in more than 50% decrease in vertebral strength. In vertebral body bone less than 40 years of age, 55% of compressive load is carried by cancellous bone. The remaining load is carried by cortical bone. Over 40 years of age, the contribution of the cancellous bone is only 35%. The cortical bone shell may be the most resistant to failure, but it has little room for adaptation due to its rigidity. On the contrary, cancellous bone is more able to manage load, since it accepts more deformation without disruption. When vertebral endplates deform, blood is forced out of the vertebra through multiple vascular foramina. This squeezing of the bone marrow and blood content results from distortion of the lattice-like trabecular bone, which accommodates the compression. Bone marrow as a hydraulic cushion has been suggested to be the main resistor to peak dynamic loads (39), absorbing energy at high rates of loading. Raising intra-abdominal pressure through contraction of abdominal muscles could also play a role by increasing intravertebral venous pressure.

Tension

Traction of 9 kg on a spine with intact ligamentous structures is sufficient to induce a 1.5 mm separation between adjacent lumbar vertebrae (7). The ability of the vertebral body to accommodate tension through elongation is negligible, and it is less resistant than under compression. The intervertebral disc is less stiff than under compression, three times stronger along the direction of annulus fibers than along the horizontal direction, and stronger in the anterior part than the posterior part (14).

When tension forces are developed, the spinal ligaments are stretched so that they become effective. Each ligament has individual properties, but all ligaments exhibit the same type of nonlinear force deformation, in which the curve slope increases with tensile forces (6). Thus deformable ligaments in physiologic ranges of motion become stiffer to resist high tensile loads. Elongation prior to failure was determined to be 34% for the posterior longitudinal ligament, 16% for the ligamentum flavum, 44.5% for the anterior longitudinal ligament, and 29.5% for the interspinous and supraspinous ligaments (6). Stronger ligaments were found at the lower thoracic or thoracolumbar level, although others (26) have drawn different conclusions. Universal agreement has not been reached regarding the relative strength of the ligaments other than that the intertransverse ligament is stronger than the interspinous ligament. Moreover, evidence of interspinous ligament rupture in patients as young as 20 years of age (21%) has been reported (28).

Time is the most important factor in mechanical properties of ligaments, since they can resist higher strains when loaded more slowly, as demonstrated for the ligamentum flavum (33). However, Twomey (38) found that, when a constant elongation force was maintained on lumbar specimens, 85% of length increase occurred immediately following weight application. Creep only accounted for a further 1- to 2-mm increase beyond the initial figure in most specimens, indicating that creep is not as important as for the intervertebral disc.

Shear

Shear forces are introduced by any load that is not perpendicular to the disc, causing one vertebra to slide on another: anteriorly during flexion, posteriorly during extension, and laterally during bending. These forces are well resisted by the disc in the horizontal plane, with high stiffness value in vitro. Facet orientation further protects the disc from abnormal displacement. In lordotic spine segments, 50% of shear resistance is attributed to the facet joints (17). Stiffness is higher during posterior shear at the lumbar level. In the anterior direction, the strong posterior muscular attachments to the superior articular processes reduce anterior translation forces on the disc. At the thoracic level, shear stiffness is the same in all directions, since the orientation and geometry of the facet joints make their contribution negligible.

According to evaluation of finite elements at the L3 level (32), during anterior bending, shear forces are important to resist since total contact force in the facet joints is mainly in the horizontal plane with almost no axial component. This study also showed that shear forces should double on the compression facet when torsion and lateral bending are added to flexion.

Torsion

Torsional stresses have received wide attention as potentially dangerous to the disc. Gordon et al. (12) recently reported that combined small values of cyclic compression, torsion, and flexion induced disc failure.

In rotational movements of the spine, motion takes place at the disc, where torsion moments generate shear and tensile stresses in the annulus that are greater at the periphery and least at the center of rotation. Removal of a 2-cm portion of the posterior annulus produces a 25% decrease in torque strength (8) while the intact disc contributes 32% of the torque resistance strength. A variation of 40% to 50% in torque strength in the isolated disc may be related to compression, since compressive loading of the disc reduces its torque strength. The disc is protected from excessive stresses and strains by the posterior elements with the mechanical advantage of their long lever arm. Their contribution is significant, since their removal from motion segments in the L1 to L4 region increases rotation by 150% (30). Their importance is even greater when torsion is associated with lateral bending and flexion–extension, especially in extension (70–80%) (23). The respective contributions of the various posterior elements to strength in resisting torsion is 15% for the articular processes, 11% for the capsule, and 7% for the interspinous ligaments (8). During torsion, the facet joints are compressed on one side and distracted on the other. Finite element evaluation at L3 (32) suggests that the tension facet remains entirely unloaded, while the compression facet supports higher contact forces during axial rotation than during extension, flexion, and lateral bending, respectively. From T7–T8 to L4, there is a continuous increase in torsional stiffness, related mainly to facet joint orientation. T12 to L5 joints are least flexible in torsion compared to flexion, extension, and lateral bending (30).

Bending

Most loads naturally imposed on the spine are applied eccentrically and generate moments that tend to bend the spine. Bending loads occurring during flexion–extension and lateral bending produce compression stresses on one side of the axis of rotation and tension on the other.

When the spine is flexed, the disc and the vertebral body are under compression and the posterior ligaments are stretched. Silver (34) demonstrated in vivo that tension in the supraspinous and interspinous L3 to L4 ligaments increases with flexion. These posterior ligaments are important in the protection of the disc (37), since the disc is less resistant in flexion than in extension (23). Flexion moments produce maximum strain in the posterior annulus fibrosus. When flexion is combined with lifting, intradiscal pressure rises (1). The posterior ligaments in the thoracic spine have a ratio of 3:1 when their lever arm is compared to the anterior portion of the vertebral body. This ratio rises to 4:1 in the lumbar spine. Experiments on isolated facet joints revealed weakness in flexion related to poor tensile resistance of capsular ligaments (41). Therefore their contribution in the posterior lever arm may be limited.

When the spine is extended, the disc is under tension, which is strongly resisted by the strength of the anterior longitudinal ligament. The posterior elements come under compression, and the osseous abutment of facet joints and spinous processes accounts for 25% to 30% in extension stiffness. In extension, the joint behaves as a stiffening spring, and this is unchanged by cutting all posterior ligaments. The disc resists extension, and the combination of the posterior spinous processes and the interspinous ligaments trapped between them (2) resists extension in the back. In rare cases of "kissing spine," extension is limited by the posterior spinous processes that abut each other. In opposition, if the spinous processes are widely spaced, the zygapophyseal joints may be damaged first. The disc can be damaged in hyperextension if the spine is subjected to high compressive forces at the same time. A sudden application of compression forces can cause an anterior disc prolapse (2).

During lateral bending, finite element evaluation (32) indicates that the tension facet is negligibly loaded with lateral bending exceeding 5° to 6°. The magnitude of the contact force generated on the compression facet remains low and is much smaller than in flexion under large rotation. According to this evaluation, removal of the facets has a negligible effect on segmental lateral flexibility.

ORGANIZATION OF THE SPINE

Curvatures of the Spine

The presence of sagittal curvatures in the normal human spine has several advantages useful in preserving the integrity of the spine. This curvature gives a 34.4% strength increase when compared to a straight construct. This is given by Euler's formula, where the cross-sectional area is elliptical compared to a circular one (15). Since the vertebrae included in the curves are oblique, vertical loads are resolved into a set of smaller compression (or tension) and shear forces, reducing the risk of failure. The smooth contour of the curves with regular, nonangular shapes are the basis for progressive change in the obliquity of the vertebrae, thereby avoiding stress concentration at a given level. Their multisegmented, articulated nature allows for a large range of motion via small movements at each level and allows multilevel stress distribution. This damping effect lessens the probability of reaching critical loads for the lower lumbar levels. Finally, in reference to the behavior of slender struts, the curves decrease the distance between the lower support of the strut in the pelvis and the upper end so that the critical buckling load of such a construct is increased.

The alternating direction of the curves (lordosis and kyphosis) adds several benefits: better distribution of the mass of the spine along the vertical axis, and variation in obliquity of intervertebral spaces, which can modify stress accordingly with only small ranges of motion necessary. The lordotic curves are the most adjustable parts of the human spine and can accept large muscle masses in their concavity. The lumbar lordosis can accommodate a muscular mass three to four times greater than the thoracic muscular mass.

External Support

The spine is an axial skeleton surrounded by the thoracic and abdominal cavities. Passive stiffening effect of the rib cage on the thoracic spine provides a fourfold increase in stability compared to the osteoligamentous spine when calculated using a mathematical model (3). Another interesting characteristic is that the content of these cavities can be constrained by muscular contraction so that the spine is no longer a slender strut but a component of a rigid-walled cylinder. This configuration decreases compressive load on the spine, but controversy exists regarding the importance of this reduction (13) (Fig. 3).

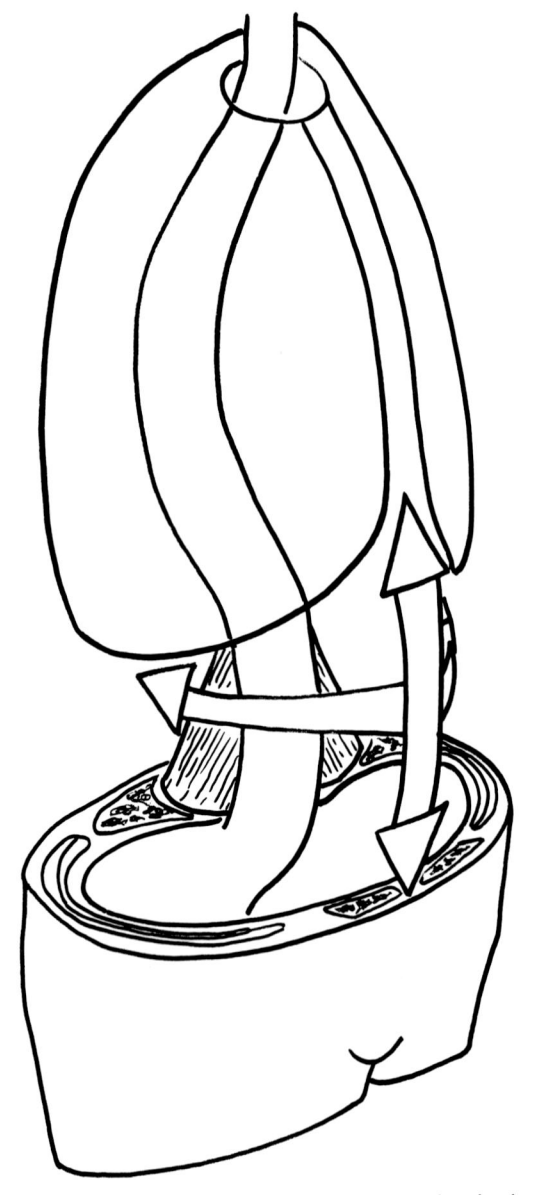

FIG. 3. Rigidification of the thoracic and abdominal cavities provides for external support.

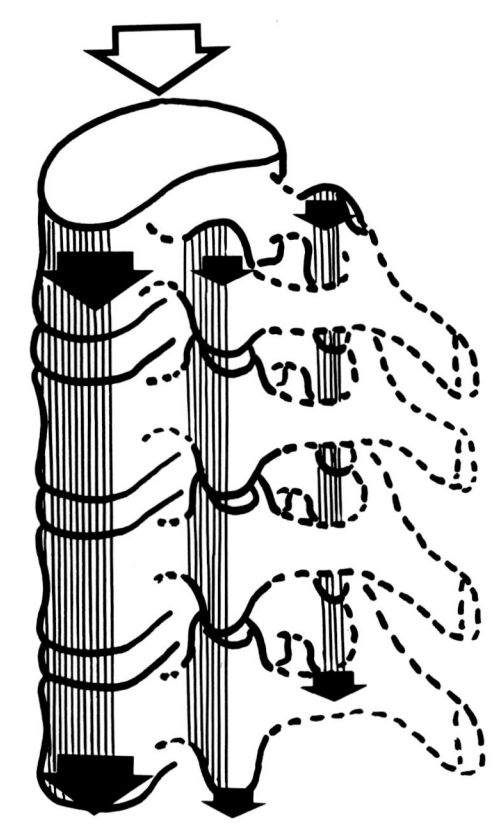

FIG. 4. Three column arrangement.

Pile Arrangement

The vertebrae in the spinal column are stacked one on top of the other in a pile arrangement with three surfaces of contact, one anterior with the disc and the vertebral body, and two posterior through the left and right facet joints. This arrangement led to the structural concept, expanded in 1973 by Louis (21), of the spine as three vertical columns connected at each level by transverse structures, lamina and pedicle (Fig. 4). The anterior column has the mechanical advantage of a large support area and has been proved to carry the major part of axial load. Depending on the eccentricity of the load, only 3% to 25% is supported by the posterior columns (41). Due to the pile arrangement, the lower segments of the spine receive larger loads than the upper ones. The progressive increase in size between the thoracic and lumbar vertebrae allows the larger load to be distributed on a larger supporting area so that stress does not become excessive. For example, the mean anteroposterior diameter is 17.7 mm at T3, 25.9 mm at T12, and 31.5 mm at L5 (31). The intercalary distribution of deformable disc material and rigid vertebral bone in the anterior column creates a flexible alignment. It also allows motion and controlled deformation at each level to facilitate energy dissipation to protect adjacent levels during impact.

STABILITY OF THE THORACOLUMBAR SPINE

The spinal column must meet the requirements of stability to prevent premature mechanical and biological deterioration of its components. Spinal stability is fundamental for protection of the spinal cord and nerve roots. It is also useful for minimizing energy expenditure.

Considering one motion segment, the intrinsic stability of the spine appears to be satisfactory. The geometric characteristics of the vertebra, with adapted facet joint orientation, as well as normal intradiscal pressure are seemingly adequate to maintain ligament tension. However, the situation is completely different when considering the vertical alignment of the thoracolumbar motion segments as a whole, since the spine buckles under a small (2-kg) vertical load. This buckling is well known in mechanical engineering for flexible beams fixed at one end. We have already seen a number of mechanisms that prevent buckling of the normal thoracolumbar spine through regularly alternating curves and external support. These biomechanical properties and mechanisms provide the foundation for understanding the stability of the thoracolumbar spine.

We can define spinal stability as the ability of the vertebrae to maintain their relationships and limit their relative displacements during physiologic postures and loads. Each motion segment must be stable, since the stability of the entire thoracolumbar spine depends on the stability of its weakest point. The challenge to spine stability is mobility, since at any time the conditions of equilibrium may change and the vertebral segments may undergo acceleration. Segmental vertebral mobility occurs with voluntary muscular contraction or is due to forces and moments generated by external loads. This takes place through deformation of the disc space and motion between facet joints. Physiologic mobility and stability require that motion be (a) within normal limits of the disc space deformation; (b) guided by the facet joints; (c) restrained by the articular capsule, the ligaments, and the muscles; and (d) contained within the limits of osseous abutments. Muscular contraction of the trunk and spine muscles, under the control of postural reflexes, provides the active part of stability. This factor is essential to allow continuous modification of forces and moments.

External support, as already mentioned, can also be modulated by muscular contractions. Axial stability is provided by the vertical alignment of the anterior column as defined by Louis (21) through the strength and shape of the vertebral bodies as well as normal function of the intervertebral discs, whose intradiscal pressures maintain ligamentous tension. Stability in the transverse direction, at each mobile segment, is established by controlled patterns of displacement. This control is based on the function of intervertebral discs, the motion and osseous abutment of the facet joints, and the capsular and ligamentous restraints that were previously described. The role of the intervertebral disc cannot be overemphasized as the common component of both axial and transverse stability.

MECHANICAL FAILURE ASSOCIATED WITH THORACOLUMBAR FRACTURES

Thoracolumbar fractures create a disruption in spinal components and introduce a weak point into the organization of the spine, which may result in a potentially dangerous instability for the spinal cord.

Disruption of Spinal Components

Various components of the thoracolumbar spine may be involved in a spinal injury. Our purpose is not to cover all aspects of these injuries but, rather, to present those that are part of a continuum of failure. This failure continuum is created by segmental component failures until all the energy of the trauma has been dissipated.

Failure Continuum with the Anterior Column Under Compression (Fig. 5)

Spinal motion segments provide greater resistance to failure when loads are applied centrally rather than eccentrically (19). Under traumatic conditions (high loads and/or high rates of loading), the intervertebral disc becomes stiffer, resulting in a decreased shock absorbing capacity with direct transmission of the load to the adjacent structures. In very excessive instances of axial compression, such as a violent fall onto the buttocks in combination with bending loads and torsion, annular fissures may occur.

The failure load for the vertebral endplate is more readily reached. The endplate is the first structure to fail, such that rupture of the vertebral endplate has been compared to a safety fuse that dissipates energy to protect the underlying bone (27). The rupture may be central, caused by the buildup of nuclear pressure resulting under axial load. Anterior failure may occur under bending load. The entire endplate may become multifragmented under the direct transmission of high compression axial load through a failed disc. In any case, rupture of the endplate may not protect adjacent bone, and further disruption may occur. Bending loads may cause simple buckling of the anterior cortex with a wedge-shaped compression fracture of the cancellous bone, while axial load may cause failure of both ends of the vertebra with a central biconcave compression fracture.

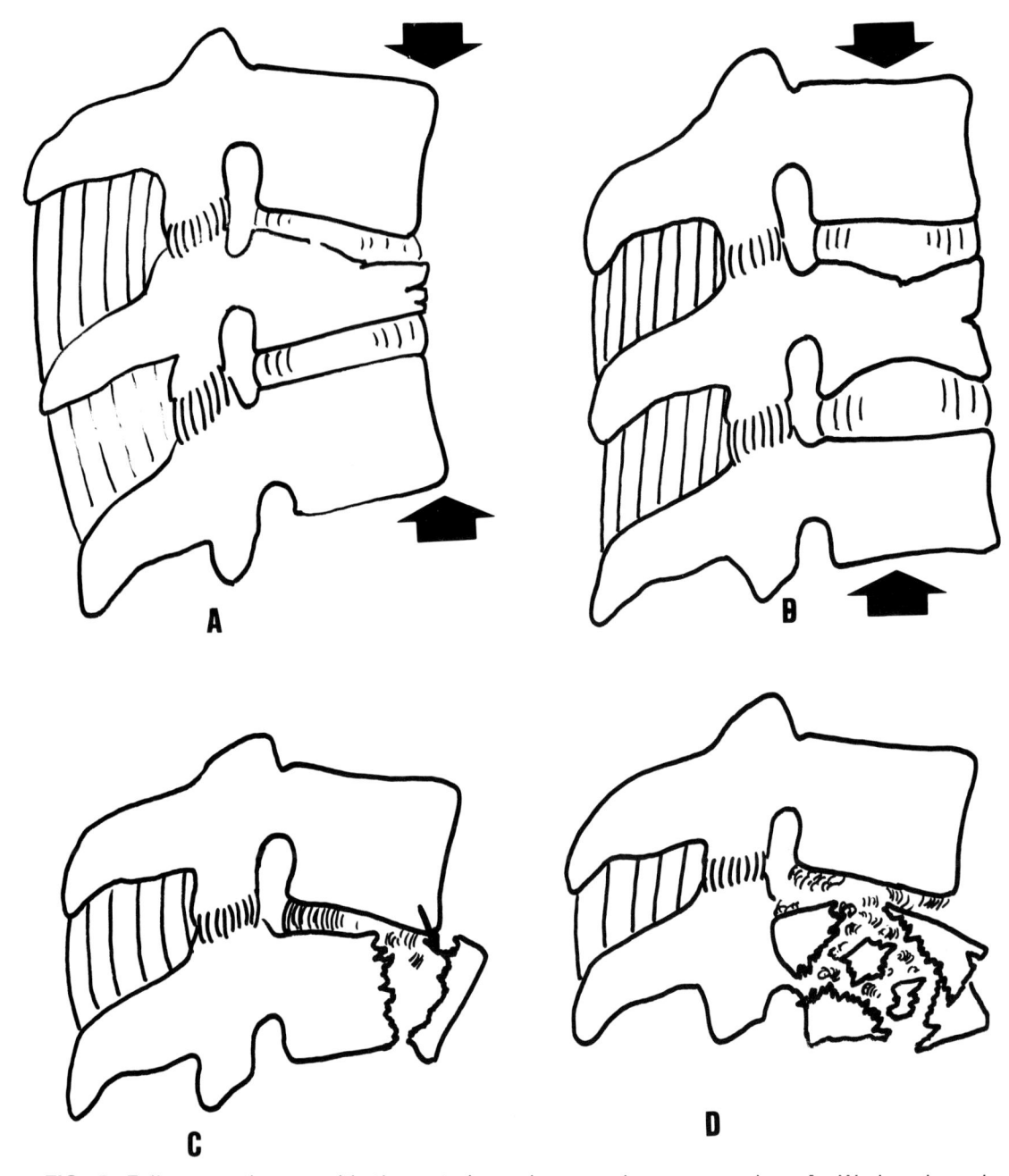

FIG. 5. Failure continuum with the anterior column under compression. **A:** Wedge-shaped compression fracture with posterior tensile stresses. **B:** Biconcave compression fracture with overload on anterior elements. **C:** Detached anterior part of vertebral body with frontal fracture line. **D:** Complete destruction of the anterior column, with nuclear material driven along the fracture lines and the spreading of bony fragments.

Once endplate disruption has occurred under bending loads, shear forces are no longer resisted through the failed disc. The forces may induce separation in the anterior part of the vertebral body with a fracture line in the frontal plane. Disc material as well as endplate fragments are driven into the vertebral bone by the anteroinferior corner of the vertebra above, further deepening the separation of the anterior part of the vertebra.

Under dynamic axial compressive loads, as demonstrated by Willen et al. (40), extensive injuries are associated with displacement of the nucleus both from the superior and inferior discs and with fragmentation of the endplates resulting in crush or burst fracture. In such cases (27), the compressive load is transmitted directly through the annulus so that peripheral injuries occur to the endplate as a result of the insertion of annulus fibers. Compressive load is also carried through the cortical shell of the vertebral body, while the cancellous bone of the vertebral body is destroyed by the penetration of endplate fragments by disc material and loss of cortical bone support. The vertebral body is no longer contained and spreads laterally, anteriorly, and posteriorly and protrudes into the spinal canal at the level of the superior and/or inferior endplates. Lindahl et al. (20), among others, found in some cases a crush fracture of the upper one-half of the vertebral body with superior disc injury combined with a sagittal fracture (cleavage fracture) of the lower one-half, bone fragments in the spinal canal, and laminar fracture.

Height loss axially on the anterior vertebral body column brings a part of the compression load onto the facet joints so that the posterior elements are involved in such fractures with a vertical laminar fracture. The facet joints sublux as a result of posterior rotation, leading to capsular stretching or rupture (41).

On the contrary, height loss anteriorly through wedging increases both the tensile stress on the posterior ligamentous structures and the shear stress resisted by the osseous abutment of the articular facets. In severe cases the interspinous and supraspinous ligaments may be damaged, and the relative weakness of the capsular ligaments may allow subluxation to take place.

Failure Continuum with Posterior Elements Under Distraction (Fig. 6)

Failure under pure axial tensile load imposed on the entire spinal column is rather rare. A more common

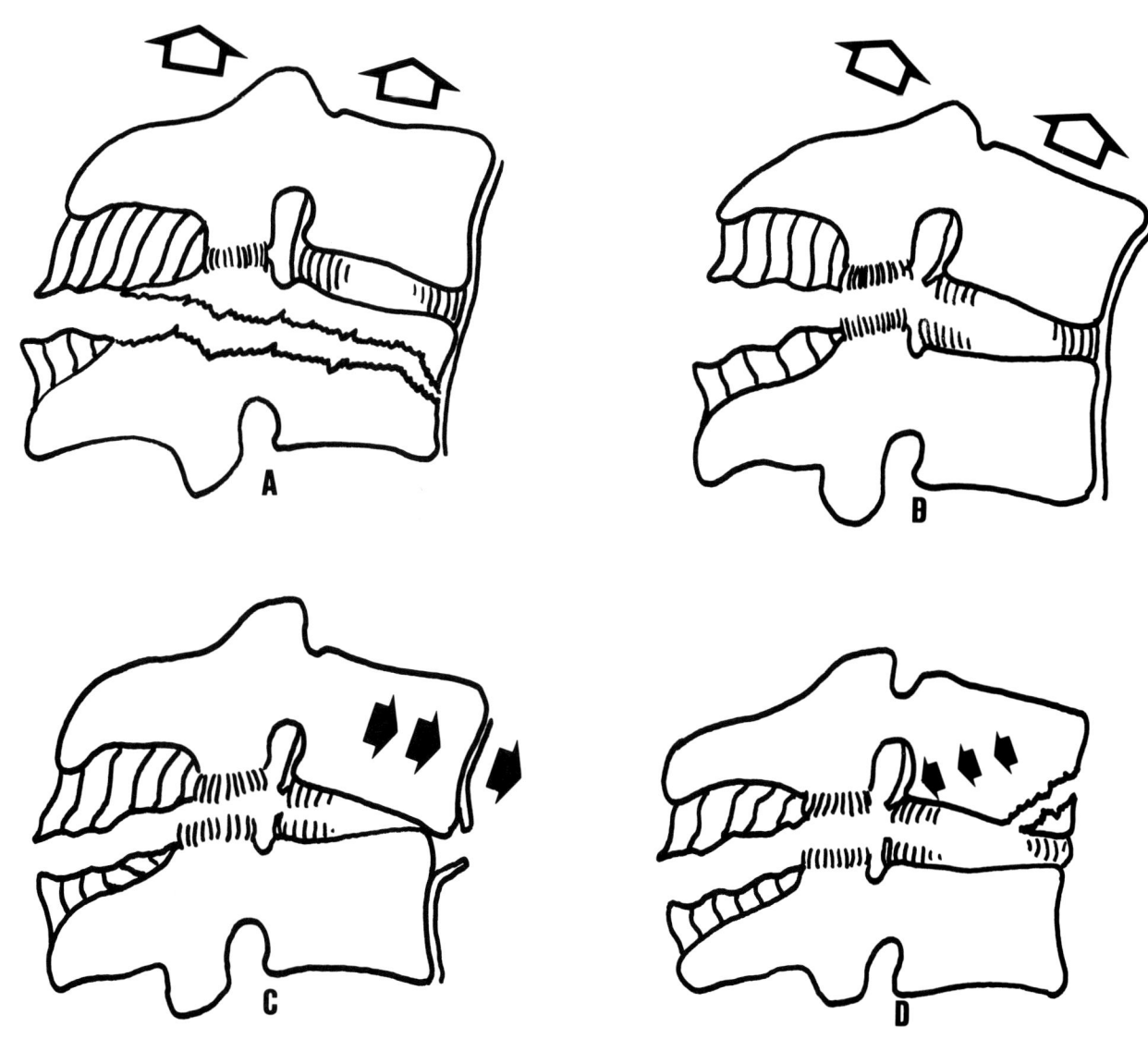

FIG. 6. Failure continuum with posterior elements under distraction. **A:** Chance fracture. **B:** Ligamentous type seat-belt fracture. **C:** Rupture of anterior longitudinal ligament and anterior translation. **D:** Teardrop fracture: fracture of the osseous abutment as a hinge for sagittal bending.

situation is met when the anterior bending moment is associated with flexion, as in a car accident in which violent deceleration accelerates the body bent over a lap-type seat belt (35). In such a case, all portions of the spinal column are posterior to the flexion axis and should be protected against major tensile stresses associated with anterior bending stresses. The ligaments are loaded so rapidly that they become rigid, and dissipation of energy cannot occur through deformation, creating abnormal stress in bony attachments and in the ligament itself. The most peripheral structures relative to the axis of rotation are subjected to higher loads than those closer, so that failure will occur either through the neural arch or through the posterior ligaments. Bone failure produces a Chance fracture that starts through the spinous process, disrupts the pedicles and the posterior part of the vertebral body, and ends in the anterior part of the vertebral body, which buckles at the hinge of the opening of the vertebra through the bone.

Failure through the ligaments produces another type of seat belt fracture with complete ligamentous rupture starting through the supraspinous and interspinous ligaments, disrupting the capsular ligaments and the posterior longitudinal ligament. This allows full distraction to be exerted on the posterior annulus, which is less resistant than the anterior annulus. Through this failure continuum, disruption may extend farther anteriorly in the intervertebral disc, with complete rupture of the annulus ending in complete separation of the intervertebral joint, allowing subluxation or dislocation to take place. Completion of the failure continuum (not accounted for in seat-belt fracture) allows anterior translation cleared by the failure of the anterior longitudinal ligament.

Teardrop fractures are another example of the failure of posterior elements under distraction with hyperflexion. Along with the tensile stresses generated by high bending moments, there is complete disruption of the posterior ligaments going to the posterior longitudinal ligament. These posterior ligaments are essential for protection of the disc in such a situation, since the disc is weaker in flexion than in extension (23). Once the posterior ligaments have been disrupted, they will no more protect the intervertebral disc, which has been shown to fail beyond 15° flexion when the posterior elements have been removed. Disc opening occurs through hinging due to the abutment of the anteroinferior corner of the vertebra above as it flexes on the vertebra below. Enough energy is left to fracture the osseous abutment so that the hinge of sagittal rotation is destroyed and the osseous fragment may disrupt the anterior longitudinal ligament. Backward translation of the rotating vertebra is then possible, leading to a dangerous posterior tilt of the vertebra during the terminal phase of flexion with protrusion into the canal.

Another fracture type, similar to the cervical teardrop fracture, occurs when osseous abutment is on the anterosuperior corner of the vertebra, with the same backward tilting of the vertebra toward the spinal canal.

Failure Continuum with Rotation Combined with Various Loads (Fig. 7)

For significant rotation to take place in the thoracolumbar spine, there must be a fracture or dislocation of the articular processes (16). Axial torque is first best resisted by the intervertebral disc, even if some damage takes place at angles greater than 3° (8). After the interspinous ligament is torn or detached from bone, further displacement is opposed by the articular processes, with one facet joint under compression and the other opened in tension. At a rotation of less than 9°, Farfan (9) noted a decrease in distance between the inferior articular processes and an increase in distance between the superior processes (3–4 mm). The compression facet is the first structure to yield; the tension facet opens as much as 0.5 to 1 cm before failure (1). The joint is fractured near the base of the articular processes and the capsule is torn, resulting in several small avulsion fractures. Further disruption occurs through the posterior longitudinal ligament and then in the intervertebral disc, where failure in torsion is reported to occur at angles of 10° to 30° (10). The anterior longitudinal ligament is the last component to fail.

In fact, torsion is often associated with compression and/or bending. With bending in flexion, subluxation of the facet joints can progress to dislocation without fracture of the articular processes, allowing the injury to progress either through the disc with an associated compression fracture of the vertebral body or through the vertebral body, detaching a slice of vertebral body and producing a fracture/dislocation as described by Holdsworth (16). Under compression, the ability of the intervertebral disc to resist the torque is reduced (8). The facet joints are locked and strongly resist torsional forces so that a fracture rather than a dislocation will occur. This fracture may go through the pedicles.

Various amounts of lateral or anteroposterior displacements are to be expected from such injuries. During the progression of failure, there are changes in hinges, freedom of movement, and a loss of stability. Furthermore, additional shear forces may be present after the fracture or dislocation has cleared the way for translation.

Potential Instability of Thoracolumbar Fractures

Changes due to injury of the normal mechanisms of axial and transverse stability may result in instability.

Various classifications with different theories exist, which try to identify stable or unstable fractures. Each is convincing but it is difficult to find agreement for a simple classification among them. As stated by Roy-Camille et al. (29), the problem of instability is to anticipate three possible situations: stable injury where no more displacement will take place, unstable injury with progressive and predictable displacement, and unstable injury with sudden, uncontrolled displacement possible at any moment.

Stable injuries are those that reflect the beginning of a failure continuum that did not progress. They are indicative of low disruptive forces with practically no associated spinal injuries.

Central compression fractures and wedge fractures with less than one-third of vertebral height loss are stable. The vertebral body is squeezed into a firm mass of disorganized osseous trabeculae, and the wedge fracture maintains 60% to 70% of its original load bearing capacity.

Supraspinous and interspinous ligamentous ruptures with subluxed facets are also stable.

Unstable injuries with sudden displacement are those that reflect the entire extent of the failure continuum, ending with a complete disruption or marked displacement. The disruptive process goes through anterior and posterior elements and is always associated with severe intervertebral disc injury.

Burst fractures with posterior element involvement have extensive bone damage with a crushed vertebral body uncontained in any direction and disruption of both intervertebral discs. These fractures are unstable due to the complete loss of anterior support. Little hope should be placed in bone healing, since the disc material driven into the bone interferes with healing and may produce a pseudarthrosis. Willen et al. (40) experimentally established the instability of such injuries.

Pure dislocation or fracture/dislocation with significant translation is indicative of extensive discoligamentous injury with major instability and high probability for neurologic damage. The most common site for this lesion is between T12 and L1, where there is very little room in the spinal canal.

Unstable injuries with progressive displacement are those that reflect a large extent of the failure continuum. They are unstable through the complete impairment of either stability system and include the intervertebral disc in all cases.

Severe wedge fractures combined with posterior ligamentous rupture are not locked posteriorly and will displace progressively due to the severity of anterior height loss. The cancellous bone may not reexpand as some authors pointed out, and the osseous tissue is necrotic.

In the frontal plane fracture of the vertebral body, a

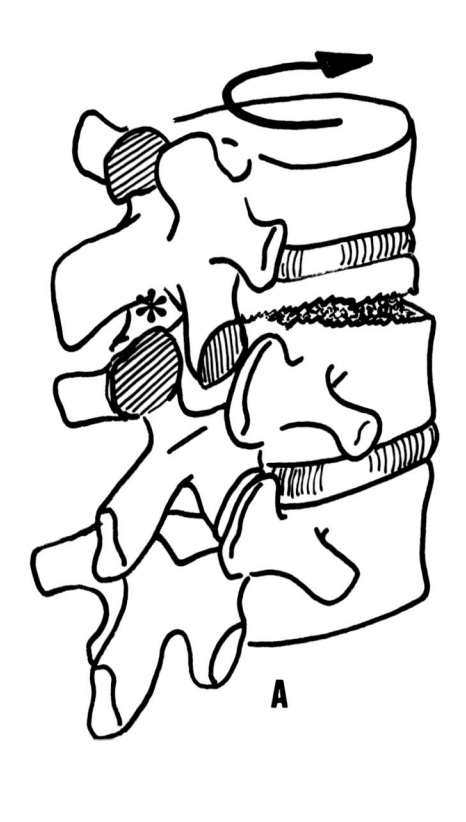

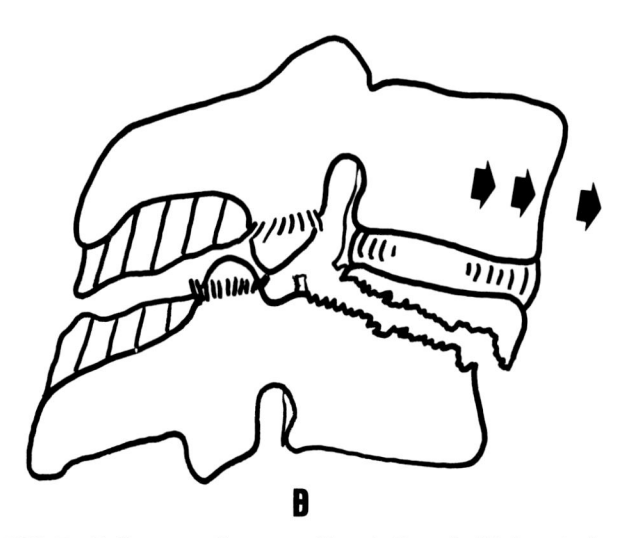

FIG. 7. Failure continuum with rotation. **A:** Dislocated articular process (*asterisk*) and progression of rotatory injury through the vertebral body. **B:** Secondary anteroposterior instability.

This will be reflected at the injured level as the risk of secondary displacement under physiological loads with potential neurological impairment. A thorough evaluation is essential to determine the nature and the extent of spinal component disruption. Discoligamentous injuries are sometimes hard to demonstrate but are essential with regard to potential instability since they heal poorly. Osseous injuries are more readily apparent, and bone healing may resolve temporary osseous instability.

gap is produced by the separation of the anterior third of the vertebral body. The vertebral body above will progressively tip, leading to gradual displacement. Since disc material is pushed into the gap, spontaneous healing will not occur, and pseudarthrosis is frequent. Louis (22) insists on the loss of stability through the loss of bone in such fractures.

The teardrop fracture has some stability through the impaction of the tilted vertebral body onto the vertebral body below, but it is mainly characterized by the complete disruption of the intervertebral joint.

Pure, complete disruption of the intervertebral joint (disc and ligaments connecting two adjacent vertebrae), as present in the ligamentous form of seat belt fracture, is the best example of pure discoligamentous instability. The same situation may result from rotatory displacement.

CONSEQUENCES OF POST-TRAUMATIC DEFORMITY

Focal deformity from thoracolumbar fractures modifies the organization of the spine with durable alteration of mechanical properties. By far, the most common problem is kyphosis resulting from the loss of vertebral body height due to either severity of compression and wedging, secondary necrosis of bone, or pseudarthrosis of a fracture with disc material scattered among bone fragments. The deformity is segmental, and the regular contour of the thoracolumbar spine is disrupted. This leads to stress concentration at this level, particularly if the shock absorbing capacity of adjacent discs is no longer present. The angular deformity reverses the gradual anterior disc space opening that is normally present so that kyphosis is globally increased, with forward displacement of the gravity line and more eccentric loading of the spine. The greater moment arm leads to greater compression stresses transmitted along the anterior column and more tensile stresses on the posterior elements. Tensile stresses have to be resisted passively by strong posterior bone and ligament elements, which may be problematic when disruptions occur, either from injury or laminectomy. Tensile stresses also have to be resisted actively through compensatory lordosis and strong muscular control to reduce forward displacement of the gravity line. Few disc spaces are available below the deformity to establish a compensatory lumbar hyperlordosis, and spinal instrumentation may definitively preclude this possibility, especially when iatrogenic flat back has been created. Muscular control may be difficult to maintain as muscles act on a shorter lever arm reduced by the deformity itself and by the reduction of lumbar lordosis; it may be completely impossible in cases of neurologic impairment. Through abnormal anatomy leading to abnormal function, residual deformities add more vulnerability to this transition area of the spine, with possible progression or pain.

CONCLUSION

The thoracolumbar spine is prone to failure under certain conditions. It is protected from such failure through its ability to adapt to load, its efficient organization, and its stability as a whole as well as at each level. Fractures that disrupt these mechanisms may cause potentially irreversible neurologic damage and progressive displacement. Knowledge of normal biomechanics is helpful in understanding the mechanism of injury, the extent of disruption, and implications for acute as well as late instability.

REFERENCES

1. Adams MA, Hutton WC, Stott JRR. The resistance to flexion of the lumbar intervertebral joint. *Spine* 1980;5:245–253.
2. Adams MA, Dolan P, Hutton WC. The lumbar spine in backward bending. *Spine* 1988;13:1019–1026.
3. Andriacchi TP, Schultz AB, Belytschko TB, Galante JO. A model for studies of mechanical interactions between the human spine and rib cage. *J Biomech* 1974;7:497–507.
4. Brinckmann P, Frobin W, Hierholzer E, Horst M. Deformation of the vertebral endplate under axial loading of the spine. *Spine* 1983;8:851–856.
5. Brown T, Hansen R, Yorra A. Some mechanical tests on the lumbosacral spine with particular reference to the intervertebral discs: a preliminary report. *J Bone Joint Surg* 1957;39A:1135–1164.
6. Chazal J, Tanguy A, Bourges M, Gaurel G, Escande G, Guillot M, Vanneuville G. Biomechanical properties of spinal ligaments and a histological study of the supraspinal ligament in traction. *J Biomech* 1985;18(3):167–176.
7. DeSeze S, Levernieux J. Les tractions vertébrales. Premières études expérimentales et résultats thérapeutiques d'après une expérience de quatre années. *Semaine des Hôpitaux (Paris)* 1951;27:2085.
8. Farfan HF, Cossette JW, Robertson GH, Wells RV, Kraus H. The effects of torsion on the lumbar intervertebral joints: the role of torsion in the production of disc degeneration. *J Bone Joint Surg* 1970;52A:468–497.
9. Farfan HF. *Mechanical disorders of the low back.* Philadelphia: Lea & Febiger, 1973.
10. Fiorini GT, McCammond D. Forces on lumbovertebral facets. *Ann Biomed Eng* 1976;4:354–363.
11. Galante JO. Tensile properties of human annulus fibrosus. *Acta Orthop Scand Suppl* 1967;100:1–91.
12. Gordon SJ, Yang KH, Mayer PJ, Mace A, Kish VL, Radin EL. Mechanism of disc rupture. *Spine* 1991;16:450–456.
13. Gracovetsky S. *The spinal engine.* Vienna: Springer Verlag, 1988.
14. Gregerson GG, Lucas DB. An in vivo study of the axial rotation of the human thoracolumbar spine. *J Bone Joint Surg* 1967;49A:247–262.
15. Guillot M, Fournier J, Scheye T, Escande G, Chazal J, Tanguy A, Vanneuville G. Justification mécanique approachée de la géométrie particulière du rachis humain soumis à contrainte verticale. Presented at the 70th Meeting, Association des Anatomistes, Paris, 1988.
16. Holdsworth FW. Fractures, dislocations and fracture–dislocations of the spine. *J Bone Joint Surg* 1970;52A:1534–1551.
17. Hutton WC, Stoot JRR, Cyron BM. Is spondylolysis a fatigue fracture? *Spine* 1977;2:202–209.

18. Janevic J, Ashton-Miller JA, Schultz AB. Large compressive preloads decrease motion segment flexibility. *J Orthop Res* 1991;9:228–236.
19. Lin HS, Liu YK, Adams KA. Mechanical response of lumbar intervertebral joints under physiological loading. *J Bone Joint Surg* 1978;60A:41–55.
20. Lindahl S, Willen J, Nordwall A, Irstam L. The crush–cleavage fracture. A "new" thoracolumbar unstable fracture. *Spine* 1983; 8:559–569.
21. Louis R. *Chirurgie du rachis*. Vienna: Springer-Verlag, 1982.
22. Louis R. Traumatisme récent du rachis dorsal sans signe neurologique in Fractures et luxations récentes du rachis. In: Roy-Camille R, ed. *Cahiers d'enseignement de la SOFCOT*. Paris: Expansion Scientifique Française, 1988;1732.
23. Markolf KL. Deformation of the thoracolumbar intervertebral joints in response to external loads. *J Bone Joint Surg* 1972;54A: 511–533.
24. Markolf KL, Morris JM. The structural components of the intervertebral disc. *J Bone Joint Surg* 1974;56A:675–687.
25. Morris JM, Markolf KL. Biomechanics of the lumbosacral spine. In: *Atlas of orthotics: biomechanical principles and applications*. American Academy of Orthopaedic Surgeons Saint Louis: Mosby, 1975.
26. Mykelbust JB, Pintar F, Maiman D. Tensile strength of spinal ligaments. *Spine* 1988;13:526–531.
27. Perey O. Fracture of the vertebral endplate in the lumbar spine. *Acta Orthop Scand* 1957;25:1–101.
28. Rissanen PM. The surgical anatomy and pathology of the supraspinous and interspinous ligaments of the lumbar spine with special reference to ligament ruptures. *Acta Orthop Scand [Suppl]* 1960;46.
29. Roy-Camille R, Saillant G, Mazel C, LaPresle P. Anatomie pathologique des lésions traumatiques du rachis. Révision de la notion d'instabilité. Fractures et luxations récentes du rachis. In: Roy-Camille R, ed. *Cahiers d'enseignement de la SOFCOT*. Paris: Expansion Scientifique Francaise, 1988;16.
30. Schultz AB, Warwick DN, Berkson MH, Nachemson AL. Mechanical properties of the human lumbar spine motion segments—part 1: responses in flexion, extension, lateral bending and torsion. *J Biomech Eng* 1979;101:46–52.
31. Scoles P, Linton AE, Latimer B. Vertebral body and posterior element morphology: the normal spine in middle life. *Spine* 1988; 13:1082–1086.
32. Shirazi-adl A. Finite element evaluation of contact loads on facets of an L2–L3 lumbar segment in complex loads. *Spine* 1991; 16(5):533–541.
33. Sikoryn TA, Hukins DWL. Mechanism of failure of the ligamentum flavum of the spine during in vitro tensile tests. *J Orthop Res* 1990;8(4):586–591.
34. Silver PHS. Direct observations of changes in tension in the supraspinous and interspinous ligaments during flexion and extension of the vertebral column in man. *J Anat* 1954;88:550.
35. Smith WS, Kaufer H. Patterns and mechanisms of lumbar injuries associated with lap seat belts. *J Bone Joint Surg* 1969;51A: 239–254.
36. Stagnara P, DeMauroy JC, Dran G, Gonon P, Costanzo G, Dimnet J, Pasquet A. Reciprocal angulation of vertebral bodies in a sagittal plane: approach to reference for the evaluation of kyphosis and lordosis. *Spine* 1982;7:335–342.
37. Twomey LT, Taylor JR. Sagittal movements of the human lumbar vertebral column: a quantitative study of the role of the posterior vertebral elements. *Arch Phys Med Rehabil* 1983;64: 322–325.
38. Twomey LT. Sustained lumbar traction: an experimental study of long spine segments. *Spine* 1985;10:146–149.
39. White AA, Panjabi MM. *Clinical biomechanics of the spine*. Philadelphia: Lippincott, 1978.
40. Willen J, Lindahl S, Irstam L, Aldman B, Nordwall A. The thoracolumbar crush fracture. An experimental study on instant axial dynamic loading: the resulting fracture type and its stability. *Spine* 1984;9(6):624–631.
41. Yang KH, King AI. Mechanism of facet load transmission as a hypothesis for low back pain. *Spine* 1984;9(6):557–565.
42. Zaki W. Aspects morphologiques et fonctionnels de l'annulus fibrosus du disque intervertébral de la colonne dorsale. *Arch Anat Pathol (Paris)* 1973;21(4):401–403.

Epidemiology of Traumatic Spinal Column and Cord Injuries

Milka Donchin

Traumatic spinal cord injury (SCI) has been described as the most catastrophic of disabling conditions. Due to the magnitude of the morbidity and mortality of traumatic SCIs and the high cost associated with these injuries, in 1987 a surveillance system was suggested in the United States by the Council of State and Territorial Epidemiologists (CSTE) (19). The purpose of this surveillance is to better define the national incidence of acute traumatic SCI, identify high-risk groups in order to target prevention strategies, determine etiologies, and evaluate services. Currently, 15 states have established SCI registries at the state level, and 12 of these have mandatory reporting (13). The Centers for Disease Control (CDC) have developed the following definition of SCI as a guideline for use in surveillance at the state level: "person who suffers an acute, traumatic lesion of neural elements in the spinal canal, resulting in any degree of sensory deficit, motor deficit, or bladder/bowel dysfunction."

The first epidemiological study on traumatic SCI was published in 1975 by Kraus et al. (15). The average annual incidence rate, for the years 1970 to 1971, was found to be 53.4 per 1 million population in 18 California counties. California used a definition similar to that of the CDC for case identification. The mortality rate was found to be 25.8 per million population, and the case fatality rate was 48.3% (number of deaths/number of cases). Seventy-nine percent of the deaths occurred prior to hospitalization (15). Survival is estimated to be only 72% in the first minute, 64% in the first hour, and 58% in the first week (9).

Using the same definitions, similar rates of traumatic SCI incidence, mortality, and case fatality were described for Olmsted County, Minnesota (8). For the 47-year period from 1935 to 1981, the average annual sex and age adjusted incidence rate was found to be 54.8 per million. The adjusted rate increased steadily during these years, especially for men, from an average of 22.2 in the time period from 1935 to 1944 to 70.8 per million person-years for the years 1975 to 1981 (Fig. 1).

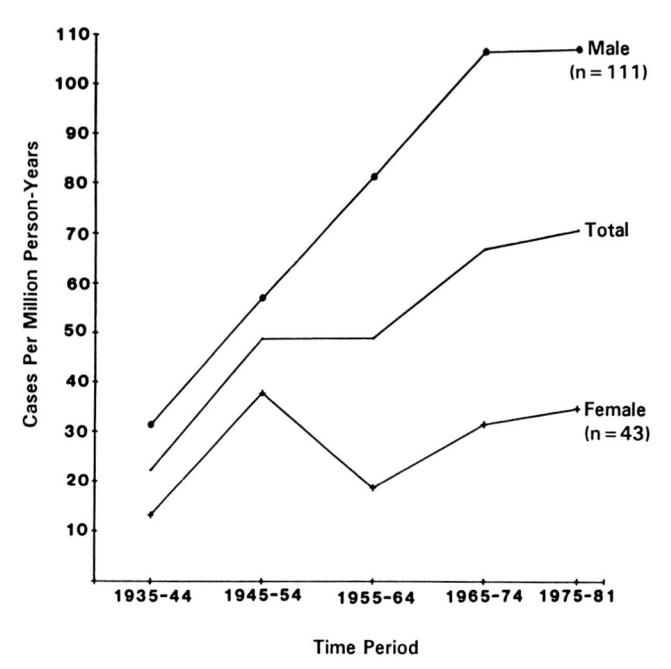

FIG. 1. Average annual age-adjusted incidence rates per million person-years for spinal cord injury, by decade and sex, Olmsted County, Minnesota, 1935 to 1981. (From ref. 8.)

M. Donchin: Department of Social Medicine, Hebrew University Hadassah School of Public Health and Community Medicine, Jerusalem 91120, Israel.

An estimated average annual rate of 40.1 per million noninstitutionalized population, based on the National Center for Health Statistics Hospital Discharge Survey (5), was consistent with the hospitalization rate in Olmsted county for the same period (8).

Prevalence rate of SCI in the United States in 1980 is estimated to be between 583 per million population (Olmsted county) (9) and 906 per million (based on National Model Spinal Cord Injury Data Base) (6). Prevalence rate in the United States in 1988 is estimated to be 721 per million (14), that is, in 1988 there were 176,965 persons. Despite the severity of the injury and associated complications, only 2.6% of all traumatic SCI patients are institutionalized (14).

VERTEBRAL COLUMN INJURIES

No similar data are available on the incidence of vertebral fractures. Only one epidemiological study, referring to the neurological damage associated with fracture, has been published (22). That study, which is part of the 18 California counties, is limited to admissions to four major hospitals in Sacramento County. The incidence of vertebral injuries could not be determined, but the estimated annual rate of occurrence of vertebral column injury resulting in hospitalization was 233 per million population.

Based on the results of a study carried out in emergency rooms in three counties in Israel (1), an estimate of the incidence in the population can be suggested. All motor vehicle injuries admitted to five emergency rooms in three consecutive months were recorded. Of a total of 2555 admissions, 21 were cases of spinal column fractures. Only two-thirds of the cases (14 injuries) were hospitalized. Assuming that indications for hospitalization are similar in Israel and the United States, an estimate of the annual incidence of spinal column fracture is 350 per million population.

Overall, the probability of neurologic damage associated with an injury to the vertebra was 14% (22). Fractures of the vertebrae were divided into two major categories (22): fractures of the vertebral bodies and fractures of the posterior elements. A dislocation was defined as any malalignment of the vertebral column greater than 2 mm. Patients who sustained only a vertebral body fracture had a 3% incidence of neurologic deficit, while patients with fractures of both body and posterior elements with some degree of dislocation had a 61% incidence of neurologic damage (22).

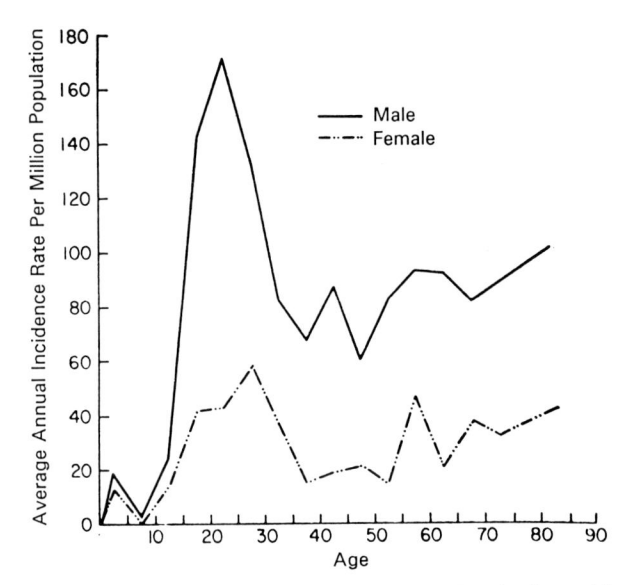

FIG. 2. Average annual incidence rate of spinal cord injury per million population: 18 California counties, 1970 to 1971. (From ref. 15.)

In a series of pediatric cases of vertebral and spinal cord injuries (11), 50% of the cases with vertebral injury had neurologic deficit. The majority of injuries in the 0- to 9-year-old group (72%) involved the cervical spine. Cervical spine fractures were more commonly associated with SCI (22). The incidence of neurologic damage with cervical spine fracture was 39%, with the highest rate of spinal cord deficit, 70%, in patients with cervical fracture–dislocation. Similar findings referring to cervical spine injuries are described in case series studies (4,10,21) of hospitalized patients with cervical spine injuries.

Fractures of the vertebral bodies are the most common spine injuries in the thoracic area. The incidence of spinal cord damage with injuries to the thoracic vertebrae was about 10% (22). In a case study in Pittsburgh (12), all patients admitted with thoracic spine injuries during the years 1973 to 1983 were included. Twelve

TABLE 1. Male to female ratio of traumatic SCI incidence in selected studies

Study	Place	Period	N	Male/female ratio
Kraus et al. (15)	California	1970–1971	619	2.9
Watson (25)	England	1961–1981	1080	4.4
Bracken et al. (5)	United States	1970–1977	430	2.4
Kuhn et al. (16)	Switzerland	1979–1981	330	2.6
Griffin et al. (8)	Minnesota	1935–1981	154	2.6
Fine et al. (7)	Alabama	1973–?	359	4.3
Biering-Sorensen et al. (3)	Denmark	1975–1984	268	3.3

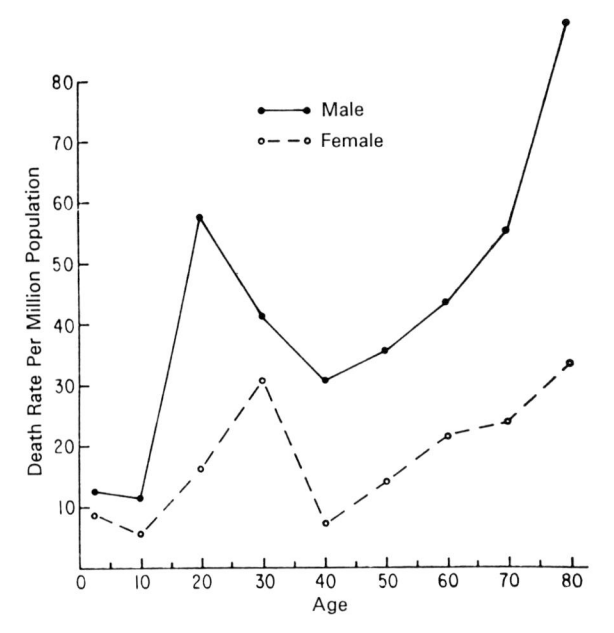

FIG. 3. Average annual spinal cord injury death rates per million population: 18 northern California counties, 1970 to 1971. (From ref. 15.)

TABLE 2. *Distribution of patients with vertebral injury, with and without neurological deficit, by external cause of injury and cause specific rate of neurological deficit*

External cause of injury	With deficit N	With deficit %	Without deficit N	Without deficit %	Cause specific deficit rate/100
Motor vehicle	20	41	136	49	13
Falls	6	12	121	44	5
Firearm	8	16	—	—	100
Recreation	13	27	17	6	43
Other	2	4	3	1	8
All causes	49	100	277	100	14

Based on ref. 22. Study took place in four major Sacramento County, California, hospitals in 1970 to 1971.

percent of cases with compression injuries had neurologic injury, compared to 90% of those with fracture/dislocation (12). Fractures in the lumbar spine are associated with neurologic deficit in only 3% of the cases (22).

The incidence rate of traumatic SCI is significantly higher for men than for women. The male to female rate ratio was found to be 2.9 in the Kraus et al. (15) epidemiological study, and 2.4 in the national study on hospital discharges (5). An excess rate for men was also described in the case series studies carried out in the United States and Europe (Table 1). Higher male to female ratios were reported also in earlier case studies reviewed by Kurtzke (17).

The peak age of incidence (Fig. 2) for men is 15 to 24 years (3,5,8,15). As for death rates (Fig. 3), the first peak is at 15 to 24 years, followed by a sharp decline, with generally increasing rates over the age of 40 (15). The average age at time of injury for men was 34.4 years; for women, it was 36.2 years (15), with the peak incidence for women about 5 years later than for men. The death rate for women was lower than for men, but the pattern was similar. For men, a similar age distribution for spinal column injuries without neurologic deficit was described when compared to SCI patients (22). For female patients without neurologic deficit, 33.6% were age 65 or older (Fig. 4).

Seasonality

A higher incidence of traumatic SCI is noticed during the summer months, with a peak number of cases in May (5) or July (7,8).

Causes of Injury

Motor vehicle accidents are the largest single cause of spine injuries (Table 2) with or without neurologic

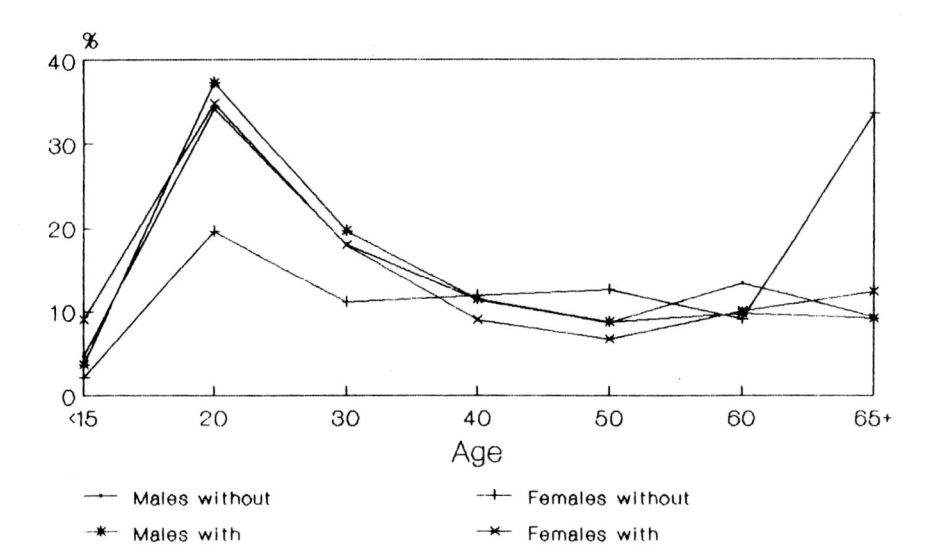

FIG. 4. Distribution (%) of cases with vertebral injury with and without neurological deficit. (Based on ref. 22.)

TABLE 3. *Distribution of the injuries by the most pronounced mechanism of the trauma and the primary area of the lesion*

Mechanism of trauma	Bony level of lesion			
	Cervical	Thoracic	Lumbar	Total
Flexion	62	22	18	102
Flexion/rotation	7	20	5	32
Extension	43	3	0	46
Compression	13	16	20	49
Direct blow	0	9	9	18
Uncertain	11	6	4	21
Total	136	76	56	268

From ref. 3.

damage (22). The studies describe the similar cause distribution for vertebral (10,21) and cord injuries (3,7,8,15,16). The proportion of vertebral fractures among hospitalizations for motor vehicle accidents was only 4.4% (1).

Among children under the age of 15 years (18,23), and more specifically under the age of 10 (11), the predominant cause of injury is falls. Similarly, falls are the main cause of thoracic or lumbar fractures in patients aged 50 and older (2). Based on radiologic patterns, a presumed mechanism of trauma at each vertebral level (Table 3) was suggested by Biering-Sorensen et al. (3).

Sport and Recreation Injuries

Among sports injuries, diving is the main cause of SCI in the adult population (3,8,15) as well as in children and adolescents (18). Several studies were conducted in specific groups, and they give an estimate of the incidence of this injury.

In 1976, the incidence of American football-related spinal cord injuries (20) in the United States was estimated to be 2.2 per 100,000 participants. Following an intervention program that adopted rules for proper use of the helmet, the incidence of SCI decreased to 0.4 per 100,000. In Wales (26), the incidence of cervical column injury among rugby players is estimated to be 30 per 30,000 players during a 20-year period. Sixty percent of these injuries were SCI cases.

In a series of 42 cases of hockey-related spinal injuries in Canada (24), all but three were in the cervical spine region. The most frequently injured levels were C5 or C6.

Flying ultralight aircraft is gaining popularity. On average, 60 deaths per year occur in the United States due to ultralight crashes. A case report describes three cases of thoracolumbar spine fractures associated with ultralight aircraft (27).

Functional Impairment

The most frequent form of impairment among patients hospitalized with SCI was quadriparesis. The rate was 9.5 per million population (15). The incidence rates for paraplegia, other forms of paralysis, paraparesis, quadriplegia, and other deficits were 7.7, 6.5, 4.7, 3.2, and 1.6 per million, respectively (15).

The type of functional impairment was related to the cause of spinal cord injury. Quadriplegia resulted mainly from motor vehicle accidents, while the risk for quadriparesis is highest for those injured in recreation-related activity, mostly diving injuries (15). In Olmsted county (8), the in-hospital case fatality ratios were 16.3% for quadriplegia–quadriparesis patients and 4.9% for paraplegia–paraparesis.

REFERENCES

1. Avitzour M. Road accidents injuries—circumstances, evacuation and outcomes. Report to the Ministry of Transport, Israel, 1992 [in Hebrew].
2. Bengner U, Johnell O, Redlund-Johnell I. Changes in incidence of vertebral fractures during 30 years. *Calcif Tissue Int* 1988;42:293–296.
3. Biering-Sorensen F, Pedersen V, Clausen S. Epidemiology of spinal cord lesions in Denmark. *Paraplegia* 1990;28:105–118.
4. Bohlman HH. Acute fractures and dislocations of the cervical spine. An analysis of three hundred hospitalized patients and review of the literature. *J Bone Joint Surg* 1979;61A:1119–1141.
5. Bracken MB, Freeman DH, Hellenbrand K. Incidence of acute traumatic hospitalized spinal cord injury in the United States, 1970–1977. *Am J Epidemiol* 1981;113:615–622.
6. DeVivo MJ, Fine PR, Maetz HM, Stover SL. Prevalence of spinal cord injury. A reestimation employing life table techniques. *Arch Neurol* 1980;37:707–708.
7. Fine PR, Kuhlemeier KV, DeVivo MJ, Stover SL. Spinal cord injury: an epidemiologic perspective. *Paraplegia* 1979–80;17:237–250.
8. Griffin MR, Opitz JL, Kurland LT, Ebersold MJ, O'Fallon WM. Traumatic spinal cord injury in Olmsted county, Minnesota, 1935–1981. *Am J Epidemiol* 1985;121:884–895.
9. Griffin MR, O'Fallon WM, Opitz JL, Kurland LT. Mortality, survival and prevalence: traumatic spinal cord injury in Olmsted county, Minnesota, 1935–1981. *J Chron Dis* 1985;38:643–653.
10. Guthkelch AN, Fleischer AS. Patterns of cervical spine injury and their associated lesions. *West J Med* 1987;147:428–431.
11. Hadley MN, Zabramski JM, Browner CM, Rekate H, Sonntag KH. Pediatric spinal trauma. Review of 122 cases of spinal cord and vertebral column injuries. *J Neurosurg* 1988;68:18–24.
12. Hanley EN, Eskay ML. Thoracic spine fractures. *Orthopedics* 1989;12:689–696.
13. Harrison CL, Dijkers M. Spinal cord injury surveillance in the United States: an overview. *Paraplegia* 1990;29:233–246.
14. Harvey C, Rothschild BB, Asmann AJ, Stripling T. New estimates of traumatic SCI prevalence: a survey-based approach. *Paraplegia* 1990;28:537–544.
15. Kraus JF, Franti CE, Riggins RS, Richards D, Borhani NO. Incidence of traumatic spinal cord lesions. *J Chron Dis* 1975;28:471–492.
16. Kuhn W, Zach GA, Kochlin P, Urwyler A. Comparison of spinal cord injuries in females and in males, 1979–1981 Basle. *Paraplegia* 1983;21:154–160.
17. Kurtzke JF. Epidemiology of spinal cord injury. *Exp Neurol* 1975;48:163–236.

18. McPhee IB. Spinal fractures and dislocations in children and adolescents. *Spine* 1981;6:533–537.
19. MMWR. Acute traumatic spinal cord injury surveillance—United States, 1987. *JAMA* 1988;259:3108.
20. MMWR. Football-related spinal cord injuries among high school players—Louisiana, 1989. *JAMA* 1989;264:1520.
21. Reiss SJ, Raque GH, Shields CB, Garretson HD. Cervical spine fractures with major associated trauma. *Neurosurgery* 1986;18:327–330.
22. Riggins RS, Kraus JF. The risk of neurologic damage with fractures of the vertebrae. *J Trauma* 1977;17:126–133.
23. Ruge JR, Sinson GP, McLone DG, Cerullo LJ. Pediatric spinal injury: the very young. *J Neurosurg* 1988;68:25–30.
24. Tator CH, Edmonds VE. National survey of spinal injuries in hockey players. *Can Med Assoc J* 1984;130:875–880.
25. Watson N. Spinal cord injury in the female. *Paraplegia* 1983;21:143–148.
26. Williams P, McKibbin B. Unstable cervical spine injuries in rugby—a 20 year review. *Injury* 1987;18:329–332.
27. Zwimpfer TJ, Gertzbein SG. Ultralight aircraft crashes: their increasing incidence and associated fractures of the thoracolumbar spine. *J Trauma* 1987;27:431–436.

Descriptive Epidemiology of Traumatic Spinal Cord Injury in New York State

John H. Relethford

Traumatic spinal cord injury is one of the most serious medical conditions, leading to loss of motor and sensory function. Given the role of the spinal cord in the nervous system, any trauma (or for that matter disease) can lead to serious disability (13). To date, there have been surprisingly few comprehensive studies of the epidemiology of traumatic spinal cord injury. The major studies have been a population-based study in northern California (5) and a nationwide survey based on data from selected centers treating spinal cord injured patients (13).

The purpose of this chapter is to present some basic epidemiologic findings on the incidence and distribution of traumatic spinal cord injury among New York State residents based on hospital discharge data. This study has the advantage of being population-based. Since the data used here were obtained from a statewide hospital discharge reporting system, case definition and selection are not as precise as that obtained in other studies from detailed examination of medical records from hospitals (5). However, use of a preexisting data source is more cost-effective. A secondary purpose of this chapter is to compare the results from New York State with other studies in order to determine the utility of hospital discharge data for surveillance of traumatic spinal cord injury.

MATERIALS AND METHODS

Data on traumatic spinal cord injuries were obtained from SPARCS (Statewide Planning and Research Cooperative System), a statewide collection system for hospital discharge data administered by the New York State Department of Health. All discharges from acute care hospitals within New York State are required to submit reports to SPARCS. Inclusion in SPARCS is limited to those patients that are actually admitted into an acute care facility. Those treated and then released from an emergency room would not be counted. The exclusion of emergency room discharges is not a serious problem when considering traumatic spinal cord injury; the severe nature of traumatic spinal cord injury dictates admission in most cases. Injured persons that die prior to admission, however, would not be included in the SPARCS data. In any case, all incidence rates described in this chapter are best thought of as estimates of the incidence of traumatic spinal cord hospitalizations.

Traumatic spinal cord injury cases were selected using the diagnosis codes provided on discharge abstracts. The SPARCS data contain a principal diagnosis code (that condition most representative of the reason for admission) and up to four additional diagnosis codes indicating other conditions that relate to the current hospital stay. All diagnosis codes use *The International Classification of Diseases, 9th Revision, Clinical Modification* (ICD-9-CM) (7).

Cases were selected where the principal diagnosis indicated traumatic spinal cord injury, or where a secondary diagnosis indicated traumatic spinal cord injury and the primary diagnosis indicated some other form of traumatic injury. The last restriction helps exclude cases where a previous spinal cord injury contributes to a noninjury event (e.g., a patient with previous spinal cord injury being admitted for pressure sores). The inclusion of cases with any traumatic injury as a principal diagnosis also helps include cases with multi-

---

J. H. Relethford: Department of Anthropology, State University of New York College at Oneonta, Oneonta, NY 13820-4015.

ple trauma (e.g., a primary diagnosis of head injury and a secondary diagnosis of spinal cord injury). In terms of the ICD-9-CM codes, traumatic spinal cord injury was defined using the codes 806 (fracture of vertebral column with spinal cord injury) and 952 (spinal cord injury without evidence of spinal bone injury). Traumatic injury was defined using standard codes (6): 800 to 959, excluding late effects (905–909), foreign bodies (930–939), and early complications (958).

Case selection was further limited to new admissions. Transfers were not included since a single injured person would be counted two or more times. Only patients that were residents of New York State were included. In order to maximize sample size a 5-year period was used defined by year of discharge (1984–1988). Pooling these years does not bias results since previous analysis has shown little trend in spinal cord injury incidence in New York State over time (11).

Data were obtained for each case for sex, ethnicity, and age at discharge. In addition to a statewide estimate, incidence rates were also computed for men and women and for whites and blacks (data on population size are not available for other ethnic groups). Annual incidence rates were derived using pooled population size estimates obtained from the Bureau of Biometrics, New York State Department of Health. In order to compare incidence rates across groups (e.g., men versus women), a measure of relative risk was computed as the ratio of age-adjusted incidence rates. Age-adjustment was performed using the direct method of adjustment (12) based on 18 age groups (0–4, 5–9, 10–14, . . . , 80–84, 85+) and using the 1980 New York State census as the reference population. The 95% confidence intervals for relative risk were obtained using the Ederer–Mantel method (2).

RESULTS

There were 3793 discharges from New York State hospitals for New York State residents with a traumatic spinal cord injury. The annual incidence rate is 4.3 per 100,000 residents, falling within the range of 2.8 to 5.3 per 100,000 observed in studies within the United States to date (4), but above the United States average of 3.1 per 100,000 (13). The age-adjusted rate is 4.2 per 100,000 (this age-adjustment was performed using the 1980 U.S. Census to allow comparability in future studies in other states).

Spinal cord injury cases are often classified as quadriplegia (the injury occurred at the cervical vertebrae) or paraplegia (occurring at the thoracic, lumbar, or sacral vertebrae). Here, a total of 1793 patients (47.3%) are classified as quadriplegic, 1785 patients (47.1%) are classified as paraplegic, and 215 (5.7%) had an unspecified location of injury. These percentages are very similar to those found in other studies; for example, Fine et al. (3) report 47.5% quadriplegic and 52.5% paraplegic in the southeastern United States.

Traumatic spinal cord injury can also be classified according to the degree of neurologic injury. Such information is useful in assessing severity and disability. Here, 300 cases (7.9%) had a complete lesion (the most severe), 697 (18.4%) had an incomplete lesion, and 2796 (73.7%) did not have sufficient information contained in the ICD-9-CM codes to assess severity. Surveillance by severity class is therefore not possible.

Of the total sample, 323 (8.5%) died while in the hospital, 55 (1.5%) left against medical advice, 845 (22.3%) were transferred to another institution (acute or long-term care), and 2570 (67.8%) were discharged home.

Of the total sample, 2601 (68.6%) are men and 1192 (31.4%) are women. A total of 2571 patients (67.8%) are white, 743 (19.6%) are black, 461 (12.1%) belong to other ethnic groups, and 18 (0.5%) are of unknown ethnicity. Annual incidence rates (crude and age-adjusted) are reported in Table 1 by sex and ethnicity. In general, age-adjustment has little effect on incidence rate. As found in other studies, the male rate is greater than the female rate (3–5), and this difference is found both within whites and blacks. For both sexes, higher age-adjusted rates are found among blacks than among whites. This ethnic difference has been seen in some, but not all, of the few studies of traumatic spinal cord injury that focus on ethnic variation (4).

Relative risks by sex and ethnicity are reported in Table 2. There is a significant sex difference ($p < 0.05$) with men being 2.6 times more likely to have a traumatic spinal cord injury resulting in hospitalization than women. The relative risk falls close to the range reported by others studies (4) in the United States (2.8–4.3). The ethnic difference is also statistically sig-

TABLE 1. Incidence rates by sex and ethnicity

Group	Number of cases 1984–1988	Annual crude incidence rate per 100,000 residents	Annual age-adjusted incidence rate per 100,000 residents[a]
Men	2601	6.2	6.3
Women	1192	2.6	2.4
Blacks	743	5.3	5.5
Whites	2571	3.6	3.5
Black men	577	9.1	9.7
White men	1659	4.8	4.9
Black women	166	2.2	2.3
White women	912	2.4	2.2

[a] Age-adjusted to the 1980 New York State population using the direct method.

TABLE 2. *Relative risk by sex and ethnicity*

Groups compared	Relative risk	95% Confidence interval
Men/women	2.63	2.45–2.82
Black/white	1.57	1.45–1.70
White men/white women	2.23	2.06–2.42
Black men/black women	4.22	3.54–5.03
Black men/white men	1.98	1.80–2.18
Black women/white women	1.05	0.89–1.24

nificant ($p < 0.05$), with blacks being almost 1.6 times more likely to have a traumatic spinal cord injury than whites. This figure is similar to the relative risk of 1.4 found in the northern Californian study (5).

As shown in Table 2, further breakdown reveals some interesting results. The sex difference is significant within both whites and blacks but is much higher (relative risk = 4.2) among blacks. The ethnic difference is clear among men (relative risk = 2.0) but is not significant among women. Overall, black men have the highest incidence rates, followed by white men, followed by women of both ethnic groups.

Age-specific incidence rates are shown for men and women in Fig. 1 using 18 five-year age groups. For both sexes, the incidence rate increases sharply after the middle teens, reaching a peak between 20 and 25 years of age. For this age group, the male rate is 4.1 times that of the female rate. After the middle 20s, the male rate declines sharply and the female rate diminishes more slowly. Both sexes show a rapid increase after age 65, resulting in the highest rates among the most elderly (85+).

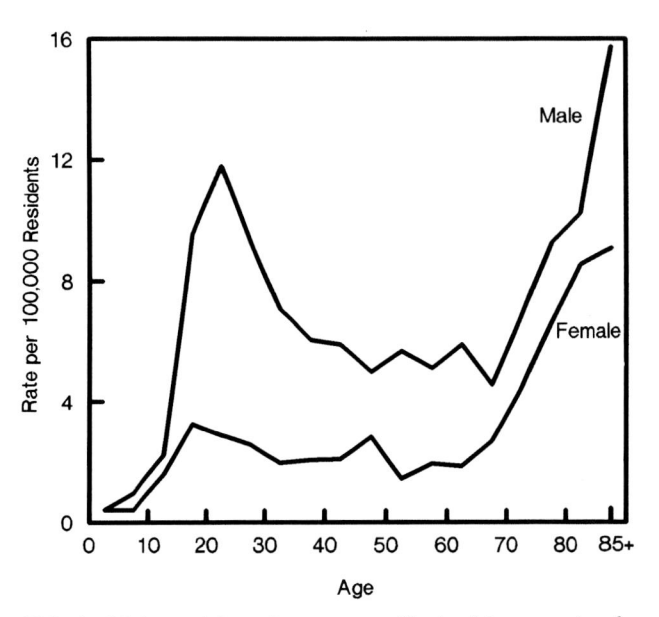

FIG. 1. Male and female age-specific incidence rates for traumatic spinal cord injury discharges among New York State residents.

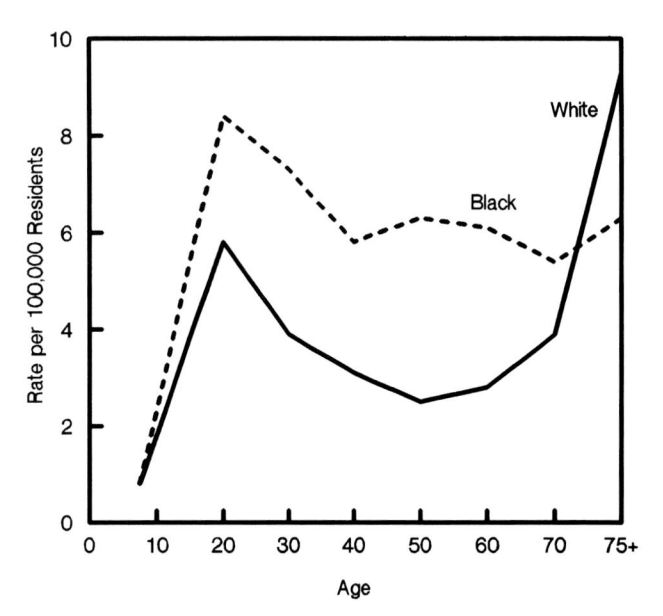

FIG. 2. Black and white age-specific incidence rates for traumatic spinal cord injury discharges among New York State residents.

Age-specific incidence rates for blacks and whites are shown in Fig. 2. Due to the small number of blacks at some age groups, eight age groups are used: 0–14, 15–24, 25–34, 35–44, 45–54, 55–64, 65–74, and 75+ years of age. Both blacks and whites show the rapid increase in the middle teens and a rapid decline afterward. Among the elderly, however, only whites show a rapid increase in incidence with age, such that the usual pattern of higher black rates is reversed after age 70.

DISCUSSION

The observed patterns of variation in incidence by sex, ethnicity, and age are in close agreement with results from other studies of traumatic spinal cord injury, showing that hospital discharge records provide a reasonable source of data for surveillance and descriptive epidemiology.

Judging from the literature to date, differences in incidence among groups most likely reflect differences in the specific cause of spinal cord injury. While few studies have detailed data on cause, a recent review shows agreement among these studies in the leading causes of spinal cord injury: motor vehicle incidents, falls, violence (especially firearm related), and sports and recreational injuries (especially those resulting from football and diving) (4).

Higher rates of traumatic spinal cord injury among men is not surprising, since men have higher rates than women for most types of injuries, especially in the late teens and early 20s (8). The large sex difference shown in Fig. 1 between ages 15 and 35 probably reflects higher injuries from motor vehicles, violence, and sports. Previous analysis of injury mortality in New York State has shown that sex differences are most pronounced at this age group for a variety of different injuries (10); possible common factors could be greater alcohol and drug use and increased risk-taking behavior among men.

The increase in incidence among the elderly in both sexes (Fig. 1) most likely reflects injuries due to falls and motor vehicle incidents. Nationwide estimates (13) show that falls are the leading cause, and motor vehicle incidents the second leading cause, of traumatic spinal cord injury after age 45. Possible contributing factors include a decrease in sensory ability and reaction times, reduction of bone mass, and overall increased fragility (14).

Black–white differences most likely also reflect variation in rates of specific cause of injury. Both nationwide estimates (13) and the northern Californian study (5) found that whites had higher proportions of spinal cord injuries due to motor vehicle incidents and sports injuries, whereas blacks had a higher proportion due to violence. The higher overall incidence of traumatic spinal cord injury among blacks may be due to overall higher rates of violence-related injuries. As shown in Table 2, this difference is apparent only among men; there is no significant difference in incidence rates between black and white women. This hypothesis is supported by a recent study of homicide in the United States (1), which found that black men had the highest death rates of any sex and ethnicity group, particularly in the late teens and early adulthood. As shown in Fig. 2, it is this age group (early 20s) where the black–white difference in spinal cord injury incidence is greatest.

The reversal of black–white rates among the elderly (Fig. 2) may reflect a greater proportion of elderly white drivers and occupants. Another possibility is that the average higher bone density among blacks (9) reduces the probability of falling, or at least the probability of spinal cord injury among those that do fall.

The variation in traumatic spinal cord injury rates by sex, age, and ethnicity is easy to document but harder to explain. Some of the suggestions made here relate to variation in specific causes of injury. In any case, these interpretations should be taken as suggestive and not conclusive. The data used in this chapter do not include cause of injury, and therefore any suggestions regarding specific cause have to be made based on inference from previous studies. While these inferences are useful for a preliminary survey, it is clear that more detailed data on cause of injury are needed specifically for New York State. Starting in 1990, all injury discharges in New York State must include the ICD-9 external cause of injury code (E-Code). When complete, these data will improve greatly the statewide surveillance and epidemiology of traumatic spinal cord injury.

ACKNOWLEDGMENT

The research described in this chapter was performed while the author was a research scientist in the Injury Control and Disability Prevention Programs, New York State Department of Health.

REFERENCES

1. Centers for Disease Control. Homicide among young black males—United States, 1978–1987. *MMWR* 1990;39(48): 869–873.
2. Ederer F, Mantel N. Confidence limits on the ratio of two Poisson variables. *Am J Epidemiol* 1974;100:165–167.
3. Fine PR, Kuhlemeier KV, DeVivo MJ, et al. Spinal cord injury: an epidemiologic perspective. *Paraplegia* 1979;17:237–250.
4. Kraus JF. Epidemiological aspects of acute spinal cord injury: a review of incidence, prevalence, causes, and outcome. In: Becker DP, Povlishock JT, eds. *Central nervous system trauma status report*. Prepared for the National Institute of Neurological and Communicative Disorders and Stroke, National Institutes of Health, 1985;313–322.
5. Kraus JF, Franti CE, Riggins RS, et al. Incidence of traumatic spinal cord lesions. *J Chron Dis* 1975;28:471–492.
6. Marganitt B, MacKenzie EJ, Smith GS, et al. Coding external causes of injury (E-Codes) in Maryland hospital discharges 1979–1988: a statewide study to explore the uncoded population. *Am J Public Health* 1990;10:1463–1466.
7. National Center for Health Statistics. *The international classification of diseases, 9th revision, clinical modification*. Ann Arbor, MI: Commission on Professional and Hospital Activities, 1986.
8. National Committee for Injury Prevention and Control. *Injury Prevention: meeting the challenge*. New York: Oxford University Press, 1989.
9. Overfield T. *Biologic variation in health and illness: race, age, and sex differences*. Menlo Park, CA: Addison-Wesley, 1985.
10. Relethford JH. Sex differentials in unintentional injury mortality in age at death. *Am J Hum Biol* 1991;3:369–375.
11. Relethford JH, Standfast SJ, DL Morse. Trends in traumatic spinal cord injury in New York, 1982–1988. *MMWR* 1991;40(31): 535.
12. Shyrock HS, Siegel JS. *The methods and materials of demography*, condensed edition. New York: Academic Press, 1976.
13. Stover SL, Fine PR, eds. *Spinal cord injury: the facts and figures*. Birmingham: The University of Alabama at Birmingham, 1986.
14. Waller JA. *Injury control: a guide to the causes and prevention of trauma*. Lexington, MA: Heath, 1985.

7

Imaging of Thoracic and Lumbar Vertebral Fractures

Richard H. Daffner

The surgeon whose patient has a suspected injury to the thoracic or lumbar vertebral column is the benefactor of new imaging technology and the improvement of existing technology (24). Until the mid-1970s, the primary diagnostic radiographic procedures available for evaluation of these patients were plain film radiography, tomography, and pantopaque myelography. One of the first applications of computerized tomography (CT), developed at that time, was the evaluation of patients with vertebral injuries. For the first time, radiologists were able to demonstrate displacement of bone fragments into the vertebral canal. In addition, it became possible to recognize recurrent patterns of fracture, thus affording us a better opportunity to study the biomechanics of injury as well as to formulate the appropriate treatment.

In the late 1970s, it became possible to perform myelography using a water-soluble contrast medium. This added a new dimension of safety in the performance of myelography, since contrast no longer had to be removed from the subarachnoid space. Further refinements in contrast regarding toxicity and osmolarity occurred in the early 1980s.

The most recent technologic innovation in the imaging field is magnetic resonance imaging (MRI). This new tool does not rely on ionizing radiation and makes it possible to see, for the first time, the spinal cord. As equipment improved, it became possible not only to demonstrate the cord, but to identify specific areas of injury, such as hemorrhage, contusion, or syringomyelia, within the cord.

Thus the surgeon has a highly sophisticated armamentarium of diagnostic studies that may be performed on patients with suspected vertebral injuries. This chapter discusses the practical applications of each of these imaging techniques, and the salient imaging findings are discussed in detail. It is my hope that this chapter will provide the reader with a better understanding of the complex field of diagnostic vertebral traumatology.

CONVENTIONAL RADIOGRAPHY

Conventional (plain film) radiography is literally the "backbone" for the diagnosis of all vertebral injuries (13,20). These studies are easy to perform, provide sufficient diagnostic information, and allow us to turn our attention to specific areas of abnormality for which more sophisticated imaging studies need to be performed.

Technical Considerations

Radiography of the thoracic and lumbar vertebral columns may be accomplished with the patient in the supine position. In our institution, an anteroposterior (AP) view of the thoracic column is obtained immedi-

---

R. H. Daffner: Department of Diagnostic Radiology, The Medical College of Pennsylvania, Allegheny Campus, and Allegheny General Hospital, Pittsburgh, PA 15212-9986.

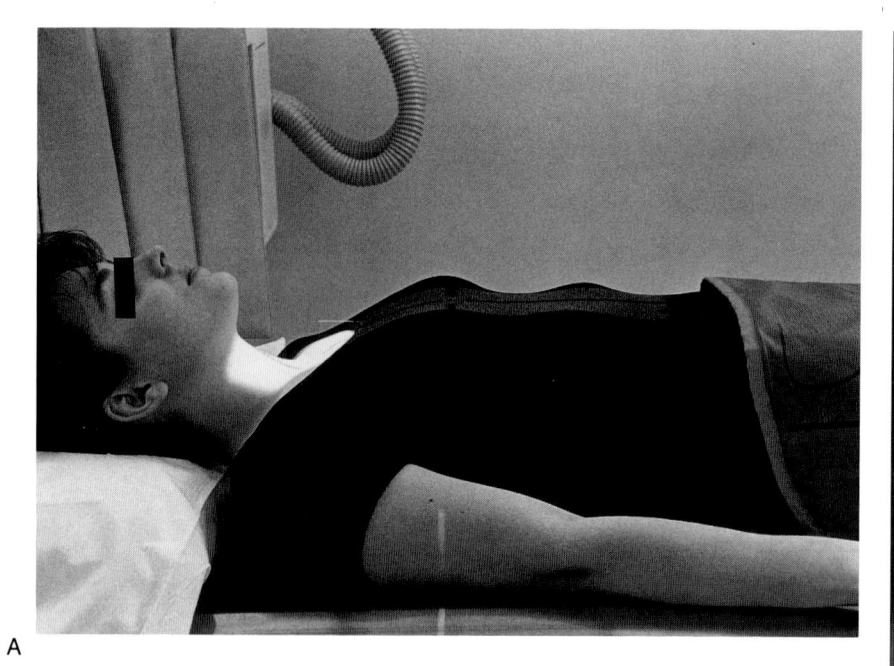

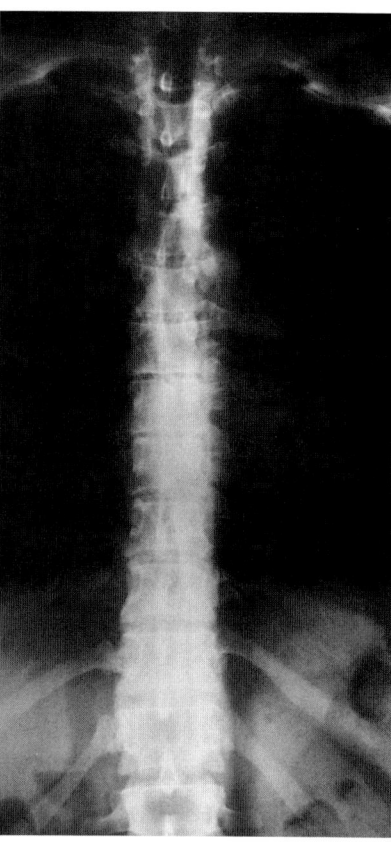

FIG. 1. Normal thoracic column, frontal view. **A:** Positioning technique. **B:** Radiographic appearance. There is normal alignment of the vertebral body margins, pedicles, and spinous processes. The interspinous spaces and interpediculate distances are uniform. The paravertebral soft tissues are normal. (From ref. 13.)

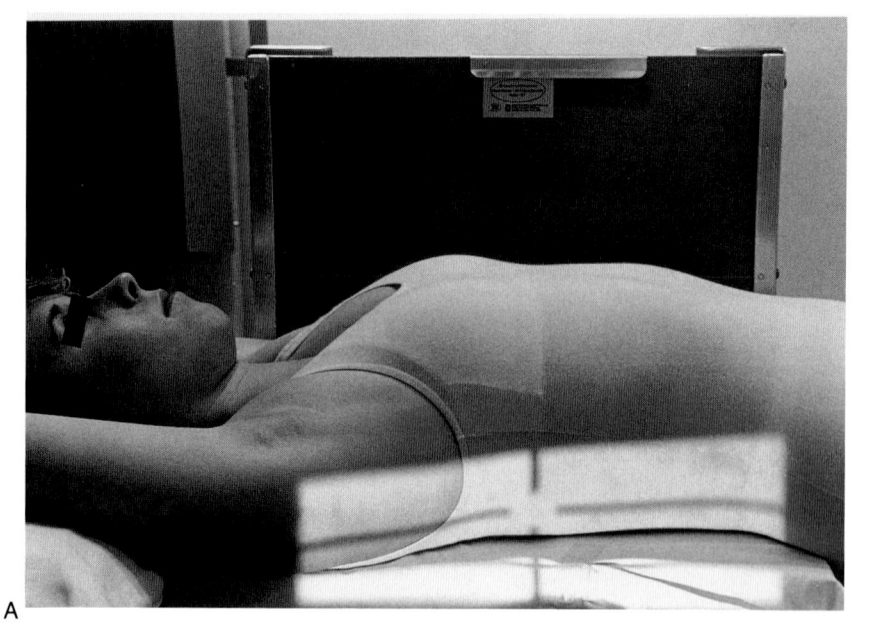

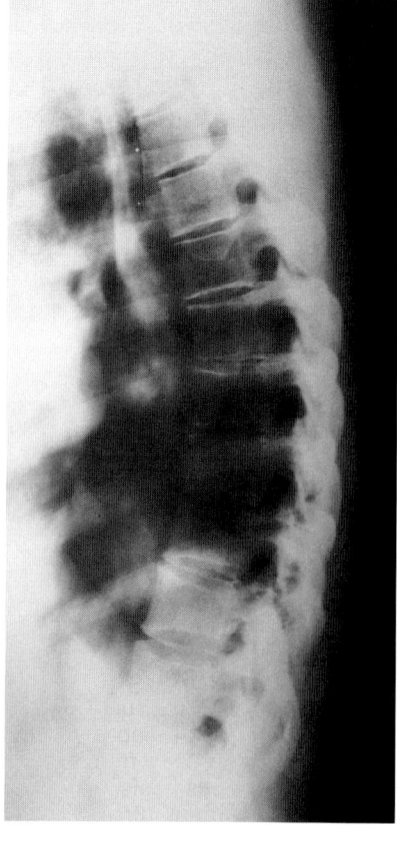

FIG. 2. Normal thoracic column, lateral view. **A:** Positioning technique, horizontal beam. **B:** Radiographic appearance. There is normal alignment with a gentle kyphosis. The disc margins are uniform. (From ref. 13.)

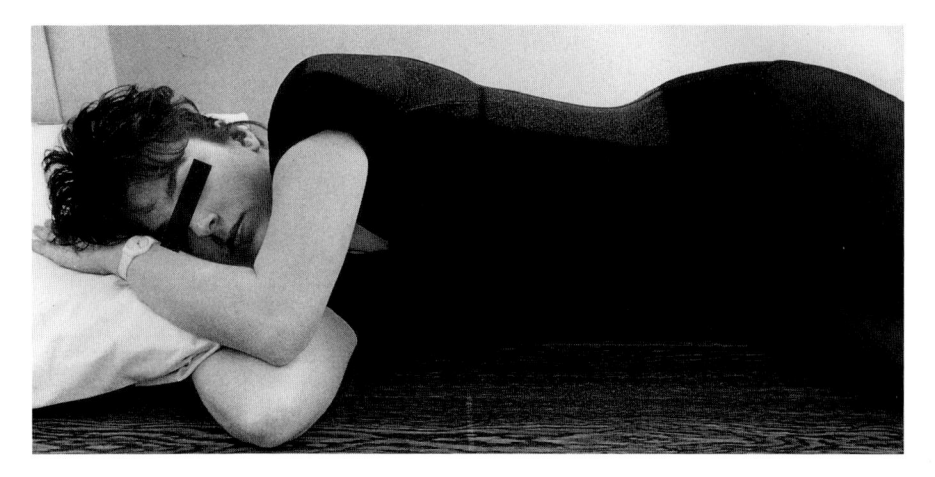

FIG. 3. Lateral thoracic radiography, vertical beam technique. (From ref. 13.)

ately after the chest radiograph (Fig. 1). Then a horizontal beam lateral radiograph is obtained (Fig. 2). Because of the shoulders and arms, demonstration of the upper thoracic region is often poor. For this reason, a modified swimmer's view may be necessary as well. An alternate method used to obtain the lateral radiograph of the thoracic column is to use a vertical beam technique, which may be obtained by carefully "log-rolling" the patient into the lateral position (13) (Fig. 3).

There is one important pitfall in radiography of the thoracic vertebrae: the upper thoracic column is frequently not demonstrated adequately on lateral films. We have found a high incidence of injury to this region in motorcyclists who are thrown from their vehicles. In these instances, it may be necessary to obtain lateral tomograms or CT scans through this region. MRI also has proved extremely useful for evaluating the cervicothoracic junction and upper thoracic column (22) (Fig. 4).

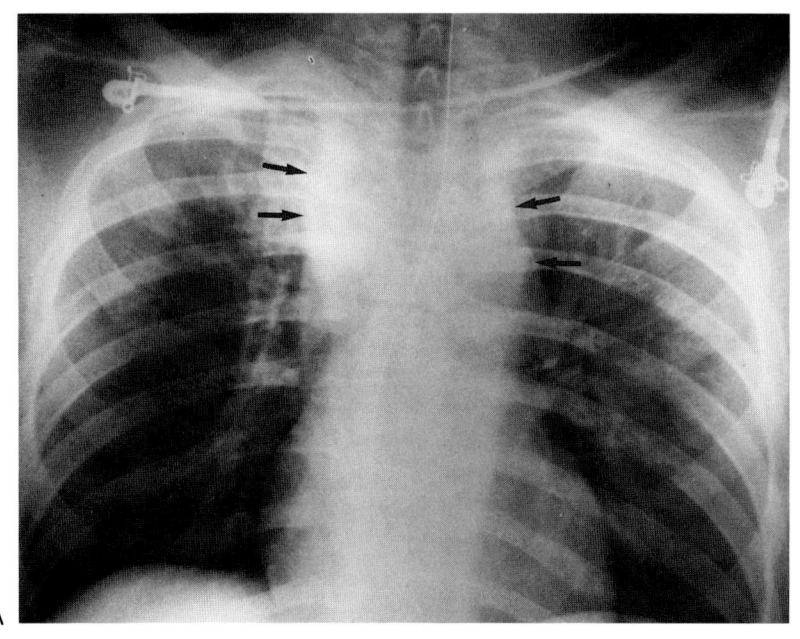

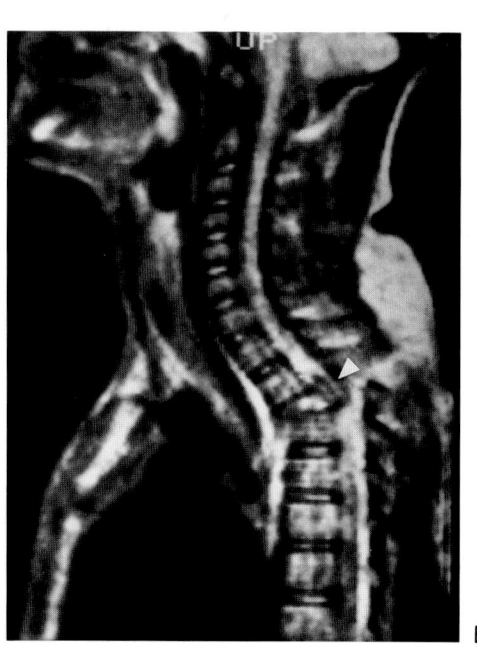

FIG. 4. T3 fracture–dislocation in a motorcyclist. **A:** Supine chest radiograph shows widening of the superior mediastinum (*arrows*). **B:** MR examination shows fragmentation of T3 and retropulsion of a bone fragment into the vertebral canal transecting the spinal cord (*arrowhead*). There is anterolisthesis of T2 on T3. MRI is excellent for demonstrating abnormalities in the cervicothoracic regions. (From ref. 10.)

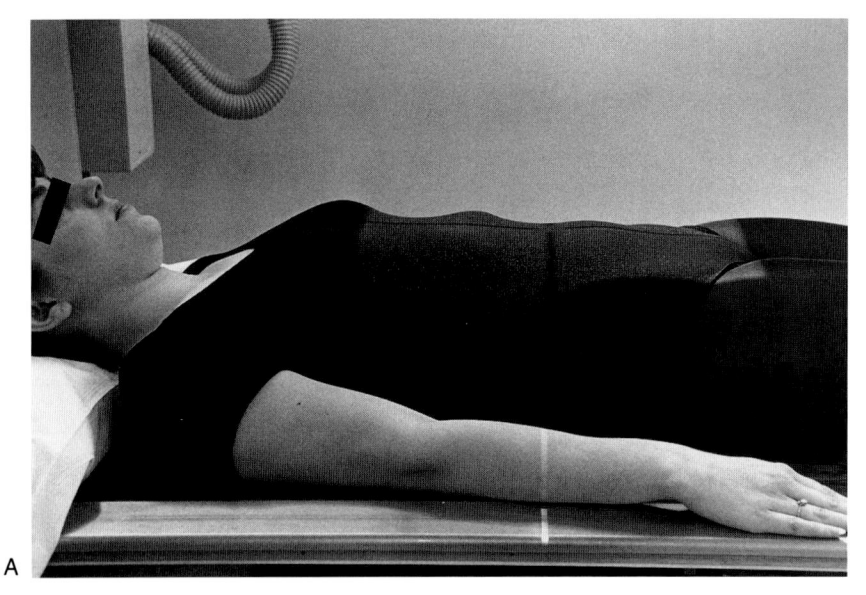

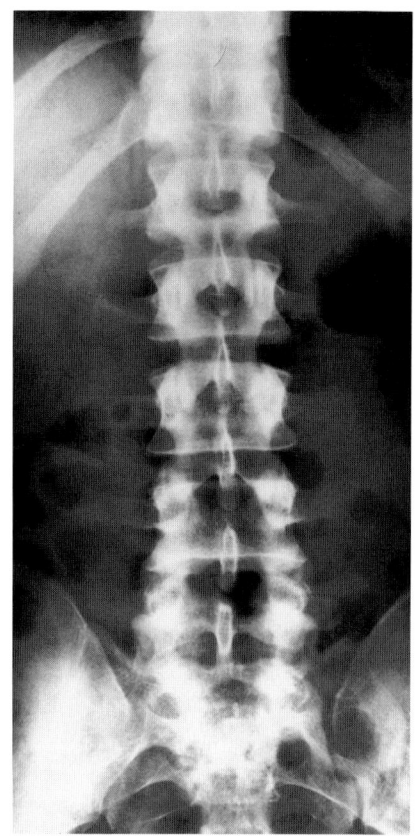

FIG. 5. Normal lumbar column, frontal view. **A:** Positioning technique. **B:** Radiographic appearance. There is normal alignment of the vertebral bodies, spinous processes, and pedicles. The interspinous spaces and interpediculate distances are uniform. (From ref. 13.)

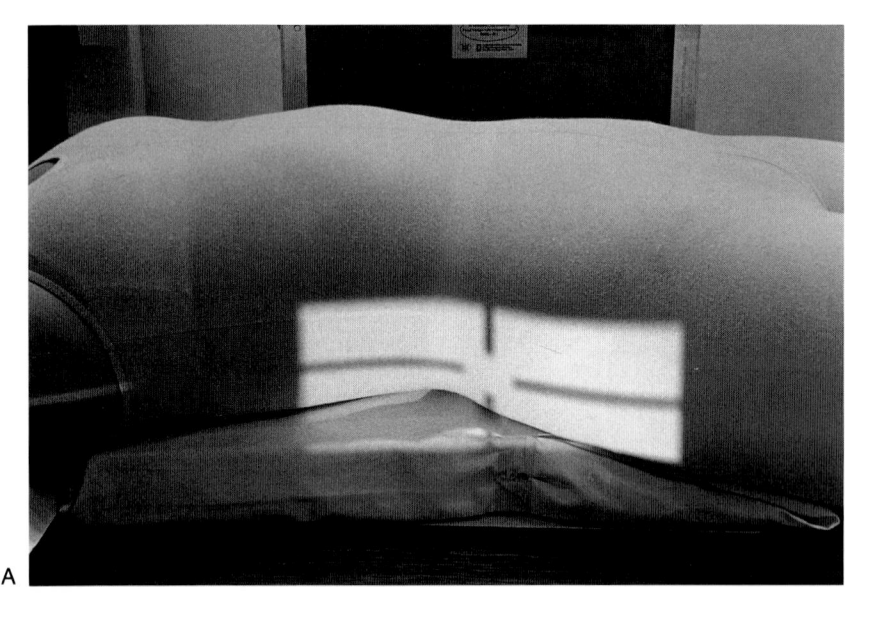

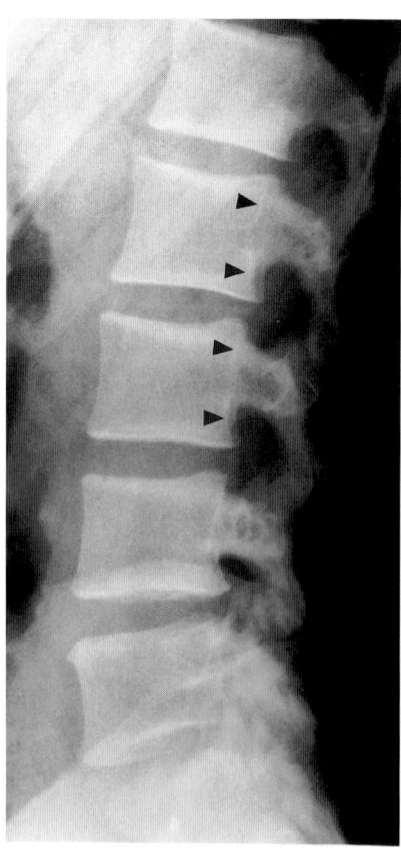

FIG. 6. Normal lumbar column. **A:** Horizontal beam technique. **B:** Radiograph. There is normal alignment of the vertebral bodies. The posterior vertebral body lines (*arrowheads*) are either single or bifid at the level of the nutrient canal. The disc spaces are uniform. (From ref. 13.)

In the lumbar region, all radiography also may be obtained with the patient in the supine position. AP supine (Fig. 5) and cross-table lateral (Fig. 6) films should be obtained. We also include, on all trauma patients, an AP view of the pelvis since we encounter a high number of pelvic injuries. Sacral injuries are generally the result of concomitant pelvic injuries. We do not obtain oblique views of the lumbar vertebrae since frontal and lateral films are usually adequate. A vertical beam lateral view of the lumbar column may also be obtained using the same careful "logrolling" technique employed for the thoracic column (13).

It is important that the entire vertebral column be radiographed in all patients who have suffered severe trauma. The incidence of multiple-level, noncontiguous vertebral fractures has been reported to be between 3% and 9% (5,41). Quite often, one fracture is very obvious and the other is less so.

Diagnostic Considerations

I use two approaches to identify fractures and dislocations of the thoracic and lumbar vertebral columns. The first is an anticipation of injuries that may be encountered based solely on the mechanism that produced the injury. This is the so-called fingerprints approach (8,13). The second is a careful analysis of the radiographs using the "ABCS" approach (13). By using these two methods, there should be no difficulty in diagnosing even subtle abnormalities.

The biomechanics of vertebral injury are described elsewhere in this book. It is sufficient to say, however, that an injury produced by a particular mechanism will result in a characteristic series of radiographic changes that can be called "fingerprints." In each instance, the precise mechanism produces a series of radiographic changes that are similar in appearance no matter where they are encountered in the vertebral column.

There are four basic mechanisms of injury to the thoracic and lumbar vertebral columns: flexion, rotation, shear, and extension (13,28,42). Some degree of flexion with an increased axial load is the common denominator in the first three mechanisms.

Flexion injuries are the most common type found throughout the entire vertebral column (8,11–13,18, 28,42). In a large series of patients who were studied, flexion mechanisms were responsible for nearly 85% of all injuries (8). All flexion injuries are variations on the same mechanical theme, combining compressive forces anteriorly and distraction forces posteriorly (18,28,42) (Fig. 7). Thus these injuries may occur when unrestrained front seat occupants of motor vehicles are force-flexed onto the steering wheel or dashboard or are ejected from the vehicle. Motorcyclists are subject to injuries of the upper thoracic column when they are ejected over the handlebars after their

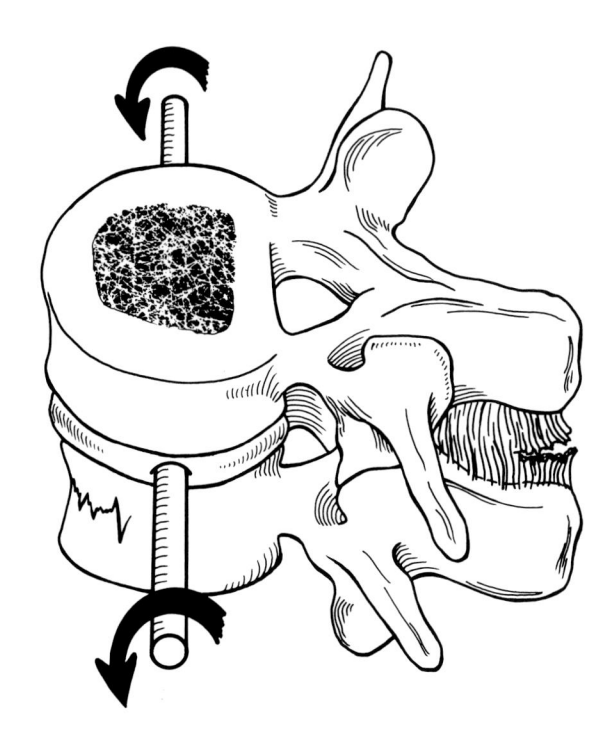

FIG. 7. Mechanism of flexion injury. Flexion occurs about a fulcrum through the middle of the intervertebral disc (*curved arrows*). Excessive compression produces fractures in the anterior and superior aspects of the vertebral body. As the force continues, the fracture propagates posteriorly, ultimately resulting in fragments that may be retropulsed into the vertebral canal, as in a burst injury. Furthermore, there is distraction of the posterior elements and subsequent tearing of the ligamentous structures. A single mechanism may produce a spectrum of injuries depending on the severity of the compressive forces and the degree of axial loading. (From ref. 13.)

cycle strikes a solid object (10,33) (Fig. 8). Rear seat vehicle occupants using a lap-type seat belt may suffer a severe disruptive flexion injury in the thoracolumbar region as a result of forces that are primarily distractive (7,11,12,43,46) (Fig. 9). These injuries, described originally by Smith and Chance, are generically referred to as Chance fractures (Fig. 10). In this particular mechanism, the seat belt moves the fulcrum of flexion from the center of the intervertebral disc to the anterior abdominal wall and accounts for the primary distraction aspect to the injury (7,8,13,43,46). I have encountered several patients with identical injuries that were sustained when the patient struck the midsection of a solid object, with subsequent forward flexion of the torso over that object, while skiing.

Pure flexion injuries may be divided radiographically into four subtypes: (a) simple, in which there is anterior compression of the superior aspect of the vertebral body with or without narrowing of the disc space above the level of injury, but with intact posterior vertebral body line and posterior ligamentous structures; (b) bursting, the most common type encountered in my practice, in which the vertebra is literally exploded by compressive forces that produce severe comminution of the vertebral body, retropulsion of fragments, and cleavage in the posterior arch (1,34,35,42,45,48) (Fig. 11); (c) distraction, with or without fracture, in which there is widening of the interspinous and interfacet dis-

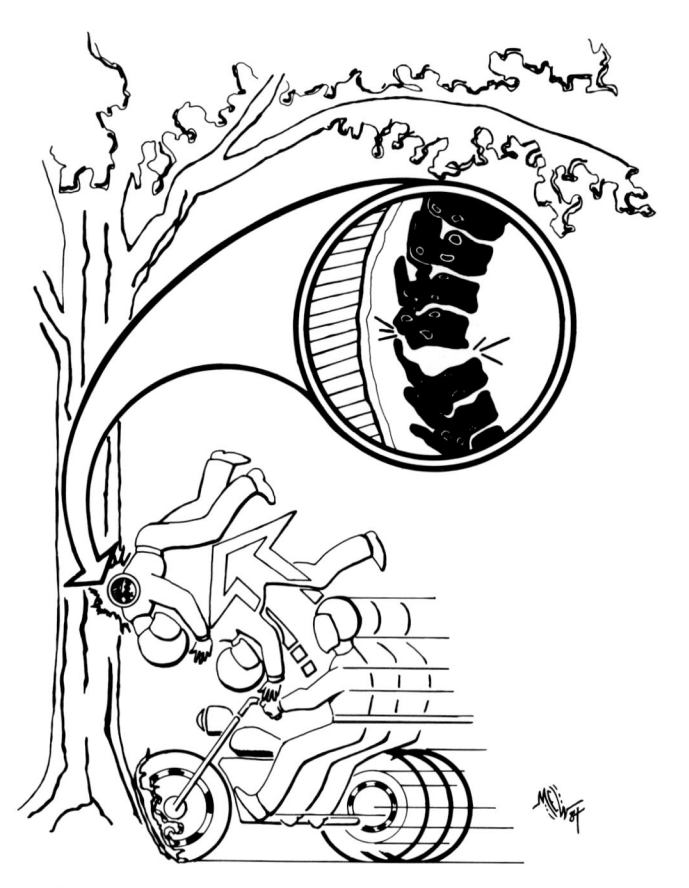

FIG. 8. Mechanism of flexion injury in motorcyclists. Sudden deceleration on impact results in the rider being catapulted over the handlebars. Forward flexion occurs in the upper thoracic region. (From ref. 10.)

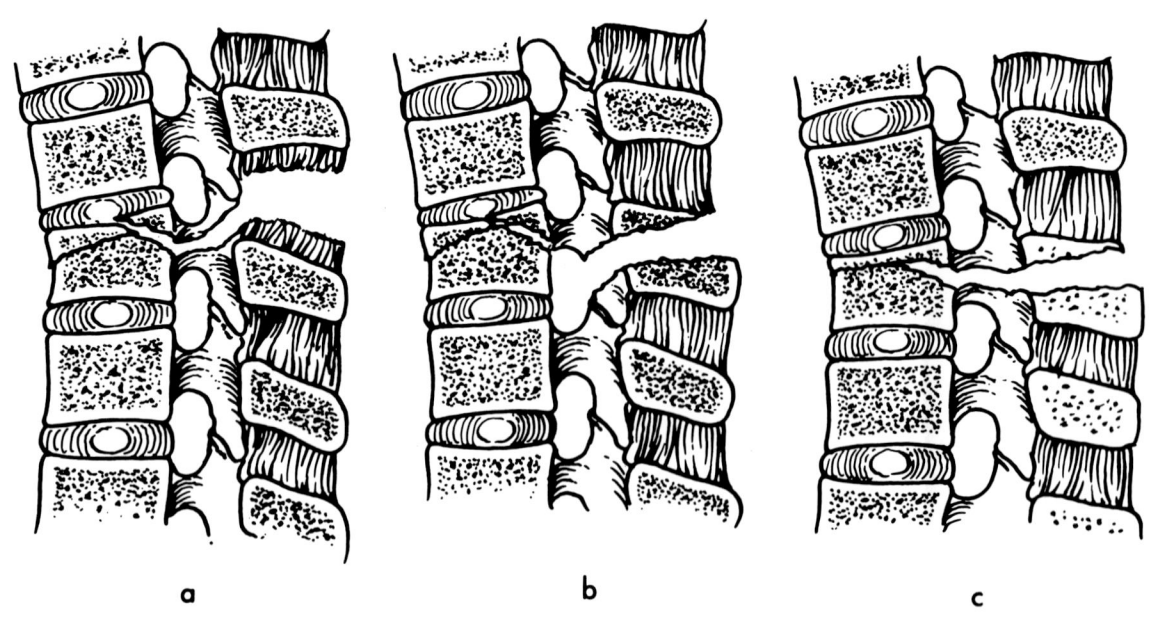

FIG. 9. Three types of flexion injuries due to the use of lap-type seat belts. **a:** Smith fracture. **b:** Chance fracture. **c:** Pure horizontal fracture. (From ref. 11.)

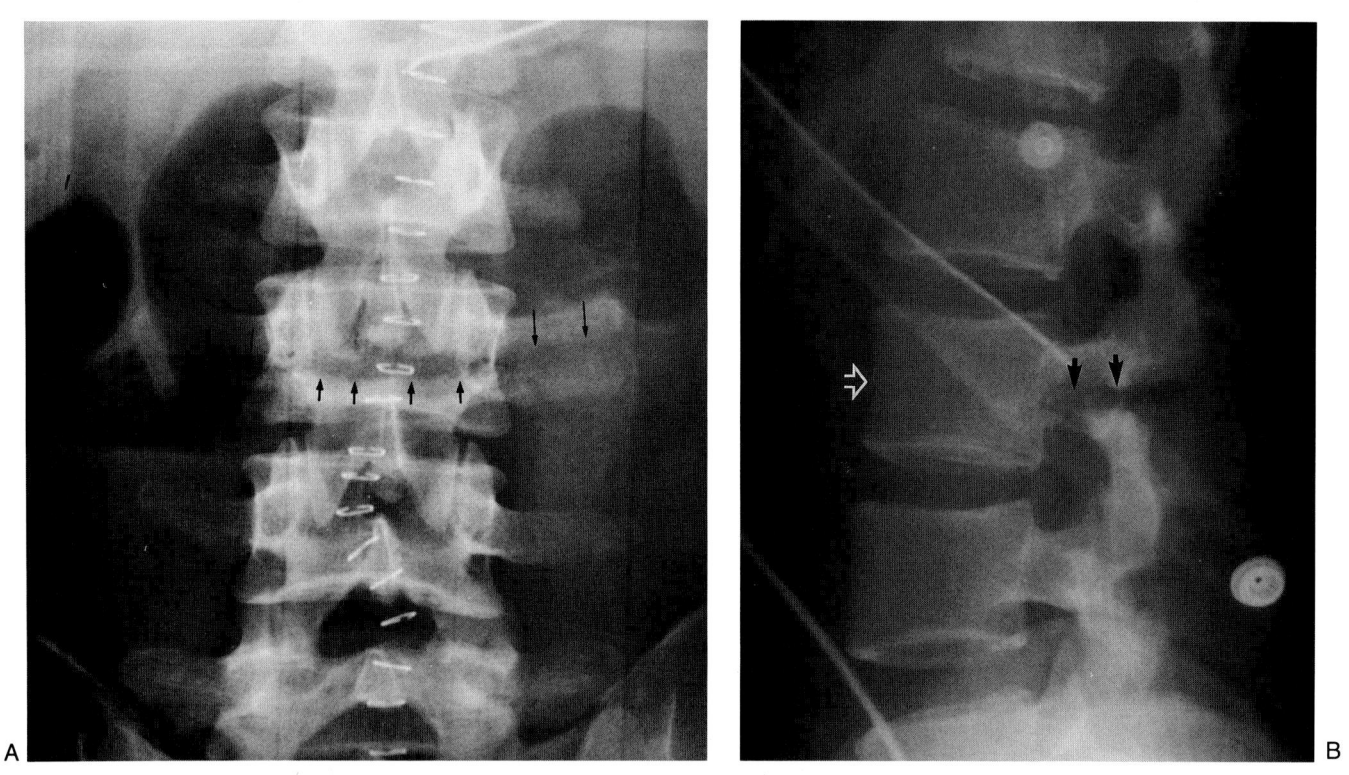

FIG. 10. Chance fracture. **A:** Frontal view shows horizontal fractures extending through the transverse processes (*long arrows*) and vertebral body and lamina (*short arrows*). **B:** Lateral view shows the fractures extending through the pedicles (*arrows*). Note the buckling of the anterior cortex of the vertebral body (*open arrow*).

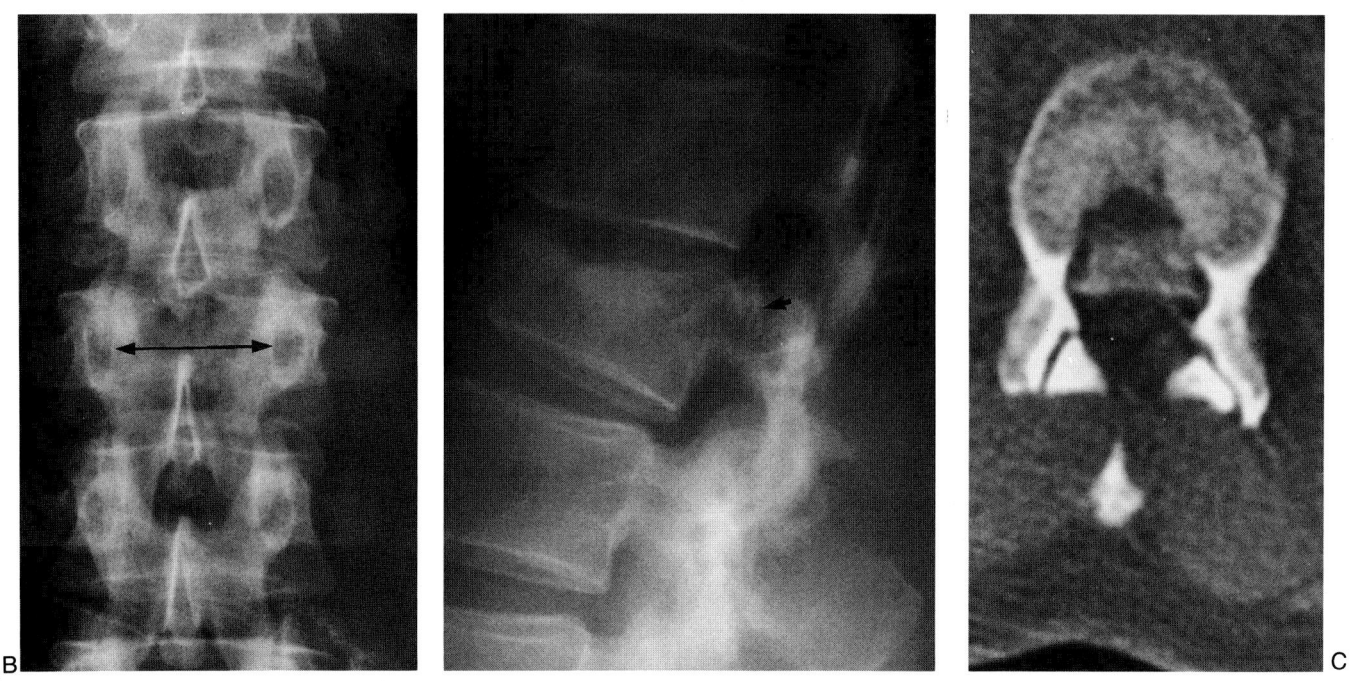

FIG. 11. Burst fracture. **A:** Frontal view shows widening of the interpediculate distance (*double arrow*). **B:** Lateral view shows marked anterior compression of the vertebral body and retropulsion of a bone fragment from the posterior vertebral body line (*arrow*). **C:** CT scan shows the retropulsed bone fragment narrowing the vertebral canal by at least 50% of its transverse diameter.

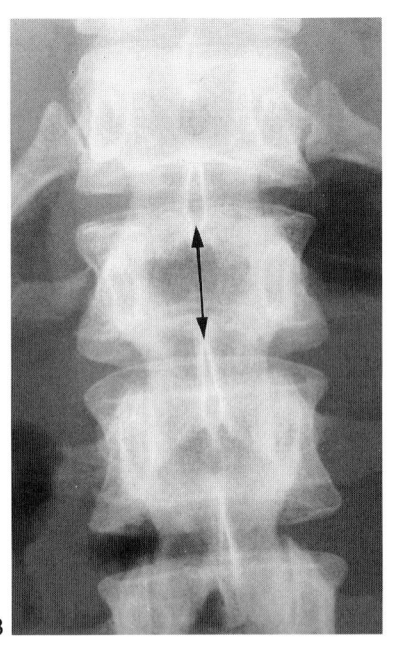

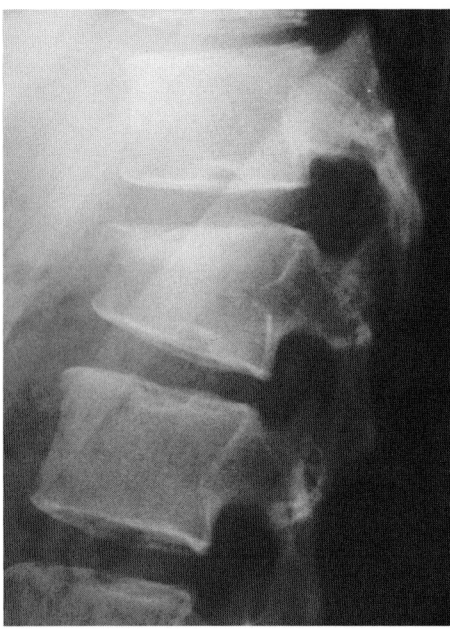

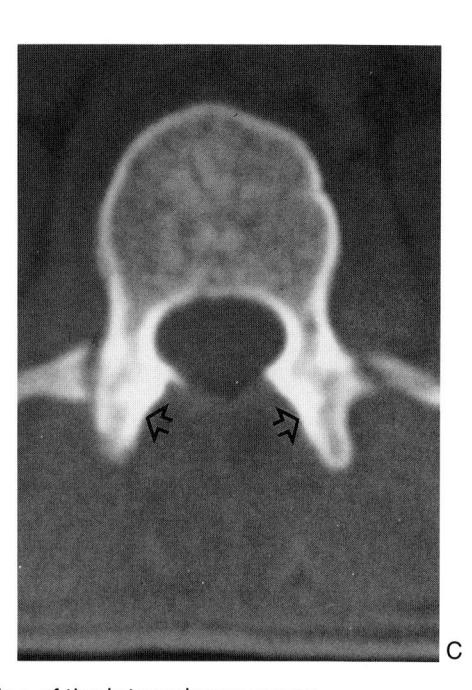

FIG. 12. Distraction injury of T12 to L1. **A:** Frontal view shows widening of the interspinous space between T12 and L1 (*double arrow*). Note the transverse process fractures laterally. **B:** Lateral view shows anterior compression of L1. The degree of distraction is not apparent on this view. **C:** CT scan shows "naked" facets (*arrows*). Note the absence of the posterior elements from T12. There are bilateral transverse process fractures.

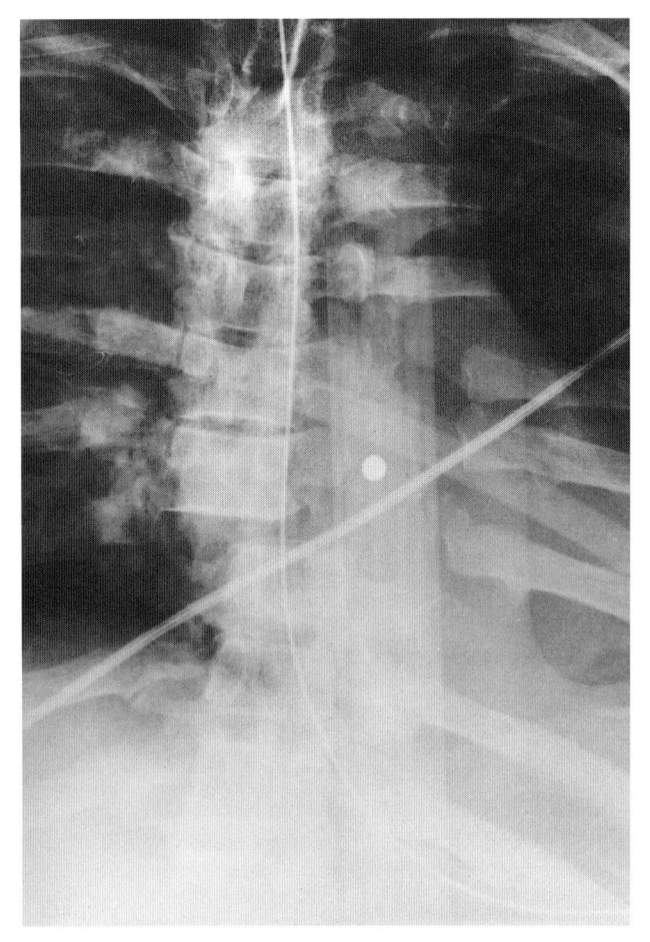

FIG. 13. Thoracic dislocation. Frontal view shows gross dislocation of T8 on T9. Note the vertebrocostal dislocations as well on the left.

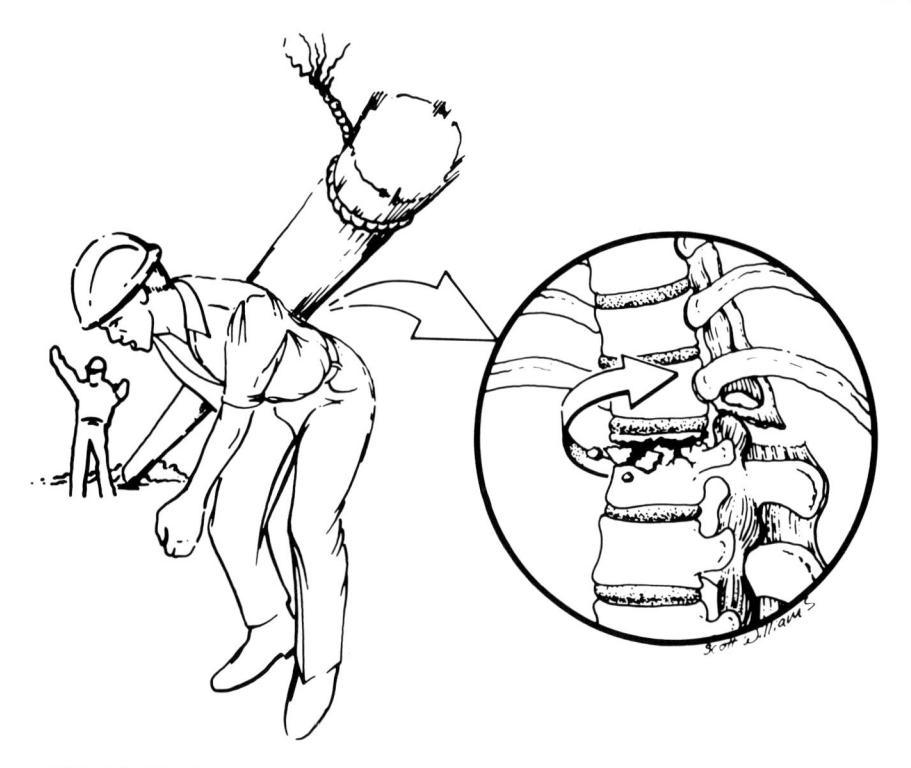

FIG. 14. Mechanism of rotary injury with forward flexion. (From ref. 13.)

tance without frank dislocation (Fig. 12); and (d) dislocation, in which a complete loss of bony continuity of the articular surfaces occurs (Fig. 13).

The "fingerprints" of flexion injuries are as follows: (a) compression fragmentation and burst of vertebral body (Fig. 11); (b) "teardrop" fragments (generally seen in the cervical region); (c) widened interlaminar or interspinous space (Fig. 12); (d) anterolisthesis; (e) disruption of the posterior vertebral body line (Figs. 10 and 11); (f) "naked" facets (Fig. 12); (g) locked facets (Fig. 13); and (h) narrowed disc space *above* the level of injury.

Rotary, or grinding, injuries are the result of a rotary or torsional force applied about the long axis of the vertebral column, usually in the presence of flexion. These are found almost exclusively in the thoracolumbar region. The characteristic mechanism is that of a heavy blow struck to the upper torso. This blow compresses the vertebral column and flexes the torso laterally; in the typical case, the lower portion of the body is fixed in position (Fig. 14). These injuries are extremely disruptive to both the vertebral body and the posterior elements as well as the ligamentous complex (8,12,13). There is generally a high incidence of neurologic deficit as a result of these injuries. The "fingerprints" of a rotary or grinding injury are (a) severe distortion of anatomy of the involved vertebrae; (b) rotation; (c) dislocation; (d) facet and pillar fractures; (e) transverse process or rib fractures; and, on CT scan, (f) circular array of fragments and unilateral wid-

Text continues on page 79.

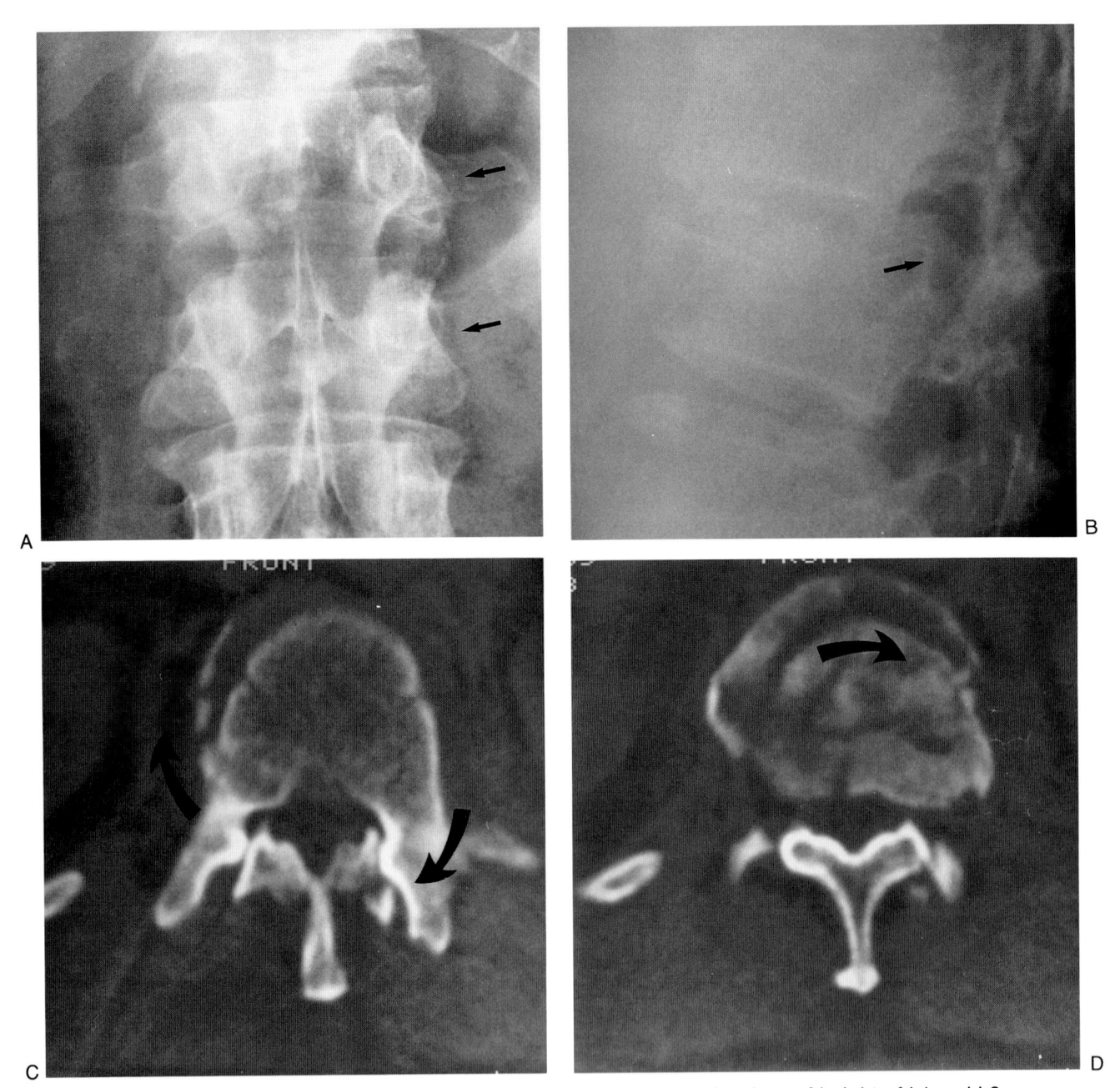

FIG. 15. Rotary ("grinding") injury of L1. **A:** Frontal view. There is a loss of height of L1 and L2. Note the transverse process fractures on the left (*arrows*). **B:** Lateral view. There is subluxation of T12 on L1. Note the fragmentation of the posterior vertebral body line of L1 (*arrow*). **C:** CT scan shows disruption of the facet joints. *Curved arrows* indicate the direction of motion to produce this injury. The facets have followed this line of motion. **D:** Another section shows a rotary distribution of fracture fragments of the vertebral body (*curved arrow*).

ening of the facet joint on the antirotational side. Figure 15 shows all these characteristic findings.

Shearing injuries result from forces that are horizontally or obliquely directed on the vertebral column. As with rotary injury, forward or lateral flexion may contribute to these findings. In the typical mechanism, the lower portion of the body is fixed, and the vertebral column in the mobile portion absorbs the blow and moves with it (8,12,13) (Fig. 16). These injuries are extremely disruptive and result in severe neurologic compromise.

The "fingerprints" of shearing injuries include (a) severe distortion of vertebral anatomy, with a "windswept" appearance to the vertebrae; (b) lateral distraction; (c) lateral dislocation; (d) transverse process and rib fractures; and, on CT scan, (e) a linear oblique array of fragments. Figure 17 shows typical radiographic findings in a shearing injury.

Text continues on page 81.

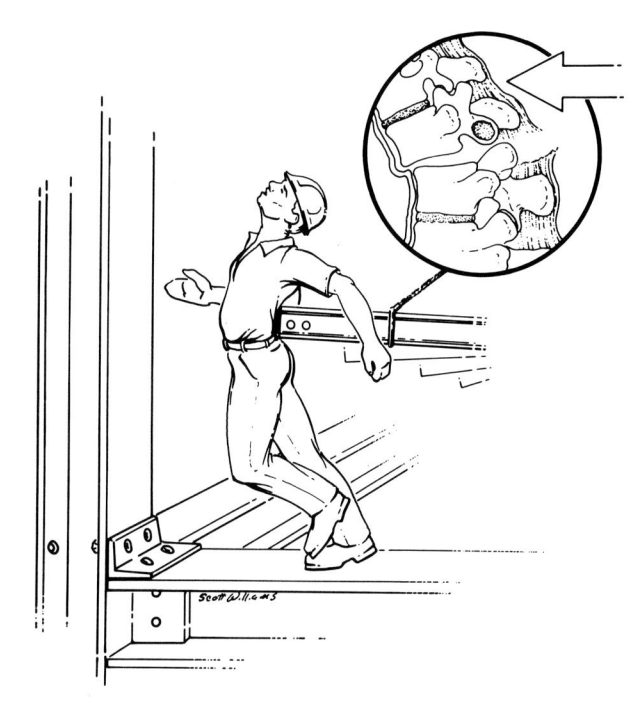

FIG. 16. Mechanism of shearing injury. (From ref. 13.)

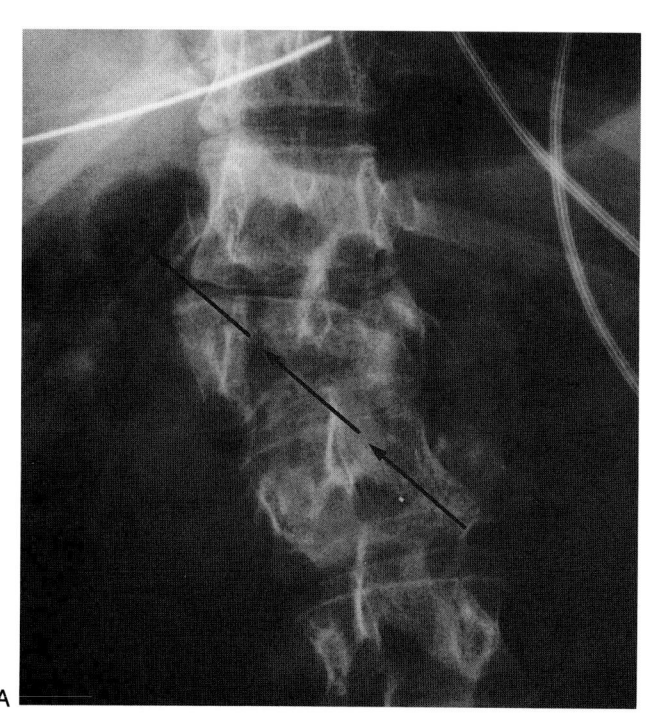

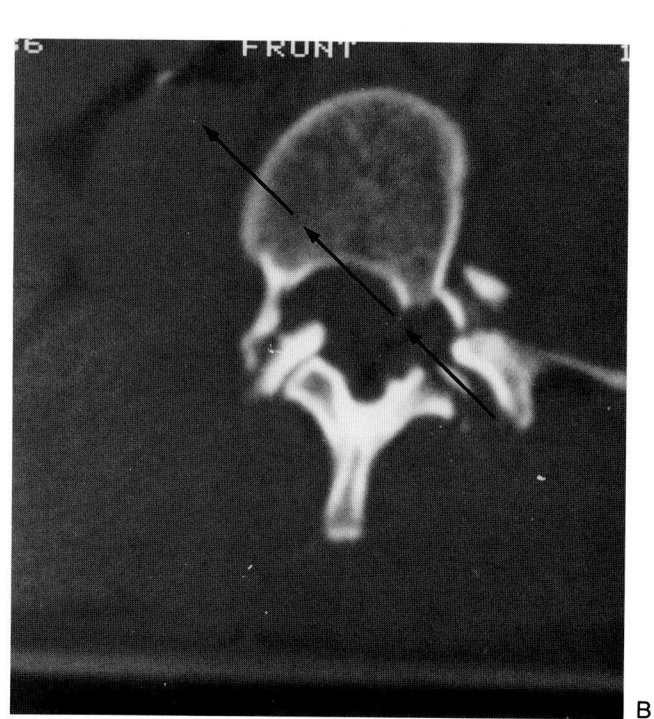

FIG. 17. Shearing injury, T12 to L2. **A:** Lateral view shows a "windswept" appearance of the vertebrae. The *arrows* indicate the direction of the shearing motion. **B:** CT scan through the region shows severe disruption again with a "windswept" appearance. The *arrows* indicate motion vector.

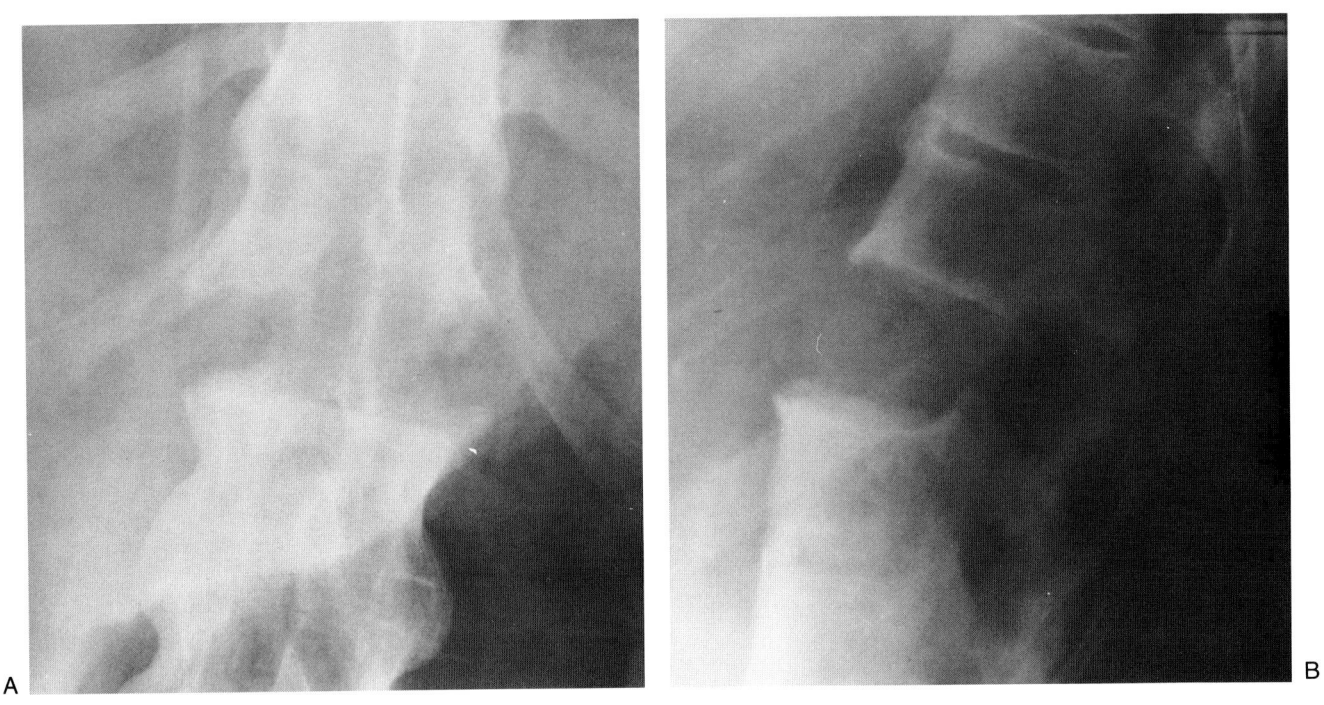

FIG. 18. Extension injury in a patient with diffuse idiopathic skeletal hyperostosis (DISH). **A:** Frontal view shows dislocation of T12 on L1 with marked widening of the intervertebral disc space. Note the ankylosis between the other vertebrae. **B:** Lateral view shows the severity of the disruption.

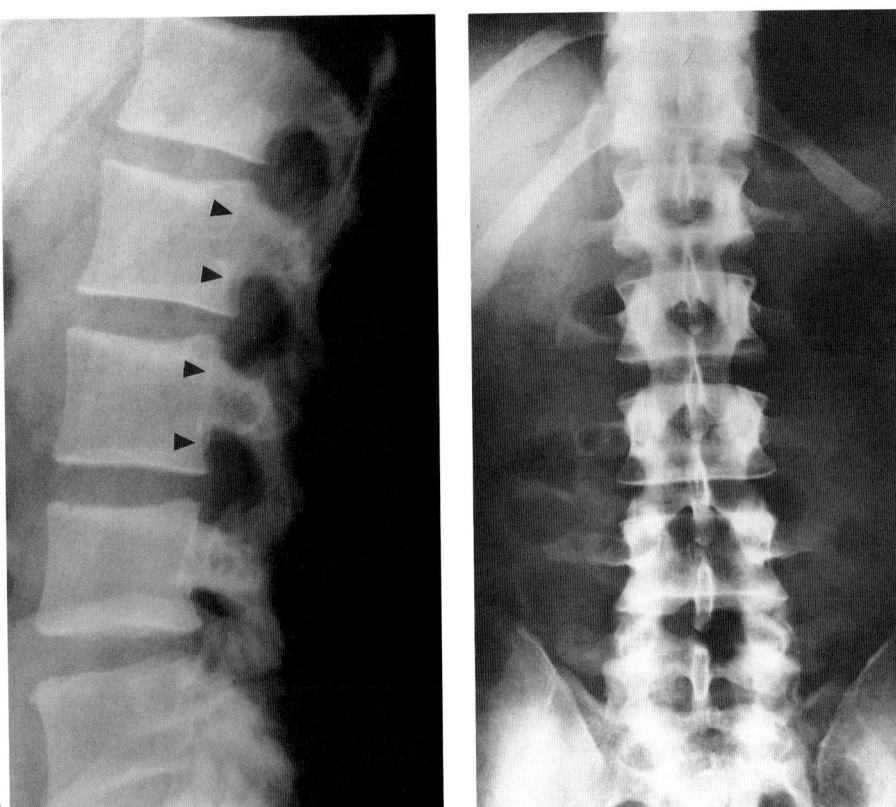

FIG. 19. Normal lumbar vertebral column. **A:** Lateral view showing the position of the posterior vertebral body lines (*arrowheads*). At L1 and L2, the central nutrient foramen interrupts these lines. **B:** Frontal view shows normal alignment, normal interpediculate distance, and normal interspinous space.

Extension injuries are not common in the thoracic and lumbar columns. In almost all instances, they are the result of the patient falling backward and hyperextending over a solid object (8,12,13). Diseases that tend to fuse the vertebrae [ankylosing spondylitis and diffuse idiopathic skeletal hyperostosis (DISH)] tend to predispose patients to this type of injury (20,21,25) (Fig. 18).

The characteristic "fingerprint" of an extension injury in the thoracolumbar region is a widening of the intervertebral disc space and possibly retrolisthesis (8,12,13) (Fig. 18).

The ABCS of the Radiologic Diagnosis of Vertebral Injuries

The evaluation of any radiographic study demands a logical approach that is both easy to follow and accurate in its conclusions. Once a diagnosis has been made on the plain film, we may turn to more sophisticated imaging studies to confirm the diagnosis as well as to elaborate on the extent of injury.

The system that I prefer to use in the evaluation of plain films is the ABCS method:

A. Alignment and anatomy abnormalities.
B. Bony integrity abnormalities.
C. Cartilage or joint space abnormalities.
S. Soft tissue abnormalities.

To recognize abnormalities of alignment and anatomy, one must have a thorough knowledge of the normal anatomy and variants that may occur within the vertebral column. Normal alignment may be assessed on both lateral and frontal radiographs. The following normal anatomic markers may be seen on the lateral view (Fig. 19): the anterior and posterior margins of the vertebral bodies, the latter of which is interrupted centrally by a nutrient foramen; the spinolaminar line; the articular pillars and their facet joints; and the interlaminar or interspinous space. Degenerative disease of the intervertebral disc or facet joints may result in minor degrees of malalignment such as anterolisthesis or retrolisthesis. In these patients, lateral flexion/extension views may be required to determine if, in fact, there is instability. On the frontal view, we observe the alignment of the lateral margins of the vertebral bodies, the interpediculate distance, the width of the facet joints, the position of the transverse processes, and the interspinous distance.

Abnormalities of alignment include disruption of the anterior or posterior vertebral body lines (Fig. 20), disruption of the spinolaminar line, rotation of spinous processes (14), and widening of the interpediculate dis-

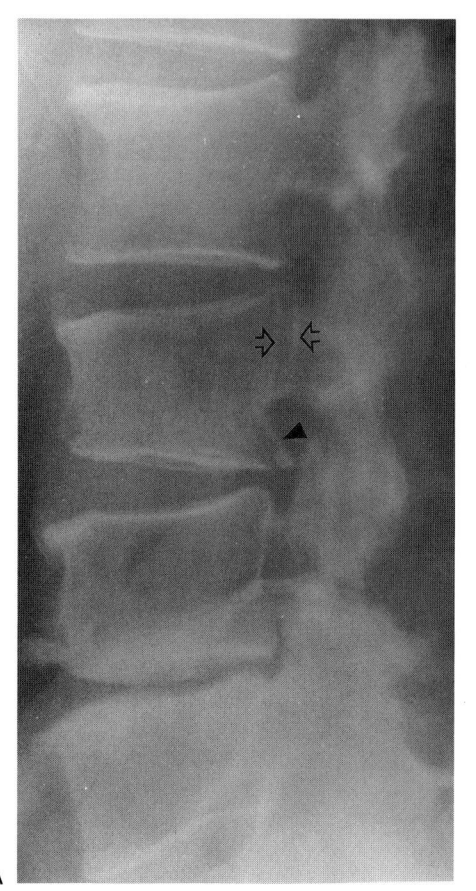

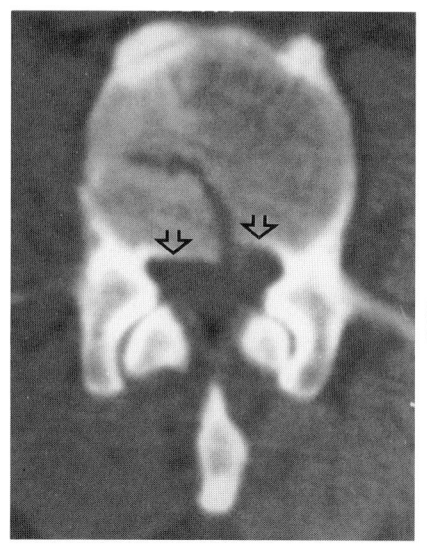

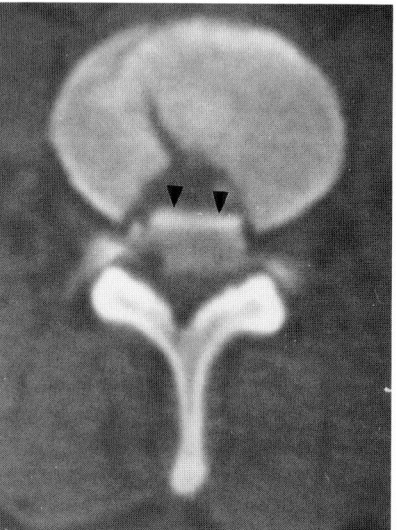

FIG. 20. Burst fracture of L3. **A:** Lateral radiograph shows anterior compression of L3. There is duplication of the upper portion of the posterior vertebral body line (*open arrows*). In addition, there is posterior angulation of the lower portion of the posterior vertebral body line (*arrowhead*). **B:** CT scan through the upper portion of L3 shows the fracture through the vertebral body. Note the retropulsion of a fragment on the right side. This retropulsed fragment combined with the undisplaced portion of the posterior vertebral body line (*open arrows*) was responsible for the upper abnormality seen on the plain radiograph. **C:** CT scan through the lower portion of L3 shows a large retropulsed fragment from the body within the vertebral canal. This fragment has rotated 180° with the posterior vertebral body line now pointing anteriorly (*arrowheads*).

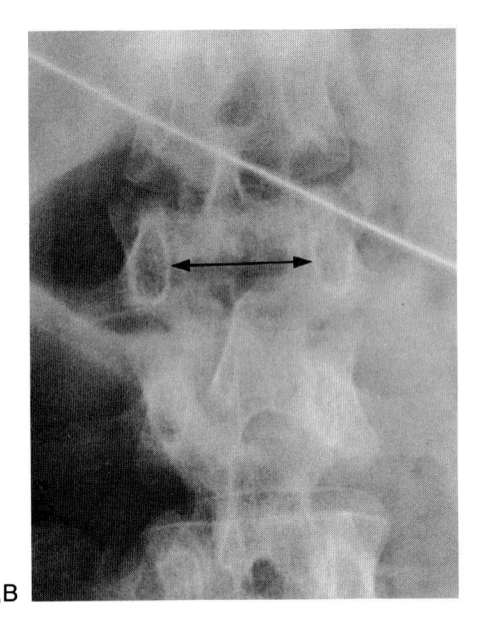

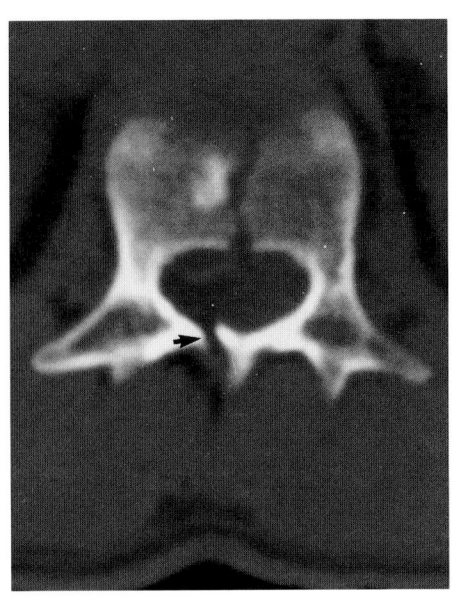

FIG. 21. Burst fracture of L1. **A:** Frontal radiograph shows widening of the interpediculate distance (*double arrow*). Compare this with the vertebrae above and below. The facet joints of L1 are clearly visible and are wider than the other levels. **B:** CT scan through the same vertebra shows the vertical fracture through the body as well as through the lamina (*arrow*).

tance (Fig. 21). Abnormalities of the posterior vertebral body line are often extremely subtle, but careful evaluation will show these findings. Any displacement, angulation, rotation, or absence of a portion or all of this structure is abnormal (9,12,13). Acute kyphotic angulation and loss of lordosis also may indicate that an abnormality is present. However, these findings are nonspecific and are of no significance when they occur by themselves.

Abnormalities of bony integrity are usually easy to detect when obvious fracture lines or displacement of normal structures occurs. However, widening of the interpediculate distance (Fig. 21) and disruption of the posterior vertebral body line (Fig. 22) may occur in the absence of more obvious changes (8,9,13).

Cartilage or joint space abnormalities generally occur more overtly than in the cervical region. A widening or narrowing of an intervertebral disc space may indicate that injury has occurred at that level. As a rule, narrowing of a disc space generally accompanies a flexion injury and occurs at the level *above* the fractured vertebra. However, since narrowing of the intervertebral disc space is an extremely common finding of degenerative disease, this sign cannot be relied on alone. Widening of the facet joint or even complete baring of the facets ("naked facets") indicates that a severe posterior ligamentous injury has occurred as the result of distractive forces (Fig. 23). These findings almost always occur with widening of the interlaminar or interspinous distance.

There are two important soft tissue abnormalities that accompany thoracic and lumbar vertebral injuries. These are the presence of a paraspinal soft tissue mass (Fig. 24) and the loss of the psoas stripe (Fig. 25). Soft

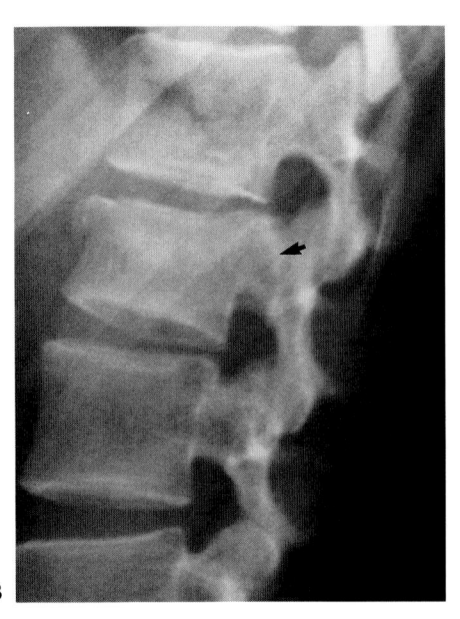

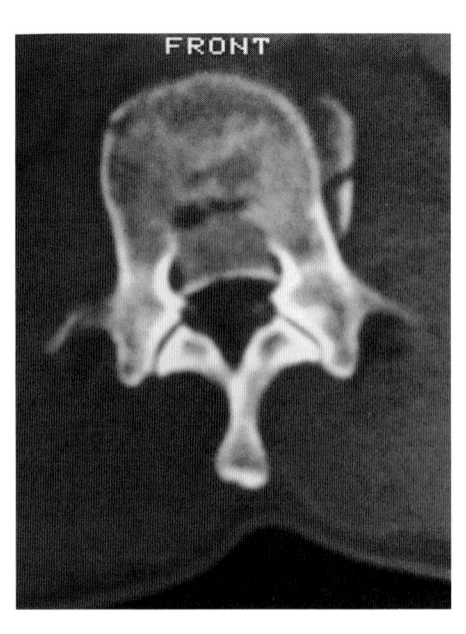

FIG. 22. Burst fracture of L1. **A:** Lateral radiograph shows anterior compression of the body of L1. The upper portion of the posterior body line is not in its anatomic position. A vague density is seen within the vertebral canal (*arrow*). **B:** CT scan shows the retropulsed fragment of the vertebral body within the vertebral canal. This accounted for the abnormality seen on the plain film.

IMAGING OF VERTEBRAL FRACTURES • 83

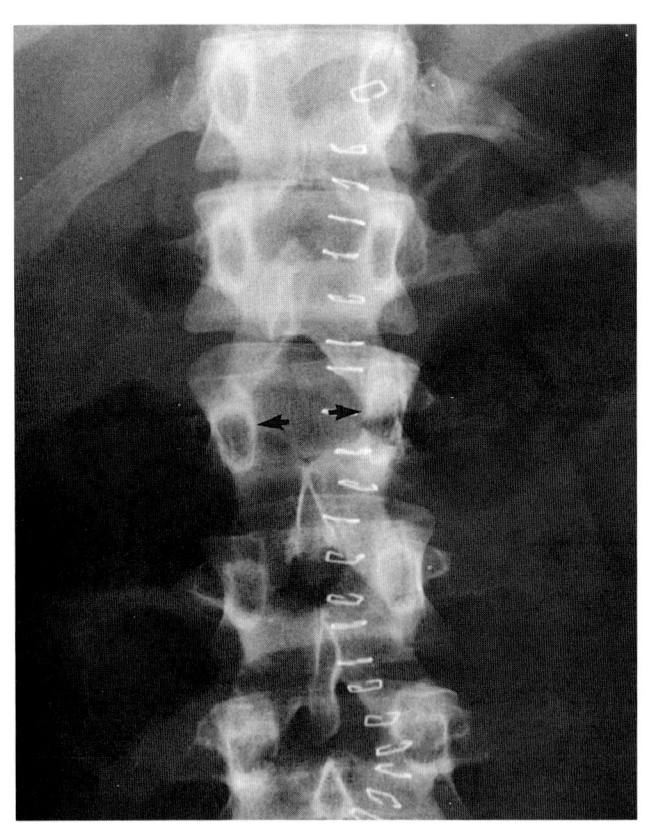

FIG. 23. Distraction injury of L1–L2. Forward flexion and posterior distraction has resulted in "naked" facets (*arrows*). Note the widened interspinous space between L1 and L2.

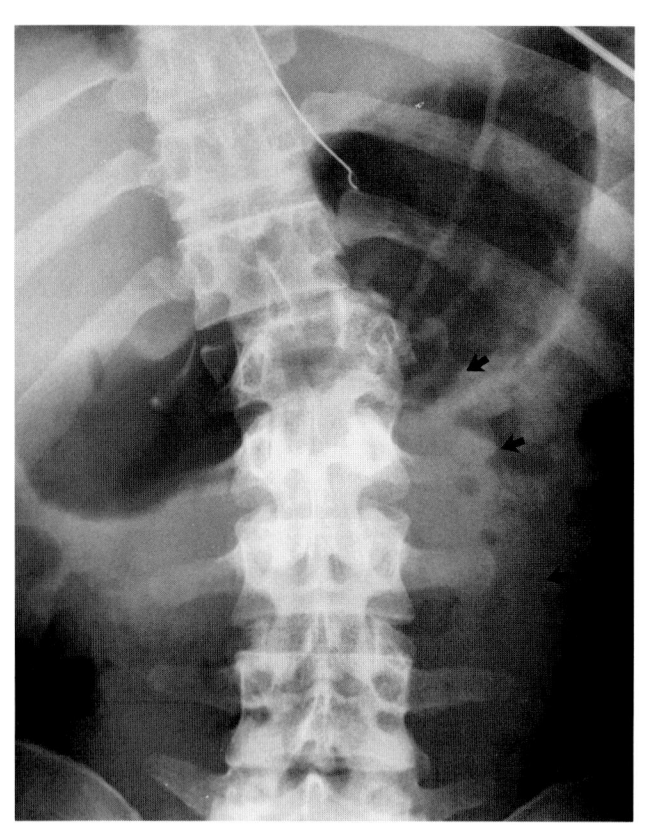

FIG. 25. Loss of the psoas stripe in a patient with a shearing fracture–dislocation of T12 to L1. The normal psoas is present on the left (*arrows*). Note the loss of this shadow on the right side.

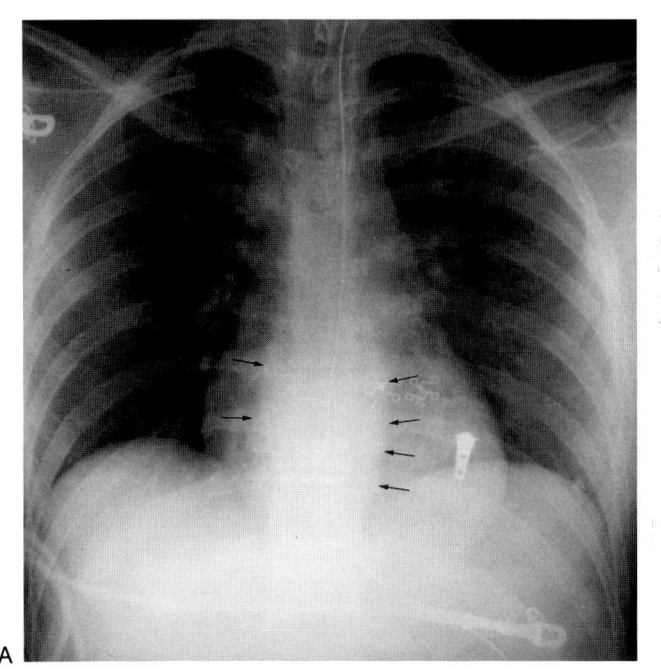

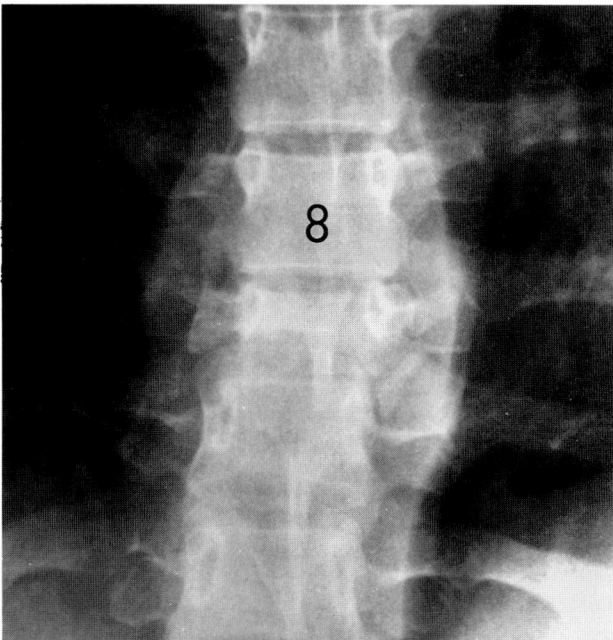

FIG. 24. Widening of the paraspinal lines in a patient with a fracture of T9. **A:** Frontal chest radiograph shows widening of the paraspinal lines in the lower thoracic region (*arrows*). **B:** A detailed view of the lower thoracic column shows the compression of T9 and laterolisthesis of T8 to the left. Note the paraspinal hematoma. (From ref. 13.)

tissue findings may be extremely useful, particularly in injuries to the thoracic vertebrae when the diagnosis may be made from an abnormality seen on a chest radiograph (12,13,20) (Fig. 24).

THE ASSESSMENT OF POST-TRAUMATIC VERTEBRAL STABILITY

The stability of the vertebral column rests on the integrity of both the skeletal and soft tissue components (2,17,38). Any injury that has caused sufficient damage to allow abnormal motion at, above, or below the site is said to be unstable. While disruption of any of the individual ligaments composing the vertebral column does not produce an unstable situation, it is the combination of these abnormalities that results in instability. From a clinical standpoint, unstable injuries have the potential to produce further neurologic deterioration and skeletal deformity.

There is considerable controversy regarding the subject of vertebral stability following injury (29). Each surgeon must apply his/her own standards to the management of these patients. It is possible, however, to define the extent of injury and to predict the *probability* of instability on the basis of radiographic findings. It is important to note that, because of the stabilizing influence of the ribs in the T1 to T8 region, the same radiographic findings that would indicate an unstable injury in the lumbar region might not have as great an impact in the midthoracic region.

Most surgeons agree on Denis' three-column concept of the vertebral column in defining stability (16,17). Denis divided the vertebral column into three distinct functional zones. The anterior zone extends from a line drawn vertically to the junction of the middle and posterior third of the vertebral body to the anterior longitudinal ligament. The middle zone extends from this line to the posterior longitudinal ligament, and the posterior zone extends from the posterior longitudinal ligament to the supraspinous ligament. By Denis' concepts, anatomic instability occurs when there is disruption of any two contiguous zones or from any injury that disrupts the middle zone (16,17).

From a radiographic standpoint, there are five signs that indicate disruption of specific zones in the vertebral column. These signs are displacement, widening of the interspinous or interlaminar space, widening of the facet joints, widening of the interpediculate distance, and disruption of the posterior vertebral body line (11–13,15,19,20). Displacement disrupts all three of Denis' zones. Widening of the interspinous or interlaminar space (Fig. 12) indicates a severe posterior disruptive injury that has ruptured the interspinous and interfacet ligaments, the ligamentum flavum, the posterior longitudinal ligament, and a portion of the posterior aspect of the intervertebral disc. Widening of the facet joints implies severe disruption of the same structures. Widening of the interpediculate distance commonly occurs in severe crush injuries of the vertebrae—usually burst fractures or rotary injuries (Figs. 11 and 15). Widening of the interpediculate distance (Fig. 21) indicates that the vertebral body is fractured in the sagittal plane and that the lamina is fractured as well. The interpediculate widening can occur only if this combination is present. Thus the finding indicates disruption of all three zones. Finally, disruption of the posterior vertebral body line is graphic evidence of disruption of the middle zone. It occurs in a variety of injuries, the most common of which are burst fractures (12,13,15) (Figs. 11 and 21).

PITFALLS OF PLAIN FILM RADIOGRAPHY

There are two main pitfalls in the use of plain films to diagnose vertebral injuries. The first of these is failure to demonstrate the abnormality, which often is the result of poor radiologic technique in which the films are either over or underpenetrated. In some instances, the injured vertebra may actually be near the very top of the film and may not be seen. It is imperative that the surgeon obtain adequate radiographs on all patients with suspected vertebral injury.

The second pitfall is failure to diagnose. Like the fourth son in the Passover Hagada, the son who does not know how to ask, injuries may easily be overlooked by one who does not know how to look. It is incumbent on each practitioner to know the normal anatomy, variations, and the subtle radiographic changes that indicate injury before treating a patient with suspected vertebral injury.

COMPUTERIZED TOMOGRAPHY

The development of computerized tomography (CT) in the early 1970s revolutionized the practice of diagnostic radiology. CT made it possible, for the first time, to obtain cross-sectional images of areas in the body that previously defied noninvasive diagnostic techniques. One of the earliest applications of CT was the evaluation of patients with vertebral trauma (3,4,26,37,40).

The CT examination of the patient with vertebral trauma is relatively easy to perform. All that is required is that the patient remain motionless for the duration of the examination. Thus, to obtain an adequate examination in an acutely injured patient, it may be necessary to pharmacologically induce immobility. In our institution, each CT examination is tailored to the specific areas of injury for each patient. The levels for study are determined for both plain films and the CT scout film. Once this is accomplished, contiguous 4- or 5-mm thick slices are obtained from one full level above the injured vertebra to one full level below. If several levels are in question and are separated by

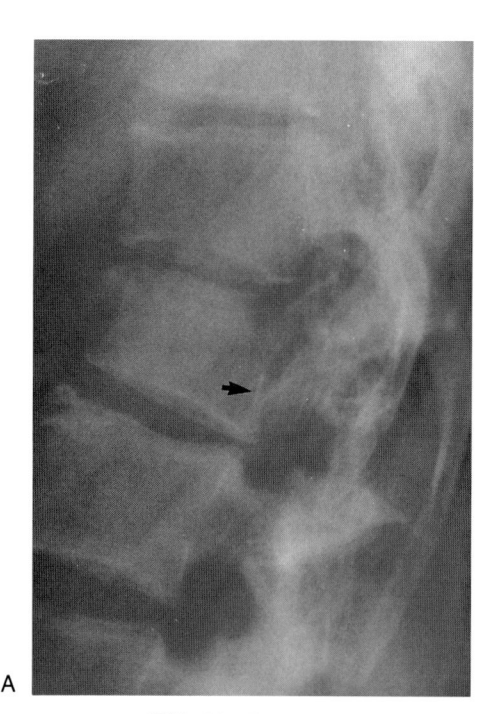

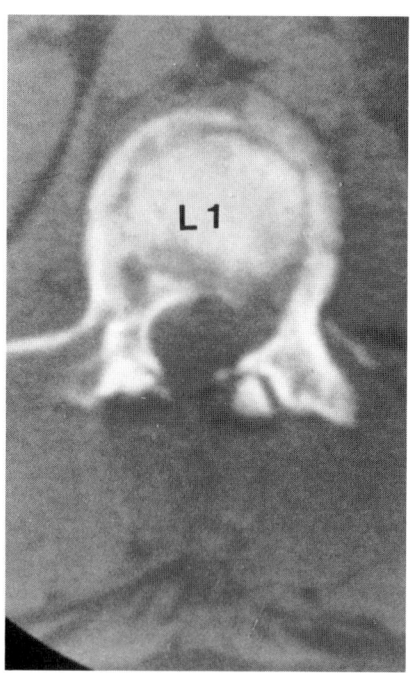

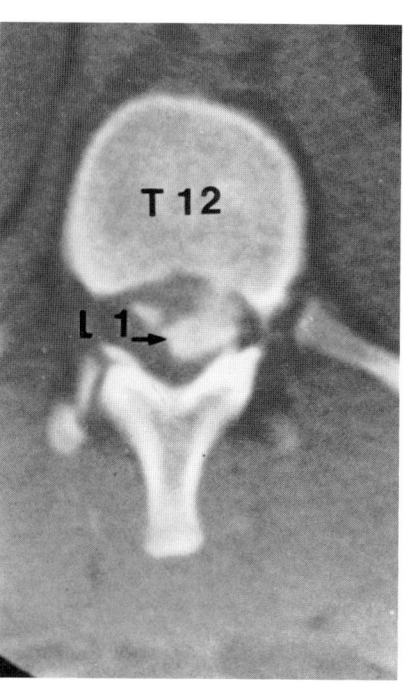

FIG. 26. Burst fracture of L1. **A:** Lateral radiograph shows disruption of the body of L1. The lower portion of the posterior vertebral body line is intact (*arrow*). The upper portion is not identified. There is, however, suggestion of bony debris at and just above the T12 disc level. **B:** CT scan through the upper portion of L1 shows absence of a portion of the posterior body line on the left. There are compression fractures through the body of L1. **C:** A scan through the inferior aspect of T12 shows bony debris within the vertebral canal. This bony debris represents the missing fragments of the posterior body line of the upper portion of L1. This case illustrates the need to obtain full, contiguous sections of all involved vertebrae.

more than two vertebrae, separate studies are performed at the same time. The bracketing is necessary because injuries that are not always apparent on plain films often occur at contiguous levels (Fig. 26). Films are made at both bone and soft tissue windows, giving us the ability to evaluate both bone and soft tissue components of an injury such as disc herniation (Fig. 27). We do not use intravenous contrast enhancement (13).

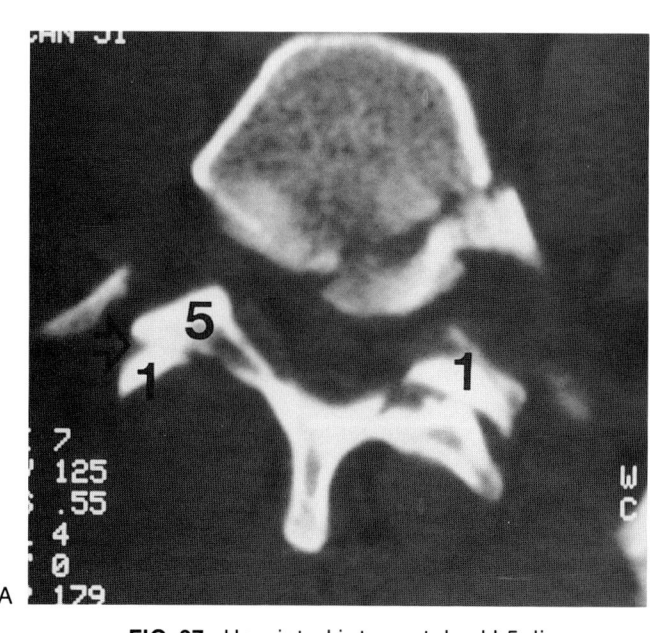

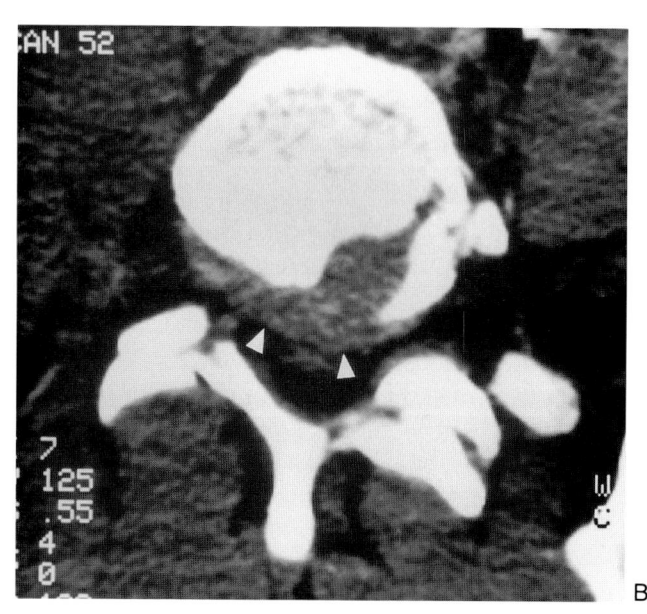

FIG. 27. Herniated intervertebral L5 disc accompanying fracture. **A:** CT scan using bone windows shows a fracture of the posterior aspect of L5. There is unilateral facet lock of L5 on S1 on the right (*open arrow*). **B:** CT scan using soft tissue windows shows herniated disc material (*arrowheads*) accompanying the fracture at L5. (From ref. 14.)

The scout films that precede the CT examination should be obtained in a manner that allows easy and rapid identification of all involved vertebrae. It is important to correlate the findings on a CT scan to a specific anatomic level. For this reason, we rely on an AP scout film if an injury is suspected from C6 to T8. If a lateral view is obtained, the presence of the shoulder girdle and heavy upper arm musculature obscures the vertebral column and precludes accurate anatomic localization. For injuries including T8 and the vertebrae below, lateral films are preferred (13).

One cannot overemphasize the need to *correlate the CT findings with those on plain films* (12,13). In an age when sophisticated imaging studies are easily avail-

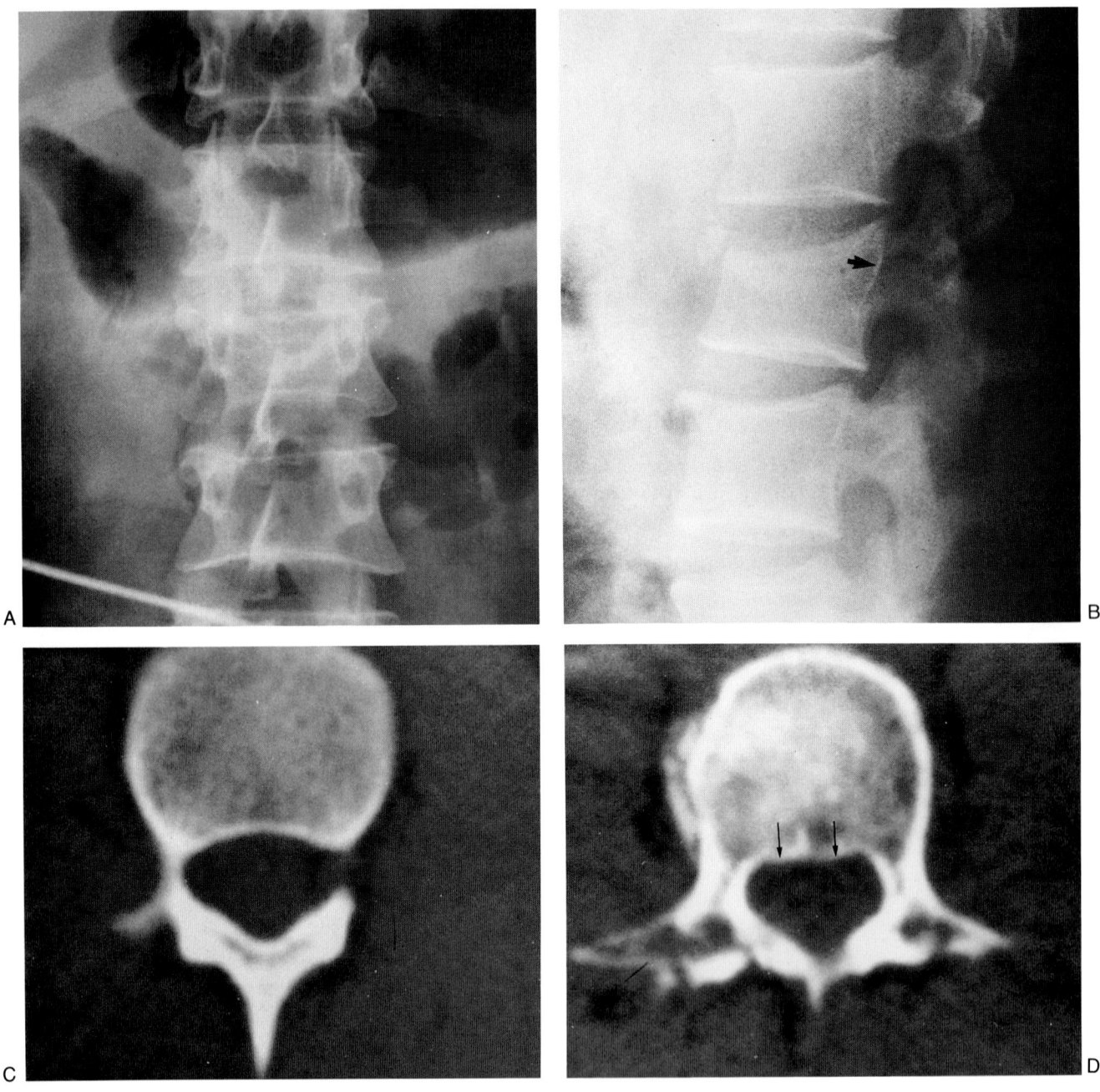

FIG. 28. Burst fracture of L2. **A:** Frontal radiograph shows compression of the body of L2. **B:** Lateral view shows compression of the superior aspects of L1, L2, and L3. There is posterior bowing of the posterior vertebral body line of L2 (*arrow*). **C:** CT scan through the middle of L2 shows no abnormality. **D:** CT scan through the upper portion of the vertebra shows compression of the anterior margin of the body on the right and a transverse process fracture on the right. There is straightening of the posterior vertebral body line (*arrows*), an extremely subtle finding. Compare with C. This case is an example of the situation in which the plain film findings are far more dramatic than on the CT scan.

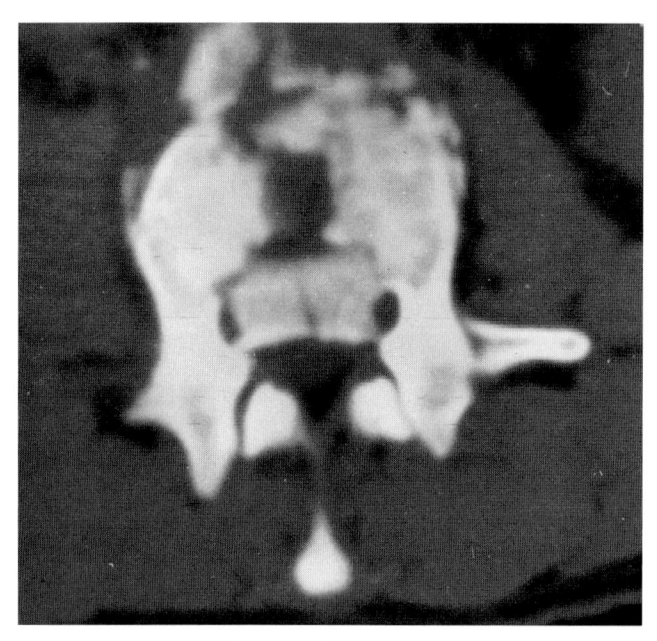

FIG. 29. CT scan of a classic burst fracture. Note the severe comminution of the vertebral body and retropulsion of a large fragment into the vertebral canal.

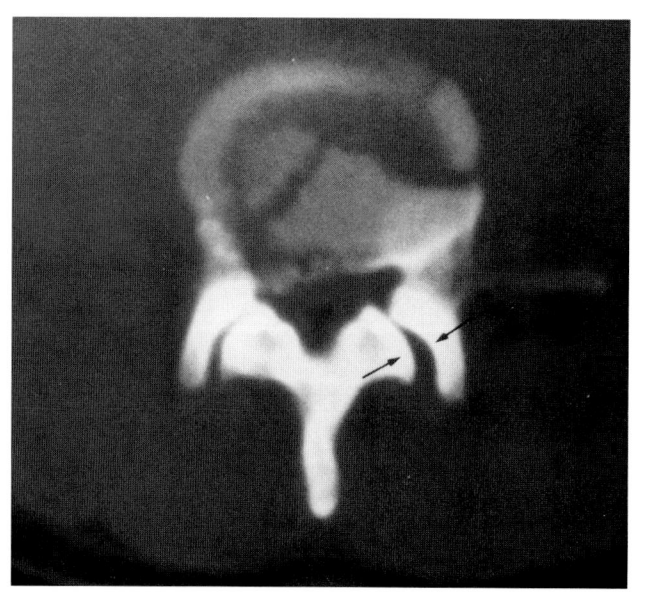

FIG. 31. Facet joint disruption in a patient with a rotary ("grinding") injury. Note the widening of the facet joint and malalignment on the left (*arrows*).

able, it is often tempting to avoid the simpler studies to proceed with a technically more sophisticated study. This is a practice to be avoided. The plain film serves as a road map to guide the radiologist and surgeon to the correct diagnosis. I have seen many instances in which a CT examination was erroneously interpreted as being normal in the presence of very obvious pathology on plain film (Fig. 28).

Computerized tomography further delineates the extent of injury and is the best method for determining the presence and degree of canal encroachment (26,34,35,45) (Fig. 29). It also is useful for demonstrating injuries to the lamina (34,45) (Fig. 30) and disruptions of the facet joints (Fig. 31). The ability to perform sagittal and coronal reconstruction, particularly at the cervicothoracic junction, is also important (12,13) (Fig. 32).

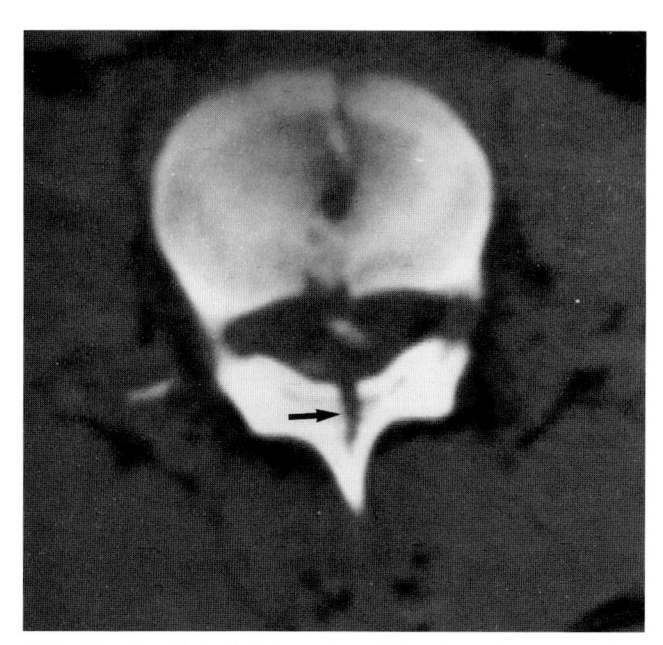

FIG. 30. Sagittal cleft-type burst fracture (same patient as Fig. 29). CT scan shows fractures through the vertebral body as well as through the lamina (*arrow*).

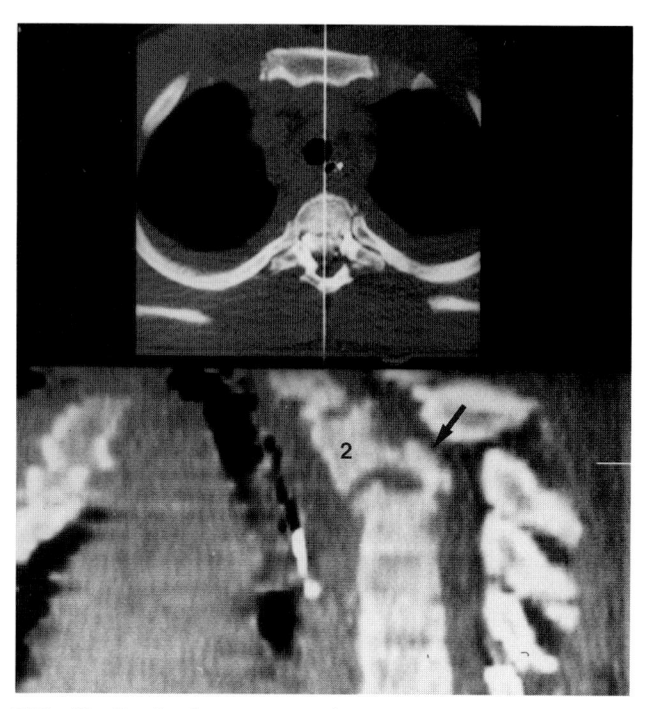

FIG. 32. Sagittal reconstruction as an aid to diagnosis (same patient as Fig. 4). Sagittal reconstruction through the midline shows the fracture–dislocation of T2 on T3. Note the large fragment of T3 within the vertebral canal (*arrow*). (From ref. 10.)

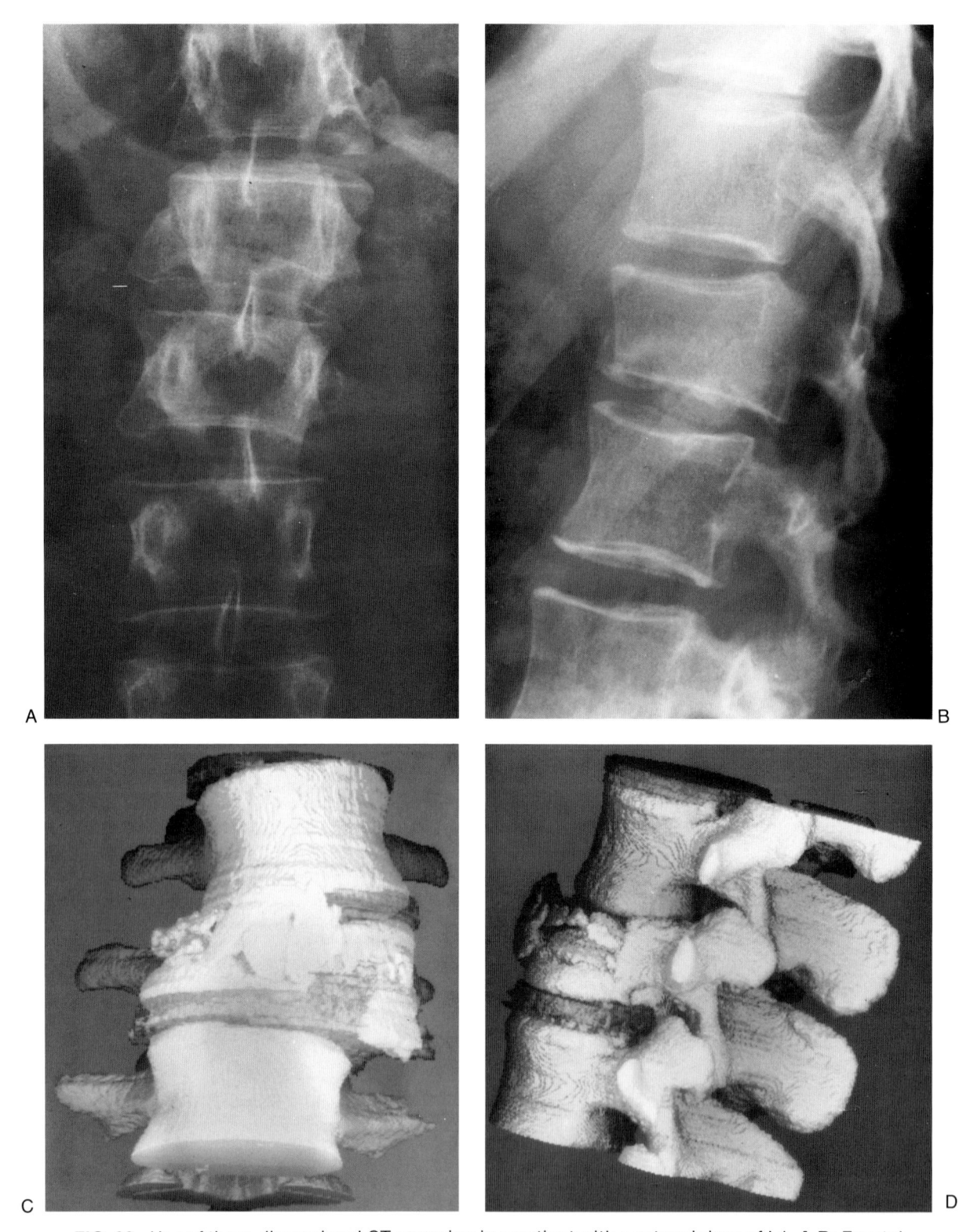

FIG. 33. Use of three-dimensional CT scanning in a patient with a rotary injury of L1. **A,B:** Frontal (A) and lateral (B) plain radiographs show a severely disruptive injury of L1. **C,D:** Frontal (C) and lateral (D) three-dimensional reconstructions of a similar injury show the spatial relationships of the bone fragments. (From ref. 13.)

In some institutions, CT scans may be combined with myelography using low osmolar water-soluble contrast (13). This study is often performed where magnetic resonance imaging is not available. Computerized tomography/myelography is useful in the cervical region for studying cervical root avulsion and post-traumatic cystic myelopathy (syringomyelia) (13,36).

Improvements in computer techniques have now made it possible to obtain three-dimensional (3-D) reconstruction from CT images. Surgeons find this technique useful to determine the spatial relationships of bone fragments. The applications to the vertebral column have been limited; most of the work has been confined to the cervical region (49). Most radiologists, including myself, do not find any particular advantage to the technique (Fig. 33).

Pitfalls of Computerized Tomography

There are several limitations and pitfalls in the use of CT scans for the evaluation of vertebral trauma. These may be categorized into patient-related and technical-related. Patient-related pitfalls are the result of motion, patient size, and artifacts from metallic implants. Motion results in blurred images and the possibility of misdiagnosis. In most instances, however, this is not a significant factor because it is possible to control patient motion pharmacologically. A more serious problem is that of the extremely large patient. Most CT scanners have a limit of 300 to 350 pounds as the maximum weight that the extended gantry can support. Furthermore, patients of extremely large girth may come in contact with the gantry wall, thus producing additional artifacts.

The presence of surgical rods or other surgical hardware from previous stabilization attempts causes artifacts that seriously detract from the CT image. In these patients, it may be necessary to perform conventional tomography for adequate evaluation.

There are three technical factors that may result in pitfalls. These are (a) the averaging effect, (b) poor level calibration, and (c) fractures in the plane of scan.

The partial volume averaging effect is a well-known pitfall in CT scans. The CT image represents an average of the radiographic densities of all the structures contained within that section of tissue. Any structure that is not completely located within the plane may be distorted or totally discarded from the final image. Most important, segments from a contiguous level may be projected onto the image with the resultant appearance of a "fracture" (Fig. 34). This is most likely to occur in a patient with severe kyphosis or scoliosis. In most instances, the partial averaging effect causes diagnostic difficulties in the cervical region. We have not found it to be a significant problem in the thoracic or lumbar region. When a partial volume effect is suspected, careful correlation with a scout film is mandated.

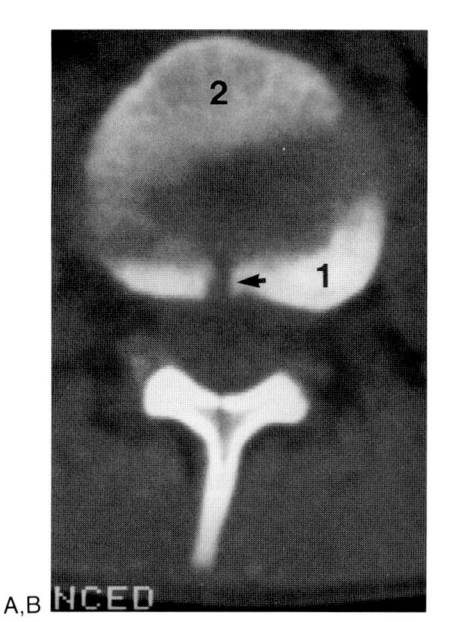

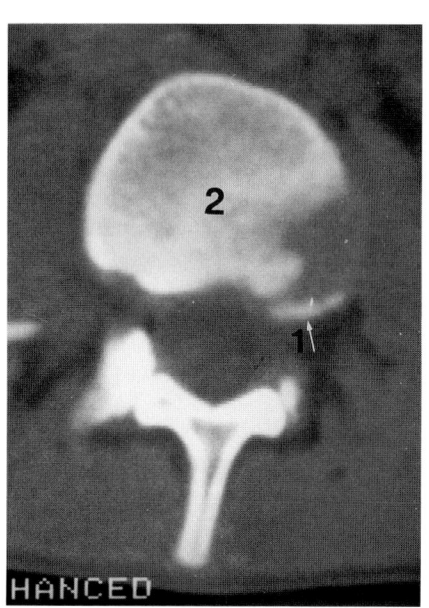

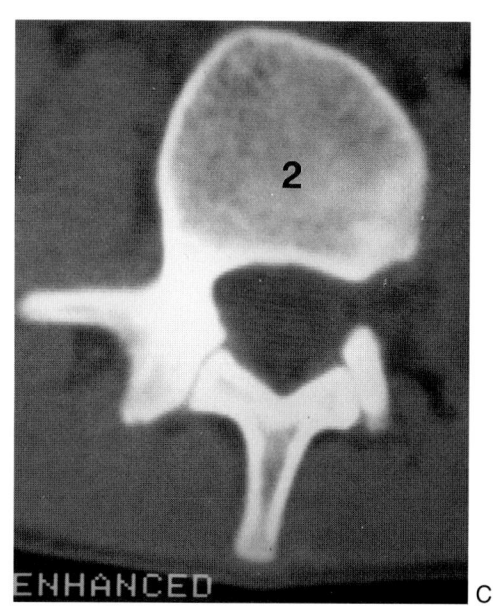

FIG. 34. Partial volume averaging effect. **A:** CT scan through the L1 disc space in a patient with an L1 burst fracture. Portions of L1 and L2 are visible on this section. The fracture is seen in the posterior aspect of L1 (*arrow*). **B:** CT scan slightly lower shows a small bony density (*arrow*) on the left. This represents a portion of L1 and is still within the plane of the scan. **C:** The scan slightly lower shows no fracture of L2. The absence of the posterior elements of L2 on the left is due to scoliosis in this patient that resulted from the injury.

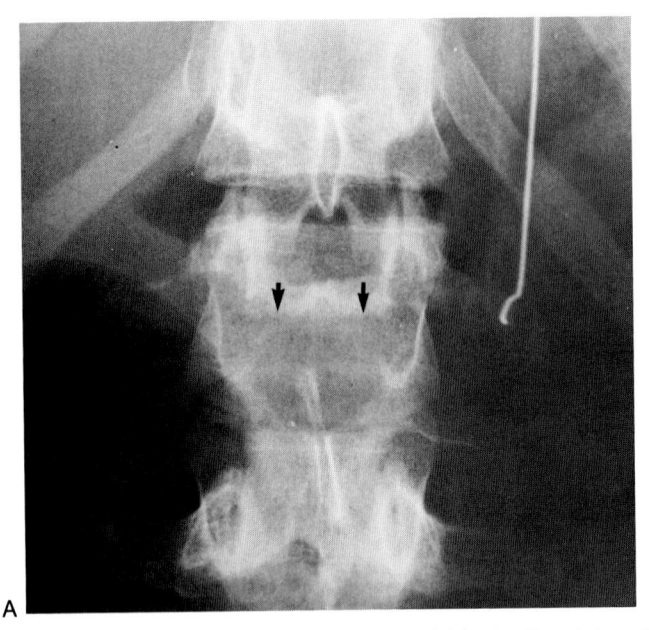

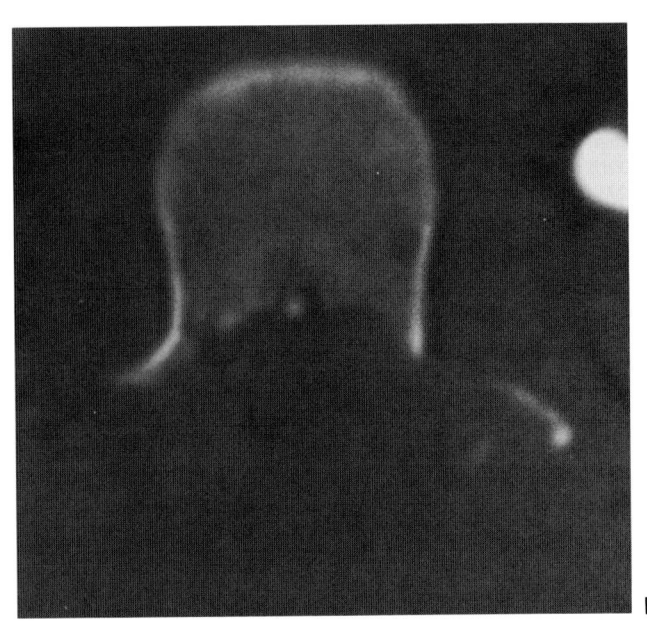

FIG. 35. Chance fracture of L1. **A:** Frontal radiograph shows the fracture through the lamina (*arrows*) and spinous process of L1. **B:** CT scan did not show the fractures as such. There is absence of the posterior element as the result of the posterior distraction. A CT scan is not useful for horizontal injuries.

Occasionally, a discrepancy in annotation on the scout film may result in erroneous information being provided about the level of injury. Again, correlation with plain films will easily overcome this pitfall.

Fractures that are oriented in the plane of the scan such as Chance type fractures may not always be demonstrated by CT scan (Fig. 35). Once again, careful correlation of plain films is recommended. It may also be necessary to tilt the gantry of the CT scanner to demonstrate the fracture. In some cases, it may be necessary to resort to conventional tomography to define the injury.

PLURIDIRECTIONAL TOMOGRAPHY

Conventional pluridirectional tomography is not used as extensively now as it was in the past because of the widespread availability of CT scanners. Nevertheless, there is still a use for this older procedure. Conventional tomography may be used to supplement plain film and CT examinations (13). Although the greatest area of use is in the cervical column, it is particularly useful for evaluating the cervicothoracic junction (Fig. 36) and the posterior elements (Fig. 37).

Pluridirectional tomography is usually performed with the patient in the lateral position. When evaluating defects of the pars interarticularis, it is necessary to obtain only lateral views, since the study will demonstrate both sides. To do dual studies in the oblique projection doubles the radiographic dose, time, and cost of the examination.

There is only one serious pitfall to conventional tomography, and that is the formation of phantom images. This phenomenon is usually caused by projection of the image of a structure located outside the plane of focus across the area of interest (Fig. 38).

MAGNETIC RESONANCE IMAGING

The development of computerized tomography paved the way for other computer-enhanced methods of diagnostic imaging. Less than a decade after computerized tomography was developed, magnetic resonance imaging (MRI) came to center stage. MRI was initially used for evaluation of the brain and spinal cord. In most vertebral studies, the initial interest was related to the diagnosis of diseases of the intervertebral disc. However, it soon became apparent that MRI

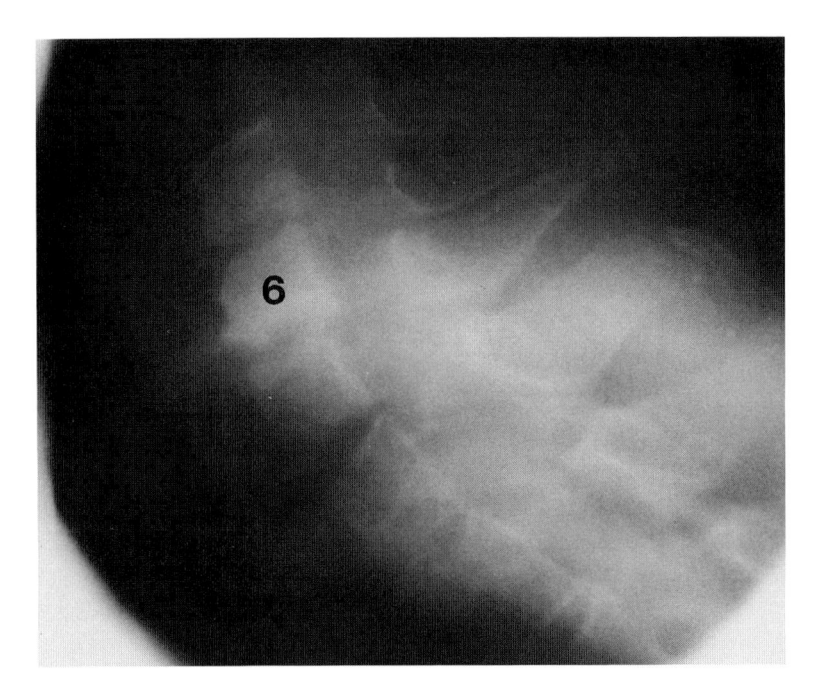

FIG. 36. The value of tomography at the cervicothoracic junction. A lateral midline tomogram of the cervicothoracic junction shows retrolisthesis of C6 on C7. This area could not be delineated on either lateral cervical films or "swimmer views." Tomography is uniquely useful in this region.

could have a great impact on the assessment of patients with acute vertebral injuries. Although plain film radiography and CT scanning have been the mainstays of diagnosis of acute vertebral injury, certain deficiencies, particularly the inability to image changes within the spinal cord, were recognized. MRI is uniquely designed to fill the void and overcome many of the pitfalls of both plain films and CT scans by its ability not only to image the spinal cord but, in certain cases, to define the internal anatomy of that structure. Furthermore, the capability of MRI to image supine patients in multiple planes—sagittal, coronal, and oblique as well as transverse—is a distinct advantage over other imaging methods. MRI also is useful in demonstrating

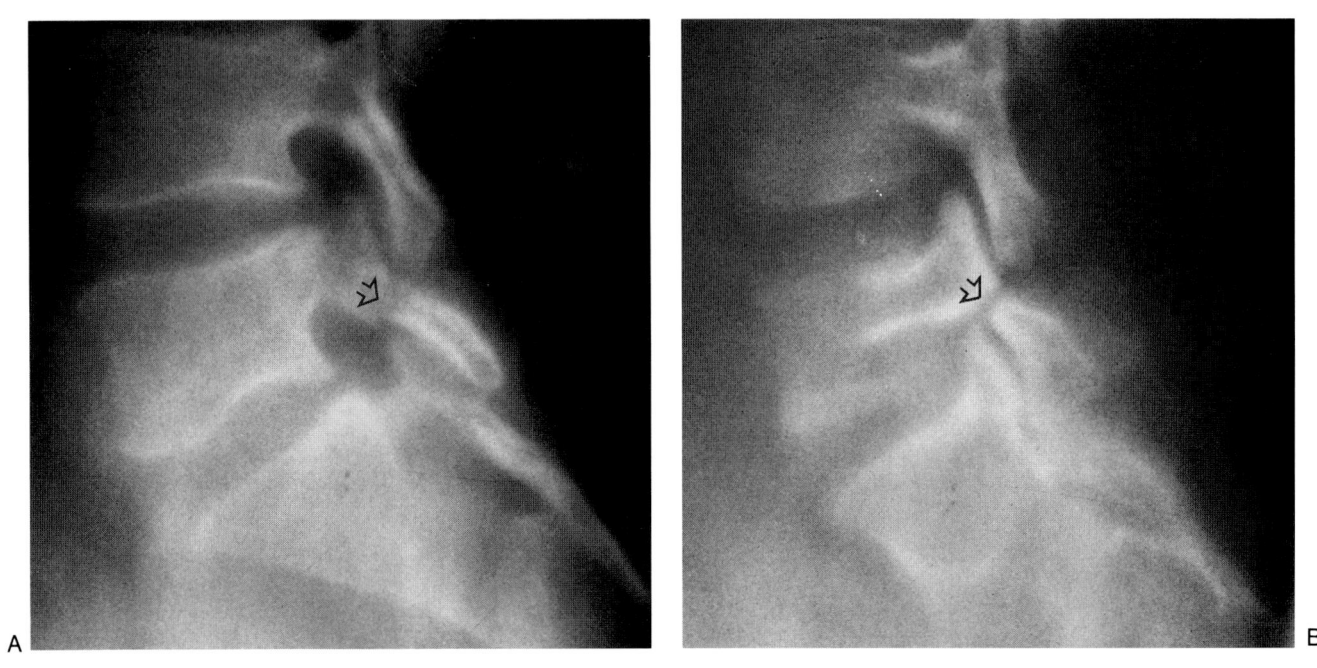

FIG. 37. Bilateral pars interarticularis defects of L5 (*open arrows*). **A:** Right side. **B:** Left side.

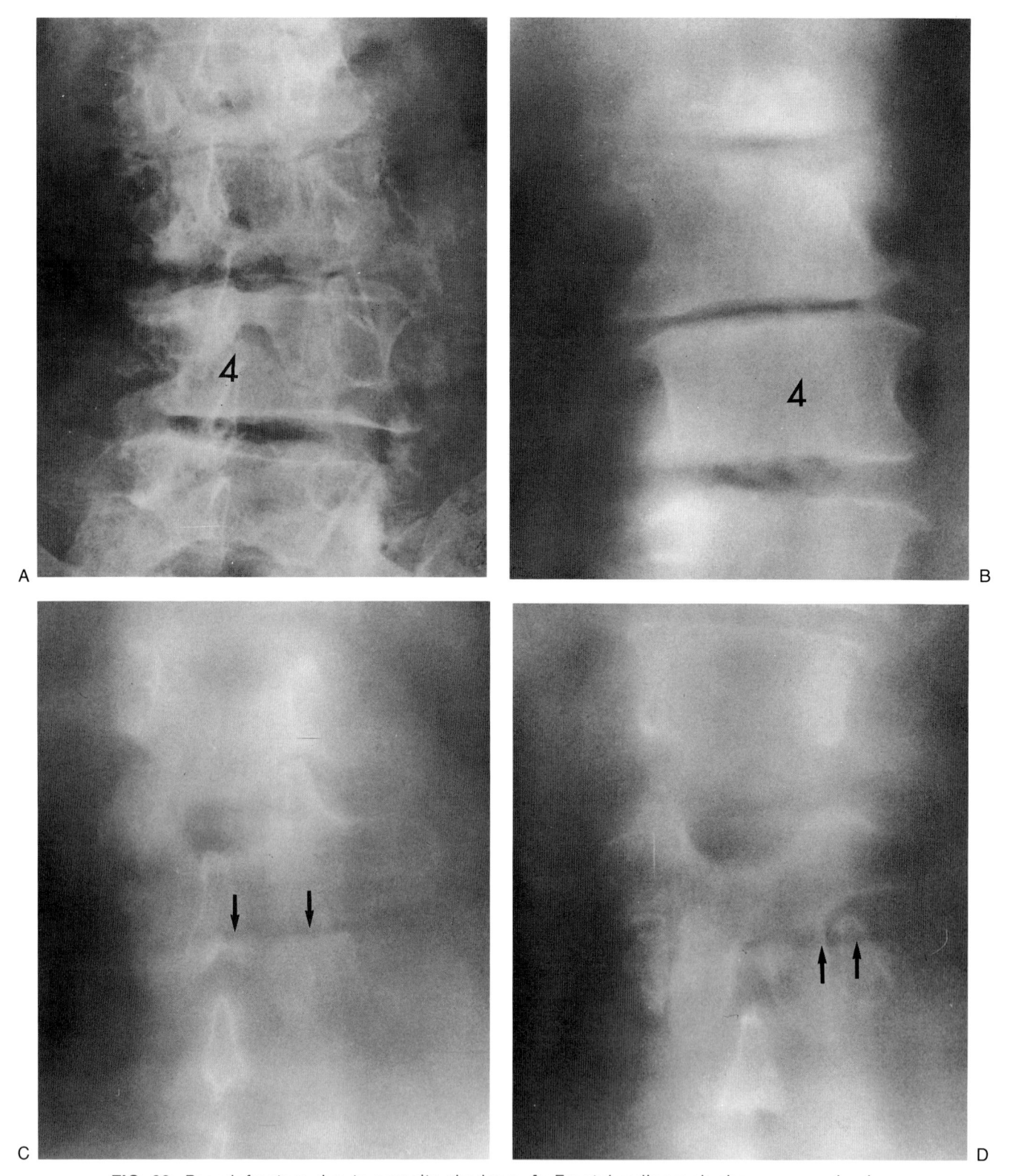

FIG. 38. Pseudofracture due to parasite shadows. **A:** Frontal radiograph shows severe lumbar spondylosis. **B:** Tomogram shows a vacuum phenomenon at the L3 disc space. **C:** Further posteriorly the tomogram shows a lucency crossing the inferior articular process of L3 on the left (*arrows*). **D:** A section slightly more anteriorly shows no evidence of fracture of the L3 inferior articular process. Note the persistent lucency that extends beyond the margin of the bones (*arrows*). This is a phantom image from the vacuum phenomenon in the L3 disc space.

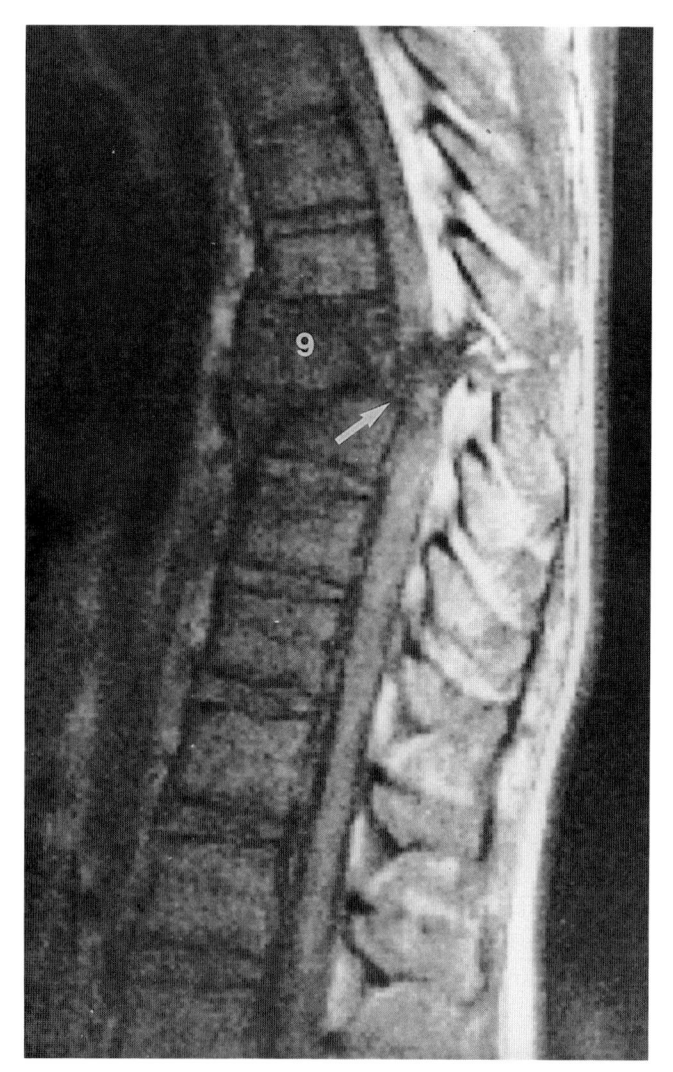

FIG. 39. Cord transection (*arrow*) demonstrated by MRI in a patient with a T9–T10 dislocation.

truding radiofrequency beam, and this energy is detected, amplified, and translated into an image based on the location of those atoms in space. The exact strength of each signal is determined by the chemical composition of the atom in question. This forms the basis for imaging using magnetic resonance. The exact appearance of the images will be dependent on such factors as strength of the magnet, the type of radiofrequency coil used, and the length of echo time (TE) and recovery time (TR).

In our institution, we use the following combination of scanning sequences to obtain specific information: a short sequence (T1-weighting) emphasizing skeletal anatomy and demonstrating vertebral alignment and bony relationships to the spinal cord. This is particularly useful for determining spinal cord compression. This sequence takes approximately 9 min and produces five slices of 5-mm thickness. A second, longer sequence (T2-weighting) is performed to evaluate the interface of the cerebrospinal fluid and extradural space, especially for suspected extradural compression from bone fragments. This sequence produces nine slices of approximately 7-mm thickness and is obtained in 9 min. Both images are produced in the sagittal plane

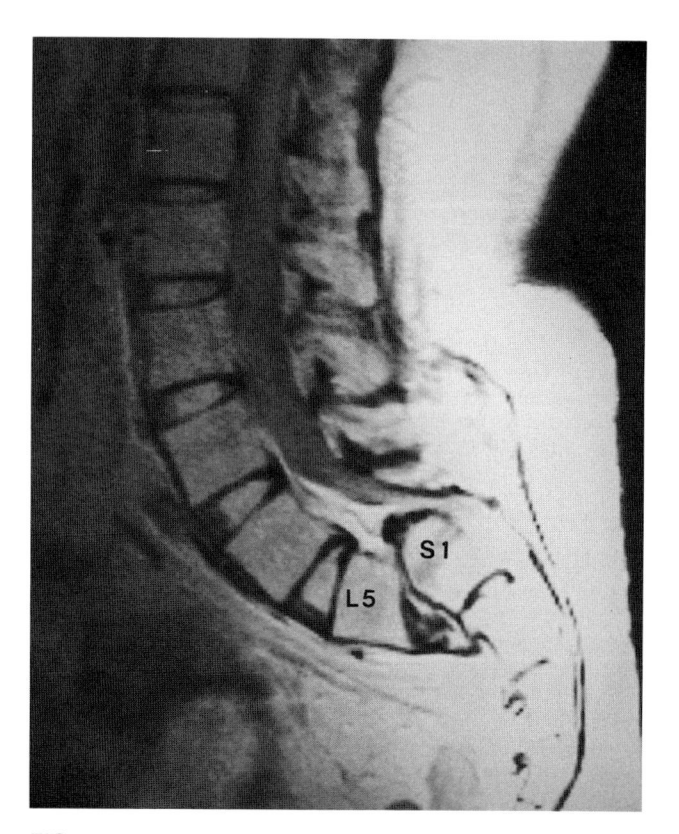

FIG. 40. Fourth degree spondylolisthesis of L5 on S1 demonstrated by MRI.

areas of spinal cord injury, abnormalities of vertebral alignment, and herniation of intervertebral discs (6,23,27,30–32,44,47) (Figs. 39–41).

An in-depth discussion of the principles of MRI is beyond the scope of this book. However, a superficial explanation is in order. Whenever a body is placed within a strong magnetic field, the nuclei of all the atoms, which are normally aligned in a random fashion in that body, orient themselves to the poles of the magnet. When a radiofrequency beam is pulsed at the body, the individual atoms are knocked off their axis of orientation for as long as the radiofrequency beam is activated. When the radiofrequency beam is turned off, the atoms return to their resting "aligned state." They give up the energy that was absorbed by the in-

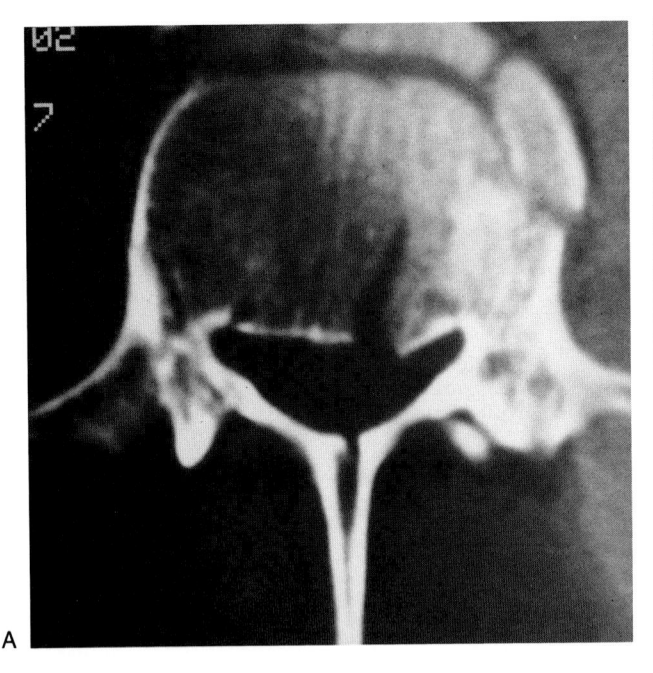

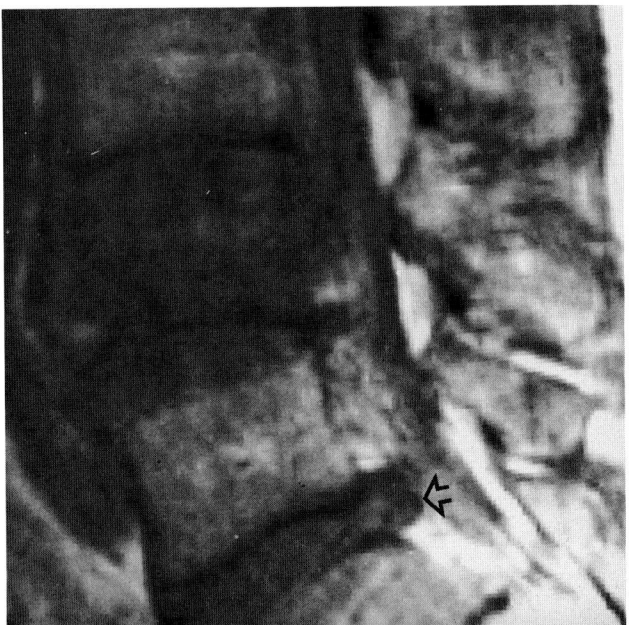

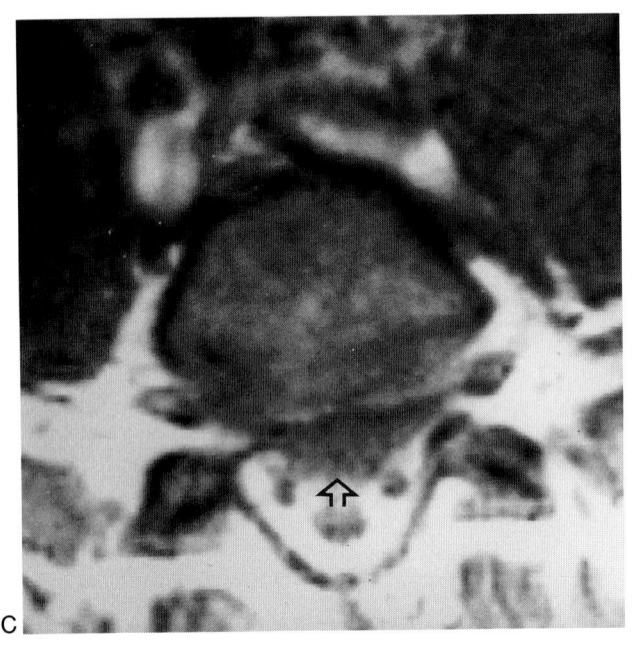

FIG. 41. Lumbar disc herniation accompanying fracture. **A:** CT scan through L4 shows typical changes of a sagittal cleft-type burst fracture. **B:** Sagittal MR image of T1-weighting shows herniated disc material (*open arrow*). **C:** Axial section at the same level again shows herniated disc material (*open arrow*).

(Fig. 42). A third "fast" sequence is obtained on high field strength magnets (1.5 Tesla) using very short scanning parameters. Images are obtained in the sagittal and transverse planes. This type of scan outlines the spinal cord because of the high signal of cerebrospinal fluid. If we are able to obtain only one set of images on a patient, we prefer the long sequence because of the clear-cut separation of spinal cord from cerebrospinal fluid (12,13).

The performance of an MR examination requires that the patient be hemodynamically stable. Life support equipment that is nonferromagnetic is now available to use on patients who require an MR examination. Also, the freedom from any deleterious effects caused by high magnetic fields allows nursing personnel to monitor the patient in the room while the study is being performed. Contraindications to MR examination include any patient who is hemodynamically unstable, any patient with a cardiac pacemaker or prosthetic heart valve, and the presence of recently implanted surgical hardware.

Applications of MRI

There are three areas where MRI excels when compared to other methods of diagnosis: extrinsic injury to the vertebral canal, intrinsic injury to the spinal cord,

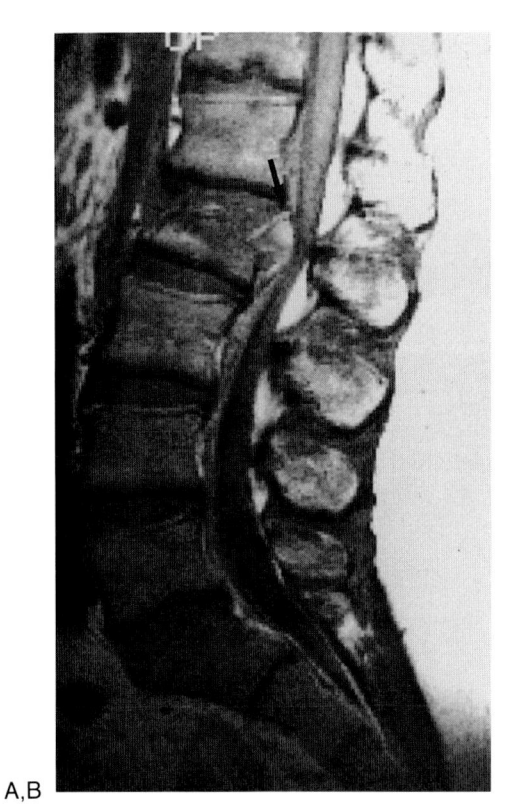

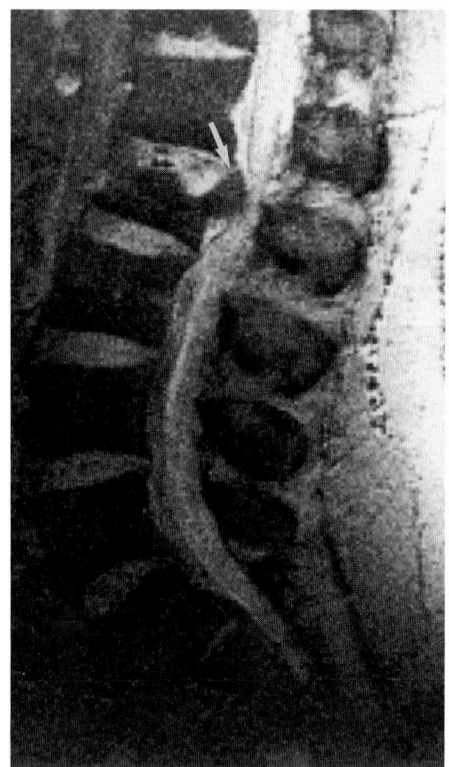

FIG. 42. Difference in appearance between T1-weighting and gradient echo-weighted images in a patient with an L2 burst fracture. **A:** T1-weighted image shows a bone fragment (*arrow*) displaced posteriorly encroaching on the thecal sac. In this study, bone marrow appears gray, the bone margins are black, and the thecal sac is a uniform gray. **B:** Gradient echo image again shows the bone fragment (*arrow*). On this image, the marrow and cortical bones are black. The thecal sac and cerebrospinal fluid are brighter.

and evaluation of the cervicothoracic junction. MRI is extremely useful in determining the relationship of bony fragments that have been displaced into the vertebral canal with the spinal cord (6,23,27,30–32,47) (Fig. 43).

MRI also can show the full extent of injury, including soft tissue damage that may not be apparent (44) (Fig. 43). Herniated intervertebral discs (Fig. 41) may be demonstrated by MRI in both sagittal and transverse planes.

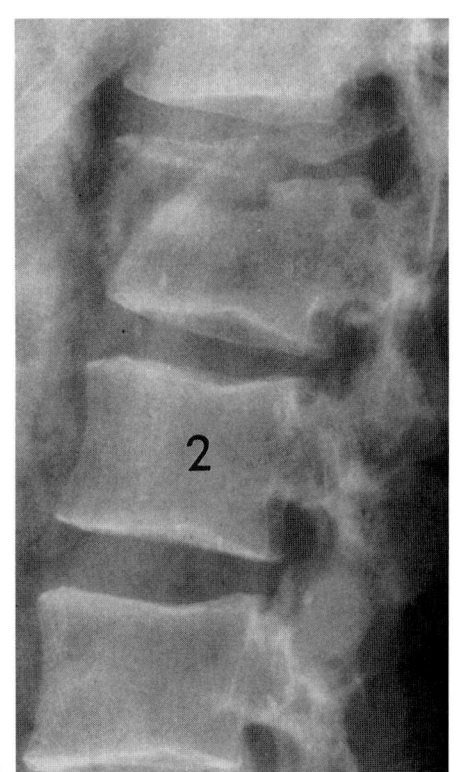

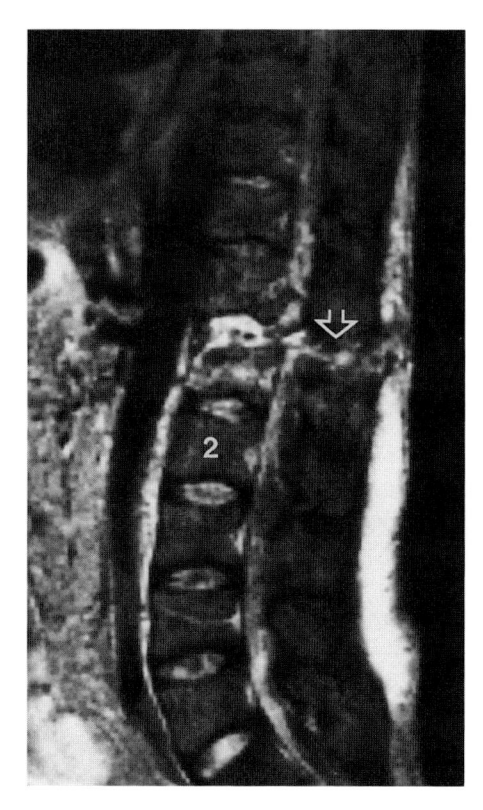

FIG. 43. Rotary ("grinding") injury of L1. **A:** Lateral radiograph shows severe disruption of the L1 vertebra. **B:** T1-weighted MR image shows a severe disruption not only of the vertebral body, but also of the posterior soft tissues (*open arrow*). The bright areas surrounding the fracture represent acute hemorrhage.

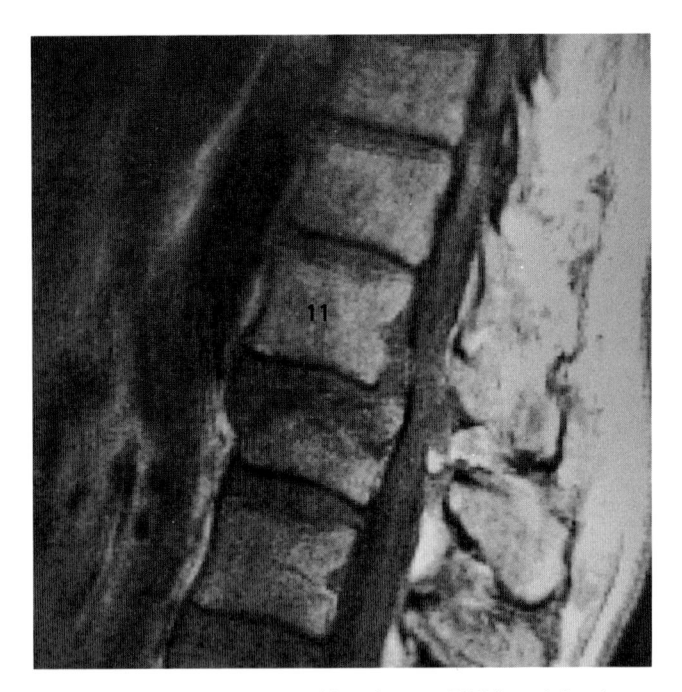

FIG. 44. Cord edema resulting from a T12 burst fracture. This T1-weighted image shows an increase in signal (brightness) adjacent to the retropulsed bone fragment encroaching on the vertebral canal at T12.

The ability of MRI to demonstrate intrinsic injury to the spinal cord has been one of its greatest assets. Recent articles have shown direct correlation between the appearance of the injured spinal cord on MRI and its relation to the recovery of neurologic function (30,31,47). Furthermore, the ability to distinguish between cord contusion, cord edema (Fig. 44), and cord hemorrhage has become more important since the results of a recent study on the use of massive doses of intravenous methylprednisolone for spinal cord-injured patients. Methylprednisolone was shown to have a significant effect on improving neurologic function or progression to complete recovery in patients with edema or contusion. Those patients with cord hemorrhage had no improvement.

The sagittal imaging capability of MRI is especially useful in evaluating the cervicothoracic junction (22). This area is nearly impossible to demonstrate because of the overlying shoulders on plain films and CT scans. MRI can readily show this region and demonstrate abnormalities that would have necessitated lateral tomography in the past (Fig. 45).

MRI has completely superseded myelography in our institution. MR scans are available 24 hours a day, 7 days a week. This should be the case at any major trauma center. It is an integral part of our diagnostic armamentarium for vertebral injuries.

MRI has several disadvantages. The first is that detailed skeletal anatomy is less than provided by CT scans, but correlation with plain films and CT examinations can easily overcome this. Another disadvantage is that patients who require cardiac pacemakers or paramagnetic life support equipment cannot be imaged. As previously mentioned, developments in equipment to allow MRI compatibility have occurred. Finally, improvements in nonmagnetic external fixation devices

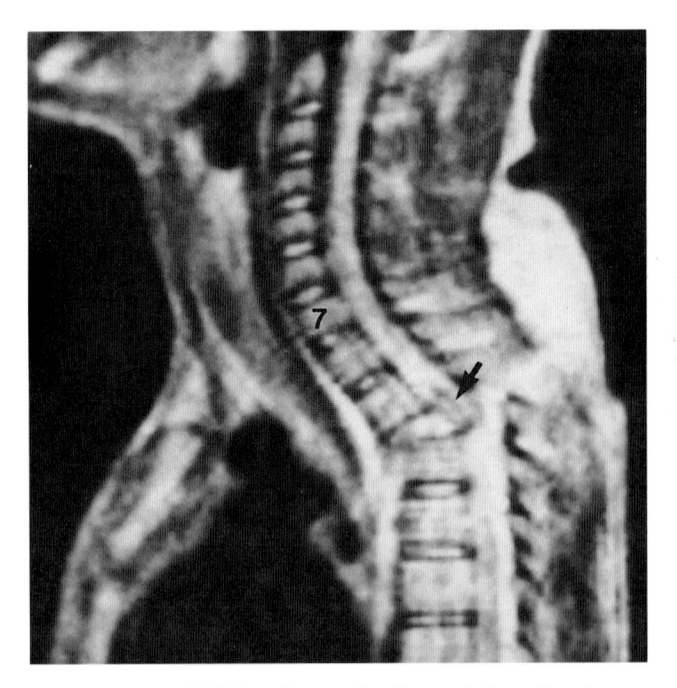

FIG. 45. Use of MRI at the cervicothoracic junction (same patient as Fig. 32). This sagittal T1-weighted image shows the bone fragment from T3 in the vertebral canal (arrow). (From ref. 10.)

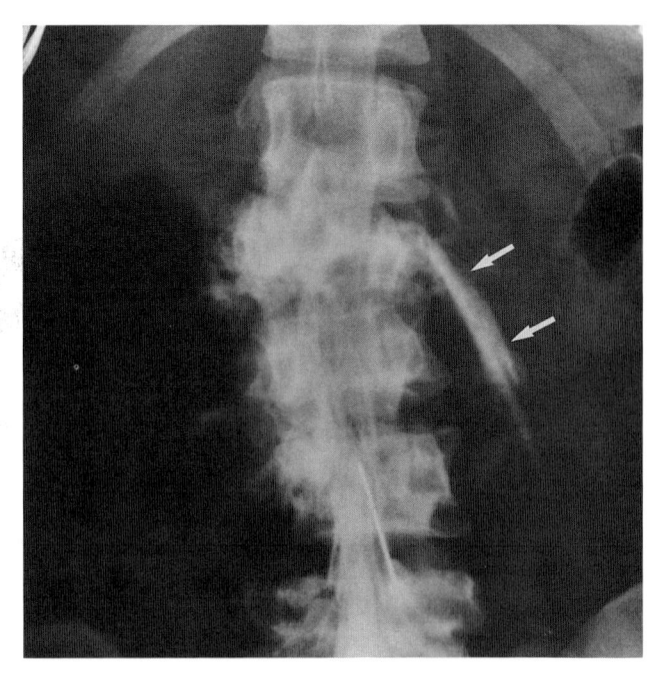

FIG. 46. Dural tear with extravasation of contrast (arrows) following myelography in a patient with a rotary injury of L2. (From ref. 13.)

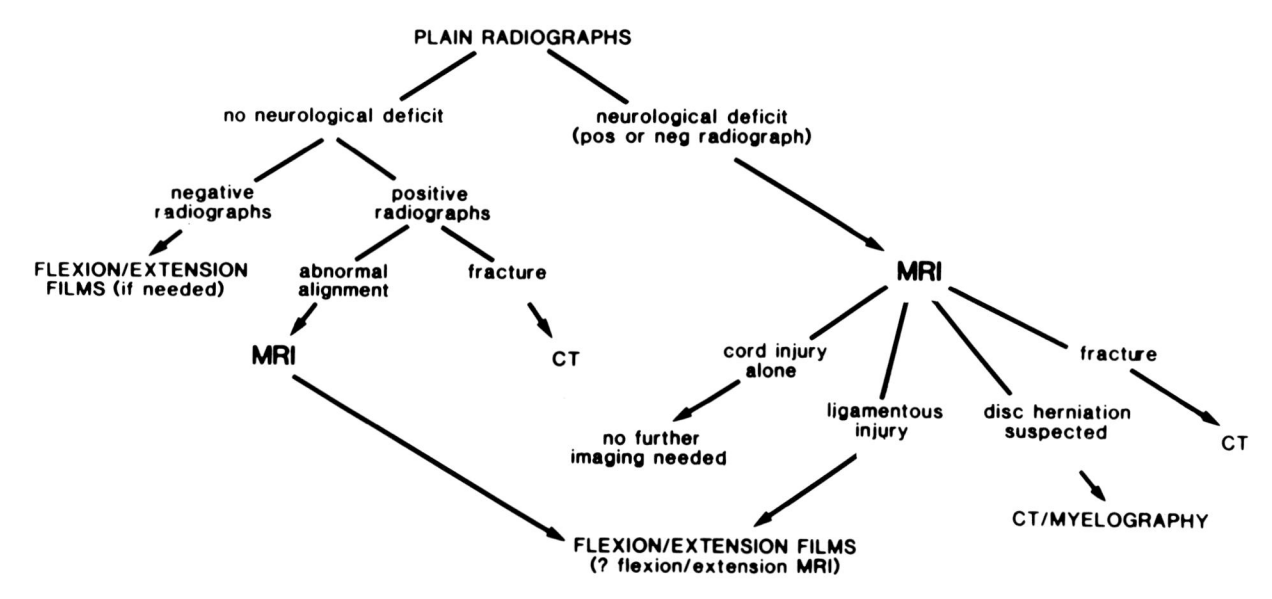

FIG. 47. Imaging algorithm for patients with vertebral injuries. (From ref. 22.)

and cervical halos have made it possible to image patients who have these devices.

MYELOGRAPHY

In the past, myelography was used extensively to determine the blockage of flow of cerebrospinal fluid by bone fragments in the vertebral canal (13,39). As previously mentioned, the use of MRI in many institutions has superseded myelography for this purpose. However, in those hospitals where MRI is not available, myelography may still be useful. In addition to diagnosing blockage of cerebrospinal fluid flow, myelography, particularly when combined with a CT scan, is useful in demonstrating extradural lesions such as herniated intervertebral discs associated with acute injury, the diagnosis of acute traumatic dural tears (36) (Fig. 46), and in the cervical region, the evaluation of nerve root avulsions. In addition, myelography in combination with a CT scan is useful for evaluating post-traumatic cystic myelopathy (syringomyelia).

SUMMARY

The surgeon caring for the patient who has suffered an injury to the thoracic or lumbar vertebral column now has at his/her disposal a large number of studies to evaluate the patient. The initial diagnosis will be made from clinical examination and plain films supplemented by more sophisticated imaging studies such as CT scans or MRI. Figure 47 shows the algorithm used in our hospital for the radiologic evaluation of patients with acute vertebral injuries. It should serve as a guideline for the clinicians who must remember that each evaluation must be tailor-made.

REFERENCES

1. Atlas SA, Regenbogen V, Rogers LF, et al. The radiographic characterization of burst fractures of the spine. *AJR* 1986;147: 575.
2. Bedbrook GM. Stability of spinal fractures and fracture dislocations. *Paraplegia* 1971;9:23.
3. Brant-Zawadzki M, Miller EM, Federle MP. CT in the evaluation of spine trauma. *AJR* 1981;136:369.
4. Brant-Zawadzki M, Jeffrey RB, Minagi H, et al. High resolution CT of thoracolumbar fractures. *AJNR* 1982;3:69.
5. Calenoff L, Chessare JW, Rogers LF, et al. Multiple level spinal injuries: importance of early recognition. *AJR* 1978;130:665.
6. Chakeres DW, Flickinger F, Bresnahan JC, et al. MR imaging of acute spinal cord trauma. *AJNR* 1987;8:5.
7. Chance GQ. Note on a type of flexion fracture of the spine. *Br J Radiol* 1948;21:452.
8. Daffner RH, Deeb ZL, Rothfus WE. "Fingerprints" of vertebral trauma—a unifying concept based on mechanisms. *Skeletal Radiol* 1986;15:518.
9. Daffner RH, Deeb ZL, Rothfus WE. The posterior vertebral body line: importance in the detection of burst fractures. *AJR* 1987;148:93.
10. Daffner RH, Deeb ZL, Rothfus WE. Thoracic fractures and dislocations in motorcyclists. *Skeletal Radiol* 1987;16:280.
11. Daffner RH. Injuries of the thoracolumbar vertebral column. In: Dalinka MK, Kaye JJ, eds. *Radiology in emergency medicine.* New York: Churchill Livingstone, 1984;317–341.
12. Daffner RH. Thoracic and lumbar vertebral trauma. *Orthop Clin North Am* 1990;21:463.
13. Daffner RH. *Imaging of vertebral trauma.* Rockville MD: Aspen Publishers, 1988.
14. Daffner RH. Case report #570. *Skeletal Radiol* 1989;18: 489–490.
15. Daffner RH, Deeb ZL, Goldberg AL, et al. The radiologic assessment of post-traumatic vertebral stability. *Skeletal Radiol* 1990;19:103.
16. Denis F. The three column spine and its significance in the classification of acute thoracolumbar spinal injuries. *Spine* 1983;8:817.

17. Denis F. Spinal instability as defined by the three-column spine concept in acute spinal trauma. *Clin Orthop* 1984;189:65.
18. Ferguson RL, Allen BL. A mechanistic classification of thoracolumbar spine fractures. *Clin Orthop* 1984;189:77.
19. Gehweiler JA, Daffner RH, Osborne RL. Relevant signs of stable and unstable thoracolumbar vertebral column trauma. *Skeletal Radiol* 1981;7:179.
20. Gehweiler JA, Osborne RL, Becker RF. *The radiology of vertebral trauma*. Philadelphia: Saunders, 1980.
21. Gelman MI, Umber JS. Fractures of the thoracolumbar spine in ankylosing spondylitis. *AJR* 1978;130:485.
22. Goldberg AL, Rothfus WE, Deeb ZL, et al. The impact of magnetic resonance on the diagnostic evaluation of acute cervicothoracic spinal trauma. *Skeletal Radiol* 1988;17:89.
23. Goldberg AL, Deeb ZL, Rothfus WE, Daffner RH. Magnetic resonance imaging in evaluation of acute spinal trauma. In: *Spine: state of the art reviews*, vol 14, no 2. Philadelphia: Hanley and Belfus, Inc. 1989;339–348.
24. Goldberg AL, Daffner RH, Schapiro RL. Imaging of acute spinal trauma: an evolving multimodality approach. *Clin Imaging* 1990; 14:11.
25. Grisolia A, Bell RL, Peltier LF. Fractures and dislocations of the spine complicating ankylosing spondylitis. *J Bone Joint Surg* 1967;49A:339.
26. Guerra J Jr, Garfin SR, Resnick D. Vertebral burst fractures: CT analysis of the retropulsed fragment. *Radiology* 1984;153: 769.
27. Hackney DB, Asato R, Joseph PM, et al. Hemorrhage and edema in acute spinal cord compression: demonstration by MR imaging. *Radiology* 1986;161:387.
28. Holdsworth FW. Review article: fractures, dislocations, and fracture–dislocations of the spine. *J Bone Joint Surg* 1970;52A: 1534.
29. Jacobs RR, Casey MP. Surgical management of thoracolumbar spinal injuries: general principles and controversial considerations. *Clin Orthop* 1984;189:22.
30. Kadoya S, Nakamura T, Kobayashi S, et al. Magnetic resonance imaging of acute spinal cord injury: report of three cases. *Neuroradiology* 1987;29:252.
31. Kulkarni MV, McArdle CB, Kopanicky D, et al. Acute spinal cord injury: MR imaging at 1.5 T. *Radiology* 1987;164:837.
32. Kulkarni MV, Bondurant FJ, Rose SL, et al. 1.5 Tesla magnetic resonance imaging of acute spinal trauma. *Radiographics* 1988; 8:1059.
33. Kupferschmid JP, Weaver ML, Raves JR, Diamond DL. Thoracic spine injuries in victims of motorcycle accidents. *J Trauma* 1989;29:593.
34. Lindahl S, Willen J, Nordwall A, Irstram L. The crush-cleavage fracture: a "new" thoracolumbar unstable fracture. *Spine* 1983; 8:559.
35. McAfee PC, Yuan HA, Lasda NA. The unstable burst fracture. *Spine* 1983;7:365.
36. Morris RE, Hasso AN, Thompson JR, et al. Traumatic dural tears: CT diagnosis using metrizamide. *Radiology* 1984;152:443.
37. O'Callaghan JP, Ullrich CG, Yuan HA, et al. CT of facet distraction in flexion injuries of the thoracolumbar spine: the "naked" facet. *AJNR* 1980;1:97.
38. Panjabi MM, Hausfield JN, White AA. A biomechanical study of ligamentous stability of the thoracic spine in man. *Acta Orthop Scand* 1981;52:315.
39. Pay NT, George AE, Benjamin MV, et al. Positive and negative contrast myelography in spinal trauma. *Radiology* 1977;123:103.
40. Post MJD, Green BA, Quencer RM, et al. The value of computed tomography in spinal trauma. *Spine* 1982;7:417.
41. Powell JN, Waddell JP, Tucker WS, Transfeldt EE. Multiple-level noncontiguous spinal fractures. *J Trauma* 1989;29:1146.
42. Roaf R. A study of the mechanics of spinal injuries. *J Bone Joint Surg* 1960;42B:810.
43. Rogers LF. The roentgenographic appearance of transverse or Chance fractures of the spine: the seat-belt fracture. *AJR* 1971; 111:844.
44. Rothfus WE, Goldberg AL, Deeb ZL, Daffner RH. MR recognition of posterior lumbar vertebral fracture. *J Comput Assist Tomogr* 1990;14:790.
45. Smith GR, Northrop CH, Loop JW. Jumper's fractures: patterns of thoracolumbar spine injuries associated with vertical plunges. *Radiology* 1977;122:657.
46. Smith WS, Kaufer H. Patterns and mechanisms of lumbar injuries associated with lap seat belts. *J Bone J Surg* 1969;51A:239.
47. Tarr RW, Drolshagen LF, Kerner TC, et al. MR imaging of recent spinal trauma. *J Comput Assist Tomogr* 1987;11:412.
48. Willen JAG, Gaekwad UH, Kakulas BA. Burst fractures in the thoracic and lumbar spine. A clinico-neuropathologic analysis. *Spine* 1990;14:1316.
49. Wojcik WG, Edeiken-Monroe BS, Harris JH. Three-dimensional computed tomography in acute cervical spine trauma: a preliminary report. *Skeletal Radiol* 1987;16:261.

8

Electrophysiology of the Normal and Diseased Spine

Jörg Herdmann and Jiří Dvořák

As described in Chapter 11 by Stauffer, fractures of the thoracolumbar spine result in a wide variety of neurological syndromes caused by damage (a) to the spinal cord, including the conus medullaris with its parasympathetic structures; (b) to the motor and sensory nerve roots, including the cauda fibers; and (c) to the paraspinal sympathetic system.

Neurophysiological examinations must help in answering the following questions:

Which neural elements are involved?
Which spinal segment is responsible for a mechanical or other irritation?
Is the lesion chronic, acute, or progressing, or has neural function improved?

In spinal trauma with severe neural malfunction, other major questions relate to the prognosis of the neurological deficit.

Another field of growing importance for neurophysiological techniques is intraoperative monitoring of cord pathways during spinal reconstructive surgery, which, however, is not the subject of this chapter.

Table 1 shows the different neurophysiological tests, together with the neural structures that they help to evaluate. Whereas somatosensory evoked potentials (SEPs) and motor evoked potentials (MEPs) are most helpful in the investigation of the central nervous system pathways, electromyography (EMG), conventional neurography, and F-wave and H-reflex studies are most useful for evaluation of the peripheral segments of the sensory and motor pathways. The different neural elements and the connecting pathways are schematically shown in Fig. 1.

Sophisticated SEP techniques allow for scrutiny of the neural elements of the sensory pathways shown: the dorsal roots, the root entry zone, the dorsal horns, the dorsal columns, the dorsal column nuclei, the lemniscal fibers, and the thalamus and its projections to the primary and secondary sensory areas of the cortex. MEPs allow for assessment of lesions that affect the upper motor neuron and lesions that affect the motor root, plexus fibers, or peripheral nerve segments of

TABLE 1. *Neurophysiological techniques used for evaluation of different neural structures*

Neurophysiological technique	Neural structures evaluated
Somatosensory evoked potentials (SEPs)	Sensory nerve fibers and dorsal roots, spinal cord dorsal columns
Motor evoked potentials (MEPs)	Corticospinal tract (lateral spinal cord), motor roots and motor nerve fibers
Neurography	Motor and sensory nerve fibers
F-wave	Motor roots, motor nerve fibers
H-reflex	Dorsal and motor roots, sensory and motor nerve fibers
Electromyography (EMG) of limb muscles	Motor roots and motor nerve fibers
of paraspinal muscles	Motor roots
Sympathetic skin response (SSR)	(Paraspinal) sympathetic system

---

J. Herdmann: Department of Neurosurgery, Heinrich-Heine-University of Düsseldorf, 4000 Düsseldorf 1, Germany.
J. Dvořák: Department of Neurology, Spine Unit, W. Schulthess Hospitals, 8008 Zürich, Switzerland.

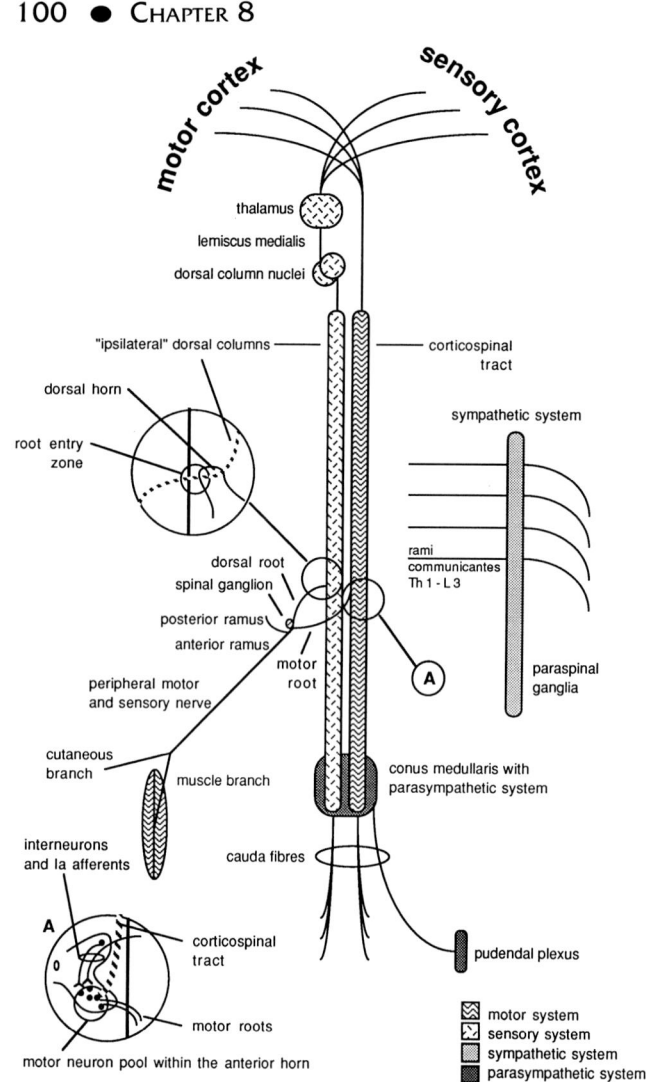

FIG. 1. Diagram of the motor, sensory, and autonomic systems with their neural elements.

the lower motor neuron. EMG of limb and paraspinal muscles allows for distinction between affection of motor roots and of more peripheral nerve elements. EMG allows for a level diagnosis and for evaluation of peripheral nerve disease and offers information regarding the age of the lesion. Neurography, F-wave, and H-reflex studies also allow for distinction between proximal root and peripheral nerve disease. Fractionated peripheral nerve stimulation helps to localize a circumscript peripheral lesion. An autonomic nervous system malfunction is difficult to assess. The sympathetic skin response (SSR) has proved helpful in the evaluation of autonomic peripheral neuropathy (91) and in differential diagnosis of erectile impotence (58). Its applicability to thoracolumbar lesions will be discussed. Clinical tests such as the pilomotor reflex, the sweat test, or thermography are often more helpful.

SOMATOSENSORY EVOKED POTENTIALS

In the context of spinal cord evaluation, only *short-latency somatosensory evoked potentials* are of relevance. These are potentials recorded from the lumbar or cervical spine as well as the first components of scalp recordings. Mid- and long-latency components of scalp recorded potentials show great inter- and intraindividual variability highly dependent on alertness and psychological factors. These components are relevant for neuropsychological evaluation.

Stimulation and Recording Techniques

SEPs are generally recorded after electric stimulation of peripheral nerves. The nerves used are the median, radial, or ulnar nerves of the upper limbs and the posterior tibial, sural, or common peroneal nerves of the lower limbs. In *neuro-urologic* involvement with bladder dysfunction or erectile impotence, SEPs can also be recorded after pudendal nerve stimulation. In radicular and in spinal disease, several nerves, which are supplied by different segments, must be stimulated for a level diagnosis. In cervical radiculopathy, digits may also be stimulated. Table 2 shows the nerves and digits that are used in a level diagnosis. Dermatomal stimulation and motor point stimulation have been proposed by several authors, but even with the absence of technical problems, these procedures revealed inconsistent results. As one can see from Table 2, there are no nerves that have been used in a thoracic level diagnosis.

TABLE 2. *Nerves stimulated and muscles recorded from in SEP and MEP studies, respectively, for evaluation of cervical and lumbosacral radiculopathies*

Segment	Nerve	Muscle
C5, (C6)	N. cutaneus antebrachii lateralis	M. deltoideus
C6, (C7)	N. radialis digit I	M. biceps brachii
C7	N. medianus digits II and III	M. abductor pollicis brevis
C8	N. ulnaris digit V	M. abductor digiti minimi
(L3), L4	N. saphenus	M. quadriceps femoris
(L4), L5	N. peroneus	M. tibialis anterior M. extensor digitorum brevis
(L4, L5), S1, (S2)	N. tibialis posterior	M. gastrocnemius
	N. suralis	M. abductor hallucis
S2–S4	N. pudendus	M. sphincter ani externus

Electric square wave pulses of 100- to 200-μsec duration are applied to the peripheral nerve by surface or needle electrodes at a rate of 3 to 5/sec. In mixed sensory and motor nerves the intensity is varied according to the motor threshold of those muscles controlled by the nerve. Most important is the patient's appreciation of the stimulus intensity. The intensity is adjusted to produce minimal movement of the fingers or toes, depending on the nerve stimulated. In most cases, a stimulator output current of 20 mA is sufficient. Inadequate stimulation (poor placement or insufficient intensity) may result in absent SEPs or scalp potentials of reduced amplitude. Stimulation of one limb at a time should be preferred to bilateral stimulation, which generally results in SEPs of larger amplitude. If bilateral stimulation is used, the normal waveforms generated by the good side conceal the abnormal evoked potentials of the bad side.

The stimulating electrodes, which are the easiest to use, are those that have two metal disks embedded in plastic and that can be held at the proper stimulus site by adhesive tape, elastic, or a Velcro band. Needle electrodes can be used to stimulate more closely to the nerve and thus reduce the amount of current flow needed for stimulation. As in conventional sensory neurography, the cathode of the pair of stimulating electrodes should be located proximal to the anode. For details and descriptions of stimulator devices see the section entitled "Nerve Conduction Studies."

Conventional EMG AC-amplifiers, which allow for an amplification of 100,000 to 500,000, may be used. Filter settings should be 1 to 20 Hz high pass (low cutoff) and 2000 to 3000 Hz low pass (high cutoff). Sweep duration should then be set to 50 or 100 msec. The sampling rate should be at least 5000 Hz; that is, a maximal dwell time of 0.2 msec should be used.

Recording electrodes are of the conventional type used for the EEG: either needle or surface electrodes can be used. Impedance should be kept below 5000 ohms. Needle electrodes often show slightly higher values than this.

An average of 100 to 500 sweeps should be taken. Sometimes up to 2000 sweeps are necessary for spinal recordings. In some scalp recordings, a clear potential can already be recognized after the first 10 to 20 sweeps. A second trial should always be performed and superimposed to verify waveform reproducibility.

Conventional SEPs are recorded from the scalp by averaging EEG activity time locked with the electric pulse. Figure 2 shows the international 10–20 system for placement of EEG electrodes. For SEPs, the electrodes are positioned above the leg or hand areas of the primary sensory cortex. These areas are located 2 to 3 cm behind Cz, behind C3 over the left hemisphere, or behind C4 over the right hemisphere. In European

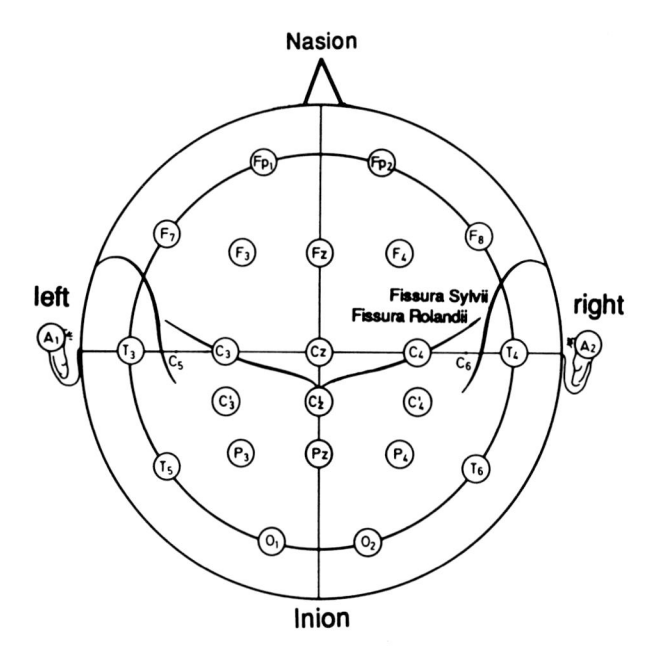

FIG. 2. International 10–20 system for electrode positions for EEG recordings. The positions used for SEP recordings (C3', Cz', and C4') are located 2 cm behind C3, Cz, and C4, respectively.

literature, these electrode positions are often marked with an apostrophe: Cz', C3', and C4'. The reference electrode is preferentially placed at Fz. In addition to scalp recordings, SEPs are also recorded from the lumbar and cervical spine.

In upper limb testing (radial, median, or ulnar nerve), a brachial plexus potential can be recorded from Erb's point. *Erb's point* is in the supraclavicular fossa approximately 2 cm above the midpoint of the clavicle dorsolateral of the sternocleidomastoid muscle. SEP components generated within the different subcortical structures shown in Fig. 1 vary greatly in amplitude and latency, even in normal subjects. For clinical purposes it is necessary to concentrate on components that can be consistently recognized in all normal subjects (6,20). This is achieved with a recording electrode placed at C2, that is, in the midline over the spinous process of the second cervical vertebra. For recordings from Erb's point as well as from C2, the reference electrode is placed at Fz as for recordings from the contralateral scalp.

In lower limb testing (saphenous, peroneal, posterior tibial, or sural nerve) a so-called lumbar potential (LP) can be recorded with the electrode placed in the midline over the L1 spinous process. The reference electrode is preferentially placed on the iliac crest. These cauda equina and lower cord potentials are more difficult to record following sural or saphenous nerve stimulation due to a lack of muscle Ia afferents in these nerves, which contribute a large part of the LP.

The use of Erb's point potential or of the LP as reference potential (reference latency) allows for largely ignoring a slowing in nerve conduction due to neuropathies or due to changes in limb temperature, and greatly diminishes the variation due to different body sizes (20).

Nomenclature, Waveforms, and Normal Values

SEP waveforms represent voltage differences between the reference electrode and the active electrode. If the active electrode is more negative than the reference electrode, a negative potential is recorded and vice versa. As in electromyography, it is agreed that negative potentials point upward. Peaks are labeled with an "N" if the potential underneath the active electrode is negative. Since a voltage difference between two electrodes—namely, the reference electrode and the active electrode—is measured, the potential underneath the reference electrode must then be comparatively more positive and the label "P/N" may also be used as in American literature. Peaks are numbered in order of appearance: N1, N2, and N3 or P1, P2, and P3, and so on. Peaks are more closely defined by adding the mean normal latency, which they are expected to have, to the N or P: for example, "N19" (= "N20" of European literature), which is the first cortical component of the median SEP, or "N/P37" (= "P40" of European literature), the first cortical component of the tibial SEP. In clinical recordings, the latencies actually measured can also be used. In order to distinguish between the observational and the theoretical terminology by latency, the latter should be set in quotation marks ("N19") or marked by a bar on top ($\overline{N19}$).

In the context of thoracolumbar spine disease, only SEPs from lower limb nerves can be expected to reveal disease-related pathology. SEPs from upper limb stimulation are used in order to exclude cervicomedullary, lemniscal, and thalamocortical disorders, which also affect lower limb SEPs. Median and tibial nerve SEP waveforms are described in detail.

Median Nerve SEPs

The median nerve is stimulated at the wrist. For a detailed analysis, recordings should be made at Erb's point, at C2, and over the contralateral scalp (Cc, i.e., C3' or C4'). The reference electrode is placed at Fz for all recordings. Figure 3 shows median SEPs from Erb's point, C2, and Cc.

The potential at Erb's point ("EP") is biphasic with an initial positivity and a large negative peak with a mean latency of about 10 msec ("N10"). The latency

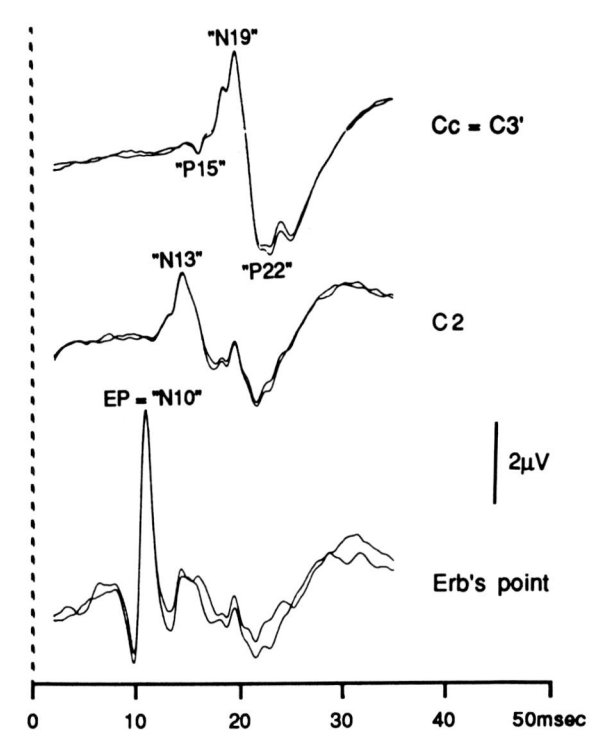

FIG. 3. Normal median nerve SEPs recorded from Erb's point, C2, and C3'.

of the initial positive peak can be used to calculate a conduction velocity of the sensory fibers of the median nerve. The potential recorded from C2 shows a negative deflection with a peak latency of about 13 msec ("N13"). The Fz reference electrode contributes positivities, while the C2 electrode contributes negativities which are generated in or around the dorsal column nuclei (7,52,59,65,71,94).

The scalp response is dominated by a negative peak at 19- to 20-msec latency ("N19") followed by a positivity at 22- to 25-msec latency ("P22"). "N19" is the first cortical response (primary sensory area) to the thalamocortical projections. If the negative peak is split, the second component must be used for measurement of "N19", the first component—usually with a latency of about 18 msec—being of subcortical origin (52,102,104). Sometimes an initial small "P15" can be distinguished, which originates in the thalamus. Amplitude is measured for the "N19" component (baseline-to-peak) or for the "N19"–"P22" wave (peak-to-peak). The "central sensory transit time" is calculated by subtracting the "N13" latency of the C2 recording from the scalp recorded "N19" latency. This is a measure for the total conduction time plus synaptic delay between the dorsal column cuneate nucleus (i.e., the termination of the first sensory neuron) and the cortical neurons of the primary sensory area.

For normal data see Table 3.

TABLE 3. Median nerve SEP: normal values of EP, "N13," "N19," "P22," and interpeak latencies

Peak	Latency (msec)		R − L difference (msec)		Amplitude (μV)		R − L difference (%)	
Study (Reference)	Mean ± SD	Mean + 3SD	Mean ± SD	Mean + 3SD	Mean ± SD	Minimum	Mean ± SD	Maximum
EP recorded from Erb's point–Fz								
Chiappa 1990 (19)	9.7 ± 0.76	12.0	0.20 ± 0.20	0.80	3.0 ± 1.86[a]	0.5		
Stöhr 1989 (93)	10.2 ± 0.88	12.8	0.15 ± 0.08	0.40	3.7 ± 2.30[b]	0.8		48[e]
"N13" = "P/N13" recorded from C2 spinous process–Fz								
Chiappa 1990 (19)	13.5 ± 0.92	16.3			2.3 ± 0.87[b]	0.8		
Stöhr 1989 (93)	13.7 ± 0.88	16.3	0.24 ± 0.20	0.84	1.6 ± 0.69[b]	0.4		38[e]
"N19" = "P/N20" = "N20" recorded from contralateral scalp (Cc, C3' or C4'–Fz)								
Chiappa 1990 (19)	19.0 ± 1.02	22.1			1.0 ± 0.56[b]	0.1	41.7 ± 33.1[d]	141[f]
Stöhr 1989 (93)	19.3 ± 1.19	22.9	0.25 ± 0.33	1.24	2.3 ± 0.99[b]	0.6		46[e]
"P22" = "P25" (European literature) recorded from contralateral scalp (Cc, C3' or C4'–Fz)								
Chiappa 1990 (19)	22.0 ± 1.29	25.9			2.2 ± 1.10[c]	0.5	25.7 ± 21.2[d]	89[f]
Stöhr 1989 (93)	23.1 ± 1.80	28.5		max. 3.3	4.9 ± 2.20[c]	0.9		45[e]
Interpeak latencies								
Chiappa 1990 (19)								
EP–N13	3.8 ± 0.45	5.2	0.2 ± 0.17	0.7				
EP–N19	9.3 ± 0.53	10.9	0.2 ± 0.21	0.8				
N13–N19	5.5 ± 0.42	6.8	0.3 ± 0.25	1.1				
Stöhr 1989 (93)								
EP–N19	9.0 ± 0.77	11.6		max. 1.0				
N13–N19	5.6 ± 0.58	7.3		max. 1.0				

[a] Peak-to-peak.
[b] Baseline-to-peak.
[c] Peak-to-peak "N19"–"P22".
[d] [(abs (R − L))/((R + L)/2)] × 100.
[e] [(abs (R − L))/larger amplitude] × 100.

Tibial Nerve SEPs

The posterior tibial nerve is stimulated behind the malleolus medialis. Recordings should be obtained from the lumbar spine and from the scalp (Cz') (Fig. 4). The lumbar potential (LP) is best recorded by an electrode placed in the midline over the L1 spinous process with a reference electrode two or three levels away or, even better, on the iliac crest, which reduces EKG artifacts. The LP is dominated by a negative peak at 20- to 22-msec latency, which is generated in the gray matter of the root entry zone (89,90) and which is sometimes called "spinal cord response" (S-component) (1). It is the reference point for latency measurements of the spinal cord sensory tracts. Stimulation of the posterior tibial nerve at the ankle usually produces a higher amplitude LP than stimulation of the common peroneal nerve at the knee due to the content of Ia afferents and to the rich innervation of the foot. The ascending potential in the cord gradually disperses due to slightly different conduction velocities of the dorsal column fibers. Its duration increases, whereas its amplitude gradually decreases so that it is usually not recordable above mid- to high thoracic levels. Only a very large number of averaged sweeps (2000–4000) in well relaxed, normal subjects (25) or the use of interspinal ligament needle electrodes (64) allow for reproducible recordings of potentials from the cervical spine after stimulation of lower limb nerves. The initial negative peak of a cervical response recorded at C2

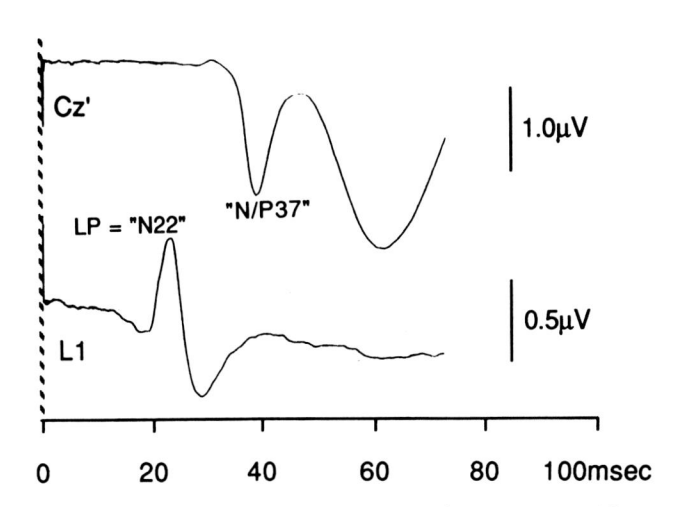

FIG. 4. Normal posterior tibial nerve SEPs recorded from L1 and Cz'.

has a latency of about 27 to 30 msec ("N30"). The site of generation is not definitively known. For these reasons this potential is not helpful in the evaluation of thoracolumbar disorders.

In the common Fz–Cz' derivation, the scalp-recorded potential, after distal stimulation of lower limb nerves, only sometimes begins with a small negative component at 32- to 36-msec latency (N1, "N33") (103). The first positive peak (P1) with latencies between 37 and 40 msec ("N/P37" = "P40" European literature) is more important, because it is always recordable in normals. In analogy to "P15" after median nerve stimulation, "N33" is thought to be generated in the thalamus or thalamocortical projections (51,88), whereas "N/P37" is generated in the parasagittal parietal cortex. Amplitude is generally measured between baseline and "N/P37," or, if the initial "N33" can be distinguished, peak-to-peak between "N33" and "N/P37." In addition to the Fz–Cz' derivation, Chiappa (19) recommends a recording between the contralateral and ipsilateral scalp (Cc–Ci) with the electrodes 2 to 3 cm behind C3 and C4, that is, at C3' and C4'. This waveform is similar to the Fz–Cz' waveform and we do not feel that this derivation provides any important additional information.

For normal data see Table 4.

The peroneal nerve is stimulated at the fibular head of the knee, and the sural nerve is stimulated behind the malleolus externus. Waveforms are similar to tibial nerve SEPs, but amplitudes are smaller. Latencies of the initial components are similar to tibial SEPs in sural nerve stimulation and are about 5 to 6 msec shorter in peroneal nerve stimulation due to the shorter peripheral pathway.

For normal data see Table 5.

Subject Factors Influencing the SEP Results

Obviously, SEP peak latencies are proportional to *body size*. With median nerve SEPs, the effect of different heights on interpeak latencies is insignificant enough that it may be disregarded. With lower limb testing, peak and interpeak latencies must be corrected for height. The following formulas can be used for calculating normalized LP (81) and "N/P37" latencies (93):

$$\text{LP [msec]} = 15.0 \text{ [msec/m]} \times \text{height [m]} - 4.6 \quad r = 0.59$$

$$\text{"N/P37" [msec]} = 17.7 \text{ [msec/m]} \times \text{height [m]} + 9.51 \quad r = 0.749$$

Gender does not significantly influence latencies or amplitudes of SEPs (69) provided that body size is normalized.

Allison et al. (4,5) have performed extensive studies of median nerve SEPs in 286 subjects in an *age* range from 4 to 95 years old. They provided detailed data on latency changes in two age groups: 4 to 17 and 18 to 95 years old. However, apart from children below the age of 10 years, age-dependent changes are only of minor clinical relevance if interpeak latencies are used, excluding peripheral conduction time, and if size is normalized. Cracco et al. (23,24) found that peripheral

TABLE 4. *Posterior tibial nerve SEP: normal values of LP, "N/P37," and interpeak latencies*

Peak	Latency (msec)		R − L difference (msec)		Amplitude (μV)		R − L difference (μV)
Study (Reference)	Mean ± SD	Mean + 3SD	Mean ± SD	Mean + 3SD	Mean ± SD	Minimum	Maximum
LP = S− (spinal) response = "N22" (European literature) recorded from T12/L1–iliac crest							
Chiappa 1990 (19)	19.9 ± 1.8	25.3	0.4 ± 0.28	1.26			
Riffel et al. 1984 (82)	21.8 ± 1.6	26.6		max. 1.20	0.6 ± 0.3[a]	0.15	0.5[b]
"N/P37" = "P40" (European literature) recorded from the scalp (Cz'–Fz)							
Chiappa 1990 (19)	36.3 ± 2.4	43.5	0.7 ± 0.37	1.78			
Riffel et al. 1984 (82)	38.8 ± 2.0	44.8		max. 2.10	1.8 ± 1.3[a]	0.35	2.5[b]
Interpeak latency							
Chiappa 1990 (19) LP–"N/P37"	16.5 ± 1.4	20.7	0.7 ± 0.42	0.84			
Riffel et al. 1984 (82) LP–"N/P37"	17.0 ± 1.7	22.1		max. 3.5			

[a] Baseline-to-peak.
[b] Mean ± 2SD.

TABLE 5. *Peroneal and sural nerve SEP: normal values of LP and "N/P34" and of LP, "N/P40," and interpeak latency*

Site of Stimulation	Peak Study (reference)	Latency (msec) Mean ± SD	Latency (msec) Mean + 3SD	R − L difference (msec) Mean ± SD	R − L difference (msec) Mean + 3SD
Peroneal nerve stimulated at fibular head at knee	*LP = S− (spinal) response recorded from T12/L1–iliac crest*				
	Chiappa 1990 (19)	10.8 ± 0.9	13.5	0.99 ± 0.14	1.41
	Philips and Daube 1980 (76)	13.0 ± 1.1	16.3		
	"N/P34" recorded from the scalp (Cz'–Fz)				
	Chiappa 1990 (19)	33.5 ± 2.4	40.7	1.1 ± 1.62	5.96
	Tsumoto et al. 1972 (103)	34.0 ± 3.3	43.9		
Sural nerve stimulated at ankle	*LP = S− (spinal) response recorded from T12/L1–iliac crest*				
	Chiappa 1990 (19)	20.2 ± 1.6	25.0	0.6 ± 0.30	1.5
	"N/P40" recorded from the scalp (Cz'–Fz)				
	Chiappa 1990 (19)	38.7 ± 2.9	47.4	0.7 ± 0.40	1.9
	Eisen and Elleker 1980 (31)	42.1 ± 1.4	46.3		
	Interpeak latency: LP–"N/P40"				
	Chiappa 1990 (19)	18.5 ± 2.0	24.5	0.9 ± 0.60	2.7

nerve conduction values reached adult levels by about 3 years of age, whereas spinal cord values did not reach adult levels until about 5 years of age (see also "Nerve Conduction Studies").

Body temperature significantly influences nerve conduction velocity. This primarily affects the peripheral nerve segment (see "Nerve Conduction Studies").

Finally, *peripheral neuropathies*, especially those of the demyelinating types, obviously affect SEP latencies. However, they have only minor influence on interpeak latencies.

These factors are of minor clinical relevance if interpeak latencies are used for SEP interpretation: LP–"N/P37" with lower limb testing or EP–"N13" and "N13"–"N19" with median nerve SEPs.

MOTOR EVOKED POTENTIALS

The method of painless magnetoelectric transcranial stimulation of the cerebral cortex was introduced in 1985 by Barker and co-workers (10,11). They applied short magnetic pulses to the scalp, which were produced by a device designed to stimulate peripheral nerves, and recorded muscle action potentials from upper and lower limb muscles: motor evoked potentials (MEPs). Stimulating currents within the nervous tissue are induced by a time-varying magnetic field (78) generated by a brief high-voltage current pulse conducted through a copper coil (9,43). The magnetic field passes through scalp and skull without attenuation. Induced currents within the tissue are inversely proportional to the resistance of the tissue: the current induced in the high-resistance scalp is of low intensity, and few (if any) pain receptors and fibers are stimulated, whereas gray matter cortical structures, with a resistance of only about 250 $\Omega\cdot$cm (36), are excited. Magnetoelectric stimulation has also proved to be suitable for stimulation of deep lying proximal segments of peripheral nerves and nerve roots (13), thus allowing for evaluation of central and proximal peripheral pathways.

The outstanding advantage of magnetoelectric stimulation over high-voltage electric stimulation introduced by Merton and Morton in 1980 (68) is the absence of pain when stimuli are applied to the conscious subject. Apart from that, electric stimulation similarly allows for examination of central motor pathways (85). In this chapter only magnetoelectric stimulation will be described in detail. If required, techniques for high-voltage electric stimulation may be obtained from Rossini et al. (84) or Rothwell et al. (85).

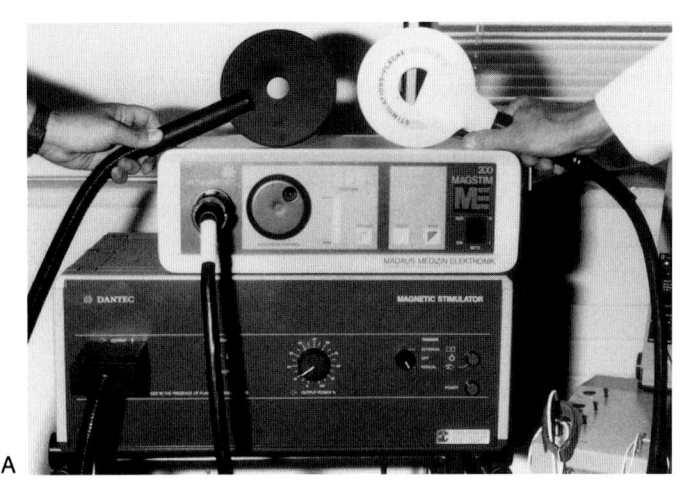

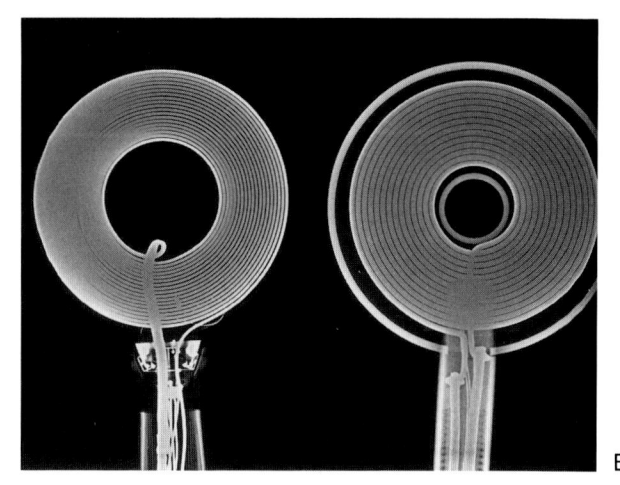

FIG. 5. A: Two magnetoelectric stimulators and their conventional stimulating coils. Top stimulator and right coil: Magstim 200 (The Magstim Company, Whitland, UK); bottom stimulator and left coil: Dantec Magnetic Stimulator (Dantec, Skovlunde, Denmark). **B:** Radiograph of the two coils. Left: Magstim; right: Dantec.

Figure 5 shows two magnetic stimulators and radiographs of their coils.

Safety Issues

Magnetoelectric stimulation has been applied to patients with various neurological, neuro-orthopaedic, and neurosurgical disorders. Besides numerous applications in adults, it has also been used in children (57,72). No negative side effects have been described thus far in animal studies (3,33,101), or human subjects (12,60), with the exception of a single case of kindling (46). Subjects with a history of seizures, or subjects with intracranial or intraocular metal objects, and patients carrying microprocessor-controlled devices (e.g., cardiac pacemakers) should be excluded from magnetic stimulation because of the risk of possible complications.

Magnetically encoded information on computer disks and credit cards or other such objects may be ruined if these are placed too close to the stimulating coil.

Stimulation and Recording Techniques

Figure 6 shows the sites at which the stimulating coil is placed in order to stimulate (A) the motor cortex, (B) the cervical nerve roots, (C) the lumbar nerve roots, and (D) the sciatic nerve trunk. Muscles generally used for recording MEPs are given in Table 2. The segmental innervation of these muscles is used for level diagnosis in analogy to the segmental distribution of the afferent nerves stimulated for SEPs.

Conventional AC amplifiers are used. Filter settings are 20 Hz high pass and 5 kHz low pass with a sample frequency of 5 kHz and a sweep duration of 50 or 100 msec. Surface recording electrodes are placed over the muscle in the belly–tendon or belly–belly fashion.

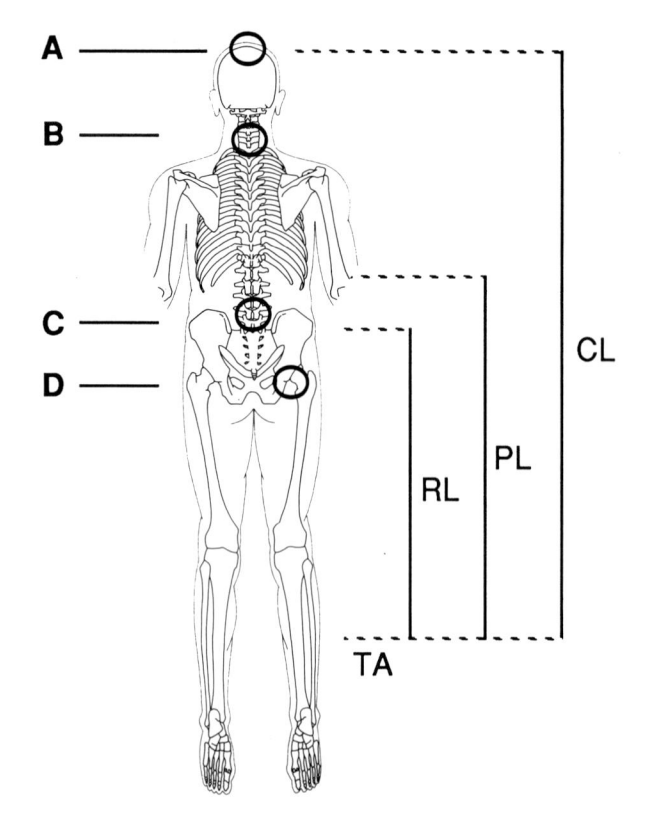

FIG. 6. Stimulation sites with magnetoelectric coils (cf. text). CL, cortical latency; RL, root latency; PL, peripheral latency; TA, anterior tibial muscle.

Transcranial Stimulation

During transcranial stimulation, upper limb muscles are preferentially activated with the center of the coil positioned above the vertex. Lower limb muscles are more easily activated if the center of the coil is moved 4 to 6 cm frontally and 2 to 3 cm contralaterally to the side from which the MEP is recorded. Most magnetic stimulators, for example, the Magstim 200 (The Magstim Company, Whitland, UK) or the Dantec Magnetic Stimulator (Dantec, Skovlunde, Denmark), use a monophasic electric pulse, which is conducted through the copper coil in one direction only. In this case, it is of great importance which side of the coil faces the patient. If the coil is positioned above the vertex and the current flow is counterclockwise when viewed from above, the induced current within the tissue flows clockwise and preferentially activates the left hemisphere (i.e., right limb muscles) and vice versa. The Cadwell MES 10 (Cadwell Laboratories, Inc., Kennewick, WA), for example, uses a polyphasic current and does not show such a preferential activation of either left or right hemisphere (22). Stimulus intensity is described as percentage of the maximal output capacity of the machine used.

The threshold of the resting muscle is determined by applying magnetoelectric stimuli of successively increasing strength. It has proved most practical to use magnetic stimuli of an intensity 50% above threshold for data collection. In addition, the subject is instructed to perform a slight voluntary contraction of the muscles from which recordings are made. This procedure is referred to as *facilitation* (43): Facilitation increases the amplitude and reduces the latency of MEPs. In order to achieve appropriate facilitation, the subjects can be asked to hold both arms in front of them and to spread the fingers or to slightly lift the feet off the ground and to dorsiflex the toes. These easy tasks, while not needing complicated force measurement devices, yield results of the same reproducibility as in force controlled studies. Voluntary innervation need not exceed 10% of the maximal voluntary force in order to achieve a maximal facilitation.

Despite an unchanged procedure, MEP onset latency and amplitude vary slightly in consecutive trials. Three to five consecutive trials should be performed and onset latency should be read from the earliest potential. The reason for this is the following: Transcranial stimulation produces several consecutive volleys that descend through the corticospinal tract. Descending volleys following cortical stimulation have been called direct (D-) and indirect (I-) waves (75). The D-wave was so-called because it is elicited by direct excitation of the initial segment or axon hillock region of the pyramidal tract axon. The later I-waves were shown to be due to transsynaptic activation of the same pyramidal tract neuron (53). Magnetic stimuli preferentially activate pyramidal tract cells transsynaptically, whereas direct activation of these cells is rare. Thus magnetic stimuli preferentially produce I-waves, the first of which, I_1, can depolarize parts of the motor neuron pool and produce an MEP if its intensity is adequate (97). If this is not the case, consecutive I-waves (I_2, I_3, and so on) produced by higher stimulus intensities lead to *temporal summation* and motor neuron pool depolarization. Facilitatory voluntary preinnervation of the muscle under study raises the spinal motor neurons nearer to their discharge threshold. This, together with the descending volleys, leads to *spatial summation*, and the initial I-wave is therefore more likely to discharge at least some motor neurons (97).

MEPs following transcranial stimulation are analyzed for onset latency (cortical latency, CL), peak-to-peak amplitude, duration, and the number of phases in analogy to motor unit action potential evaluation in EMG studies. In order to allow for interindividual comparison, amplitude and duration are related to M-wave amplitude and duration, respectively, and are expressed as ratios (see "M-Wave and F-Wave Evaluation").

Root Stimulation

For motor root stimulation over the cervical or lumbar spine, the intensity of the stimulator is adjusted so that a potential with a steep negative rise can be recorded. With this the onset latency is not critically dependent on the positioning of the coil or the stimulation strength (13). The excitation site of the nerve root is most likely in the region of the root exit from the intervertebral foramen (13) and does not differ from that suggested for electric stimulation over the spine (70). This is probably due to a "channeling" of the current flow within the foramina, creating depolarizing currents as shown in Fig. 7 (18).

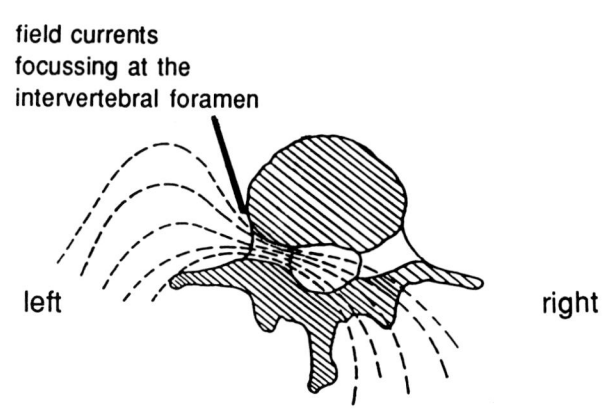

FIG. 7. Channeling of currents induced by magnetoelectric stimulation within and near the intervertebral foramen.

Although the orientation of the current flow within the coil is not as essential as in transcranial stimulation, clockwise orientation, when viewed from behind, produces somewhat larger MEPs in the muscles on the left side and vice versa. To obtain the largest response in a particular limb muscle, the coil is best placed with the coil windings overlying the appropriate nerve roots: the large coil of the Magstim 200 stimulator that we used is best centered over the C7 spinous process in order to record MEPs from the biceps muscle, over the C3/4 spinous process for the hand muscles, over the L2 spinous process for the quadriceps femoris, and over the S3 level for the anterior tibial or extensor digitorum brevis muscles.

MEPs following motor root stimulation are analyzed for onset latency (root latency, RL) only. Since it is not possible to achieve supramaximal stimulation as in electric stimulation of the peripheral nerves (13,21), amplitude and other waveform measurements are not of any help. Nevertheless, latency measurements are reliable, since the fastest conducting fibers should also have the lowest thresholds.

M-Wave and F-Wave Evaluation for the Interpretation of MEPs

In order to judge the MEP waveform, it is also necessary to obtain an M-wave recording by means of conventional neurography. The M-wave is the response to a supramaximal stimulus of the peripheral nerve and thus an electric measure of muscle "size" (79). It is used as a reference signal with which post-transcranial stimulation MEP amplitude and duration are compared; that is, MEP amplitude and duration are expressed as ratios of M-wave amplitude and duration, respectively.

F-wave recordings allow for determination of a total peripheral conduction time (peripheral latency, PL) from the anterior horn cell to the muscle, which thus includes the conduction over the motor root to its exit from the intervertebral foramen. Calculation of PL (see "F-Wave") is especially important in lumbar spine disorders where motor roots measure 10 to 20 cm (40) and contribute considerably to PL, and when this procedure may help to localize the site of lesion (30).

Normal Values

Latencies and amplitudes of MEPs following cortical or root stimulation are measured in a manner identical to that in peripheral nerve conduction studies. Onset latency is measured at the point of first deflection of the trace from the baseline. If several sweeps have been recorded, the shortest reliable latency measurement is taken. Central motor latency (CML) is calculated in two ways: (a) CL minus RL using MEPs following magnetoelectric stimulation only, or (b) CL minus PL, using transcranial magnetoelectric stimulation and the F-wave technique. The result of the first is abbreviated CML-M, and the result of the second is abbreviated CML-F.

MEPs after cortical (i.e., transcranial) stimulation are also analyzed for their amplitudes, duration, and number of phases. Due to the sometimes unstable baseline while performing facilitatory preinnervation for cortical stimulation, amplitudes are measured peak-to-peak rather than baseline-to-peak. This becomes obvious in severely pathological MEPs. The highest reliable amplitude is used. Amplitude and duration are expressed as ratios of the M-wave amplitude and duration after supramaximal electric peripheral nerve stimulation.

Normal values of MEP latencies (CL, RL, CML-M, CML-F, and CML-M minus CML-F) for the biceps brachii (BB), abductor pollicis brevis (APB), abductor digiti minimi (ADM), quadriceps femoris (QF), anterior tibial (TA), and extensor digitorum brevis (EDB) muscles are given in Table 6. Amplitudes (MEP/M-wave ratio), duration (MEP/M-wave ratio), and number of phases are given in Table 7. Neither M- nor F-waves can be obtained from the BB or QF muscles. Therefore, instead of ratios, absolute amplitudes and durations are given.

TABLE 6. *Motor evoked potentials: normal values of CL, RL, CML-M, CML-F, and [CML-M − CML-F]*

Muscle recorded from	CL (msec)		RL (msec)		CML-M (msec)		CML-F (msec)		CML-M minus CML-F (msec)	
	Mean ± SD	Mean + 2SD	Mean ± SD	Mean + 2SD	Mean ± SD	Mean + 2SD	Mean ± SD	Mean + 2SD	Mean ± SD	Mean + 2SD
BB	13.0 ± 1.4	15.8	7.9 ± 1.3	10.5	5.1 ± 1.0	7.1				
APB	20.7 ± 1.3	23.3	15.6 ± 1.2	18.0	5.2 ± 0.6	6.4	4.3 ± 0.8	5.9	0.9 ± 0.8	2.5
ADM	20.0 ± 1.5	23.0	14.9 ± 1.5	17.9	5.2 ± 0.9	7.0	4.0 ± 0.8	5.6	1.1 ± 0.9	2.9
QF	22.3 ± 2.0	26.3	9.3 ± 1.5	12.3	13.0 ± 1.4	15.8				
TA	29.5 ± 2.5	34.5	16.1 ± 2.3	20.7	13.3 ± 1.5	16.3	11.6 ± 0.9	13.4	2.8 ± 1.0	4.8
EDB	38.2 ± 2.6	43.4	24.6 ± 2.1	28.8	13.4 ± 1.7	16.8	11.3 ± 1.7	14.7	2.5 ± 1.4	5.3

TABLE 7. *Normal values of the MEP amplitude/M-wave amplitude ratio, MEP duration/M-wave duration ratio, and number of phases of the MEPs after cortical stimulation*

Muscle	Amplitude MEP/M-wave ratio		Duration MEP/M-wave ratio		Number of phases (counts)	
	Mean ± SD	Minimum	Mean ± SD	Mean + 2SD	Mean ± SD	Maximum
BB[a]	4.5 ± 3.2 mV	0.6 mV	27.4 ± 7.0 msec	41.4 msec	1.2 ± 0.4	3
APB	0.43 ± 0.17	0.20	2.7 ± 1.0	4.7	2.3 ± 1.2	4
ADM	0.50 ± 0.25	0.09	2.5 ± 0.9	4.3	1.9 ± 0.9	4
QF[a]	5.3 ± 3.0 mV	2.0 mV	30.4 ± 8.5 msec	47.4 msec	1.9 ± 0.9	4
TA	0.59 ± 0.30	0.29	1.4 ± 0.3	2.0	2.6 ± 1.3	5
EDB	0.35 ± 0.31	0.03	3.0 ± 1.1	5.2	3.6 ± 1.4	6

[a] M-waves and F-waves cannot be recorded from the BB or QF muscles; absolute values of MEP amplitude and duration are therefore given.

BB, biceps brachii; APB, abductor pollicis brevis; ADM, abductor digiti minimi; QF, quadriceps femoris; TA, anterior tibial; EDB, extensor digitorum brevis muscles.

NEUROGRAPHY AND ELECTROMYOGRAPHY

This chapter offers a brief review of the basics of clinical neurography and electromyography. It does not, however, offer a detailed description of the elaborated techniques, which must remain the domain of experienced electromyographers. It is the electromyographer who must decide on the tests to be performed, guided by the clinical findings and by the request of the referring physician. For detailed descriptions see refs. 27, 55, 62, and 73. These references also contain a large number of tables with normal values for all parameters described below.

Neurographic Studies

Neurapraxia, Axonotmesis, and Neurotmesis

Seddon (86,87) defined three degrees of nerve injury: neurapraxia, axonotmesis, and neurotmesis. This classification can also be applied to nerve root injuries within the lumbar spinal canal.

Neurapraxia is characterized by conduction failure without structural changes in the axon. Fibers usually regain function promptly. Short-term changes in nerve conduction within the affected nerve segment (reduced conduction velocity by as much as 30% and finally complete conduction block) are probably caused by anoxia due to ischemia. Prognosis for complete recovery is excellent and there are generally no electromyographic changes. Voluntary innervation of reduced interference is temporary. There are no signs of denervation (e.g., spontaneous activity).

Axonotmesis results in loss of continuity of the axons, with immediate conduction block across the site of nerve injury. There is subsequent Wallerian degeneration of the distal segment. After 4 or 5 days following acute interruption, the distal segment becomes inexcitable. Preceding conduction failure, there is neither change in the maximal conduction velocity of the efferent motor potential or of the afferent sensory nerve action potential, nor is it possible to distinguish axonotmesis from neurapraxia on the basis of distal nerve excitability. Recovery depends on regeneration of nerve fibers, a process that takes place at a rate of 1 to 3 mm/day, therefore taking months and perhaps years.

Neurotmesis is the state of transsection of the entire nerve, including myelin sheath and connective tissue. The nerve must be sutured. Regeneration is often poorly oriented, and regenerating nerve fibers do not regain their original number or diameter. Initial neurographical findings are identical to those in axonotmesis. In both, axonotmesis and neurotmesis, EMG shows positive sharp waves 8 to 14 days and fibrillation potentials 14 to 20 days after nerve injury. Whereas reduced voluntary activity may be preserved in axonotmesis, this is not the case in neurotmesis.

Commonly Tested Nerves and Their Segmental Innervation

Commonly tested nerves and their segmental innervation are shown in Table 8. In upper limb testing, the radial, median, and ulnar nerves are generally examined. Different nerves derived from the brachial plexus fibers can be tested by stimulating the trunks of the brachial plexus at Erb's point and recording muscle action potentials (M-waves) from the biceps (n. musculocutaneus), deltoid (n. axillaris), triceps (n. radialis), supraspinatus, and infraspinatus muscles (both n. suprascapularis).

The tibial, the common and deep peroneal, the superficial peroneal, and the sural nerves are those commonly studied in lower limb testing. Other nerves accessible to neurography are the femoral, saphenous,

TABLE 8. *Nerves studied neurographically, the roots from which they are derived, and various muscles they innervate*

Nerves	Roots	Muscles
N. phrenicus	C3–C4	Diaphragm
N. suprascapularis	C5–C6	M. supraspinatus
		M. infraspinatus
N. axillaris	C5–C6	M. deltoideus
N. musculocutaneus	C5–C6	M. biceps brachii
N. radialis	C5–C8	M. triceps brachii
	(T1)	M. brachioradialis
		Hand and finger extensors
N. medianus	C6–T1	M. flexor carpi radialis
		M. abductor pollicis brevis (thenar)
		Finger flexors
N. ulnaris	C8–T1	M. flexor carpi ulnaris
		M. abductor digiti minimi (hypothenar)
		Finger flexors
N. cutaneus femoris lateralis	L2–L3	
N. femoralis	L2–L4	M. quadriceps femoris
N. obturatorius	L2–L4	Leg adductors
N. peroneus communis (= lateral popliteal nerve)	L4–S1	M. tibialis anterior
		M. extensor digitorum brevis
		Foot and toe extensors
N. tibialis (= medial popliteal nerve)	L4–S3	M. gastrocnemius
		M. soleus
		M. abductor hallucis
		Foot and toe flexors
N. suralis	L4–S3	
N. pudendus	S1–S4	M. sphincter ani externus

and lateral femoral cutaneous nerves. The deep lying lumbosacral plexus fibers are not accessible by percutaneous electric stimulation. Measurements can be derived from indirect conduction studies, for example, F-wave (see "F-Wave") or H-reflex studies (see "H-Reflex") or by means of magnetoelectric stimulation (see "Transcranial Stimulation").

Nerve Conduction Studies

The conduction velocity of motor fibers was originally measured by Helmholtz (37), who recorded the mechanical response of a muscle. The muscle action potential was first used for this purpose by Piper in 1909 (77). The compound muscle action potential (CMAP) following supramaximal electric stimulation of the supplying motor fibers is called M-wave (see also "M-Wave and F-Wave Evaluation").

Surface recording electrodes are arranged over the muscle belly (active electrode) and over its tendon (reference electrode) so that the initial deflection of the M-wave is negative (i.e., pointing upward). The latency is measured at the onset of the first negative deflection. Amplitude is either measured baseline-to-peak of the first negative wave or peak-to-peak. For reasons explained in the section "Normal Values" (page 108) peak-to-peak measurements should be used.

Stimulating electrodes consist of an anode (positive pole, "attracting anions") and a cathode (negative pole, "attracting cations"). Generally, both are placed over the nerve trunk. As the current flows from the anode to the cathode, negative charges accumulate between the surface of the nerve and the cathode, depolarizing the nerve under the cathode. Under the anode it is hyperpolarized, and an anodal block of impulse propagation may occur at this point. The cathode must therefore be located closer to the recording site, that is, distal in motor conduction studies and proximal in orthodromic sensory conduction studies or SEPs (see "Stimulation and Recording Techniques," page 100) with the distance to the anode being 2 to 3 cm. In calculating conduction velocities, the distance is measured either between consecutive cathodal points or from the cathode to the active recording electrode.

Constant-current electric stimulators should be used rather than constant-voltage stimulators, even though there is no difference between the action potentials recorded (if intensity of nerve stimulation is the same). Comparison between stimulus intensities is facilitated by use of constant-current stimulators because it allows one to speak in terms of milliampere of current used. This is the unit most closely related to the amount (number and size) of nerve fibers stimulated.

Age significantly influences peripheral nerve conduction velocity. Sensory and motor conduction velocities reach their maximum values between 5 and 15 years of age (35). After approximately 30 to 40 years of age they gradually decline. Consequently, F-wave latencies gradually increase. Normal values can be found in Ludin (62). Action potential amplitudes also slowly decline with increasing age.

Temperature significantly influences sensory and motor conduction velocity. A decrease of 1°C in temperature reduces conduction velocity by 1.2 to 2.4 m/sec (16,63). On the other hand, local reduction of temperature has been shown to increase CMAP amplitude (80).

Safety Issues

There is no particular risk applying electric stimuli of the intensity described below to the skin of healthy subjects. As a rule, the ground electrode should be placed between stimulus and recording site on the limb stimulated. A cardiac pacemaker could be inhibited by such currents in its vicinity and central venous catheters may direct the currents to the cardiac tissue. Care must therefore be taken and patients in these cases should be excluded from routine nerve conduction studies.

Motor Nerve Conduction

In motor conduction studies, a square wave pulse of 0.05- to 1.0-msec duration is applied. In general, full activation (i.e., supramaximal stimulation of a nerve) is achieved with surface stimuli of 0.2-msec duration and 20- to 40-mA intensity. However, 60 to 80 mA may be required in diseased nerves with reduced excitability. Animal experiments have shown that large-diameter fibers are activated at lower stimulus intensities than axons of a smaller diameter (32,95). In vivo, however, with submaximal stimuli, the onset latency can vary considerably from one trial to the next due to the spatial distribution of the nerve fibers relative to the stimulating electrodes and to the different lengths of the axon terminals. Thus it is essential not only for amplitude measurements but also for latency measurements to apply supramaximal stimuli, that is, stimuli of an intensity greater than maximal stimuli, which activate all the axons.

The nerve is stimulated at two or more points along its course. The CMAP is recorded using surface electrodes placed over the belly of the muscle (active electrode) and over the tendon (indifferent electrode), that is, in the belly–tendon fashion. The recorded response should then be a simple biphasic potential with initial negativity. If this is preceded by a small positivity, the recording electrode should be repositioned. The latency between the stimulus and the onset of the CMAP includes (a) nerve conduction from the stimulus point to the nerve terminal of the fastest conducting fibers, and (b) neuromuscular transmission, including the time required to depolarize the muscle fibers. The latency after the most distal stimulation of the motor nerve is called *distal motor latency* (DML). Calculating the difference between the latencies after stimulation of the nerve at two points at least 10 cm apart reveals the conduction time over the nerve segment between the stimulating points only, while allowing for calculation of a motor conduction velocity by the formula

velocity [m/sec] = distance [mm]/(proximal latency [msec] - distal latency [msec])

Kimura (55) defines three basic types of abnormalities commonly encountered in motor nerve conduction studies if the nerve is stimulated proximal to the site of the presumed lesion: (a) reduced amplitude with normal or slightly increased latency; (b) increased latency with relatively normal amplitude; and (c) absent response. Nerve lesions in thoracolumbar spine fractures, however, are located proximal to the possible sites of stimulation of leg nerves. Neurapraxia will not cause changes in the CMAP if the nerve is stimulated distal to the lesion. Four to five days after nerve injury (i.e., root injury causing axonotmesis or neurotmesis), when degenerating nerves distal to the lesion show reduced and subsequently absent excitability, CMAP amplitude is reduced and then absent. Distal excitability remains normal only in neurapraxic lesions.

Sensory Nerve Conduction

Sensory nerve conduction studies allow for distinction between radicular lesions proximal of the sensory ganglion and plexopathy or neuropathy distal of the ganglion. The cell body of the sensory axon lies in the ganglion; therefore lesions distal to it lead to centrifugal axonal degeneration (in analogy to motor axon degeneration with reduced CMAP amplitude or absent response to peripheral nerve stimulation). Thoracolumbar spine fractures affecting the nerve roots proximal to the ganglion, however, do not affect sensory nerve conduction of the peripheral nerves.

Sensory nerve conduction can be studied orthodromically (i.e., recording electrodes placed proximal to the stimulating electrodes) or antidromically (i.e., recording electrodes placed distal to the stimulating electrodes). The results are basically the same. Electric square wave stimuli of 0.1- to 0.2-msec duration are applied. As in motor nerve conduction studies, stimulus intensity must be supramaximal: this can be defined as fourfold the sensory threshold (measured in mA) (16). More practical is an intensity 30% to 50% above the intensity, at which a clear sensory nerve action potential (SNAP) is seen in single trials. Averaging 10 to 30 trials distinctly increases the signal-to-noise ratio and allows for precise measurements. The orthodromic potential recorded with the active electrode on the nerve is triphasic or tetraphasic and generally shows initial positivity. Antidromic recordings usually begin with a negative deflection. Latency is measured at the initial positive peak or at the onset of the negative deflection in orthodromic and antidromic recordings, respectively. The amplitude of the SNAP is generally measured peak-to-peak.

Large-diameter sensory fibers have lower thresholds and conduct faster than motor fibers by 5% to 10% (26). Whereas a motor latency includes neuromuscular transmission, sensory latency is identical to the nerve conduction time from the stimulating cathode to the active recording electrode. Therefore stimulation of sensory fibers at a single site allows for calculation of the sensory nerve conduction velocity.

For sensory conduction in lower limbs, antidromic sensory potentials of the sural nerve (S1 root) are recorded using surface electrodes placed dorsal and below the lateral malleolus. The sural nerve is stimulated on the calf slightly lateral to the midline about 10 cm from the proximal (active) recording electrode.

The sensory fibers of the superficial peroneal nerve (L5) can be stimulated by placing the electrodes laterally against the anterior edge of the tibia at a fixed distance of 12 cm from the active recording electrode, located at the ankle just medial to the lateral malleolus. The reference electrode is placed 2 to 3 cm more distally.

F-Wave

Motor conduction of the proximal roots and cauda fibers can be assessed more directly by measurement of the F-wave first described by Magladery and McDougal (66). It is a late CMAP that results from the backfiring of antidromically activated anterior horn cells after supramaximal peripheral stimulation of a motor nerve, which was first explored in detail in patients with Charcot–Marie–Tooth neuropathy by Kimura (54).

Recurrent activation of anterior horn cells occurs in only a minority of alpha motor neurons, preferentially in the larger motor neurons with faster conducting axons. Thus the minimal F-wave latency is a measure of the fastest conducting fibers. However, the latency variability of consecutive F-waves is high because with successive supramaximal stimuli, recurrent discharges occur in different groups of motor neurons.

The stimulating cathode should be placed proximal to the anode to avoid anodal block of the antidromic volley. Amplifier gain is about 10 times higher than for M-wave recordings and sweep duration should be set to 50 or 100 msec. Ten clearly identifiable F-waves should be recorded on a screen. The minimal onset latency of the negative going potential is determined. A slight voluntary contraction of the recording muscle facilitates the response and results in larger amplitudes.

The conduction time from the spinal cord to the muscle (total peripheral latency, PL) can be calculated from the formula (54)

PL [msec] = (minimal F-wave latency [msec] + M-wave latency [msec] − 1 [msec])/2

The estimated delay for the turn-around time of the antidromic volley at the anterior horn cell is 1 msec.

The F-wave is usually normal in mild cases of radiculopathy. Distinct delay of the F-wave or a reduced number of clearly distinguishable F-waves after a given number of supramaximal peripheral stimuli, yet normal distal motor conduction studies, is a sign of a proximal lesion. Only in conjunction with MEPs, however, is it possible to determine conduction times for cauda fibers (i.e., motor roots), which may be affected in lumbar spine fractures (see "M-Wave and F-Wave Evaluation" and "Normal Values," page 108).

H-Reflex

The H-reflex was first described by Hoffmann (47). The H-wave is a CMAP elicited by electric stimulation of large low threshold sensory nerve fibers (Ia muscle spindle afferents), which monosynaptically excite a motor neuron pool that innervates the muscle (from which the H-wave is recorded) via the same nerve. It is a monosynaptic reflex activity comparable to the tendon jerk, yet bypassing the muscle spindles.

In adults it is usually only recordable in a limited group of physiologic extensors, particularly in the calf muscles (S1 root) and in the flexor carpi radialis. Slight voluntary preinnervation facilitates the H-response (92). Stimulation of the tibial nerve at the knee (cathode showing proximal) with slowly increasing intensity from subthreshold to submaximal levels allows for recording of H-responses of growing amplitude from the soleus muscle. Further increase of stimulus intensity elicits M-waves of increasing size, while the H-reflex diminishes progressively and is eventually replaced by the F-wave with supramaximal stimulus intensity. H- and F-waves are of similar latency. S1 sensory or motor root affection reduces H-responses and increases their latency. Interside latency differences are a sensitive indicator of unilateral S1 radiculopathies.

In contrast to F-waves, H-reflexes are identical in response to repetitive stimuli as each trial transsynaptically activates the same motor neurons. H-reflex and F-wave amplitudes depend on stimulus intensity and on the excitability of the alpha motor neurons. Myelopathy (e.g., due to cervical or thoracic spine disease) leads to increased motor neuron excitability with paraspasticity and results in enhanced H-responses.

Electromyographic Studies

Electromyography must be considered an extension of the physical examination rather than simply a laboratory procedure. The muscles to be tested are selected according to clinical findings. The knowledge of physiologic mechanisms underlying normal muscle contraction is a prerequisite for understanding the electrophysiologic abnormalities found in various disorders of the motor system. Electromyographers must also be thoroughly familiar with multiple factors that can significantly affect the outcome of recordings (55).

Needle myography is not free of pain. However, the experienced examiner learns to perform this technique in a manner that is well tolerated by most patients, including children. Care should be taken in patients with coagulopathies (bleeding tendencies) and high susceptibility to recurrent systemic infections.

Recording Technique

Four principal steps delineate the electromyographic study of a muscle:

1. *Insertional activity* is evaluated with the placement and each repositioning of the needle electrode in the muscle.
2. After stationary and stable positioning of the needle electrode, the recording is evaluated at rest for detection of *spontaneous activity*.
3. Single *motor unit action potentials* (MUAPs) are recorded with a mild voluntary contraction of the muscle and examined with respect to amplitude, duration, and number of phases.
4. *Motor unit recruitment* and the *interference pattern* are recorded with a gradual increase of voluntary muscle contraction and maximal voluntary contraction, respectively.

Filters of the EMG amplifiers should be set to 10 to 20 Hz low cutoff (high pass) and 10 kHz high cutoff (low pass). Gain is set to 50 to 100 μV/division for studying insertional and spontaneous activity, and between 100 μV and 1 to 10 mV/division for assessment of single MUAPs with a sweep speed of 5 to 10 msec/division. Sweep speed is reduced to 100 msec/division and gain is set to 1 or 2 mV/division for analysis of the interference pattern.

Since its introduction by Adrian and Bronk (2), the standard concentric (coaxial) needle electrode has been the most commonly used electrode for recording from inside the muscle. It is a stainless steel cannula with a nichrome, silver, or platinum wire of about 0.1 mm in diameter in the center of the shaft. The potential difference between the needle tip (leading-off surface) and the shaft is recorded. A separate ground electrode is required.

Since a needle electrode registers ("sees") MUAPs from a limited area in the nearest vicinity of its leading-off surface only, it is necessary to record from many different areas within the muscle by repositioning the needle, moving its tip at least 2 mm perpendicular to the muscle fibers each time. Ten distinct areas should be sampled.

With thoracolumbar fractures of the spine, EMG studies are aimed at delineating damage to the lower motor neuron, that is, axonal injury in terms of axonotmesis or neurotmesis of the motor roots with muscular denervation. In normal muscles, MUAPs are elicited only in response to neural discharges. Denervated muscle fibers become unstable, as they are no longer under neural control, and individual muscle fibers will fire in the absence of neural stimuli. This uncontrolled activity results in (a) increased insertional activity, (b) increased endplate activity, and (c) spontaneous activity. These signs of denervation in the EMG can be spotted at the earliest about 8 days after the injury. They are termed as *acute* signs of denervation. The different types of spontaneous activity are described in the section entitled "Spontaneous Activity." The analysis of single MUAPs may also reveal changes that are typical but not specific of lower motor neuron damage (e.g., radiculopathy): increased amplitude, increased number of phases, and increased duration. These changes are seen only after reinnervation or sprouting of nonaffected fibers has taken place. They are therefore termed as *chronic* signs of denervation and are described in the section entitled "Single MUAP Analysis." Changes of motor unit recruitment and discharge are also seen in radiculopathy and are described in the section entitled "Motor Unit Recruitment and Discharge Pattern."

Commonly Tested Muscles and Their Segmental Innervation

Localization of the lesion with respect to the motor roots affected is supported by the examination of a variety of muscles innervated by different motor roots. If motor roots on their intraspinal course or the spinal nerve trunks within the intervertebral foramen are affected by the lesion, the paraspinal musculature, which is supplied by the posterior ramus from the spinal nerve, may also show the typical EMG changes otherwise found only in limb muscles or muscles of the anterolateral body wall supplied by the anterior ramus. Due to the short nerve segment, spontaneous activity can already be detected by the fifth day after the injury (61). Normal findings in paraspinal musculature, however, do not exclude root damage. Furthermore, the difficulty many patients have in completely relaxing back muscles often hinders lucid results.

Both upper and lower limb muscles commonly tested in EMG studies are listed in Table 9 together with their segmental innervation and the nerves by which they are supplied. Detailed descriptions for localizing these muscles and positioning the needle electrode are given by Delagi and Perotto (27).

Spontaneous Activity

Action potentials recorded at rest after insertional activity has subsided and when there is no voluntary

TABLE 9. *Spinal segments and the muscles and nerves mainly innervated*

Segment	Muscles	Nerves
C4	Diaphragm	N. phrenicus
C5	M. supraspinatus	N. suprascapularis
	M. deltoideus	N. axillaris
C6	M. biceps brachii	N. musculocutaneus
	M. brachioradialis	N. radialis
C7	M. pectoralis major	Nn. pectorales medialis and lateralis
	M. triceps brachii	N. radialis
	M. abductor pollicis brevis	N. medianus
C8	M. abductor digiti minimi	N. ulnaris
	M. flexor digiti superficialis	N. medianus
L2	M. iliopsoas	N. femoralis
L3	Mm. adductor longus and brevis	N. obturatorius
L4	M. quadriceps femoris	N. femoralis
L5	M. tibialis anterior	N. peroneus
	M. extensor digitorum brevis	N. peroneus
	M. tibialis posterior	N. tibialis
S1	Mm. gastrocnemius and soleus	N. tibialis
	M. biceps femoris caput longum	N. tibialis
	M. biceps femoris caput breve	N. peroneus communis
S2	M. abductor digiti minimi pedis	N. tibialis
S3	M. sphincter ani externus	N. pudendus

contraction or external stimulus are called *spontaneous activity*. Spontaneous activity, if reproducible in at least two muscle sites, is an unequivocal sign of abnormality and one of the most useful findings in clinical electromyography. It is usually seen in the denervated muscle but may also occur in certain primary muscle diseases. As a rule, spontaneous activity is not found in paretic limbs of patients with upper motor neuron disorders or disuse atrophy (55). However, fibrillation potentials and positive sharp waves have also been reported in hemiplegic patients (49).

Spontaneous activity is due to an increased sensitivity of muscle fibers to acetylcholine (ACh) within the first 2 weeks after denervation. Denervation hypersensitivity to ACh is as much as 100-fold (14,67,98) and is not limited to the endplate zone (8). It results in spontaneous discharges of single muscle fibers (not motor units) as responses to small quantities of circulating ACh (28).

There are four basic types of spontaneous activity: fibrillation potentials, positive sharp waves, fasciculation potentials, and complex repetitive discharges. Fibrillation potentials and positive sharp waves are the first to appear after nerve injury. The larger the distance between the site of the lesion and the muscle, the longer is the time interval between nerve injury and initial electromyographic changes (61).

Fibrillation potentials are discharges from single muscle fibers of 1- to 5-msec duration and 20- to 200-μV amplitude when recorded with a concentric needle electrode (17,83). They are initially positive and biphasic or triphasic. However, if the leading-off surface of the needle is near the endplate zone, fibrillation potentials appear biphasic with initial negativity and are difficult to differentiate from physiologic endplate spikes. Regular discharges occur at a rate of 1 to 30 impulses per second with an average frequency of 13 Hz (17). Motor units fire more irregularly, and only in severe demyelinating neuropathy at rates below 5 to 8 Hz (79). Fibrillation potentials produce a crisp clicking noise in the loudspeaker (Fig. 8A).

Positive sharp waves probably represent potentials from single muscle fibers recorded from an injured area. They show an initial positive spike of less than 5-msec duration and up to 1 mV in amplitude, which may be followed by a negative wave of 10- to 100-msec duration and low amplitude, and recur in a uniform, regular pattern at a rate of 2 to 50 Hz (17). Positive sharp waves tend to appear a little earlier than fibrillation potentials after nerve injury (Fig. 8B).

Fasciculation potentials are spontaneous discharges of groups of muscle fibers belonging to a motor unit, most likely the entire motor unit. They occur sporadically as single discharges with an average interval of 3.5 sec (99). They are associated with visible twitching of muscle bundles if not restricted to the depth of the muscle (45). Fasciculation potentials are predominantly found in diseases of the anterior horn cells but may also occur in lesions of the roots or peripheral nerves. In myelopathy, fasciculations have also been observed in lower limb muscles (50,56), where they may disappear after successful surgical decompression.

Complex repetitive discharges have also been termed *bizarre high-frequency discharges* or *pseudomyotonia*. They represent a group of muscle fibers discharging in near synchrony at rates between 5 and 100 Hz and they are 50 μV to 1 mV in amplitude and up to 50 to 100 msec in duration. Despite their superficial resemblance to myotonic discharges, they lack the waxing and waning quality but resemble the sound of a machine gun with an abrupt beginning, constant firing rate, and abrupt cessation. This type of spontaneous discharge is seen in a wide variety of myopathic and lower motor neuron disorders including long-standing radiculopathy (100) (Fig. 8C).

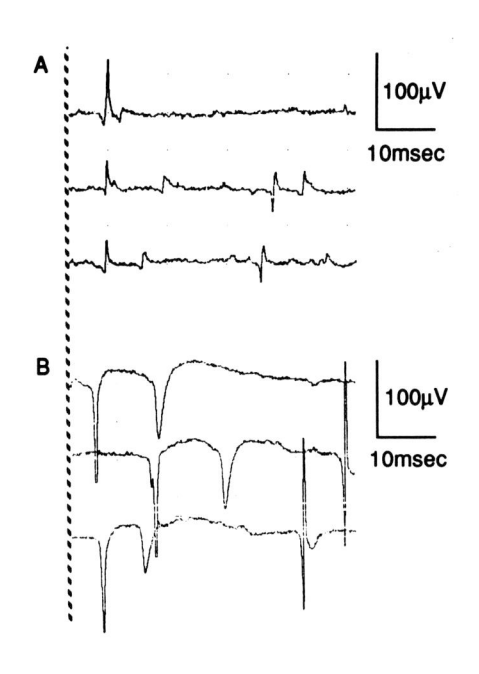

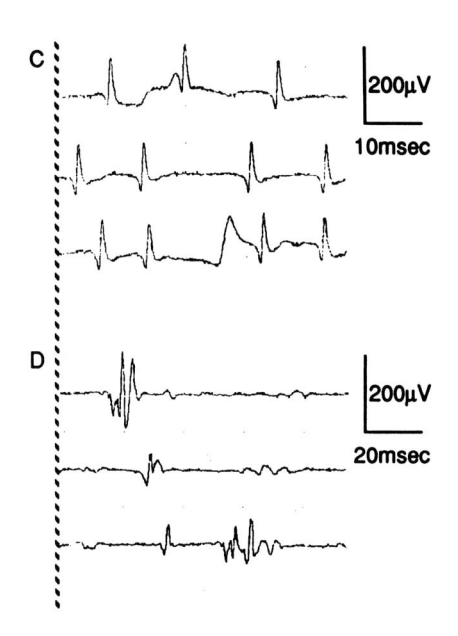

FIG. 8. Fibrillation potentials (**A**), positive sharp waves and two fibrillation potentials (**B**), complex repetitive discharges (**C**), and polyphasic MUAPs (**D**) from the anterior tibial muscle of a patient with an acute L5 root compression syndrome due to discal herniation and a 10-year history of low back pain.

Single MUAP Analysis

A motor unit potential is defined by its amplitude, rise time, duration, number of phases, stability, and territory. In neuropathy, radiculopathy, or anterior horn cell disease, MUAPs are normal or larger than normal in size but reduced in number, reflecting functional or structural loss of axons.

The amplitude of the MUAPs varies greatly with the position of the needle electrode relative to the discharging unit. Only MUAPs with a rise time of less than 500 μsec, preferably less than 200 μsec, qualifying the leading-off surface of the needle as close enough to the unit should be analyzed.

The duration of the MUAPs is an indicator of motor unit territory: distant muscle fibers, while not contributing to the amplitude of the negative spike, significantly add to the MUAP duration, increasing the time of the initial and terminal positivity. Sprouting of terminal nerve branches and reinnervation result in longer duration. For assessment, the duration of MUAPs must be compared with the normal range for the same muscle in the same age group (15).

The majority of MUAPs are biphasic or triphasic. In healthy muscle 5% to 15% may be polyphasic, having four or more phases (Fig. 8D). Polyphasia indicates increased temporal dispersion of muscle fiber potentials within the motor unit and may be the result of different conduction times within the terminal branches of the nerves (e.g., during reinnervation) or over the muscle fiber membrane. An increased number of polyphasic motor units can be seen either in myopathy, neuropathy, radiculopathy, or motor neuron disease.

Motor Unit Recruitment and Discharge Pattern

According to the size principle, small motor units are recruited before large units (38). EMG studies revealed a strong positive correlation between MUAP amplitude and the threshold force of recruitment of a motor unit (39). If the number of recruitable motor units is reduced due to motor neuron disease or disorders of the root or of the peripheral nerve, a limited number of motor units can be recruited and larger units of higher thresholds are recruited earlier. The increased MUAP amplitudes due to sprouting and reinnervation contribute to the picture of an early recruitment of large-amplitude units in chronic axonal lower motor neuron disease (42). Furthermore, the recruitment order may appear deranged (41). Maximal voluntary contraction will, in any case of a reduced number of motor units, reveal an incomplete interference pattern. A failure of descending impulses or reduced motor unit discharge rates, as in demyelinating neuropathy (79), would also contribute to the picture of an incomplete interference pattern. In extreme instances, single motor units produce a so-called picket fence interference pattern at maximal effort. Impaired force generation in lower motor neuron disorders is the result of an interplay of changes in motor unit recruitment and in firing rate modulation (79).

EMG of the External Anal Sphincter

The external anal sphincter is innervated from the anterior divisions of the S2 to S4 spinal nerves through the pudendal nerve. Unlike peripheral skeletal muscle, the anal sphincter always maintains a basic tonus with isolated motor units continuously discharging at low rates. During sleep, discharge rate is less than during consciousness. It is increased by coughing, speaking, and body movements of the trunk (34). It is therefore difficult to detect abnormal spontaneous activity in the partially denervated muscle.

In central paralysis, voluntary activity is reduced or absent, although the muscle can be activated via reflexes (simply elicited by digital examination of the anal sphincter). Reduced voluntary activity produces an incomplete interference pattern. If voluntary activity is completely lost, the basic low-frequency discharges at rest are unchanged during maximal effort to contract the muscle and may also remain unchanged during defecation maneuvers, thereby prohibiting normal defecation.

In incomplete peripheral paralysis caused by lesions in the cauda equina, few motor units with polyphasic potentials of long duration can be volitionally activated to discharge at high frequency. If axonal degeneration occurs, fibrillation potentials, positive sharp waves, or complex repetitive discharges can be seen.

Traumatic injuries of the conus medullaris result in a mixture of central and peripheral paresis. Both voluntary and reflex activities are markedly reduced or absent. Isolated high-frequency discharges of few motor units may be seen in response to stretch. Spontaneous activity can be recorded.

AUTONOMIC EVALUATION

Shanhani et al. (91) described a biphasic skin DC potential shift from hand or foot in response to electric stimuli. This response is mediated through unmyelinated C fibers derived from the paraspinal sympathetic plexus and is called *sympathetic skin response* (SSR). It allows for an assessment of sympathetic autonomic dysfunction due to peripheral neuropathy (91) and proved to be helpful in the evaluation of erectile impotence (58), which may also occur after thoracolumbar fractures.

Supramaximal electric square wave stimuli are applied to the skin over the median or tibial nerve. Other *unexpected* stimuli can also be applied but are more difficult to standardize. Recordings are taken with surface electrodes fixed to the volar, that is, plantar and dorsal sides of the contralateral hand or foot, respectively. Total sweep duration is set to 5 sec, gain to 100 to 500 μV/division, and filters are set to 3 Hz to 3 kHz. A biphasic potential is expected after 1.5 to 3.0 sec. Twenty seconds should elapse between consecutive stimuli to avoid habituation. Only an absent response can be judged as pathological.

Neuro-urological involvement, however, always calls for subtle urological assessment. This is especially important in cases of disturbances of bladder function and its result, chronic renal failure, which may be fatal in paraplegic patients.

PROGNOSIS OF SPINAL CORD TRAUMA

Despite several reports of neurophysiological assessment (i.e., SEP or MEP studies) in patients or animals after spinal cord trauma (29,74,96), there is no clarity about the significance of the results for either short- or long-term prognosis of spinal cord trauma. Ducker and co-workers (29) performed a study on SEPs following stimulation of the sural nerve in experimental spinal cord trauma in monkeys. In animals rendered completely paraplegic, only 8% had preserved SEP responses at 5 min after injury. A transient recovery of SEPs often occurred at 2 to 3 hr after injury before they were eventually lost in 85% of the animals. In 40% to 60% of the animals with paraparetic outcome, it was possible to record SEP responses, although generally abnormal. Of those animals able to stand or run, initially only a few (8%) showed absent responses. SEPs were obtainable in all animals of the latter group at 2 to 3 hr after injury. Naturally, MEPs reflect integrity of the motor pathways more precisely than SEPs (96). However, results of MEPs after transcranial magnetoelectric stimulation in the acute stage after cord trauma are difficult to interpret. Since transcranial stimulation is never supramaximal, absent responses are not necessarily a pathological finding; they may also be absent due to an increased threshold level or an absence of temporal or spatial summation. Preserved responses of reduced amplitude and increased latencies can be interpreted in analogy to preserved SEPs: the lesion is incomplete and recovery is possible. Interpretation of the results beyond this point appears questionable. With respect to prognostic significance of MEPs, further studies are necessary. MEPs are most helpful, however, in demonstrating preservation of central and peripheral motor pathways in patients showing a pseudoparesis owing to inappropriate voluntary activation of muscles (48).

CASE STUDY

Patient C.C. (male, 46 years old) dropped 5 m onto his feet, resulting in a severe compression trauma. Radiographs and CT scans showed a compression fracture of L2 (Fig. 9). The patient showed paresis of the knee extensors (L4, grade 2–3) more severe on the right side. Feet and toes were paralyzed on both sides. Light touch and pinprick sensation were lost below the

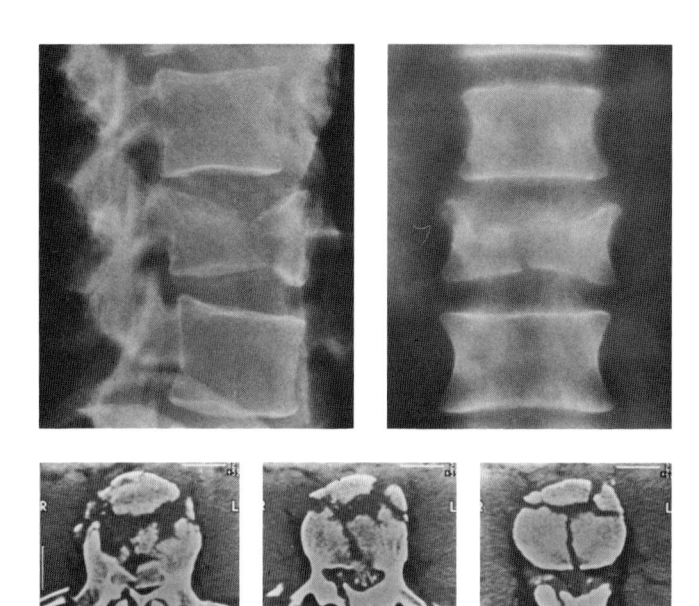

FIG. 9. Radiographs and CT scans showing compression fracture of L2 with severe confinement of the spinal canal.

L4 dermatome. There was loss of bladder tonus with overflow voiding, erectile impotence, and loss of control over bowel voiding. Sweating was normal upon examination.

Motor Nerve Conduction and Motor Evoked Potentials

Motor nerve conduction velocities and compound muscle action potential (CMAP) amplitudes of peroneal and tibial nerves on both sides were normal at 24 hr after the accident. Fifteen days later no CMAP could be recorded following peroneal or tibial nerve stimulation (Fig. 10A). F-waves were all absent.

Fifteen days after the accident, motor evoked potentials (MEPs) from the left quadriceps femoris muscle showed normal latencies and amplitudes after transcranial as well as after root stimulation (Fig. 11A). MEP amplitudes from the right quadriceps femoris muscle following transcranial stimulation were markedly reduced and latencies were distinctly increased. After root stimulation, MEPs showed normal latencies but reduced amplitudes (Fig. 11B). No reproducible MEPs could be recorded from either left or right anterior tibial or gastrocnemius muscles. Control responses from the right abductor digiti minimi muscle were normal.

Sensory Nerve Conduction and Somatosensory Evoked Potentials

Antidromic sural nerve conduction on both sides was normal at 24 hr and at 15 days after the accident

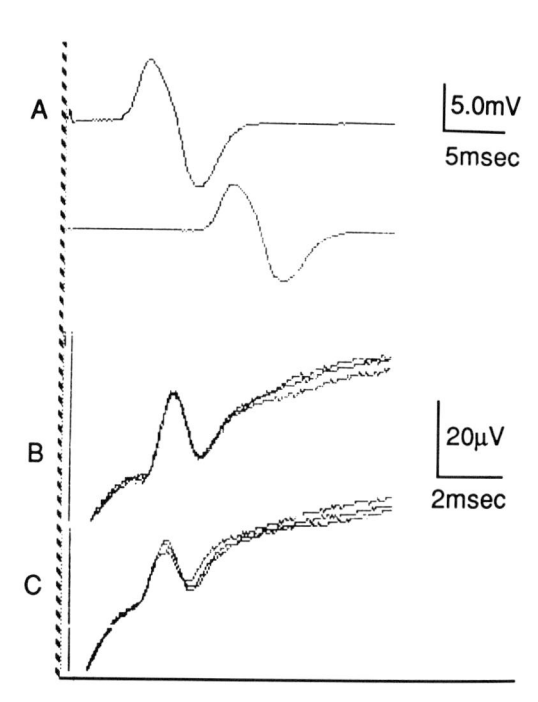

FIG. 10. A: Compound muscle action potential from the right extensor digitorum brevis muscle after stimulation of the peroneal nerve at the ankle (top trace) and below the knee (bottom trace) 24 hr after the accident (cf. text). Antideromic sensory nerve action potential from the right sural nerve 24 hr (**B**) and 15 days (**C**) after the accident.

(Fig. 10B). SEPs after peroneal or posterior tibial nerve stimulation, however, could not be recorded from L1 or from the scalp at any time. Median nerve control SEPs were normal.

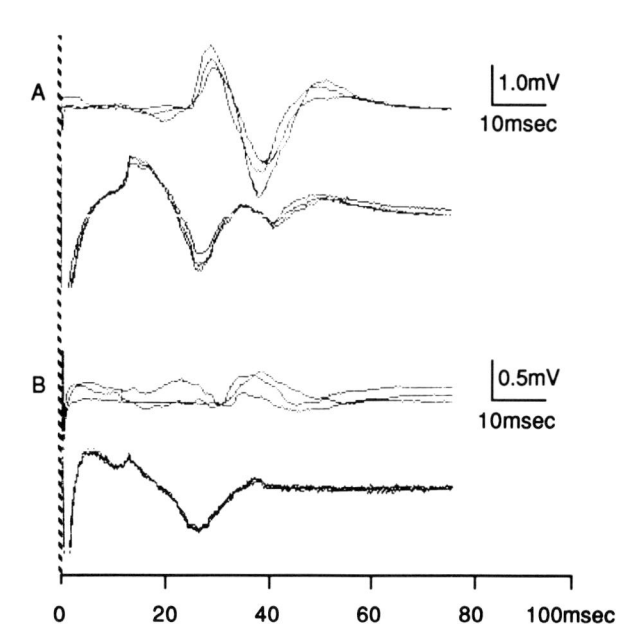

FIG. 11. MEPs recorded from the left (**A**) and right (**B**) quadriceps femoris following cortical (*top trace*) and motor root stimulation (*bottom trace*) (cf. text).

Electromyography

Fifteen days after the accident electromyography was performed from the iliopsoas, quadriceps femoris, anterior tibial, and gastrocnemius muscles on the right side. Spontaneous activity was found in all but the iliopsoas muscles, being most pronounced in the anterior tibial muscle (Fig. 12). Whereas voluntary motor unit activity with incomplete interference pattern (the so-called picket fence interference pattern) could be recorded on maximal effort from the quadriceps, no voluntary activity was found in either the anterior tibial or in the gastrocnemius muscles.

Interpretation

Initial normal motor nerve conduction studies distal to the lesion and inexcitability of the same motor nerves 15 days later are signs of axonotmesis or neurotmesis with wallerian degeneration (cf. "Neurapraxia, Axonotmesis, and Neurotmesis" and "Motor Nerve Conduction"). Normal sensory nerve conduction studies at the initial examination and 15 days later indicate that the lesion was located proximal to the sensory ganglia (cf. "Sensory Nerve Conduction") because distal sensory fibers did not degenerate. The inexcitability of F-waves indicates a lower motor neuron affection but does not allow for a more precise location of the lesion (cf. "F-Wave"). A normal central motor latency in the MEPs recorded from the left quadriceps femoris muscle excluded a bilateral spinal cord lesion above the L4 segment. Together with the increased central motor latency and the reduced amplitude in the MEPs recorded from the right quadriceps, these results were compatible with a root lesion on the right side at the L4 level. Reduced amplitudes from the right quadriceps femoris muscle after magnetoelectric root stimulation indicated an incomplete lesion of the right L4 root or femoral nerve motor fibers (a neurography of the femoral nerve was not performed). The immediate loss of SEPs (LP and scalp potential) after peroneal and posterior tibial nerve stimulation indicated a lesion at or distal to the root entry zone of the L5 and S1 sensory roots. EMG findings indicated acute denervation of the L4, L5, and S1 muscles. Voluntary activity could only be recorded in the quadriceps muscle with reduced interference, indicating incomplete denervation of the L4 segment. Normal findings in the iliopsoas muscle showed that the L2 root was not affected. Additional evidence for a root lesion, as compared to a plexus or peripheral nerve lesion, could have originated from an EMG of the paraspinal muscles, where spontaneous activity should have been present at 5 days after injury (cf. "Commonly Tested Muscles and Their Segmental Innervation"). The necessary operation for decompression and stabilization by dorsal instrumentation, however, rendered evaluation of these muscles useless. Information on sudorimotor (sympathetic) function might have come from a sweat test or from the sympathetic skin response. Neither test was performed, since sweating appeared normal upon examination.

In summary, these findings were in favor of an acute structural lesion (axonotmesis or neurotmesis) of the L4, L5, and S1 cauda fibers. Clinical findings also showed involvement of the S2, S3, and S4 fibers.

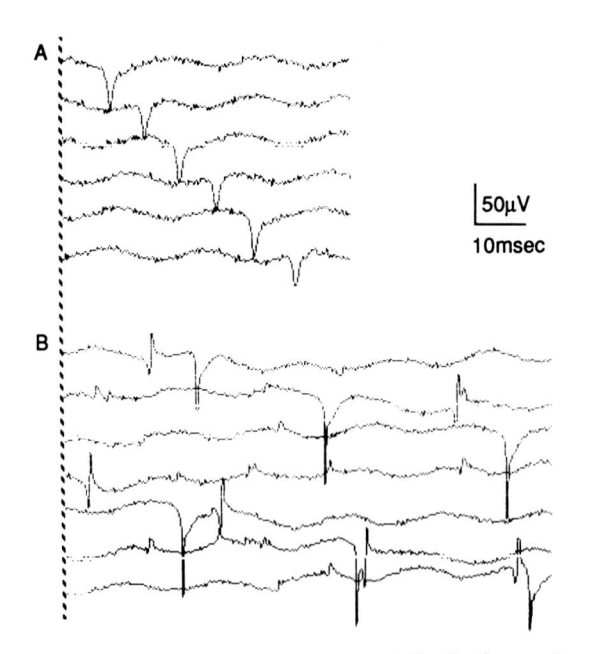

FIG. 12. Positive sharp waves (**A**) and fibrillation potentials (**B**) from the right anterior tibial muscle (cf. text).

ACKNOWLEDGMENTS

The authors thank E. Kunesch, Department of Neurology, and M. Krzan, Department of Neurosurgery, Heinrich-Heine-University Düsseldorf, for their valuable advice and criticism and gratefully acknowledge the editorial work of S. J. Bockover, B.A. Public Communication/German.

REFERENCES

1. Abbruzzese M, Favale E, Leandri M, Ratio S. Spinal components of the cerebral somatosensory evoked response in normal man: the "S wave." *Acta Neurol Scand* 1978;58:213–220.
2. Adrian ED, Bronk DW. The discharge of impulses in motor nerve fibres. Part II. The frequency of discharge in reflex and voluntary contractions. *J Physiol* 1929;67:119–151.
3. Agnew WF, McCreery DB. Considerations for safety in the use of extracranial stimulation for motor evoked potentials. *Neurosurgery* 1987;20:143–147.
4. Allison T, Hume AL, Wood CC, Goff WR. Developmental and

aging changes in somatosensory, auditory and visual evoked potentials. *Electroencephalogr Clin Neurophysiol* 1984;58: 14–24.
5. Allison T, Wood CC, Goff WR. Brain stem auditory, pattern-reversal visual, and short-latency somatosensory evoked potentials: latencies in relation to age, sex, and brain and body size. *Electroencephalogr Clin Neurophysiol* 1983;55:619–636.
6. Anziska B, Cracco RQ. Short latency somatosensory evoked potentials: studies in patients with focal neurological disease. *Electroencephalogr Clin Neurophysiol* 1980;49:227–239.
7. Anziska B, Cracco RQ. Short latency SEPs to median nerve stimulation: comparison of recording methods and origin of components. *Electroencephalogr Clin Neurophysiol* 1981;52: 531–539.
8. Axelsson J, Thesleff S. A study of supersensitivity of denervated mammalian skeletal muscle. *J Physiol* 1957;149:178–193.
9. Barker AT, Freeston IL, Jalinous R, Jarratt JA. Magnetic stimulation of the human brain and peripheral nervous system: an introduction and the results of an initial clinical evaluation. *Neurosurgery* 1987;20:100–109.
10. Barker AT, Freeston IL, Jalinous R, Merton PA, Morton HB. Magnetic stimulation of the human brain. *J Physiol* 1985;369: 3P.
11. Barker AT, Jalinous R, Freeston IL. Non-invasive magnetic stimulation of the human motor cortex. *Lancet* 1985;1: 1106–1107.
12. Bridgers SL, Delaney RC. Transcranial magnetic stimulation: An assessment of cognitive and other cerebral effects. *Neurology* 1989;39:417–419.
13. Britton TC, Meyer B-U, Herdmann J, Benecke R. Clinical use of the magnetic stimulator in the investigation of peripheral conduction time. *Muscle Nerve* 1990;13:396–406.
14. Brown GL. The actions of acetylcholine on denervated mammalian and frog's muscle. *J Physiol* 1937;89:438–461.
15. Buchthal F. *An introduction to electromyography*. Copenhagen: Scandinavian University Books, 1957.
16. Buchthal F, Rosenfalck A. Evoked action potentials and conduction velocity in human sensory nerves. *Brain* 1966;3:1–119.
17. Buchthal F, Rosenfalck P. Spontaneous electrical activity of human muscle. *Electroenceph Clin Neurophysiol* 1966;20: 321–336.
18. Cadwell J. Principles of magnetoelectric stimulation. In: Chokroverty S, ed. *Magnetic stimulation in clinical neurophysiology*. Boston: Butterworths, 1989;13–32.
19. Chiappa KH. Short-latency somatosensory evoked potentials: methodology. In: Chiappa KH, ed. *Evoked potentials in clinical medicine*, 2nd ed. New York: Raven Press, 1990;307–370.
20. Chiappa KH, Choi S, Young RR. Short latency somatosensory evoked potentials following median nerve stimulation in patients with neurological lesions. In: Desmedt JE, ed. *Progress in clinical neurophysiology*, vol 7. Basel: Karger, 1980; 264–281.
21. Chokroverty S, Spire JP, DiLullo J, Moody E Jr, Maselli R. Magnetic stimulation of the human peripheral nervous system. In: Chokroverty S, ed. *Magnetic stimulation in clinical neurophysiology*. Boston: Butterworths, 1989;249–273.
22. Claus D, Murray NMF, Spitzer A, Flügel D. The influence of stimulus type on the magnetic excitation of nerve structures. *Electroencephalogr Clin Neurophysiol* 1990;75:342–349.
23. Cracco JB, Cracco RQ, Graziani LJ. The spinal evoked response in infants and children. *Neurology* 1975;25:31–36.
24. Cracco JB, Cracco RQ, Stolove R. Spinal evoked potentials in man: a maturational study. *Electroencephalogr Clin Neurophysiol* 1979;46:58–64.
25. Cracco RQ. Spinal evoked responses; peripheral nerve stimulation in man. *Electroencephalogr Clin Neurophysiol* 1973;35: 379–386.
26. Dawson GD. The relative excitability and conduction velocity of sensory and motor nerve fibres in man. *J Physiol* 1956;131: 436–451.
27. Delagi EF, Perotto A. *Anatomic guide for the electromyographer*, 2nd ed. Springfield: CC Thomas, 1982.
28. Denny-Brown D, Pennybaker JB. Fibrillation and fasciculation in voluntary muscle. *Brain* 1938;61:311–334.
29. Ducker TB, Salcman M, Lucas JT, Garrison WB, Perot PL. Experimental spinal cord trauma, II: blood flow, tissue oxygen, evoked potentials in both paretic and plegic monkeys. *Surg Neurol* 1978;10:64–70.
30. Dvořák J, Herdmann J, Theiler R, Grob D. Magnetic stimulation of motor cortex and motor roots for painless evaluation of central and proximal peripheral motor pathways. Normal values and clinical application in disorders of the lumbar spine. *Spine* 1991;16:955–961.
31. Eisen A, Elleker G. Sensory nerve stimulation and evoked cerebral potentials. *Neurology* 1980;30:1097–1105.
32. Erlanger J, Gasser HS. *Electrical signs of nervous activity*. Philadelphia: University of Pennsylvania Press, 1937.
33. Eyre JA, Flecknell PA, Koh THHG, Miller S. Acute effects of electromagnetic stimulation of the brain on cortical activity, cortical blood flow, blood pressure and heart rate in the cat: an evaluation of safety. *J Neurol Neurosurg Psychiatry* 1990;53: 507–513.
34. Floyd WF, Walls EW. Electromyography of the sphincter ani externus in man. *J Physiol* 1953;122:599–609.
35. Gamstorp I. Normal conduction velocity of ulnar, median and peroneal nerves in infancy, childhood and adolescence. *Acta Paediatr Scand Suppl* 1963;146:68–76.
36. Geddes LA, Baker LE. The specific resistance of biological material. *Med Biol Eng Comput* 1967;5:271–293.
37. Helmholtz H. Vorläufiger Bericht über die Fortpflanzungsgeschwindigkeit der Nervenreizung. *Arch Anat Physiol Wiss Med* 1850;71.
38. Henneman, E. Relation between size of neurons and their susceptibility to discharge. *Science* 1957;126:1345–1347.
39. Herdmann J, Büdingen HJ, Reiners K, Berger W, Freund H-J. The dependence of the motor unit action potential amplitude on its threshold force of recruitment: implications for clinical electromyography. *EEG EMG* 1986;17:140–146.
40. Herdmann J, Dvořák J, Rathmer L, Theiler R, Peuschel K, Zenker W, Lumenta CB. Conduction velocities of pyramidal tract fibres and lumbar motor nerve roots: normal values. *Zentralbl Neurochir* 1991;52:197–199.
41. Herdmann J, Reiners K, Freund H-J. Motor unit recruitment order in neuropathic disease. *Electromyogr Clin Neurophysiol* 1988;28:53–60.
42. Herdmann J, Reiners K, Freund H-J. Disturbance of motor unit recruitment and firing rate modulation in polyneuropathies. In: Lovelace RE, Shapiro HK, eds. *Charcot–Marie–Tooth disorders: pathophysiology, molecular genetics, and therapy*. Neurology and neurobiology, vol 53. New York: Wiley-Liss, 1990; 141–146.
43. Hess CW, Mills KR, Murray NMF. Magnetic stimulation of the human brain: facilitation of motor responses by voluntary contraction of ipsilateral and contralateral muscles with additional observations on an amputee. *Neurosci Lett* 1986;71: 235–240.
44. Hess CW, Mills KR, Murray NMF. Methodological considerations for magnetic brain stimulation. In: Barber C, Blum T, eds. *Evoked potentials III*. London: Butterworths, 1988;456–461.
45. Hjorth RJ, Walsh JC, Willison RG. The distribution and frequency of spontaneous fasciculations in motor neurone disease. *J Neurol Sci* 1973;18:469–474.
46. Hömberg V, Netz J. Generalised seizures induced by transcranial magnetoelectric stimulation of motor cortex. *Lancet* 1989; 2:1223.
47. Hoffmann P. Über die Beziehung der Sehnenreflexe zur Willkürlichen Bewegung und zum Tonus. *Z Biol* 1918;68:677–694.
48. Janssen BA, Grob D, Dvořák J: Are motor evoked potentials a useful diagnostic tool in verifying a psychogenic paresis? Presented at the *Annual Meeting of the International Society for the Study of the Lumbar Spine*, Heidelberg, Germany, 1991.
49. Johnson EW, Denny ST, Kelley JP. Sequence of electromyographic abnormalities in stroke syndrome. *Arch Phys Med Rehabil* 1975;56:468–473.
50. Kadson DL. Cervical spondylotic myelopathy with reversible fasciculations in the lower extremities. *Arch Neurol* 1977;34: 774–776.
51. Kakigi R, Shibasaki H. Scalp topography of the short latency somatosensory evoked potentials following posterior tibial

nerve stimulation in man. *Electroencephalogr Clin Neurophysiol* 1983;56:430–437.
52. Katayama Y, Tsubokawa T. Somatosensory evoked potentials from the thalamic sensory relay nucleus (VPL) in humans: correlations with short latency somatosensory evoked potentials recorded at the scalp. *Electroencephalogr Clin Neurophysiol* 1986;65:249–259.
53. Kernell D, Wu Chien P. Responses of the pyramidal tract to stimulation of the baboon's motor cortex. *J Physiol* 1967;191:653–672.
54. Kimura J. F-wave velocity in the central segment of the median and ulnar nerves: a study in normal subjects and patients with Charcot–Marie–Tooth disease. *Neurology* 1974;24:539–546.
55. Kimura J. *Electrodiagnosis in diseases of nerve and muscle: principles and practice*, 2nd ed. Philadelphia: FA Davis, 1989.
56. King RB, Stoops WL. Cervical myelopathy with fasciculations in the lower extremities. *J Neurosurg* 1963;20:948–952.
57. Koh THHG, Eyre JA. Maturation of corticospinal tracts assessed by electromagnetic stimulation of the motor cortex. *Arch Dis Child* 1988;63:1347–1352.
58. Kunesch E, Reiners K, Müller-Mattheis V, Strohmeyer T, Ackermann R, Freund H-J. Neurological risk profile in organic erectile impotence. *J Neurol Neurosurg Psychiatry* 1992;55:275–281.
59. Lesser RP, Lueders H, Hahan J, Klem G. Early somatosensory potentials evoked by median nerve stimulation: intraoperative monitoring. *Neurology* 1981;31:1519–1523.
60. Levy WJ, Walter J, Tucker D. Safety of magnetic transcranial stimulation. Presented at the Congress of the International Medical Society of Motor Disturbances (ISMD), Rome, 1988.
61. Luco JV, Eyzaguirre C. Fibrillations and hypersensitivity to ACh in denervated muscle: effect of length of degenerating nerve fibres. *J Neurophysiol* 1955;18:65–73.
62. Ludin HP. *Praktische Elektromyographie*, 3rd ed. Stuttgart: F Enke Verlag, 1988.
63. Ludin HP, Beyeler F. Temperature dependence of normal sensory nerve action potentials. *J Neurol* 1977;216:173–180.
64. Lueders H, Andrish J, Gurd A, Weiker G, Klem G. Origin of far-field subcortical potentials evoked by stimulation of the posterior tibial nerve. *Electroencephalogr Clin Neurophysiol* 1981;52:336–344.
65. Lueders H, Lesser R, Hahn J, Little J, Klem G. Subcortical somatosensory evoked potentials to median nerve stimulation. *Brain* 1983;106:341–372.
66. Magladery JW, McDougal DB. Electrophysiological studies of nerve and reflex activity in normal man. 1. Identification of certain reflexes in the electromyogram and the conduction velocity of peripheral nerve fibres. *Bull Johns Hopkins Hosp* 1950;86:265–290.
67. Maillis AG, Johnstone BM. Observations on the development on muscle hypersensitivity following chronic nerve conduction blockage and recovery. *J Neurol Sci* 1978;38:145–161.
68. Merton PA, Morton HB. Stimulation of the cerebral cortex in the intact human subject. *Nature* 1980;285:227–228.
69. Mervaala E, Paakkonen A, Partanen JV. The influence of height, age and gender on the interpretation of median nerve SEPs. *Electroencephalogr Clin Neurophysiol* 1988;71:109–113.
70. Mills KR, Murray NMF. Electrical stimulation over the human vertebral column: which neuronal elements are exited? *Electroencephalogr Clin Neurophysiol* 1986;63:582–589.
71. Møller AR, Jannetta PJ, Burgess JE. Neural generators of the somatosensory evoked potentials: recording from the cuneate nucleus in man and monkeys. *Electroencephalogr Clin Neurophysiol* 1986;65:241–248.
72. Müller K, Hömberg V, Lenard H-G. Magnetoelectric stimulation of motor cortex and nerve roots in children. I: Maturation of cortico-motoneuronal projections. *Electroencephalogr Clin Neurophysiol* 1991;81:63–78.
73. Mumenthaler M, Schliack H. *Läsionen Peripherer Nerven*, 5th ed. Stuttgart: G Thieme Verlag, 1987.
74. Owen JH, Jenny AB, Naito M, Weber K, Bridwell KH, McGhee R. Effects of spinal cord lesioning on somatosensory and neurogenic-motor evoked potentials. *Spine* 1989;14:673–682.
75. Patton HD, Amassian VE. Single and multiple unit analysis of cortical stage of pyramidal tract activation. *J Neurophysiol* 1954;17:345–363.
76. Phillips LH, Daube JR. Lumbosacral spinal evoked potentials in humans. *Neurology* 1980;30:1175–1183.
77. Piper H. Weitere Mitteilungen über die Geschwindigkeit der Erregungsleitung im markhaltigen menschlichen Nerven. *Pflügers Arch Ges Physiol* 1909;127:474.
78. Polson MJR, Barker AT, Freeston IL. Stimulation of nerve trunks with time varying magnetic fields. *Med Biol Eng Comput* 1982;20:243–244.
79. Reiners K, Herdmann J, Freund H-J. Altered mechanisms of muscular force generation in lower motor neuron disease. *Muscle Nerve* 1989;12:647–659.
80. Ricker K, Hertel G, Stodieck G. Increased voltage of the muscle action potential of normal subjects after local cooling. *J Neurol* 1977;216:33–38.
81. Riffel B, Stöhr M. Spinale und subkortikale somatosensorisch evozierte Potentiale nach Stimulation des N. tibialis. *Arch Psychiatr Nervenkr* 1982;232:251–263.
82. Riffel B, Stöhr M, Körner S. Spinal and cortical evoked potentials following stimulation of the posterior tibial nerve in the diagnosis and localization of spinal cord diseases. *Electroencephalogr Clin Neurophysiol* 1984;58:400–407.
83. Rosenfalck P, Buchthal F. Studies on fibrillation potentials of denervated human muscle. *Electroencephalogr Clin Neurophysiol Suppl* 1962;22:130.
84. Rossini PM, Caramia MD, Zarola F. Mechanisms of nervous propagation along central motor pathways: noninvasive evaluation in healthy subjects and in patients with neurological disease. *Neurosurgery* 1987;20:183–191.
85. Rothwell JC, Thompson PD, Day BL, Dick JPR, Kachi T, Cowan JMA, Marsden CD. Motor cortex stimulation in intact man. 1. General characteristics of EMG responses in different muscles. *Brain* 1987;110:1173–1190.
86. Seddon HJ. Three types of nerve injury. *Brain* 1943;66:237–288.
87. Seddon HJ. *Surgical disorders of peripheral nerves*, 2nd ed. Edinburgh: Churchill Livingstone, 1975.
88. Seyal M, Emerson RG, Pedley TA. Spinal and early scalp-recorded components of the somatosensory evoked potential following stimulation of the posterior tibial nerve. *Electroencephalogr Clin Neurophysiol* 1983;55:320–330.
89. Seyal M, Gabor AJ. The human posterior tibial somatosensory evoked potential: synapse dependent and synapse independent spinal components. *Electroencephalogr Clin Neurophysiol* 1985;62:323–331.
90. Seyal M, Gabor AJ. Generators of human spinal somatosensory evoked potentials. *J Clin Neurophysiol* 1987;4(2):177–187.
91. Shahani BT, Halperin JJ, Boulu P, Cohen J. Sympathetic skin response: a method of assessing unmyelinated axon dysfunction in peripheral neuropathies. *J Neurol Neurosurg Psychiatry* 1984;47:536–542.
92. Stanley EF. Reflexes evoked in human thenar muscles during voluntary activity and their conduction pathways. *J Neurol Neurosurg Psychiatry* 1978;41:1016–1023.
93. Stöhr M. Somatosensible Reizantworten von Rückenmark und Gehirn (SEP). In: Stöhr M, Dichgans J, Diener HC, Buettner UW, eds. *Evozierte Potentiale*, 2nd ed. Berlin: Springer, 1989;23–277.
94. Stöhr M, Riffel B. Short latency somatosensory evoked potentials to median nerve stimulation: components N13–P13, N14–P14, P15, P16 and P18 with different recording methods. *J Neurol* 1982;228:39–47.
95. Tasaki I. Electrical stimulation and the excitatory process in the nerve fiber. *Am J Physiol* 1937;125:380.
96. Thompson PD, Dick JPR, Asselman P, Griffin GB, Day BL, Rothwell JC, Sheehy MP, Marsden CD. Examination of motor function in lesions of the spinal cord by stimulation of the motor cortex. *Ann Neurol* 1987;21:389–396.
97. Thompson PD, Rothwell JC, Day BL, Dressler D, Maertens de Noordhout A, Marsden, CD. Mechanisms of electrical and magnetic stimulation of human motor cortex. In: Chokroverty S, ed. *Magnetic stimulation in clinical neurophysiology*. Boston: Butterworths, 1989;121–143.

98. Trojaborg W. Early electrophysiologic changes in conduction block. *Muscle Nerve* 1978;1:400.
99. Trojaborg W, Buchthal F. Malignant and benign fasciculations. *Acta Neurol Scand* 1965;41(suppl 13):251–254.
100. Trontelj JV, Stålberg E. Bizarre repetitive discharges recorded with single fibre EMG. *J Neurol Neurosurg Psychiatry* 1983;46:310–316.
101. Tsubokawa T, Yamamoto T, Nakamura S. Electrophysiological and morphological consequences of repeated magnetic stimulation of the brain and peripheral nerve. Presented at the 1989 International Motor Evoked Potential Symposium, Chicago, 1989.
102. Tsuji S, Shibasaki H, Kato M, Kuroiwa Y, Shima F. Subcortical, thalamic and cortical somatosensory evoked potentials to median nerve stimulation. *Electroencephalogr Clin Neurophysiol* 1984;59:465–476.
103. Tsumoto T, Hirose N, Nonaka S, Takahashi M. Analysis of somatosensory evoked potentials to lateral popliteal nerve stimulation in man. *Electroencephalogr Clin Neurophysiol* 1972;33:379–388.
104. Yamada T, Kayamori R, Kimura J, Beck DO. Topography of somatosensory evoked potentials after stimulation of the median nerve. *Electroencephalogr Clin Neurophysiol* 1984;59:29–43.

Intraoperative Ultrasonography in Spinal Trauma

Nathan H. Lebwohl and Parley W. Madsen

Real-time sonography is an important technique for evaluating the contents of the spinal canal during surgery for spine trauma. Modern, high-resolution scanners allow the intraoperative display of fine, anatomic detail, which permits the surgeon to identify and localize the compression of neural elements by bone or metal fragments as well as soft tissue. Sonography is extremely accurate in the evaluation of parenchymal lesions of the spinal cord including cysts and myelomalacia. The portability of ultrasound equipment allows its use intraoperatively to provide real-time imaging, whereas computerized tomography (CT) or magnetic resonance imaging (MRI), although highly accurate, are not similarly available intraoperatively. Sonography provides higher resolution than intraoperative myelography without exposure of the patient to the risks associated with intrathecal contrast agents. Additionally, there is no radiation exposure to the patient or to the operative staff when sonography is used instead of myelography.

BASIC PHYSICS

Ultrasound images are produced by measuring the reflection of sound waves in tissue (2). Audible sound waves have a frequency of 16 to 20 kHz. Ultrasound waves have higher frequencies. Spinal sonography typically employs a 7.5- or 10-MHz frequency probe. The sonography waves are generated by a piezoelectric crystal in the ultrasound probe. Reflections occur whenever the ultrasound beam passes through an interface between tissues of different density. Ultrasound is exquisitely sensitive to small differences in tissue density. Water, blood, fat, and connective tissue all have different tissue densities and will create an interface adequate to generate a reflection.

Ultrasound is more sensitive than CT scanning to differences in tissue density. However, large differences in tissue density will create large reflections, attenuating the beam so that no information can be obtained from deeper structures. At soft tissue–bone interfaces, about 70% of the beam is reflected, and at soft tissue–air interfaces, 99% of the beam is reflected. Thus, in spinal ultrasound, a laminotomy is required to provide a window through bone. The wound is filled with saline to provide a path through which the beam can travel.

TECHNIQUE

Several manufacturers supply high-frequency ultrasound transducers that are small enough to allow their use in an operative wound. At Jackson Memorial Hospital, a 7.5-MHz ATL scanner (Advanced Technology Laboratory, Bellevue, WA) is currently the sonographic machine most frequently employed for intraoperative scanning. Prior to scanning, the probe is placed in a sterile, plastic sheath filled with sterile lubricant (K-Y Jelly, Johnson & Johnson, New Brunswick, NJ) (Fig. 1). Care is taken to eliminate any air bubbles adjacent to the transducer, since this will otherwise result in image degradation.

A laminotomy is performed over the area of interest, and an opening of at least 1 cm in length and 1.5 cm in

---

N. H. Lebwohl: Department of Orthopaedics and Rehabilitation, University of Miami/Jackson Memorial Medical Center, Miami, FL 33101.

P. W. Madsen: Department of Neurological Surgery, University of Miami School of Medicine, Miami, FL 33101.

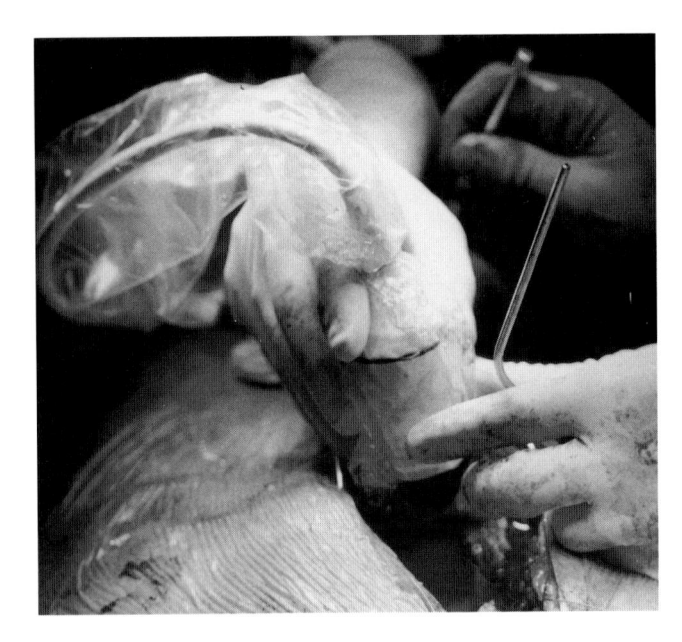

FIG. 1. The transducer in its sterile plastic sleeve is positioned in saline filled wound.

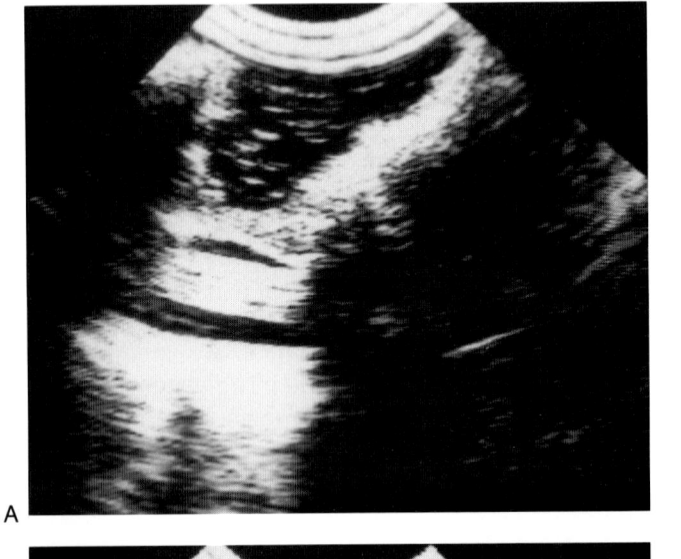

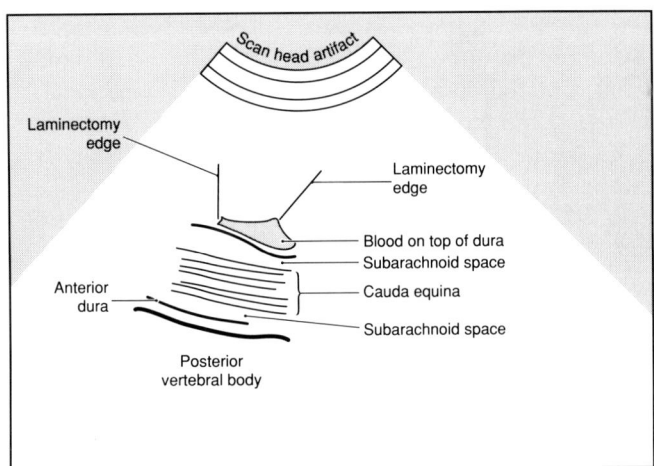

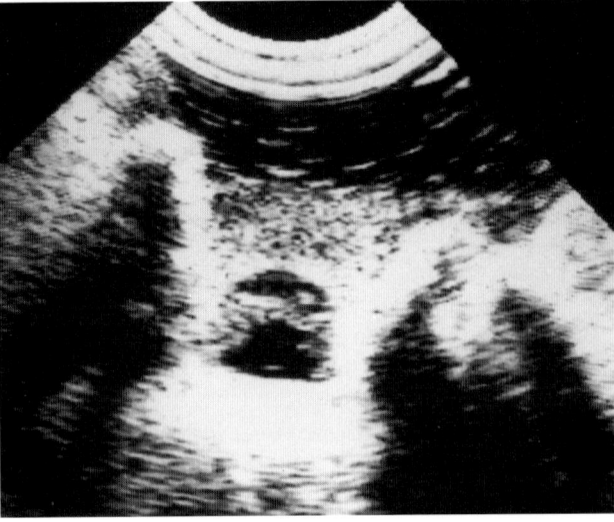

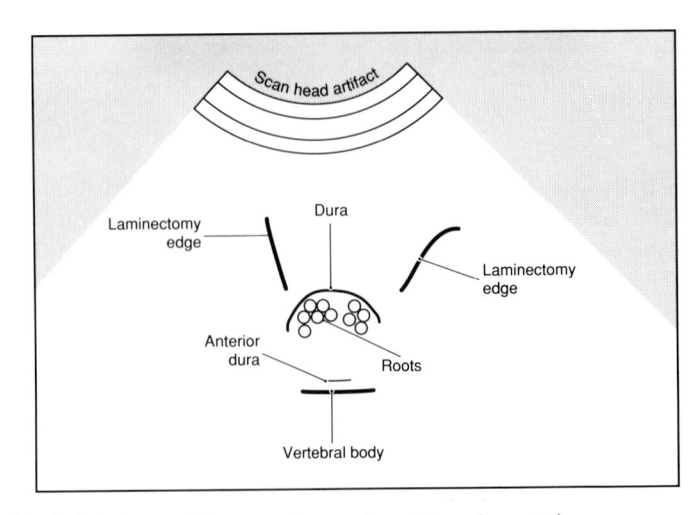

FIG. 2. A: Sagittal view of the cauda equina. **B:** Axial view of the cauda equina. The clumped roots suggest arachnoiditis.

width is created. The surgical wound is then filled with plain saline, avoiding the antibiotics frequently mixed with the irrigation saline. The use of plain saline will minimize formation of air bubbles, which degrade the image quality of the sonogram. The probe is then inserted into the saline, taking care to avoid contact with the dura, and positioned so that the area of interest is properly focused. Transverse and sagittal images are routinely obtained by merely rotating the transducer 90°. As blood mixes with the saline bath, it reflects the ultrasound waves and degrades the image with artifacts. Replacing the saline in the operative site will restore the image quality.

Ultrasonic evaluation of the spine can be performed from an anterior approach through a corpectomy or discectomy defect. As with the posterior approach, the wound is filled with saline.

NORMAL ANATOMY

The scans are displayed with the scanhead artifact at the top of the image. With the patient prone, structures displayed top to bottom are situated posterior to anterior. On the transverse scan, the posterior dura is seen as a line convex to the scanhead (9). The bony margins of the laminectomy are seen as bright echoes laterally with no detail below them. The spinal cord is seen below the dura closest to the transducer. The central canal provides a bright reflection visible as a dot or small circle. This is an important landmark that is particularly useful when the anatomy is distorted. Surrounding the cord is the fluid subarachnoid space, which generates no reflections (Figs. 2 and 3).

At the conus, the cord is visualized tapering down to the filum terminale. Below the conus, the roots of

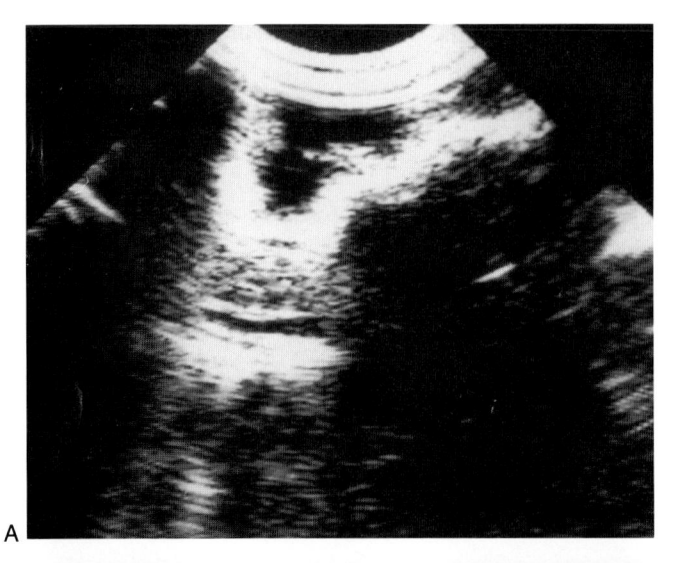

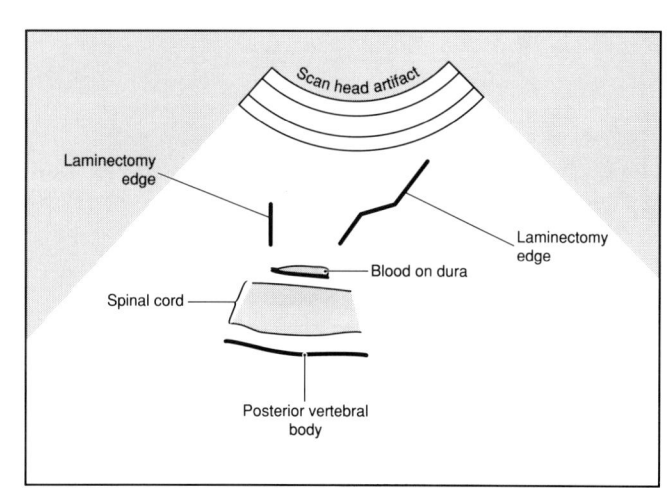

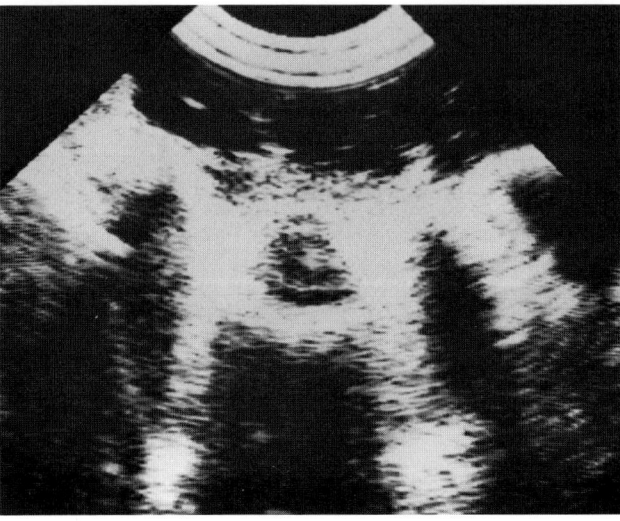

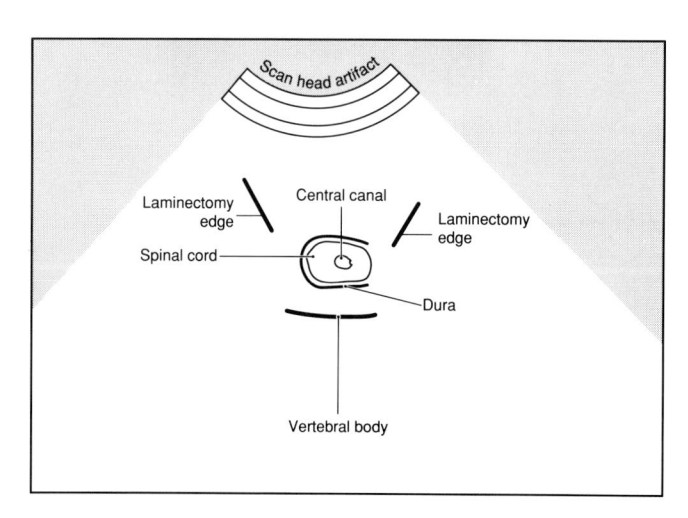

FIG. 3. A: Sagittal view of the spinal cord. **B:** Axial view of the spinal cord (S.C.). Note prominent central canal (C.C.).

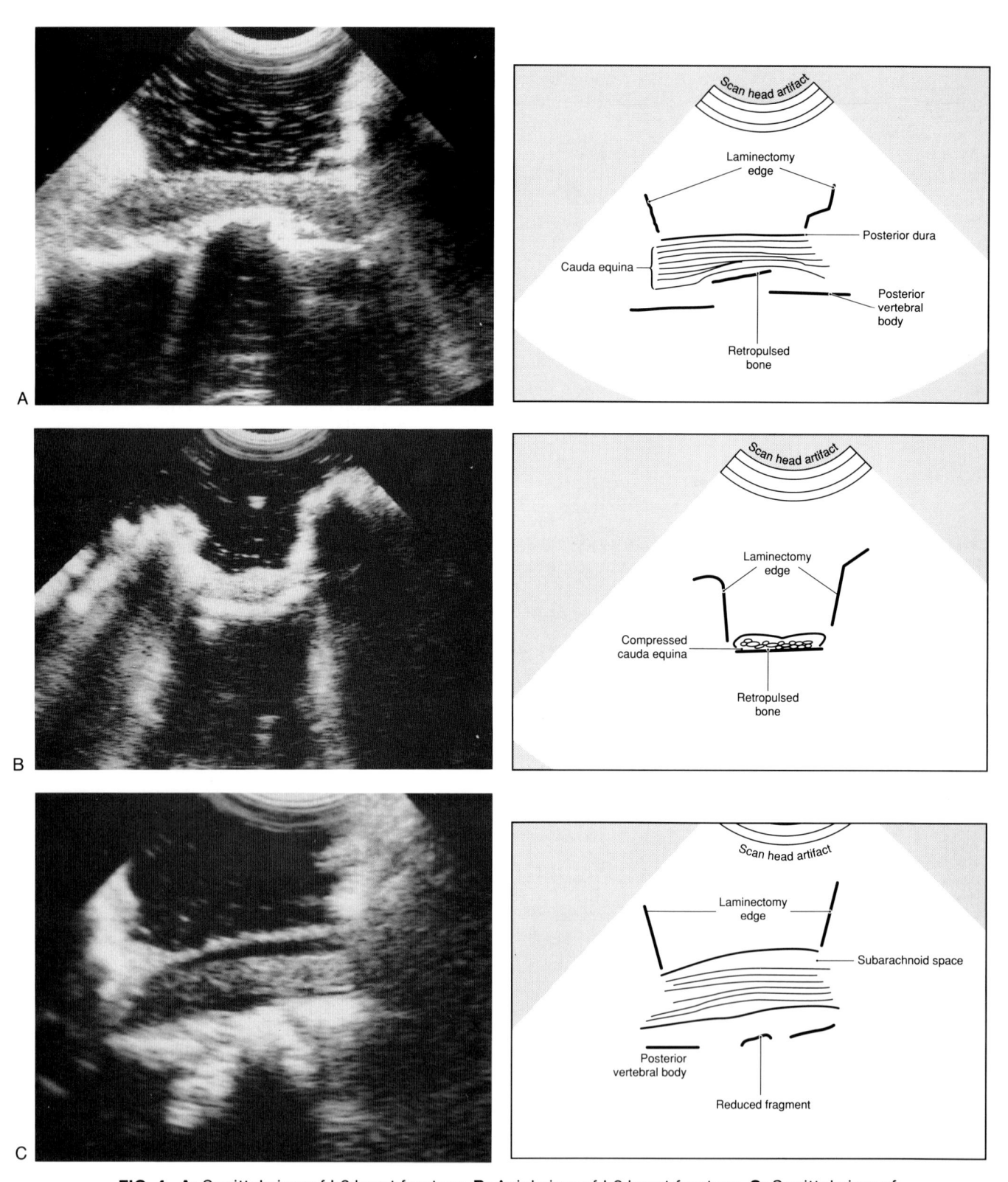

FIG. 4. A: Sagittal view of L2 burst fracture. **B:** Axial view of L2 burst fracture. **C:** Sagittal view of L2 burst fracture after decompression. Note restoration of anterior subarachnoid space.

the cauda equina are seen distributed in the subarachnoid space.

During real-time sonography, the anterior spinal artery is visible as a pulsating structure that cannot be visualized on static films. The bone of the posterior vertebral body generates a bright reflection and structures anterior to the vertebral bodies cannot be visualized. Intervertebral discs are less echogenic and are visualized as dark bands between the bright reflections of the posterior vertebral bodies.

DECOMPRESSION OF THE SPINAL CANAL

Intraoperative visualization of neural compression by a fracture deformity, retropulsed bone, or a foreign body is easily accomplished with ultrasound imaging. Preoperative radiographic studies are critical to assist in localization so that a limited laminotomy can be performed overlying the region of compression. In patients with fractures of the spinal column, neural compression is visualized as absence of the subarachnoid space and deformation of the neural elements. Bone fragments are visualized as highly reflective elements within the canal.

Metallic foreign bodies such as bullet fragments are easily located as they have a characteristic appearance on ultrasound imaging. The sound energy causes the metal to resonate, sending multiple echoes back to the transducer. The echoes appear behind the reflecting object as a series of bright lines, which has been described as a "comet tail" (9).

Although the ability to document neural compression with intraoperative sonography is useful, the ability to confirm adequate decompression at surgery is of more significance. Ultrasound imaging allows evaluation of the anterior spinal canal through a posterior portal without retraction of the neural elements and makes feasible intraoperative evaluation of indirect decompression techniques performed from the posterior approach (5) (Fig. 4).

Using a Harrington rod distraction technique, Eismont et al. (4) demonstrated persistent compression of neural elements with intraoperative sonography in 12 of 23 patients treated with distraction alone. Posterolateral decompression was then performed with relief of the neural compromise as documented by sonography. Follow-up CT scan in nine patients revealed adequate restoration of canal diameter in all but one patient. In that patient, significant canal compromise was noted at a level remote from the intraoperatively visualized level. This case demonstrated the importance

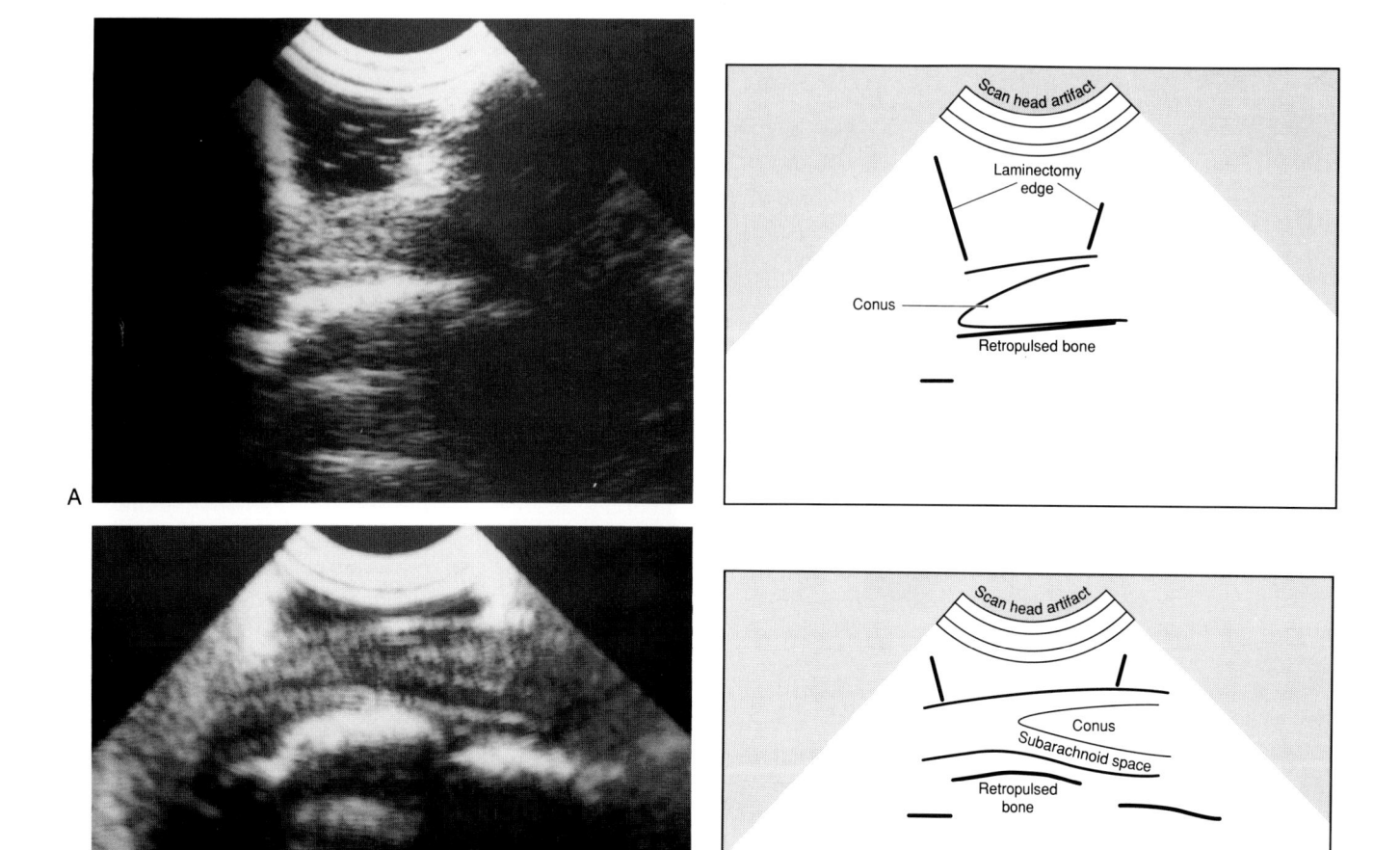

FIG. 5. A: L1 burst fracture with compression of conus (sagittal view). **B:** Harrington distraction instrumentation partially reduces retropulsed bone. Note appearance of anterior subarachnoid.

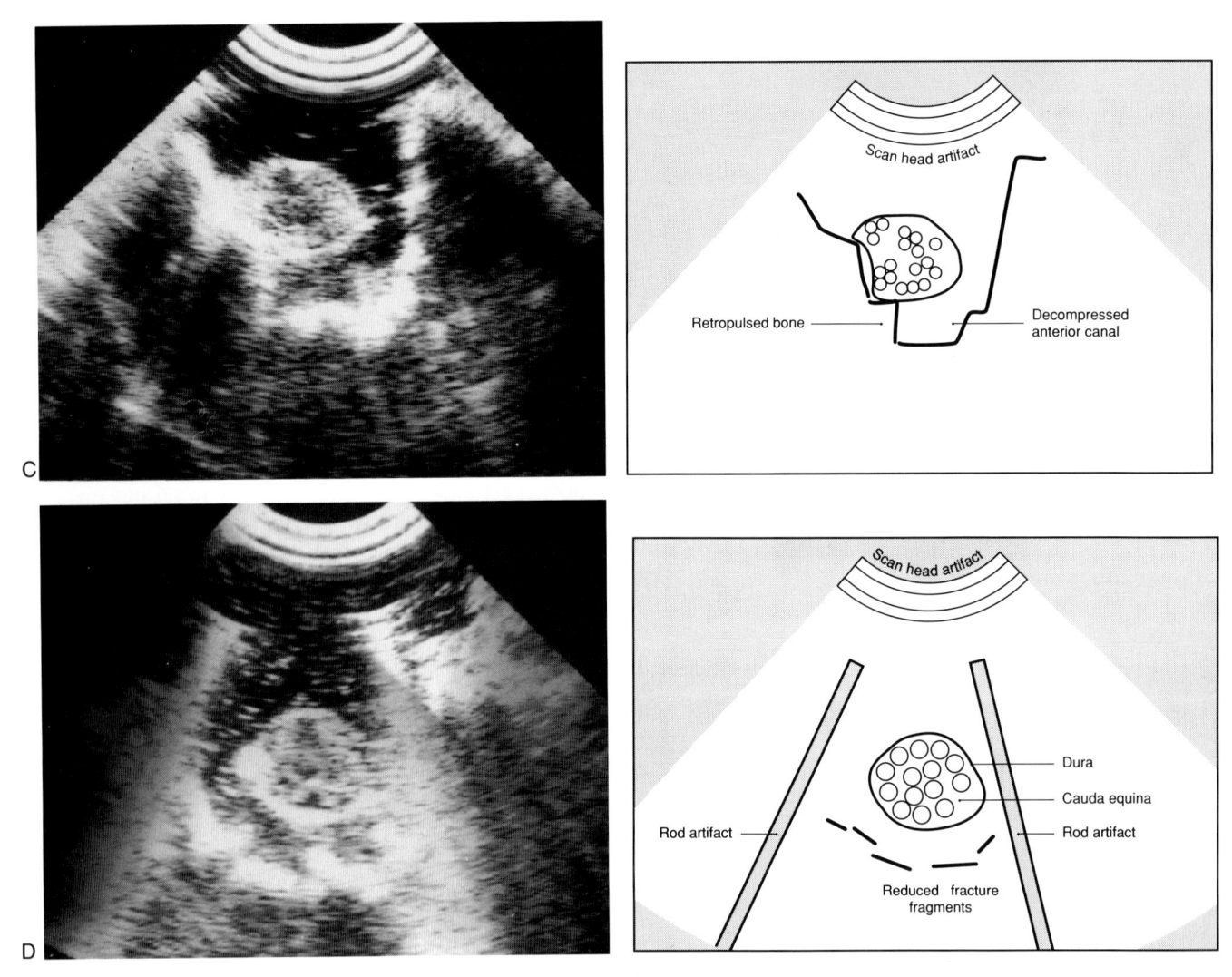

FIG. 5. *(Continued)* **C:** One side of the spinal canal has been decompressed through a transpedicular approach. **D:** Axial view after complete transpedicular decompression. Note artifact from rods.

of preoperative imaging for adequate evaluation of the spinal canal and proper placement of the laminotomy. Vincent et al. (11) also used intraoperative sonographic imaging to evaluate the reduction of canal compromise after the placement of distraction rods and a posterior lateral decompression. The adequacy of the decompression was confirmed with postoperative CT scanning (Fig. 5).

Additional uses for intraoperative ultrasound imaging in the trauma patient include the visualization of subligamentous hematoma, the localization of residual bone in the spinal canal, and the identification of herniated intravertebral disc material in the spinal canal. The identification of the latter entity is of particular significance in patients who undergo compression instrumentation of fracture dislocations of the spine. In reducing the dislocation the disc can be forced into the spinal canal with resultant damage to the underlying neural tissue. Sonographic imaging can obviate this iatrogenic injury by demonstration of the mass and the subsequent modification of surgical technique (3).

CYSTIC MYELOPATHY

Spinal cord cysts are more accurately evaluated by intraoperative ultrasound than by any other imaging technique. Sonography is superior to CT myelography, delayed myelography, and MRI in the detection of septations or of small additional cysts (6,8,10). In the nontrauma patient ultrasound may also demonstrate soft tissue nodules in the wall of a cyst, suggesting tumor as the etiology of the lesion (Fig. 6).

In addition to characterization of a spinal cord cyst, intraoperative ultrasound aids the surgeon in cyst localization and in the identification of the optimal site

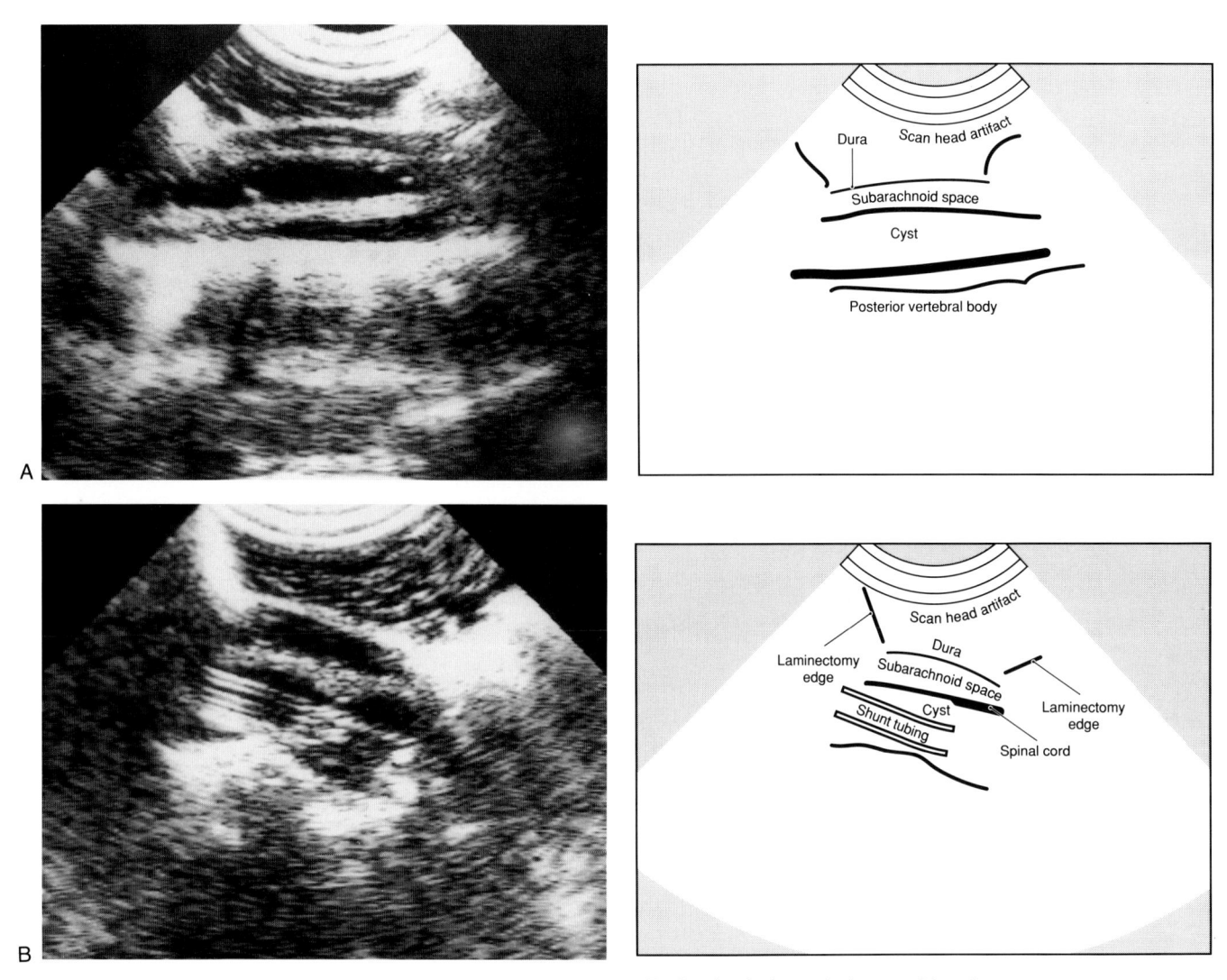

FIG. 6. A: Sagittal view of spinal cord cyst. **B:** Sagittal view of shunt tubing in cyst.

for myelotomy. Sonography can also confirm effective decompression of the cyst. In the case of a multiloculated cyst, communication between the cyst cavities can be verified, thereby obviating the need for additional shunt catheters. Doppler ultrasound may allow the confirmation of flow through a functional shunt.

EVALUATION OF CORD TRAUMA

Intraoperative ultrasound reliably detects parenchymal abnormalities within the spinal cord following trauma. Mirvis and Geisler (7) studied 30 patients with acute spinal cord injury who underwent surgical decompression. They performed intraoperative ultrasound following corpectomy or laminectomy and evaluated the extent of cord abnormality. The degree of cord abnormality correlated significantly with both the initial American Spinal Injury Association motor score as well as the motor score at follow-up.

In infants with incompletely ossified posterior elements, the cord can be evaluated by transcutaneous ultrasound. In a group of four neonates with birth trauma to the cord, three autopsy specimens showed good correlation with ultrasound in the evaluation of cord edema and hemorrhage (1).

SUMMARY

Intraoperative ultrasound evaluation of the spine allows the surgeon to evaluate the contents of the spinal canal with little risk of iatrogenic morbidity. Sonography allows the identification and localization of foreign bodies, bone fragments, hematoma, and parenchymal abnormalities of the cord. The real-time images provided by intraoperative ultrasonography are important information for the surgeon. The adequacy of decompression procedures can be verified. Sonography is rapid and easily set up, allowing frequent repetition to assess the progress of surgery. This imaging technique is superior to intraoperative myelography and eliminates the risks of intrathecal contrast and x-ray exposure.

REFERENCES

1. Babyn PS, Chuang SH, Daneman A, Davidson GS. Sonographic evaluation of spinal cord birth trauma with pathologic correlation, *AJR* 1988;151:736–766.
2. Bartrum RJ, Crow HC. *Real-time ultrasound,* 2nd ed. Philadelphia: Saunders, 1983.
3. Chadduck WM, Flanigan S. Intraoperative ultrasound for spinal lesions. *Neurosurgery* 1985;16(4):477–83.
4. Eismont FJ, Green BA, Berkowitz BM, Montalvo BA, Quencer RM, Brown MB. The role of intraoperative ultrasonography in the treatment of thoracic and lumbar spine fractures. *Spine* 1984; 9(8):782–787.
5. Eismont FJ, Green BA. Surgical treatment of spinal injuries: anterior versus posterior approaches. *Adv Orthop Surg Rev* 1984;24–34.
6. Gebarski ST, Maynard FW, Gabrielsen TO, Knake JE, Latack JT, Hoff JT. Posttraumatic progressive myelopathy. *Radiology* 1985;157:379–385.
7. Mirvis SE, Geisler FH. Intraoperative sonography of cervical spinal cord injury: results in 30 patients. *AJNR* 1990;11:755–761.
8. Quencer RM, Morse BMM, Green BA, Eismont FJ, and Brost P. Intraoperative spinal sonography: adjunct to metrizimide CT in the assessment and surgical decompression of posttraumatic spinal cord cysts. *AJR* 1984;142:593.
9. Rubin JM, Chandler WF. The use of ultrasound during spinal cord surgery. *World J Surg* 1987;11:570–578.
10. Rubin JM, Dohrmann GJ. The spine and spinal cord during neurosurgical operations: real-time ultrasonography. *Radiology* 1985;155:197–200.
11. Vincent KA, Benson DR, McGahan, JP. Intraoperative ultrasonography for reduction of thoracolumbar burst fractures. *Spine* 1989;14(4):387–390.

10

Classification of Thoracolumbar Spine Fractures

Claude Argenson and Pascal Boileau

The spine's complex anatomy and biomechanical properties allow it to bear deforming forces of great amplitude and sustain loads of high magnitude. When these exceed a certain level, either in axial loading, flexion, extension, rotation, or shear, a host of injuries are likely to occur. Since Boehler (9) in 1929, many authors have established the relationship between excessive moments of force applied to the spine and the resulting injuries, which are described in multiple classifications. Unlike the fracture patterns of long bones, which usually do not evolve over time, the pattern of spine fractures may be progressive, resulting in increased deformity. Compromise of the neural elements, which are normally protected by the intact, bony spinal canal, may develop. The question of instability as raised by Watson-Jones (48), Nicoll (38), and others has been prominent in classification schemes that were successively proposed.

HISTORIC PERSPECTIVE

Each author contributed to the knowledge of each specific injury and its consequences on the neural tissues. It is essential to go back in history to review the most important landmarks in this educational process.

The first classification, of Boehler (9) in 1929, included five types:

1. Compression fracture with vertebral body injuries.
2. Fracture by anterior flexion, anterior injury due to compression, and posterior injury due to distraction.
3. Fracture by extension, with injury to the anterior and posterior longitudinal ligaments, and posterior arch injuries.
4. Shear fractures following application of force, whose moment is perpendicular to the spine's long axis, with subsequent, large sagittal displacement.
5. Fractures by torsion, which are responsible for asymmetric injuries.

The next relevant classification was made by Watson-Jones in 1931. For the first time, the Watson-Jones classification introduced the concept of "instability," which he related to ligamentous injuries of the spine.

Nicoll, in 1949, redefined this concept of instability when he described acute and secondary displacements after attempted reduction, which, according to his work, were due to the following:

1. A "bony gap" inside the vertebral body when the vertebral fracture was comminuted.
2. A disc injury that did not heal.
3. A torn anterior ligament.

Holdsworth's classification (25,26) has been adopted largely since 1963, when he described injuries as classified into six groups:

1. Anterior wedge compression.
2. Dislocation.
3. Fracture/dislocation by rotation (slice fracture).
4. Injury due to extension.
5. Comminuted fractures (burst).
6. Shear fractures.

C. Argenson: Department of Orthopaedic Surgery, Service de Chirurgie Orthopedique et Traumatologique, Centre Hospitalier Regional et Universitaire de Nice, St. Roch University Hospital, 06000 Nice, France.
P. Boileau: Department of Orthopaedic Surgery, St. Roch University Hospital, 06000 Nice, France.

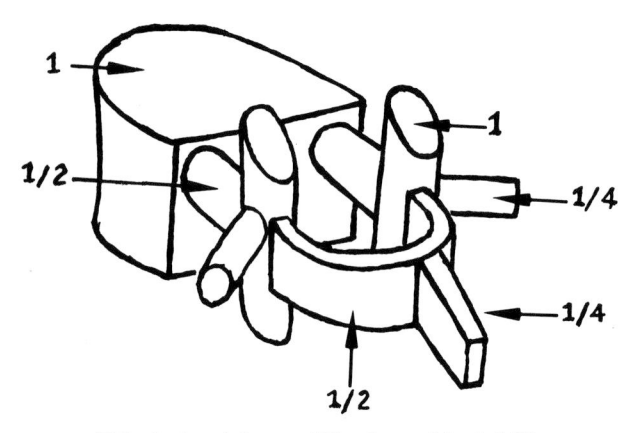

FIG. 1. Louis' quantification of instability.

Holdsworth was the first to introduce the concept of the burst fracture in which the nucleus of the disc penetrates the endplate of the vertebral body. This injury was seen as stable in spite of multiple fragments because the posterior ligamentous complex and the interspinous ligaments, articular facet capsules, and ligamentum flavum remained intact. Wedge fractures were also seen as stable. In contrast, the four other fractures were found to be unstable.

In 1958, Decoulx and Rieunau (15) refined the Watson-Jones classification and incorporated the concept of instability as described by Nicoll. The emphasis they placed on the posterior wall and posterior disc annulus and ligament complex deserved more credit. The posterior part of the vertebral body and the annulus fibrosus are lined by the posterior longitudinal ligament: injuries of these elements are responsible for fracture instability. Unfortunately, the literature has retained only the Decoulx–Rieunau theory of the posterior wall of the vertebral body as the element responsible for fracture instability; the disc and ligament complex were totally forgotten. The significance of disc and ligament injury to instability is now well recognized.

The first notion of "spinal columns" came with Kelly and Whitesides (27) in 1968. These authors assimilated the spine to a system made up of two columns: one was anterior, composed of disc and verte-

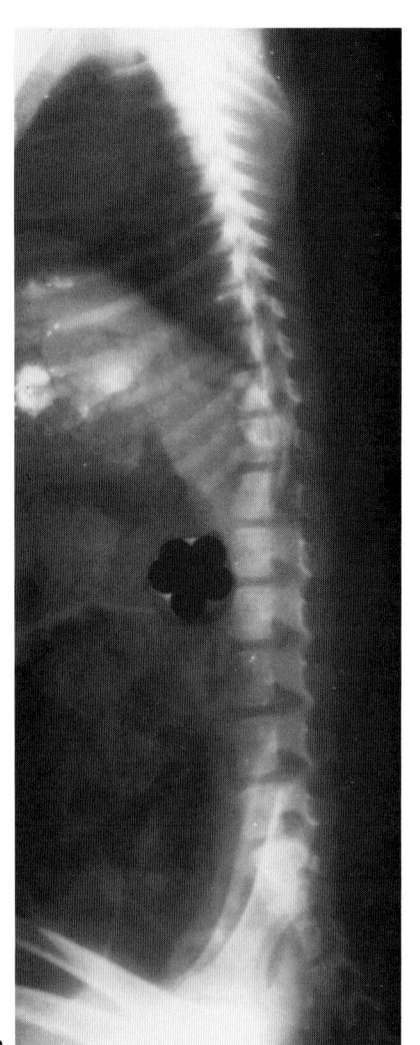

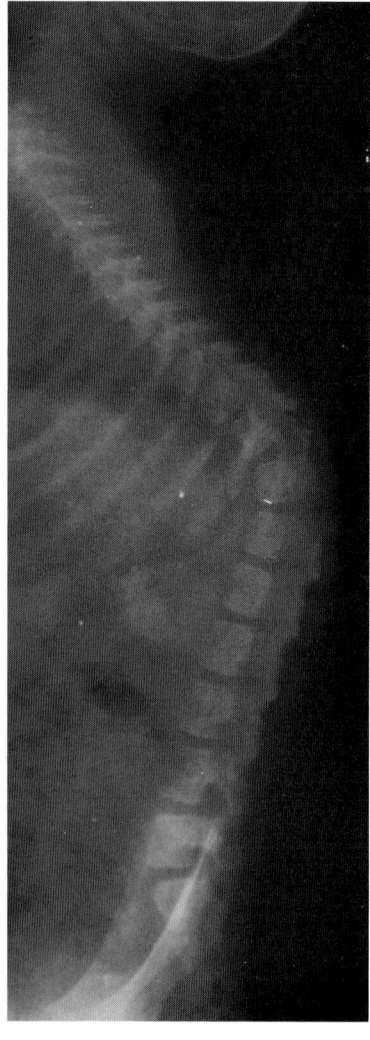

FIG. 2. Experimental section of posterior part of annulus fibrosus and posterior longitudinal ligament on monkeys (4). **A:** Postoperative day. **B:** Tenth postoperative day.

bral body, which work under load in compression; the other was the posterior column, which works under tension. Kelly and Whitesides also demonstrated bony fragments retropulsed from the body of the vertebra into the spinal canal in comminuted fractures, which gave these fractures a high potential for instability. They were the first to recommend removal of these fragments by anterior approach to the spine.

Roberts and Curtiss (40) corroborated the concept of late displacement of compression fractures by establishing neurologic findings in patients who were initially intact, or diagnosed as intact. These fractures could have been burst injuries.

Roy-Camille and co-workers (41,42) in 1970, emphasized the "intermediate vertebral segment," constituted by the posterior part of the disc, annulus fibrosus, and the posterior longitudinal ligament as well as the pedicles and posterior articular processes.

In 1973, Louis (32) described the architecture of the spine as a three-column system: one column is anterior, composed of the discs and vertebral bodies; two other columns are posterior and composed of the facets, articular processes, and the isthmus. These two posterior columns are connected by two arches, the two pedicles, which are similar in function to buttresses between each posterior column and the anterior column. The neural arc consists of the laminae and the posterior processes. With the help of this classification, it is possible to quantify instability, in which each column counts as 1.0, the arcs count as 1/2, and the other elements as 1/4. Instability is defined by a score of 2 or greater than 2 (32,33) (Fig. 1).

In 1976, Argenson and Dintimille (4) carried out experiments on monkeys, the only animal erect during the postoperative period and thus closest to the human condition. They demonstrated that the most unstable injuries, and therefore those prone to become worse, were injuries of the posterior ligaments and the posterior part of the annulus fibrosus (Fig. 2). The experimental transection of successive ligamentous and disc structures confirmed the studies of Bedbrook (7) and Roy-Camille and co-workers (41,42) on cadavers and helped to establish the concept of disc and ligament late instability, related to their tendency to heal poorly. In contrast, the bony structures, responsible only for instability of short duration, carry a good prognosis because of bony healing. Instability was found to be progressive, similar to the instability encountered after extensive laminectomies or fracture treated by conservative means.

Denis (17), in 1983, did a retrospective study of 412 thoracolumbar injuries. Fifty-three of these injuries were studied with CT scan. He proposed a new, biomechanical, three-column concept of the spine and ventured a new classification (Fig. 3).

The anterior column is formed by the anterior longitudinal ligament, the anterior part of the disc annulus fibrosus, and the anterior part of the vertebral body.

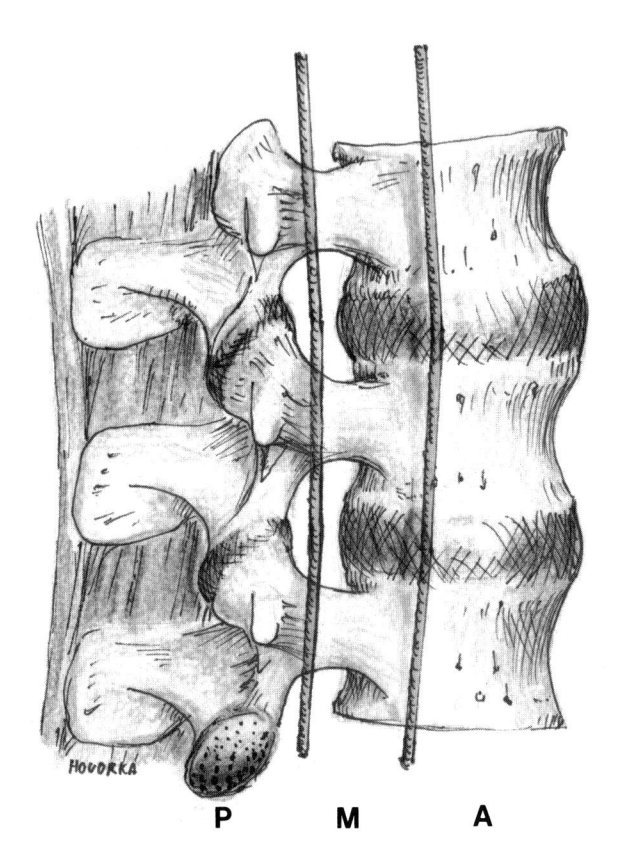

FIG. 3. The three-column spine: anterior (A), middle (M), and posterior (P) columns (17).

TABLE 1. *Modified Denis classification as used at the University of Nice*

Type	Mechanism	Preferred localization	Definition	Stability[a]	Denis classification	Late aspects
I—Compression fracture	Flexion (% compression)	Thoracic	AC = Height decreased MC = Intact PC = None or horizontal lesions (ligamentous > bony)	STABLE Anterior wedge < 50% No posterior lesions UNSTABLE Multiple lesions Anterior wedge > 50% Ligamentous posterior lesions	Type I B, C, D (A) A (B, C, D)	Kyphosis by angulation
II—Burst	Compression (% flexion)	T12–L1 L5 Lumbar	AC = Height decreased MC = Height decreased PC = Vertical lesions (bony > ligamentous)	STABLE Posterosuperior fragment (PSF) < 30% Sagittal index[b] (SI) 20% UNSTABLE PSF ≥ 30–50% ≤ SI 20–35 ± Posterior lesions UNSTABLE[c] PSF > 50%	Type II A (B–C) B–C (A) B–C (A)	 Kyphosis and subluxation Pseudarthrosis Kyphosis Neurological impairment Pseudarthrosis
III—Seat belt	Flexion–distraction	T12–L1	AC = Intact or disrupted MC = Increased Height PC = Increased Height	STABLE Osseous horizontal lesion UNSTABLE Discoligamentous horizontal lesions AC = disrupted	Type III A (Chance) Type III B, C, D Type IV C	Pseudarthrosis
IV—Dislocations	Translation (% every movement)	All the spine	AC = MC = PC = disrupted All possible lesions	ALL UNSTABLE Osseous instability Discoligamentous instability	Type IV A (through bone) D[d] Type II D–E Type IV A (through disc) B	Dislocation

[a] Stable = unstable = by conservative treatment.
[b] See Farcy et al. (18)
[c] Mechanical and neurological instability.
[d] See text.
AC, anterior column.
MC, middle column.
PC, posterior column.

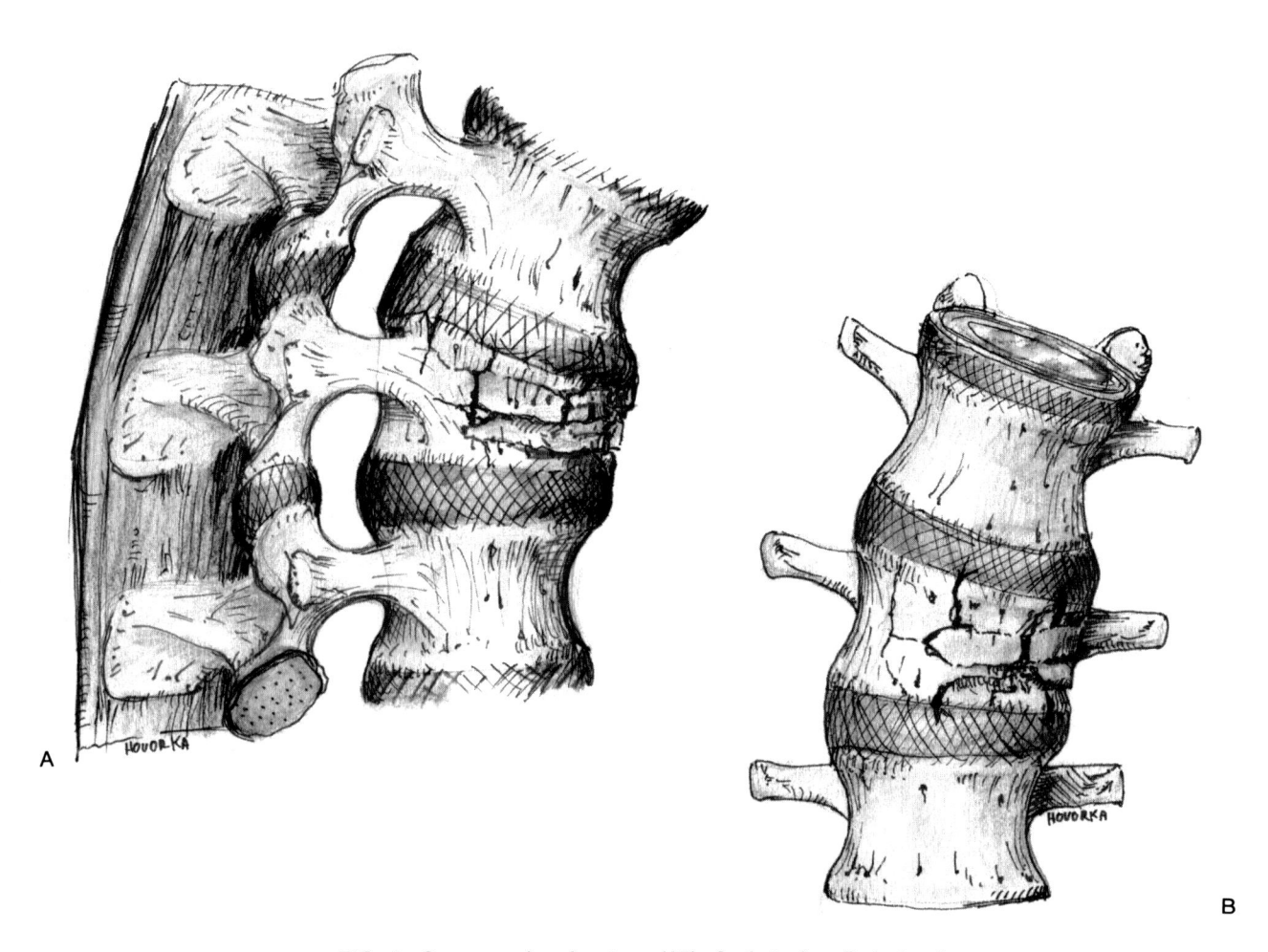

FIG. 4. Compression fracture (17). **A:** Anterior. **B:** Lateral.

The middle column is formed by the posterior longitudinal ligament, the posterior annulus fibrosus, and the posterior wall of the vertebral body. The posterior column is essentially the same as described by Holdsworth and is formed by the posterior bony complex, which is composed of the posterior arc as well as the posterior ligamentous complex, supraspinous ligament, interspinous ligament, capsule of the facet joint, and ligamentum flavum.

The classification of Denis is based on four main types related to the injury of the three columns. His distinction is based on the mechanism of injury; it can be seen in Table 1.

Miscellaneous types of fractures, minor in nature, are listed also by Denis but form a less significant part of the classification. These include transverse process fractures, isolated fractures of the articular processes, spinous process fractures, and pars interarticularis fractures.

The major types in Denis' classification are:

Compression fractures result from failure of the anterior column; the middle column remains intact. In severe cases, there may be a partial tension failure of the posterior column. The compression is anterior or lateral (Fig. 4B). Four subtypes can also be described (Fig. 5).

Burst fractures exhibit a combination of failure of the anterior and middle columns, which are under compression. Different types of burst fractures are described: the types depend on the mode of failure and the site at which the fracture occurs (Fig. 6).

Seat belt type fractures is the term preferred by Denis instead of "flexion–distraction injury," even though many of these lesions do not result from wearing a seat belt (Fig. 7).

Fracture/dislocation is used to describe failure of all columns under compression, tension, rotation, or shear; this leads to subluxation or dislocation (Fig. 8).

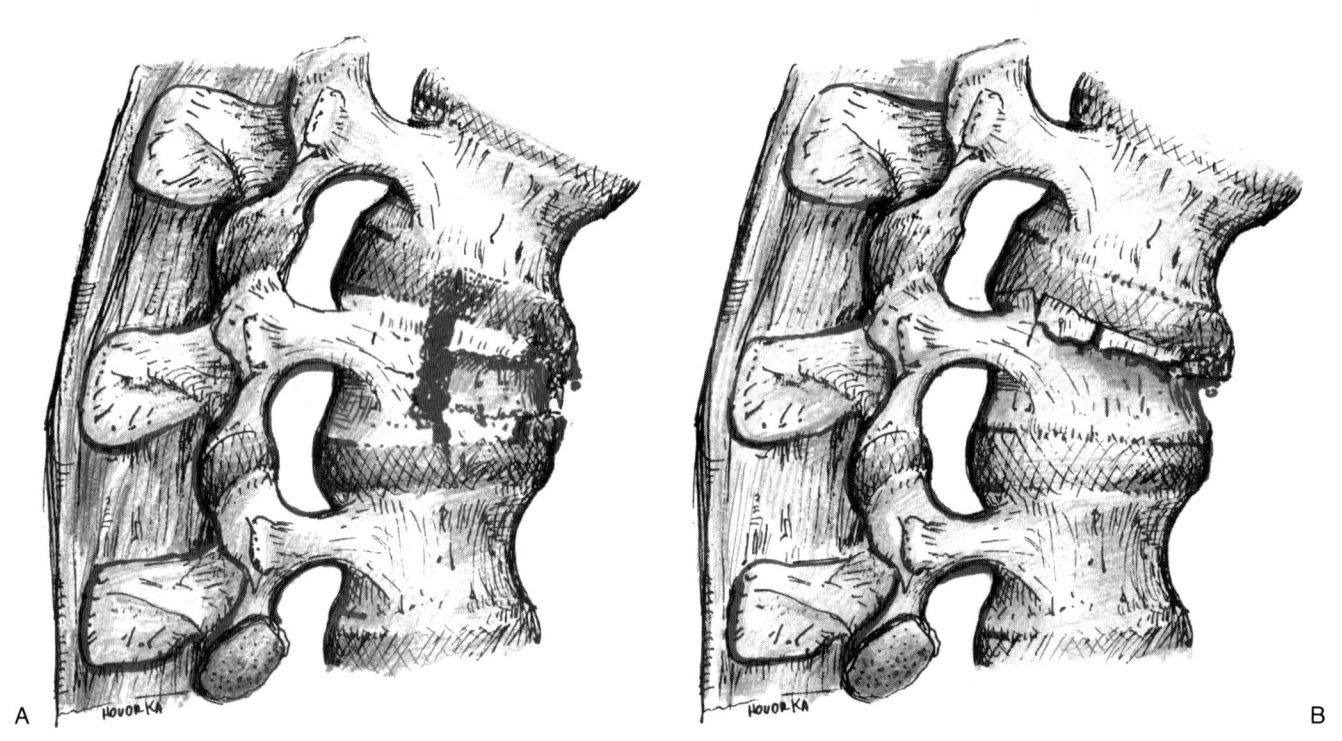

FIG. 5. Denis' Type I: compression fractures (17). **A:** Fracture in the frontal plane. **B:** Fracture of the anterior upper endplate.

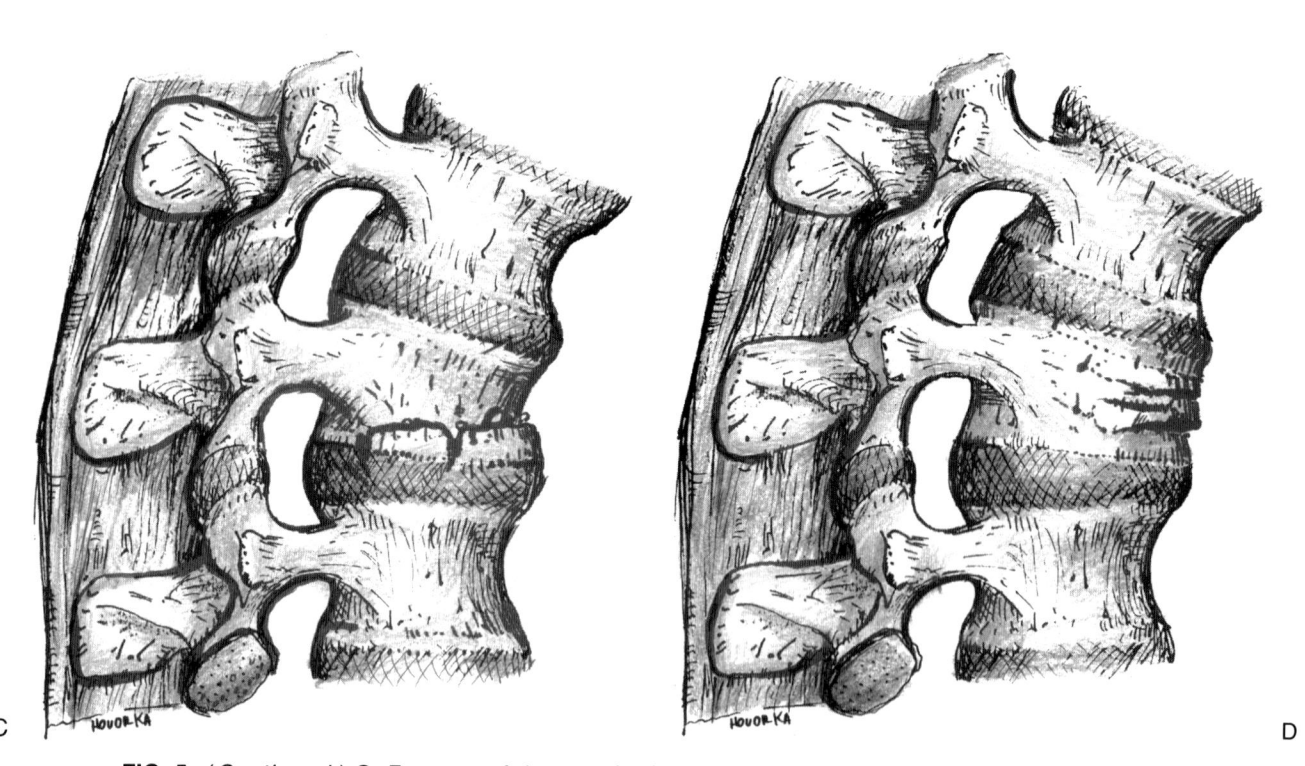

FIG. 5. (*Continued.*) **C:** Fracture of the anterior inferior endplate. **D:** Failure of both endplates.

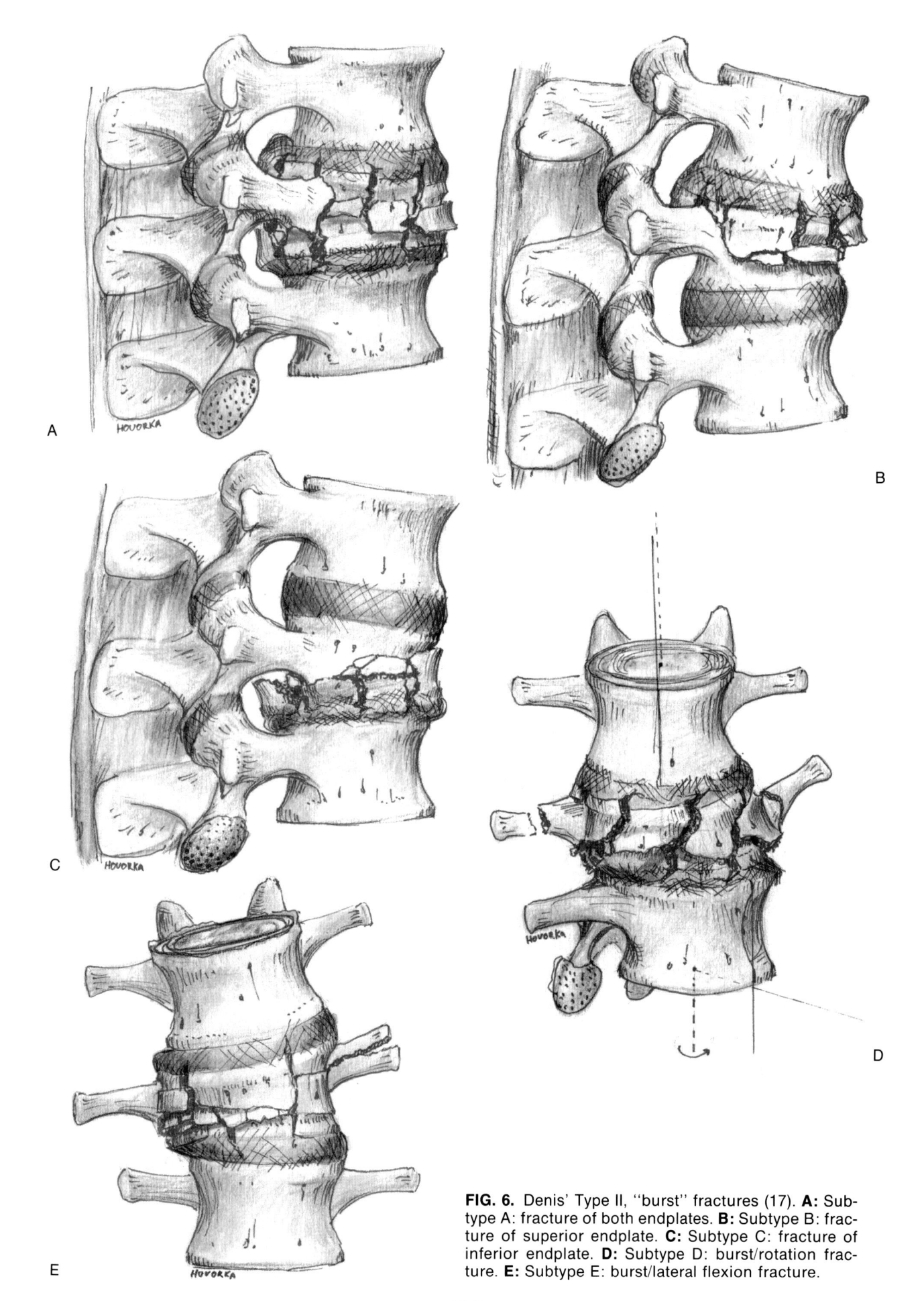

FIG. 6. Denis' Type II, "burst" fractures (17). **A:** Subtype A: fracture of both endplates. **B:** Subtype B: fracture of superior endplate. **C:** Subtype C: fracture of inferior endplate. **D:** Subtype D: burst/rotation fracture. **E:** Subtype E: burst/lateral flexion fracture.

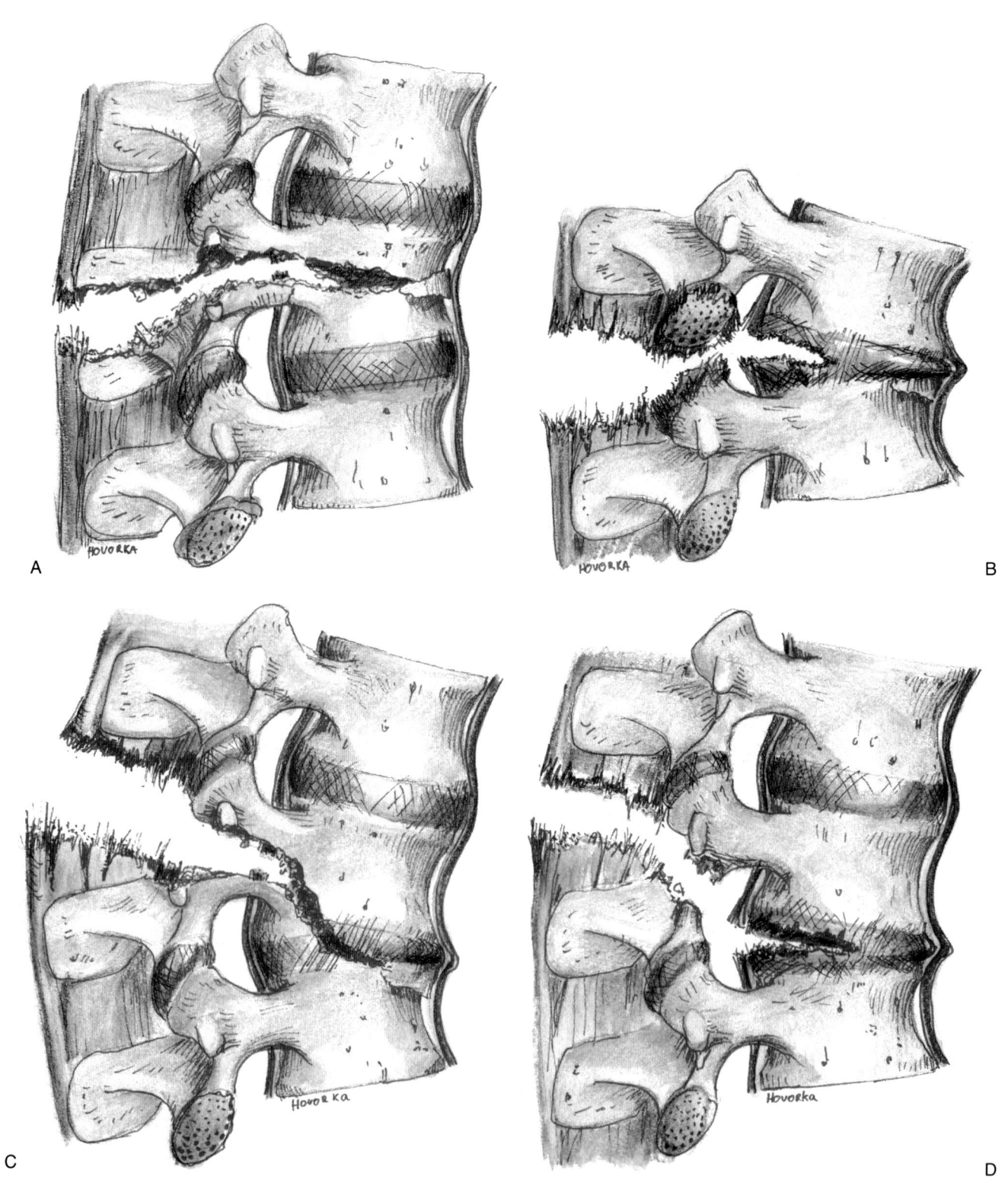

FIG. 7. Denis' Type III, "seat belt" fractures (17). **A:** One level "Chance" fracture with bone disruption. **B:** One-level discoligamentous disruption. **C:** Two-level fracture with bone and ligamentous disruption. **D:** Two-level ligamentous disruption.

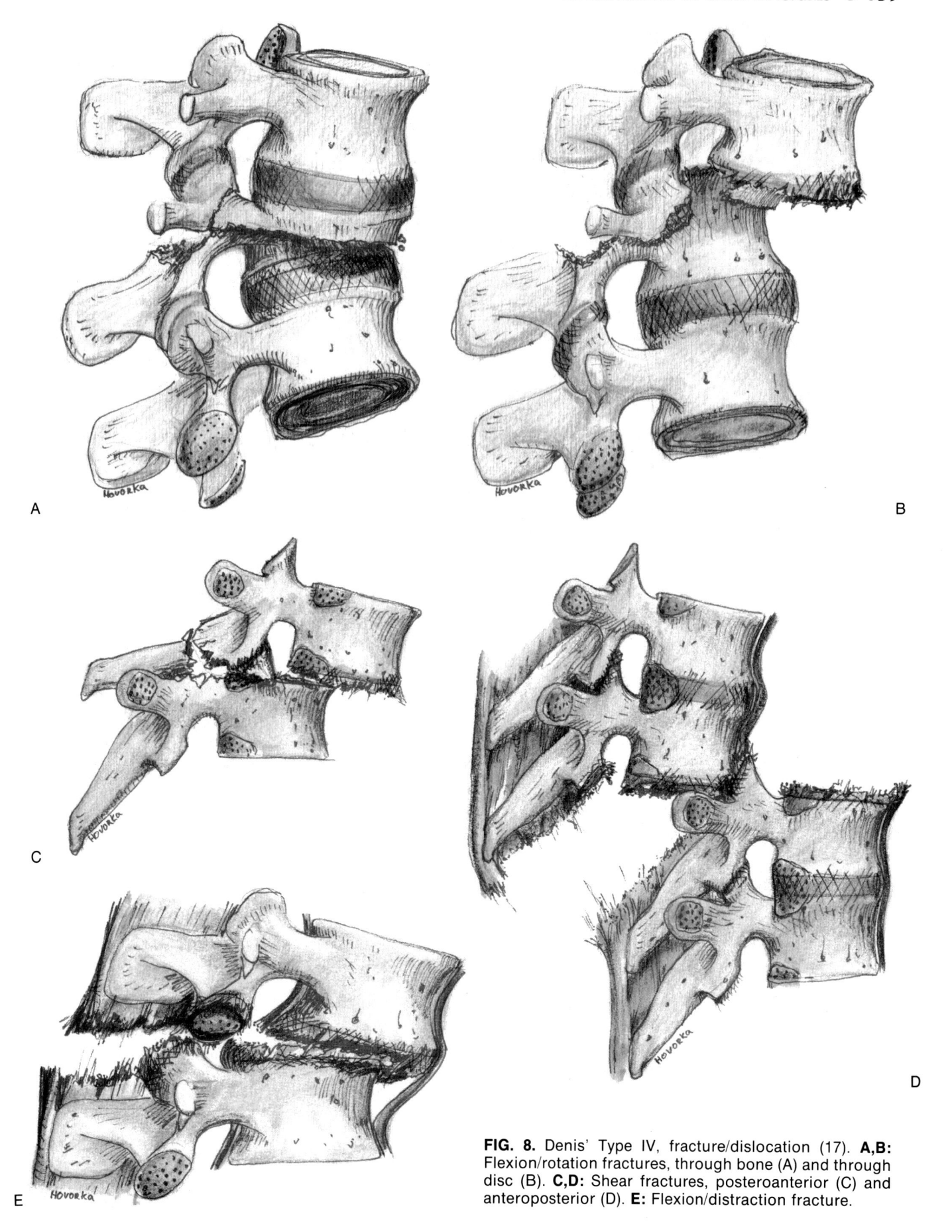

FIG. 8. Denis' Type IV, fracture/dislocation (17). **A,B:** Flexion/rotation fractures, through bone (A) and through disc (B). **C,D:** Shear fractures, posteroanterior (C) and anteroposterior (D). **E:** Flexion/distraction fracture.

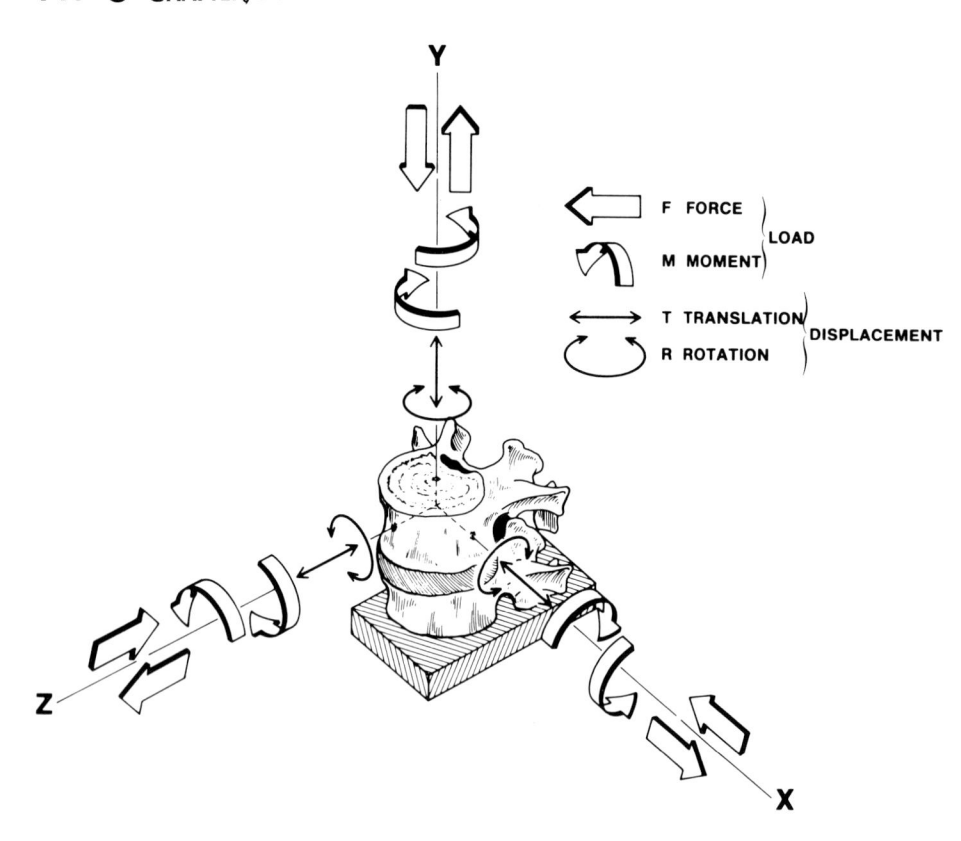

FIG. 9. The individual components of a complex spinal injury can be analyzed with reference to the X, Y, and Z axes. Along the X axis there are three mechanisms of injury: flexion, extension, and left and right lateral translation. Along the Y axis, there are axial compression, axial distraction, and clockwise and counterclockwise rotation. Along the Z axis, there are lateral flexion to either side and anterior or posterior translation. Axial compression, axial distraction, and translation are of prognostic significance and correlate with specific patterns of injury. (From ref. 49.)

McAfee et al. (34) adopted the three-column concept and made a major contribution to the understanding of middle-column injuries. Systemic evaluation of the middle column by CT scan correlated with the biomechanical studies of White and Panjabi (49). Each fracture was defined in terms of a moment of force acting on a vertebra, with reference to its application to the three spatial axes, X, Y, and Z, as shown in Fig. 9. There are six degrees of freedom in spine mobility: compression/distraction and rotation occur along the Y axis; flexion/extension and lateral translation occur along the X axis; and lateral flexion and anteroposterior translation occur along the Z axis.

Combining the advantages of Denis' classification and the other classifications, McAfee and co-workers developed a simplified scheme based on three forces as they act to injure the middle column: axial compression, axial distraction, and translation within the horizontal plane. They defined six types of injuries.

1. *Wedge compression fracture* results from forward flexion and causes an isolated failure of the anterior column. It is rarely associated with neural compromise, except when it occurs on multiple adjacent vertebral levels.
2. *Stable burst fracture* is described as a failure in compression of both the anterior and middle columns; the posterior column is unaffected (25,35).
3. *Unstable burst fracture* is described as failed in compression, lateral flexion, or rotation. It frequently results in late kyphosis with progressive neurologic impairment.
4. *Chance fracture,* as described elsewhere, is due to the application of strong tensile forces with the axis of rotation in front of the anterior longitudinal ligament, creating a horizontal transection of the vertebral body.
5. *Flexion/distraction injuries* occur when the axis of rotation is posterior to the anterior longitudinal ligament. The flexion/distraction results in failure in compression of the anterior column and failure in tension of the posterior and middle columns. Subluxation and/or dislocation of the facets may be associated.
6. *Translational injuries* occur when shear forces cause failure of all three columns, resulting in displacement of all structures in the horizontal plane.

In 1984, Ferguson and Allen (19) proposed a biomechanical classification in which a new notion of hydraulic "blow out" is introduced in an attempt to explain how the disc material under high energy axial load will penetrate the vertebral body and "blow out" the cancellous bone, leaving an empty vertebra surrounded by an "egg shell" cortex. They stated that compression alone could not account for the mechani-

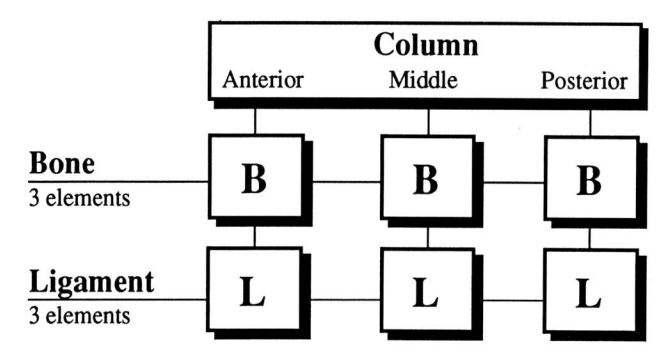

FIG. 10. Evaluation of instability: each of the columns of the spine (anterior, middle, posterior) includes a bony (B) and a ligamentous (L) component—a total of six elements. Injury to any three or more of these elements results in instability. A burst fracture generally involves injury to the B and L of the anterior and middle columns, resulting in grade 4 instability (two B + two L). A compression fracture generally involves the B and L of the anterior column (B + L) and results in grade 2 instability. A Chance injury includes any three of the components (grade 3): three L, three B, two L + B, or two B + L. A fracture/dislocation involves all six elements (grade 6).

cal failure, since this would shorten the height of the posterior vertebral body wall. When the posterior body wall is shortened, the deformity is less likely to progress than when the wall height is preserved and a marked angular deformity is present.

Finally, Farcy et al. (18) (Fig. 10) modified the Denis classification to include expression of both bone and soft tissue injuries in each of the three columns of a mobile segment, thereby developing a scheme that shows instability graded from 1 to 6. They noted that injuries greater than or equal to grade 3 were unstable. Magnetic resonance imaging is useful to evaluate ligamentous or disc disruption (18).

INSTABILITY

All the classifications reviewed so far have attempted to analyze the instability concept. However, the definition of "instability" is multifaceted.

For Nicoll (38), stable fractures were those in which there is neither increased deformity over time nor neurologic deficit.

For Whitesides (50), an unstable spine is a spine in which deformity progressively leads to increasing neurologic compromise.

For White and Panjabi (49), "clinical instability is defined as a loss in the ability of the spine under physiologic loads to maintain relationships between vertebrae in such a way that there is neither damage nor subsequent irritation to the spinal cord or nerve roots. In addition, there is no development of incapacitating deformity or pain due to structural changes."

Denis described three degrees of instability (16).

First degree instability is seen in severe compression fractures. The posterior elements allow the spine to buckle around the hinge, which is the middle column. In a seat belt injury, flexion allows buckling around the hinge of the anterior column; both of the other columns have already been disrupted.

Second degree instability, or neurologic instability, is typical of burst fractures. It happens in 20% of patients treated conservatively and results in progressive canal stenosis due to the retropulsion of bony fragments from the posterior wall.

Third degree instability is a combination of mechanical and neurologic instability. Fracture/dislocation and severe burst fractures with neurologic deficits have major secondary displacement; progression of neurologic symptoms may occur in both.

The term "late instability" for both mechanical and neurological consequences of fracture appears more often in the recent literature (8,30,52). We prefer the term "progression" of deformity to the term "instability."

ATTEMPTS AT UNIFICATION

The classifications of Holdsworth (1963) and Denis (1983) are the most frequently used to understand and treat thoracolumbar spine fractures. Holdsworth's classification, based on a mechanical concept of the two-column spine, has been criticized by Denis, who disagrees with instability caused by injuries to the posterior ligamentous structure. The middle column is reminiscent of the Decoulx–Rieunau posterior wall. Denis' classification is widely used, not only in the English-speaking literature but also in Europe (2). The apparent complexity of Denis' classification has prompted discussion by some authors (34,52).

Our experience is based on 750 patients, 250 of whom were treated surgically (2,5), and 30 patients with late kyphosis whose natural history could be traced (1). In light of this experience and recent studies, we modified Denis' classification (F. Denis, *personal communication*) (see Table, page 134).

Denis Type I: Compression Fracture

The *middle* column's integrity should be enough to ascertain stability. As recognized by Denis, there are some severe compression fractures that can progress to post-traumatic kyphosis. This progression already had been noted by Nash et al. (37) and Sutherland et al. (45) regarding multiple injuries of the thoracic spine

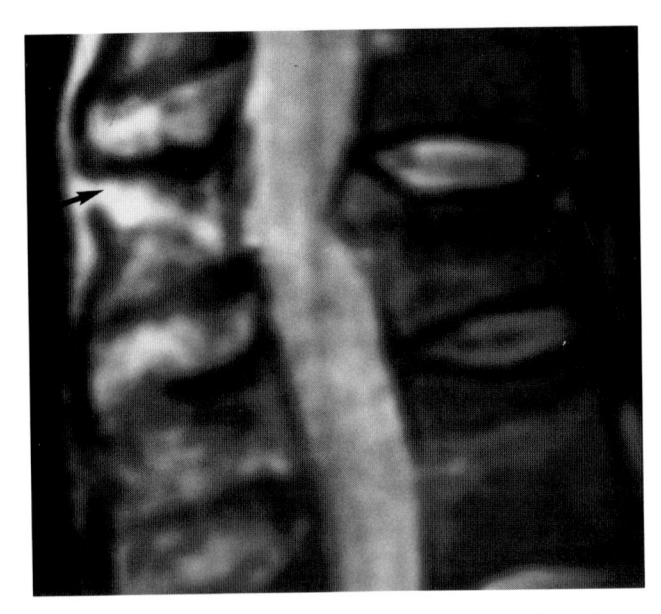

FIG. 11. A posterior ligamentous lesion *(arrow)* as shown on MRI.

in young patients. We have treated two thoracic malunions in kyphosis with neurologic symptoms resulting from injuries that were labeled "compression fractures." However, we must recognize that, among all the cases reported by Nash et al. (37), Sutherland et al. (45), and Argenson et al. (3), there were no CT scans available.

According to Ferguson and Allen (19), the possibility of progressive lesions due to "eccentric, compressive forces exists even though the middle column is intact, if compression the anterior part of the body is more than 50% of the total body height." Ferguson and Allen called this fracture the "compressive flexion fracture." In addition, progressive late deformity in kyphosis may occur following surgical treatment for scoliosis if a posterior ligamentous surgical lesion was created above the instrumentation.

Allen and Ferguson have stressed the importance of the flexion mechanism that Daffner et al. (14) have found to be the cause of 85% of thoracolumbar fractures. This flexion takes place on an axis at the level of the middle column that has been left intact and may cause posterior ligamentous damage. It is important to recognize that posterior ligamentous injury is the main factor that determines stability in compression fractures, mainly at the thoracic level. This concept, described by Whitesides (50) and White and Panjabi (49), was confirmed by Plaue (39) and Lindahl et al. (30) through experiments. They have shown that an isolated body fracture carries few hazards for worsening and can resist to loads similar to those of an intact vertebral body; when increased sagittal deformity develops, it will take place at the level of the discs adjacent to the injured vertebra. Displacement within the discs is due to posterior ligamentous disruption. Thus, in dealing with type I fractures, it is essential to evaluate anterior compression and posterior ligamentous injury by evaluating the interspinous process space, which will be increased on the lateral radiograph or, better, by evaluation of the MRI scan (18) (Fig. 11).

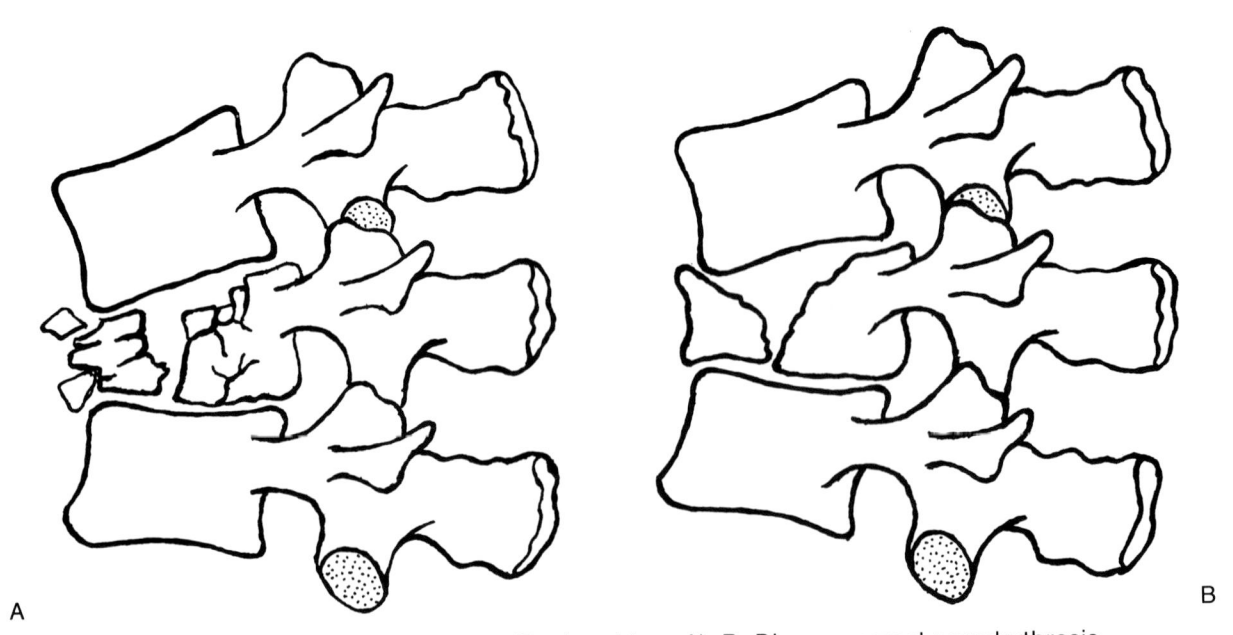

FIG. 12. A: Compression fracture (Denis subtype A). **B:** Discocorporeal pseudarthrosis.

Flexion-Compression

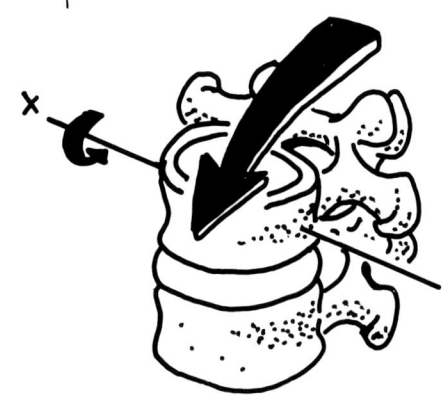

FIG. 13. Compression fracture, type I.

Subtype A as described by Denis (Fig. 12) may be related to a progressive lesion due to injury of the discs above and below the fractured vertebra. The typical fracture line is in the back of the midportion of the vertebral body and can result in an extremely rare body pseudarthrosis. This lesion was first described in the lumbar spine by Roy-Camille and Lelievre (41).

In summary, in compression fractures, the flexion axis is the middle column (Fig. 13). There is a direct relationship between the amount of anterior column compression and posterior ligamentous damage: if anterior wall compression is equal to or greater than 50%, ligamentous injuries in the posterior column are likely to be present.

Denis Type II: Burst Fracture

Since Holdsworth (25) introduced the term "burst," controversies based on the stability of this injury have developed. It is defined as a compression injury of both the anterior and middle columns; "the posterior column remains intact, except for a green stick-type fracture" of the lamina. The compression injury is due to a perpendicular load applied to the endplate (Fig. 14). This explains why similar injuries are often found at T12 and L5, both of which are aligned on the gravity line. However, because of the spine's contour, compression forces can be associated with a flexion moment at the thoracolumbar level; at the lumbar level, the force can be applied more posteriorly (53), causing bony injury at the level of the posterior elements with a vertical fracture line.

Middle-column injuries are most typical for these types of fractures. An evaluation is made by the decreased height of the posterior body wall and adjacent discs. Thus, along with the decrease in height of the posterior wall, there is a retropulsion of almost the entire posterior wall in subtype A (fracture of both endplates) or a retropulsion of the upper part of the posterior wall as a free fragment, in subtype B (the most frequent). The retropulsed fragment infrequently may come from the inferior part of the vertebral wall (subtype C) (Fig. 6). With regard to subtype D (burst/rotation) and subtype E (burst/lateral flexion), (Fig. 6), we think they belong to the fracture/dislocation type IV, as they present with a posterior articular lesion with dislocation. This explains why Denis found a prevalence of 14% burst fractures, while other series found only 4% to 5%, with a low of 1.5% found in McAfee's series. Bursting of the vertebral body can be seen in different fracture types, not only in type II but also in some cases of type IV (subtype A, through the bone) or, as advocated by Gertzbein and co-workers (21,22), in some fractures of type III.

The inability to evaluate instability in terms of "burst" is a source of controversy (36) (Fig. 15). Evaluation of instability, for Holdsworth, McAfee, and others, is directly related to injury of the posterior element. However, for Denis, it is related only to medial column injury. CT scan, on which ligament injury cannot be evaluated, has shown a prevalence of posterior bony injuries (6,24); in contrast, Kilcoyne et al. (28) have reported some unstable fractures with intact posterior elements. Review of the literature and the results of our clinical experience, with special emphasis on patients who were treated conservatively by a plaster cast, confirms our feeling that, at the thoracolumbar level, the criteria for instability at the level of the middle column depend on the integrity of both its bony and ligamentous structures (1,4,18). Denis (17) stressed the bony injury and recognized stability for the subgroup A; he did not elaborate on the disc and ligament injuries, even when he recognized their importance and compared them to the cruciate ligament of the knee.

The post-traumatic kyphosis is similar to a progressive anterior subluxation, typical at the level of the

Axial Load

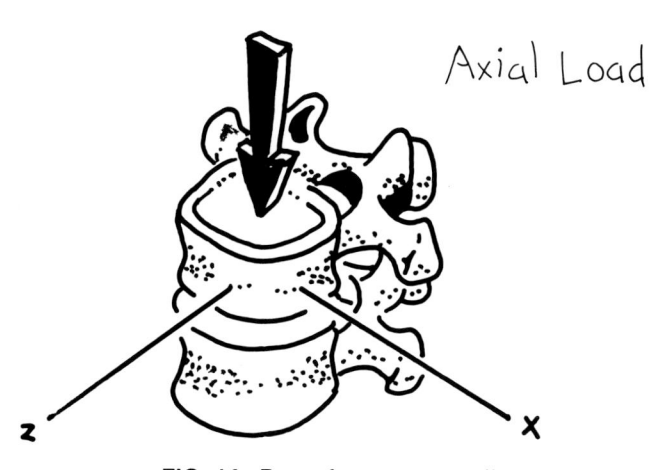

FIG. 14. Burst fracture, type II.

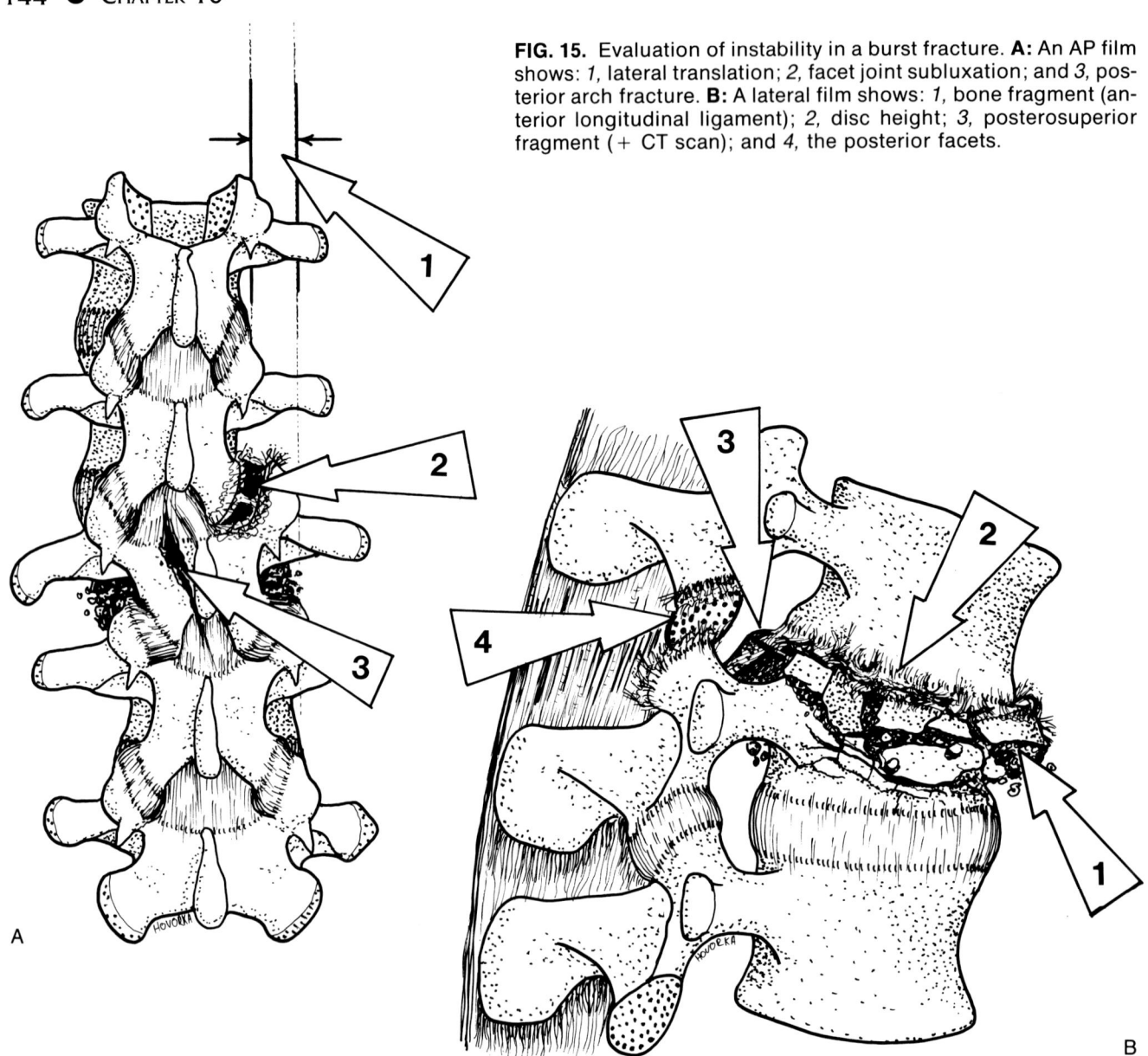

FIG. 15. Evaluation of instability in a burst fracture. **A:** An AP film shows: *1*, lateral translation; *2*, facet joint subluxation; and *3*, posterior arch fracture. **B:** A lateral film shows: *1*, bone fragment (anterior longitudinal ligament); *2*, disc height; *3*, posterosuperior fragment (+ CT scan); and *4*, the posterior facets.

thoracolumbar spine, and presents in a manner similar to a knee subluxation due to an anterior cruciate ligament disruption. This finding implies a posterior longitudinal ligament disruption. The posterior longitudinal ligament is pivotal in spine stability, as we demonstrated in 1976 in monkeys (4). Its importance in spine stability as well as in choice of management of acute fracture has been pointed out in two recent papers (24,53).

Guerra et al. (24), on a series of 40 patients, have studied the posterior fragment of the posterior wall. For them, it always comes from the superior part of the body (subtype B) under the action of a compressive axial load with some degree of hyperflexion. Sagittal reconstruction has shown evidence that, under a rotational moment, this fragment will rotate on itself (Fig. 16) and its cartilage-covered part will face anteriorly one of every three times. This rotation happens, according to Guerra et al. (24), under the action of axial compression, which causes "the posterior longitudinal ligament to tear, destabilizing the posterior corner of the vertebra." In some rare instances, the bony fragment can be totally detached from the ligament. Different authors have stressed the difficulty of reduction of this fragment because it has rotated or moved in a cranial or caudal direction, as in instances of failed ligamentotaxis under distraction with Harrington rods.

Next, Willen and co-workers (51,53) reported on studies about the posterosuperior fragment, evaluating bony and ligamentous injuries in eight fresh fractures and 12 old fractures on anatomic specimens after autopsy. In 16 cases, the fracture was subtype A (Denis' classification: fracture of the two endplates of the vertebra); a mid-sized posterosuperior fragment was at-

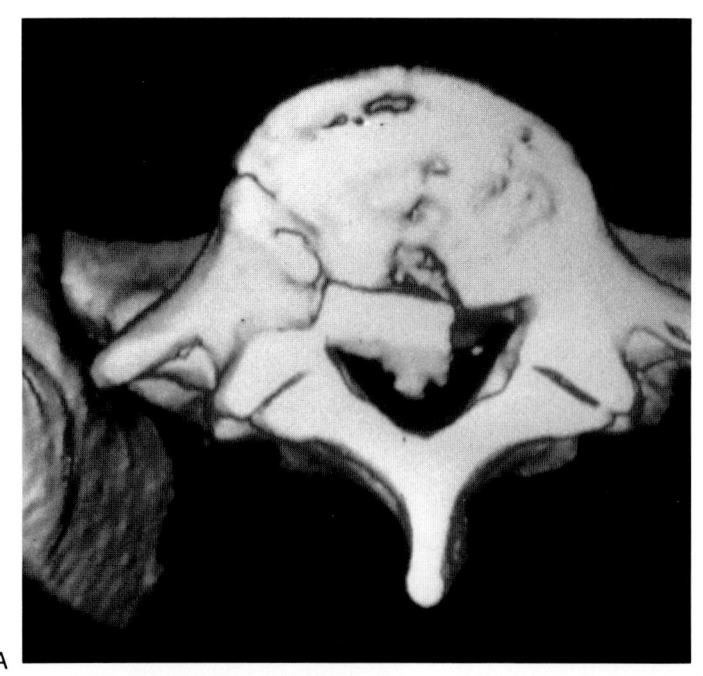

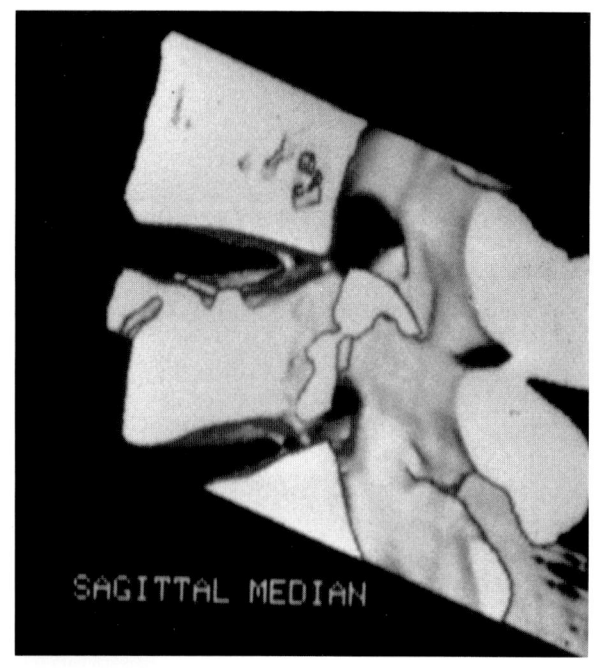

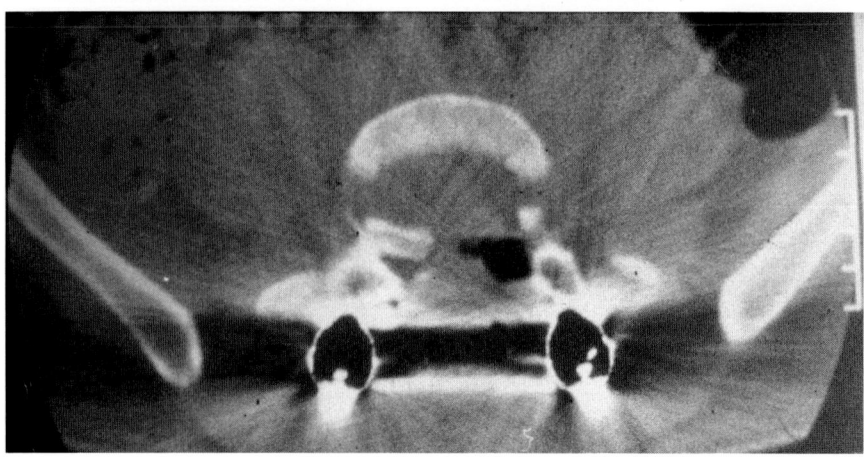

FIG. 16. Burst fracture of L5. **A:** Radicular signs are present. The posterosuperior fragment has rotated on itself. **B:** At surgery, the posterior longitudinal ligament was completely torn, with the fragment free in the canal; it was removed.

tached to the posterior longitudinal ligament that was only stretched or partially torn. In contrast, in four cases of fractures classified subtype B or D by Denis, a posterior ligament rupture was found, as well as a large bony fragment that turned on itself because connection with the ligament was lost.

Critical Role of the Posterior Longitudinal Ligaments Integrity

Based on their studies, Willen et al. (53) have correlated the size of the posterosuperior fragment of the body wall with a posterior longitudinal ligament injury. This posterior longitudinal ligament injury appears to be the main factor in instability, as developed above.

When the ligament has sustained only a partial injury and is still attached to the posterosuperior bony fragment, it will be reduced with the other fragments by ligamentotaxis with use of lordosis, as reported by Boehler (Fig. 17). This fracture may be assessed as stable and treated conservatively. On the contrary, when the ligament is completely torn, the posterosuperior fragment is free inside the canal and will not respond to ligamentotaxis maneuvers. This type of fracture can be considered unstable.

The same phenomenon happens after surgical treatment. Shuman et al. (44) have shown that distraction with Harrington rods can improve the correction of all subtype A fractures by ligamentotaxis because the ligament is only partially torn. In contrast, only three of the eight fractures classified subtype B improved with regard to canal stenosis by use of Harrington distraction, implying that those three cases had only a partially torn ligament. Crutcher et al. (13) reported similar results.

Last, the relationship between the size of the posterosuperior fragment and the injury of the posterior lon-

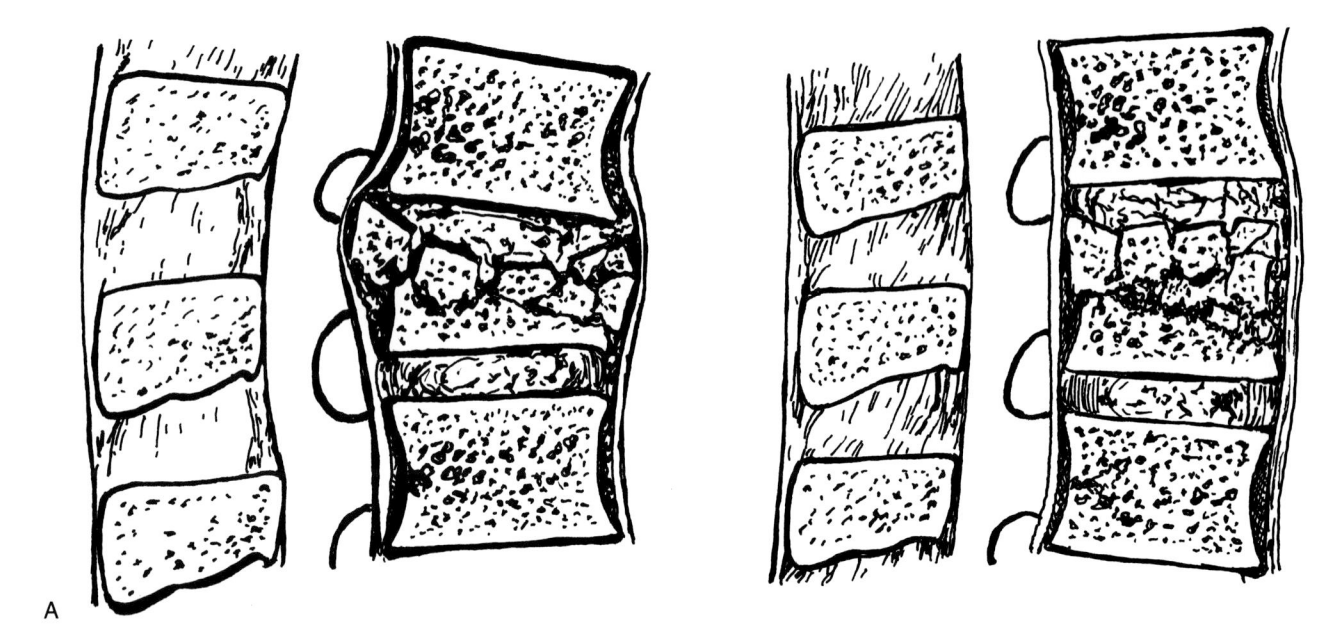

FIG. 17. Burst fracture. **A:** The posterolongitudinal ligament is intact. The spinal canal diameter is compromised only 30%. **B:** Restoring lordosis is sufficient to reduce fragments by ligamentotaxis. This is a stable fracture under conservative treatment.

gitudinal ligament was confirmed by Willen's studies on fragment resorption. In all specimens with posterior longitudinal ligament disruption, only one showed partial resorption of the posterior wall fragment. Willen et al. (51–53) concluded that burst fractures, especially severe Denis subtypes B and D with narrowing of the spinal canal that exceeds 50%, have a great risk of neurologic instability. In this type of fracture, posterior longitudinal ligament rupture and subsequent rotation of bone fragments may be responsible for the nonresorption of the bony fragments.

In our experience, indications for treatment were derived from our studies, as follows.

With the exception of patients with neurologic com-

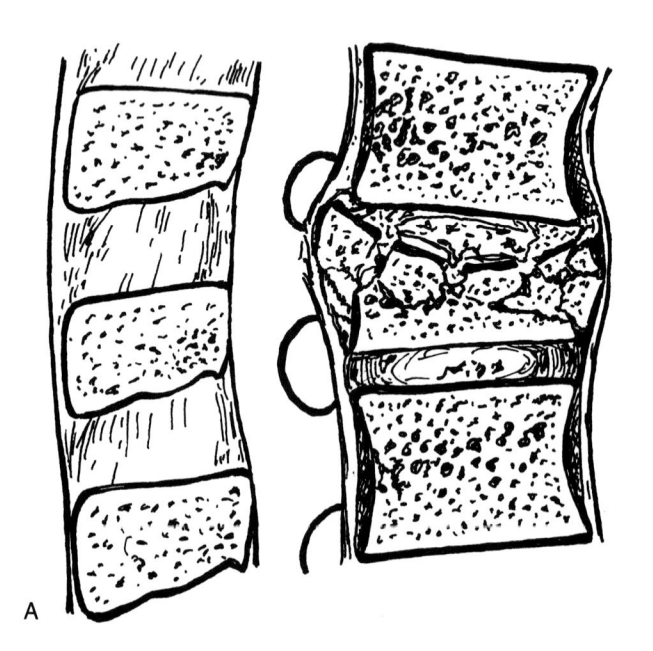

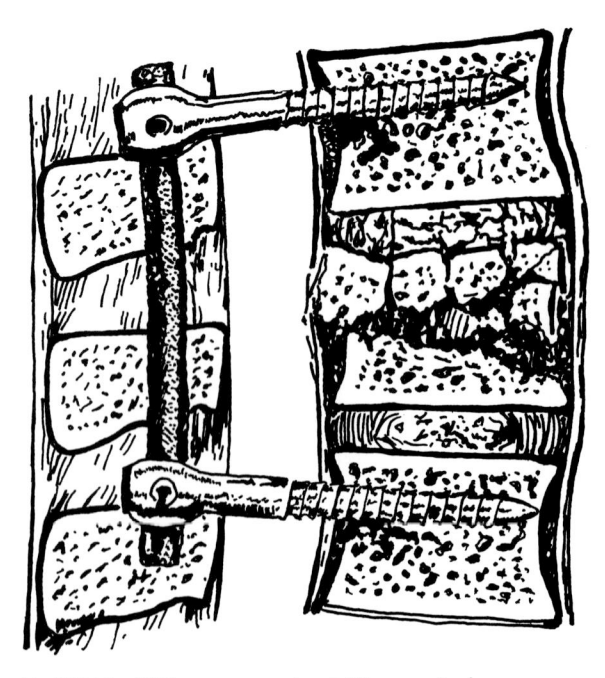

FIG. 18. Burst fracture. **A:** Diameter of the spinal canal is 30% to 50% compromised. The posterior longitudinal ligament is partially torn. **B:** Internal fixation allowed efficient ligamentotaxis for reduction.

promise, on whom decompression and stabilization take precedence (43), the burst fractures (Denis subtype A or B) are treated conservatively when the diameter of the spinal canal is compromised to only 30% as evaluated by CT scan. This is because we are convinced, since the ligament is intact and bone healing will occur, that restoring lordosis is sufficient to reduce the fragment in the canal with use of posterior longitudinal ligament ligamentotaxis (Fig. 17).

When the diameter of the spinal canal is 30% to 50% occupied by bone fragments, in our opinion the posterior longitudinal ligament is partially torn and, using conservative means, we will not be able to obtain reduction by ligamentotaxis; surgical fixation in distraction may be considered (Fig. 18), depending on the age of the patient, body shape, and the patient's physical activities. Residual kyphosis above 25° at the thoracolumbar level, which corresponds to a Farcy Sagittal Index (18) of 25, will progress to a poor, functional late result. The Boehler technique of reduction and cast immobilization is only partially efficient at the thoracic level and not really efficient at the lumbar level.

When 50% of the spinal canal diameter is occupied by bone fragments, we presume that the ligament is almost completely torn, and internal stabilization should be accomplished, as for patients with neurologic compromise (Fig. 19). In these cases, a "direct" decompression is advocated.

At the Lumbar Level (L3, L4, L5)

Other than at L5, it is very rare to find the typical posterosuperior fragment of the vertebral body. Due to lordosis, which displaces the line of gravity posteriorly, one-third of the load in compression is applied to the posterior articular processes. In trauma, axial load is applied to a point located mid-distance between the vertebral body and the posterior arch, and this explains the high rate of bony injury of the three columns. The fracture lines are vertical at the level of the posterior column.

Lindahl et al. (31) demonstrated that axial disc injury leads to multiple disc fragments impacted in the disrupted bone, preventing good bony healing. This injury can cause a "bow tie" shape of the body after it has been penetrated by disc fragments from above and below, resulting in a "body pseudarthrosis" (41). Besides a few rare subtype A fractures with minor retropulsion of the posterior wall, at the lumbar level one must be concerned about a progressive kyphosis in all lumbar burst fractures. In this case, the loss of anatomic lordotic contour can account for low back pain and radiculopathy and can require eventual surgical correction.

Evaluation of the stability of lumbar burst fractures (20) cannot be based solely on the posterior injuries, which are almost always found. Rather, the evaluation

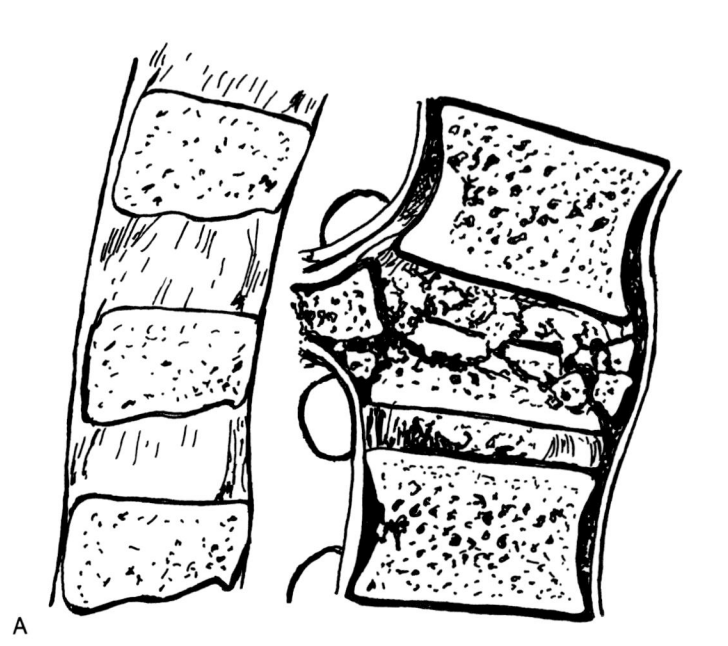

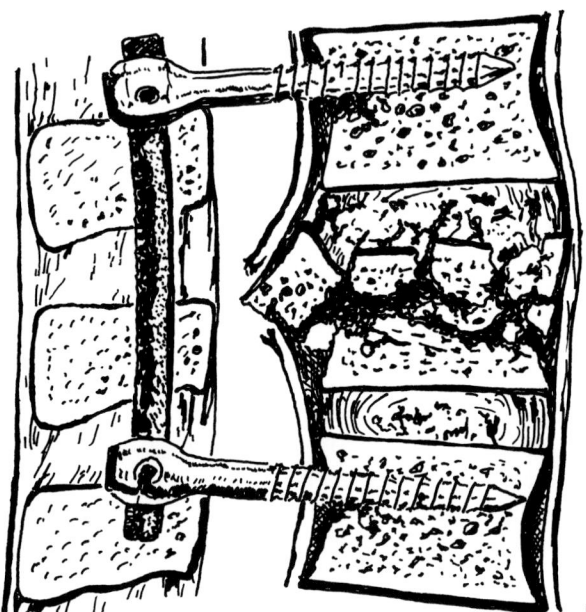

FIG. 19. Burst fracture. **A:** Diameter of the spinal canal is compromised more than 50%. The posterior longitudinal ligament is completely torn. **B:** The fragment could not be reduced by ligamentotaxis; therefore, direct decompression is advocated.

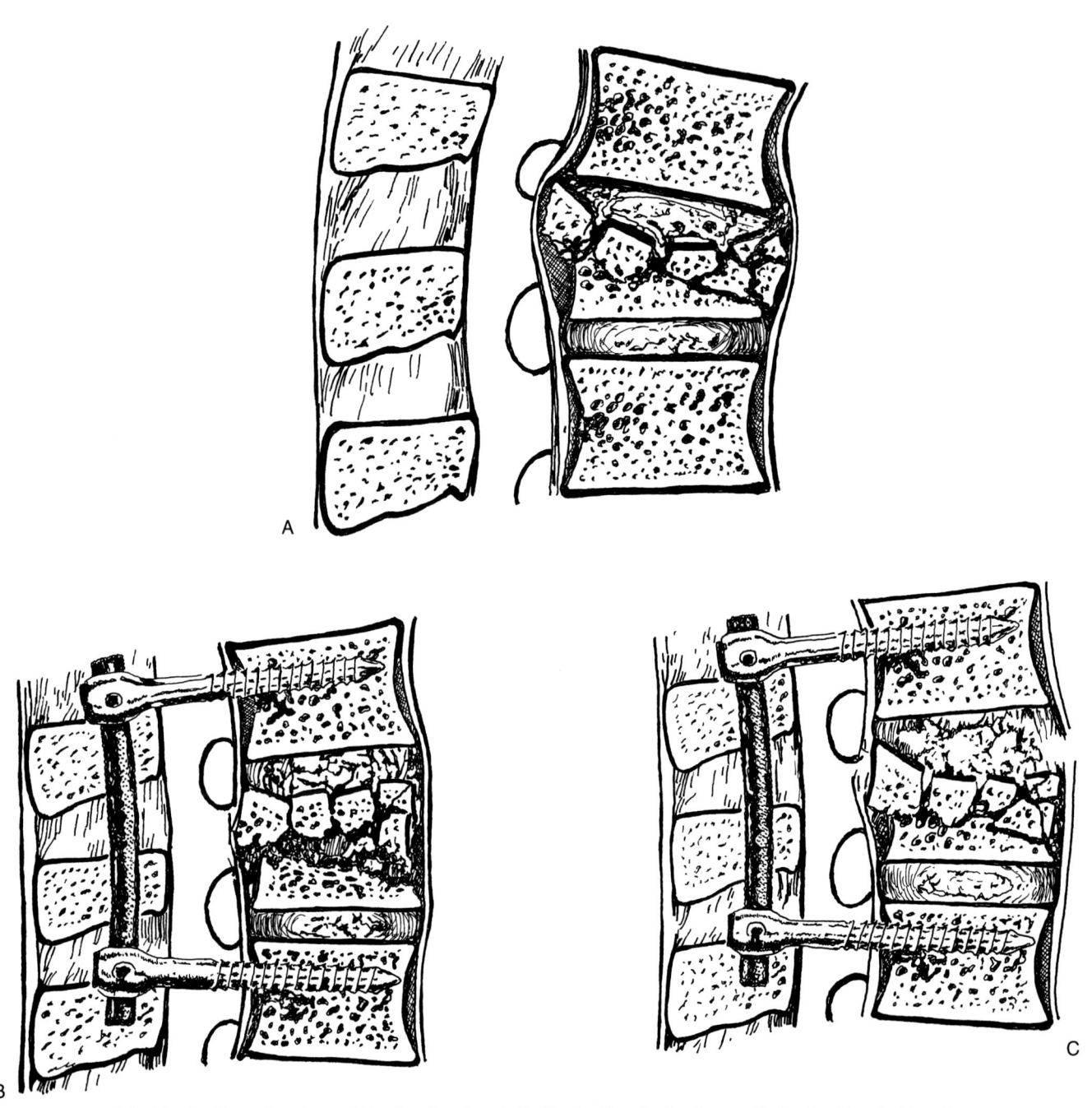

FIG. 20. A: Burst fracture at the lumbar level. **B:** Reduction in the bone. **C:** Reduction in the disc, with risk of late collapse.

must be based on the magnitude of body disruption and disc injury at the level of the anterior and middle columns. One must keep in mind the "too good looking" disc reconstructions (2) that mean, rather, a complete transection of the annulus and anterior and posterior longitudinal ligaments (Fig. 20). In the latter case, risk of late collapse is emphasized; anterior bone grafting is often necessary (10).

Denis Type III: Seat Belt Injuries

Not all injuries described by this name result from wearing a seat belt. A biomechanical definition such as "flexion/distraction injury" (12) is perhaps more accurate for all the injuries that show a characteristic posterior opening, described by Denis in the four subtypes of type III and in subtype C of type IV (fracture/dislo-

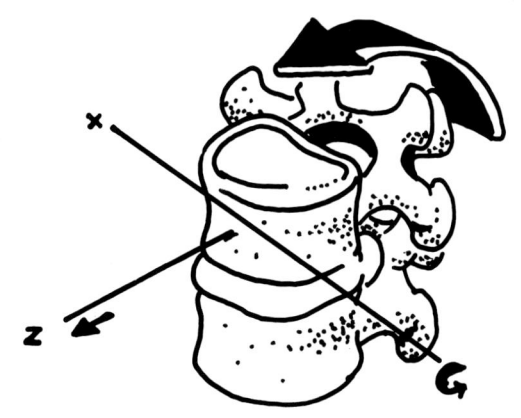

FIG. 21. Type III, "seat belt" fracture.

cation due to flexion/distraction), since they result from the same mechanism (Figs. 7 and 8).

This mechanism is forced flexion, the axis of rotation of which is on the anterior column of the spine (Fig. 21). In this type, the difference is due to the location of the fracture line, which can pass *through the bone* from the spinous process, the lamina, or the pedicle to the vertebral body, as in the classic Chance fracture (11) (50% of cases). In this fracture, bony instability does not last longer than the time required for bone healing; conservative treatment or a short compression fixation will provide for predictable healing (Fig. 22A). However, if the fracture line passes *through the discoligamentous space*, with or without partial bony involvement, a long-lasting instability may be anticipated, resulting in delayed healing or even pseudarthrosis (Fig. 22B,C,D).

In this case, according to the abruptness and magnitude of the initial trauma, the anterior ligament may be normal or may present with partial to total disruption. In the latter case, as described by Denis in subtype C of type IV, instability is greater.

In conclusion, we prefer to include in this type III all the lesions that result from a flexion/distraction force, such as the four subtypes of type III and subtype C of type IV (Fig. 22). The presence of either an osseous or ligamentous lesion seems the most important, decisive factor of stability.

Denis Type IV: Fracture/Dislocations

Denis elected to define three subtypes, which are defined by a three-column disruption, according to a biomechanical mechanism (Fig. 8).

Subtype A. Flexion/rotation injuries are the most frequent, well-known since Holdsworth's description and are divided into lesions through the bone and lesions through the disc.

Subtype B. Shear injuries are anteroposterior or posteroanterior, following dislocation. They are very rarely "real dislocations" at the thoracolumbar level but are more often associated with a facet joint fracture/dislocation.

Subtype C. Flexion/distraction injuries can be confused with subtype B of type III because they are caused by the same mechanism and present the same ligamentous injuries at the levels of the posterior and middle columns. As stressed by Denis, the anterior column rupture creates an obviously unstable fracture; as seen above, we prefer to include this subtype in type III.

Subtype D. Besides the shear mechanism in the transverse plane as described by Denis, we feel that some injuries can be the result of a shear or shear forces exerted in an oblique plane.

We have seen one lumbar and five thoracic injuries (3) that were difficult to classify in any of the subtypes of Denis' classification (17). They all presented common parameters: following high-velocity injury; running through three or more levels; association with other injuries such as fracture of the scapula, or multiple rib fractures associated with a thoracic spine lesion; and pelvic fracture associated with a lumbar spine lesion. All were without neurologic damage in spite of very large displacement of the bony elements (Figs. 23 and 24).

Reviewing the literature, we nevertheless found three similar cases: one in a paratrooper described by Gertzbein and Offieski (23), and one each in the series of Vichard et al. (47) and Uriarte et al. (46). The analysis of these cases, when compared to ours, defines a biomechanical shear force directed obliquely due to the presence of counterpressure on the opposite side of the trunk (Fig. 25), as described by Gertzbein and Offieski in their case report. Vichard and co-

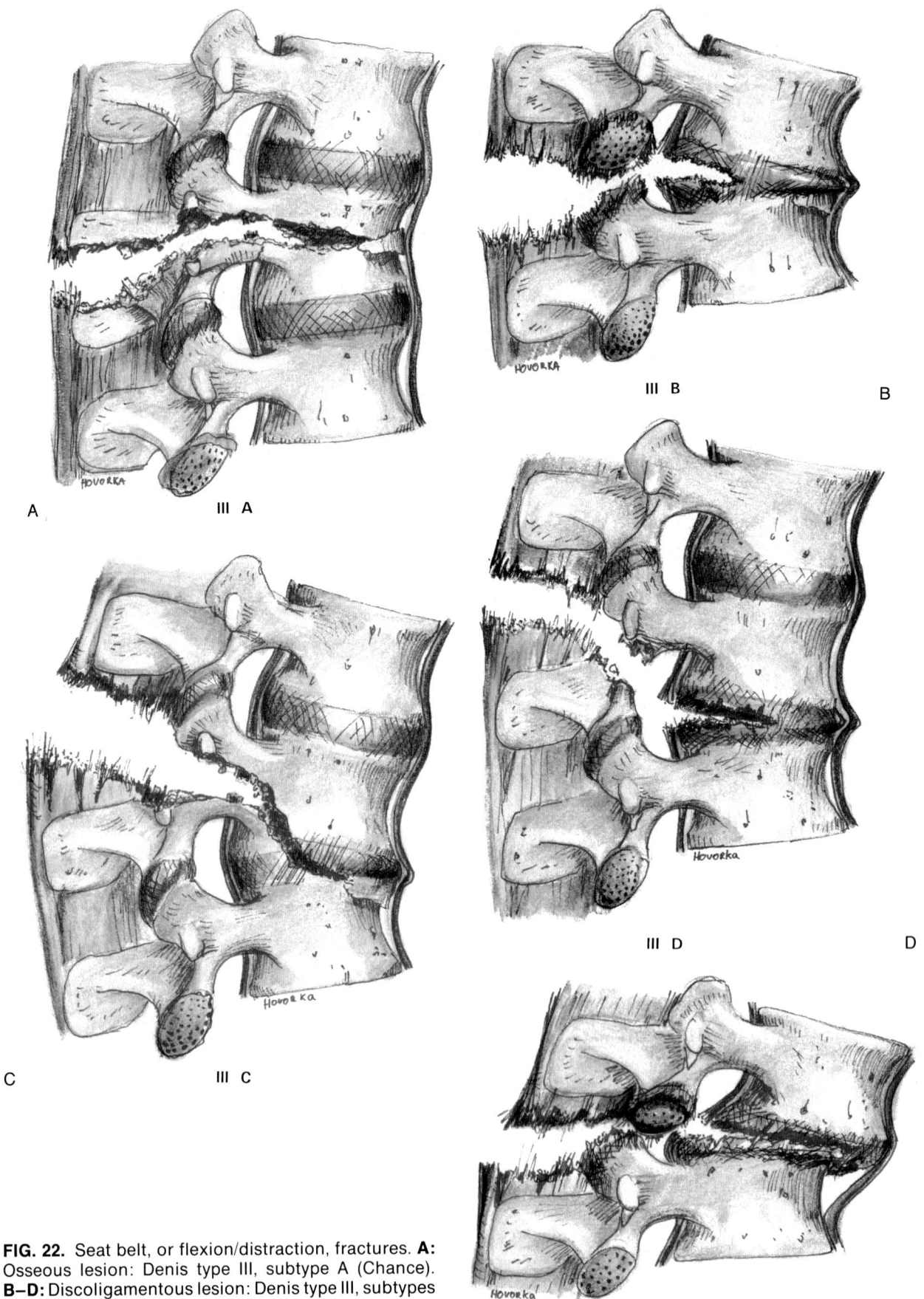

FIG. 22. Seat belt, or flexion/distraction, fractures. **A:** Osseous lesion: Denis type III, subtype A (Chance). **B–D:** Discoligamentous lesion: Denis type III, subtypes B, C, and D. **E:** Denis Type IV, subtype C.

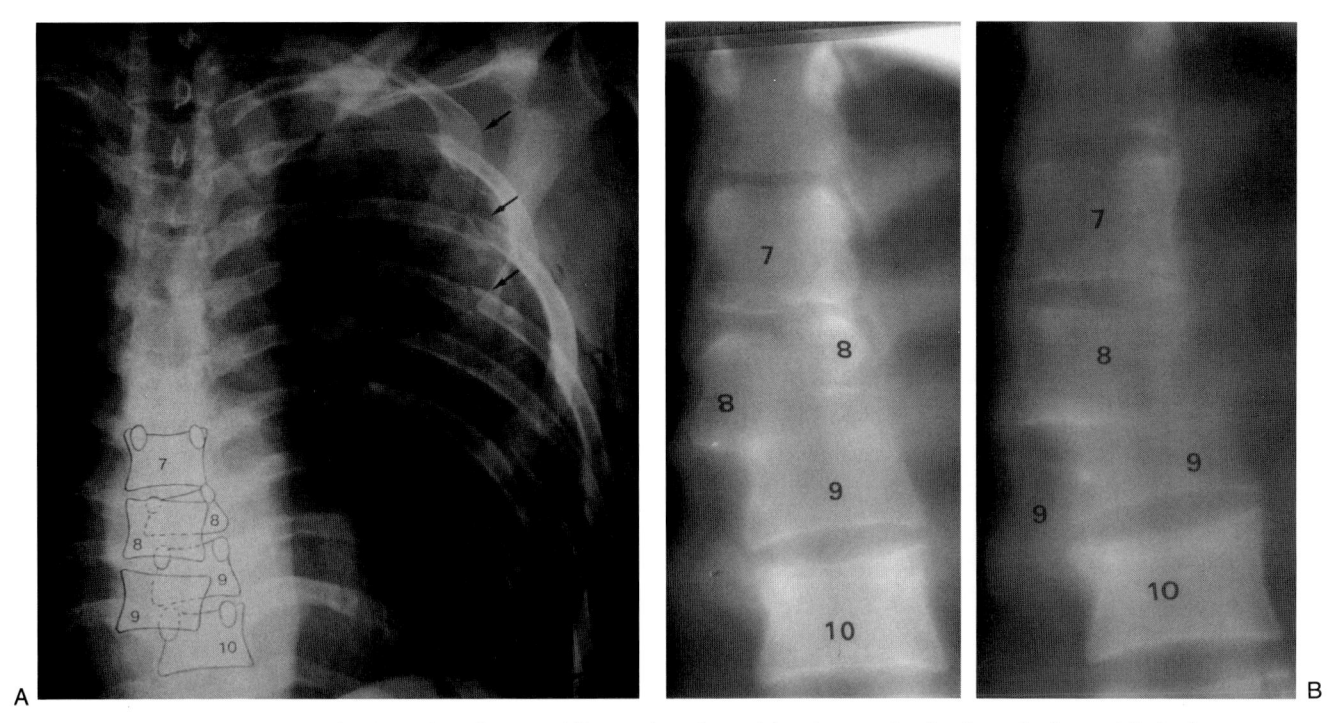

FIG. 23. Fracture/dislocation due to oblique shearing without neurologic signs (subtype D). **A:** A 50-year-old pedestrian knocked over by a car had associated thoracic and shoulder lesions. **B:** Tomography.

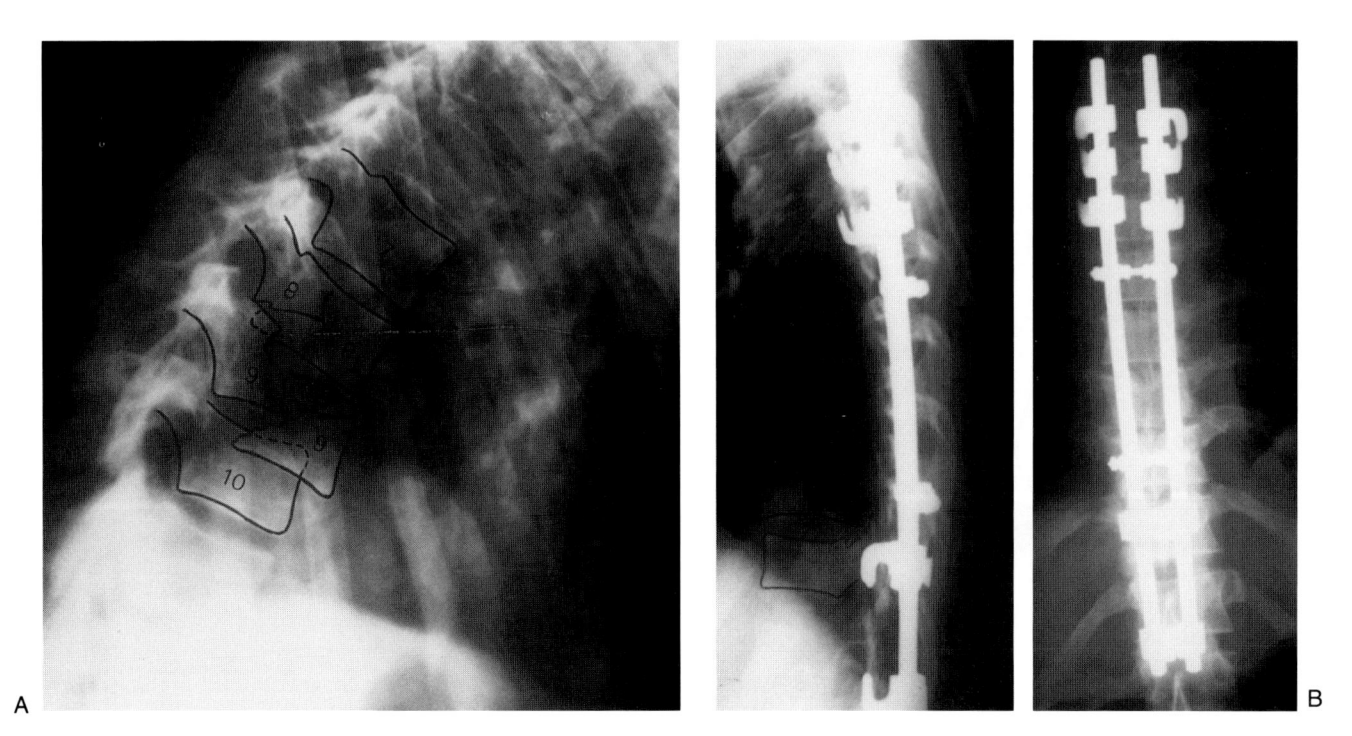

FIG. 24. Fracture/dislocation due to oblique shearing; without neurologic signs (subtype D). **A:** Lateral film. **B:** Reduction and fixation by CD instrumentation in distraction.

workers demonstrated that the fracture line is in an oblique plane, posterior through the uppermost vertebra and anterior through the lowest vertebra. This provides an opening in the ring of the vertebral canal, resulting in a "natural medullary decompression," well-seen on CT scan (Fig. 26). This would account for the integrity of the neurologic elements in this patient. We therefore considered these lesions as a separate subtype D.

All these type IV fracture/dislocations are unstable and could be described better as type IV dislocations with either dominant bony injury or dominant discoligamentous injury.

Subtype A: dominant osseous lesion. We include here the Denis type IV, subtype A, flexion/rotation through the bone, and subtype D, as we described above, as well as the two subtypes D and E of Denis type II (burst fracture) (18) (Fig. 27). All these injuries present a bony lesion of the two anterior columns and a fracture of the posterior articular facets.

Subtype B: dominant discoligamentous injury. We include here the Denis type IV subtype A, flexion/rotation through the disc, and subtype B, shear fracture.

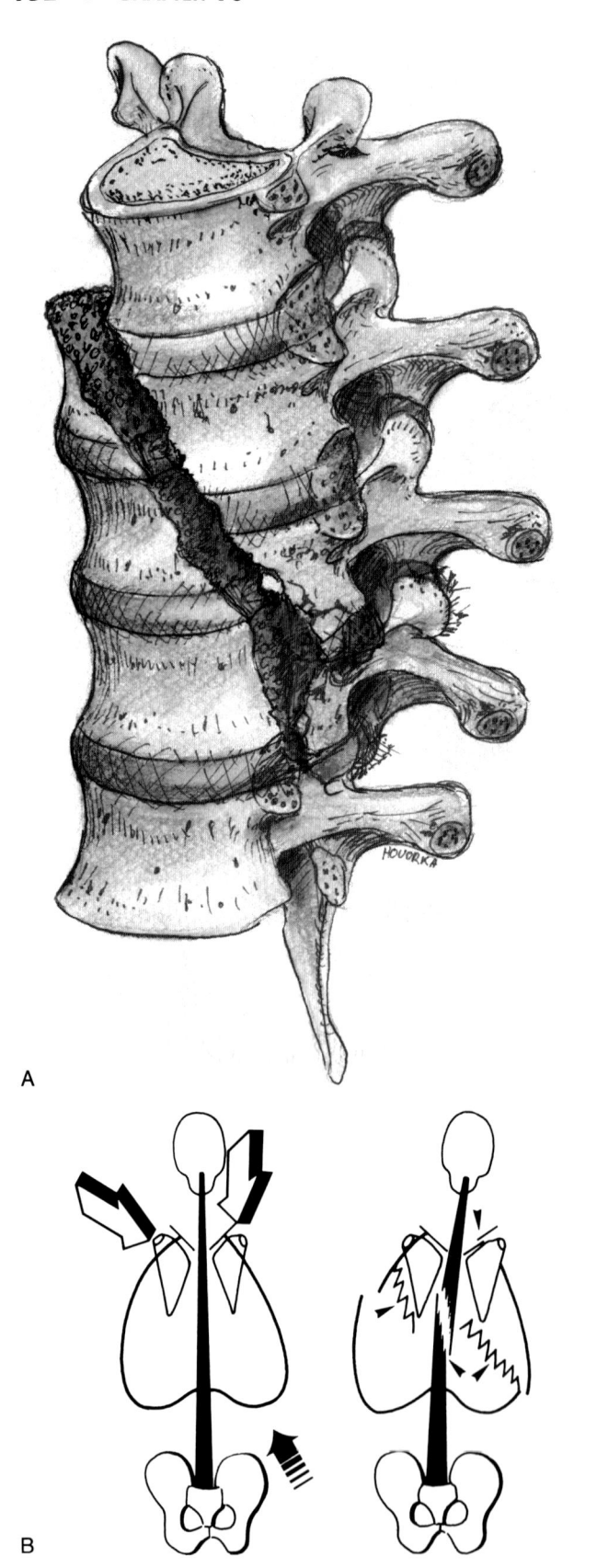

FIG. 25. A: Type IV, subtype D. **B:** Shear force directed obliquely, with a counterpressure on the opposite side of the trunk.

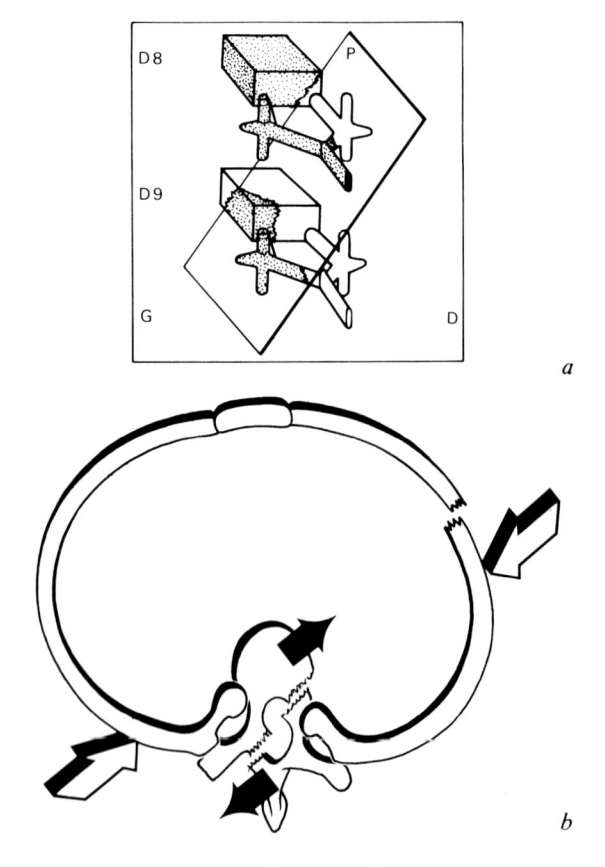

FIG. 26. A fracture line in an oblique plane causes an opening of the ring of the vertebral canal.

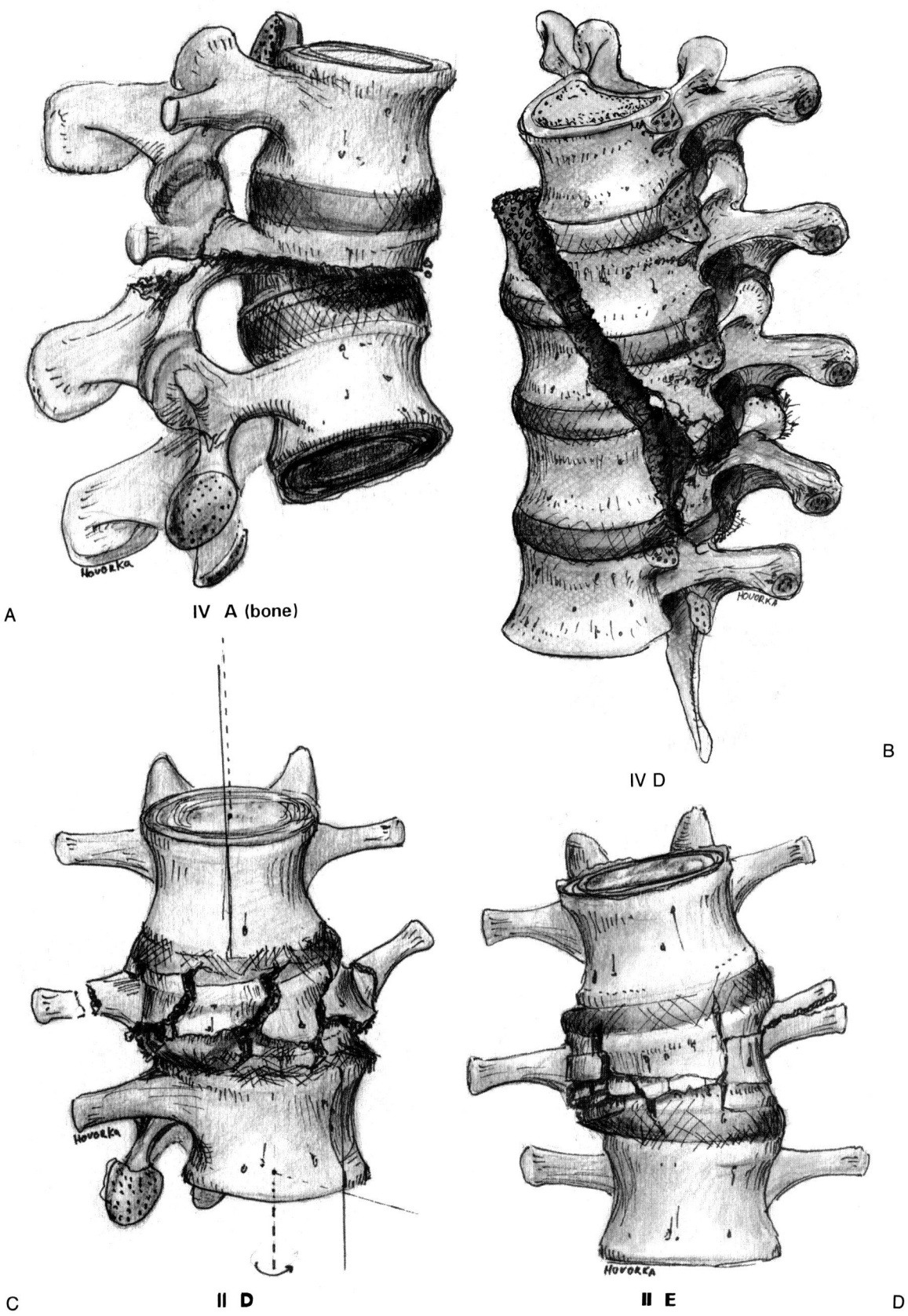

FIG. 27. Fracture/dislocation (type IV) with dominant bony injury. **A,B:** Denis type IV, subtype A (flexion/rotation through the bone) and subtype D (oblique shear force). **C,D:** Denis type II, burst/rotation, subtype D, and burst/lateral flexion, subtype E.

FIG. 28. Fracture/dislocation (type IV) with dominant disco-ligamentous injury. **A:** Denis type IV, subtype A: flexion/rotation through the disc. **B:** Denis type IV, subtype B, posteroanterior. **C:** Anteroposterior shear fracture.

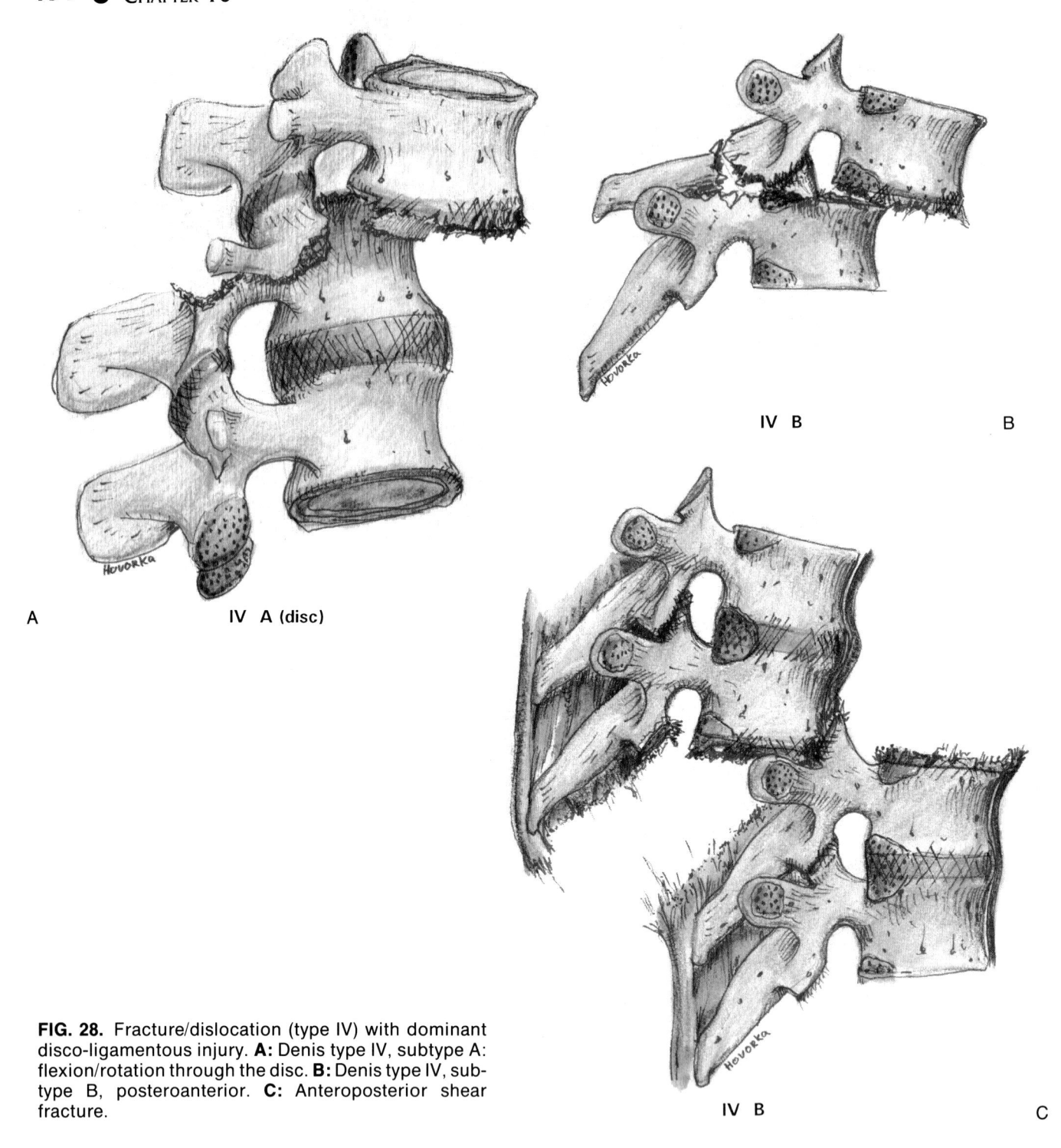

Both present with the same appearance of dislocation and require the same treatment (Fig. 28).

In conclusion, Denis' classification is the basis of the understanding of traumatic injury of the thoracolumbar spine. The four types, corresponding to a dominant causative force (29), include a variety of stable and unstable lesions.

It is important to recognize the middle column's discoligamentous injuries, since these lesions may have potential for late instability.

The amount of kyphosis due to the lesion of the vertebral body and the adjacent disc (18) (Fig. 29) has also to be taken into account for evaluation of the degree of instability.

Kyphotic Deformity — Normal Contour = Sagittal Index (SI)

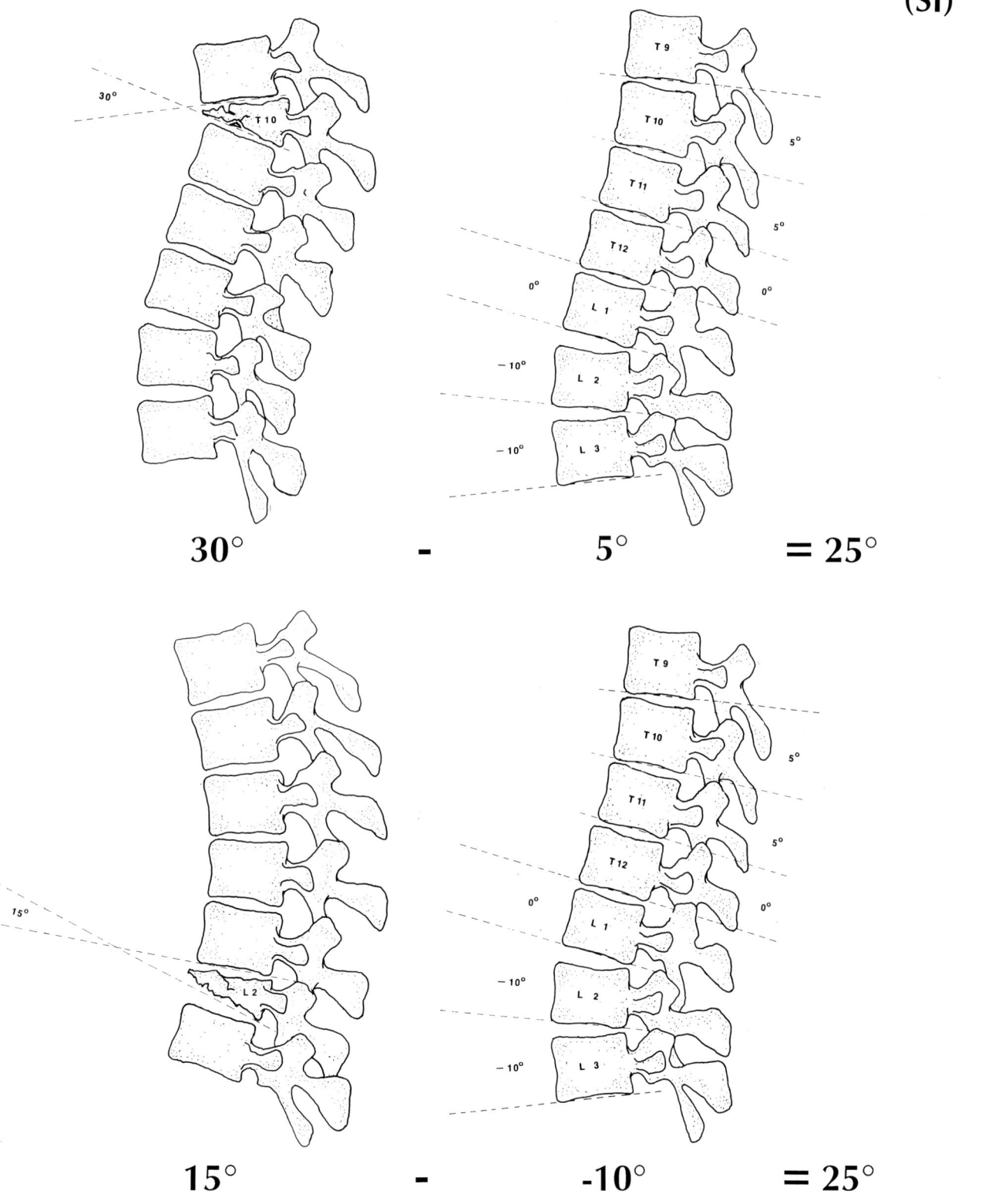

30° − 5° = 25°

15° − -10° = 25°

FIG. 29. Sagittal index (18).

Table 1, which recaps all the precedent considerations, may be helpful in selecting the best-adapted treatment, according to the degree of "immediate instability" and risk of "late deformity."

REFERENCES

1. Argenson C. Cals vicieux et pseudarthroses du rachis thoracolombaire. In: *Cahiers d'Enseignement de la SOFCOT*. Paris: Expansion Scientifique Francaise, 1990;205–236.
2. Argenson C. Traitement des fractures du rachis dorso-lombaire chez l'adulte. In: *Cahiers d'Enseignement de la SOFCOT*. Paris: Expansion Scientifique Francaise, 1984;5–27.
3. Argenson C, Boileau P, de Peretti F, Lovet J, Dalzotto H. Fractures of the thoracic spine (T1–T10). A review of 105 cases. *Fr J Orthop Surg* 1989;3(3):238–254.
4. Argenson C, Dintimille H. Lésions traumatiques expérimentales du rachis chez le singe. *Rev Chir Orthop* 1977;63:430–431.
5. Argenson C, Lovet J, de Peretti F, Cambas PM, Griffet J, Boileau P. Treatment of spinal fractures with C-D instrumentation: results of 85 cases. SRS-ESDS Combined Meeting. Amsterdam, Holland, Sept 17–22, 1989.
6. Atlas SW, Regenbogen V, Rogers LF, Kim KS. The radiographic characterization of burst fractures of the spine. *AJR* 1986;147:575–582.
7. Bedbrook GM. Stability of spinal fractures and fracture dislocation. *Paraplegia* 1971;9:23–32.
8. Benson DR. Unstable thoracolumbar fractures with emphasis on the burst fracture. *Clin Orthop* 1988;230:14–29.
9. Boehler L. *Technique de traitement des fractures de la colonne dorsale et lombaire* (translated by M Boppe). Paris: Masson, 1944;149.
10. Bridwell KH, DeWald RL, eds. *The textbook of spinal surgery*. Philadelphia: Lippincott, 1991.
11. Chance GO. Note on a type of flexion fracture of the spine. *Br J Radiol* 1948;21:452–453.
12. Court-Brown CM, Gertzbein SD. Flexion–distraction injuries of the lumbar spine: mechanism of injury and classification. *Clin Orthop* 1988;227:52–60.
13. Crutcher JP, Anderson PA, King KA, Montesano PX. Indirect spinal canal decompression in patients with thoracolumbar burst fractures treated by posterior distraction rods. *J Spinal Disord* 1991;1:30–48.
14. Daffner RK, Deeb ZL, Rothfus WE. "Fingerprints" of vertebral trauma. A unifying concept based on mechanisms. *Skeletal Radiol* 1986;15:518.
15. Decoulx P, Rieunau G. Les fractures du rachis dorso-lombaire sans troubles neurologiques. *Rev Chir Orthop* 1958;44:254.
16. Denis F. Spinal instability as defined by the three column spine concept in acute spinal trauma. *Clin Orthop* 1984;189:65–70.
17. Denis F. The three column spine and its significance in the classification of acute thoracolumbar spinal injuries. *Spine* 1983;8(6):817–831.
18. Farcy JPC, Weidenbaum M, Glassman SD. Sagittal index in management of thoracolumbar burst fractures. *Spine* 1990;15(9):958–965.
19. Ferguson RL, Allen BL. A mechanistic classification of thoracolumbar spine fractures. *Clin Orthop* 1984;189:77–88.
20. Floman Y. *Disorders of the lumbar spine*. Rockville, MD: Aspen Publishers, 1990.
21. Gertzbein SD, Court-Brown CM. Flexion/distraction injury of the lumbar spine: mechanism of injury and classification. *Clin Orthop* 1988;227:52.
22. Gertzbein SD, Court-Brown CM, Marks P, et al. The neurologic outcome following surgery for spinal fractures. *Spine* 1988;13:641–644.
23. Gertzbein SD, Offieski C. Complete fracture–dislocation of the thoracic spine without spinal cord injury. *J Bone Joint Surg* 1979;61A:449–451.
24. Guerra J, Garfin SR, Resnick D. Vertebral burst fractures: CT analysis of the retropulsed fragment. *Radiology* 1984;153:769–772.
25. Holdsworth FW. Fractures, dislocations, and fracture-dislocations of the spine. *J Bone Joint Surg* 1963;45B(1):6–20.
26. Holdsworth FW. Fractures, dislocations, and fracture–dislocations of the spine. *J Bone Joint Surg* 1970;52A(8):1534–1551.
27. Kelly RP, Whitesides TE. Treatment of lumbodorsal fracture–dislocations. *Ann Surg* 1968;167(5):705–717.
28. Kilcoyne RF, Mack LA, King HA, Ratcliffe SS, Loop JW. Thoracolumbar spine injuries associated with vertical plunges: reappraisal with computed tomography. *Radiology* 1983;146:137–140.
29. Laulan J, Rosset M, Favard L, Burdin M, Castaing J. Lesions traumatiques du rachis dorsolombaire de l'adulte. *Rev Chir Orthop* 1990;76(S1):100.
30. Lindahl S, Willen J, Irstam L. Computed tomography of bone fragments in the spinal canal: an experimental study. *Spine* 1983;8:181–186.
31. Lindahl S, Willen J, Nordwall A, Istam L. The crush–cleavage fracture. A "new" thoracolumbar unstable fracture. *Spine* 1983;8(6):559–569.
32. Louis R. *Surgery of the spine*. Berlin: Springer-Verlag, 1983.
33. Louis R, Goutallier D. Fractures instables du rachis. *Symp Rev Chir Orthop* 1977;63:415–481.
34. McAfee PC, Hansen AY, Fredrickson BE, Lubicky JP. The value of computed tomography in thoracolumbar fractures. *J Bone Joint Surg* 1983;65A:461–473.
35. McAfee PC, Yuan HA, Lasda NA. The unstable burst fracture. *Spine* 1982;7(4):363–373.
36. McEvoy RD, Bradford DS. The management of burst fractures of the thoracic and lumbar spine. Experience on 53 patients. *Spine* 1985;10:631–637.
37. Nash CL, Schatzinger LH, Brown RH, Brodkey J. The unstable thoracic compression fracture. *Spine* 1977;2(4):261–265.
38. Nicoll EA. Fractures of the dorsolumbar spine. *J Bone Joint Surg* 1949;31B(3):376–394.
39. Plaue R. The mechanics of compression fractures in the spine. *Zentralbl Chir* 1973;90:761.
40. Roberts JB, Curtiss PH. Stability of the thoracic and lumbar spine in traumatic paraplegia following fracture or fracture–dislocation. *J Bone Joint Surg* 1970;52A(6):115–130.
41. Roy-Camille R, Lelievre JF. Pseudarthrose des corps vertébraux du rachis dorsolombaire. *Rev Chir Orthop* 1975;61:249–257.
42. Roy-Camille R, Saillant G. Rachis dorsolombaire traumatique non neurologique. In: *2es Jounées d'Orthopédie de la Pitié*. Paris: Masson, 1980.
43. Roy-Camille R, Saillant G. Rachis traumatique neurologique. In: *3es Journées d'Orthopédie de la Pitié*. Paris: Masson, 1983.
44. Shuman WP, Rogers JV, Sickler ME, Hanson JA, Crutcher JP, King HA, Mack LA. Thoracolumbar burst fractures: CT dimension of the spinal canal relative to post surgical improvement. *AJR* 1985;145:337–341.
45. Sutherland CJ, Miller F, Wang GJ. Early progressive kyphosis following compression fractures. Two case reports from a series of "stable" thoracolumbar compression fractures. *Clin Orthop* 1983;173:217–220.
46. Uriarte E, Elguezabal B, Tovio R. Fracture–dislocation of the thoracic spine without neurologic lesion. *Clin Orthop* 1987;217:261–265.
47. Vichard P, de la Salle R, Tropet Y, Runge M. Fracture-luxation complete D8-D9 sans complications neurologiques. Description lésionnelle. Déductions thérapeutiques. *Rev Chir Orthop* 1983;69:645–648.
48. Watson-Jones R. *Fractures and other bone and joint injuries*. Edinburgh: E & S Livingstone Ltd, 1940.
49. White AA, Panjabi MM. Clinical biomechanics of the spine. Philadelphia: Lippincott, 1978.
50. Whitesides TE. Traumatic kyphosis of the thoracolumbar spine. *Clin Orthop* 1977;128:79–92.
51. Willen J, Anderson J, Toomoka K, Singer K. The natural history of burst fractures of the thoracolumbar junction. *J Spinal Disord* 1990;7:39–45.
52. Willen JAC, Gaekwad VH, Kakulas BA. Burst fractures in the thoracic and lumbar spine. A clinico-neuropathologic analysis. *Spine* 1989;14(12):1316–1323.
53. Willen J, Lindahl S, Nordwall A. Unstable thoracolumbar fractures. A comparative clinical study of conservative treatment and Harrington instrumentation. *Spine* 1985;10(7):111–122.

11

Neurologic Injuries

Syndromes, Diagnosis, and Prognosis

E. Shannon Stauffer

Fractures in the thoracic, lumbar, and sacral levels of the spine may cause injuries to the spinal cord, nerve roots, or cauda equina, which may result in varying degrees of paralysis. The paralysis may be mild and temporary or severe and permanent. Each level of the spine has a distinct pattern of neurologic deficit associated with injuries to the neurologic elements. It is important to understand the anatomy of the bony spinal column and the relationship of the spinal cord and nerve roots within the spinal canal.

ANATOMY

Upper Thoracic Spine

The upper thoracic spine consists of small vertebral bodies held rigidly in place by short ribs attached to the sternum. Fractures of the T1–T2 and T3 level are rare. This area is difficult to visualize on routine radiographs and fractures are often missed unless attention is drawn to this area by an attending neurologic deficit. Due to the great amount of energy required to disrupt the spine in this area, the injury is usually sufficient to cause a complete spinal cord lesion injury (Fig. 1A).

Midthoracic Spine: T4 to T10

This area is also a very stable area of the spine. The circular connections of the ribs and sternum provide resistance against disruption of the spine by rotation and flexion forces. Flexion compression injuries may cause compression fractures of the vertebral body without translation and without spinal cord injuries. Most serious injuries in this area are from shear forces causing fracture dislocations. The spinal canal is quite narrow and there is little epidural space around the spinal cord. If there is enough translation of the vertebra to cause neurologic damage, this most frequently results in a complete spinal cord lesion.

Lower Thoracic Spine: T11 and T12

This area of the spine is the least stable of the thoracolumbosacral axis. This is due to the transition from the upper stable ribs to the lower floating ribs without firm sternal attachment, and the coronal orientation of the facet joints.

Neurologic injuries at this level are mostly spinal cord injuries just above the conus (supraconus) and involve few levels of upper lumbar nerve roots.

Thoracolumbar Junction: T12–L1

This is the level of the thoracolumbar spine most likely to fracture. This level lacks the support of the ribs of the upper thoracic level and has smaller vertebral bodies and facets than the lower lumbar vertebrae. Due to the abrupt change of orientation of coronal facets at the superior aspect of T12 to sagittal facets at the inferior aspect of T12, flexion rotation forces frequently cause a fracture through the superior facet of L1 and down through the vertebral body, causing a

---

E. S. Stauffer: Department of Orthopaedic Surgery, Southern Illinois School of Medicine, Springfield, IL 62794.

FIG. 1. A: Bony stability of thoracolumbar spine—lateral and posterior view of vertebrae. **B:** Coronal facet joints of thoracic spine allow rotation motion. The abrupt change to a sagittal configuration at T12–L1 blocks rotation. Continued rotation of dorsal element produces a fracture dislocation of T12–L1. **C:** Spinal cord segment in relation to skeletal level.

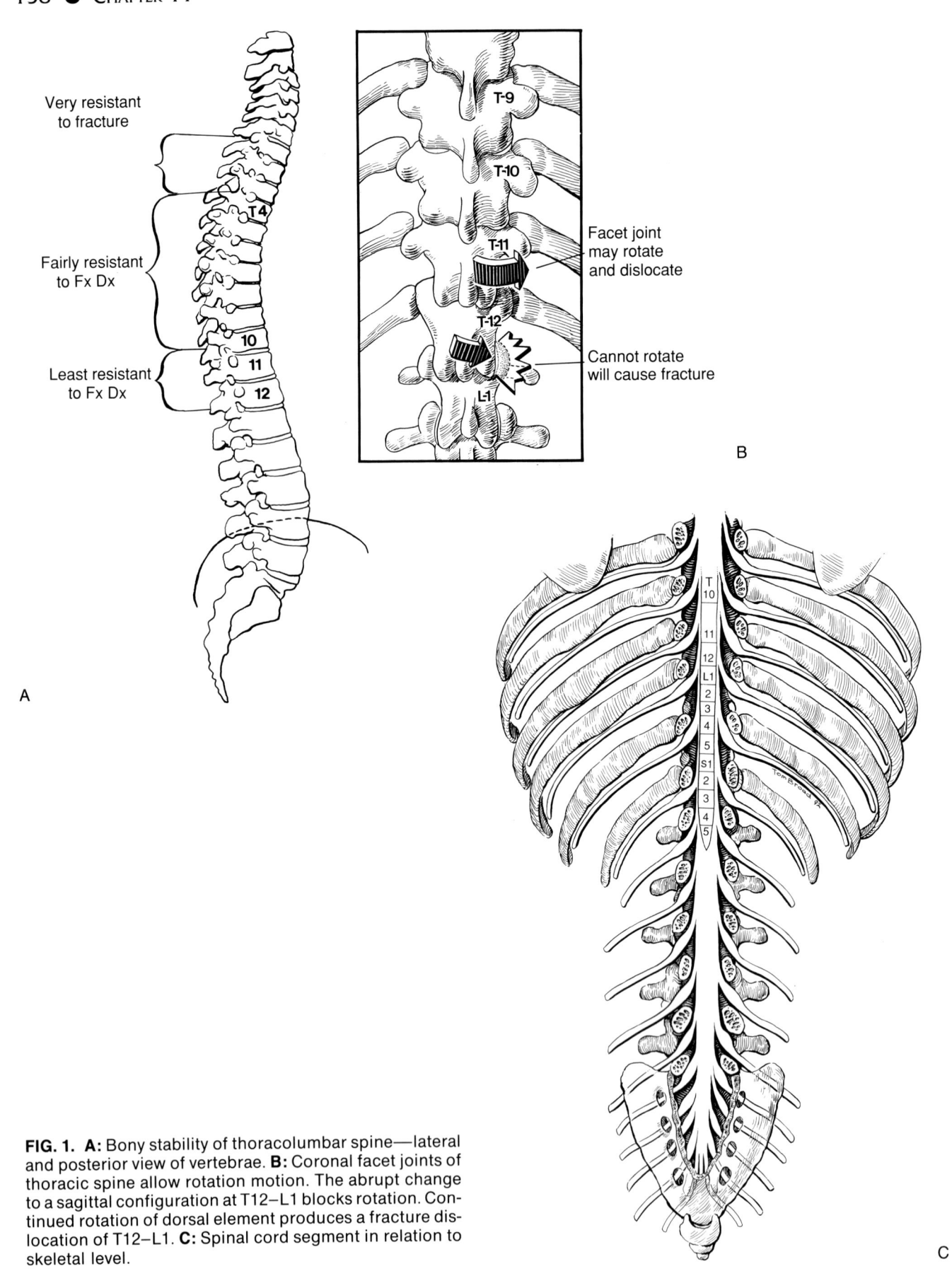

grossly unstable fracture dislocation that frequently causes injury to the neural elements (Fig. 1B).

The spinal cord behind T12 consists of the supraconal area of cord segments L5 and S1. The neural elements behind the body of L1 consist of the conus (sacral cord elements S2 and S3) plus all the lumbar roots; therefore the neurologic examination of patients with injury at the T12–L1 junction must specifically address the evidence for or against a cord injury of the sacral innervated segments and a root injury of the lumbar innervated skin and muscles of the lower extremities (Fig. 1C).

Lumbar Spine: L2 to L5

Injuries in the L2 to L5 area are most frequently burst fractures. Fracture dislocations with sagittal shear forces are less common and dislocations without fracture are most rare. The neural elements in this level of the spinal canal consist of the cauda equina only and are usually partial lesions. The spinal canal gets progressively larger from L2 down through L5. The neural injuries are usually less severe as one descends the spinal canal from L2 down through L5.

NEUROLOGIC INJURIES

Upper Thoracic Spine T1 to T10 Vertebral Fracture

Paraplegia is defined as the loss of sensibility and paralysis of the voluntary muscles of the lower extremities. Depending on the level of the neurologic injury, this may also include a portion of the trunk involving the thoracic, abdominal, and spinal musculature. The severity is classified by the Frankel classification (4) (Table 1).

Frankel A. A complete lesion paraplegia exists when there is no sensibility or voluntary motor power detectable below the level of the injury including bowel and bladder control and perianal sensibility.

TABLE 1. *Frankel classification of patients with spinal cord injuries*

A	Sensibility and voluntary motor function absent
B	Sensibility present, motor function absent
C	Sensibility present, voluntary motor function present but not useful (grade 1/5–2/5)
D	Sensibility present, motor function present and useful (grade 3/5–4/5)
E	Sensibility normal and motor function normal (grade 5/5) (reflexes may be abnormal and paresthesias may be present)

Frankel B, C, and D. A partial lesion (paraparesis) is present when either sensibility recognition or voluntary motor power is evident in the muscles distal to the level of injury including the bowel and bladder sphincters.

The intercostal, abdominal, spinal, and extremity muscles are segmentally innervated. The muscles and the skin over them are innervated by the same nerve root levels.

Physical Examination of the Apparent Neurologically Intact Person with a Fracture of the Thoracic Spine

A. Motor Examination

1. Ask the patient to take a deep breath; then observe and palpate the intercostal muscle contraction.
2. Palpate the abdominal muscles and ask the patient to cough (do not attempt a situp).
3. Examine the lower extremity muscle power beginning distally.
4. Document the grade of the toe flexors and extensors, the ankle flexors and extensors, the quadriceps, and the hip internal rotators, external rotators, and adductors. If these all appear normal and do not cause increased back pain, you may then attempt to test the hip abductors and flexors of one leg while stabilizing the pelvis by holding the opposite leg in extension. Examination of hip musculature may be painful and documentation inaccurate due to pain with contraction of the iliopsoas or abductor muscles at the fracture level of the spine.

B. Sensibility

Pinwheel examination from the forehead down over face, shoulders, trunk, lower extremities, and toes will be normal.

C. Reflexes

Deep tendon reflexes are intact, and plantar responses are negative.

D. Rectal

Rectal and perianal sensation are intact with voluntary sphincter contraction and a positive bulbocarvernosus reflex.

Before a diagnosis of a normal neurologic examination is confirmed, the patient must demonstrate a continence of urine and must be able to void voluntarily; in addition, the male patient should be able to get a penile erection. A mild occult lesion of the conus at the vertebral level of T12–L1 may cause occult irregularities in the bladder sphincter control and erection reflexes in a patient with an otherwise normal neurologic evaluation.

Complete Paraplegia: Physical Examination (Fig. 2)

A. Motor

1. Examine the muscle strength of the upper extremity to assure patient understanding and cooperation and assess the patient's overall strength and discomfort.
2. Observe for intercostal muscle contraction and rib elevation with breathing.
3. Palpate abdominal muscles as you ask the patient to cough.
4. Examine for and document the muscle grade of voluntary function of the lower extremities starting distally, with the patient supine: toe flexors, toe extensors, ankle flexors, ankle extensors, quadriceps, hamstrings, hip adductors, and hip flexors (Fig. 2B).

B. Sensibility

"Sensibility" is a more precise term than "sensation" to describe the patient's ability to accurately perceive stimuli of the skin and deep tissue. The term sensation has many diverse connotations. Patients with a complete paraplegia may have "sensations" in their lower extremities consisting of burning, stinging, dysesthesias, or phantom pains. Immediately after an injury to the spinal cord, the patient may have many "sensations" due to the irritation and injury of the spinal cord itself.

Sensibility to sharp/dull discrimination and deep pressure should be tested separately. Beginning with a pinwheel over the forehead and proceeding down over the face and shoulders, the patient will appreciate the difference between the sharp and dull stimuli. Mark the level of decreased sensibility, then start over the toes and feet and work up to the level of the lesion to confirm the level and identify any area of partial sensibility (Fig. 2C). There will often be a "zone of injury" at the level of the injury, which will have present but altered sensibility. After the sharp/dull discrimination test, proceed with the test for appreciation of deep pressure and proprioception sensibility by forcibly flexing and extending the toes and squeezing the tendo-Achilles area.

C. Reflexes

Deep tendon reflexes initially are depressed or absent due to spinal shock but may recover within 2 or 3 days. After cord reflexes return, the deep tendon reflexes will become hyperactive over a 2- to 6-week period.

The plantar response may be neutral or may cause toe flexion for the first several days, but then it reverts to the typical upgoing Babinski.

D. Rectal Exam

The most important examination to confirm a suspected complete paraplegia is the perineal exam for perianal sensibility, rectal sensibility, rectal sphincter control, and the bulbocarvernosus reflex (2).

Perianal sensibility may be the only finding of voluntary sensibility present in an otherwise apparent complete paraplegia. If the patient has the ability to discriminate sharp/dull sensibility around the perineum, this places him/her in the incomplete lesion category and has a good prognosis for some progressive recovery. Following the perianal sensibility examination, a rectal examination with a gloved finger is performed to detect any deep sensibility that may be present in the rectum and to evaluate the tone and any voluntary contraction of the rectal sphincter. The third part of the perianal evaluation is the bulbocarvernosus reflex. When the glans penis is squeezed or the mons pubis is tapped or a catheter is gently tugged against the trigon of the bladder, this normally will cause an involuntary reflex contraction of the anal sphincter through a spinal cord mediated reflex. If this reflex is absent, the patient may be in spinal shock from a thoracic cord injury or may have a lower motor neuron lesion of the conus medullaris area of the spinal cord or an injury to the cauda equina. This reflex is the first cord reflex to return, signifying the end of spinal shock in the complete lesion paraplegic with a supraconus lesion. Therefore if this reflex is absent during the first several hours or days, the patient may be in spinal shock and the complete lesion cannot be confirmed because he/she may show some progressive recovery of voluntary neurologic function during the first 24 to 48 hr. The bulbocarvernosus reflex may return anytime after 4 to 6 hr following the injury. Therefore if the bulbocarvernosus reflex is negative, a definitive diagnosis cannot be made. If the bulbocarvernosus reflex is positive and there is no sign of any voluntary motor control or sensibility in the lower extremities, including the perianal and rectal area, the diagnosis of complete lesion is confirmed and there is no anticipation of functional, distal neurologic recovery in the future.

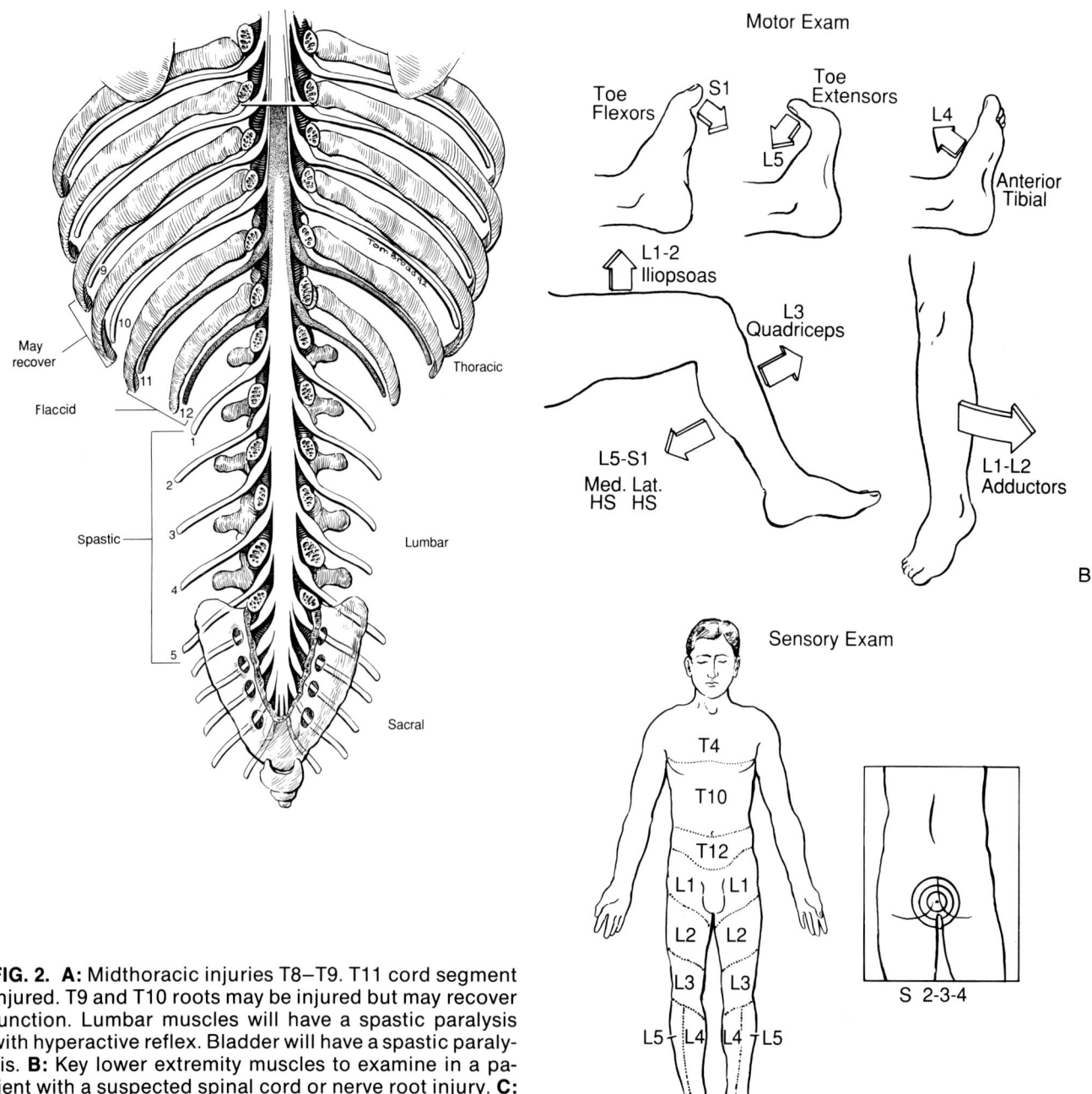

FIG. 2. A: Midthoracic injuries T8–T9. T11 cord segment injured. T9 and T10 roots may be injured but may recover function. Lumbar muscles will have a spastic paralysis with hyperactive reflex. Bladder will have a spastic paralysis. **B:** Key lower extremity muscles to examine in a patient with a suspected spinal cord or nerve root injury. **C:** Sensibility dermatomes for documentation of level paraplegia.

During the perianal examination it is important to recognize that the scrotal skin is innervated by the sacral 2-3 nerve roots and it is appropriate to test the scrotal skin along with the skin of the penis for sacral sparring. However, the testes in the scrotum receive their nerve supply from their original intrapelvic level, which is above the T12 spinal cord segment. Therefore one should not be confused if a patient presents with a complete T12 functional level paraplegia with complete anesthesia of the scrotum but retains deep pressure sensibility when squeezing the testicle. This is not a sign of an incomplete lesion.

Urodynamic studies performed during the period of spinal shock will demonstrate a flaccid bladder; however, after spinal reflex activity recovers, urodynamic examination will demonstrate a lack of bladder sensibility of filling and a reflex spasticity of the bladder musculature. All spinal cord segments below the zone of cord injury will regain involuntary reflex activity to provide reflex bowel and bladder emptying and spasticity of the paralyzed lower extremity and trunk muscles.

Diagnosis of the Level of the Paraplegia: Complete Paraplegia T1 to T11

A. Motor

The functional level of paraplegia is defined as the level of the lowest functioning muscle. The intercostals document T2 through T9; the upper abdominals document T10 and the lower abdominals T12.

B. Sensibility

The sensory level is described as the level of lowest sensibility of sharp versus dull discrimination. The "zone of injury" may have one or two root levels of altered sensibility.

C. Reflexes

All deep tendon reflexes (DTRs) are absent while in spinal shock. They usually recover between 3 days and 3 weeks following injury.

D. Rectal

No rectal voluntary contraction can be palpated. No rectal or perianal sensibility is found. The bulbocarvernosus reflex is negative while in spinal shock (first 4–24 hr) and becomes positive after spinal shock is over.

E. Urodynamics

There is no sensibility of bladder filling. There are no voluntary sphincter contractions. The bladder has a flaccid paralysis for several days; then the bladder develops spasticity after 1 to 2 weeks.

Incomplete Thoracic Lesions: T1 to T11

If any sensibility perception or voluntary motor power is found below the zone of injury, even though it is abnormal, this indicates a partial lesion paraplegia (paraparesis).

Browne-Séquard Syndrome

This syndrome results from an injury limited to one side of the spinal cord (Fig. 3). This injury will cause a motor paralysis and loss of proprioception on the ipsilateral side of the body and a loss of sensibility to

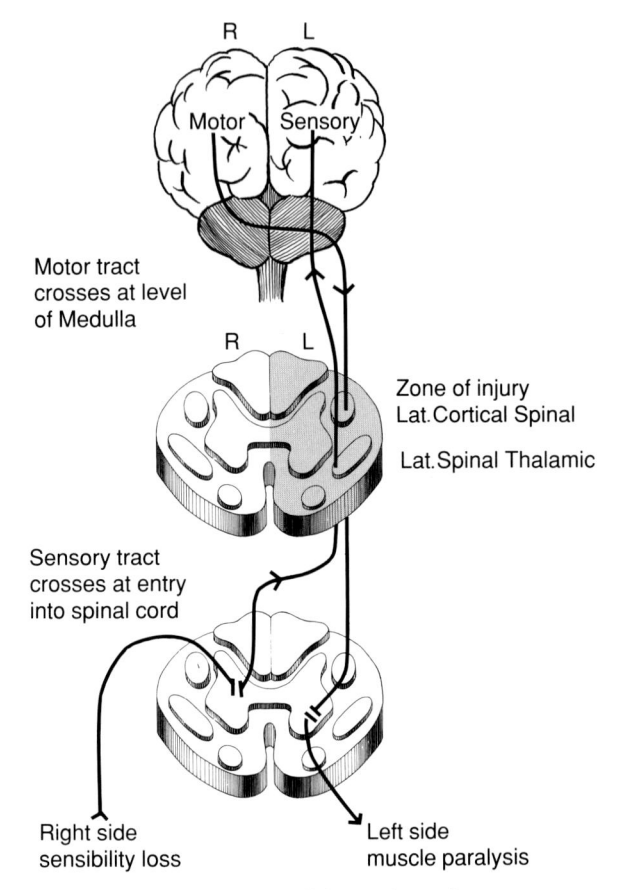

FIG. 3. Browne–Séquard syndrome.

pain and temperature on the contralateral side. The descending motor tracts cross at the cephalad aspect of the cord and descend on the contralateral side of the cord from the brain. The sensory fibers cross at the distal portion of the cord and travel up the spinal cord on the ipsilateral side of the destination in the brain. The prognosis for ambulation and bladder control recovery is good due to the retained unilateral innervation of motor on one side and sensibility on the opposite side (1).

Central Cord Syndrome

This is the most common incomplete thoracic cord syndrome (Fig. 4). The motor exam may demonstrate complete paralysis below the zone of injury, but the rectal exam will demonstrate perianal sensibility sparing with the presence of sharp/dull discrimination (5). There may be some voluntary sphincter control and toe flexor power present, but these are not required for this diagnosis. This syndrome has a 50% chance of good functional recovery. The motor recovery usually begins distal with toe flexors as the first voluntary motor power detected and proceeds proximally. How much recovery will occur cannot be predicted early; however, as long as the patient continues to have im-

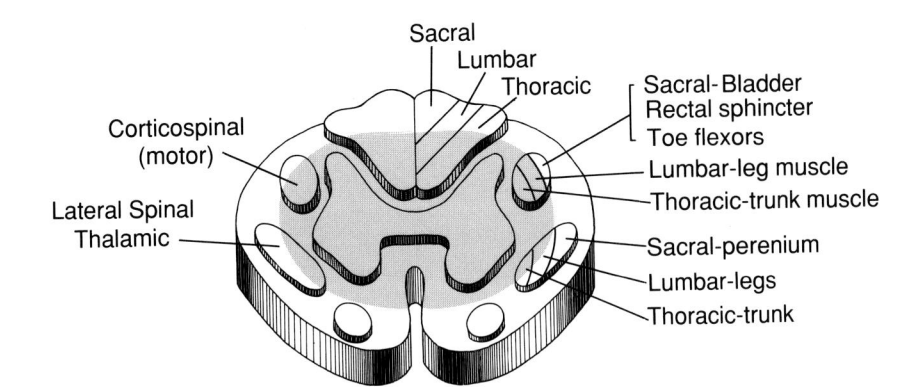

FIG. 4. Central cord syndrome.

provement with new muscles being found, the prognosis remains good. When the patient reaches a plateau and no new muscles are detected, the prognosis for future muscle recovery becomes guarded. However, the muscles that are present may continue to get stronger for several months. Patients may show progressive functional improvement for 12 to 18 months (7).

Anterior Cord Syndrome

This is a severe incomplete spinal cord injury with complete motor paralysis and only the dorsal column sensibility function remaining intact (6) (Fig. 5). This patient will have only touch and deep pressure sensibility perception with no sharp/dull discrimination below the level of the injury. Prognosis is poor (10–15%) for any future functional recovery.

The key to differentiation between the central cord syndrome with a good prognosis and the anterior cord syndrome with a poor prognosis is the presence of sacral sparing consisting of perianal sharp and dull sensibility discrimination. Any voluntary sacral motor function consisting of sphincter control or toe flexor control also places the patient in the category of the central cord syndrome with its better prognosis.

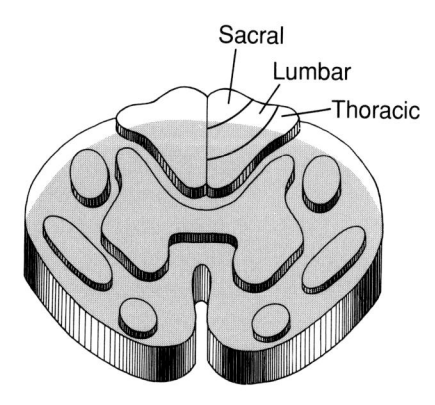

FIG. 5. Anterior cord syndrome.

Complete Cord Lesions

Injuries at the T11–T12 Vertebral Level

The neural elements in the spinal canal at this level consist of low lumbar cord segments (L4–L5) and upper lumbar nerve roots (L1, L2, L3). Following a

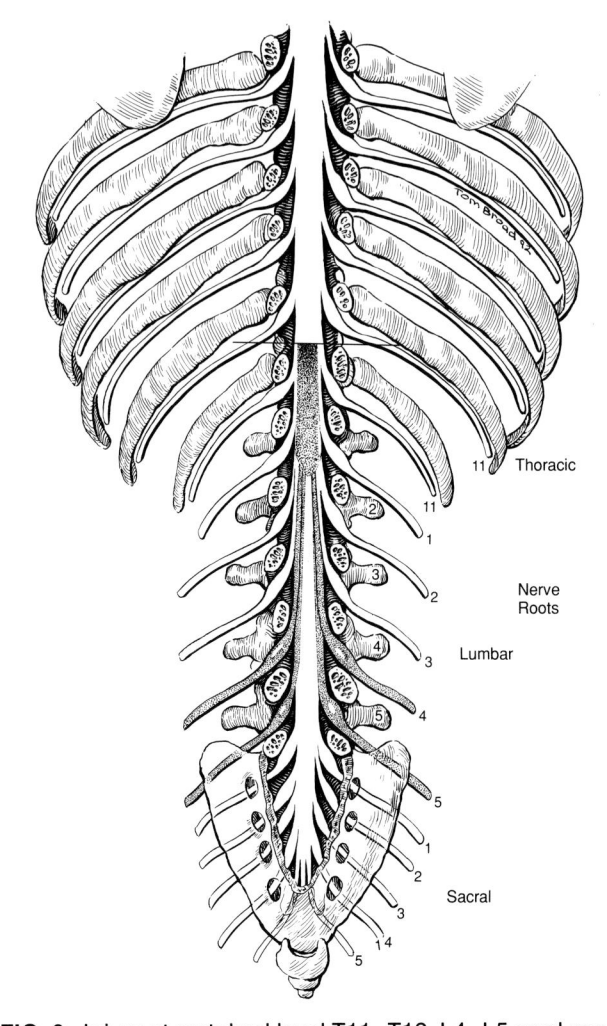

FIG. 6. Injury at vertebral level T11–T12. L4–L5 cord segment injuries. T12–L1–L2–L3 roots may be injured but may recover.

complete cord injury, the L4–L5 innervated areas will be permanently flaccid, whereas T12–L1, L2, and L3 nerve roots may demonstrate recovery from root injuries (Fig. 6). The sacral segments below this level will remain paralyzed but regain reflex emptying of the bladder and bowel.

Injuries at the T12–L1 Vertebral Level

A complete cord injury at this level will consist of an injury to the conus medullaris (Fig. 7). Injury of the S2–S3 segments will cause permanent flaccid paralysis of the bowel and bladder. All the lumbar nerve roots, L1 to L5, may be fully functional (root escape) or they may be injured with a neurapraxia or axonotmesis and demonstrate recovery over a 6- to 12-month period. Severely injured roots (neurotmesis) will not demonstrate recovery.

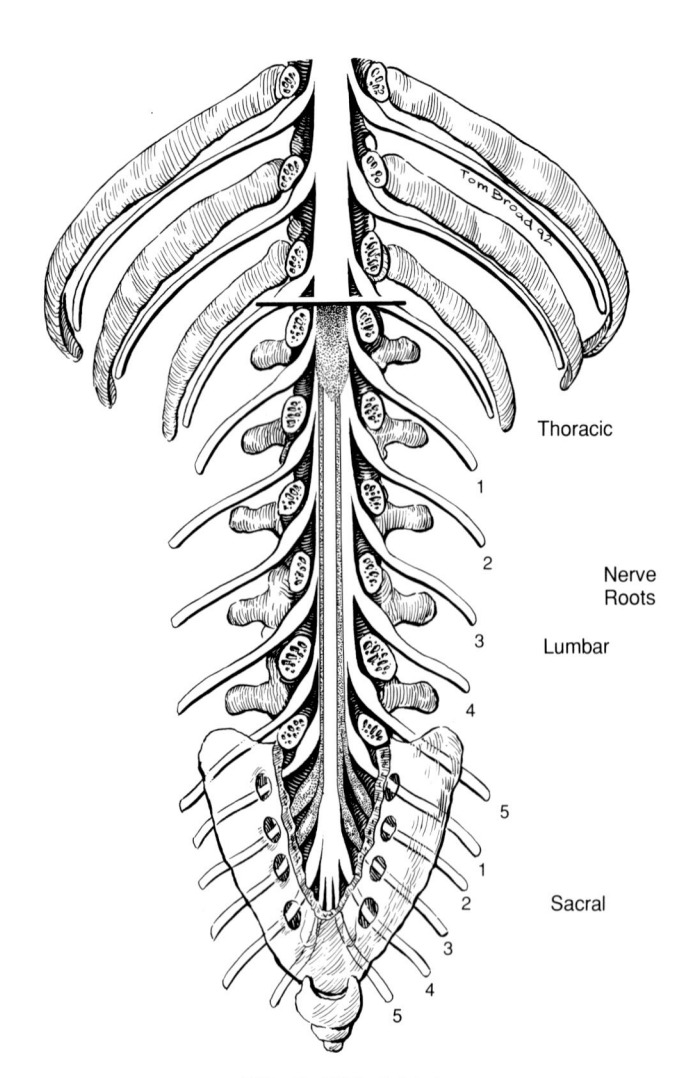

FIG. 7. T12–L1 injury.

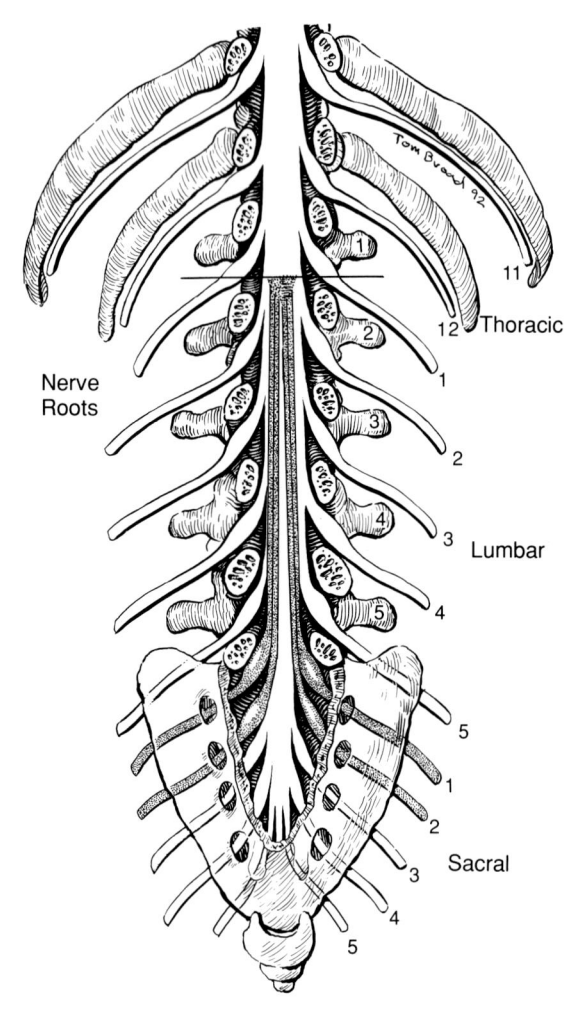

FIG. 8. L2 injury.

L2 Burst Fractures

There is no cord lesion at this level since the spinal cord ends at the L1 vertebral level (Fig. 8). In a complete lesion, the hip flexors and adductors will be the lowest muscles that are intact. The cauda equina lumbar and sacral nerve roots may be injured to varying degrees. Partial lesions usually demonstrate some progressive recovery of leg muscle power as well as bladder control.

L3–L4–L5 Fracture

Injuries to the neural canal contents at this level consist of injury to cauda equina nerve roots (Fig. 9). With a burst fracture of L3 causing a complete cauda equina lesion, the L2 roots supplying hip flexors and adductors will be the lowest function nerve roots. With a burst fracture of L4, the L3 nerve root supplying the quadriceps will be the lowest functioning roots. A fracture at the L5 level causing a complete cauda equina lesion will demonstrate the L4 innervated anterior tibialis as the lowest voluntary muscle. An injury to the nerve roots in the lower cauda equina may be documented by an L5 injury causing toe extensor paralysis, S1 causing toe flexor and gastrocnemius weakness, and S2 and S3 causing bladder control paralysis.

The further down the lumbar spine the injury occurs, the less likelihood of neurologic damage. L4 and L5 vertebral burst fractures frequently have little or no neurologic damage even with large amounts of bone fragments in the canal as demonstrated by a CT scan. The further down the lumbar canal the injury occurs, the greater the likelihood of progressive spontaneous recovery of nerve root injuries.

Sacral Fractures

Sacral fractures may be transverse or longitudinal (Fig. 10). The longitudinal sacral fractures are more common and usually occur through or just adjacent to the sacral foramina (3). These injuries are usually significant for persistent pain; however, the functional loss is usually slight due to the intact opposite side for bowel/bladder control and sensibility.

The transverse fractures are more rare and usually occur across the level of the lower sacral nerve root foramina. If the fracture is below the S2 nerve roots, there is little functional deficit and bladder and bowel control is usually preserved by the functioning S2 nerve roots.

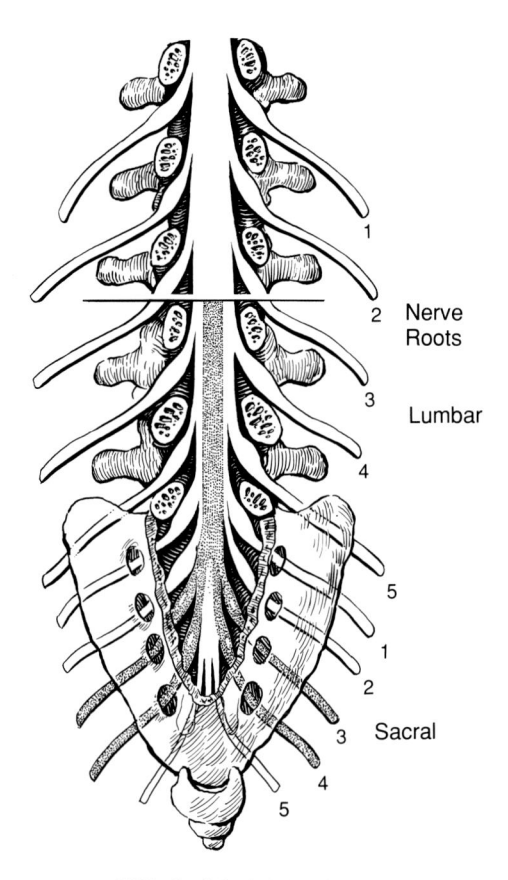

FIG. 9. L3–L4–L5 injury.

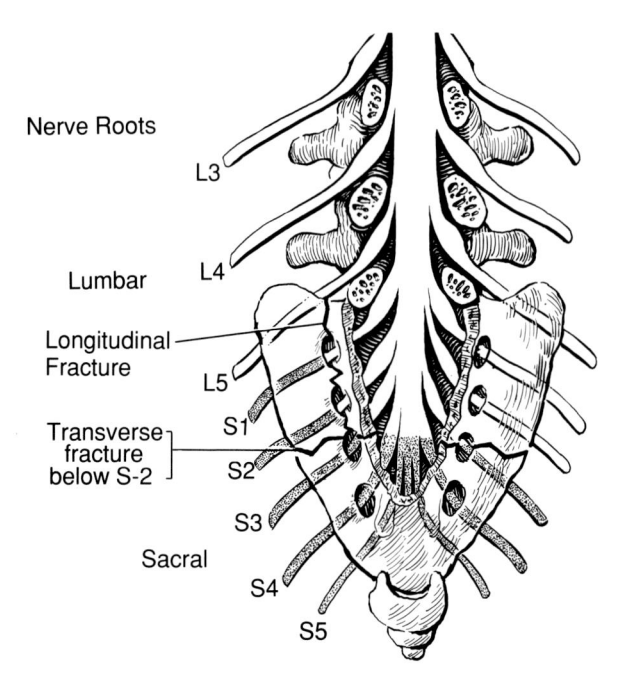

FIG. 10. Sacral fracture: transverse longitudinal.

REFERENCES

1. Bosch A, Stauffer ES, Nickel VL. Incomplete traumatic quadriplegia, a 10 year review. *JAMA* 1971;216:473.
2. Chusid JG. *The spinal nerves. Correlative neuroanatomy and functional neurology,* 19th ed. 1985;134.
3. Denis F, Stevens D, Comfort T. Sacral fractures, 236 cases. *Clin Orthop* 1988;27:67–81.
4. Frankel HL. The value of postural reduction in the initial management of closed injuries of the spine with paraplegia and tetraplegia. *Paraplegia* 1969;7:179–192.
5. Schneider RC. The syndrome of acute central cervical spinal cord injury. *J Neurosurg* 1954;11:546–577.
6. Schneider RC. The syndrome of acute anterior cervical spinal cord injury. *J Neurosurg* 1955;12:95–122.
7. Stauffer ES. Diagnosis and prognosis of the acute cervical spinal cord injury. *Clin Orthrop* 1975;112:9–15.

12

Intensive Care of the Spinal Cord Injured Patient

Reuven Pizov, Leonid Eidelman, and Yizhar Floman

The management of patients with spinal cord injuries (SCIs) is a long and complicated process. The last two decades have witnessed a greatly improved prehospital care with the introduction of standard guidelines and training of personnel administering care at the scene of the accident. In addition to the utilization of skilled prehospital care providers, trauma centers and spinal cord injury units were introduced.

There are five phases of prehospital care: evaluation, resuscitation, immobilization, extrication, and transport. Immobilization, extrication, and transport are no less important than resuscitation since Podolsky et al. (18) have noted that SCI may occur or be exacerbated after the initial event, for example, during extrication or transport and even later on. After immobilization at the scene of the accident, and early on clinical evaluation, the patient is transferred to a spinal cord injury unit or intensive care unit. Such centers contain facilities for adequate imaging, intensive care, and surgery as well as rehabilitation. This aggressive approach in managing SCIs, has brought about remarkable improvement in survival rates and quality of life for these individuals (5,9).

The spinal cord carries integrated neural activity from the brain to the periphery, that is, the rest of the body. Interruption in this cycle causes not only motor and sensory loss but also pertubation of the autonomic activity. This may lead to cardiovascular, respiratory, gastrointestinal, genitourinary, neurologic, and musculoskeletal system impairments. In a complete lesion, total interruption of communication across the injury level occurs. In addition to the original injury inflicted, neurologic deterioration may occur in about 5% of the patients with SCI during the early hospital stay (16).

This chapter deals with intensive care management of patients with thoracolumbar injuries, especially with complete high thoracic cord lesions.

INDICATION OF ADMITTANCE TO INTENSIVE CARE UNIT

Since SCI leads to dysfunction of many organ systems, the appropriate management of these patients requires admission to the intensive care unit. Whereas intensive care management of patients with cervical SCI is an absolute necessity, there are no clear guidelines with which patients with lower SCIs should be managed in the intensive care unit. Since the sympathetic system is regulated mostly by thoracic cord segments, any lesion above T7 may create severe cardiovascular and other systems dysfunction. Therefore patients with a cord lesion above T7 should be initially managed in an intensive care unit.

SPINAL CORD RESUSCITATION

The neurological deficit resulting from a spinal cord injury depends on the immediate morphologic damage inflicted to the cord, and secondary deleterious effects due to vascular and biochemical changes that follow the injury. Therefore the final neurologic deficit resulting from spinal cord trauma may be influenced by ma-

---

R. Pizov: Intensive Care Unit, Department of Anesthesiology, Hadassah University Hospital, Jerusalem 91120, Israel.
L. Eidelman: Departments of Anesthesiology and Critical Care Medicine, Hadassah University Hospital, Kiryat Hadassah, Jerusalem 91120, Israel.
Y. Floman: Department of Orthopaedic Surgery and Spine Surgery Unit, Hebrew University–Hadassah Medical School, Hadassah University Hospital, Jerusalem 91120, Israel.

nipulating these vascular and biochemical changes, that is, early "cord resuscitation." Cord resuscitation is time dependent and the optimal time for pharmacologic intervention is usually within the first hours after injury.

The secondary pathologic processes within the cord that follow trauma include ischemia and impairment of the cord's autoregulation. These changes make the spinal cord vulnerable to reduction in perfusion and oxygenation, processes frequently occurring after cord injury (10,20). Adequate oxygenation should be evaluated by continuous pulse oximetry or periodic analyses of arterial blood gases. Oxygen saturation above 95% and PaO_2 above 80 torr should be maintained during acute periods of spinal cord injury.

The estimation of local spinal cord perfusion pressure is complicated. The pressure might be expressed as a difference between mean arterial pressure and one of the following: cerebrospinal fluid (CSF) pressure, spinal venous pressure, or spinal cord interstitial pressure (6). The recommended level of spinal cord perfusion pressure is about 60 to 70 mmHg. Even though this parameter is not used as widely as the cerebral perfusion pressure, maintenance of mean arterial pressure at least at normal levels may be in the patient's best interest.

Although there is a lack of clinical studies, theoretically, the use of mannitol to decrease spinal cord edema is justified. Mannitol also causes a vigorous osmotic diuresis and adequate intravascular volume must be maintained to ensure spinal cord perfusion.

Hyperbaric oxygen therapy to elevate low oxygen levels in the area of the cord injury has been used in some experimental models as well as in clinical studies. The theory behind this treatment is to preserve marginally injured neuronal elements in the spinal cord through reversal of focal tissue hypoxia. However, there is a possibility that hyperbaric oxygenation might exacerbate unwarranted ongoing lipid peroxidation that occurs after injury. Thus its use is not recommended at this time.

Local profound hypothermia by perfusion of the subarachnoid space was introduced by Albin et al. (1) in 1961. Theoretically, the technique has much to recommend itself: a "decompressive" laminectomy and durotomy are required, both of which may improve spinal cord perfusion. Whether cooling by itself to 10°C is more protective against the secondary cord damage than its adverse effects remains to be determined. In practice, cord cooling has enjoyed only sporadic clinical success (6,10). In the same context, body temperature elevation for any reason should be treated vigorously during the acute period of cord injury.

There is a list of different agents that have had beneficial results in experimental cord injury but did not get through the clinical trials. This list contains dimethyl sulfoxide, naloxone, and thyrotropin-releasing hormone. A limited number of these drugs still have clinical relevance. Naloxone was very popular during the previous decade not only in spinal cord injuries but in different brain injuries and shock. It was administered to block the deleterious effects of endorphins, released after injury. With today's knowledge, there is no reason to use naloxone in spinal cord injury (3).

Total calcium levels have been found significantly elevated in the area of SCI. This fact justified studies evaluating the effect of Ca^{2+} channel blockers (such as diltiazem hydrochloride or nifedipine) in post-ischemic hypoperfusion syndrome (22). Recently, the interest of researchers turned to a new group of agents—lazaroides (2). Lazaroides are 21-aminosteroids that lack glucocorticoid or mineralocorticoid activity and are very potent inhibitors of lipid peroxidation, which is one of the biochemical mechanisms of the secondary neurologic injury. Both Ca^{2+} channel blockers and lazaroides still did not come through clinical trials.

It has taken more than 20 years to prove the efficacy of glucocorticoids in the treatment of acute spinal cord injury (3). In NASCIS I (National Acute Spinal Cord Injury Study), using 1000-mg infusion of methylprednisolone with 100 mg given as a bolus and daily administration for 10 days, there was no relative difference from the placebo group. NASCIS II protocol dictated administration of 30 mg per kilogram of methylprednisolone given as an i.v. bolus and maintenance dose of 5.4 mg per kilogram per hour i.v. for 23 hr (3). In this study, patients who received glucocorticoids within 8 hr of injury showed significant improvement in motor function and sensation compared to the controls. The improvement in the neurologic outcome with the latter protocol may be explained by inhibition of lipid peroxidation and hydrolysis at the site of injury by the very high doses of glucocorticoids. The administration of high doses of methylprednisolone for 1 day did not increase the risk for wound infection and gastrointestinal bleeding. Methylprednisolone was not effective if treatment began more than 8 hr after injury (3). Therefore it is mandatory that patients with spinal cord trauma (SCT), arriving at the hospital within 8 hr after injury, should receive methylprednisolone, according to the above-mentioned protocol.

Recently, administration of GM_1 ganglioside after spinal cord injury showed promising clinical results (4). Gangliosides are a complex of acidic glycolipids that are present in high concentrations in the central nervous system. Experimental studies have shown that gangliosides stimulate the growth of nerve cells and the regeneration of damaged nerve tissues. Patients treated with GM_1 had significantly better recovery of neurologic function than the control groups. An advantage of this treatment is the possibility of delaying its administration after the injury up to 3 days.

CARDIOVASCULAR PROBLEMS

In addition to sensory and motor loss, SCI leads also to autonomic nervous dysfunction. The autonomic nervous system involvement in SCI leads to a host of cardiovascular complications. The critical spinal level above which significant hemodynamic changes will occur is T5 to T7 (6,14,23). Most SCI patients will present in the acute phase with varying degrees of hypotension and bradycardia. This phase, which is a manifestation of spinal shock, is characterized by significant vasodilatation and bradycardia due to lack of sympathetic mediated increase in heart rate and cardiac contractility. These patients are extremely sensitive to any changes in their positioning or posture, due to loss of orthostatic and other vasopressor reflexes. In addition, ECG abnormalities may be present at this acute stage such as ST-T changes and various types of dysrhythmia.

Management of hypotension in the acute stages of SCI and "spinal shock" is dictated by the physiologic changes that produced it. If hypotension occurs together with significant bradycardia, then care should be taken first to correct the bradycardia. A starting dose of 0.5 mg atropine intravenously is recommended in case of significant bradycardia. The need for long-term vagolytic therapy is very rare. The existence of hypotension with normal heart rate will require volume loading. It is usually preferable to combine crystalloids and colloid solutions administration during the first 24 hr after SCI. The hemodynamic insult in high thoracic SCI usually presents with both bradycardia and vasodilatation, which necessitate the use of sympathomimetic drugs with combined α- and β- adrenergic properties. We recommend starting with small doses of ephedrine (5 mg) intravenously or, in selected cases, with 25 to 50 mg of ephedrine subcutaneously every 4 to 6 hr. This regimen will assure stable hemodynamics

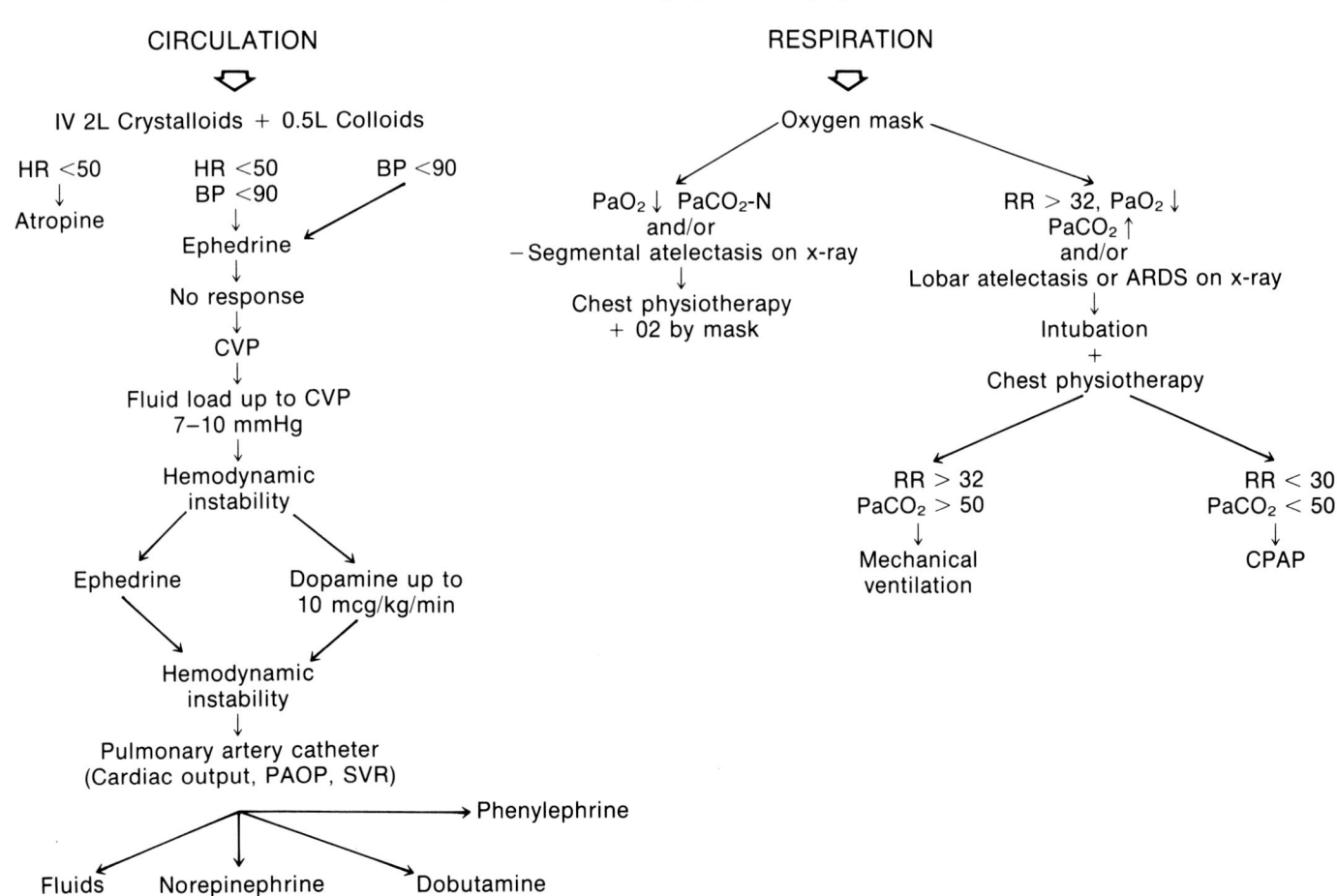

FIG. 1. An algorithm of the non-operative management of acute spinal cord injuries. SCI, spinal cord injury; HR, heart rate; BP, blood pressure; CVP, central venous pressure; PAOP, pulmonary artery occlusion pressure; SVR, systemic vascular resistance; RR, respiratory rate; CPAP, continuous positive airway pressure; ARDS, adult respiratory distress syndrome.

in mild "spinal shock." In cases of a more severe hemodynamic dysfunction, we administer dopamine, phenylephrine hydrochloride, or norepinephrine. If hypotension necessitates the administration of large doses of vasopressors, hypovolemia or reduced heart contractility should be suspected. Therefore we recommend the insertion of a pulmonary artery catheter, which allows measurement of cardiac output, estimation of heart preload, and calculation of the vascular resistance. In view of these pressure findings, fluid and/or catecholamines may be chosen more accurately (Fig. 1).

When "spinal shock" ends, about 2 to 6 weeks after injury, reflexes reappear. This may lead to autonomic dysreflexia (AD) causing nasal obstruction, facial tingling, piloerection, headaches, shortness of breath, nausea, and blurred vision. Bradycardia, arrhythmia, sweating, and occasionally loss of consciousness and seizures (13). Patients with lesions above T6 have at least a 50% chance of developing this syndrome. Autonomic dysreflexia occurs because of uninhibited reflex outflow over the entire sympathetic chain below the injury level. Triggering mechanisms may be an occluded urinary catheter or fecal impaction. Management of AD is achieved with ganglionic blockers, α-adrenergic blockers, and vasodilators.

RESPIRATORY COMPLICATIONS

Depending on the level and degree of SCI, respiration may be impaired by paralysis of the intercostal or abdominal muscles. Patients with thoracic SCI have a preserved diaphragmatic and accessory muscle function; nevertheless, pulmonary function tests will be significantly affected in lesions above T7. Thoracic SCI may also cause paradoxic inward rib cage movement during inspiration, secondary to loss of the intercostal muscle function (15). Paralyzed abdominal musculature may further compromise respiratory mechanics by moving the diaphragm to the caudal direction, which impairs its fiber length–tension relationship.

Prompt respiratory evaluation should focus on the respiratory rate, volume of breathing, and accurate examination of the different groups of respiratory muscles. Arterial blood gases should be measured as soon as possible, although further respiratory monitoring would be better followed with a pulse oximeter. The pulse oximeter, which is a very sensitive and accurate oxygenation monitor, enables effective warning of forthcoming ventilatory problems, particularly if the patient is not breathing a gas mixture with high oxygen concentration.

Respiratory complications are the most common cause of death in acute SCI (15). In order to prevent pulmonary complications in these patients, there should be a strict adherence to the standard protocol, which includes a change in the patient's position in bed every 2 hr; assisted coughing and chest percussion if needed every 4 hr; bronchodilators to combat bronchospasm; and fiberoptic bronchoscopy if atelectasis is diagnosed (14,23). Patients with a high thoracic SCI are prone to pulmonary complications especially during the first week following injury. Inadequate coughing as a result of paralyzed intercostal and abdominal musculature predisposes these patients to atelectasis, which by itself will increase paradoxical rib cage movement by the increased inspiratory effort.

Some of the patients, even with solitary high thoracic injury or with combined injuries, may require an artificial airway or mechanical ventilation. Endotracheal intubation in thoracic SCIs is less problematic than in cervical SCIs. Most of these patients can be intubated easily by a blind nasotracheal or by direct laryngoscopy. We prefer to anesthetize and paralyze these patients with short-acting drugs for intubation. There is no contraindication to use succinylcholine in paraplegic patients in the first 2 to 3 days. In a more anatomically complicated airway, a fiberoptic bronchoscope or a retrograde technique may be utilized. Intubated patients who maintain normal ventilation should receive a low level of continuous positive airway pressure to prevent atelectasis. Patients who show signs of respiratory fatigue should be assisted with mechanical ventilation. There is no evidence that any particular ventilatory mode (e.g., pressure support or intermittent mandatory ventilation) is preferable for such patients. Once the decision to ventilate the patient is made, we utilize a mode of ventilation that provides close to full respiratory support for the first couple of days, until the major cause of respiratory embarrassment, such as pneumonia, pulmonary edema, or adult respiratory distress syndrome, show signs of resolution.

The time of weaning from mechanical ventilation depends on the patient's general condition and lung functions. Usually, pulmonary function improves after stiffening of the chest wall. It is unreasonable to make a weaning attempt in a patient with uncontrolled pneumonia, high fever, or severe electrolyte and metabolic disturbances. Bedside spirometry might be helpful in monitoring ventilatory function during the weaning period. Forced vital capacity should be at least 1 liter or more to allow effective coughing, and maximal minute ventilation should be above 10% of the predicted value to make weaning efforts reasonable. In addition, spirometry might be helpful in elucidation of a bronchoconstriction component, if present. There are controversial data as to whether or not theophylline is beneficial in increasing diaphragmatic function in these kinds of patients (14,15).

Pulmonary mechanics usually improve 2 to 3 weeks

after the SCI. Whenever the patient meets the weaning criteria, the weaning techniques themselves are less important. There are two classical techniques: T-tube trials and intermittent mandatory ventilation. To our knowledge there are no data showing an advantage of one technique over the other. Lately, with the introduction of pressure support ventilation, we utilize this technique to wean spinal cord injured patients. Because of possible laryngeal incompetence after prolonged intubation, we suspend enteral feeding for 2 to 3 hr before extubation and at least 12 hr after. Following successful weaning, patients should be transferred to oral feeding gradually. It is preferable to begin oral feeding with jelly, which is easier to swallow than clear fluids.

ELECTROLYTE DISORDERS

Hypokalemia occurs very frequently in the early post-injury period. Usually K^+ does not reach dangerously low levels (below -3 mEq/liter) and maintenance with balanced fluids enriched with electrolytes will correct this disturbance. Only in a more severe hypokalemia or when cardiac arrhythmias occur is there an indication for the more aggressive K^+ replacement. It should be remembered that rapid K^+ correction requires ECG monitoring and that high K^+ concentrations are very irritating to veins.

After the primary resuscitation, patients with SCI may frequently present with the syndrome of inappropriate antidiuretic hormone secretion (SIADH). This syndrome is characterized by excessive vasopressin secretion, without relation to the serum's osmolality, and results in free fluid reabsorption and hyponatremia. Most of the clinical features associated with SIADH are related to hyponatremia, but the early signs will be expressed only by high urinary sodium concentrations. Other laboratory findings supporting the diagnosis of SIADH are low serum level of BUN and creatinine, low plasma osmolality, and high urine osmolality (19). Hyponatremia may cause brain edema, manifested by weakness, mental confusion, and even progression to convulsions and coma. It is important to differentiate oliguria in SIADH from oliguria caused by other origins because the management is completely different and contradictory.

PREVENTION OF THROMBOEMBOLISM

The incidence of deep vein thrombosis in SCI patients varies from 15% to 100% (7,17). Awareness of this potentially lethal complication has resulted in active prophylaxis and decrease in its frequency. Early prophylaxis includes physical therapy, frequent movement of the patient, calf-compression boots, and the administration of heparin and warfarin. Recently, low molecular weight heparin has been shown to be superior to standard heparin. Low molecular weight heparin is not only more effective in preventing thrombosis, but it also has significantly lower incidence of causing bleeding (8). Inferior vena cava filters, such as the Greenfield filter, should be inserted in patients with high risk to anticoagulant therapy or failure to prevent thromboembolism under anticoagulation (11).

NUTRITION AND GASTROINTESTINAL FUNCTION

Almost all patients with high thoracic SCIs develop gastric atony and paralytic ileus, which last from 1 to 3 weeks (6,14). A nasogastric tube is obligatory, even in patients who breath spontaneously. Metaclopramide may improve gastrointestinal motility in some patients, but most require nasogastric drainage until the spontaneous return of autonomic function. In a solitary high thoracic cord lesion and combined injuries, we prefer early parenteral nutrition, followed by enteral tube feeding once the gastric atony and intestinal ileus resolve spontaneously. In a patient with prolonged gastric atony, introduction of a feeding tube into the small bowel may help to avoid parenteral nutrition, or shorten its period.

Gastrointestinal (GI) bleeding is a very frequent complication in patients with SCI (12). Active prophylaxis is justified in these patients, particularly if the injury is combined with hemodynamic instability, respiratory distress, surgery, or steroid treatment. We practice pharmacological prophylaxis of GI bleeding in every patient with SCI. During the last few years our first choice has been sucralfate, 1 g every 6 hr, and H_2 blockers as an additional treatment if GI bleeding occurs.

GENITOURINARY FUNCTION

During acute paraplegia, the urinary bladder is denervated, which requires catheterization. Catheterization should prevent bladder distension and the triggering of sympathetic reflexes. Another reason for urinary bladder catheterization is to monitor the urinary output. Adequate urinary output (not less than 0.5 ml/kg/hr) is accepted as a sign of proper tissue perfusion.

SUMMARY

SCI creates dysfunction in many "target" systems; the extent of involvement does not always correlate with the injury level. This necessitates close monitoring for the purpose of early detection of organ dysfunction. Prompt diagnosis and aggressive treatment are required in SCI. The recommended approach presented in this chapter has led to increased survival rates in these patients.

REFERENCES

1. Albin MS, White RJ, Donald DE, et al. Hypothermia of the spinal cord by perfusion cooling of the subarachnoid space. *Surg Forum* 1961;12:188.
2. Anderson DK, Branghler JM, Hall ED. Effects of treatment with N-74006F on neurological outcome following experimental spinal cord injury. *J Neurosurg* 1988;69:562.
3. Bracken MB, Shephard MJ, Collins WF, et al. Randomized, controlled trial of methylprednisolone or naloxone in the treatment of acute spinal cord injury. *N Engl J Med* 1990;322:1405.
4. Geisler FH, Dorsey FC, Coleman WP. Recovery of motor function after spinal cord injury—a randomized, placebo controlled trial with GM-1 ganglioside. *N Engl J Med* 1991;324:1829.
5. Geisler WO, Jonsse HT, Wynne-Jones M, Breithampt O. Survival in traumatic spinal cord injury. *Paraplegia* 1983;21:364.
6. Gilbert J. Critical care management of the patient with acute spinal cord injury. *Crit Care Clin* 1987;3:(3):549.
7. Green D, Lee MY, Ito WT, et al. Fixed adjusted heparin in the prophylaxis of thromboembolism in spinal cord injury. *JAMA* 1988;260:1255.
8. Green D, Lee MY, Lim AC, et al. Prevention of thromboembolism after spinal cord injury using low molecular weight heparin. *Ann Intern Med* 1990;113:571.
9. Heinemann AW, Yarkony GM, Roth EJ, et al. Functional outcome following spinal cord injury: a comparison of specialized spinal cord injury center vs general hospital short-term care. *Arch Neurol* 1989;46:1098.
10. Janssen L, Hansebout RR. Pathogenesis of spinal cord injury and newer treatments. A review. *Spine* 1989;14:23–32.
11. Kanter B, Moser KM. The Greenfield vena cava filter. *Chest* 1989;93:170.
12. Kiwersky J. Bleeding from the alimentary canal during the management of spinal cord injury. *Paraplegia* 1986;24:92.
13. Lindau R, Jainer E, Freehater AA, Mazel C. Incidence and clinical features of autonomic dysreflexia in patients with spinal cord injury. *Paraplegia* 1980;18:285.
14. Luce JM. Medical management of spinal cord injury. *Crit Care Med* 1975;13:126.
15. Mansel JR, Norman JR. Respiratory complications and management of spinal cord injuries. *Chest* 1990;97:1446.
16. Marshall CF, Knowlton S, Garfin SR, et al. Deterioration following spinal cord injury: a multicenter study. *J Neurosurg* 1987;66:400.
17. Myllynen P, Kammonen M, Rokkanen P, et al. Deep venous thrombosis and pulmonary embolism in patients with acute spinal cord injury: a comparison with non-paralyzed patients immobilized due to spinal fractures. *J Trauma* 1985;25:541.
18. Podolsky S, Baraff LJ, Simo RR. Efficiency of cervical spine immobilization methods. *J Trauma* 1985;23:462.
19. Rossi NF, Schvier RW. Hyponatremic states. In: Maxwell MH, et al, eds. *Clinical disorders of fluid and electrolyte metabolism.* New York: McGraw-Hill, 1987;461.
20. Sandler AN, Tator CH. Review of the effect of spinal cord trauma on the vessels and blood flow in the spinal cord. *J Neurosurg* 1976;45:638.
21. Soderstrom CA, Brumback RJ. Early care of the patient with cervical spine injury. *Clin Orthop North Am* 1986;17:3–13.
22. Stokes BT, Fox P, Hollinden G. Extracellular calcium activity in the injured spinal cord. *Exp Neurol* 1983;80:561.
23. Troll GF, Dohrmann GJ. Anesthesia of the spinal cord injured patient: cardiovascular problems and their management. *Paraplegia* 1975;13:162.
24. Winsplow EBJ, Lesch M, Talano JJ, Meyer PR Jr. Spinal cord injuries associated with cardiopulmonary complications. *Spine* 1986;11:809.

Early Management of Spinal Cord Injury

Paul C. McCormick and Bennett M. Stein

Traumatic injury to the spinal cord occurs at an annual incidence of 20 to 40 per million in most industrialized countries (9). In the United States, there are between 8000 and 10,000 cases of spinal cord injury per year with a prevalence of about 900 per million. Thus there are nearly one-quarter million patients in the United States with traumatic spinal cord injury. One-half of these injuries are complete. Motor vehicles accidents account for over 40% of spinal cord injuries and is followed in decreasing frequency by falls, assaults, and sports-related (e.g., diving) activities. Young healthy men between the ages of 16 and 26 are by far the most commonly affected (80%).

The individual lifetime direct and indirect costs of spinal cord injury is estimated at about $1.5 million but the personal and psychological costs to the patients and their families are much more profound. Despite intensive development and implementation of prevention programs, such as the National Head and Spinal Cord Injury Prevention Program, there does not appear to be as yet an appreciable decline in the incidence of spinal cord injury. While advances in critical care, comprehensive spinal cord injury management protocols, and aggressive physical medicine programs have reduced the early morbidity and mortality from spinal cord injury and improved functional outcome, very little effective therapy directed at the injured spinal cord has been developed.

In this chapter, the early management of the spinal cord injured patient is reviewed. It should be recognized that optimal treatment has yet to be standardized and that there are many controversies of early management.

PRINCIPLES OF EARLY MANAGEMENT

The main goals of management of the spinal cord injured patients include prevention of further injury and restoration or maintenance of the optimal environment for spinal cord recovery. Early post-traumatic morbidity and mortality resulting directly from spinal cord injury or from complications of paralysis as well as associated injuries to other organ systems must also be minimized. Early management of these patients is initiated at the scene of the injury. An assumption of spinal cord injury is made in the patient with impaired motor/sensory function or in the unconscious patient, particularly if there is evidence of head injury. Emergency resuscitative efforts aimed at airway maintenance, cardiovascular stabilization, and control of hemorrhage should be administered in a manner that minimizes movement of the spine. These emergency procedures are not only life saving but also maintain or restore the metabolic environment of the spinal cord and perhaps limit the extent of injury. The patient is then transported to the hospital on a backboard. Additional neck support can be provided by sandbags. A Trendelenburg position may enhance central venous return and diminish the risk of aspiration.

The initial emergency room clinical and radiological evaluations are performed by a multidisciplinary team for identification of associated head, limb, visceral, or vascular injury. The extent of injury and the need for further imaging or treatment are prioritized and implemented. An early lateral cervical spine plane film will determine whether intubation, if required, can be performed routinely or via a fiberoptic nasal route. An

---

P. C. McCormick and B. M. Stein: Department of Neurological Surgery, Columbia–Presbyterian Medical Center, New York, NY 10032.

emergency cricothyroidotomy may have to be performed in some cases. Once the patient has been stabilized, a thorough neurological examination must be performed and documented. Serial examinations to note any change in neurological status must also be recorded. If there is clinical evidence of spinal cord injury, then methylprednisolone is administered according to protocol (30 mg/kg bolus, 5.4 mg/kg/hr × 23 hr), provided that the injury is less than 8 hr old (1,2). Plane films of the spine are obtained to screen for spinal injury. The entire spine may need to be imaged because of the 15% incidence of noncontiguous multiple spine fractures. High-resolution computerized tomography scanning of any abnormality may then be performed. Preliminary experience of low field magnetic resonance imaging (MRI) for imaging of spinal cord injury has been encouraging. Advantages include visualization of the spinal cord as well as any intracanal soft tissue such as herniated disc or hematoma. MRI may also give some insight into ligamentous integrity.

Following stabilization and management of their acute injuries, patients with spinal cord injury should be enrolled in a comprehensive spinal cord protocol aimed at the prevention of the complications of spinal cord injury and optimized functional outcome. The unstable spinal segment must be effectively immobilized to prevent further injury to the spinal cord. In one case a patient with a paraparesis from an L1 burst fracture was rendered paraplegic following a portable chest radiograph. There had been unsupervised patient manipulation for radiograph cassette placement by a technician. This emphasizes the importance of a skilled vigilant nursing staff as an integral part of the care team.

Parenteral alimentation may be considered in many patients because of the hypermetabolic state and prolonged ileus frequently associated with thoracolumbar trauma. Institution of oral alimentation may be further delayed if major surgery is required, particularly from an anterior route. A bowel regimen that includes a high-fiber diet, stool softeners, and periodic nighttime laxatives, combined with postprandial bowel training and digital stimulation will usually result in adequate bowel function in the majority of spinal cord patients. Intermittent bladder catheterization according to volume/interval protocol should be instituted promptly to enhance the return of bladder tone, minimize the risk of infection and hydronephrosis, and avoid reflex autonomic phenomena, typically associated with bladder overdistention and infection. Intermittent pneumatic compression stockings are applied to prevent deep venous thrombosis. Subcutaneous low-dose heparin administration is also begun if clinically appropriate. A weekly noninvasive Doppler study is conducted on all patients with lower extremity paralysis. Positive studies are treated with full-dose heparin and are followed by coumadin anticoagulation. One frequently encountered problem is the patient with spinal cord injury who has a concomitant lower extremity fracture. In our experience, this paralyzed fractured limb dramatically increases the risk and complications associated with deep venous thrombosis. It is difficult to monitor these patients because they are immobilized in a cast and intermittent pneumatic stockings cannot be applied. Anticoagulation or placement of a Greenfield filter may be considered in these patients until active mobilization has been achieved. Pressured decubiti to insensate skin overlying a bony prominence, particularly the sacrum and the heels, must be prevented. An air mattress and frequent (every 2 hr) side-to-side positioning are usually adequate prophylaxis. Frequent passive range motion exercises should be performed for each paralyzed joint to prevent contractures.

MEDICAL MANAGEMENT OF SPINAL CORD INJURY

Most of the pharmacological agents used for the direct treatment of spinal cord injury have been developed as a result of experimental models of spinal cord injury. Most have been specifically tailored to counteract the effects of secondary injury. The initiating event of secondary injury is presumed to be ischemia, although direct injury to neuronal membranes may also contribute to delayed deleterious effects. Following a short period of hyperemia, spinal cord blood flow (SCBF) rapidly reduces to potentially ischemic levels within minutes of the injury. The possible causes include mechanical disruption of spinal cord microvasculature, vasospasm, increased blood viscosity, or thrombosis caused by prostaglandin-induced platelet aggregation or thrombosis. Autoregulation of SCBF may also be impaired for variable periods after injury, which results in direct variation of SCBF with systemic pressures (8,10). Thus postinjury hypotension, typically from hemorrhage or neurogenic shock, may exacerbate local spinal cord ischemia. The predominantly fibrous pia mater likely resists spinal cord expansion, which occurs as a result of intramedullary hemorrhages and white matter edema. This may further reduce perfusion pressures as intramedullary tissue pressure rises and is perhaps similar to the limb compartment syndromes.

It is widely held by many investigators that the duration and severity of ischemia may institute or contribute to a cascade of biochemical, metabolic, and membrane effects that have a deleterious effect on neuronal function and viability. It has been proposed that the initial metabolic failure impairs the integrity of ionic membrane pumps, which leads to potassium efflux and massive calcium influx into neuronal cells, which ultimately contributes to cell death. These secondary changes are further elucidated by Farcy and Rawlins (Chapter 3).

Over the years, numerous pharmacological agents have been utilized in the treatment of spinal cord injury. Most of these drugs were studied in the laboratory and were shown to exhibit under variable conditions some beneficial effects on spinal cord injury. Agents that enhanced SCBF [such as corticosteroids, thyroid releasing hormone (TRH), and naloxone], diminish spinal cord edema [e.g., corticosteroids, diuretics, osmotic agents, dimethy sulfoxide (DMSO)], achieve membrane stabilization and lipid peroxidation inhibitors (corticosteroids, DMSO), and calcium channel blockers have all been studied in human trials. In addition, other treatments such as hyperthermia or hyperbaric oxygen delivery have also been evaluated.

Despite enormous investigational support, the clinical significance of secondary injury has been questioned because delayed, permanent neurological deterioration following an incomplete injury, other than from an identifiable structural cause, is rarely witnessed. The failure of any pharmacological agent to alter the clinical course of spinal cord injury has posed further doubts. It is possible that these secondary phenomena may convert a physiologic but potentially reversible clinically complete (i.e., dyscomplete) injury into a permanent injury.

Evidence in support of the clinical relevance of secondary injury came in the recent publication of the North American Spinal Cord Injury Study (NASCIS) (2). In this prospective, randomized, and double-blinded trial, patients receiving methylprednisolone, 30 mg/kg intravenous bolus followed by a 23-hr continuous infusion at 5.4 mg/kg/hr, experienced a statistically significant improvement in neurological examination over those receiving placebo. No benefit was seen, however, if the steroids were not begun within 8 hr of the injury.

This study has been criticized because of the method of neurological assessment and the relatively short follow-up. Recently published data, however, indicate that early neurologic improvement associated with steroids is maintained at 1 year, postinjury (1). In fact, there was no significant improvement in functional (e.g., change in Frankel grade) status associated with steroid use. Nevertheless, although the clinical implications of steroids are unclear, this study is crucial because it represents the first clinical evidence that supports the wealth of investigational data concerning secondary injury. The massive dose of steroids required to produce a clinical effect also suggests that these effects are probably not mediated through known steroid receptors and most likely are exerting their effect through their inhibition of lipid peroxidation.

The current and future directions of spinal cord injury research are directed not only at pharmacological methods to limit secondary injury but also at modifying the response of the spinal cord to injury, diminishing glial scarring, which serves as a barrier to axonal growth, and enhancing reparative and regenerative capabilities within the central nervous system. In one recent prospective and double-blinded study, for example, spinal cord injury patients treated with GM_1 ganglioside, which experimentally has induced neuronal regeneration and neurite outgrowth, have a statistically greater motor recovery than the matched control group (4).

SURGERY

The role of surgery in the management of acute spinal cord injury remains controversial. While early decompression and stabilization are indicated in patients with progressive neurological deficit and documented spinal cord impingement, the role and timing of surgical intervention for fixed partial or complete deficits are not as clear. Arguments in favor of early emergent decompression for complete injuries are frequently based on the surgeon's philosophical orientation and supported by anecdotal reports of significant recovery in temporal relation to early surgical decompression. It must be noted, however, that perhaps 1% to 3% of patients with initial documented complete deficit will exhibit significant recovery without surgical intervention. It is therefore possible that early surgery may simply take advantage of a prolonged concussive event (11). In fact, numerous studies have failed to demonstrate any statistically significant correlation between either the performance or timing of surgery and neurological outcome (3,5,6).

The one clear benefit of early surgery is that the management and avoidance of complications associated with spinal cord injury are more effective in the patient who can be mobilized following surgical stabilization (6). Early enrollment into an aggressive physical medicine program following stabilization may also improve functional, albeit not neurological, outcome. The advantages of early surgical intervention, however, must be weighed against a possibly increased morbidity of early operation. Increased cardiopulmonary and vascular lability, concomitant injury to other organ systems, and metabolic derangements all contribute to the increased risk of general anesthesia and surgery in the acute post-traumatic setting. The deleterious effects of hypotension/hypovolemia on spinal cord blood flow in the presence of impaired autoregulation, surgical manipulation of the injured and swollen spinal cord, and dural tears may also increase neurological morbidity.

It is our belief that the prognosis of traumatic spinal cord injury is determined predominantly by the amount of energy absorbed by the spinal cord (i.e., hysteresis) at the time of the injury. The primary responsibility of management must therefore be prevention of further injury to the spinal cord and other organ systems, which may contribute to additional morbidity or even mortality. Decisions on the timing, type, and appropriateness of surgical intervention are based not only on the severity of spinal cord injury but also on other organ injuries, systemic derangements, and associated morbid and premorbid factors. Contrary to some reports, for example, dural tears do not represent an indication for early surgery but, in fact, complicate it. Loss of tamponading effect of an intact subarachnoid space on the epidural veins may result in excessive blood loss during spinal canal decompression. Persistent cutaneous, pleural, or dead space fistulas as a consequence of surgery, along with associated complications (e.g., meningitis), may further increase postoperative morbidity.

It is this institution's experience that in most cases, however, early surgery optimizes the comprehensive management of the spinal cord injured patient for reasons already listed. Priority of early intervention for incomplete injury is particularly high for two reasons. First, the risk and consequence of further injury from an unstable spine with canal encroachment are significant. Second, incomplete injuries tend to be (but are not always) associated with less severe systemic injuries. Early reduction of vertebral dislocation is also aggressively pursued by postural, distractive, or operative methods because of the sustained axial tension within the spinal cord.

The goals of surgical intervention in spinal cord injury are spinal stabilization that prevents further spinal cord injury and allows early mobilization as well as reestablishment of the spinal canal. Spinal canal decompression is performed on almost all patients with significant canal compromise, irrespective of the severity of the neurologic deficit. The benefit of decompression for incomplete spinal cord injuries is well established and may be independent of the timing of intervention. While the same benefit cannot be claimed with complete injury, canal reconstruction in these patients may prevent ascending sensorimotor paralysis from syrinx formation. This is often secondarily due to spinal cord tethering and impaired cerebrospinal fluid circulation at the site of the injury. This complication is seen in approximately 15% of spinal cord injury patients left with significant spinal cord compression (Fig. 1).

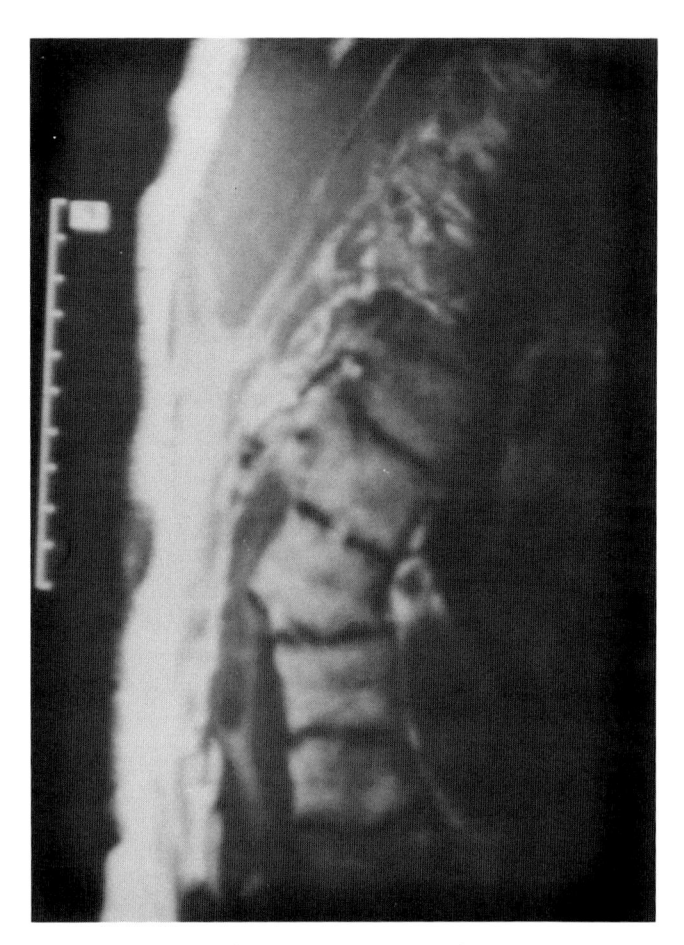

FIG. 1. Sagittal MRI scan shows persistent spinal cord compression with syrinx formation in a 62-year-old man, 10 years after a T10–T11 fracture dislocation. Worsening paraparesis and ascending loss were associated with syrinx.

The requirement for decompression and stabilization can create a management dilemma because while most spinal instrumentation systems are applied posteriorly, spinal cord compression is usually ventral in origin. The lateral extracavitary approach to the thoracic and lumbar spine is quite useful in these cases because it allows single-stage ventral and dorsal exposure for decompression and circumferential bone/instrument stabilization through a single incision (Fig. 2) (7). The

FIG. 2. Lateral radiograph **(A)** and CT scan **(B)** show L1 flexion–compression injury with spinal cord compression in a 28-year-old man with incomplete injury who had been involved in a motor vehicle accident. Operative photograph **(C)** shows neutral prone position and "hockey-stick" incision. Operative photograph **(D)** following completion of ventral decompression, posterior instrumentation, and anterior fusion with autologous bone graft. Postoperative CT scan **(E)** shows complete central decompression and bone graft. Lateral radiograph **(F)** shows stable construct with C-D rods and correction of kyphotic deformity.

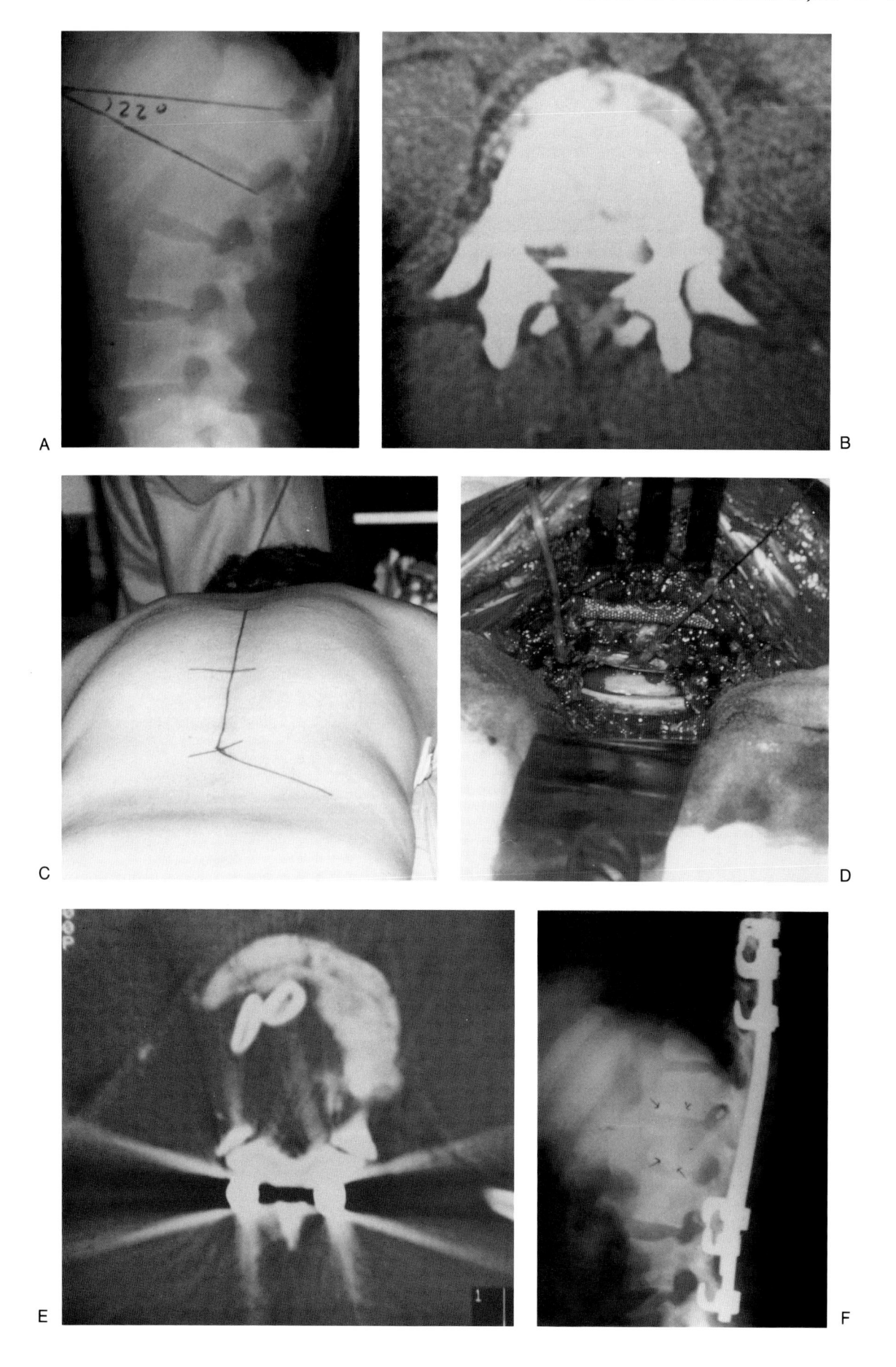

A

B

C

D

E

F

major advantages of this approach include a safe, neutral position for the unstable spine, avoidance of pleural/peritoneal cavity entry and diaphragm takedown, and direct visualization of the spinal cord/pathology interface during the entire dissection. The patient is placed in the prone position with the arms at the sides. A hockey-stick incision is centered over the spinal pathology. The skin/superficial muscle/fascia are elevated laterally as a single flap to expose the lateral border of the longitudinally oriented paraspinal muscles on one side. The paraspinal muscles are elevated medially off the ribs at the thoracic level and the quadratus lumborum and psoas muscles at the lumbar level. The ribs and/or transverse processes at the operative level are removed. Segmental nerves are identified and traced proximally to their respective foramina. The pedicle is then removed, providing a parallel, unimpeded view of the ventral spinal canal and thecal sac. A ventral subperiosteal displacement of the pleural and psoas muscles exposes the entire lateral body of the thoracic and lumbar vertebrae, respectively. A near complete corpectomy and discectomy of up to three levels can be performed with maintained vision of the lesion–dura interface. Following canal decompression, a subperiosteal dissection of the paraspinal muscles from the posterior vertebral elements is performed with placement of posterior instrumentation. Any force required for reduction or realignment may now be applied safely since the cord has been fully decompressed. An interbody graft is then placed ventrally following placement of spinal instrumentation, and the wound is closed in layers. Since the pleural and retroperitoneal cavities are not entered, drainage of these spaces is not necessary.

REFERENCES

1. Bracken MB, Shepard MJ, Collins WF, et al. Methylprednisolone or naloxone treatment after acute spinal cord injury: 1-year follow-up data. Results of the Second National Acute Spinal Cord Injury Study. *J Neurosurg* 1992;76:23–31.
2. Bracken MB, Shepard MJ, Collins WF, et al. A randomized, controlled trial of prednisolone or naloxone in the treatment of acute spinal cord injury. Results of the Second National Acute Spinal Cord Injury Study. *N Engl J Med* 1990;322:1405–1411.
3. Donovan WH, Dwyer AP. An update on the early management of traumatic paraplegia (non-operative and operative management). *Clin Orthop* 1984;189:12–21.
4. Geisler FH, Dursey FC, Coleman WP. Recovery of motor function after spinal cord injury—a randomized, placebo-controlled trial with GM-1 ganglioside. *N Engl J Med* 1991;324:1829–1838.
5. Heiden JS, Weiss MJ, Rosenberg AW, et al. Management of cervical spinal cord trauma in Southern California. *J Neurosurg* 1975;43:732–736.
6. Levi L, Wolf A, Rigamonti D, et al. Anterior decompression in cervical spine trauma: does the timing of surgery affect the outcome? *Neurosurgery* 1991;29:216–222.
7. McCormick PC. The lateral extracavitary approach to the thoracic and lumbar spine. In: *Spinal instability*. New York: Springer-Verlag (*in press*).
8. Sontag VKH, Douglas RA. Management of spinal cord trauma. *Neurosurg Clin N Am* 1990;1(3):729–750.
9. Stover SL, Fine PR. *Spinal cord injury. The facts and figures.* Birmingham: University of Alabama, 1986.
10. Tator CH, Fehlings MG. Review of secondary injury theory of acute spinal cord trauma with emphasis on vascular mechanisms. *J Neurosurg* 1991;75:15–26.
11. Zwimper TJ, Bernstein M. Spinal cord concussion. *J Neurosurg* 1990;72:894–900.

14

Orthopaedic Principles of Surgical Management

Claude Argenson

Optimizing neurologic recovery by attempting to provide the best chance for return to normal or close to normal function is the hallmark of thoracolumbar fracture treatment. Most authors recognize that surgical management is the best way to meet this challenge (13,16,31,38,44,45,47). However, the least invasive procedures for each specific case are advocated. The choice of fixation device should be based on reliability, versatility, and stiffness to enable the surgeon to optimize correction of anatomic contour and allow early physical therapy for rehabilitation. Although bony fusion is of utmost importance, the shortest fusion possible will ensure the best functional recovery.

Our indications for treatment were based on evaluation of 750 vertebral fractures treated in the Department of Orthopaedic Surgery at the University of Nice, France, from 1978 to 1990 (5,7).

CONSERVATIVE TREATMENT

Two-thirds of these patients received conservative treatment that was either:

1. Bed rest until the patient was pain free, followed by early ambulation with a light brace for 2 months. Physical therapy based on the principles of lumbar locking and isometric exercise were started immediately. (In Europe, this type of treatment is called "functional treatment.")
2. The "method of Boehler" (9) always combines reduction, immobilization, and isometric exercise. With radiograph control, reduction is done in traction, in a lordotic position with the patient awake and positioned on a Risser–Cotrel frame. Immobilization is carried out by casting after satisfactory reduction. A body jacket with sternum and pubic rests is fabricated with a front opening. This body jacket must be extended by a cervical collar in cases of upper thoracic fracture or, in cases of lumbosacral injury by a "pantalon" on one side. Isometric exercises are started immediately, as is early ambulation. After 6 weeks, rehabilitation will be facilitated by a custom-made plastic brace to replace the cast for another 6 to 8 weeks. The total period of immobilization must be at least 4 months. Application of the Boehler method must be delayed until return of normal bowel sounds or, better, the first spontaneous bowel movement to avoid paralytic ileus in a patient with a cast. After cast application, surveillance cannot be relaxed because a cast syndrome with acute gastric dilatation can occur and must be diagnosed and treated by cast removal.

Indications for either functional treatment or the Boehler method will be discussed later in this chapter.

The remaining 250 patients were treated surgically. During this 12-year period, we followed the same principles: postural reduction and internal fixation, with decompression when deemed necessary. In the same period, the first 122 cases were treated with Harrington instrumentation at the thoracic level (6) and with Roy-Camille plates (5,44–46) available since 1970, at the thoracolumbar and lumbar levels. Since April 1986, the other 128 patients have been treated with Cotrel–Dubousset (C-D) instrumentation regardless of level (7).

C. Argenson: Department of Orthopaedic Surgery, Service de Chirurgie Orthopedique et Traumatologique, Centre Hospitalier Regional et Universitaire de Nice, St. Roch University Hospital, 06000 Nice, France.

Our surgical indications are based on the neurologic status of the patient at the time of admission as well as the fracture type as described in Chapter 10.

FRACTURES WITH NEUROLOGIC COMPROMISE

Immediate, acute treatment according to Bracken's recommendations should be initiated as early as possible and carried out during the first few days, according to the recommendations of the National Institutes of Health press release of March 31, 1990 (12). The patient, having been admitted to the hospital, is placed under surgical care in a surgical intensive care unit (ICU) (see Chapter 12).

Timing of Surgery

In the case of a complete lesion as defined by Frankel type A, in which lack of reflexes and complete medullary impairment are obvious, we must wait until the end of the period of medullary shock to evaluate a possible future return of function. When there is still a complete lesion after the end of spinal shock, the chances of return are nil. These patients, mainly with high thoracic lesions, are hemodynamically unstable, and we prefer to stabilize the patient's hemodynamic and ventilatory functions before surgery. Sometimes pressure from the family, under the delusion that emergency surgery is more suitable for their relative's re-

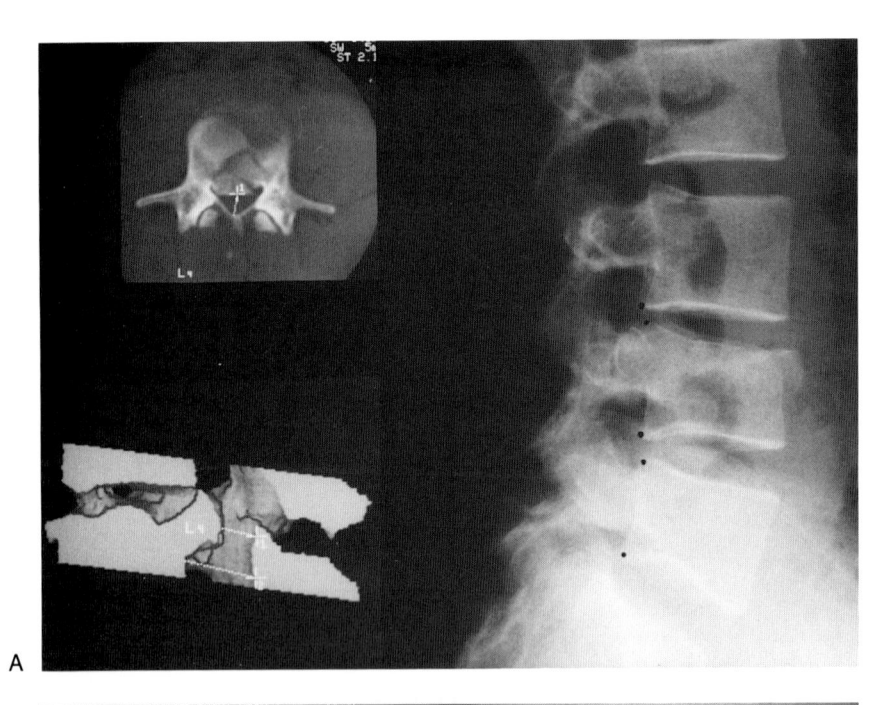

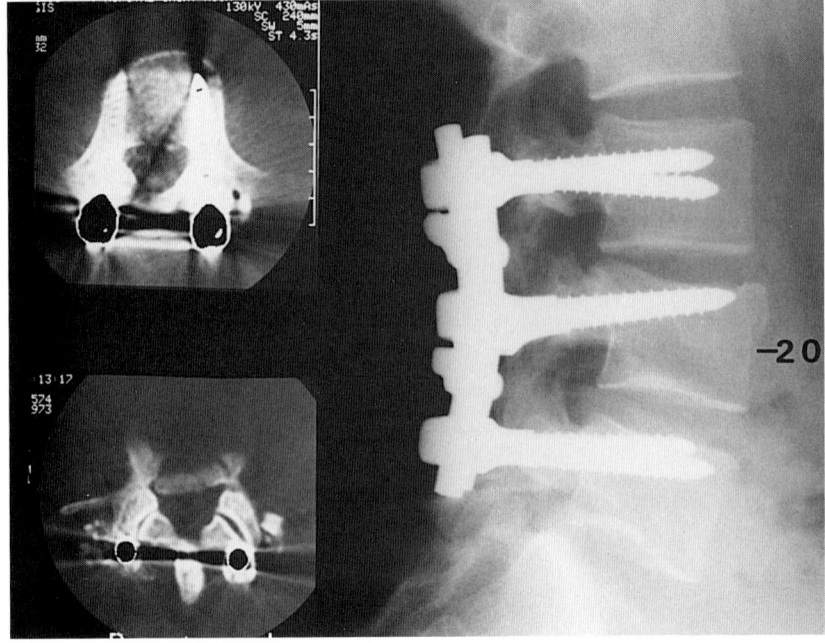

FIG. 1. A: Burst fracture of L4; canal compromise is less than 50%. **B:** Decompression by distraction only.

covery, creates difficult situations that require explanation and a very compassionate approach.

In cases of incomplete neurologic compromise, alignment by positioning is recommended on admission. Among other reasons to delay emergency surgery are the amount of bleeding from the peridural venous plexus and from the bone of the vertebral body when surgery is done on an emergency basis, creating a life-threatening problem. This blood loss at the operative site prevents complete, satisfactory decompression when emergency surgery is performed. We have elected to schedule surgery under the best technical conditions, with a fully staffed operating room and a stable patient. The average time elapsed before operating on fractures with mainly bony injury is 24 to 48 hr after admission; this delay seems to be the same in a majority of reports. However, in a case with multiple trauma, when long bone fractures are surgically fixed immediately, we recommend stabilizing the thoracolumbar fracture in the same session.

During this period of time, a complete clinical workup and imaging are performed. The shear fractures, Denis type IV, subtype B, have less tendency to bleed during reduction and stabilization, and they can be operated on earlier. No difference in neurologic recovery was found when we elected not to treat burst fractures in emergency. Conversely, Kostuik (35,36) claimed neurologic improvement that was directly related to the time interval between injury and decompression.

Technique

Many authors have advocated anterior decompression for burst fractures in cases of neurologic compromise (1,11,13,32,36). Evaluation of these fractures, preoperative planning, CT scan, and development of new fixation techniques that allow elective distraction have made us choose the posterior approach (40,44,54). In these cases with neurologic compromise, fixation after reduction in distraction by C-D instrumentation is performed; the technique is detailed in Chapter 15.

This appears to be efficient for all acute spinal stenosis having 30% to 50% canal occupancy, since in this case bursting of the entire posterior wall (subtype A) or the posterosuperior extruded fragment (subtype B) is still connected to the posterior longitudinal ligament and therefore enable an effective ligamentotaxis (see Fig. 17, Chapter 10). According to Frederickson et al. (23), distraction is the most effective mechanism to obtain reduction of the fracture fragment and takes precedence over the correction of kyphosis (Fig. 1). Two clinical studies using internal fixation in distraction have shown the difference between the two burst fracture types. In the Crutcher et al. series (15), stenosis was reduced from a preoperative mean of 62.5% to 19.2% in subtype A, and from 66.3% to 38.9% in subtype B; no attempt was made to reduce by directly addressing the fragment. Anderson et al. (3) have reported canal stenosis reduced from 61% to 21% in subtype A, and from 67% to 41% in subtype B.

When there is 50% or greater canal occupancy, or when the fragment appears to be rotated on the CT scan, we perform a laminectomy in order to remove or to push forward the fragment, which appears to be "free" in the canal, without ligamentous connection (Fig. 2).

At the thoracic level and at the thoracolumbar junction, the laminectomy must be enlarged laterally to gain

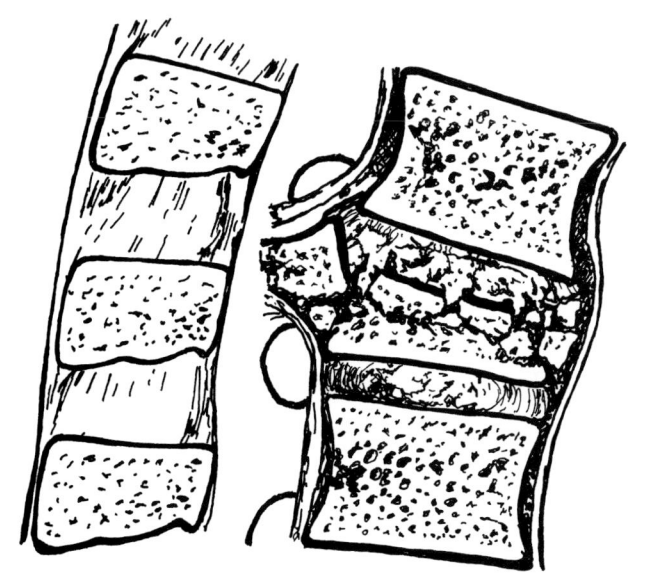

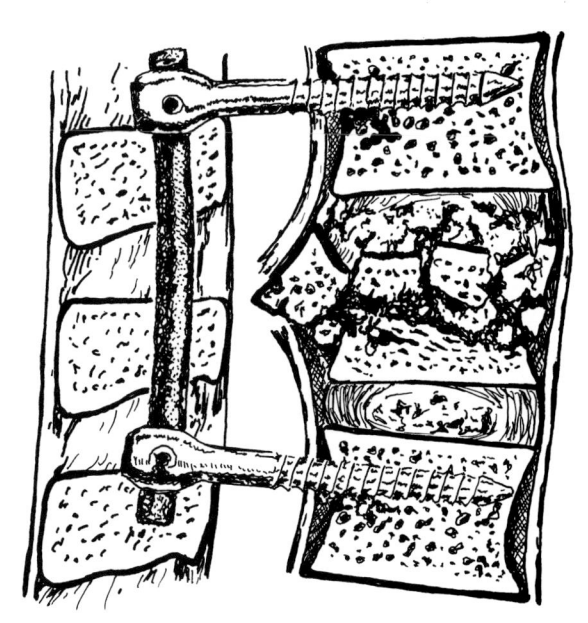

FIG. 2. A: Canal diameter is compromised more than 50%, with complete tear of the posterior longitudinal ligament (PLL). **B:** Reduction by direct decompression is advocated, using either posterolateral or anterior approach.

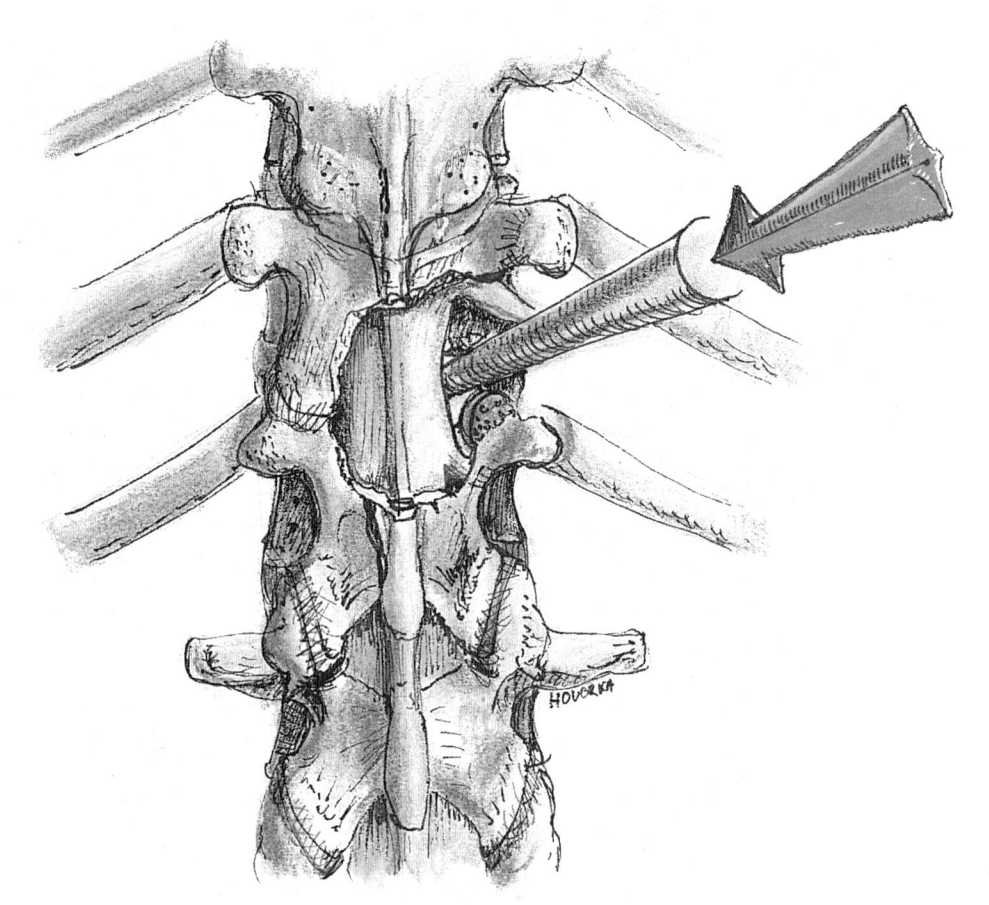

FIG. 3. Decompression at the thoracolumbar level.

access to the fragment without any manipulation of the cord (Fig. 3). The enlargement of the laminectomy is made through the articular processes, pedicles, and even the transverse processes. In subtype B, the laminectomy must be extended cranially to the vertebra above. We have found no neurologic complication related to this technique in our series (5,7) (Figs. 4 and 5).

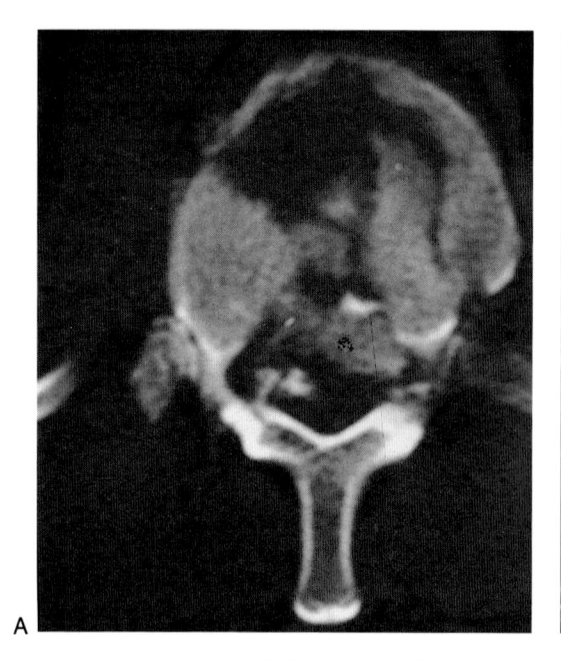

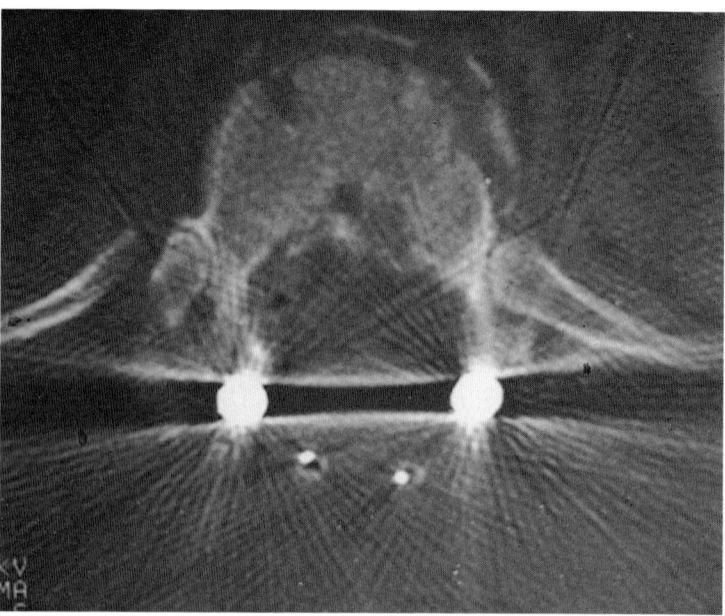

FIG. 4. A: Patient is a 50-year-old man injured in a paragliding accident. T12 burst fracture, subtype C, Frankel grade B. **B:** Posterior decompression by posterior lamino-arthrectomy, the fragments being pushed forward or removed. C-D fixation. Recovery to Frankel D.

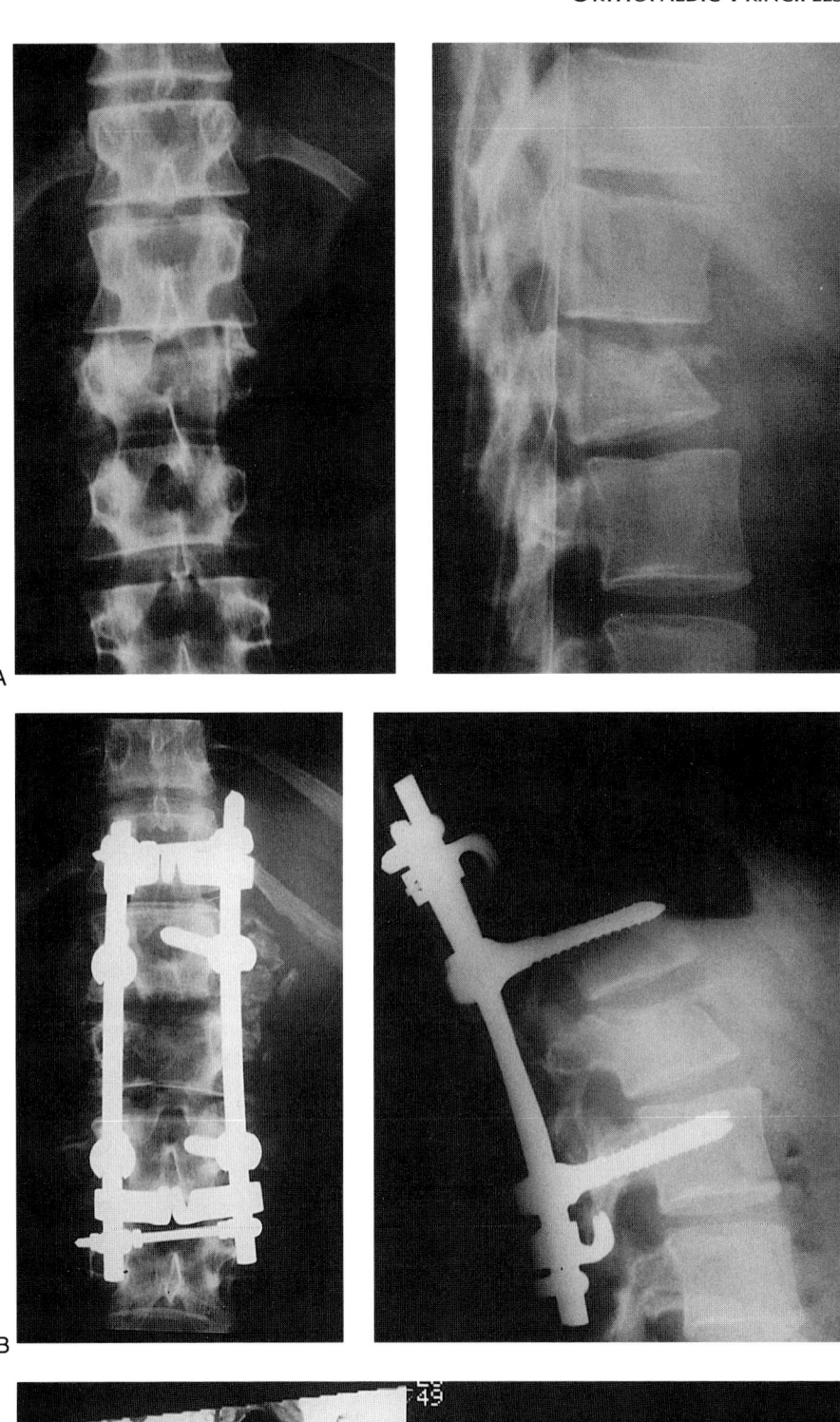

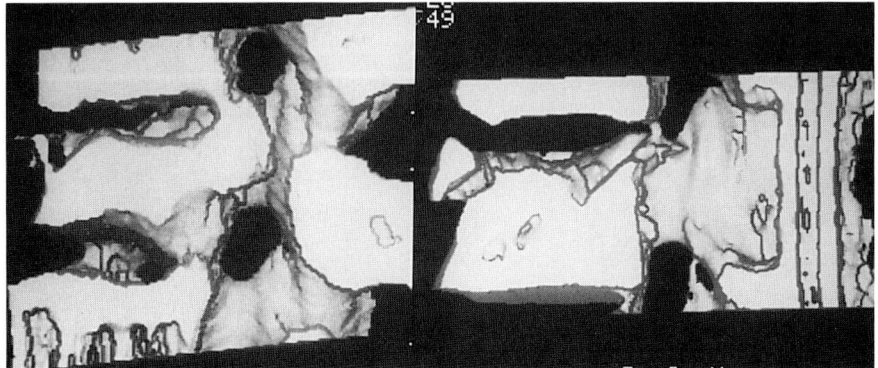

FIG. 5. A: Burst fracture, subtype C, of L2; the lesion was graded Frankel C. **B:** Posterior decompression by posterolateral approach and posterior fixation. **C:** Sagittal reconstruction after the posterosuperior fragment had been pushed forward.

Some authors have documented the amount of decompression by intraoperative myelogram or sonogram (43,49,50). The intraoperative sonogram monitoring is reported by Vincent et al. (50), who presented a series of patients treated by Benson. The retropulsed fragment in the spinal canal was monitored during distraction and fracture impaction. It resulted in a reduction of the average preoperative canal compromise from 66.5% to 18.7%, and no anterior approach was necessary (see also Chapter 9).

Without this technology, posterior decompression appeared to be less effective. Willen et al. (53) obtained reduction of canal stenosis from 45% to 26%. In our series, reduction was from 52% to 27%; two anterior approaches for further decompression were indicated.

Posterior approaches, including enlarged laminectomies, represent an important cause of destabilization of the injured spine and require fusion with corticocancellous posterolateral bone graft in addition to internal fixation. The internal fixation techniques are described in Chapter 15 according to each spine level.

Postoperative high-resolution CT scan or myelography assesses the quality of the posterior decompression, and clinical follow-up must evaluate the residual degree of stenosis. When excessive fragments or disc material is found in a patient whose neurologic status failed to improve, we advocate a second decompression by an anterior approach.

Canal occupancy of 30% at the thoracic level, 40% at the thoracolumbar level, and 50% at the lumbar level are the guidelines for second stage surgery, as per the Trafton–Boyd (49) report and our own anatomic research (see Chapter 1). The second-stage surgery will be an anterior operation to complete the decompression (Fig. 6) and is performed promptly, on an elective basis. Some authors, including Roy-Camille and Saillant (45), advocate an arteriogram to explore the blood supply left intact after the initial procedure. The second-stage surgery is performed on a patient whose stabilization has already been achieved, and whose nursing care was made easier by fixation done previously, which was secure enough to mobilize the patient in bed.

A right axillary approach, through a thoracotomy in the third intercostal space, is needed for the upper thoracic vertebrae. This provides good access to the second and third vertebral bodies. In recent fractures, we never have had an indication to split the sternum, with ligation of the brachialis venous trunk, as might be the case for late deformities in kyphosis or tumors. At the other thoracic levels, we elected a transpleural approach rather than a retropleural approach. To gain access to the thoracolumbar junction, a thoracodiaphragmatic access with retroperitoneal spine dissection was preferred. A retropleural/retroperitoneal approach, to address the first and second lumbar levels and below, is used for slender patients. This approach can be done by removing the 12th rib without transection of the diaphragm. The lumbar spine is exposed by lumbotomy (Fig. 7), and L5 exposure is made by a transperitoneal approach.

Following anterior decompression the procedure is completed by an interbody fusion with bone graft. We have opted to use an iliac tricortical graft rather than a fibula strut graft, which is used only for late kyphosis. An A-O plate with two screws in each adjacent vertebra is used to fix the construct. Anterior surgery indicated for neurologic reasons has been performed in 5% of our patient population.

The concept of spontaneous resorption of bony fragments in the canal following a burst fracture may lead to revision of our indications for decompression. Chakera et al. (14), in a study of 13 cases, were the first to call attention to spontaneous resorption. Fidler (21), Weinstein et al. (51), Edwards et al. (17), and Willen et al. (52) discussed similar cases (see Chapter 16).

We found this decrease of canal stenosis over time with three-dimensional CT reconstruction in 19 of 60 cases in which CT scans were performed before and after treatment for burst fractures. In all these cases, resorption happened when anterior bony healing, constituting spontaneous fusion, occurred in patients treated conservatively (Fig. 8) as well as in patients who had had surgical stabilization (Fig. 9). Conservative treatment, which generally cannot correct the deformity perfectly, will trigger more bone remodeling than will correction to anatomic contours. Remodeling appears to be correlated, in our study, with the amount of kyphotic deformity left after reduction and fixation. Thus only 4% of remodeling was obtained with complete deformity reduction; 41% was obtained with a residual kyphosis of 5° or more. Willen et al. (53) correlated the size of the fragments to the amount of remodeling: small fragments remodeled more quickly and completely than did large fragments. Fidler (21) speculated about bony remodeling and ventured that pulsation of neural elements within the bony canal mediated the remodeling. We favor the term "bone remodeling" to "resorption" because the same process can be seen in long bones, where large callus slowly remodels in time. Complete maturation of the healed initial injury appears to be one of the essential factors that allows bone remodeling in the direction of resorption.

Frost's theory on "adapted remodeling" (24–26) can be used to explain this phenomenon.

Text continues on page 188.

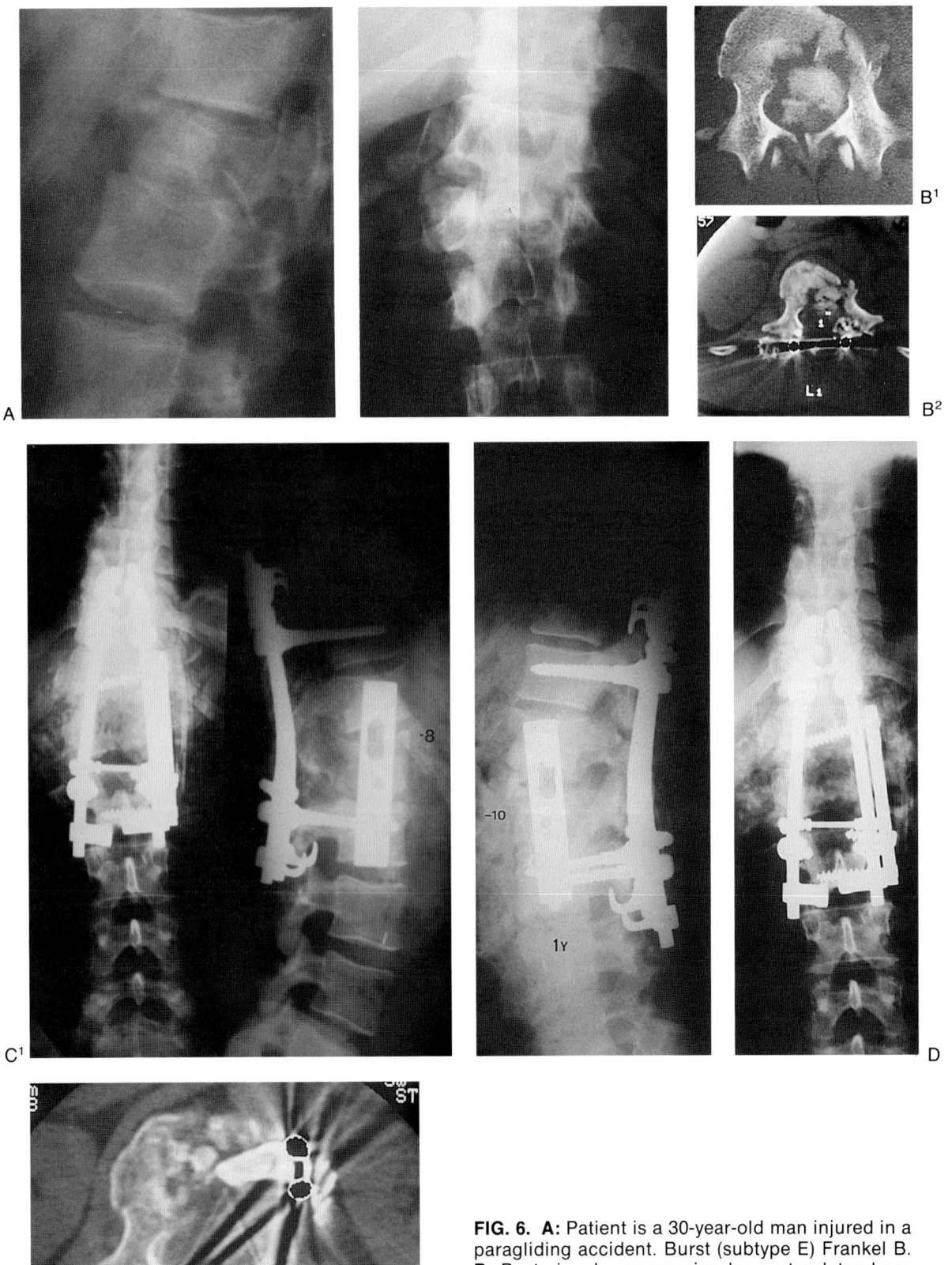

FIG. 6. A: Patient is a 30-year-old man injured in a paragliding accident. Burst (subtype E) Frankel B. **B:** Posterior decompression by posterolateral approach and removal of the fragments. Post operative canal clearance was incomplete. **C:** Complete canal clearance was gained by a second anterior stage; iliac bone graft and plate fixation. **D:** One year later—Frankel D. No loss of correction.

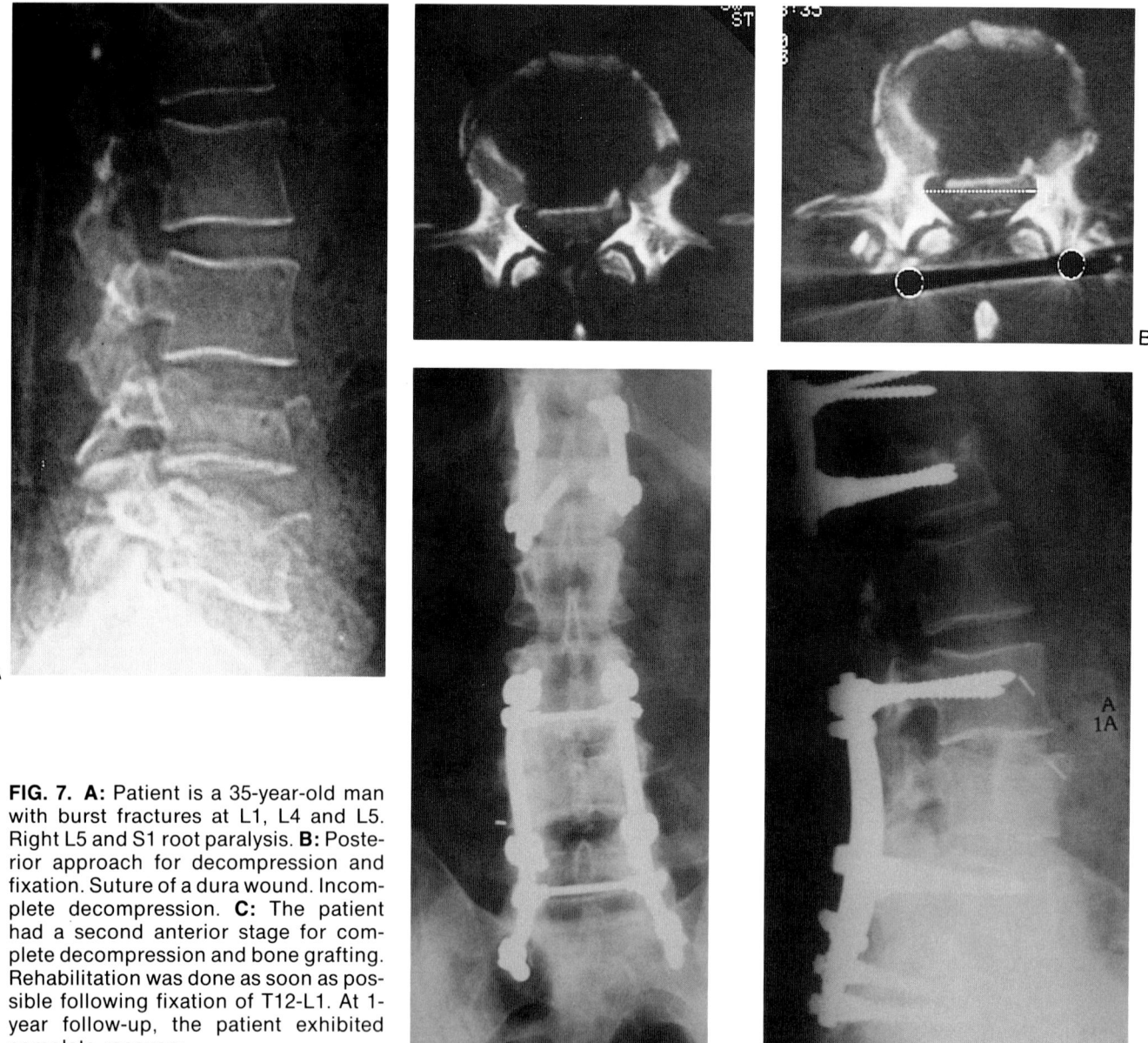

FIG. 7. A: Patient is a 35-year-old man with burst fractures at L1, L4 and L5. Right L5 and S1 root paralysis. **B:** Posterior approach for decompression and fixation. Suture of a dura wound. Incomplete decompression. **C:** The patient had a second anterior stage for complete decompression and bone grafting. Rehabilitation was done as soon as possible following fixation of T12-L1. At 1-year follow-up, the patient exhibited complete recovery.

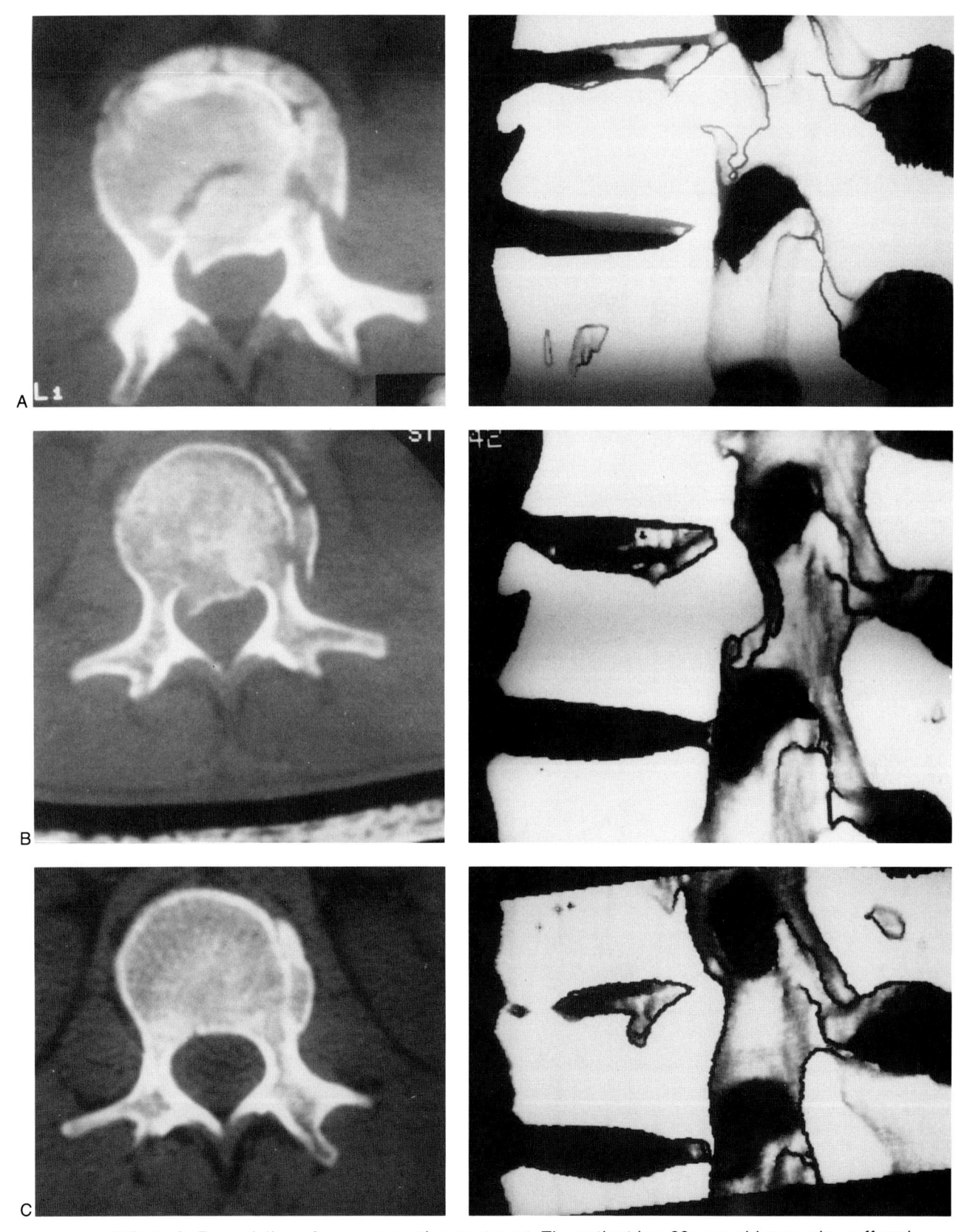

FIG. 8. A: Remodeling after conservative treatment. The patient is a 32-year-old man who suffered a burst fracture, subtype B, of L1, in a parachute jump. Neurologic grade was Frankel E. The canal diameter was initially reduced 20%. **B:** At initiation of the Boehler method, the canal diameter remained reduced by 20%. **C:** Compromised canal diameter, after follow-up of more than 1 year, was 4%.

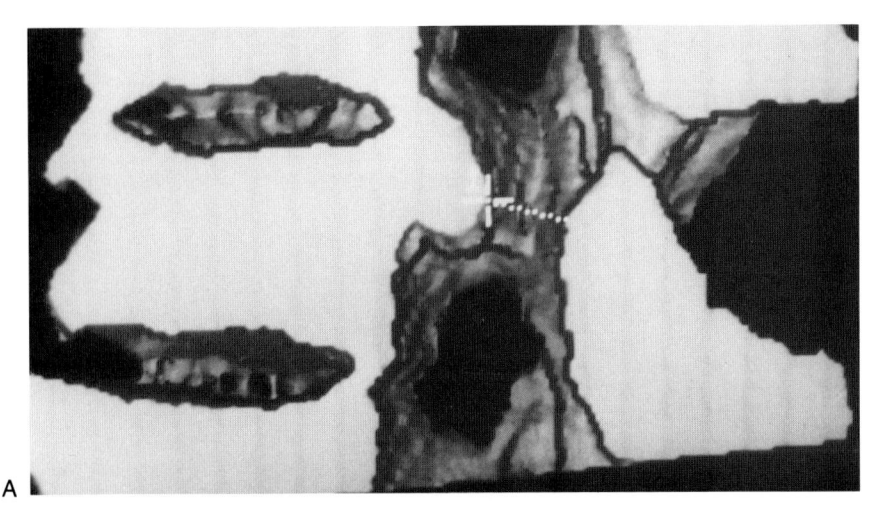

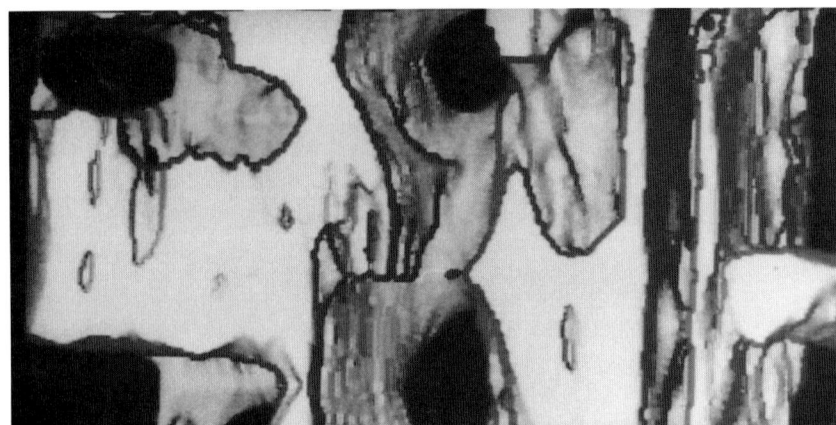

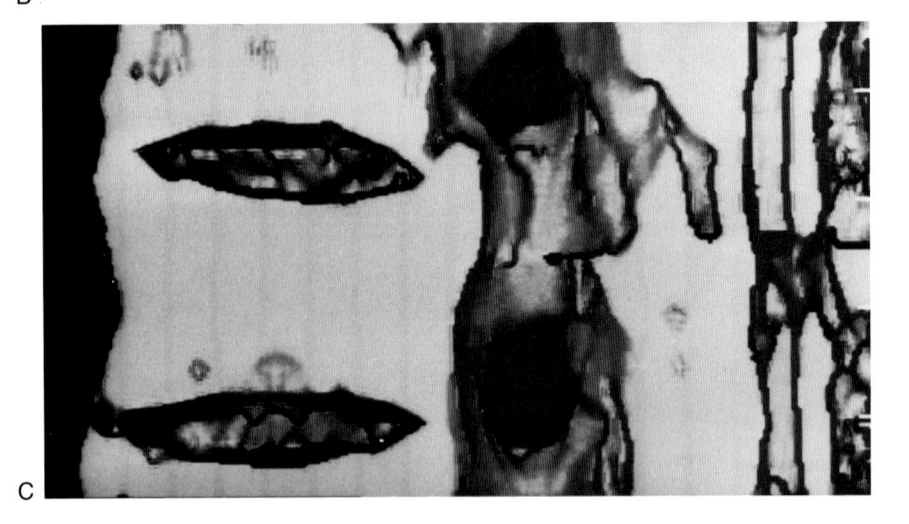

FIG. 9. Remodeling after surgical treatment. The patient is a 25-year-old man who had a T12 burst fracture, subtype B, as a result of a motorcycle accident. The patient was graded Frankel D. **A:** The initial reduction of canal diameter was 55.5%. **B:** After posterior decompression and Cotrel–Dubousset instrumentation, the reduction of the canal diameter was 42.8%. **C:** The final reduced canal diameter was 29.7%.

FRACTURES WITHOUT NEURAL COMPROMISE

The fracture type is one of the most important factors in determining the mode of management.

Compression Fractures

When the anterior height of the vertebral body is reduced by only one-third, "functional" treatment is the best choice (see above). A compression fracture that involves 50% of the anterior body height is treated by the Boehler method described earlier in the chapter. This method is most efficient at the thoracolumbar level.

There are some rare surgical indications for this type of fracture: in young patients when several vertebrae are involved at the thoracic level; when the sagittal deformity in kyphosis is greater than 15°; and/or when

50% of the anterior height of the vertebra is lost, implying a posterior ligamentous lesion.

In these cases, MRI can be used to assess the posterior injury.

Burst Fractures

Controversies in the literature abound regarding burst fracture treatment, underlining the complexity of management decision-making. As we stressed in Chapter 10, "Classification of Thoracolumbar Spine Fractures" there are stable and unstable burst fractures. For us, middle column involvement is not a formal indication for surgery. In the absence of neurologic compromise, we elect to operate on the burst fracture at the thoracolumbar level with instability as described in subtype B if more than 30% protrusion can be found inside the canal. The technique of distraction is sufficient to reduce the posterior wall of the body by ligamentotaxis up to 50% of canal diameter occupancy. Decompression by direct approach to the bone fragment through a laminectomy is performed when canal narrowing exceeds 50% and is followed by stable fixation. All other stable fractures, such as subtype A or stable subtype B, are treated by Boehler's method. However, it must be recognized that the final deformity will closely resemble the initial deformity (Fig. 10).

There are borderline cases in which both conservative treatment and surgical management may be advocated. In final decision-making, one must evaluate other factors, such as the age of the patient (i.e., the elderly patient with osteoporosis that could generate a complete vertebral collapse and in whom it is neither feasible nor acceptable to implement the Boehler technique), the noncompliant patient, or level of the spine fracture, since the Boehler technique is not very efficient at the low lumbar level.

Flexion/Distraction Fractures (Seat Belt Type)

Casts and braces are used to treat stable fractures, that is, when the fracture line is in the bony structures. In unstable lesions in which the injury involves the ligamentous elements, surgery is performed. In patients with multiple injuries, a stable, internal fixation is the best route to effective nursing and early rehabilitation. The technique used is a short compression fixation to provide stabilization.

Flexion/distraction injuries may include severe disc injury that results in neurologic deficit, as observed in one of our patients. Careful pre- and postoperative evaluation with CT scan or myelogram will avoid the need for further removal of the disc and grafting by secondary anterior approach.

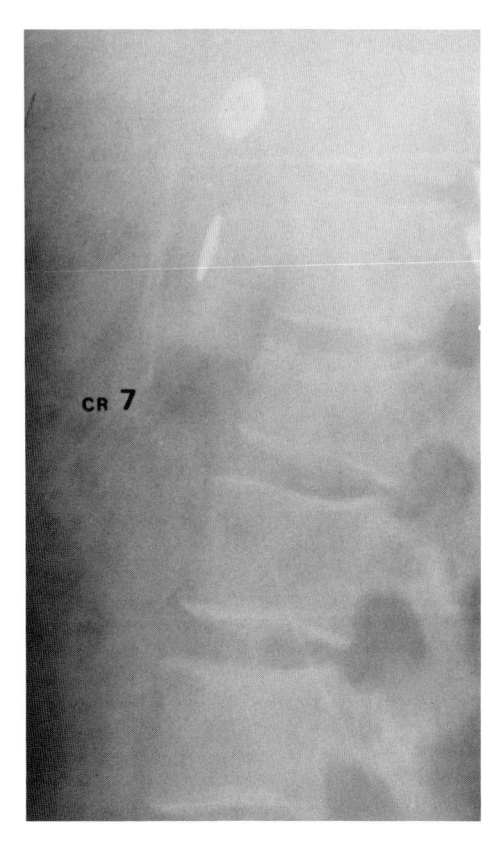

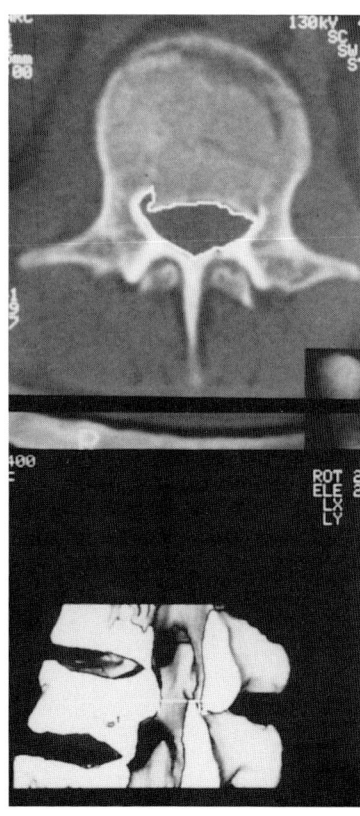

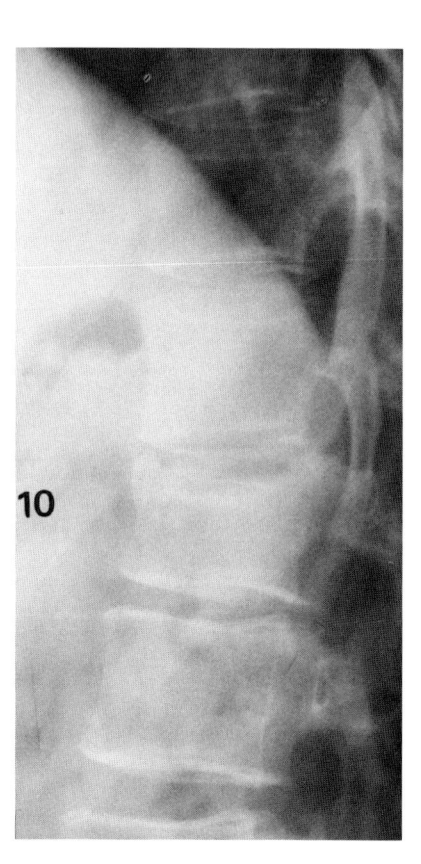

FIG. 10. Burst fracture treated by the Boehler method. Initial and final kyphotic angulation are similar.

Fracture/Dislocation

These fractures are always managed surgically, but it should be noted that caution is required when two adjacent vertebrae are injured, since it may be necessary to use a longer construct than anticipated. In two recent cases without neurologic compromise, the translation displacement was so extreme that it was reduced by progressive skeletal traction using bilateral femoral pins to obtain alignment prior to internal fixation (Fig. 11).

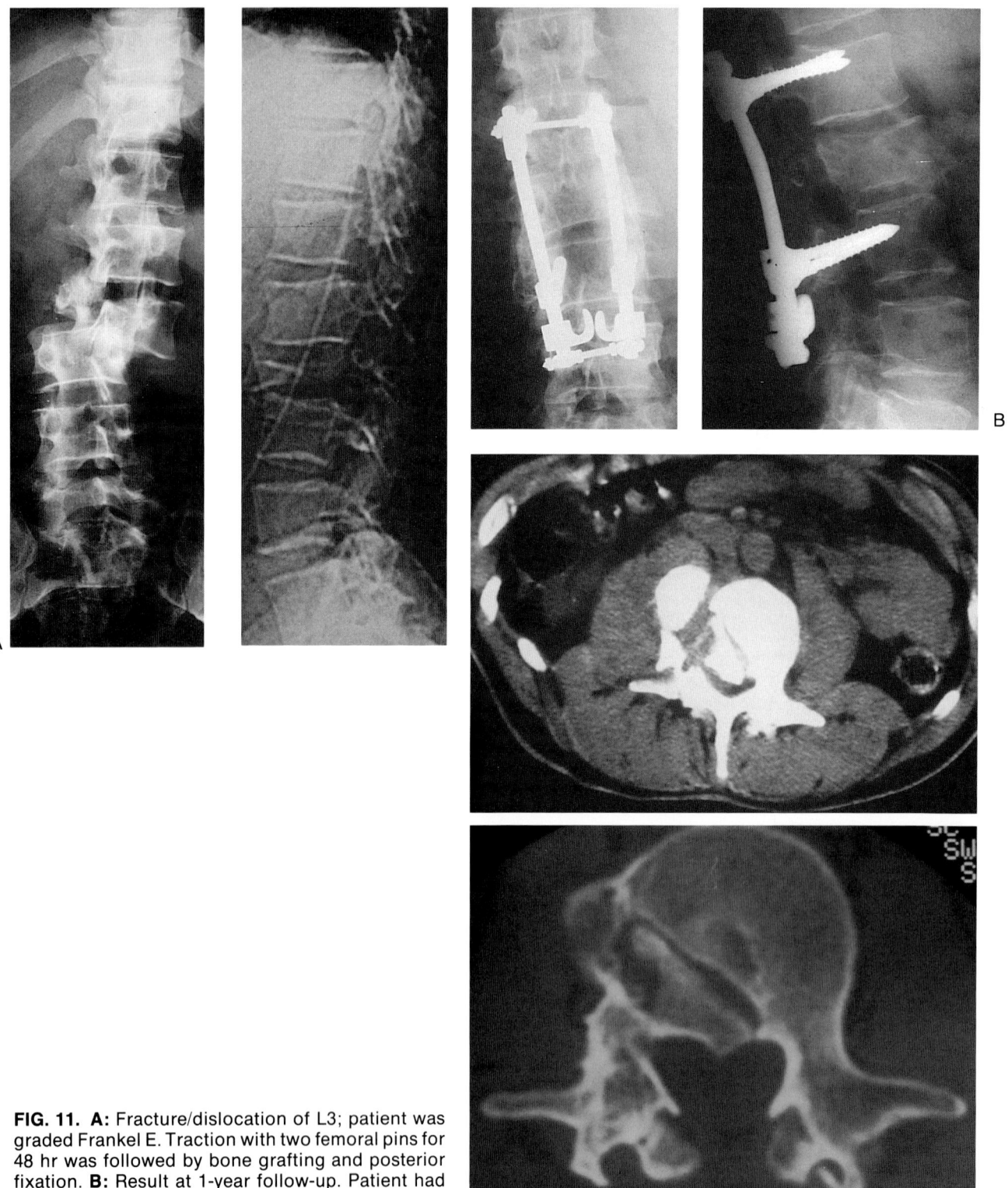

FIG. 11. A: Fracture/dislocation of L3; patient was graded Frankel E. Traction with two femoral pins for 48 hr was followed by bone grafting and posterior fixation. **B:** Result at 1-year follow-up. Patient had normal function. **C:** Preoperative and late CT scans.

RESULTS

Results can be evaluated by neurologic recovery and achievement of stable reduction.

Neurologic Evaluation

Neurologic symptoms are present in approximately 40% of thoracolumbar spine fractures and can be related to two mechanisms.

The magnitude of the initial injury is the essential cause of neural damage, on which we can have very little surgical influence; however, the consequences of the injury may be influenced pharmacologically. The second mechanism involves mechanical compression due to spinal canal narrowing, either due to malalignment or bony and disc retropulsion. These latter mechanisms can be addressed surgically. Proper radiologic evaluation, especially using CT scan, is mandatory before embarking on surgical treatment.

The issue of canal stenosis versus neurologic deficit is controversial. For Keene et al. (33,34) and other authors (8,51), there is no correlation between canal stenosis and the severity of neurologic deficit. Hashimoto et al. (30), in a study of 112 thoracolumbar burst fractures, related canal stenosis of more than 35% at the T11–T12 level, 45% at L1, and 55% lower in the lumbar spine to a significant risk of neurologic compromise. Trafton and Boyd (49), in a study of 48 cases, found that canal encroachment greater than 50% carries a risk of neurologic impairment, with a significant correlation ($\chi^2 p < 0.07$).

In our study of 60 patients, we also have found that a canal stenosis ranging from 41% to 52% at the level of the thoracolumbar junction had a significant correlation with neurologic deficit. Quantifying canal occupancy in terms of surface rather than diameter is more accurate in predicting neurologic impairment (0.0048 > 0.025).

There is now a general consensus that decompression provides the best environment for recovery of the nervous tissue (3). Decompression of the spinal canal is better performed by surgical means than by conservative measures, as reported by Jacobs and Casey (31) and Gertzbein and co-workers (27,28).

Kaneda et al. (32) reported that anterior decompression achieved 92% neurologic improvement in 67% of patients with incomplete paralysis; Kostuik (35–37) obtained a similar success rate. It appears that, from the anatomic point of view, anterior decompression is more complete in achievement of canal clearance (6% residual stenosis as opposed to 26% residual stenosis by posterior approach) (28). However, the clinical results are somewhat similar in both approaches (18,29). Since it is impossible to have a prospective double-blind study to compare posterior distraction alone, distraction and posterior decompression, and anterior decompression plus posterior or anterior instrumentation, it would be interesting to obtain multicenter participation in a study employing specific protocol management. It is our opinion that a better evaluation of the neurologic deficit is obtained by the use of the motor index score (M.I.S.) than by grading according to Frankel grades. When a patient is entered as Frankel C or D, we used the M.I.S., which provided an initial numeric value.

Decompression of neural tissue, either the cord, conus, or roots, may be efficient even if performed after considerable delay (10,37–39,41). In one series, McAfee et al. (40) obtained 70% improvement after 2 months; Kostuik and Matsusaki (37) claimed improvement in all their patients, even in those treated late. In our experience with anterior decompression for late neurologic deficits, the results were identical.

Functional Results

We were disappointed with our conservative treatment results, including reduction and Boehler cast, because satisfactory results were not always obtained. With this type of treatment, we have encountered a 20% failure rate, manifested by pain and stiffness.

The relationship between residual kyphosis and functional results has been related by different authors with different perspectives. Albassir (2) reviewed 100 patients treated conservatively in the same manner. He found that 47% had "painful stiffness" and 19% had progressive kyphosis over a 5-year follow-up. Soreff et al. (48) reviewed 147 patients with 8 to 20 years follow-up; they found no more than 30% who were asymptomatic and, in 40%, they found an increased kyphosis. Nicoll (42) found 73% good results at 7 years after injury and 34% with progressive kyphosis. His series consisted of a group of young individuals who were miners. He, as well as Weinstein et al. (51), found no correlation between residual kyphosis and back pain. For other authors (17,27,28,54), there is a direct relationship between the degree of late kyphosis and the functional result.

The explanations for late pain may be stretching of the posterior muscles, disc degeneration at the level of

TABLE 1. *Muscle force necessary to compensate for a kyphotic deformity according to the injured level*

Level	Kyphosis angle	Force (kg)
L2	15°	160
L2	45°	379
L4	15°	355
L4	45°	476

From ref. 22.

the injury, and compensatory hyperlordosis below the lesion. Table 1 shows that hypolordosis is associated with increased muscle exertion (22).

Numerous unsatisfactory results observed after in situ arthrodesis in cases of post-traumatic kyphosis confirm the necessity to restore the sagittal contour. Kostuik and Matsusaki (37) related a case report that illustrates this concept. A 34-year-old woman sustained a burst fracture of L1 and, 3 years after injury, underwent posterior fusion; the pain remained the same. She had surgical reexploration 7 years after injury, and the fusion was found to be solid. She then underwent anterior release and decompression over four levels; her kyphosis was reduced from 64° to 24°, with total relief of her back pain. In our own experience of 44 cases who underwent surgical correction (4), painful late deformities were related to a scoliosis of 15° or a kyphosis of 20° or more at the level of the thoracolumbar junction (Fig. 12).

C-D instrumentation (19), which we have used since 1986, provides a stable construct and results in a pain-free patient who can participate in early physical therapy. We were surprised by the magnitude of the patients' activity due to lack of pain, and we are now obliged to tell patients that they must delay strenuous activity until fracture healing has occurred.

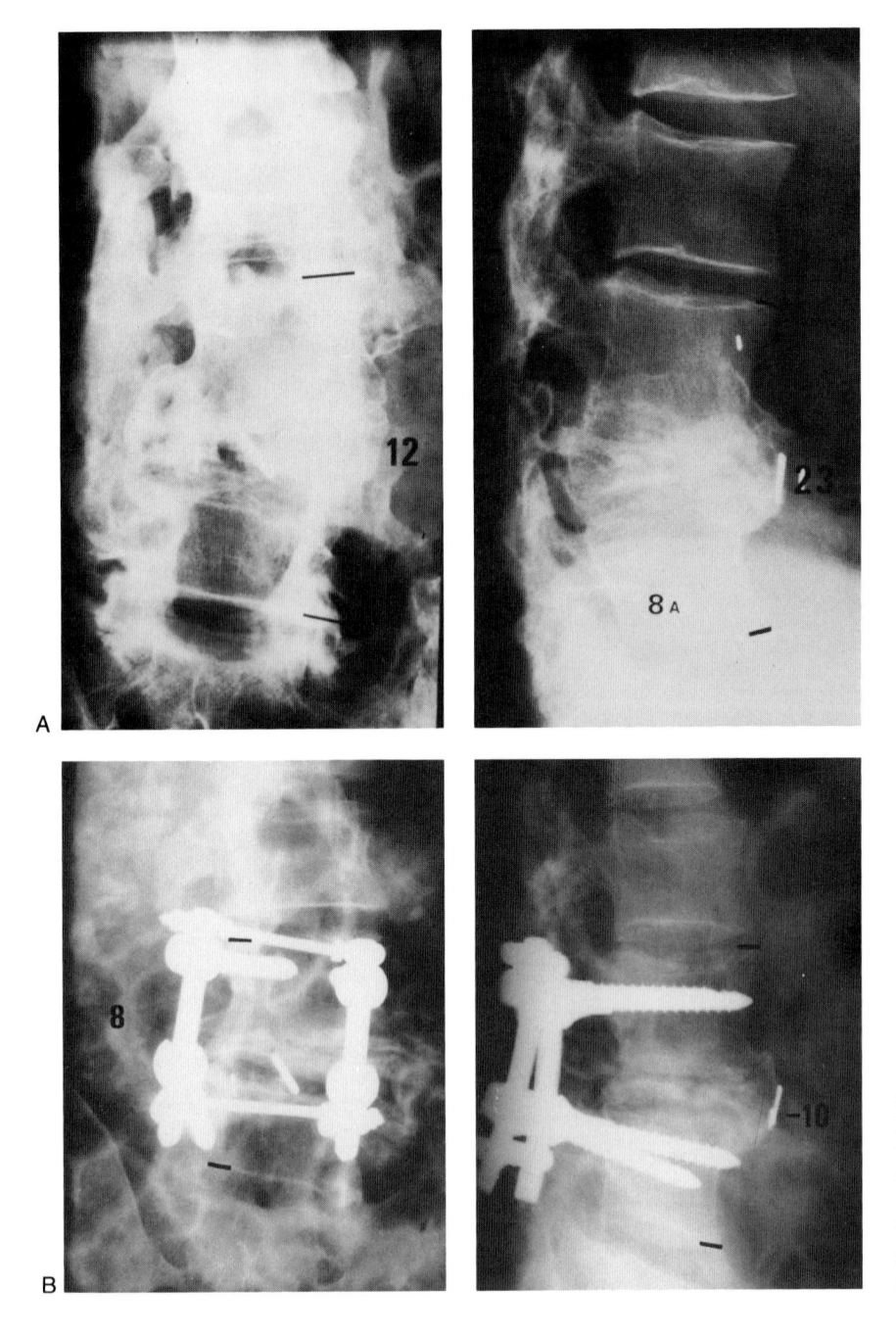

FIG. 12. A: The patient complains of low back pain and radiculopathy due to post-traumatic lumbar kyphosis. The patient was anteriorly decompressed and fused. **B:** Wedge posterior closed osteotomy fixed by C-D instrumentation in compression. Patient had relief of pain and sciatica.

Long-term good results seem to correlate with restoration of normal anatomic contour of the spine, mainly in the sagittal plane at the lumbar level. We contend that restoration of the anatomic contour is essential and can be provided by appropriate contour of the hardware. This contour must be appropriate for each different spinal level, as described in the Sagittal Index (20) (see Chapter 31).

Under these conditions, data on surgical results show more than 80% excellent (return to sports) or good results. A generalized decrease in labor compensation time was demonstrated by a study we conducted with insurance companies. A study with long-term follow-up must be documented.

Aggressive early decompression, with solid fixation that will promote good arthrodesis, has improved the neurologic recovery of patients with incomplete nerve compromise following spine fracture. Patients who are neurologically intact will present a better long-term result because of the restoration of the anatomic contour of the spine.

REFERENCES

1. Aebi M, Etter C, Kehl T, et al. The internal skeletal fixation system. A new treatment of thoracolumbar fractures and the other spinal disorders. *Clin Orthop* 1988;227:30–43.
2. Albassir A. Fractures du rachis dorsal et lombaire sans troubles neurologiques. *Acta Orthop Belg* 1979;45:509–520.
3. Anderson PA, Krengel WF, Henley MB. Neurologic recovery in patients with incomplete paraplegia due to thoracic level spinal cord injury. Fifty-Seventh Annual Meeting, American Academy of Orthopaedic Surgeons, New Orleans, Louisiana, February 8–13, 1990.
4. Argenson C. Cals vicieux et pseudarthroses du rachis thoracolombaire. In: *Cahiers d'Enseignement de la SOFCOT*. Paris: Expansion Scientifique Francaise, 1990;205–236.
5. Argenson C. Traitement des fractures du rachis dorso-lombaire chez l'adulte. In: *Cahiers d'Enseignement de la SOFCOT*. Paris: Expansion Scientifique Francaise, 1984;5–27.
6. Argenson C, Boileau P, de Peretti F, Lovet J, Dalzotto H. Fractures of the thoracic spine (T1–T10). A review of 105 cases. *Fr J Orthop Surg* 1989;3(3):238–254.
7. Argenson C, Lovet J, dePeretti F, Cambas PM, Griffet J, Boileau P. Treatment of spinal fractures with C-D instrumentation: results of 85 cases. SRS-ESDS Combined Meeting, Amsterdam, Holland, September 17–22, 1989.
8. Bedbrook GM. Spinal injuries with tetraplegia and paraplegia. *J Bone Joint Surg* 1979;61B:267–284.
9. Boehler L. *Technique de traitement des fractures de la colonne dorsale et lombaire* (translated by M Boppe). Paris: Masson, 1944;149.
10. Bohlman HH. Late progressive paralysis and pain following fractures of the thoracolumbar spine. *J Bone Joint Surg* 1976; 58A:728.
11. Bohlman HH, Eismont FS. Surgical technique of anterior decompression and fusion for spinal cord injuries. *Clin Orthop* 1987;154:57–67.
12. Bracken MB, et al. A randomized, controlled trial of methylprednisolone or naloxone in the treatment of acute spinal cord injury. *N Engl J Med* 1990;20:1405–1411.
13. Bradford DS, McBride GG. Surgical management of thoracolumbar spine fracture with incomplete neurologic deficits. *Clin Orthop* 1987;218:201–216.
14. Chakera TM, Bedbrook G, Bradley CM. Spontaneous resolution of spinal canal deformity after burst dispersion fracture. *AJNR* 1988;9:779–785.
15. Crutcher JP, Anderson PA, King KA, Montesano PX. Indirect spinal canal decompression in patients with thoracolumbar burst fractures treated by posterior distraction rods. *J Spinal Disord* 1991;1:30–48.
16. Denis F, Armstrong GWD, Matta L. Acute thoracolumbar burst fractures in the absence of neurologic deficit. A comparison between operative and nonoperative treatment. *Clin Orthop* 1984; 189:142–149.
17. Edwards CC, Rosenthal MS, Fouad G, Levine AM. The fate of retropulsed bone following thoracolumbar burst fractures: late stenosis or resorption? *Orthop Trans* 1989;13:119.
18. Esses SI, Botsford JD, Kostuik JP. Evaluation of surgical treatment for burst fractures. *Spine* 1990;15:667–673.
19. Farcy JPC, Weidenbaum M. A preliminary review of the use of Cotrel–Dubousset instrumentation for spinal injuries. *Bull Hosp Jt Dis Orthop Inst* 1988;48:1.
20. Farcy JPC, Weidenbaum M, Glassman SD. Sagittal index in management of thoracolumbar burst fractures. *Spine* 1990;15(9): 958–965.
21. Fidler MW. Remodeling of the spinal cord after burst fracture. *J Bone Joint Surg* 1988;70B:730–732.
22. Fourrier P, Bert G. Evaluation de la compensation lombaire des tassements rachidiens par fracture. *Rev Chir Orthop* 1972;58(2): 131–136.
23. Fredrickson BE, Mann KA, Yuan HA, Lubicky JP. Reduction of the intracanal fragment in experimental burst fractures. *Spine* 1988;13:267–271.
24. Frost HM. A determinant of bone architecture: the minimum effective strain. *Clin Orthop* 1983;175:286–292.
25. Frost HM. Mechanical determinants of bone modeling. *Metab Bone Dis Rel Res* 1982;4:217–229.
26. Frost HM. The mechanostat: a proposed pathogenic mechanism of osteoporoses and the bone mass effects of mechanical and nonmechanical agents. *Bone Miner* 1987;2:73–85.
27. Gertzbein SD, Court-Brown CM. Flexion/distraction injury of the lumbar spine: mechanism of injury and classification. *Clin Orthop* 1988;227:52.
28. Gertzbein SD, Court-Brown CM, Marks P, et al. The neurologic outcome following surgery for spinal fractures. *Spine* 1988;13: 641–644.
29. Gertzbein SD, McMichael D, Tile M. Harrington instrumentation as a method of fixation in fractures of the spine: a critical analysis of deficiencies. *J Bone Joint Surg* 1977;64B:745.
30. Hashimoto T, Kaneda K, Abumi K. Relationship between traumatic spinal canal stenosis and neurologic deficits in thoracolumbar burst fractures. *Spine* 1988;13:1268–1272.
31. Jacobs RR, Casey MP. Surgical management of thoracolumbar spinal injuries. *Clin Orthop* 1984;189:22–35.
32. Kaneda K, Abumi K, Fujiya M. Burst fractures with neurologic deficits of the thoracolumbar spine. *Spine* 1984;9:788–795.
33. Keene JS, Fischer SP, Vanderby R, Drummond DS, Turski PA. Significance of acute post traumatic bony encroachment of the neural canal. *Spine* 1989;14:799–802.
34. Keene JS, Wackwitz DL, Drummond DS, Breed AL. Compression–distraction instrumentation of unstable thoracolumbar fractures: anatomic results obtained with each type of injury and method of instrumentation. *Spine* 1986;11(9):895–902.
35. Kostuik JP. Anterior fixation for fractures of the thoracic and lumbar spine with or without neurologic involvement. *Clin Orthop* 1984;189:103–115.
36. Kostuik JP. Anterior spinal cord decompression for lesions of the thoracic and lumbar spine, techniques, new methods of internal fixation, results. *Spine* 1983;8(5):512–531.
37. Kostuik JP, Matsusaki H. Anterior stabilization instrumentation and decompression for post traumatic kyphosis. *Spine* 1989; 14(4):379–396.
38. Maiman DJ, Larson SJ, Benzel EC. Neurological improvement associated with late decompression of the thoracolumbar spinal cord. *Neurosurgery* 1984;143:302–307.
39. Malcolm BW, Bradford DS, Winter RB, Chou SN. Post traumatic kyphosis. A review of forty-eight surgically treated patients. *J Bone Joint Surg* 1981;63A(6):891–899.
40. McAfee PC, Yuan HA, Fredrickson BE, Lubicky JP. The value of computed tomography in thoracolumbar fractures. *J Bone Joint Surg* 1983;65A:461–473.

41. McBride GG, Bradford DS. Vertebral body replacement with femoral neck allograft and vascularized rib strut graft. A technique for treating post traumatic kyphosis with neurologic deficit. *Spine* 1983;8(4):406–415.
42. Nicoll EA. Fractures of the dorsolumbar spine. *J Bone Joint Surg* 1949;31B(3):376–394.
43. Quencer RM, Montalvo BM, Eismont FJ, et al. Intraoperative spinal sonography in thoracic and lumbar fractures. Evolution of Harrington rod instrumentation. *Am J Neuroradiol* 1985;6:353–359.
44. Roy-Camille R, Saillant G. Rachis dorsolombaire traumatique non neurologique. In: *2es Journées d'Orthopédie de la Pitié*. Paris: Masson, 1980.
45. Roy-Camille R, Saillant G. Rachis traumatique neurologique. In: *3es Journées d'Orthopédie de la Pitié*. Paris: Masson, 1983.
46. Roy-Camille R, Saillant G, Mazel C. Internal fixation of the lumbar spine with pedicle screw plating. *Clin Orthop* 1986;203:7–17.
47. Shuman WP, Rogers JV, Sickler ME, Hanson JA, Crutcher JP, King HA, Mack LA. Thoracolumbar burst fractures: CT dimension of the spinal canal relative to post surgical improvement. *AJR* 1985;145:337–341.
48. Soreff J, Exdorph G, Bylund P, Odeen I, Olerud S. Treatment of patients with unstable fractures of the thoracic and lumbar spine: a follow up study of surgical and conservative treatment. *Orthop Scand* 1982;53:369–381.
49. Trafton PG, Boyd CA. Computed tomography of thoracic and lumbar spine injuries. *J Trauma* 1984;24(6):506–515.
50. Vincent KA, Benson DR, McGahan JP. Intraoperative ultrasonography for reduction of thoracolumbar burst fractures. *Spine* 1989;4:387–390.
51. Weinstein JN, Collalto P, Lehmann TR. Thoracolumbar "burst" fractures treated conservatively: long term follow up. *Spine* 1988;13:33–38.
52. Willen J, Anderson J, Toomoka K, Singer K. The natural history of burst fractures of the thoracolumbar junction. *J Spinal Disord* 1990;7:39–45.
53. Willen JAC, Greakwad VH, Kakulas BA. Burst fractures in the thoracic and lumbar spine. A clinico-neuropathologic analysis. *Spine* 1989;14(12):1316–1323.
54. Willen J, Lindahl S, Nordwall A. Unstable thoracolumbar fractures. A comparative clinical study of conservative treatment and Harrington instrumentation. *Spine* 1985;10(7):111–122.

15

Specific Injuries and Management

Claude Argenson and Pascal Boileau

Management of thoracolumbar fractures requires knowledge of three different areas with regard to both anatomic and functional characteristics and the resultant impact on neurologic outcome:

Thoracic, from T1 to T10
Thoracolumbar, from T11 to T12, L1 and L2
Lumbar, from the L2–L3 disc to L5

THORACIC LEVEL

This corresponds to the vertebrae that constitute the thoracic "cage" or thoracic "cylinder," which is formed by the sternum and the 10 pairs of ribs laterally. T11 and T12 are not included in the cylinder. The normal sagittal contour of the thoracic spine is 25° to 50° of kyphosis.

The thoracic vertebra is characterized by: a body that has a transverse diameter equal to that of the anteroposterior diameter; a narrow, circular vertebral canal; thin pedicles; bulky transverse processes; and, above all, articular processes in the frontal plane. This composite structure allows wide mobility in flexion, extension, and rotation, which are partially limited by the thoracic cage.

The thoracic cage's rigidity explains the high energy that is necessary to cause displaced fractures and associated lesions, such as multiple level fractures (30%), chest wall injuries (27%), or intrathoracic injuries (32%). There is a high rate, up to 30%, of neurologic involvement associated with thoracic spine injuries (9). Complete paraplegia results in 20% of these cases.

Lesions and Their Mechanisms

A retrospective study of 105 patients presenting with one or more fractures of the thoracic spine was conducted in the Orthopaedic and Trauma Department of Nice University Hospital from October 1978 to July 1987 (4). The patients' ages ranged from 15 to 90 (average 38). The fractures were classified according to Denis's classification (15); bony lesions were more common than ligamentous injuries. Five cases of fracture/dislocation failed to fit into any Denis classification subtype. They were called "fracture/dislocations due to an oblique shear force." There is a peak incidence at the apex of the thoracic kyphosis, T6, T7, and T8. The distribution of the different fractures is summarized in Fig. 1.

Mechanism and Description of Injury

Compression fractures (type I) (54.2%) were usually due to a fall from a moderate height.

Burst fractures (type II) (20%) were more often due to axial injury, shown by their prevalence in falls from a great height. They were frequently associated with head injuries (one-half of the cases) and injury to one or both shoulder girdles (one-third). In our series, burst fractures were not uncommon (20%), as opposed to Eskay's series (18,24). The occurrence of a compression lesion of the middle column is not precluded by the natural kyphosis (47) because the vertebrae are fixed by the thoracic ribs and bear the applied load

---

C. Argenson: Department of Orthopaedic Surgery, Service de Chirurgie Orthopedique et Traumatologique, Centre Hospitalier Regional et Universitaire de Nice, St. Roch University Hospital, 06000 Nice, France.
P. Boileau: Department of Orthopaedic Surgery, St. Roch University Hospital, 06000 Nice, France

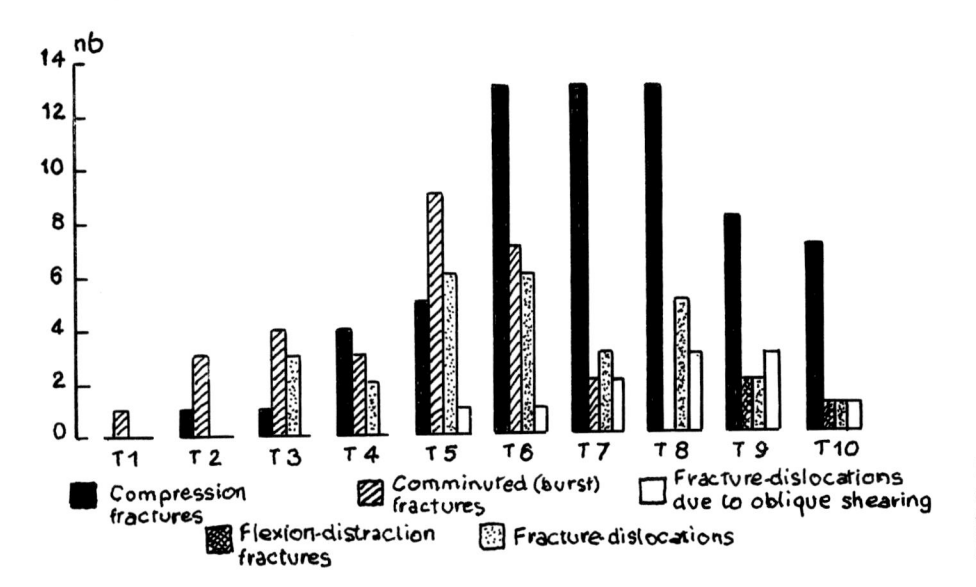

FIG. 1. Localization of fractures of the thoracic spine according to type (taking into account multilevel fractures).

through the apex of the thorax and the shoulder girdle (Fig. 2). Burst fractures were subtype A or B and were associated with neurologic deficit related to a bony fragment of the middle column, clearly displaced into the spinal canal on CT scan.

Seat belt fractures (type III) are uncommon at the thoracic level. They are seen mainly at the thoracolumbar junction. Denis and Eskay reported no cases in their series; three of our cases corresponded to flexion/distraction fractures. All three were located at the T9–T10 level, which is close to the thoracolumbar junction (Fig. 3). We must stress the value of tomography or sagittal CT reconstruction when treating this type of fracture.

The frequency of *fracture/dislocations* (type IV) already has been mentioned by Roy-Camille and Saillant (43) attesting to the inadequacy of the protection afforded by the ribs. They are caused by a variety of injuries, always of great severity; 83% presented with multiple injuries. Associated chest injuries (50% of cases) were frequent and related to horizontal and tangential shear to the rib cage (Fig. 4). The most common lesion was in flexion and rotation (subtype A, through the bone). Eskay and Hanley (18,24) considered that thoracic fracture/dislocations are due mainly to anteroposterior shear forces caused by a direct blow. The intact rib cage and sternum limit rotation of the spine. When the ribs or sternum are fractured, there no longer is any structure that can protect the thoracic spine from shear forces. This explains the frequency of flexion/rotation injury at this level, favored by the parallel and semicircular orientation of the posterior facet joints (28,32). This lesion, which involves the three-columns of the spine, is highly unstable.

Five of our cases of fracture/dislocation would not fit into Denis' subtypes and were designated as "oblique shear." (See Chapter 10.)

Associated Lesions

Hemomediastinum

Twenty percent of the patients had an abnormal appearance of the mediastinum in the chest radiographs,

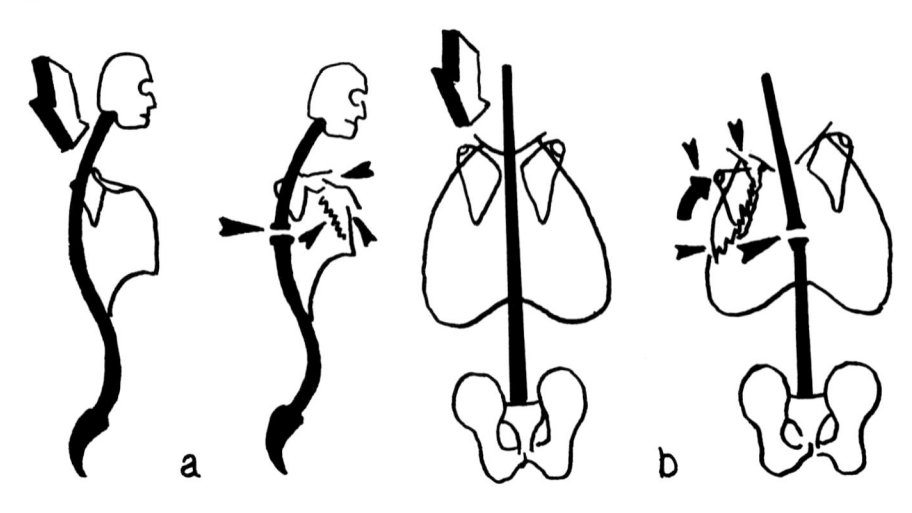

FIG. 2. Burst fracture. **a:** Direct blow on summit of thorax. **b:** Direct blow on the shoulder.

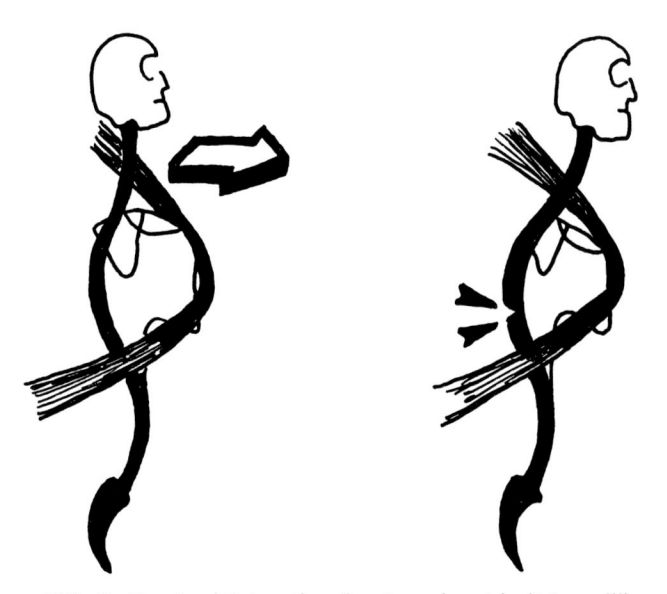

FIG. 3. Flexion/distraction fracture (seat belt type III).

suggestive of a posterior mediastinal blood effusion. Mediastinal blood effusions can exist in the absence of fracture of the ribs or sternum, thereby confirming their origin in fracture hematomas of the spine. These hematomas diffuse rapidly along the anterior longitudinal ligament to form a true hemomediastinum, which can, in turn, diffuse to the chest and present as an hemothorax (43). The diagnosis is made by unusual mediastinal appearance in the posteroanterior (PA) chest roentgenogram. A tapered image centered on the lesion creates a double contour with the aortic shadow, particularly clear in fractures of the upper thoracic spine. They are rather comparable to those described in abscesses. Even though the appearance is not as well defined, the shadow is still rounded, with hazy margins. Only tomograms can show the relationship with the fractured vertebrae. Magnetic resonance imaging (MRI), when possible, or even computerized tomography (CT) scan will document it.

Massive mediastinal effusion due to rupture of one of the great vessels is of great concern. This led us, in two cases, to perform emergency angiography, which was negative. A review of the literature confirmed that the combination of a fracture of the thoracic spine with a rupture of the aorta is rare. Meinecke (34) found only four aortic ruptures in 340 thoracic paraplegias; Roy-Camille and Saillant (43), in 41 fractures of the thoracic spine, described one case of aortic damage found at autopsy. Eskay and Hanley (18,24) found no cases, and Motin et al. (36), in a series of 36 thoracic aorta ruptures, found that only 3% were associated with spine fractures. Nevertheless, the possibility of a ruptured aorta should be considered in all fractures of the thoracic spine and should lead to a search for significant clinical and radiologic signs: a difference in blood pressure in the upper and lower limbs, a left hemothorax, poor visualization of the aortic shadow, deviation of the trachea to the right, and downward displacement of the left bronchus (36). A CT scan usually shows the aorta enlargement.

Hemothorax

Hemothorax, or hemopneumothorax, was also a frequent complication of fractures of the thoracic spine, although the incidence in our series (19%) was some-

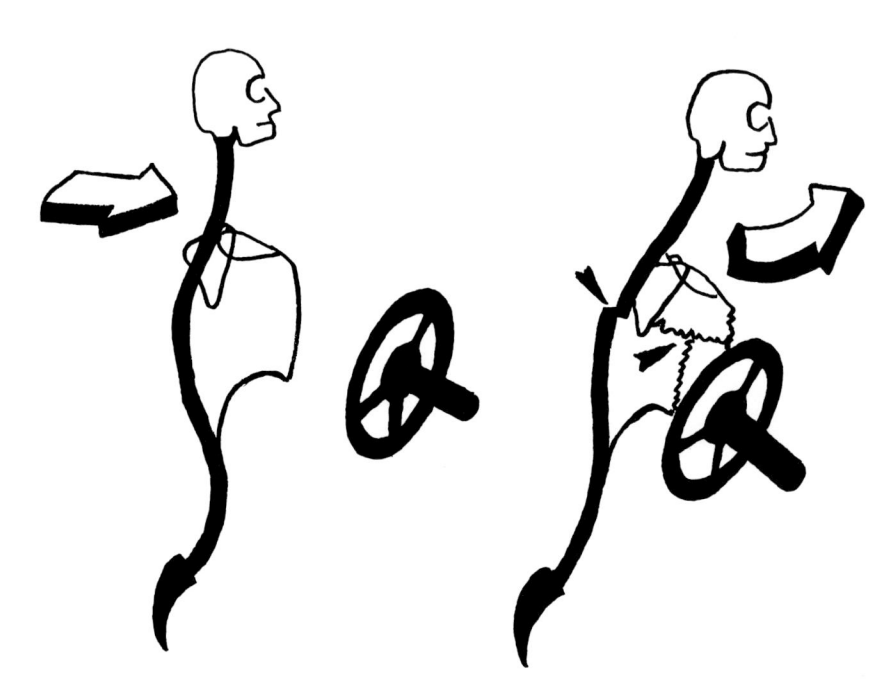

FIG. 4. Flexion/rotation fracture/dislocation through the disc (type IV-B).

what less than reported in the literature: 30% in the series of Schulte et al. (45). There are several mechanisms for hemothorax: in 13 cases, it was due to a chest wall fracture (multiple rib fractures, fractures of the clavicle, fractures of the scapula) causing damage to the intercostal, mammary, or pulmonary vessels. In seven cases, it was due to the fracture of the thoracic spine itself, either because there were no fractured ribs (six cases) or because unilateral fractures of the ribs were associated with a contralateral hemothorax (one case). The passage of blood into the pleura probably occurs, as in hemomediastinum, by diffusion of the fracture hematoma along the anterior longitudinal ligament and the mediastinal pleura, or directly if the ligament is penetrated by splinters of bone.

Pericardial Effusion

We have seen five cases of an enlarged heart in radiographs taken immediately after injury. Our five cases were associated with fractures of the lower part of the thoracic spine (T8–T9). We believe this condition is due to perforation of the pericardium by bone splinters and fracture hematoma. In our series, these hemopericardia had little clinical significance. Roy-Camille and Saillant (43) reported one death due to cardiac tamponade, and one patient who needed emergency aspiration. We have never seen signs of pericarditis, pericardial rupture, myocardial contusion, or necrosis or ruptured valves as described by other authors (50).

Hemopneumomediastinum

The presence of air in the mediastinum suggested a tracheobronchial or esophageal rupture in two of our patients. However, this was ruled out by esophagoscopy and bronchoscopy.

Neurologic Status

The susceptibility to neural damage in fractures of the thoracic spine was confirmed in our own series: neurologic impairment was present in 30% (52% of Eskay's cases). Paraplegia was more often complete (62%) than incomplete (38%). The lesions were usually severe because of the narrowness of the spinal canal, the precariousness of the blood supply, and the limited mobility of the spinal canal at this level (32). A study of the correlation with the anatomic type of fracture clearly showed that fracture/dislocations were the most frequent cause of complete paraplegia (13 of our 20 cases). However, the neural damage was associated with comminuted (burst) fractures in five cases. Apart from the anatomic factors already mentioned, the damaging role of the thoracic cage needs to be considered.

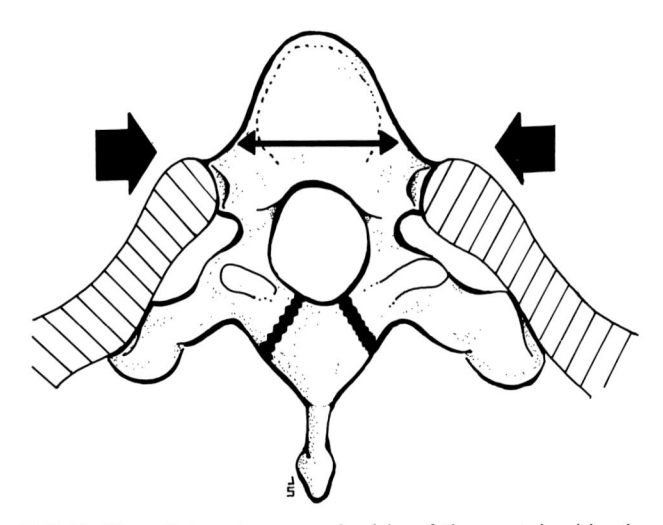

FIG. 5. The rib heads on each side of the vertebral body act like a vice and expel the fragments into the sagittal plane.

The rib heads on each side of the vertebral body act like a vice on each side of the thoracic vertebrae and forcefully expel the fragments into the sagittal plane (Fig. 5). This is facilitated by the thoracic kyphosis (Fig. 6). Paradoxically, a certain number of fracture/dislocations, particularly those due to "oblique shear," do not show any neurologic signs; no neurologic deficits were found.

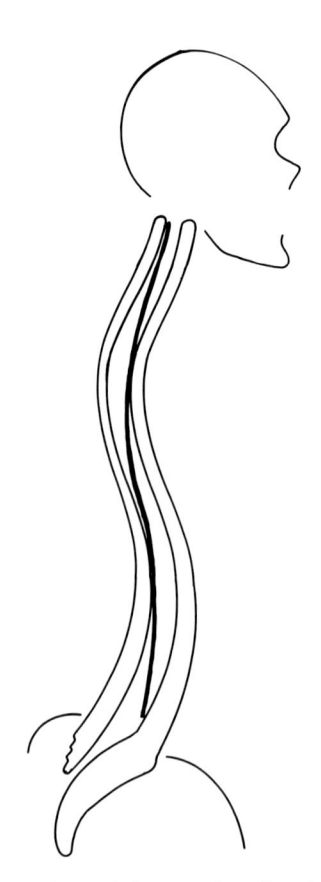

FIG. 6. Localization of the cord at the thoracic level.

Treatment

Early ambulation with a light brace for 2 months combined with physical therapy was possible in all solitary or multiple compression fractures in which the compression was less than 50%.

Conservative, nonoperative treatment by reduction on a Risser–Cotrel frame followed by a Minerva plaster jacket (Boehler method) was rarely applicable in the thoracic spine, that is, only in young patients who showed a loss of height of the anterior border of the vertebral body greater than one-half but less than two-thirds in fractures located between T5 and T10. The average duration of immobilization was never less than 4 months for adults and was sometimes longer for young people as well. After the first 45 days, the plaster cast was replaced by a plastic body jacket.

Decompression of the Neural Elements

In cases of incomplete paraplegia, posterior decompression by wide laminectomy and stabilization by rigid internal fixation are performed as early as possible. Laminectomy is only the first step of the treatment. The posterior approach is particularly justified in thoracic lesions, where the fractures often are at multiple levels, both anterior and posterior, with impaction of the laminae into the spinal cord. A wide laminectomy allows all the posterior compressive elements to be removed, and any possible anterior fragments can be displaced without retracting the spinal cord by a strictly perimedullary approach; after the first 24 hr, this posterior approach is less hemorrhagic. If residual anterior compression is shown by postoperative CT scan or myelogram, we do not hesitate to perform a second-stage anterior decompression.

In contrast to the general suggestion (12) that decompression surgery should not be performed in cases of complete paraplegia, we think that decompression should be the most complete possible, given the possible development of post-traumatic syringomyelia (2,52) (Fig. 7). A syrinx is more likely to develop if compression persists (37,40) and is encountered in 2% to 4% of patients with complete paraplegia (16).

Laminectomy, even wide, does not "destabilize" the spine as long as solid fixation and bony fusion are performed. Because it is not associated with significant motion loss, long fixation can be used in the thoracic spine. Some authors (9–11,27,30) prefer to perform this decompression and fixation by an anterolateral approach; however, 20% of second-stage posterior fixation was reported in the series of Kostuik (30). Anterior approach is the treatment of choice in cases of late decompression (2).

Our experience confirms the lack of recovery in patients with Frankel A. However, in the rare patient with incomplete neural deficit, recovery was the same as for injured patients at other levels of the spine; six of eight patients rated Frankel B improved to Frankel D or E.

Choice of Internal Fixation in the Thoracic Spine

Although the requirements for implants for fixation of the spine are well known, the anatomic peculiarities of the thoracic spine deserve attention.

Harrington rods are a useful solution (17,26,53), since they are easily inserted, taking purchase on hooks and allowing significant distraction, which is important given the limited possibilities for reduction by positioning at this level. They provide secure fixation as long as they encompass two or three vertebrae above and two or three below the lesion (41).

For all these reasons, we considered the Harrington instrumentation to be the implant of choice for performing posterior fusions in the thoracic spine. However, it has been the subject of criticism in recent publications (1,22,33). Since the Harrington instrumentation failed to protect the spine from rotational instability, a high rate of loosening (20–30%) or loss of correction (23) was encountered. Luque wiring (13), meant to increase stability, instead created new hazards due to the combination of the two techniques (42).

Roy-Camille plates and screws, which we have used almost exclusively for 13 years at other levels (3), seem to be more difficult to fix to the thoracic spine because of the small difference between the diameter of the screws (3.5 or 4 mm) and that of the pedicles: their transverse diameter is 5 mm, and their vertical diameter is 7 mm. The same restriction applies to the Dick fixator, which we do not use. Therefore, at this level, we prefer fixation by hooks rather than screws.

Cotrel–Dubousset (C-D) instrumentation has been used for the last 5 years for the treatment of spine injuries (4,5). In our opinion, it has all the advantages of the Harrington instrumentation, without the disadvantages: absence of rotational instability due to the C-D transverse rod and rod contouring; diminution of shear with use of pediculolaminar grips; and the possibility for multilevel fixation. C-D instrumentation also has eliminated cumbersome orthoses, thus allowing easy nursing care in the postoperative period and early rehabilitation in cord injury-paralyzed patients.

At recent follow-up of 29 cases treated by C-D instrumentation, there were only two hook dislodgements (one of these happened after a transfer from Europe to the United States), and an average loss of correction of only 3° in the angle of kyphosis. At the thoracic level, C-D instrumentation by hooks appears

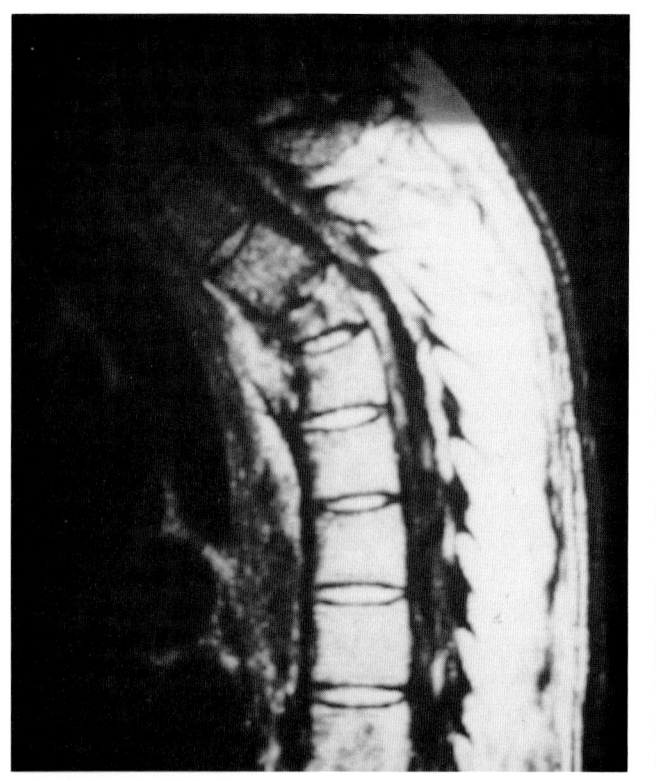

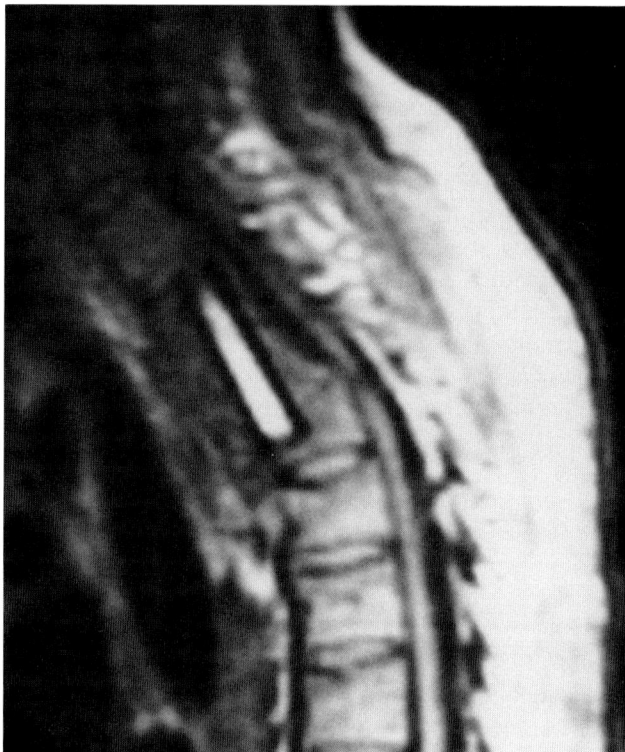

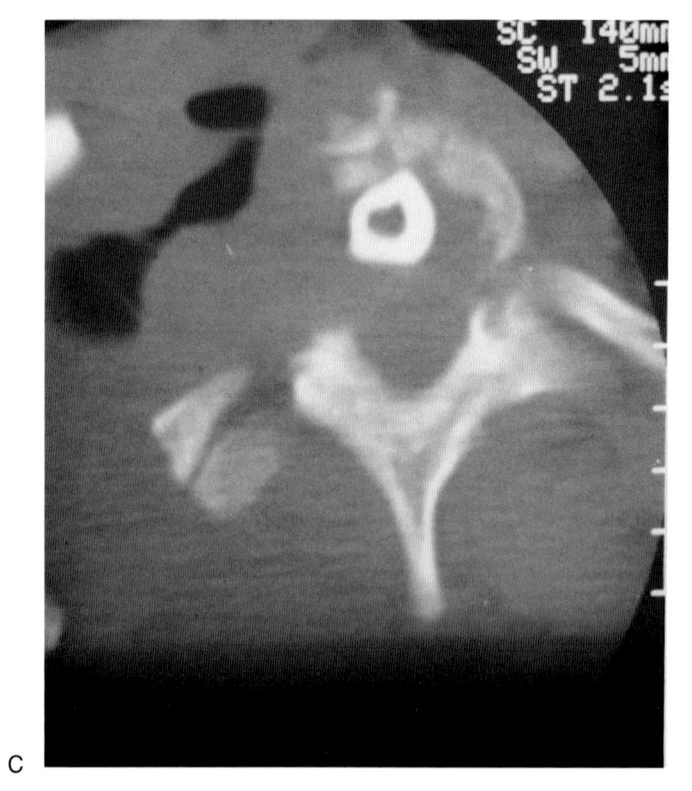

FIG. 7. Post-traumatic syringomyelia in a 19-year-old man: Frankel A. **A:** Pain and progression of spasticity 1 year after initial trauma. **B:** Anterior decompression and reduction (45° to 35°) Fibula graft + posterior fixation by C-D instrumentation. **C:** Follow-up: Frankel A. Improvement in pain and spasticity.

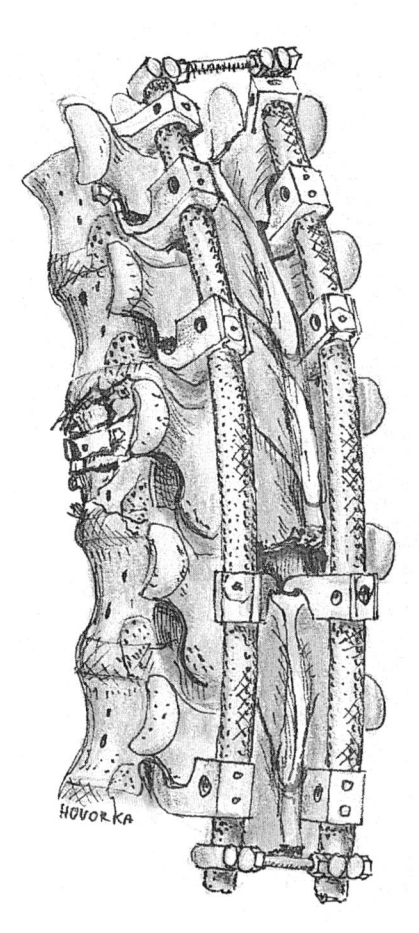

FIG. 8. The C-D construct with pediculolaminar claw above the fracture and laminolaminar claw below.

to be a very useful device that allows the surgeon to bend the rods to create distraction (Fig. 8).

THORACOLUMBAR LEVEL (T11, T12, L1, L2)

Anatomic and Physiologic Considerations

The thoracolumbar spine is the most mobile segment, where the curvature between the thoracic and lumbar spine changes, and where the gravity line bisects the T12–L1 disc. The thoracolumbar vertebrae have specific characteristics: the facet joints change orientation, from the frontal to the sagittal plane; the posterior processes become shorter and more horizontal and show transitional change between the posterior processes—oblique and downward at the level of the thoracic spine, becoming slightly oblique and upward at the level of the lumbar spine. T12 is the swivel and is therefore called the "transitional vertebra." T11 or L1, instead of T12, could be transitional, but this is far less frequent.

The thoracolumbar junction has the poorest muscular stays and therefore less efficient protection from injury. The posterior muscles extend from the posterior arches of the thoracic vertebrae and bridge T12 to gain attachment at the levels of the sacrum and the iliac crest. Combined with the change in shape and its position, located between a somewhat rigid thoracic segment and a very supple lumbar segment with large discs, the thoracolumbar junction is the most vulnerable to trauma (60% of all thoracic and lumbar fractures).

The Injuries

All types of fractures can be encountered at the level of the thoracolumbar junction. The fact that the gravity line goes through the vertebral body of T12 and then L1 explains why injuries happen more often in compression/flexion. Burst fractures show both body and ligamentous injuries, which account for instability, at the levels of the middle and posterior columns. Also, it is at the level of the thoracolumbar spine that we can find the flexion/distraction injury (type III) or the fracture/dislocation (type IV). The percentage of spinal canal occupancy by the cord goes from 30% at the upper thoracic level to 20% at T12, and to only 2% at the conus medullaris, at the level of L1, where the cauda equina roots account for 28% of the canal diameter. This partially explains the incomplete neurologic deficits and the differing rates of recovery for conus and cauda equina compression when appropriate treatment is instituted; cauda equina injury has a much greater potential for recovery. The treatment guidelines include decompression of the neural elements, reduction of deformities, and fixation in the reduced position.

As developed above, we advocate a posterior approach for decompression and fixation with use of rigid hardware. Use of only the posterior approach yielded canal clearance ranging from 52% to 27.8%. Two of 63 thoracolumbar burst fracture cases required complete decompression by a second, anterior procedure. There was no neurologic deterioration, and all patients improved one or two Frankel grades.

Fixation

Since 1986, we have used only the Cotrel–Dubousset instrumentation (6,19,20). The first 49 patients operated on with C-D instrumentation had either a short construct with one screw and one hook at either side of the lesion, or a long construct using two levels above and two levels below the lesion. The short constructs showed inconsistent results because of some hardware loosening and loss of correction. The long constructs were efficient, but they fixed segments as long as Har-

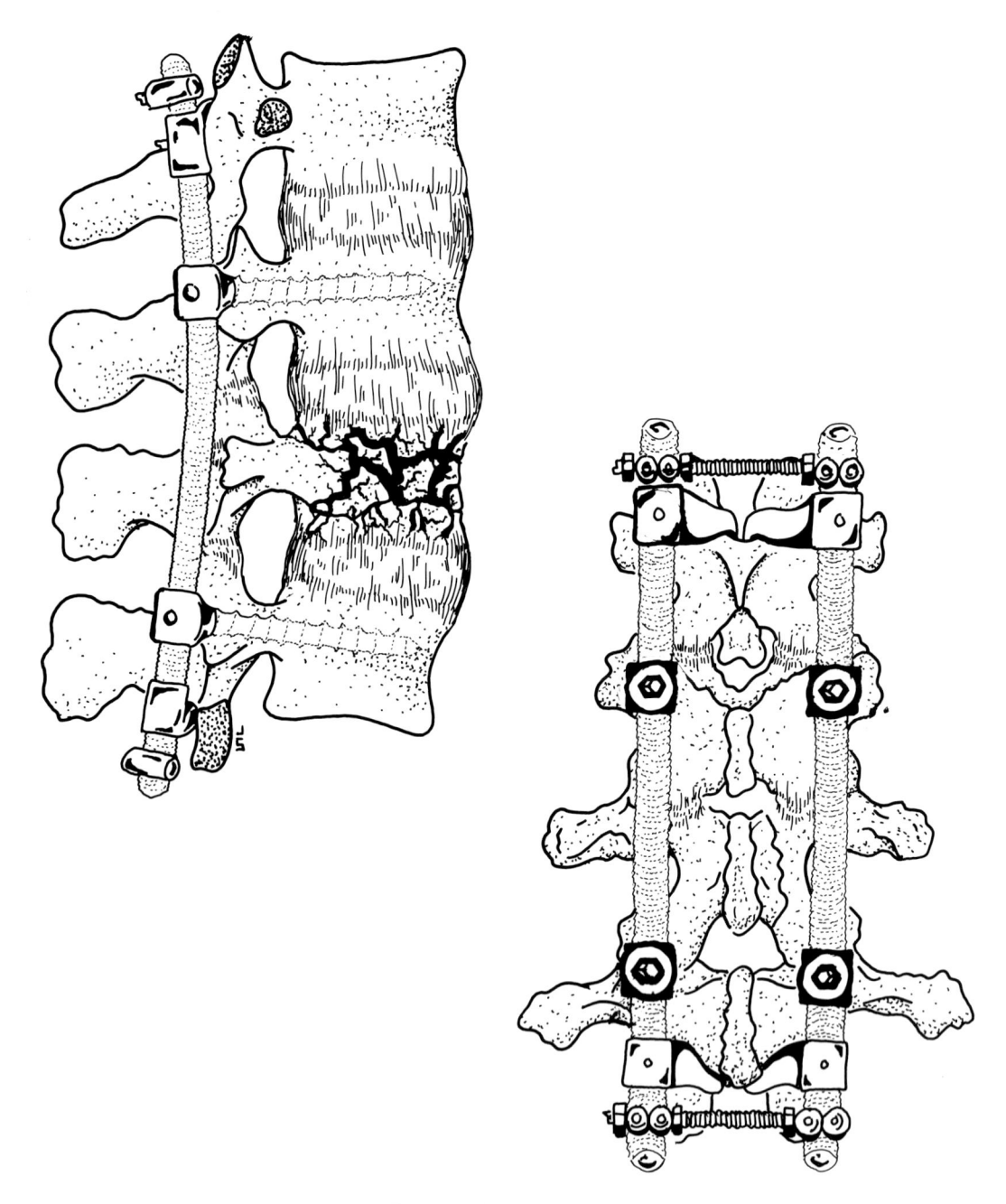

FIG. 9. Modular construct.

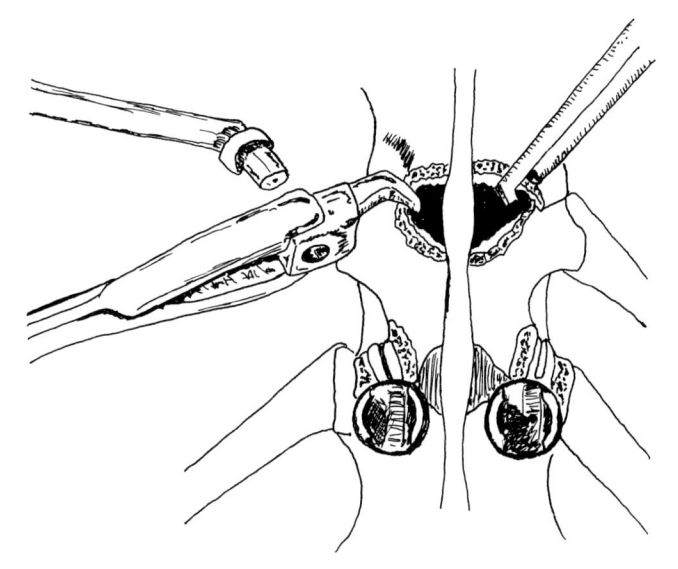

FIG. 10. Partial resection of the articular facet.

rington instrumentation. We found that when screws were used at the extremities of the construct, some of them broke. The screws that broke failed because of stress concentration on the screw as a result of a long bending moment.

In the last 40 cases, we improved the construct, made up of screws and hooks, to create variable rigidity that tapers at both the cranial and caudal ends. The advantage of this "modular construct" (5) (Fig. 9) is that only a single lumbar level is fixed below the lesion, at the caudal extremity of the construct. The screws dissipate the compression forces, and the hooks oppose pullout forces that are very strong at this level, especially when we elect not to use an orthosis. At the level of the upper vertebrae, the screws are placed in the pedicles of the first vertebra above the lesion, and a "thoracic hook" or an "eccentric hook" overrides the lamina of the second vertebra above, facing caudally. It is advantageous to locate this fixation as lateral as possible; to do so, partial resection of the articular facets at the extremities of the construct is necessary (Fig. 10).

The Rods

A rod of the appropriate length is contoured to match the lumbar lordosis, which is calculated as $-10°$ for each level (5,21,47,51). The rods are introduced into the C-D "tulip" screw heads and wiggled into the hooks. According to the type of lesion, moderate distraction is applied between the screws (Fig. 11). We must note that the distraction must not be too strong, because it can create screw loosening or favor a kyphotic deformity around the hinge that is provided by an almost always intact anterior longitudinal ligament.

For seat belt-type lesions, type III, or dislocations, type IV, subtype B (anteroposterior shear or posteroanterior shear), a short construct with one screw and one hook applied on the vertebra on either side of the lesion appears sufficient when it is placed under compression. For more complex lesions affecting two or more adjacent vertebrae, a longer construct is recommended (Fig. 12), as is a postoperative orthosis. In all cases, a bilateral posterolateral bone graft is performed using a mixture of corticocancellous iliac crest bone graft and allograft from the bone bank; we now use transpedicular grafting only in cases of laminectomy.

When the patient is intact, early physical therapy out of bed with immediate rehabilitation makes a return to normal activity possible over a short period of time.

The results on the last 40 patients with a modular construct have shown no neurologic complications. No screws have loosened or failed. Two deep wound infections were revised, with later healing. There was one hardware removal followed by loss of correction. Postoperative kyphosis was 3°, excluding the case that required removal of hardware. The average loss of correction was 5.7° at last follow-up (Fig. 13).

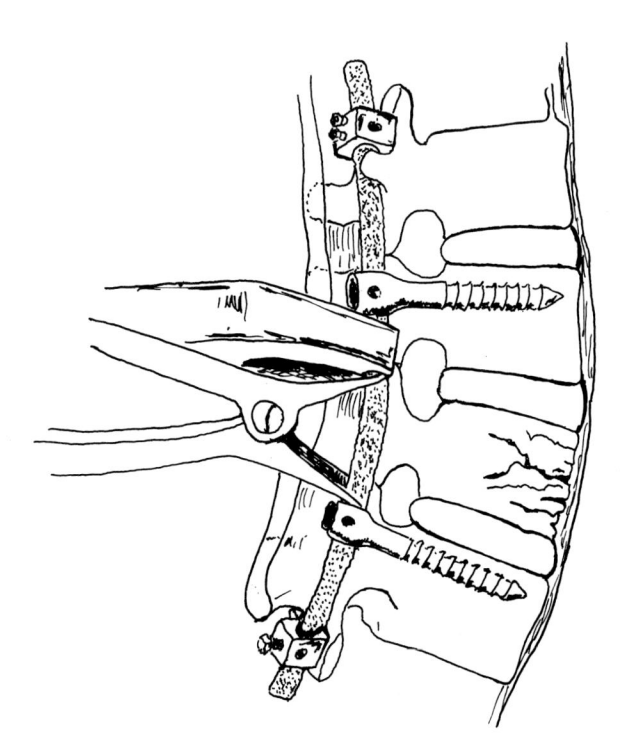

FIG. 11. Moderate distraction for burst fracture.

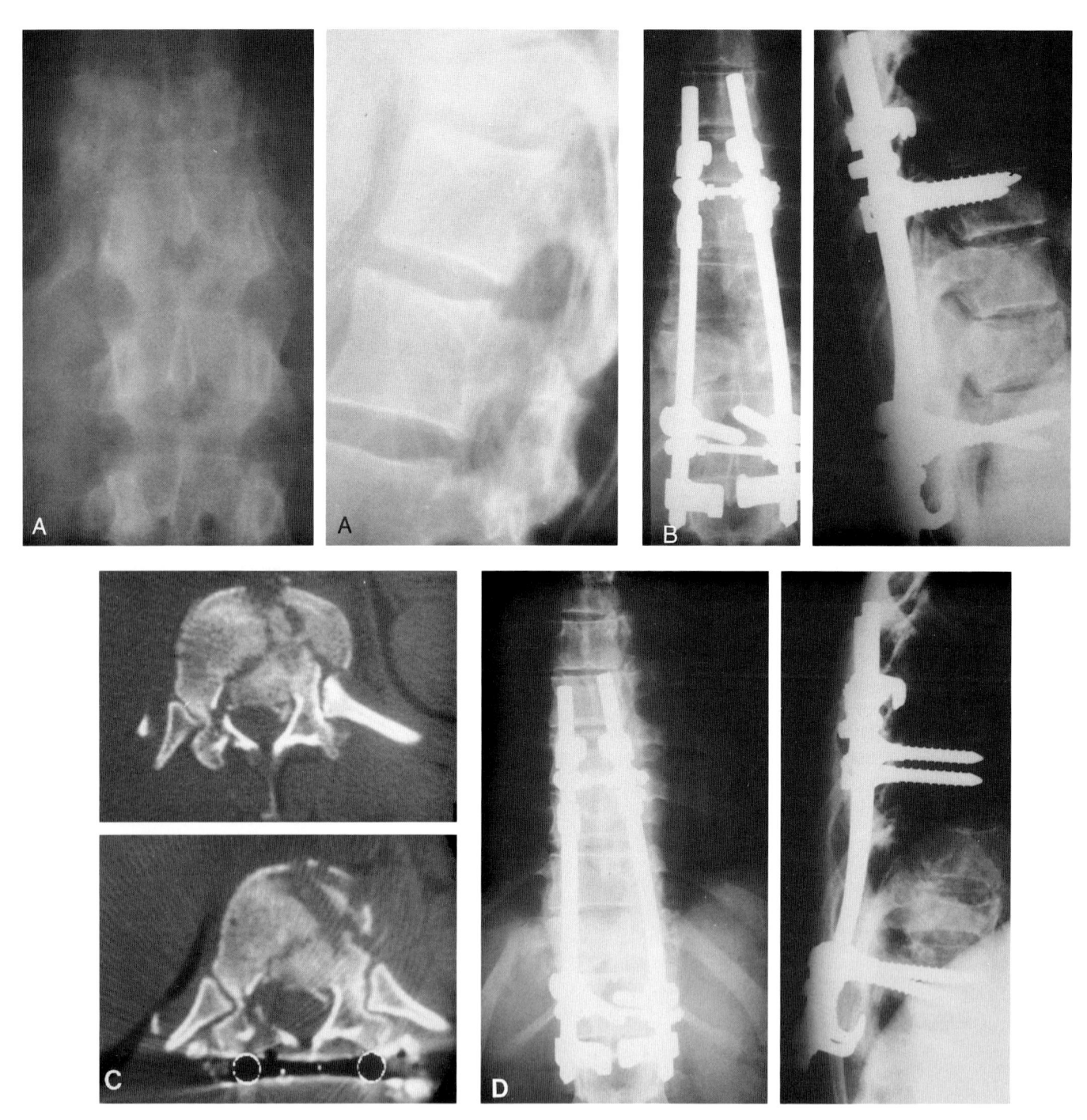

FIG. 12. A: Patient is a 30-year-old woman who had a sport accident. T11 and T12 burst fractures. Frankel E. **B:** Decompression by wide posterolateral approach. Fixation by C-D. **C:** Pre- and postoperative CT scans. **D:** Excellent functional result at 18 months. There was some loss of vertebral height without kyphotic deformity.

SPECIFIC INJURIES AND MANAGEMENT • 205

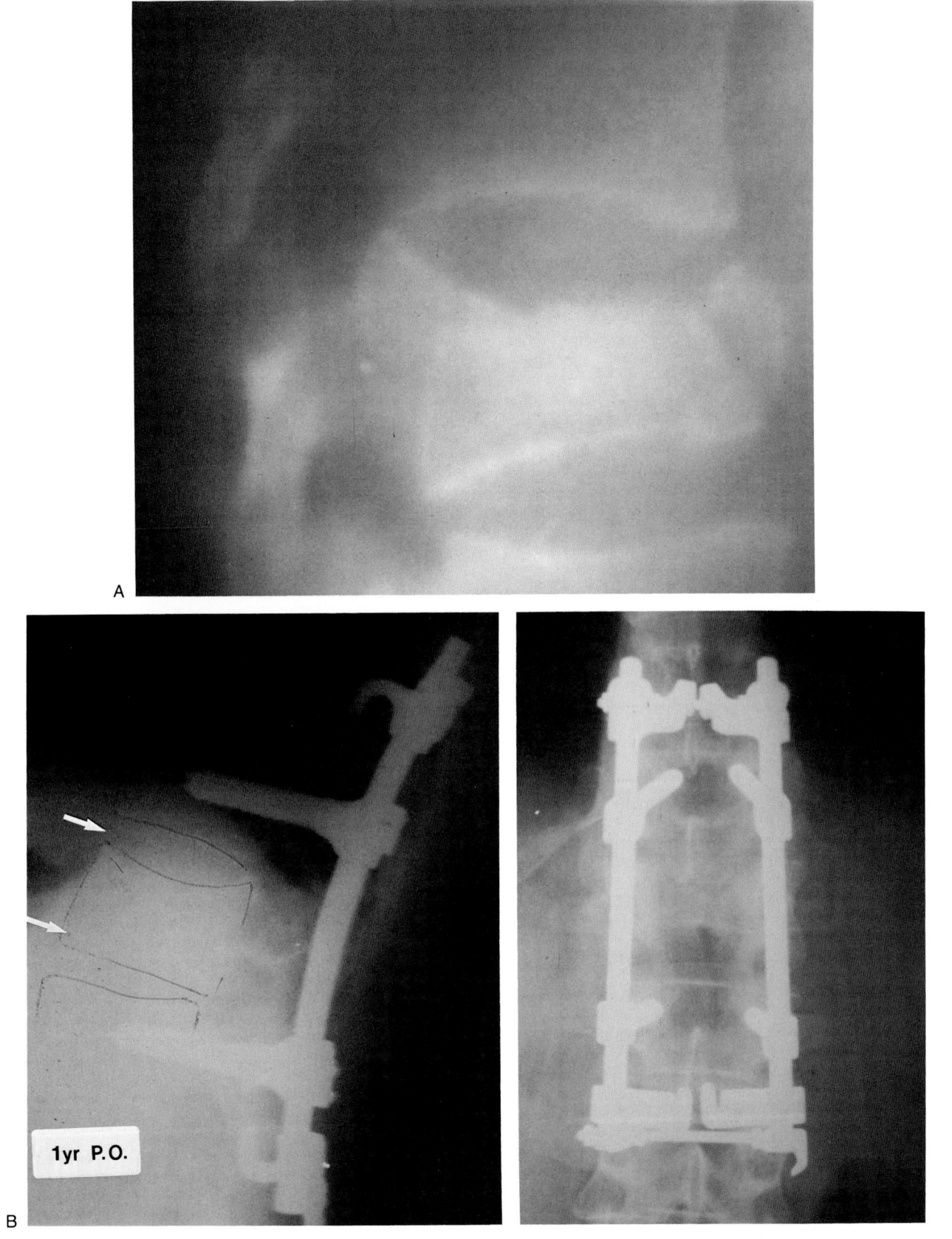

FIG. 13. A: Burst (subtype B) fracture. **B:** No loss of correction at 1 year follow up.

LUMBAR SPINE (L3, L4, L5)

Specific Anatomy and Physiology of the Lumbar Spine

The lumbar vertebrae are larger than the thoracic or thoracolumbar vertebrae. The lumbar vertebral body is quadrilateral, with two large pedicles in the back. The pedicles are directed obliquely and medially. The articular processes end in facets shaped as segmental cylinders and are located in the sagittal plane (zygapophyseal joint). The spinous processes are narrow but high, and their direction is horizontal. The lumbar lordosis, maximal at the level of L3, is such that the gravity line falls behind the bony elements of the spine.

The third lumbar vertebra's fundamental function is as a point of insertion for multiple muscles. The spinous process of this vertebra show more development for the insertion of the spinalis muscles, from which the lumbar portion of the latissimus dorsalis inserts before it expands to the iliac crest (25). This double insertion of the muscles is like a violin bow string that contains the tension of the lumbar lordosis.

The body of the fifth lumbar vertebra is higher in front than in back and cuneiform (i.e., like a trapeze) in shape. This vertebra is a swivel that is located between the vertical spine above and the oblique sacrum below. L5 sits on the sacrum at an angle of 30° to the horizontal plane, as the wedge between L5 and the sacrum is inclined 30° to the horizontal plane. Lumbar spine mobility is maximal in flexion/extension, less in lateral bending, and limited in rotation because of the sagittal orientation of the facet joints.

The first sacral vertebra must be considered to be part of the lumbar spine, since fixation often will be extended to the sacrum. Our anatomic studies, as well CT scan studies, have shown the sacral ala to be full of fatty bone marrow, in which the pedicular screws have a poor purchase (7) (see Chapter 2).

Our experiments on the pullout strength of sacral screws (7-mm diameter) were performed on 12 fresh cadavers (7). The pullout strength in the axis of the screw was 40 kg when the screw was inserted oblique and laterally, 50 kg when the screw was inserted strictly in the sagittal plane, and 70 kg when the screw was inserted oblique, medially, and slightly upward, to rest in contact with the S1 endplate. Similar experiments have been conducted by Asher and Strippgen (8), Steinman et al. (49), and Zindrick et al. (54).

At the lumbar level, the vertebral canal contains six pairs of nerve roots (L3, L4, L5, S1, S2, and S3 constitute the cauda equina) and takes a triangular shape. Nerve root mobility is limited by the point of perforation of the dural sac by the nerve roots (38).

The Lesions

In a retrospective study of 120 lumbar fractures, there were 65 fractures at L3, 36 fractures at L4, and 19 fractures at L5. Seventeen patients presented with lesions at multiple levels. Forty-nine of the cases were burst fractures and 10 fracture/dislocations were type IV. Among the fracture/dislocations, one fracture was characteristic of oblique shear, subtype D, as described above. Twenty percent of the patients presented with neurologic symptoms.

Treatment

Because of poor results of conservative treatment, surgical correction was used more often at the lumbar level than at the thoracolumbar level. Laminectomy performed routinely in cases of neurologic deficit allowed repair of eight cases of vertical dural lacerations that were always associated with bony injury of the posterior arch in burst fractures (Fig. 14). The dural tears were repaired primarily with dural allograft. Camissa et al. (14), Miller et al. (35), and Pickett and Blumenkopf (39) studied these dural wounds, and Silvestro et al. (46) found them in 16 of 25 burst fractures approached posteriorly. For Miller and Pickett, there is a significant association between a posterior element fracture and a dural laceration ($\chi^2 < 0.02$). A similar significance was found between the presence of severe laceration and severe neurologic deficit ($\chi^2\ p < 0.01$). According to these authors, the dural tears are found equally at low thoracic and lumbar levels. We found a greater frequency in the lumbar area; there were eight lumbar but only five thoracic dural tears. These tears were related to stretching of the cauda equina on the retropulsed bony fragment.

It is necessary to reduce and reinsert the herniated nerve roots and to achieve a water seal closure of the dural wound. Sometimes this can be achieved only with a dural graft. Pickett and Blumenkopf (39) reported chronic and persistent pain following conservative treatment; they treated the pain with neurolysis of the cauda equina roots that were trapped in scar tissue. To deal with pain from a neural origin related to scar tissue between the nerve roots and the posterior arch, Pickett et al. (39) and Silvestro et al. (46) favor a posterior surgical approach for lumbar burst fractures when a dural wound is suspected on imaging.

In our experience, two patients with large displacement who were neurologically intact were managed by bony realignment before internal fixation with use of progressive, 48-hr skeletal traction with bilateral femo-

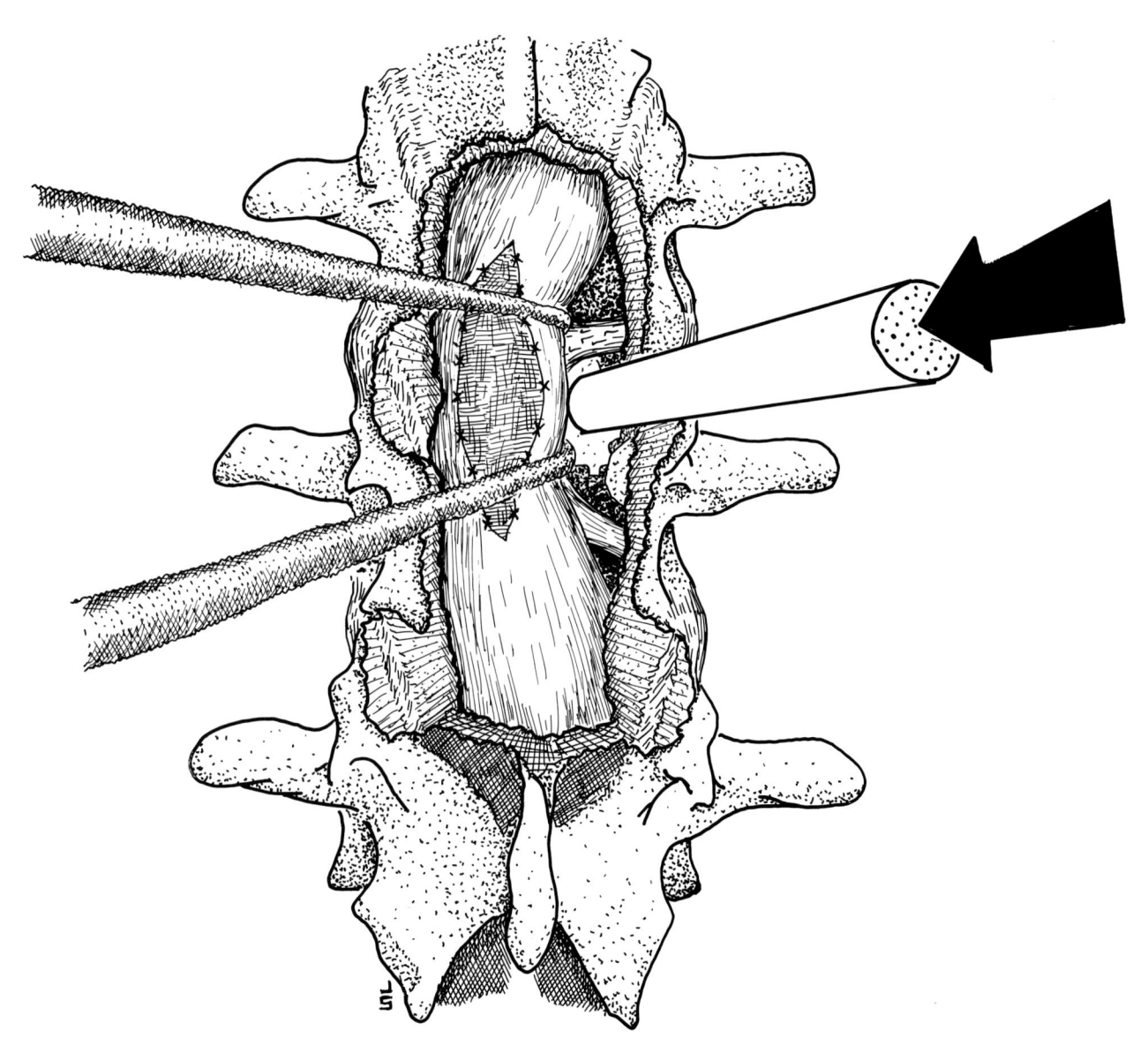

FIG. 14. Decompression at lumbar level. (Note the patch on the dural wound.)

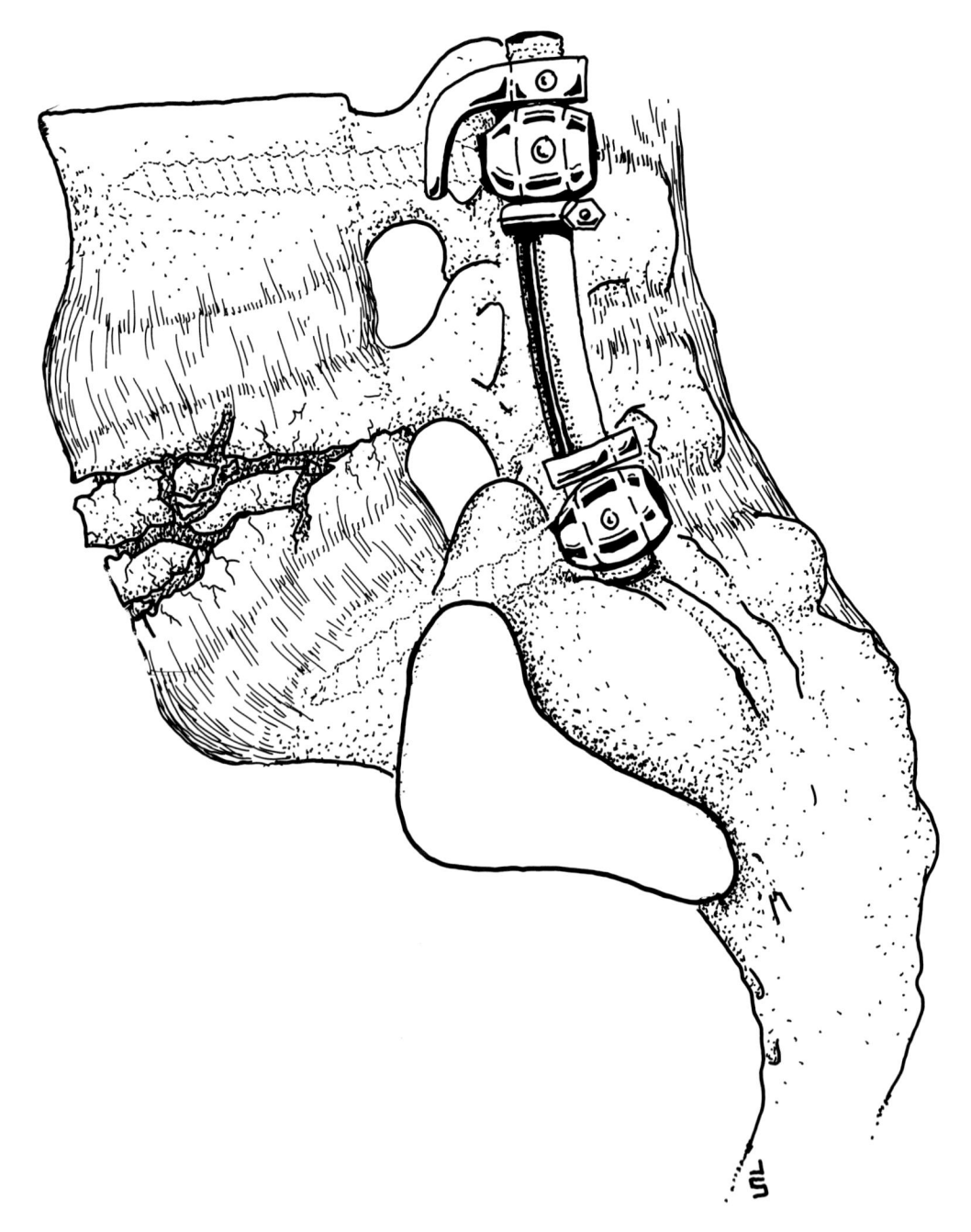

FIG. 15. Insertion of the sacral screw.

ral pins. In a similar case, in which traction was not used, the attempt at surgical reduction was hampered by a large hemorrhage, and complete reduction could not be achieved.

Fixation

Only bent rods or plates (21,31,44,48,51) fixed by pedicular screws are able to restore lumbar lordosis. The large pedicular diameter, 10 mm in the transverse plane and 15 mm in the vertical plane, allows safe insertion of screws into the pedicles. This is normally done after partial resection at the base of the transverse process with a Leksell rongeur, followed by a small curette manipulated to find the pedicle with a direction of 10° medially. For the first sacral vertebra, one solid anchorage will be obtained with careful application of medial obliquity in screw insertion, which will be in the direction of the sacral endplate with its threads jammed into subchondral bone (see Chapter 2) (Fig. 15).

In the lumbar spine, it is very important to save as many mobile segments as possible; this necessitates using a construct that is as short as possible, with one single vertebra on either side of the injured vertebra fixed by pedicular screws. We also note that the vertebra that is fractured can also be fixed if the pedicle is not fractured. The stability of the construct can be increased by adding two hooks; one hook is placed anteriorly around the transverse process at the level of the vertebra above (Fig. 16). Its function is not to create a claw, as at the thoracic level, but rather to oppose

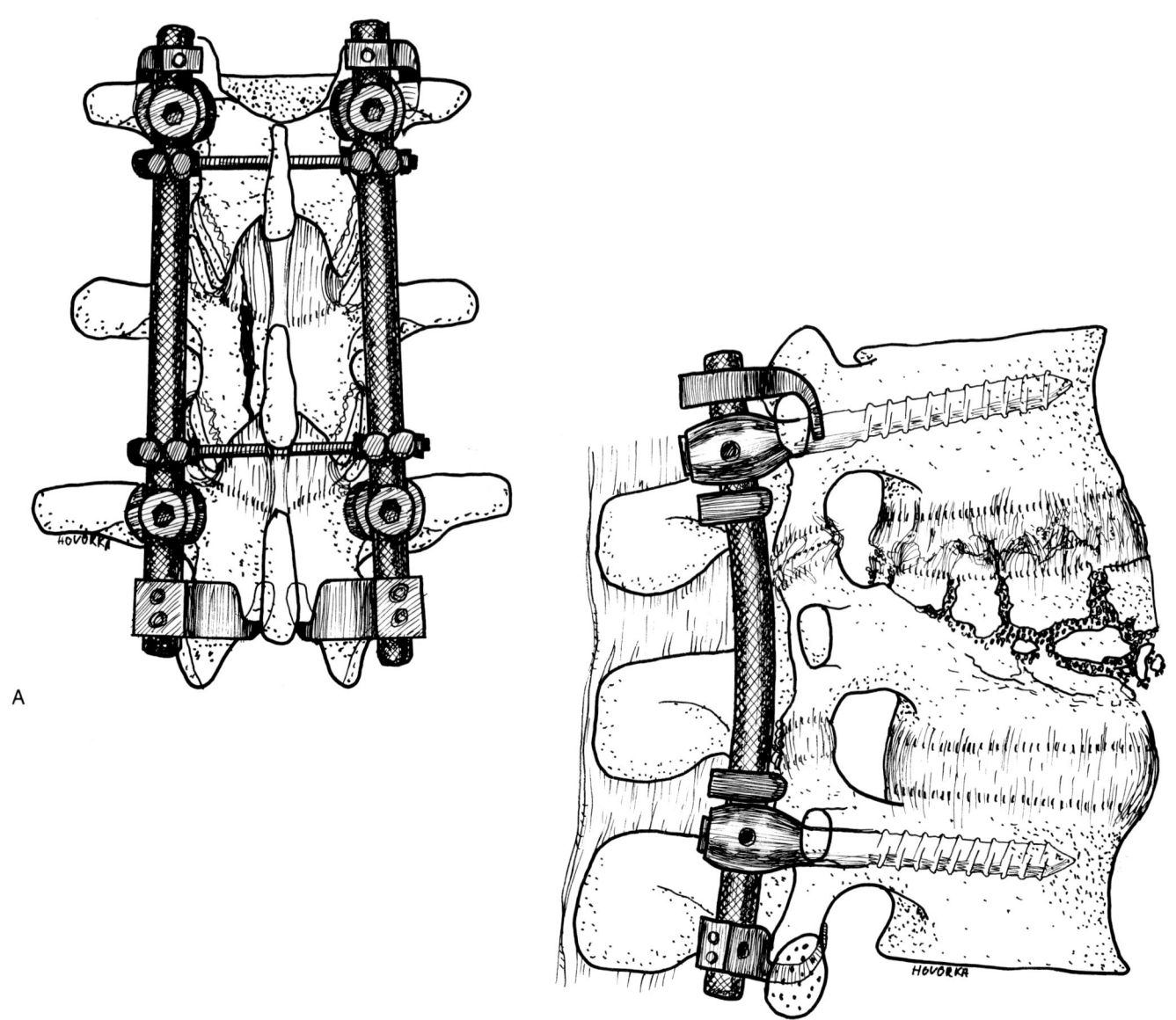

FIG. 16. The C-D construct at the lumbar level.

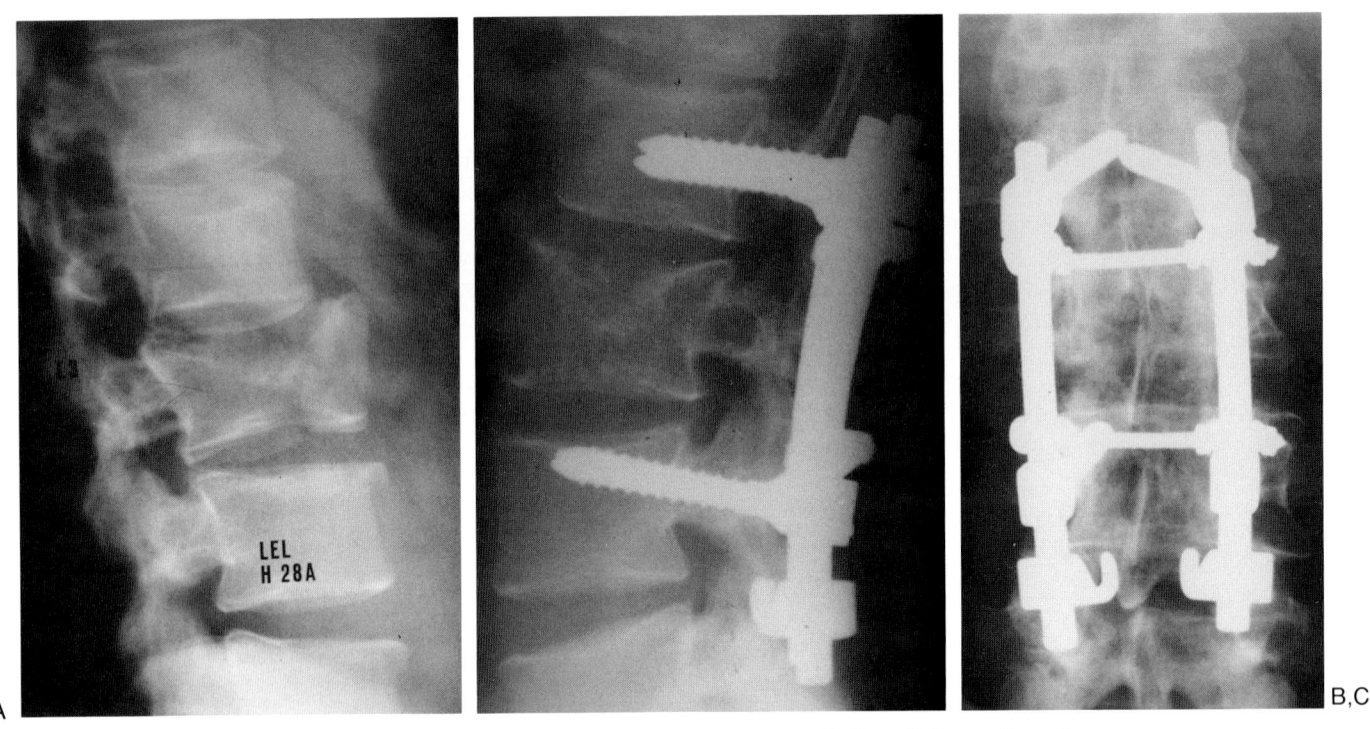

FIG. 17. A: Burst fracture of L3. **B:** Short construct. **C:** Result 9 months later.

pullout as a suspender might, in case of flexion of large amplitude. The other hook is placed under the lamina below, facing cranially, to guarantee the fixation against pullout. At this level more than at any other, there are two fundamental conditions required to obtain bony healing with normal sagittal alignment: moderate distraction must be applied to restore the height of a normal functional segment in both the sagittal and frontal planes, and the rods or plate must be contoured before screw application to obtain the desired sagittal balance (Fig. 17). It is possible to apply a slight, in situ complementary correction when necessary. If reduction and fixation fail to match the normal anatomic contour of the lumbar spine, the construct that is posterior to the load application will be submitted to a bending moment and will be responsible for secondary loosening, screw failure, or hook pullout.

In our group of 26 lumbar fixations with C-D instru-

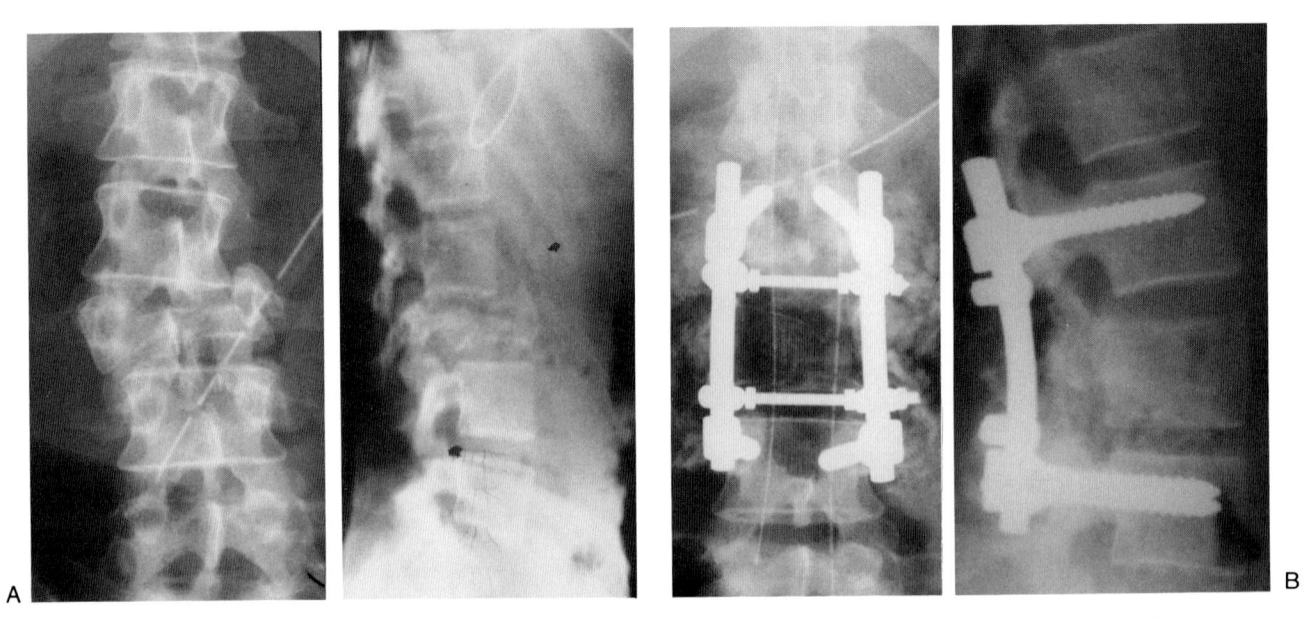

FIG. 18. A: Burst fracture of L3: Frankel E. Patient is a 35-year-old woman. **B:** Reduction, decompression by laminectomy and fixation by short C-D construct and bone grafting.

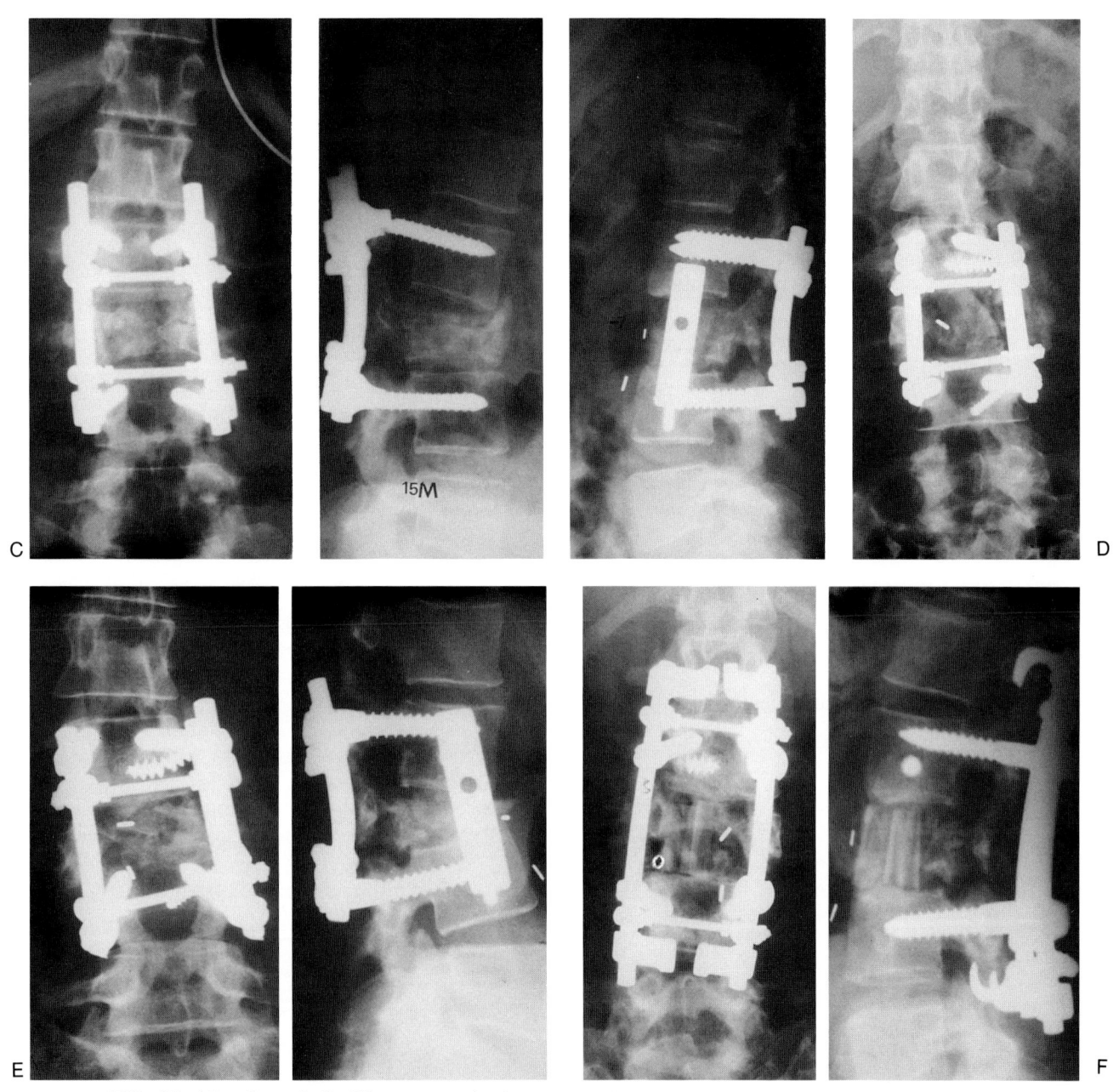

FIG. 18. (*Continued*) **C:** Fifteen months later, pseudarthrosis with pain and radiculopathy. **D:** Two-stage reconstruction: anterior iliac bone grafting + A-O plate; 6-mm screws are replaced by 7-mm (sacral) screws. **E:** Twelve months later, pain and radiculopathy at L4 and L5 roots; the fibular bone graft did not revascularize. **F:** Reconstruction in the same operative procedure: new posterior fixation (one vertebra above is included in the construct) and anterior fibular and iliac grafts. There was immediate postoperative clinical improvement.

mentation, we had two patients with loss of correction and two with pseudarthrosis at the level of the vertebral body fracture (29) (Y. Floman, *personal communication*). Both of the pseudarthroses were treated by anterior approach, with anterior iliac bone graft. In one of the two cases in which an additional anterior A-O plate was inserted, a necrosis developed at the level of the bone graft. This could have been caused by the stress shielding due to the two plates; perhaps vascular insult due to both approaches was responsible as well (Fig. 18).

For severe bone comminution and discoligamentous injury, like Bridwell and DeWald (12) and other surgeons, we recommend an anterior approach for supplementary bone grafting in addition to the posterior procedure (Fig. 19). When the reduction has taken place

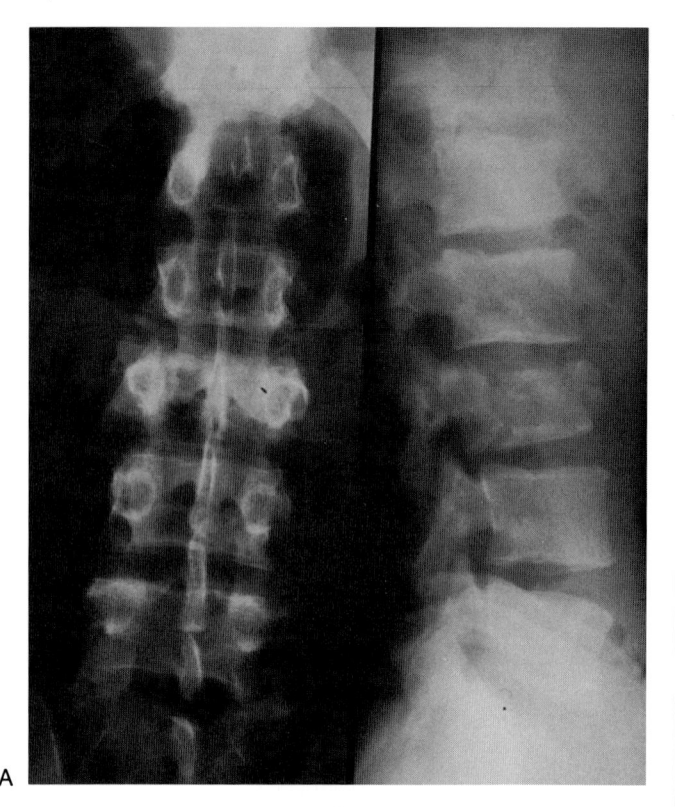

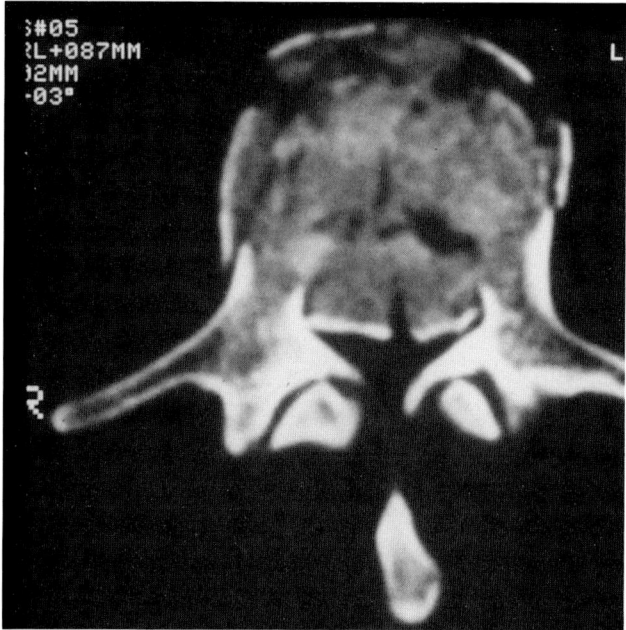

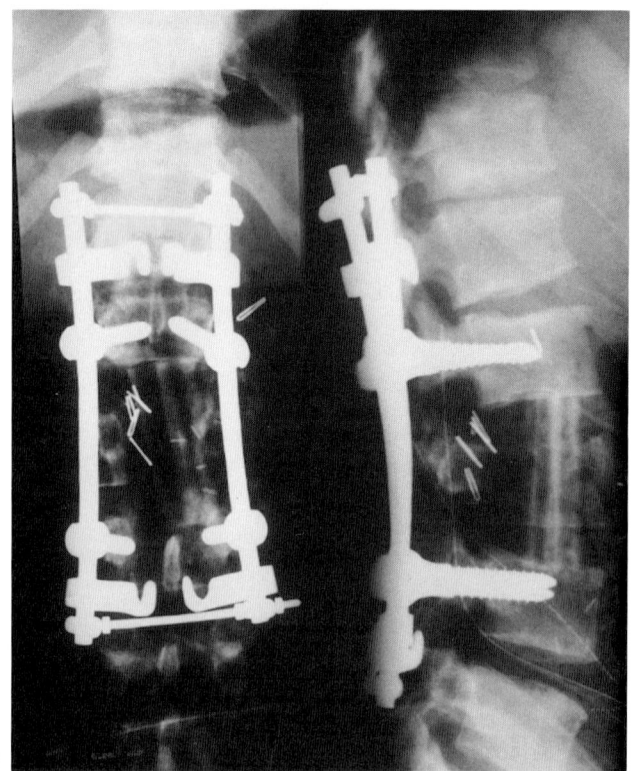

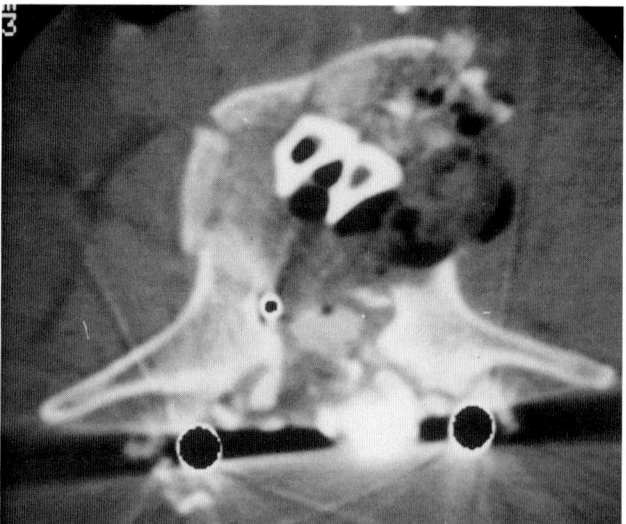

FIG. 19. A: L3 burst fracture. **B:** Pre- and postoperative CT scan: posterior procedure was done first, followed by anterior surgery. **C:** Final construct (fibular graft).

in the disc space, it means that the disc has been injured badly and, since we know it won't heal, an anterior graft is necessary (see Chapter 10).

The management in the postoperative period is very similar to the management of lumbar scoliosis for which, besides restriction of sitting position for 3 to 4 weeks, it does not appear that orthosis is very efficient.

REFERENCES

1. Aebi M, Etter C, Kehl T, Thalgott. The internal skeletal fixation system. A new treatment of thoracolumbar fractures and the other spinal disorders. *Clin Orthop* 1988;227:30–43.
2. Argenson C. Cals vicieux et pseudarthroses du rachis thoracolombaire. In: *Cahiers d'Enseignement de la SOFCOT*. Paris: Expansion Scientifique Francaise, 1990;205–236.
3. Argenson C. Traitement des fractures du rachis dorso-lombaire chez l'adulte. In: *Cahiers d'Enseignement de la SOFCOT*. Paris: Expansion Scientifique Francaise, 1984;5–27.
4. Argenson C, Boileau P, de Peretti F, Lovet J, Dalzotto H. Fractures of the thoracic spine (T1–T10). A review of 105 cases. *Fr J Orthop Surg* 1989;3(3):238–254.
5. Argenson C, Lovet J, Cambas PM, Griffet J, Barraud O. Osteosynthesis of thoracolumbar spine fracture with C-D instrumentation. In: *Fifth Proceedings of 1988 G.I.C.D.* Montpellier: Sauramps Medical, 1989;75–82.
6. Argenson C, Lovet J, de Peretti F, Cambas PM, Griffet J, Boileau P. Treatment of spinal fractures with C-D instrumentation: results of 85 cases. SRS-ESDS Combined Meeting. Amsterdam, Holland, September 17–22, 1989.
7. Argenson C, de Peretti F, Frehel M, Omar F, Lovet J. Lumbosacral arthrodesis. In: *Sixth Proceedings of 1989 G.I.C.D.* Montpellier: Sauramps Medical, 1989;75–82.
8. Asher MA, Strippgen WE. Anthropometric studies of the human sacrum relating to dorsal transsacral implant designs. *Clin Orthop* 1986;203:58.
9. Bohlman HH. Traumatic fractures of the upper thoracic spine with paralysis. *J Bone Joint Surg* 1979;56A:1299.
10. Bradford DS, Behrooz AA, Winter RB, Seljeskag EL. Surgical stabilization of fracture dislocation of the thoracic spine. *Spine* 1977;2:185–196.
11. Bradford DS, McBride GG. Surgical management of thoracolumbar spine fractures with incomplete neurologic deficits. *Clin Orthop* 1987;218:201–216.
12. Bridwell KH, DeWald RL, eds. *Spinal surgery*. Philadelphia: Lippincott, 1991.
13. Bryant CE, Sullivan JA. Management of thoracic and lumbar spine fractures with Harrington distraction rods supplemented with sequential wiring. *Spine* 1983;8:532–537.
14. Camissa FP, Eismont FJ, Green BA. Dural lacerations occurring with burst fractures and associated laminar fractures. *J Bone Joint Surg* 1989;71A:1044–1053.
15. Denis F. The three column spine and its significance in the classification of acute thoracolumbar spinal injuries. *Spine* 1983;8(6):817–831.
16. Eismont FJ, Barth A, Green BA, Quenler RM. Post traumatic spinal cord cyst. *J Bone Joint Surg* 1984;66A(4):614–617.
17. Erickson DL, Leider LL, Brown WE. One stage decompression for thoracolumbar fractures. *Spine* 1977;2:53–56.
18. Eskay ML, Hanley EN. The thoracic spine fractures. Fifty-Second Annual Meeting, American Academy of Orthopaedic Surgeons, Las Vegas, Nevada, 1985.
19. Farcy JPC, Weidenbaum M, Michelsen CB, Hoeltzel DA, Athanasiou KA. A comparative biomechanical study of spinal fixation using Cotrel-Dubousset instrumentation. *Spine* 1987;12:877–881.
20. Farcy JPC, Weidenbaum M. A preliminary review of the use of Cotrel–Dubousset instrumentation for spinal injuries. *Bull Hosp Jt Dis Orthop Inst* 1988;48:1.
21. Farcy JPC, Weidenbaum M, Glassman SD. Sagittal index in management of thoracolumbar burst fractures. *Spine* 1990;15(9):958–965.
22. Gertzbein SD, McMichael D, Tile M. Harrington instrumentation as a method of fixation in fractures of the spine: a critical analysis of deficiencies. *J Bone Joint Surg* 1977;64B:745.
23. Greenwald TA, Keen JS. Results of Harrington instrumentation in type A and B burst fractures. *J Spinal Disord* 1991;2:149–156.
24. Hanley E, Eskay M. Thoracic spine fractures. *Orthopaedics* 1989;12:689–695.
25. Jackson RP, Hamilton A. C-D screws with oblique canals for improved screw fixation. In: *Proceedings of the Seventh Annual G.I.C.D.* Montpellier: Sauramps Medical, 1991.
26. Jacobs RR, Casey MP. Surgical management of thoracolumbar spinal injuries. *Clin Orthop* 1984;189:22–35.
27. Johnson JR, Leatherman KD, Holt RT. Anterior decompression of the spinal cord for neurological deficit. *Spine* 1983;8:395–405.
28. Kapandji IA. *Articular physiology*. Paris: Maloine Editions, 1982.
29. Kinley MM, Obenchain TG, Roth KD. Loss of correction in case of posterior transpedicular decompensation. In: *Sixth Proceedings of the 1989 G.I.C.D.* Montpellier: Sauramps Medical, 1990;37–39.
30. Kostuik JP. Anterior spinal cord decompression for lesions of the thoracic and lumbar spine, techniques, new methods of internal fixation, results. *Spine* 1983;8(5):512–531.
31. Louis R. Internal fixation of the lumbar and sacral spine by internal fixation with screw plates. *Spine* 1986;203:18–34.
32. Louis R. *Surgery of the spine*. Berlin: Springer-Verlag, 1983.
33. McAfee PC, Bohlman HH. Complications following Harrington instrumentation for fracture of the thoracolumbar spine. *J Bone Joint Surg* 1985;67A:672–686.
34. Meinecke FW. Frequency and distribution of associated injuries in traumatic paraplegia and tetraplegia. *Paraplegia* 1968;5:196.
35. Miller CA, Dewey RC, Hunt WE. Impaction fracture of the lumbar vertebrae with dural tear. *J Neurosurg* 1980;53:765–771.
36. Motin J, Latarjet J, Coonet JB. Diagnostic des ruptures traumatiques de l'aorte. *Nouv Presse Med* 1980;9:2823–2327.
37. Mudge K, Van Dolson L, Lake A. Progressive cyclic degeneration of the spinal cord following spinal cord injury. *Spine* 1984;9:253–255.
38. de Peretti F, Micallef JP, Bourgeon A, Argenson C, Rabischong P. Biomechanics of the lumbar spinal nerve roots and the first sacral root within the intervertebral foramina. *Surg Radiol Anat* 1989;11:221–225.
39. Pickett J, Blumenkopf B. Dural lacerations and thoracolumbar fractures. *J Spinal Disord* 1989;2:99–103.
40. Privat JM, Privat L, Martinazzo J, Gros C. *Interet des decompressions medullaires secondaires et tardives dans les paraplegies traumatiques. Actualities en Reeducation*. Paris: Masson, 1985;156–165.
41. Purcell G, Markolf K, Dawson E. Twelfth thoracic first lumbar stability after Harrington rod instrumentation. *J Bone Joint Surg* 1981;63A:71–78.
42. Rossier AB, Cochran TP. The treatment of spinal fractures with Harrington compression rods and sequential sublaminar wiring. A dangerous combination. *Spine* 1984;8:796–789.
43. Roy-Camille R, Saillant G. Rachis traumatique neurologique. In: *3es Journées d'Orthopédie de la Pitié*. Paris: Masson, 1983.
44. Roy-Camille R, Saillant G, Mazel C. Internal fixation of the lumbar spine with pedicle screw plating. *Clin Orthop* 1986;203:7–17.
45. Schulte AM, Esch J, Vlajic I, et al. Mediastinal und pleuraengusals folge frische fraxturen der brust-wirbelsaulf. *Chirurg* 1975;45:36–40.
46. Silvestro C, Francaviglia N, Bragazzi R, Piatelli G, Viale GL. On the predictive value of radiological signs for the presence of dural lacerations related to fractures of the lower thoracic or lumbar spine. *J Spinal Disord* 1991;1:49–53.
47. Stagnara P, deMauroy JC, Dran G, Gonon DP, Costanzo G, Dimnet J, Pasquet A. Reciprocal angulation of vertebral bodies in a sagittal plane. Approach to references for the evaluation of kyphosis and lordosis. *Spine* 1982;7(4):335–342.
48. Steffee AD, Biscup RS, Sitkowski DJ. Segmental spine plates with pedicle screw fixation. A new internal fixation device for

disorders of the lumbar and thoracolumbar spine. *Clin Orthop* 1986;112:512–518.
49. Steinman JC, Mirkovic S, Abitbol JJ, Massie J, Subbaia P, Garfin SR. Radiographic assessment of sacral screw placement. *J Spinal Disord* 1990;3:232–238.
50. Viale JP, Rousselet B. *Les atteintes cardiopericardiques des traumatismes thoraciques fermes. Reanimation et Medecine d'Urgence.* Paris: Expansion Scientifique Francaise, 1984; 165–179.
51. Weidenbaum M, Farcy JPC. Surgical management of thoracic and lumbar burst fractures. In: Bridwell KH, DeWald RL, eds. *The textbook of spinal surgery*. Philadelphia: Lippincott, 1991.
52. Yanlon W. Ascendant myelopathy. *Spine* 1989;10:1084–1089.
53. Yosipovitch Z, Robin G, Makin M. Open reduction of unstable thoracolumbar spinal injuries and fixation with Harrington rods. *J Bone Joint Surg* 1977;59A:1003–1015.
54. Zindrick MA, Wiltse LL, Widell EH, Thomas JC, Holland R, Field BT, Spencer CW. A biomechanical study of intrapedicular screw fixation in the lumbosacral spine. *Clin Orthop* 1986;203: 99–110.

16

Conservative Management of Burst Fractures

Joseph E. Mumford and James N. Weinstein

Failure of the spinal column in trauma is a function of applied load and the ability of the various bony and soft tissue elements to resist that load. Load can vary by magnitude (high or low), type (blunt versus penetrating), and vector (compression, distraction, rotation, and shear). The ability of the bony elements to resist load can be altered by a variety of disease states, including tumor and metabolic processes. By incorporating these general principles, thoracolumbar spine fractures may broadly be classified as follows:

1. Low-energy blunt trauma, producing stable injuries without neurologic deficit.
2. High-energy blunt trauma, producing stable or unstable injuries with or without neurologic deficit.
3. Penetrating spine injury, most commonly from gunshot wounds.
4. Pathologic fractures, associated with tumors or metabolic disease (31).

This chapter focuses on the nonoperative management of the first two groups of patients; penetrating spine injury and pathologic fractures are discussed in separate chapters of this text.

CONTROVERSIAL ASPECTS

The goals in caring for patients with thoracolumbar spine fractures include preserving life, protecting neurologic function, minimizing the risk of further spinal column or neurologic injury, and restoring and maintaining the stability of the spine (4,12). The means chosen to achieve these goals are simple and universally agreed on in some injury patterns, such as simple anterior column compression fractures without neurologic deficit, but challenging and often controversial with other injury patterns, such as two- and three-column fractures with or without neurologic deficit.

With respect to management of the more controversial injury patterns (unstable burst fractures with or without neurologic deficit), nonoperative advocates would argue that (a) canal encroachment does not correlate with initial neurologic exam (23,29,35); (b) residual deformity does not correlate with neural recovery rate or symptoms at follow-up (2,3,8,19,37); (c) post-traumatic spinal stenosis either does not occur (1) or is an unusual sequela of nonoperative management (3,42); and (d) high complication rates (54% in one series) (17) have been reported with surgical management.

Operative advocates conclude that surgically treated groups have shorter hospitalization, earlier rehabilitation, and decreased spinal deformity (10,30). In comparative studies of operative and nonoperative management, neither approach has convincingly shown an improvement in overall neurologic recovery when compared to the other (6,16,45).

STABILITY

With spinal injury, the terms "stable" and "unstable" have no precise definitions. Rather, they are relative terms that depend on the anatomy of the injury and the loads applied to the injured area prior to and after successful healing (20). Accurate clinical and radiographic assessment of stability is critical to prevent displacement that may lead to neurologic deterioration.

A spinal fracture may be considered unstable if, during healing, fragment displacement occurs, resulting in possible neurologic deterioration. Using this defini-

---

J. E. Mumford: Orthopedic Associates, Topeka, KS 66606.
J. N. Weinstein: Department of Orthopaedic Surgery, and Spine Diagnostic and Treatment Center, University of Iowa Hospitals and Clinics, Iowa City, IA 52242-1088.

tion, one must define the treatment parameters that affect spinal loading during the period of healing. If nonoperative management is chosen, critical issues include definition and duration of recumbency as well as type and duration of bracing.

Computerized tomography (CT) has greatly enhanced the accurate visualization of fracture anatomy, formerly unavailable from plain films and tomography (15,23,41). The CT scan particularly enhances visualization of the neural canal and posterior elements. This increased knowledge of fracture anatomy has led many American and European authors to base clinical decisions largely on empiric radiographic criteria with relatively little regard to other patient data (Table 1). Great emphasis has been placed on rigid internal fixation of those fractures that would otherwise displace with early mobilization (11,13,14,22).

On the other hand, many authors in England and Australia advocate bed rest with or without postural reduction for these injuries (2,3,6,8,19,37). They would argue that a comminuted three-column fracture can be "stable" and the fragments can maintain their position if the patient completes a satisfactory period of recumbent management. Thereafter, the patient may be safely mobilized with some form of external support. This argument is logical, since the principles of spine fracture healing are the same that exist for healing in long bone injuries (40). Recumbency, analogous to casting a long bone fracture to prevent early angulation, is used until the fracture is "sticky" and able to support loading in an upright, braced position.

Since many clinical studies have documented healing of spinal fractures with or without operative intervention, the clinician must decide whether the potential benefits of surgery (shorter hospitalization, earlier mobilization, decreased residual deformity) is a significant advantage over the risks associated with recumbent management. In the younger patient with an isolated spinal injury, several weeks of bed rest represents virtually no long-term morbidity (32). Conversely, several groups of patients may benefit with surgical instrumentation to allow earlier and safer mobilization. These include the noncompliant patient (from head injury, poor intellect, or recalcitrance), the polytraumatized patient, the complete spinal cord injured patient, or the patient with a grossly displaced spine without bony opposition (20).

TABLE 1. *Surgical indications based on radiographic criteria*

Series	Criteria
Bohlman (4)	Loss of 40% body height
Brown (5)	1-cm retropulsion
Denis et al. (9)	Unstable type B fractures with "severe" obstruction of neural canal
Dewald (10)	All burst fractures; add anterior decompression if canal diameter is less than 10 mm
Dunn (12)	50% canal compromise
Ferguson and Allen (17)	"Tension blowout," middle column failure
Garfin (21)	50% compression–thoracic fracture; compression–lumbar fracture
Jacobs and Casey (25)	Any neurologic deficit, fracture that may result in neurologic deficit, evidence of posterior ligament disruption, or loss of 40% body height
Kostuik (30)	Significant retropulsion
Krompinger et al. (33)	Neurologic compromise (excluding sensory changes confined to a single root or loss of one grade of motor power), rotational fracture, dislocations, translational injuries, fractures with greater than 50% canal compromise and more than 30 degrees of kyphosis
Roy-Camille et al. (39)	Any neurologic deficit, any fragment producing dural compression greater than one-third body collapse
Weitzman (43)	Fracture subluxations with rupture of the interspinous ligaments, lamina and pedicle fractures of L4 and L5, any neurologic deficit, 50% wedging of the vertebral body
Willen et al. (44)	50% canal compromise, 50% compression of anterior column

FRACTURE GROUPS

Low-Energy Blunt Trauma Producing Stable Injuries Without Neurologic Deficit

Fortunately, 95% of all thoracolumbar fractures are not associated with neurologic deficit. These patients enjoy brief disability and excellent long-term prognosis (28). The injuries include anterior column compression of varying degrees, usually not exceeding 50% (21,43–45). Stricter criteria, including up to 40% (5,25) or 33% (39) loss of anterior body height have been used to define stability without need for surgical stabilization.

Isolated fractures of the spinous and transverse processes are also included in this group. In these injuries, the middle and posterior columns are intact, and radiographic features that include interpedicular widening, displacement of the posterior cortex of the body, interspinous widening, translation and facet fractures, and subluxations or dislocations are absent. On physical exam, no neurologic deficits are identified, and there is no palpable evidence of disruption of the interspinous ligaments.

The chief problem with these injuries is pain, which may be severe and often is accompanied by an ileus. Strict bed rest and adequate analgesics are prescribed. Standard hospital beds are generally adequate. Log rolling is permitted initially and upright sitting and mobilization are started when pain subsides, usually in 2 to 5 days. Ileus may require nasogastric suction and intravenous fluids. Thromboembolic prophylaxis is recommended, particularly if risk factors are present (previous thromboembolism, edema or paresis of a lower extremity, varicose veins, hypertension, cardiac disease, and obesity). Bedside physical therapy to strengthen the paraspinous muscles is prescribed.

When ambulation is initiated, external spine supports (braces or corsets) are not mandatory, though many patients do expect a supporting garment of some sort. Simple corsets, with or without stays, are inexpensive, nonconfining, and entirely suitable for this purpose (28).

High-Energy Blunt Trauma Producing Unstable Injuries With or Without Neurologic Deficit

These injuries fortunately comprise no more than 10% of all spinal injuries (28). Not only is the anterior column involved, but middle and/or posterior column injury is present. Interpedicular widening, displacement of the posterior cortex of the vertebral body, interspinous widening, sagittal translation, and facet injury may be seen. Physical examination may reveal neurologic deficits and palpable evidence of posterior ligament disruption.

If subjected to early physiologic upright loading, even if braced, these injuries may displace and cause neurologic deterioration. Advocates of nonoperative management contend these injuries may be rendered "stable" after an appropriate period of recumbency followed by bracing. Excellent functional results of this form of management have been presented in several series (2,3,6,8,19,37,42).

When choosing nonoperative management, the clinician must answer the following: What is the optimum duration of recumbency and bracing? What are the risks of recumbent management? What radiographic changes occur over time, particularly, what is the fate of the unreduced intracanal fragment? What clinical outcome can be expected?

Duration of Bed Rest and Bracing

Duration of recumbency and bracing, as outlined in other studies, appears to be largely empiric. Wide ranges of management have been described. Weitzman (43), an advocate of early ambulation, noted some patients do poorly, which "appears to be proportional to the length and duration of treatment." His series supports the concept of shortening bed rest in "stable" fractures to an average of 8 days. This regimen is followed by physiotherapy without a brace, for a total mean treatment time of 38 days. His criteria defining stable fractures (up to 50% body collapse) was based on plain film criteria alone. Most likely, he allowed inclusion of some middle column failures with retropulsion of fragments in the bony canal, yet he reported uniformly excellent results with this method.

Nicoll (37), writing in the pre-CT era, treated his "stable" fractures, that is, "wedge" fractures without rupture of the interspinous ligament, with 3 to 4 weeks of bed rest followed by ambulation without a brace. His excellent results support his hypothesis: good functional results do not depend on good anatomical results. It is probable that some of the fractures treated in this fashion also may have had middle column failure and retropulsion of fragments into the bony canal.

Bedbrook (3) felt clinical "stability" is rapidly achieved after 2 to 3 weeks of recumbent management of unstable injuries. Though recollapse of the vertebral body was common with mobilization at this time, major redisplacement was not. He therefore recommended maintenance of postural reduction and bed rest for a total of 6 to 8 weeks, at which time paravertebral callus is usually evident on radiograph. No bracing was necessary following this period; strong paravertebral muscles, conditioned by vigorous physiotherapy during recumbency, provided satisfactory support.

Gaines and Humphreys (20), who felt "clinical stability does not solely depend on abnormal anatomy of the fracture but is also dependent on the amount of loading that is applied," advocated 4 to 6 weeks of bed rest followed by bracing. Holdsworth (24) recommended a longer period of recumbency for unstable fractures—8 to 12 weeks in a plaster bed followed by a few weeks in a light jacket. Krompinger et al. (33) set forth more specific criteria regarding management of burst fractures. If the canal compromise is less than 50%, patients are managed with 3 to 4 days of bed rest followed by bracing. If the canal compromise is greater than 50%, bed rest was extended to 4 to 6 weeks, followed by bracing.

We evaluated nonoperative management of 41 burst fractures without neurologic deficit (J. E. Mumford et al., *unpublished data*). Mean canal compromise was 37% (range 16–66%), and mean percent narrowing of the midsagittal diameter was 37% (range 16–74%) at time of injury. Satisfactory clinical and radiographic results were seen following a mean duration of 4 weeks bed rest followed by 12 weeks of bracing. These time frames represent our current recommendations for nonoperative management of unstable thoracolumbar fractures.

Complications Related to Closed Management

Recumbent management is not entirely benign; several conservative series have reported varying incidences of complications, including neurologic deterioration, decubiti, deep venous thrombosis, cord infarction, and painful gibbus, instability, or stenosis, related to closed management, which required subsequent surgery (1,8,9,19,42).

Weinstein et al. (42) found no progression of neurologic deficits related to conservative treatment in 41 patients followed a mean of 20.2 years. Two of 34 patients (6%) in the Davies et al. (8) conservative series developed temporary neural deterioration that subsequently recovered to a level of function greater than before the postural reduction, enabling them to walk. Frankel et al. (19) had two neurologic deteriorations in their conservative series of 205 injuries at the thoracolumbar junction. Denis et al. (9), in their series of 29 patients with burst fractures managed nonoperatively, identified six patients (21%) who developed neurologic complications and four (14%) who exhibited objective deficit. Aglietti et al. (1) noted transient root symptoms in 15 of 222 patients (7%) who initially presented neurologically intact. No mention of neurologic deterioration is made in other conservative series (8,33,43).

Thus it appears from review of the literature that neurologic deterioration following recumbent management can occur. Should neurologic deterioration evolve over the course of management, decompression early, as we advocate, or late, as shown by Maiman et al. (34), has resulted in good recovery.

Bedbrook (3) reported a 1% to 2% incidence of decubiti and a 12% to 20% incidence of deep venous thrombosis in his experience. Davies et al. (8) had a 32% complication rate, including cord infarction, gibbus requiring spinous process excision, pulmonary embolism, and temporary neural deterioration, in their series of 32 conservatively managed burst fractures.

Late operation was required in several series for instability or stenosis. In the Weinstein et al. (42) long-term study, 7% required late operation, including one decompression for stenosis. Frankel et al. (19) had a 1% operation rate for instability, and 11% of the patients in the Willen et al. (44) conservative series required late decompression and/or stabilization within 3 to 16 months of injury.

In our experience, nonoperative management of selected burst fractures has resulted in very little morbidity.

Radiographic Changes Over Time Following Nonoperative Management

Many studies have evaluated various radiographic parameters over time following recumbent management. Variables of particular interest have included body collapse, kyphosis, and intracanal anatomy (particularly cross section of the canal area) as demonstrated by CT scan.

In the Willen et al. (44) conservative series of 54 burst fractures at T12 and L1, kyphosis had increased an average of 6° and anterior body compression had increased an average of 7% six months after injury. After 1 year, changes in either measurement were small, suggesting stabilization of the deformity. In the Krompinger et al. (33) series, 36% of the injuries at the thoracolumbar junction progressed 10° or more of kyphosis at follow-up; no thoracic and only one lumbar fracture progressed 10° or more. Aglietti et al. (1) attempted postural reduction in 93 of 222 patients in their series. At follow-up, reduction was held within 5° in 24 cases and lost to some degree in 44. In only nine cases was follow-up kyphosis angle greater than the initial measurement at injury. In the 129 patients in whom reduction was not attempted, only 29 showed a greater than 5° increase in the kyphosis angle at follow-up. Furthermore, neither the degree of kyphosis nor loss of body height could be correlated with symptoms at follow-up, a finding that has been duplicated in other series (8,36,42).

Thus it appears that bony deformity (kyphosis, body collapse), as measured by plain films, progresses marginally over time following nonoperative management. In addition, remaining residual deformity does not correlate with symptoms at follow-up.

Fate of Unreduced Intracanal Bony Fragments

Several articles have discussed fragment resorption following both nonoperative (7,18,26,33,39,42,44) and operative (5,26,27) management of burst fractures. In general, the degree of remodeling in these reports has not been accurately measured, nor has any attempt been made to correlate remodeling with other radiographic and clinical variables.

Krompinger et al. (33) noted bony remodeling in 11 of 14 patients who had greater than 25% canal compromise on initial evaluation. Clinically, five of six patients with 50% canal compromise at injury were employable, and four were actively working. The degree of remodeling was not stated. However, the remodeling process was felt to be time and age dependent, "following expected principles of bone remodeling to applied stress."

Olmstead (38) followed 22 patients an average of 42 months following nonoperative management of burst fractures. Three patients had follow-up CT scans that showed remodeling from 66% to 20% compromise. Using plain films, Willen et al. (44) demonstrated fragment resorption to some degree in 20 of 39 patients (51%) who had initial canal narrowing of less than 50%. However, larger fragments that narrowed the spinal canal more than 50% did not appear to resorb. Our data do not support this finding. We observed significant remodeling in virtually all canals with greater than 50% compromise (J. E. Mumford et al., *unpublished data*).

Chakara et al. (7) noted fragment resorption in 13 of 15 burst fractures managed conservatively at a follow-up ranging 3 months to 14 years. Cross-sectional areas of selected CT slices were determined manually by simple graphic integration after optical enlargement. Comparison of injury and follow-up studies showed "spontaneous resolution of the previously measured spinal canal stenosis," though quantitative data were not reported. Johnsson et al. (26), in their series of both operative and nonoperative burst injuries, demonstrated a mean reduction of canal compromise from 29% to 14% at an average of 31 months postinjury. Canal areas and percent compromise were "visually estimated" from CT scans. It appears from their data that remodeling occurs regardless of management, either operative or nonoperative.

Using computer digitization techniques, the mean canal compromise at injury in our series was calculated at 37% (range 16–66%). This improved to 14% (range 3–40%), a mean of 32 months after injury (J. E. Mumford et al., *unpublished data*). The pattern of remodeling was remarkably consistent throughout the series. The majority of cases demonstrated, to some degree, a "heart-shaped" spinal canal at follow-up, with preferential resorption of bone laterally and preservation of a midsagittal spike of bone (Fig. 1). This pattern of remodeling most likely accounts for the rather impressive canal remodeling compared to the small improvement in midsagittal diameter at follow-up. Some cases, with multiple CT scans at follow-up, eventually demonstrated resorption of the midsagittal spike of bone (Fig. 2).

The basis for this remodeling pattern is unclear. Anatomically, the lateral areas of maximal bone resorption correspond to the paired longitudinal channels of the anterior internal vertebral venous plexus, located in the epidural space. Perhaps these vessels exert a mechanical (via pulsations) and/or humeral influence on fragment resorption.

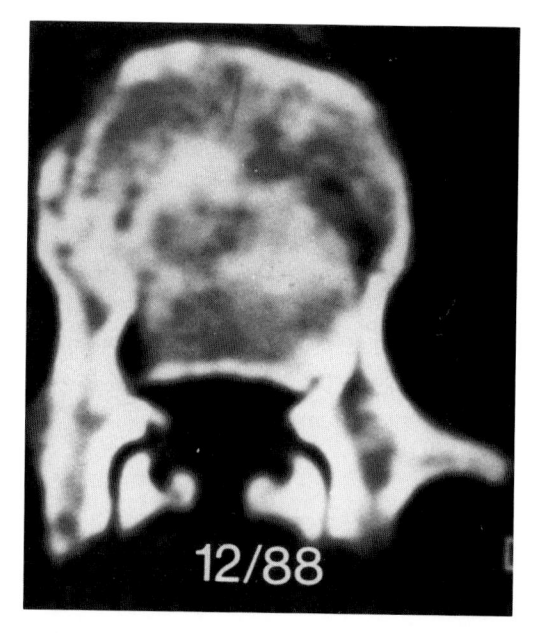

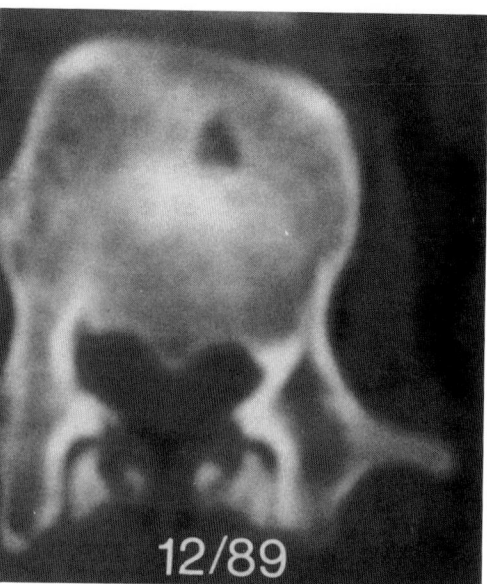

FIG. 1. Eighteen-year-old woman who sustained an L1 burst fracture following a motor vehicle accident. At the time of injury (December 1988), canal compromise and percent narrowing of midsagittal diameter measured 62% and 61%, respectively. One year later (December 1989), canal compromise and percent narrowing of midsagittal diameter measured 26% and 53%, respectively. Note the "heart-shaped" pattern of remodeling.

CLINICAL OUTCOME

The clinical outcome of nonoperative management in thoracolumbar spine fractures has generally been favorable in several large series. Outcome measures common to most studies include work status and pain.

Aglietti et al. (1) followed 222 patients for a mean of 9 years; 212 of 222 (95%) returned to work, 81% to a

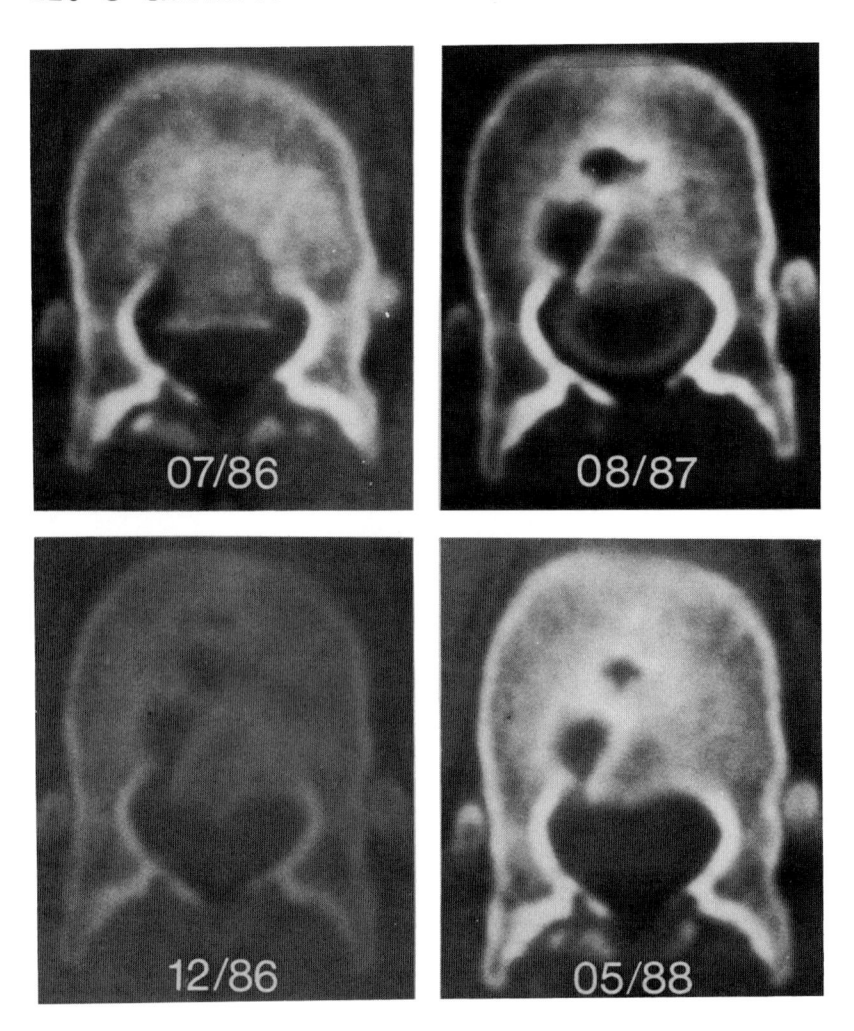

FIG. 2. Thirty-eight-year-old woman who sustained a T12 burst fracture following a fall off a one-story roof. Canal compromise at injury (July 1986) measured 34%, which improved to 9% at most recent follow-up (May 1988). Note resorption of the midsagittal spike of bone between December 1986 and August 1987.

previous job and 14% to another line of employment; only 3% were unable to return to work because of back pain. Eighty-nine percent of the patients in Nicoll's series (37) of 152 coal workers returned to mining. Roughly one-third of these patients returned to heavy labor, and two-thirds returned to lighter duty.

In the Weinstein et al. (42) long-term follow-up study, 88% of the patients were, at some time after their injury, able to work at their preinjury occupation or capacity. In our series (J. E. Mumford et al., *unpublished data*), 63% of the patients reported a same or better work status at follow-up, 23% were working but at a lower level, and 15% were unable to work. However, only 9.7% (4/41) of the patients were unable to return to work because of back complaints.

It appears from these data and the body of conservative literature that excellent functional results, as indicated by work status, can be achieved following nonoperative management of burst fractures.

At mean follow-up of 20.2 years, 38 of 42 patients (90%) in the Weinstein et al. (42) study reported some pain; the majority (62%), however, rated their pain as very little. Nicoll (37) had a 59% incidence (89 of 152) of residual pain in his series. This pain was felt either at the fracture site (40%) or low back (60%); no mention was made of radicular pain. In the Aglietti et al. (1) series, 33% of the patients (73 of 222) were pain free, 26% (58 of 222) had pain only with sports, and 32% (71 of 222) had pain that in some way impaired their work capacity at mean follow-up of 9 years. The overall incidence of some degree of back pain at follow-up in our series was 74% (J. E. Mumford et al., *unpublished data*). With few exceptions, the degree of pain was mild and did not interfere significantly with activities of daily living and work; 56% rated their pain as little or none.

Thus some degree of pain is common following conservative management of spinal injuries, though the degree of pain generally is low. This finding is supported by excellent return to work rates.

CONCLUSIONS

Nonoperative treatment of spine fractures remains a viable option and is the best approach in many instances. Appropriate clinical and radiographic assessment will often lead to a nonoperative treatment plan

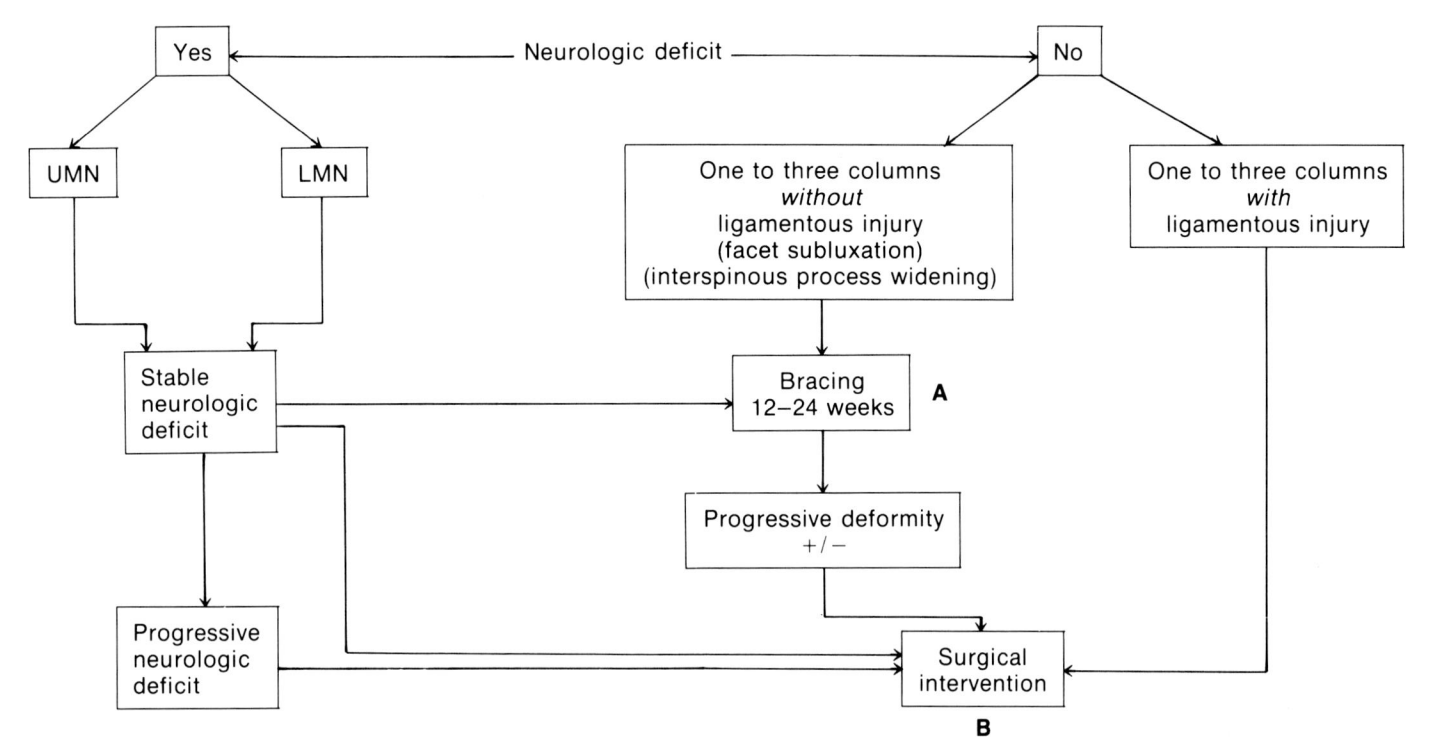

FIG. 3. An algorithm for management of thoracolumbar fractures (T11–L5). **A:** Many fractures can be managed nonoperatively. **B:** Injuries that result in progressive neurologic deficit and/or deformity and injuries with significant ligamentous injury require surgical intervention. * Canal compromise not generally correlated with neurologic deficit or outcome.

(Fig. 3). A short, 2- to 6-week course of bed rest followed by bracing in a thoracolumbar orthosis for 12 to 24 weeks in many instances yields an acceptable clinical and radiographic outcome. In our experience, nonoperative treatment, even with several weeks of hospitalization, is as cost effective or more cost effective as operative treatment.

REFERENCES

1. Aglietti P, DiMuria GV, Taylor TKF, Ruff SJ, Marcucci M, Novembri A, Innocent M. Conservative treatment of thoracic and lumbar vertebral fractures. *Ital J Orthop Traumtol (Suppl)* 1983;9:83–105.
2. Bedbrook GM. A balanced viewpoint in the early management of patients with spinal injuries who have neurological damage. *Paraplegia* 1985;23:8–15.
3. Bedbrook GM. Treatment of thoracolumbar dislocation and fractures with paraplegia. *Clin Orthop* 1975;112:27–43.
4. Bohlman HH. Current concepts review. Treatment of fractures and dislocations of the thoracic and lumbar spine. *J Bone Joint Surg* 1985;67A:165–169.
5. Brown GA. Bone resorption in the canal following a thoracolumbar fracture with a displaced diaphyseal fragment. *Iowa Orthop J* 1989;9:69–71.
6. Burke DC, Murray DD. The management of thoracic and thoracolumbar injuries of the spine with neurological involvement. *J Bone Joint Surg* 1976;58B:72–78.
7. Chakara TMH, Bedbrook G, Bradley CM. Spontaneous resolution of spinal canal deformity after burst dispersion injury. *AJNR* 1988;9:779–785.
8. Davies WE, Morris JH, Hill V. An analysis of conservative (nonsurgical) management of thoracolumbar fractures and fracture dislocations with neural damage. *J Bone Joint Surg* 1980;62A: 1324–1328.
9. Denis F, Armstrong GWD, Searls K, Matta L. Acute thoracolumbar burst fractures in the absence of neurologic deficit. A comparison between operative and nonoperative treatment. *Clin Orthop* 1984;189:142–149.
10. Dewald RL. Burst fractures of the thoracic and lumbar spine. *Clin Orthop* 1984;189:150–161.
11. Dickson JH, Harrington PR, Ewin WD. Results of reduction and stabilization of the severely fractured thoracic and lumbar spine. *J Bone Joint Surg* 1978;60A:799–805.
12. Dunn HK. Thoracolumbar spine trauma. In: Fitzgerald RH, ed. *Orthopedic knowledge update 2*, Park Ridge IL: American Academy of Orthopaedic Surgeons, 1986;295–301.
13. Dunn HK. Anterior spine stabilization and decompression for thoracolumbar injuries. *Orthop Clin North Am* 1986;17(1): 113–119.
14. Edwards CC, Levine AM. Early rod-sleeve stabilization and decompression for thoracolumbar injuries. *Orthop Clin North Am* 1986;17(1):121–145.

15. Faerber EN, Wolpert SM, Scott RM, Belkin SC, Carter BL. Computed tomography of spinal fractures. *J Comput Assist Tomogr* 1979;3(5):657–661.
16. Fang D, Loeng JCY, Cheung HC. The treatment of thoracolumbar spinal injuries with paresis by conservative versus surgical methods. *Ann Acad Med* 1982;11(2):203–206.
17. Ferguson RL, Allen BL. An algorithm for the treatment of unstable thoracolumbar fractures. *Orthop Clin North Am* 1986;17(1):105–112.
18. Fidler MW. Remodeling of the spinal canal after burst fracture: a prospective study of two cases. *J Bone Joint Surg* 1988;70B(5):730–732.
19. Frankel HC, Hancock DO, Hyslop G, Melzek J, Michaelis LS, Ungar GH, Vernon DS, Walsh JJ. The value of postural reduction in the initial management of closed injuries of the spine with paraplegia and tetraplegia. *Paraplegia* 1969;7:179–192.
20. Gaines RW, Humphreys WG. A plea for judgment in management of thoracolumbar fractures and fracture dislocations. A reassessment of surgical indications. *Clin Orthop* 1984;189:36–42.
21. Garfin SR. Thoracolumbar spine trauma. In: Poss R, ed. *Orthopedic knowledge update 3*. Park Ridge IL: American Academy of Orthopaedic Surgeons, 1990;425–440.
22. Gertzbein SD, MacMichael D, Tile M. Harrington instrumentation as a method of fixation in fractures of the spine. *J Bone Joint Surg* 1982;64B:526–529.
23. Gertzbein SD, Court-Brown CM, Marks P, Martin C, Fazl M, Schwartz M, Jacobs RR. Neurological outcome following surgery for spinal fractures. *Spine* 1988;13(6):641–644.
24. Holdsworth F. Fractures, dislocations and fracture–dislocations of the spine. *J Bone Joint Surg* 1970;53A:1534–1559.
25. Jacobs RR, Casey MP. Surgical management of thoracolumbar spinal injuries. *Clin Orthop* 1984;189:22–35.
26. Johnsson R, Herrlin K, Hagglund G, Stromquist B. Spinal canal remodeling after thoracolumbar fractures with intraspinal bone fragments. *Acta Orthop Scand* 1991;62(2):125–127.
27. Karlstrom G, Olerud S, Sjostrom L. Transpedicular fixation of thoracolumbar fractures. *Contemp Orthop* 1990;20(3):285–300.
28. Kaufer H, Kling T. Part II: The thoracolumbar spine. In: Rockwood CA, Green DP, eds. *Fracture in adults*. Philadelphia: Lippincott, 1984.
29. Keene JS, Goletz TH, Lilleas F, Alter AJ, Sackett JF. Diagnosis of vertebral fractures. *J Bone Joint Surg* 1982;64A:586–595.
30. Kostuik JP. Anterior fixation for fractures of the thoracic and lumbar spine with or without neurologic involvement. *Clin Orthop* 1984;189:103–115.
31. Kostuik JP, Hulor RJ, Esses SI, Stauffer ES. Thoracolumbar spine fractures. In: Frymoyer JW, ed. *The adult spine: principles and practice*. New York: Raven Press, 1991;1269–1325.
32. Kottke FJ. The effects of limitation of activity upon the human body. *JAMA* 1966;296:117.
33. Krompinger WJ, Frederickson BE, Mino DE, Yuan HA. Conservative treatment of fractures of the thoracic and lumbar spine. *Orthop Clin North Am* 1986;17:161–170.
34. Maiman DJ, Larson SJ, Benzel EC. Neurologic improvement associated with late decompression of the thoracolumbar spine. *Neurosurgery* 1984;14(3):302–307.
35. McAfee PC, Yuan HA, Frederickson BE, Lubicky JP. The value of computed tomography in thoracolumbar fractures. *J Bone Joint Surg* 1983;65A:461–473.
36. McEvoy RD, Bradford DS. The management of burst fractures of the thoracic and lumbar spine. Experience in 53 patients. *Spine* 1985;10:631–637.
37. Nicoll EA. Fractures of the dorsolumbar spine. *J Bone Joint Surg* 1949;31B:376–394.
38. Olmstead TG. Nonoperative management of thoracolumbar burst fractures. Presented at the Canadian Orthopaedic Association, June 5, 1990.
39. Roy-Camille R, Saillant G, Mazel C. Plating of thoracic, thoracolumbar and lumbar injuries with pedicle screw plates. *Orthop Clin North Am* 1986;17:105–112.
40. Schmorl G, Junghans H. *The human spine in health and disease*. New York: Grune & Stratton, 1971;290–291.
41. Tadmor R, Davis KR, Roberson GH, New PFJ, Taveras JM. Computed tomographic evaluation of traumatic spinal injuries. *Radiology* 1978;127:825–827.
42. Weinstein JN, Collalto P, Lehman TR. Thoracolumbar "burst" fractures treated conservatively: a long-term follow-up. *Spine* 1988;13:33–38.
43. Weitzman G. Treatment of stable thoracolumbar spine compression fractures by early ambulation. *Clin Orthop* 1971;76:116–122.
44. Willen J, Anderson J, Toomoka K, Singer K. The natural history of burst fractures at the thoracolumbar junction. *J Spinal Disord* 1990;3(1):39–46.
45. Willen J, Lindahl S, Nordwall A. Unstable thoracolumbar fractures: a comparative clinical study of conservative treatment and Harrington instrumentation. *Spine* 1985;10(2):122.

17

Low Lumbar (L3–L4–L5) Burst Fractures

Keith H. Bridwell

Treatment and management considerations for low lumbar burst (disruption of middle column) (6) fractures are somewhat different than for the rest of the axial skeleton. In this area of the spine, one is dealing entirely with the cauda equina and nerve roots with no spinal cord in the usual circumstance. The only case in which one will be dealing with spinal cord in this area is if the patient has a chronically tethered cord. Burst fractures of the low lumbar spine often involve significant displacement of the posterior elements with vertical laminar fractures in which the dura and posteriorly displaced nerve roots are trapped (4,7). Often the cause of the neurologic deficit may in fact be displacement of nerve roots through the vertical lamina fracture rather than from direct anterior compression from the retropulsed bony fragments (see Case 2).

Fixation of low lumbar spine fractures has been a problem (2,5). In the past there have been advocates of either nonoperative treatment or treatment with casts rather than internal fixation (8). Certainly not all burst fractures require surgical treatment (12). The recent popularization of pedicle fixation has revolutionized the approach to low lumbar fractures.

TREATMENT CONSIDERATIONS

Sagittal Profile

The majority (76%) of lumbar lordosis exists between L3 and the sacrum. There is wide variation in what is considered normal (3). However, an average total lumbar lordosis is 40° to 60° (3,10). The most lordotic segments are L3–L4, L4–L5, and L5–S1 (Fig. 1). Some of this lordosis exists within the vertebral bodies but much also comes from the disc spaces (Table 1) (10). With spinal fractures and burst fractures in particular, there is loss of anterior column height not

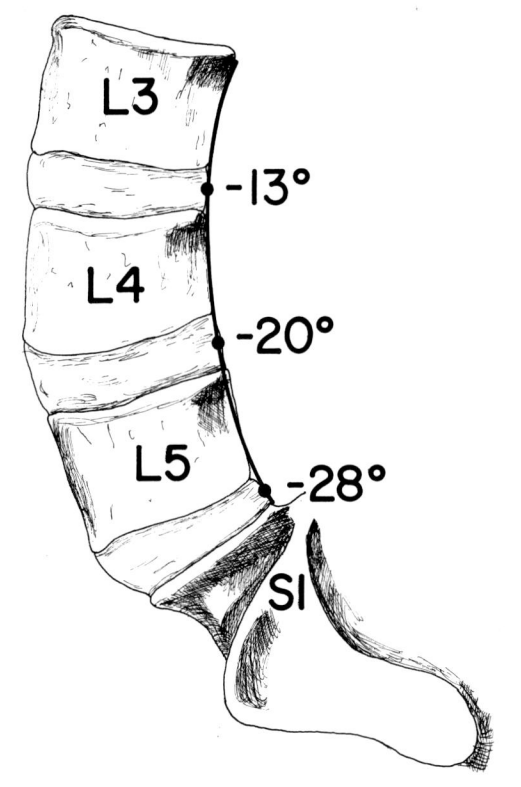

FIG. 1. Adjusted mean segmental angulations. (From ref. 3.)

TABLE 1. *Mean segmental distribution of lumbar lordosis*

Discs	Degrees	Vertebra	Degrees
L3–L4	−9°	L3	−2°
L4–L5	−11°	L4	−4°
L5–S1	−11°	L5	−10°

The mean sagittal Cobb angle from L4 to S1 is −36°. From ref. 10.

K. H. Bridwell: Division of Orthopaedic Surgery, Washington University School of Medicine, St. Louis, MO 63110.

only from reduction of anterior and posterior vertebral body height but also from reduction of disc height (Table I and Fig. 1) (see also Case 3).

One of the goals of treatment of spinal fractures is to restore the sagittal profile to a nearly normal configuration. This is not particularly easy for low lumbar burst fractures. One of the problems is that it is very difficult to brace or cast this area of the axial skeleton. The only feasible form of external immobilization is a cast or brace with one or both thighs incorporated. Although this is useful in some cases, it is cumbersome. Patients cannot sit and cannot use the toilet very well with this device, although they are able to ambulate satisfactorily with one thigh incorporated.

Initial attempts at fixation with contoured Harrington rods, with and without wire fixation in the form of either Wisconsin or sublaminar wires, were not particularly helpful. The usual scenario was one of immediate postoperative reconstitution of vertebral body height. However, with time, this would usually be lost and quite often an iatrogenic flat back would be created. A rod long fuse short type of construct would do the least amount of harm. However, at present, the use of Harrington instrumentation for a low lumbar burst is obsolete.

Presently, pedicle fixation offers an alternative fixation of these fractures. Although segmental hook rod devices such as the Texas Scottish Rite and C-D instrumentation offer advantages (11) for thoracic and upper lumbar burst fractures, Harrington instrumentation can still provide satisfactory results. In the low lumbar spine, a device consisting of hooks and rods has its limitations due to the thin L5 and sacral laminae. Even with the use of pedicle fixation, it is quite difficult to adequately control and restore the sagittal plane. Levine and Edwards (9) found that if one pedicle is attached to the vertebral body at the level of the burst, fixing a pedicle screw at the level of the burst is helpful in maintaining lordosis. The most efficient method to restore and maintain sagittal profile for these fractures is a combination of middle column decompression, posterior pedicle fixation with a tension band compression effect, and an anterior lengthening/strut (see Case 4).

If it is a burst fracture without subluxation or wide displacement of the posterior elements, then quite often a construct of one above to one below is satisfactory. However, if there is a forward listhesis/subluxation through the burst, it is often necessary to have two fixation points below and one above. Likewise, if there is a retrolisthesis through the burst fracture, it is necessary to have two fixation points above and one below to first reduce the subluxation component that is associated with the burst fracture. A subluxation component mandates posterior instrumentation and reduction before anterior decompression (Case 1).

CASE 1. Patient has a burst subluxation at L3–L4 (Fig. 2). There is a relative retrolisthesis of L3 on L4. The patient also has a relatively stable burst fracture (no subluxation) of L1 with a significant amount of bony retropulsion. For this kind of fracture at L3–L4 it is mandatory to approach the spine posteriorly first and to reduce the subluxation. In this case, reducing the subluxation is accomplished by two proximal points of fixation and one distal point of fixation. The displacements of the posterior elements and pedicles are great enough that it is not possible to safely apply pedicle screws at L4. It is not necessary to instrument down to the sacrum because the subluxation is a retrolisthesis. The subluxation is reduced by contouring the Cotrel–Dubousset (C-D) rods and engaging them into the open pedicle screws. No distraction or compression force is applied. Disruption of the dura extends all the way from the pedicle of L4 to the pedicle of L5. Prior to reduction of the subluxation, the nerve roots are replaced into the thecal sac and the dura is repaired at L4. The patient's neurologic deficit is quadriceps and anterior tibialis weakness of the right side. It appears that there is no neurologic deficit from the L1 burst fracture although there is significant bony retropulsion at this level. Should we not have instrumented the L1 fracture? We instrumented the spine from T11 to L5 and only fused L3 to L5. Eventually this patient had an anterior fusion from T12 to L1 and from L3 to L5. Removal of the posterior instrumentation is planned 6 to 12 months postoperatively. The anterior procedure was staged because the patient had very extensive deep burns throughout her trunk and abdomen and developed intraoperative disseminated intravascular coagulation (DIC) during the posterior procedure.

Neural Decompression

Appropriate decompressions are posterior, posterolateral, and anterior. If the nerve roots and dura are trapped in a vertical laminar fracture, it is mandatory that the fracture be approached posteriorly first. Bursts with displaced posterior element fractures through both cortices (anterior and posterior) and vertebral body retropulsion that seems to virtually touch the lamina (Cases 1 and 2) are strong clues. Therefore computerized tomography (CT) scans with axial cuts are mandatory for low lumbar burst fractures. One has to exercise care in stripping the spine to be sure that the nerve roots are not injured during exposure. In this situation it is quite important to atraumatically reduce the nerve roots inside the thecal sac and to repair the sac. Repair can be accomplished with direct suturing or with a piece of fascia (either allograft or autograft). Usually the dural lacerations are vertical/longitudinal. It is important to surround the area of dural tear before

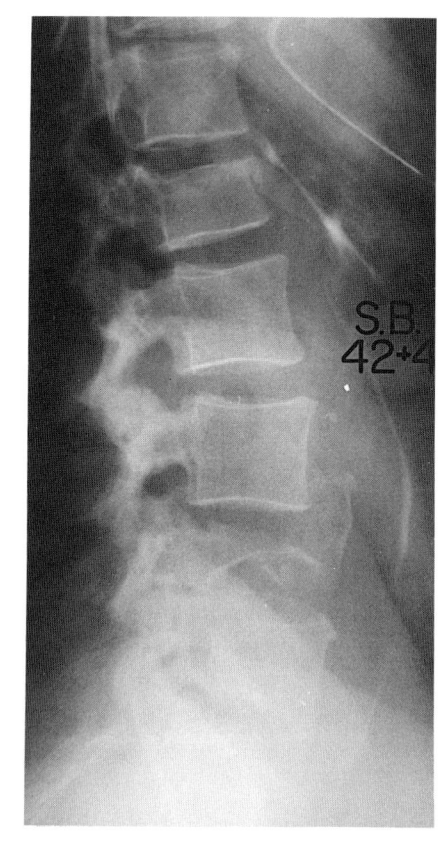

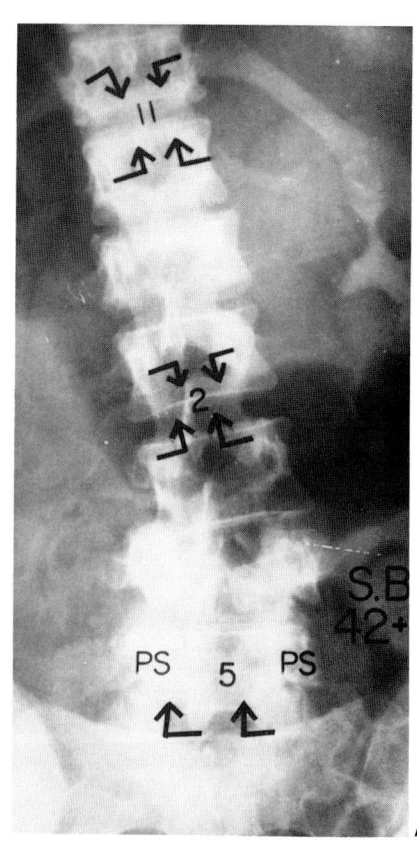

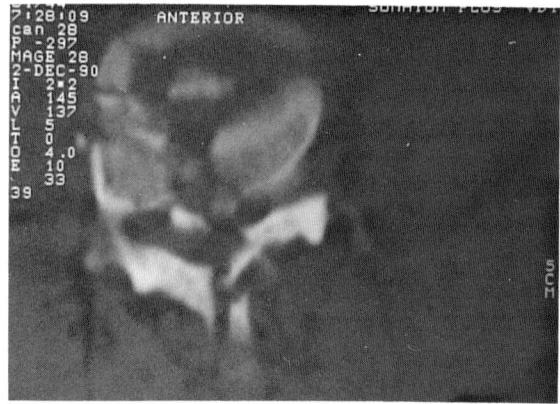

FIG. 2. (Case 1) **A,B:** Burst dislocation at L3–L4 and a stable burst fracture at L1. Note that the L3 vertebral body sits posterior to the L5 vertebral body in the sagittal plane. **C:** Note the widely displaced posterior element fractures at L4. **D:** Note the amount of bony retropulsion at L1. Note the improvement in the coronal **(E)** and sagittal **(F)** deformities. The subluxation at L3–L4 has been reduced and the L4 vertebral body takes on a more nearly normal appearance. Reduction of deformity is entirely from rod contouring and engagement into the hooks and screws. Posterior spinal fusion is performed from L3 to L5. **G:** Anterior spinal fusion (ASF) with fibular (autogenous) struts L3–L5. ASF was also done at T12–L1.

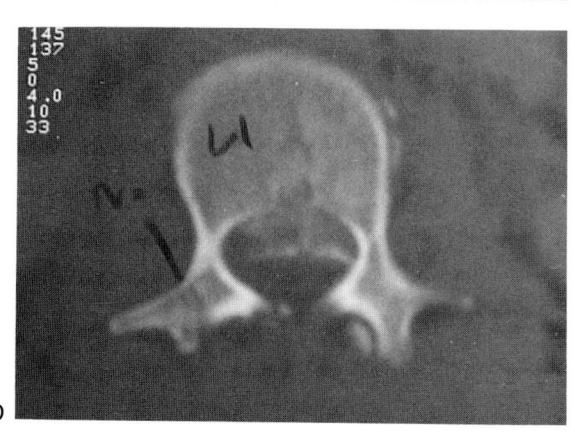

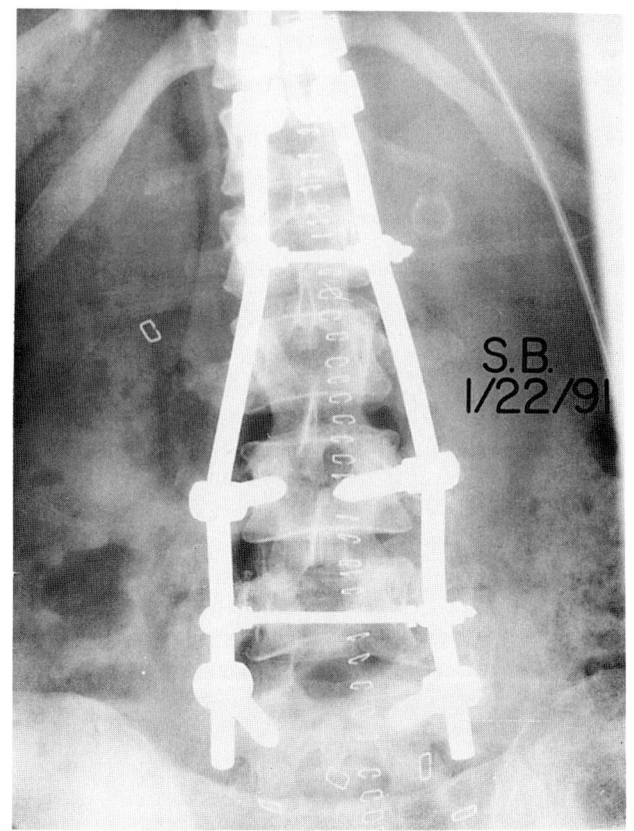

Figure continues on page 226.

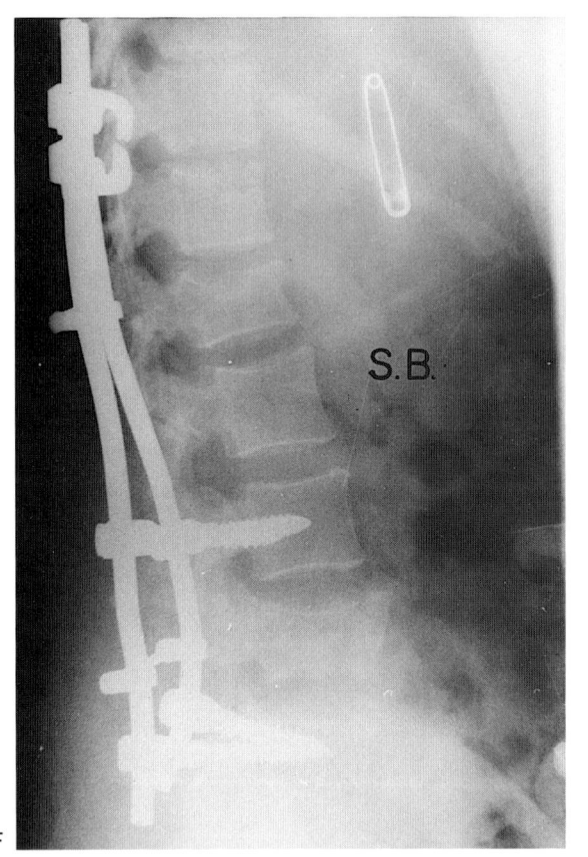

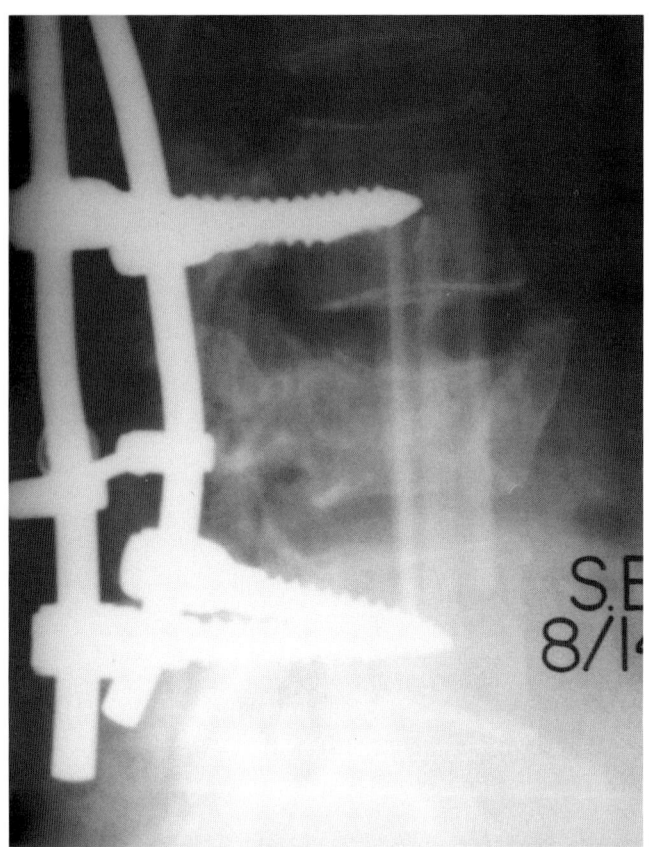

FIG. 2. (Case 1) *Continued.*

trying to repair the dura and replace the nerve roots. This can be performed by either enlarging the laminectomy defect that has been created by the fracture or by performing a laminoplasty. Either way, it is important not to initially place a Kerrison rongeur directly into the fracture site. It is important to start well away from the vertical fracture and work the ends to the middle to avoid inadvertently injuring a nerve root. Once the dura has been repaired and the nerve roots replaced, one can proceed with fixation of the spine and reduction of the deformity.

CASE 2. Patient has a burst fracture of L4 with bony retropulsion and displacement of the vertical laminar fracture (Fig. 3). There is no subluxation but note the left L3–L4 joint. The patient's neurologic deficit involves distal sacral roots with perianal and perigenital numbness and some difficulty with bowel and bladder control. This points to the patient's neurologic deficit being caused by displacement of his posterior nerve roots through the laminar fracture rather than by compression of the more anteriorly placed L4 and L5 nerve roots. At the time of the posterior procedure, the nerve roots are carefully replaced into the thecal sac. The dural tear is repaired with interrupted 5-0 suture. The fracture is then stabilized with pedicle fixation from L3 to L5 and a posterior spinal fusion is performed with posterior autogenous iliac bone graft. Should an anterior decompression be performed? The patient's neurologic deficit appears to be entirely from injury to more posteriorly displaced nerve roots. Should compression be applied to the posterior column and should the anterior column be grafted? It would be unsafe to apply compression to the posterior column without first decompressing the middle column. So some loss of sagittal profile was accepted in this case.

At L5 it is quite common for the retropulsed bone to be asymmetrical and unilateral. If this is the case, there is a role for a unilateral posterolateral decompression. This requires a laminotomy on the side of the retropulsed bony fragments with identification of the cauda equina and L5 nerve root and retraction of it over the retropulsed fragments. If they are a problem, anterior epidural veins are controlled with a bipolar. Then either directly removing the retropulsed fragment(s) or drilling a hole in the vertebral body anterior to the fragments and pushing bone anteriorly is accomplished. The decompression should continue until the cauda equina and L5 nerve root are free enough that they are easily retractable with a Penfield elevator (Case 3).

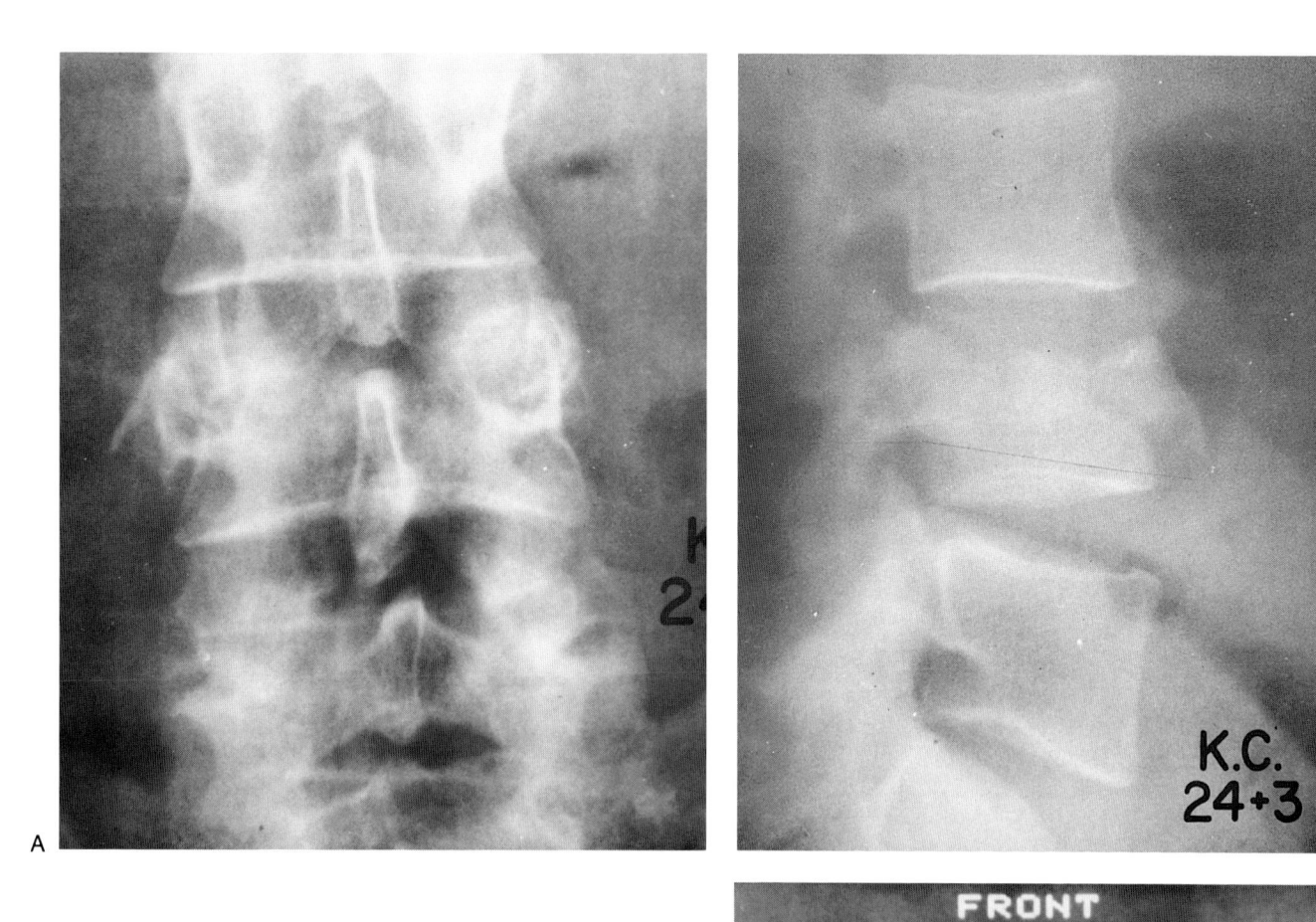

FIG. 3. (Case 2) **A,B:** Burst fracture of L4. No apparent subluxation in either the coronal or sagittal plane. Disruption of the superior endplate at L4 but the inferior endplate and L4–L5 disc appear preserved. Note on the AP radiograph the disruption of the L3–L4 facet joint on the left side. **C:** CT scan showing significant retropulsion of bone into the spinal canal and a displaced vertical laminar fracture on the left side. The nerve roots are trapped in this vertical laminar fracture.

Figure continues on the following page.

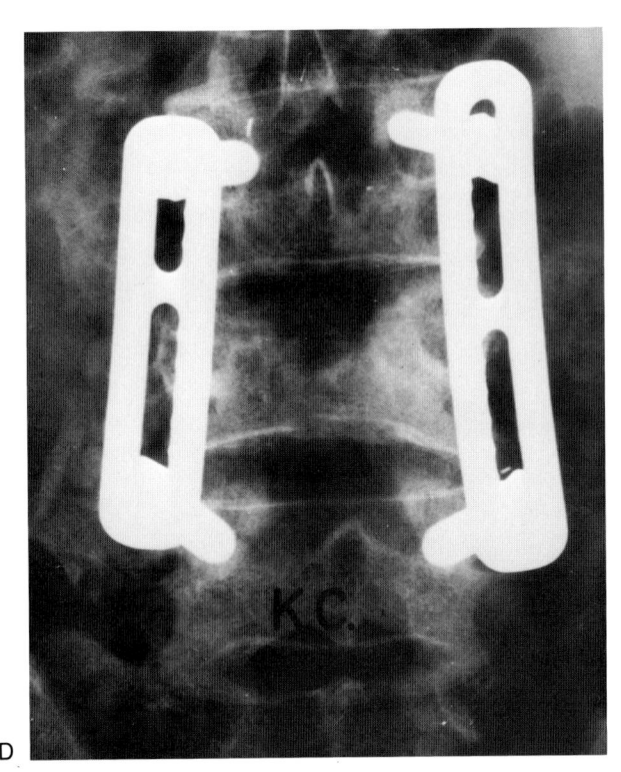

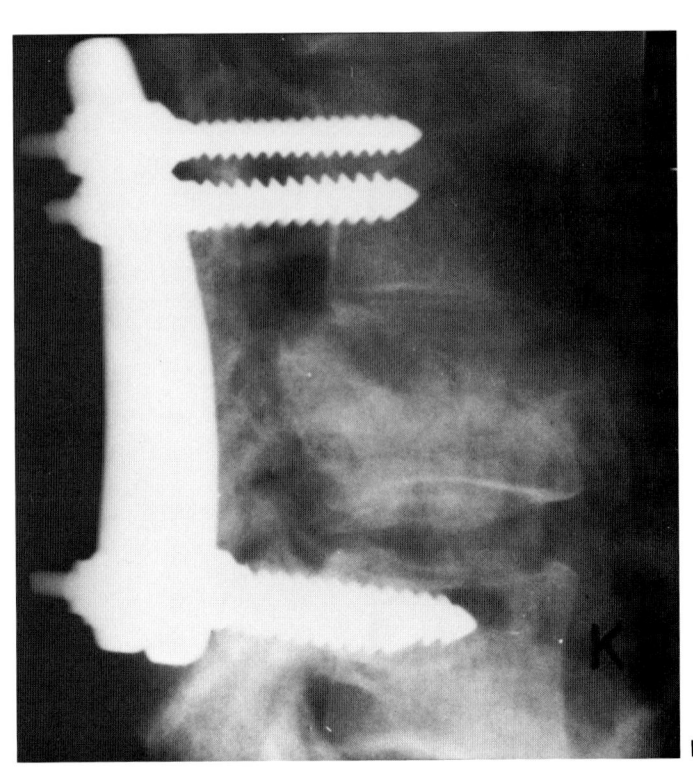

FIG. 3. (Case 2) (*Continued*) **D,E:** AP and lateral radiographs at 1 year postoperatively showing a solid spine fusion. No change in the sagittal angle from L3 to L5. The sagittal Cobb angle is roughly 0°. There is no actual kyphosis but there is relative kyphosis compared to the lordosis that normally exists between L3 and L5. The sagittal angle is not worse than it was preoperatively, but there has been settling through the L3–L4 disc space. In this case it might have been possible to safely perform transpedicular fixation at L4 on the right side to further control the sagittal plane.

CASE 3. A 15-year-old girl has a burst fracture of L5 demonstrating considerable loss of anterior column height both through bone and through disc (Fig. 4). She has weakness of her anterior tibialis, extensor hallucis longus, and a very pronounced sciatic nerve tension sign on the right side. Note on the computerized tomography (CT) scan that the retropulsion is mainly on the right side. She is therefore treated with a right unilateral posterolateral decompression at L5. After the decompression we considered pedicle fixation from L4 to the sacrum. However, any pedicle fixation in L4 runs a concern of disruption of the L3–L4 facet joint. In such a young patient we have to concern ourselves with the long-term morbidity of our fixation. In this case, we probably could have used pedicle fixation in L5 on the left side as well as L4 and S1 bilaterally. Pedicle fixation would have only been helpful if coupled with an anterior strut grafting to increase anterior column height. We performed posterior fusion in situ and placed the patient in a hyperextension cast initially with both thighs incorporated for the first 6 weeks and then ambulated the patient with one thigh incorporated for the ensuing 6 weeks. Her clinical results have been quite good but note that she has healed with a significant kyphosis from L4 to the sacrum. She does not have any clinical deformity from this and at this point has no pain. Will this kyphotic deformity predispose her upper and middle lumbar segments to prematurely degenerate?

A direct anterior decompression is considered if the retropulsion of bone is evenly distributed. If there are widely displaced posterior element fractures and a subluxation in either the coronal or the sagittal plane, it is mandatory that the fracture be approached posteriorly first. The anterior approaches to the spine can be anterolateral or directly anterior through retroperitoneal flank, retroperitoneal paramedian, or transperitoneal approaches.

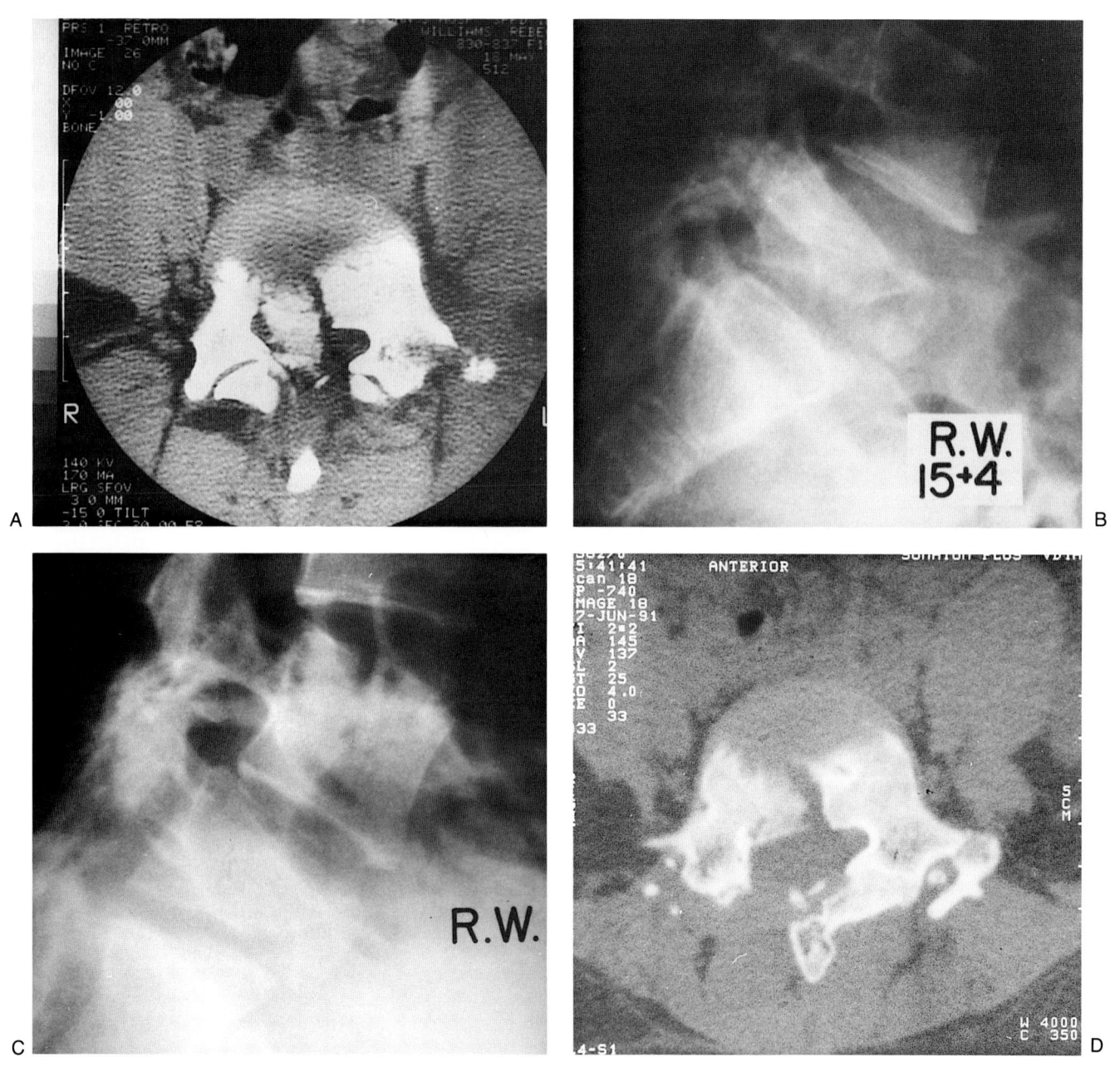

FIG. 4. (Case 3) **A:** CT scan at L5. The retropulsion of bone is asymmetrical. **B:** Preoperative lateral radiograph on the supine patient. Note reduction of both superior and inferior disc heights and reduction of anterior vertebral body height. Loss of the physiologic lordosis from L4 to the sacrum. **C:** The patient at 1 year postoperatively. Solid posterior spine fusion from L4 to sacrum. However, further collapse into kyphosis has occurred through the L4–L5 disc. Perhaps an anterior fusion should have been performed at least at L4–L5 through that disc space to prevent the further kyphotic collapse that occurred. **D:** The CT scan 13 months postoperatively showing the decompression.

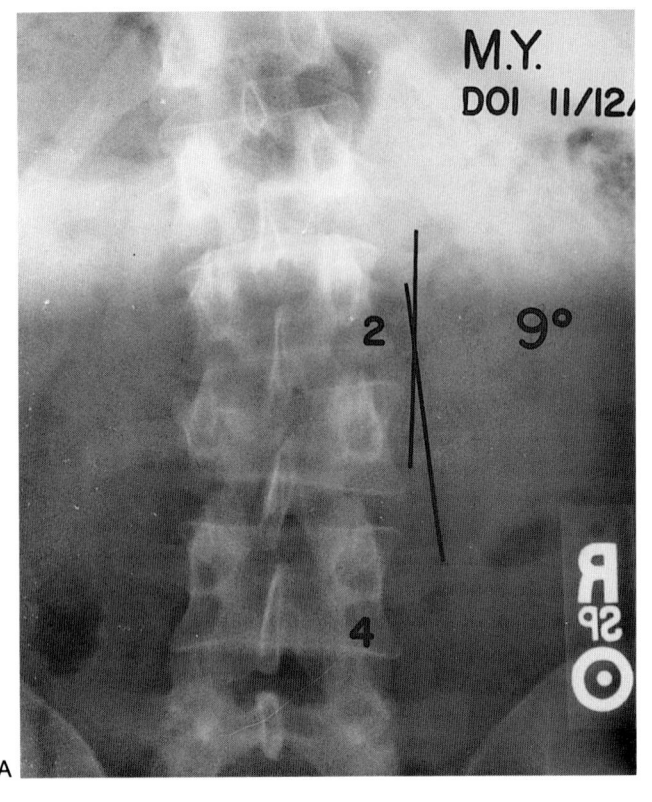

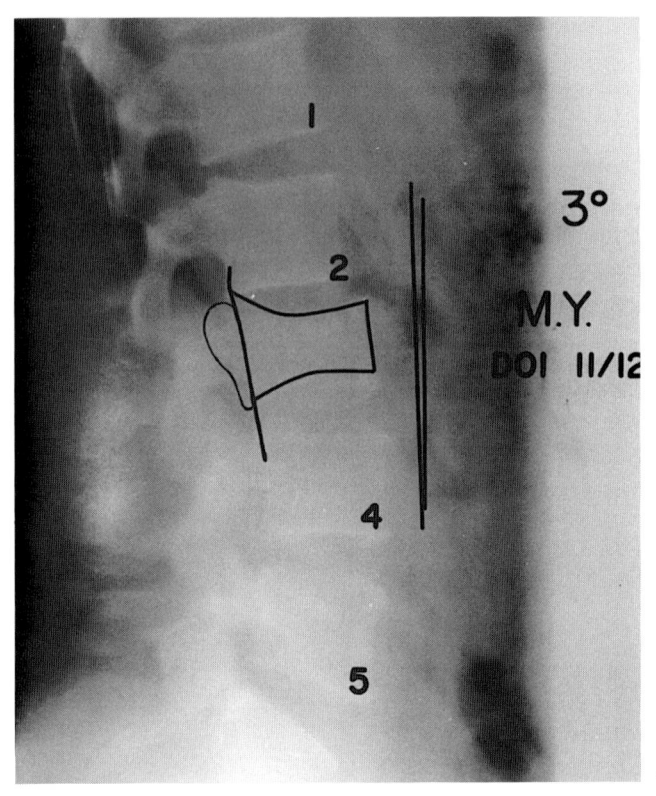

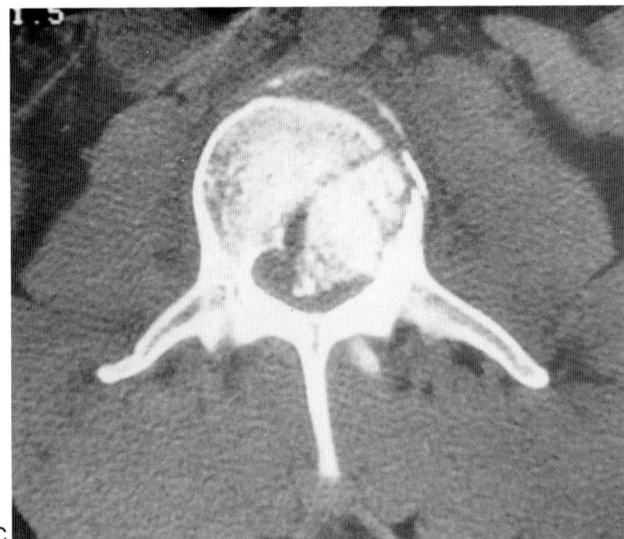

FIG. 5. A,B: Burst fracture of L3. Preoperative coronal and sagittal radiographs. **C:** Preoperative CT scan. **D,E:** Postoperative radiographs demonstrating solid spine fusion.

ANTERIOR APPROACH

Retroperitoneal Flank Approach

The retroperitoneal flank approach is applicable to fractures that require exposure to L5. If only the lumbar spine needs to be exposed, a flank incision through the tip of the 12th or 11th rib is most appropriate. Resecting the tip of either of these ribs allows one to enter into the retroperitoneum. Once the external oblique muscle and the tip of the rib have been incised, the next step is entering into the retroperitoneum through the bed of that rib. Then one sweeps the peritoneum off the undersurface of the transversus abdominis muscle and incises the internal oblique and transversus abdominis muscles parallel to the skin incision. The next step is to sweep the peritoneum off the psoas muscle and to mobilize the ureter and kidney anteriorly. Next is identification of the interval between the great ves-

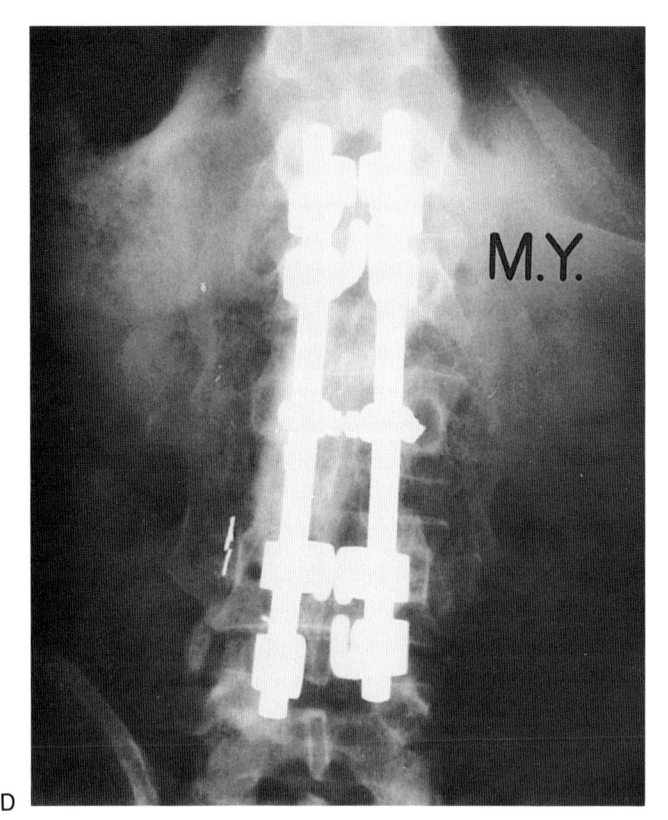

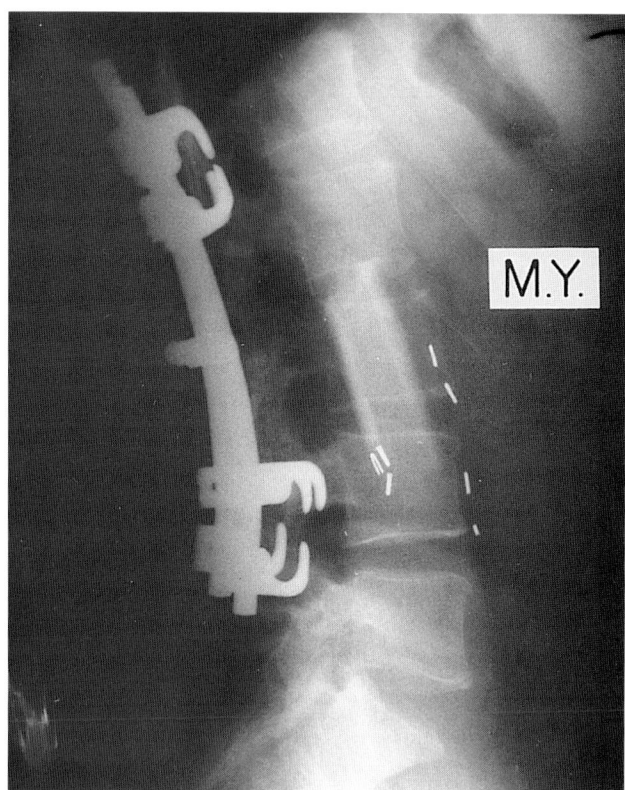

FIG. 5. (Case 4) Continued.

sels and psoas muscle and then finally identification, ligation, and cutting of the segmental vessels at the level of the fracture and one above and one below. Exposure of the vertebral bodies needs to extend anteriorly around to the other side and posteriorly back to the pedicles. Either malleable retractors or sponge sticks are placed anteriorly between the great vessels and vertebral bodies. One needs to take care in retracting the psoas muscle posteriorly. Too vigorous retraction can stretch the femoral nerve.

CASE 4. This is a stable burst fracture of L3 with an incomplete neurologic deficit (Fig. 5). There is no subluxation in either the coronal or sagittal plane. The patient is treated with an anterior decompression and strut grafting performed through an anterolateral approach. It is important to decompress the middle column before applying compression through the posterior column. After the decompression, the spine is supported anteriorly with a fresh frozen tibial allograft with the marrow cavity packed with the patient's own cancellous bone (the resected vertebral body). It is fixed posteriorly with the C-D claw technique. Pedicle fixation would be reasonable as well. Anterior column height is maintained with a strut graft and instrumentation maintains a posterior tension band effect.

This exposure works quite well down to L5, even down to the L5–S1 disc in most cases. There are problems with anterior instrumentation through the anterolateral approach at L5 and the sacrum. It is difficult to place screws anteriorly in L5 because the ilium complicates the placement of screws in the correct orientation. Also, screws in L5 may contact the great vessels after the retractors have been removed. However, at L5 the tendency is for the vein to fall over the instrumentation rather than the artery. Anchoring the strut graft into L5 presents no problem with this approach. Anchoring a strut into the sacrum is technically difficult with the anterolateral approach.

Retroperitoneal Paramedian Approach

For this approach the patient is positioned supine. The interval between the rectus and oblique muscles is identified distally. The interval between the posterior fascia and the peritoneum is developed and the peritoneum is swept off the iliac fossa. The peritoneum is then swept off the psoas muscle and the anterior fascia is divided the rest of the way from distal to proximal. This provides direct midline anterior exposure of the spine (1). The psoas muscle is less of an obstacle with this than the anterolateral approach. This approach is ideal for exposure of L5–S1 below the vascular bifurcation. It can provide exposure up to L2–L3. It is difficult to expose any higher than L2–L3 without having to swing the incision obliquely toward the rib cage. The kidney limits the proximal extent of the exposure.

For anterior decompression of an L5 fracture, this exposure is quite useful. At times, to facilitate midline exposure, it is helpful to incise some of the rectus fascia transversely. One limitation of this exposure is that any decompression involves removing the anteriormost portion of the vertebral body. In the anterolateral approach, it is possible to leave an anterior shell and the anterior longitudinal ligament (ALL) to help revascularization of the bone graft. However, with a direct anterior approach that anterior shell and the ALL, to some extent, are sacrificed, although the lateral vertebral body walls can be preserved. The direct anterior approach is preferable when it is necessary to place a strut graft from L4 into the sacrum. The strut graft should be taller anteriorly than posteriorly to preserve lordosis. One limitation of the midline anterior approach is fixation. However, it is possible to place flat plates such as the Yuan plate from L4 to the sacrum. If one places a plate directly anteriorly from L4 to the sacrum, the vein tends to fall back on the plate rather than the artery. However, if the screws back out they are going to be in immediate contact with the great vessels! Perhaps the Yuan plates can be modified to be self-locking as are the A-O (Morscher) cervical plates.

Any anterior exposure of the spine at L5–S1 runs a risk of damaging the sympathetic plexus and causing retrograde ejaculation in the male. Trying not to use the Bovie, isolating the sympathetic chain with a vascular loop, and careful retraction are helpful. When extensive exposure around the sacrum is needed, it is best to place vessel loops entirely under the bifurcation and the limb of the left iliac artery and vein. At times, this requires ligation of several sacral veins, which can be troublesome. The sacral veins are often quite short and run directly from the left common iliac vein into the sacrum.

Transperitoneal Anterior Approach

The transperitoneal anterior approach provides the same exposure as a paramedian retroperitoneal approach. One disadvantage is that the peritoneum cannot be retracted as a single sac, which complicates exposure. Entering the peritoneum increases the morbidity of the surgery and increases the potential for intra-abdominal adhesions. The lumbosacral junction can be exposed in a retroperitoneal fashion. One indication for a transperitoneal approach is if there is ongoing surgery in the peritoneum; for example, if general surgeons are inside the peritoneum to repair a ruptured spleen and the spine surgeon is contemplating a corpectomy at the same anesthesia.

INDICATIONS FOR ANTERIOR APPROACH

Sagittal Profile

If the patient's spine has not fallen into much kyphosis and if a large posterolateral or anterolateral decompression is not necessary, then the sagittal plane may be controlled entirely with posterior pedicle screw fixation. However, if the patient's spine has fallen into significant kyphosis, the only way to restore lordosis is with a combined anterior–posterior approach. The first step of the approach is to decompress the cauda equina and remove any retropulsion of bone and disc on the anterior neural elements. Once this is performed, posterior compression forces can safely be applied. It is then mandatory to maintain and restore anterior height with some form of strut graft (Fig. 6). If any subluxation exists or if one suspects that the nerve roots are trapped in the posterior elements, it is mandatory to approach the spine posteriorly first.

Decompression

For decompression purposes, the anterior approach is considered when an incomplete neurologic deficit is caused by the retropulsion of bony fragments and disc. If the retropulsion is asymmetric and unilateral, it is often easier to address this with a posterolateral approach. If bony retropulsion extends all the way across the pedicles, the decompression is probably best done anteriorly. Other indications for anterior reconstruction are loss of anterior column height by the initial fracture and/or by a wide anterior or posterolateral decompression, which begs for additional anterior support.

Difficulties

It is more difficult to control the sagittal plane in the lower lumbar spine than in the thoracic and upper lumbar spine. Problems with controlling the sagittal plane in the lower lumbar spine include difficulties with the anterior exposure and difficulties with fixation to the sacrum (controlling the distal moment arm). Generally, with any fixation of the sacrum, it is necessary that the sacral screws either penetrate the anterior cortex or penetrate the anterior–superior endplate of the sacrum. In some instances, it may be advisable to use four sacral screws instead of two. A standard TLSO or low profile TLSO may actually increase the stresses at

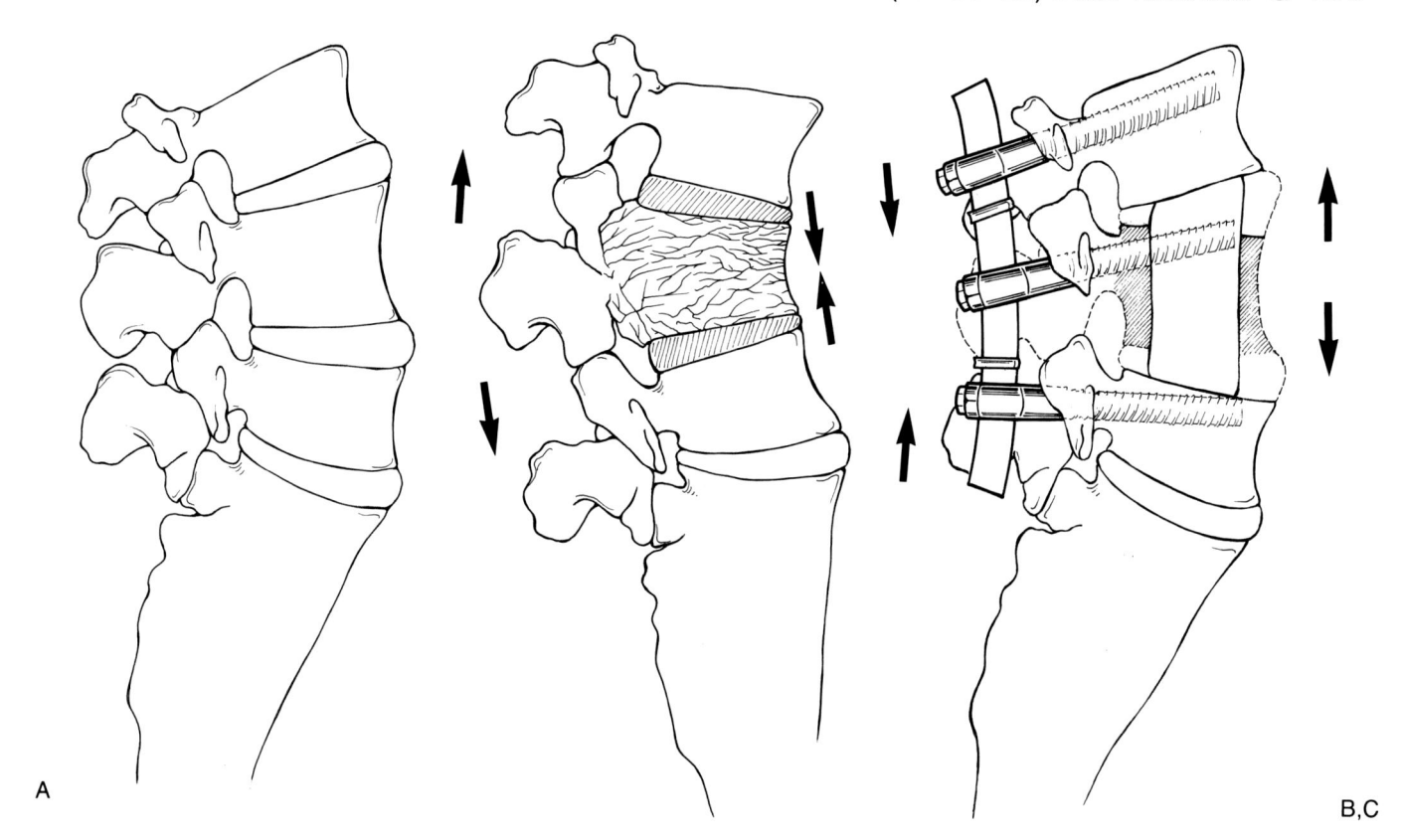

FIG. 6. A: Normal sagittal contour. **B:** Kyphosis from collapse of the L4 vertebral body and L3–L4 and L4–L5 discs. **C:** Middle column decompression, posterior tension band pedicle fixation, restoration of anterior column height with the strut. Note the strut is taller anteriorly than posteriorly.

L5–S1. A cast or brace with one thigh incorporated will help control motion at the lumbosacral joint but this will pose social problems for the patient.

SUMMARY

For low lumbar burst fractures it is important to initially realize whether there is an associated subluxation and/or a suggestion that the thecal sac and posterior nerve roots are trapped within the laminar fracture. If so, an initial posterior surgical approach to the spine is mandatory. We have entered into a phase in which low lumbar burst fractures are being treated surgically rather than nonsurgically because of the evolution of pedicle fixation. However, it remains to be seen whether or not pedicle fixation will provide a better sagittal contour for this part of the spine. Fixation to the sacrum both anteriorly and posteriorly is somewhat difficult and tenuous. Complications and difficulty with exposure anteriorly around the lumbosacral joint are greater than they are proximally in the spine. An ideal result after surgical treatment is one in which the neural elements are circumferentially decompressed, a minimum of segments are fused, and the spine is held in a physiologic coronal and sagittal position.

REFERENCES

1. Allen BT, Bridwell KH. Paramedian anterior approach to the lumbar spine. In: Bridwell KH, Dewald RL, eds. *Textbook of spinal surgery*. Philadelphia: Lippincott, 1991.
2. An HS, Vaccaro A, Cotler JM, Lin S. Low lumbar burst fractures: comparison among body casts, Harrington rod, Luque rod and Steffee plate. *Spine* 1991;16(8S):440–444.
3. Bernhardt M, Bridwell KH. Segmental analysis of the sagittal plane alignment of the normal thoracic and lumbar spines and thoracolumbar junction. *Spine* 1989;14(7):717–721.
4. Cammisa FP, Eismont FT, Green BA. Dural laceration occurring with burst fractures and associated lamina fractures. *J Bone Joint Surg* 1989;71-A:1044–1052.
5. Court-Brown CM, Gertzbein SD. Management of burst fractures of the fifth lumbar vertebra. *Spine* 1987;12:308–312.
6. Denis F. The three column spine and its significance on the classification of acute thoracolumbar spinal injuries. *Spine* 1983;8:817–831.
7. Denis F, Burkus JK. Diagnosis and treatment of cauda equina entrapment in the vertical lamina fracture of lumbar burst fractures. *Spine* 1991;16(8S):433–439.
8. Fredrickson BE, Yuan HA, Miller H. Burst fractures of the fifth lumbar vertebrae: a report of four cases. *J Bone Joint Surg* 1982;64-A:1088–1094.

9. Levine AM, Edwards CC. Low lumbar burst fractures: reduction and stabilization using the modular spine fixation system. *Orthopedics* 1988;11:1427–1432.
10. Wambolt A, Spencer DL. A segmental analysis of the distribution of lumbar lordosis of the normal spine. *Orthop Trans* 1987;11:92–93.
11. Weidenbaum M, Farcy JP. Surgical management of thoracic and lumbar burst fractures. In: Bridwell KH, Dewald RL, eds. *Textbook of spinal surgery*. Philadelphia: Lippincott, 1991.
12. Weinstein JN, Collalto P, Lehmann TR. Thoracolumbar burst fractures treated conservatively: a long-term follow-up. *Spine* 1988;13:33–38.

18

Considerations in Management of Facet Joint Injuries

Mark Weidenbaum and Jean-Pierre C. Farcy

ANATOMY AND BIOMECHANICS

Spine stability is the result of the harmonious anatomic arrangement of bone and soft tissue. Located on the posterior arch, the paired facet joints are diarthrodial joints with hyaline cartilage overlying subchondral bone. The facet joints play a role in determining range of motion and distributing axial, rotational, and shear forces (6,9). They maintain static stability. Dynamic stability is provided by soft tissue attachments, including the facet capsule, ligamentum flavum, interspinous ligament, supraspinous ligament, longitudinal ligament, intervertebral disc, and muscles.

The thoracic facets are oriented primarily in the coronal plane and are adjacent to short, wide laminae; the laminar widths increase caudally (36,45). The thoracic facets are anatomically unique because they are further stabilized by rib attachments. The costovertebral joints provide stability in flexion, although the posterior ligaments contribute to this as well.

In the thoracic spine, facet orientation gently shifts to a more sagittal orientation in the lower thoracic spine, which progresses into the lumbar spine. This is accompanied by reduction in rotational freedom and increased motion in the sagittal plane. The presence of a much larger interlaminar space facilitates lumbar extension, which contributes to the lordosis of the lumbar spine (22). This is in marked contrast to the thoracic spine, where minimal interlaminar spaces are present, and overlapping laminae and spinous processes inhibit extension and contribute to gentle kyphosis.

The stability and function of the facet capsules depend to some extent on complementary functions of the anterior and posterior longitudinal ligaments. The anterior longitudinal ligament (ALL) stretches in extension; the posterior longitudinal ligament (PLL) stretches in flexion. The ALL increases in tensile strength at the thoracolumbar junction and, in combination with the intervertebral disc, provides rotational and translation stability.

In the thoracic region, the facet capsules are thin and provide little resistance to kyphosis if the ligamentum flavum is disrupted. The facet capsules are stronger in the thoracolumbar region, and the ligamentum flavum is stronger in the lower thoracic region. Following multiple thoracic laminectomies, the usual support provided by the flavum is lost, predisposing these levels to kyphosis (46).

Capsule and posterior ligament function depend on maintenance of their appropriate length as determined by the proper heights of disc and vertebral body. Reduction in these heights results in capsular laxity. Rotation stretches the ipsilateral upper and lower capsules but relaxes the contralateral ones (23,44).

In the lumbar spine, the capsules are well developed and play a major role in stabilization. At these levels, the interspinous ligaments and posterior longitudinal ligaments are thin and do not contribute substantively to clinical stability (41). The supraspinous ligaments increase in strength from the upper thoracic to the lumbar region (36).

Facet range of motion depends in part on orientation.

J.-P. C. Farcy: Department of Orthopaedics, Columbia University College of Physicians and Surgeons, and Columbia–Presbyterian Medical Center, New York, NY 10032.
M. Weidenbaum: Department of Orthopaedic Surgery, College of Physicians and Surgeons, Columbia–Presbyterian Medical Center, New York, NY 10032.

In the thoracic spine, the facets lie in a coronal orientation tilted forward, which permits flexion, extension, and rotation but limits lateral bending. White and Hirsch (45) measured range of motion in the thoracic spine by comparing intact segments with those in which posterior elements were removed. They noted a 50% to 80% increase in flexion/extension in the upper thoracic spine, but only a 15% increase in the lower thoracic region. However, axial rotation increased by 40%.

The annulus' resistance to rotation far exceeds that of the facet joint, either alone or in combination with other structures (21). Adams and Hutton (1) showed the damaging effect of excessive offset loading and the potential effect of chronic rotational stress resulting from facet joint asymmetry. However, although the facets do act as a "positive stop" to axial rotation, variations of facet geometry do not affect this function in the lumbar spine (2).

All lumbar facets are oriented primarily in the sagittal plane, allowing flexion and extension as well as lateral bend but limiting torsion. Sullivan and Farfan (43) showed that axial rotation of more than 30° caused failure of the neural arch. Markolf (32) demonstrated increasing torsional stiffness from T7–T8 to L3–L4, with a corresponding decrease in these values after facetectomy.

The lumbar facets bear approximately 16% to 18% of axial load in the erect posture (1,37). Nachemson (37) also confirmed a marked increase in intradiscal pressure in the sitting position when compared to standing. Similarly, King et al. (27) showed a range of 0% to 33% load carried through the facets depending on posture. These studies correlate reduction in facet load with changes in center of gravity and load transfer to the disc.

Several investigators have confirmed that degeneration increases facet load (31,48). Because of their close proximity to the nerve roots, the lumbar facets contribute significantly in development of spinal stenosis (16).

When axial load is steadily increased, force measured at the facet surface rises, reaches a plateau, and drops (31). This is probably due to the rotation of the almost vertically oriented joint surfaces as the inferior facet swivels, stretching the joint capsule. Thus the capsule and its attachment on the pars interarticularis, rather than the facet joint, take the increasing load (48).

In a biomechanical analysis, Jacobs et al. (26) correlated mechanism of injury with resulting structural failure. Axial distraction led to facet capsule disruption, rotation resulted in facet fracture, and flexion led to facet capsule disruption with or without body fracture. Hence facet fracture–dislocation requires excessive axial rotation in conjunction with flexion.

The combination of facet geometry and the relative strengths of static bone and dynamic soft tissues determine the mechanism and extent of injury.

COMPLETE BILATERAL THORACOLUMBAR FACET DISLOCATION

Bilateral facet dislocation accounts for 11% of unstable thoracic and lumbar spine trauma (3,28). Disruption of the posterior structures alone via sudden flexion/distraction is inadequate to allow the translation necessary for dislocation (12). Dislocation is entirely a soft tissue injury in which there is no fracture of bone and is thus distinguished from fracture–dislocation. Translation and instability arise from complete disruption of all posterior ligamentous structures in addition to disruption of the PLL and the annulus. Nagel et al. (38) showed that anterior flexion of 20° or lateral flexion of 10° disrupts all posterior ligaments and some portion of the annulus fibrosus. Panjabi et al. (40) showed that instability results when all ligaments posterior to and including the posterior one-half of the discs were cut; the ALL may remain in continuity, but it is stripped from the anterior aspect of the inferior vertebra. McAfee et al. (34) noted that the axis of rotation for this injury lies posterior to the ALL.

Fifty-one percent of these dislocations (30) occur at the thoracolumbar junction as a result of four anatomic considerations: (a) transition from kyphosis to lordosis, (b) loss of the stability that was provided by the rib cage, (c) increased segmental sagittal mobility, and (d) transitional facet orientation (29).

The diagnosis of dislocation is often apparent on a lateral radiograph, with anterior translation of the vertebra and slight anterior compression but minimal loss of posterior vertebral body height. Anterior column fracture may not be present when the mechanism is pure flexion distraction with ALL rupture or in low lumbar facet fractures (28). AP films are notable for the absence of interpedicular widening and for marked increase in distance between the spinous processes. CT scanning, particularly when combined with sagittal reconstruction, will clearly elucidate the "empty facet sign" (18), the "double body sign" (39), and a marked reduction in canal diameter as measured from the inferior facet proximally to the posterosuperior aspect of the vertebral body inferiorly. Canal compromise results from shear and malalignment, rather than retropulsion of bone or soft tissue into the canal. A gibbus is often clinically evident. A small crack extending cephalad may be visible in the pedicle on an AP radiograph. The lateral film may show a crack at the level of the superior facet or a discontinuity in the line of the facet joint. If there is even the slightest suspicion of facet injury, a CT scan should be obtained. Flexion/extension films may be useful as well. MRI scanning does not show facet fractures as well as CT scans do but may better demonstrate capsular injuries.

When the spine is flexed and shear forces are applied, there may be soft tissue disruption with or without accompanying osseous fracture. This leads to multidirectional instability.

Closed postural reduction for bilateral facet dislocation is ineffective (15), and disruption of the posterior ligamentous structures in addition to the annulus leads to chronic instability with deformity (25,47). On rare occasions, it may be possible to reduce some thoracolumbar or lumbar facets, but this is never successful in the thoracic region (11,15); if reduction can be achieved, stabilization cannot be accomplished by closed means due to the extensive soft tissue injury.

In view of the failure of conservative management, surgical management consists of (a) reduction, (b) decompression, and (c) stabilization. Reduction is done by recreating the deformity and distracting the proximal vertebra while the distal level is stabilized and gently pushed forward. When displacement recurs after reduction, one must look for a fracture and/or another dislocation. After exposure and removal of the disrupted facet capsule, interspinous ligament, and ligamentum flavum, reduction is performed by placing towel clips on the spinous processes on either side of the dislocation (28). Fractures of the pars interarticularis and/or articular processes are often associated. Facet resection to facilitate reduction should be minimized, since intact facet architecture is necessary to maintain stability following reduction.

Following reduction, compression instrumentation is used. Caution must be exercised if the anterior longitudinal ligament has been disrupted, since this may allow hyperextension and anterior opening with posterior compression. In addition, compression may exacerbate prolapse of the disrupted disc, leading to untoward neurologic events unless the disc was inspected prior to compression.

Prophylactic discectomy should precede compression instrumentation in patients who are intact or who have incomplete neurologic injury. Canal patency is best evaluated with myelography or MRI both before and after surgery. Anterior surgery is contraindicated, since it disrupts the only remaining intact column and is not helpful in reduction and decompression (33).

The timing of surgery depends on neurologic status. Immediate complete paraplegia with no spinal shock is irreversible, and surgery can be scheduled electively. Associated visceral injuries may be difficult to diagnose in this setting. An incomplete neurologic deficit warrants immediate intervention if medically feasible. Reduction of canal diameter of 50% is associated with cord compression (3). This correlates with 33% translation in the thoracic spine.

ISOLATED UNILATERAL FACET DISLOCATION AND FRACTURE/DISLOCATION

Most isolated unilateral facet dislocations and fracture/dislocations occur in the cervical spine, where the bony architecture and soft tissue attachments allow significant motion. These injuries are rare in the thoracic, lumbar, or lumbosacral spine, where there is far less motion than the cervical spine.

Unilateral thoracic facet dislocation, or "jumped facet," has been reported (4), but it is rare because of the laminar overlap, thin discs, and dual rib articulations. Multiple contralateral rib fractures must be present to allow the rotatory motion in flexion distraction that causes the dislocation to occur. The anterior vertebral body displacement is less than 30% of body width. Unlike bilateral thoracic or thoracolumbar facet fractures, where complete paraplegia is usually associated, neurologic function may be preserved in unilateral thoracic facet dislocations (18,28).

Most facet injuries result from a combination of flexion, rotation, and shear. Garin et al. (17) reported a fracture/dislocation of L1 that occurred from pure rotation, resulting in disruption of the inferior growth plate with unilateral facet subluxation. This unusual type of pure rotatory injury was facilitated by the cartilaginous growth plate.

At the lumbosacral level, the mechanism of unilateral facet fracture/dislocation is flexion and rotation (5,10) or hyperflexion in conjunction with compression and rotation (42). Neurologic status may be normal due to the large spinal canal and the relative paucity of neural elements at this level. Early treatment options include bed rest and attempts at closed reduction (5,49). Miz and Engler (35) recommend early open reduction and fusion with casting, while Carl and Blair (7) advocate the addition of pedicle fixation to facilitate rapid mobilization.

CLINICAL CONSIDERATIONS

If recognized early, isolated facet or pars fractures may be treated with closed immobilization for 6 to 12 weeks. Diagnosis is made with judicious use of MRI, tomography, and myelogram/CT scan. These injuries are often self-limited and do not present management difficulties. However, the situation is quite different when injuries go unrecognized in the presence of other, more obvious spine trauma.

Numerous classifications, fully detailed elsewhere in this text, exist for spine fractures and fracture/dislocations. Many of these injuries may be accompanied by disruption of thoracic or lumbar facets, leading to subluxation or dislocation.

In general, flexion rotation injuries include failure of the posterior and middle columns under tension and rotation and anterior column failure under compression in rotation (25,42). Shear injuries may occur in any direction. Some apparent lateral dislocations are actually burst rotation injuries (13). Although Chance injuries involve flexion–distraction (8), sudden, subsequent axial loading may result in an associated compression or burst fracture. Furthermore, the path of injury may occur through or between the spinous processes, disrupting varying amounts of bone and soft tissue (19,20).

Regardless of mechanism or classification, fracture/dislocation of the thoracic spine nearly always results in catastrophic injury with complete neurologic loss. The tight fit of the spinal cord within the thoracic canal results in minimal free space, and retropulsion of bone or soft tissue into the canal and/or translation in the sagittal or frontal plane results in direct damage to the spinal cord. These grossly unstable injuries mandate reduction, fusion, and internal fixation.

It is essential to emphasize that a unilateral facet fracture, subluxation, or dislocation as well as a unilateral pars fracture may not be recognized initially. These injuries may occur in conjunction with other more obvious injuries and lead to significant late instability with pain and deformity if not recognized and properly treated. Late deformity with malunion may require complete anterior and posterior osteotomies to achieve realignment, which would have been possible with a simpler, single procedure at the time of injury.

Progressive deformity often occurs in compression fractures of the vertebral body when the height of the anterior vertebral body is less than one-third that of the posterior wall and the Sagittal Index (SI) is greater than 35° (14). Segmental deformity of this magnitude is generally accompanied by tearing of the supraspinous and interspinous ligaments as well as the facet capsules, resulting in facet subluxation (see Fig. 1). This is no longer a stable compression fracture with isolated injury to the anterior column. Rather, an unstable injury exists with compression fracture of the anterior column and soft tissue damage to the middle and posterior columns; the loss of anterior support differentiates this situation from the typical flexion–distraction injury. The potential for late deformity is due to the loss of both anterior structural integrity and posterior tensile stabilization. In the presence of an intact posterior vertebral body wall, the reduction, stabilization, and fusion necessary to prevent progressive deformity are applied via posterior compression.

When facet injury or severe posterior ligamentous damage is present, distinguishing between burst and compression fractures is crucial for two reasons. First, in burst fractures, compression instrumentation cannot be used because the posterior body wall is broken and cannot be used as a fulcrum. Second, distraction instrumentation cannot be used, since posterior column soft tissues have been torn and can no longer tether and prevent overdistraction. In this setting, neutralization instrumentation may be preferred, since it stabilizes the posterior column before the burst component is addressed.

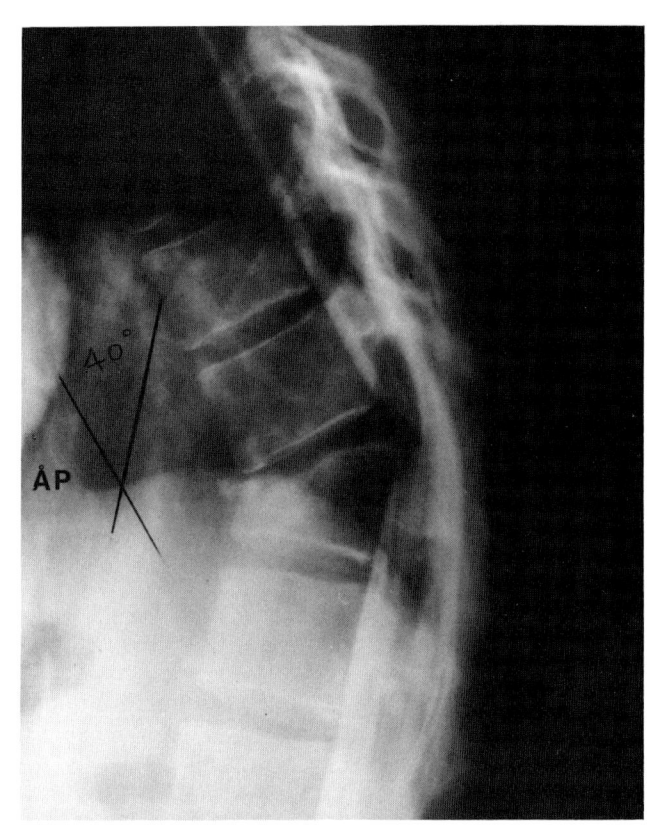

FIG. 1. Compression fracture of T12 with a 40° segmental kyphosis on a lateral myelogram view of the thoracolumbar spine. The injury was not recognized initially and the patient developed progressive pain and deformity that required anterior and posterior osteotomies and fusion.

Isolated unilateral facet fracture in conjunction with limited, lateral vertebral body compression may lead to long-term rotational instability with subsequent scoliosis. Unilateral pars fracture may result in late kyphosis and/or scoliosis. Acute bilateral pars fracture may be reconstructed without fusion; if this fracture is accompanied by anterior injury, a single-level fusion can be performed.

CASE 1. Facet fracture/subluxation: patient is a 26-year-old woman, who sustained a fracture of the right L3 superior articular facet with L2–L3 facet subluxa-

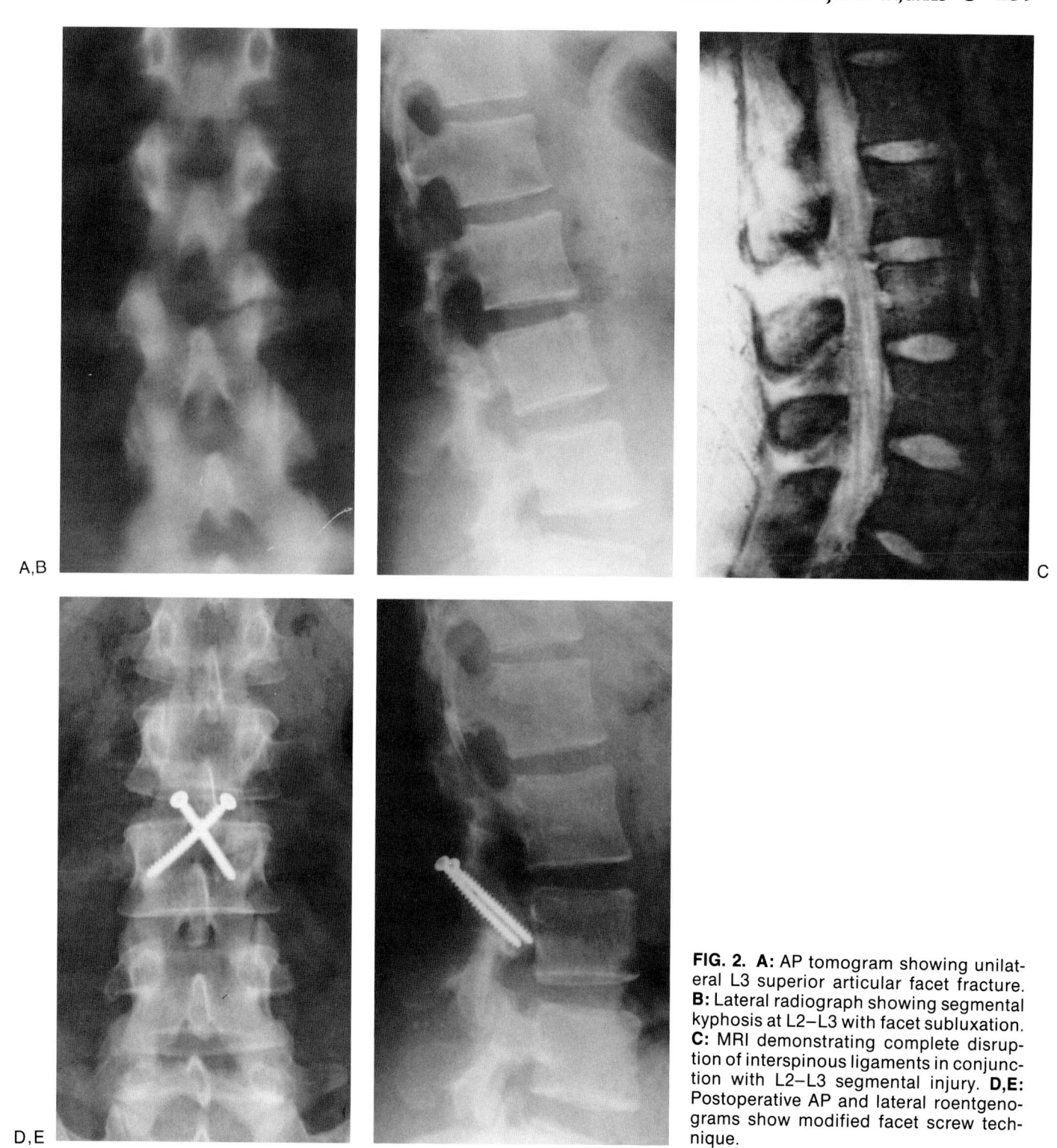

FIG. 2. A: AP tomogram showing unilateral L3 superior articular facet fracture. **B:** Lateral radiograph showing segmental kyphosis at L2–L3 with facet subluxation. **C:** MRI demonstrating complete disruption of interspinous ligaments in conjunction with L2–L3 segmental injury. **D,E:** Postoperative AP and lateral roentgenograms show modified facet screw technique.

tion and segmental kyphosis. The facet fracture is well visualized on AP tomogram. MRI clearly shows disruption of the interspinous and supraspinous ligaments. Patient underwent ORIF with modified translaminar facet screws (24) using crossed A-O 3.5-mm screws from the inferior facet of L2 into the pars of L3. The screws broke at 3 months but there was complete pain resolution (Fig. 2).

CASE 2. Facet subluxation: patient is a 31-year-old woman, who sustained an L2 Chance fracture with facet subluxation and instability at L2–L3. Following abdominal surgery, she underwent reduction at L2 and L3 using heavy merseline suture to compress the spinous processes, followed by fixation with a DC plate, using 4.5-mm A-O screws in the pedicles of L2 and L3. She was braced for 4 months (Fig. 3).

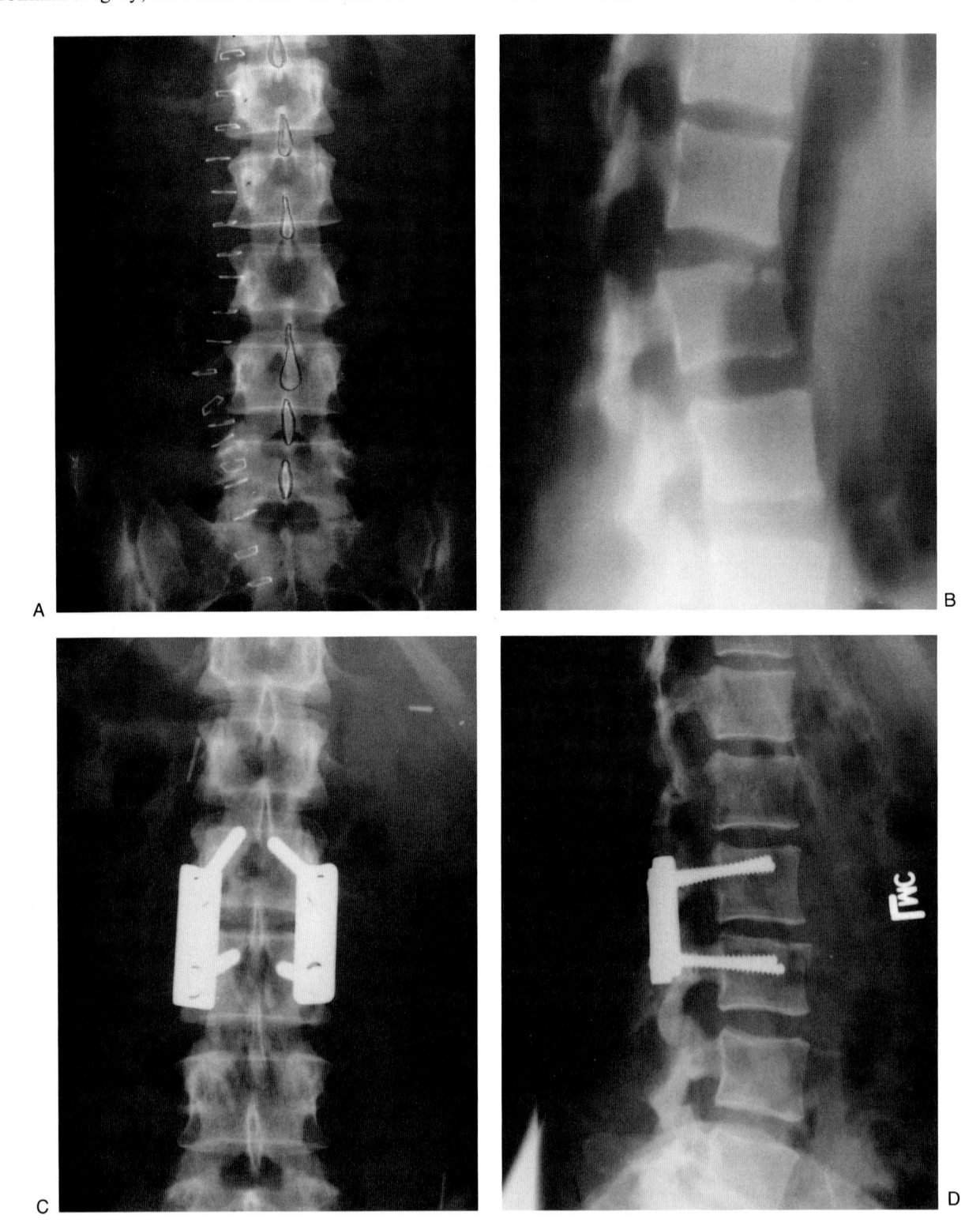

FIG. 3. A: AP view of L2–L3 Chance injury with splitting of the L3 spinous process. Clips are from previous abdominal exploration. **B:** Lateral tomogram shows slight anterior vertebral body compression with subluxed (perched) facets bilaterally. **C,D:** Postoperative AP and lateral views following open reduction with merseline suture, fixation with A-O plate, and single-level fusion.

CASE 3. Malunion: patient is a 16-year-old boy, who sustained a rotation–flexion injury at L2–L3, which was initially braced. At presentation 1 year later, there was a fixed 41° segmental kyphosis with anterior rotation and subluxation of the right L2 inferior facet. Correction to kyphosis of 12° required anterior and posterior osteotomies and fusion and with instrumentation from L1 to L4 (Fig. 4).

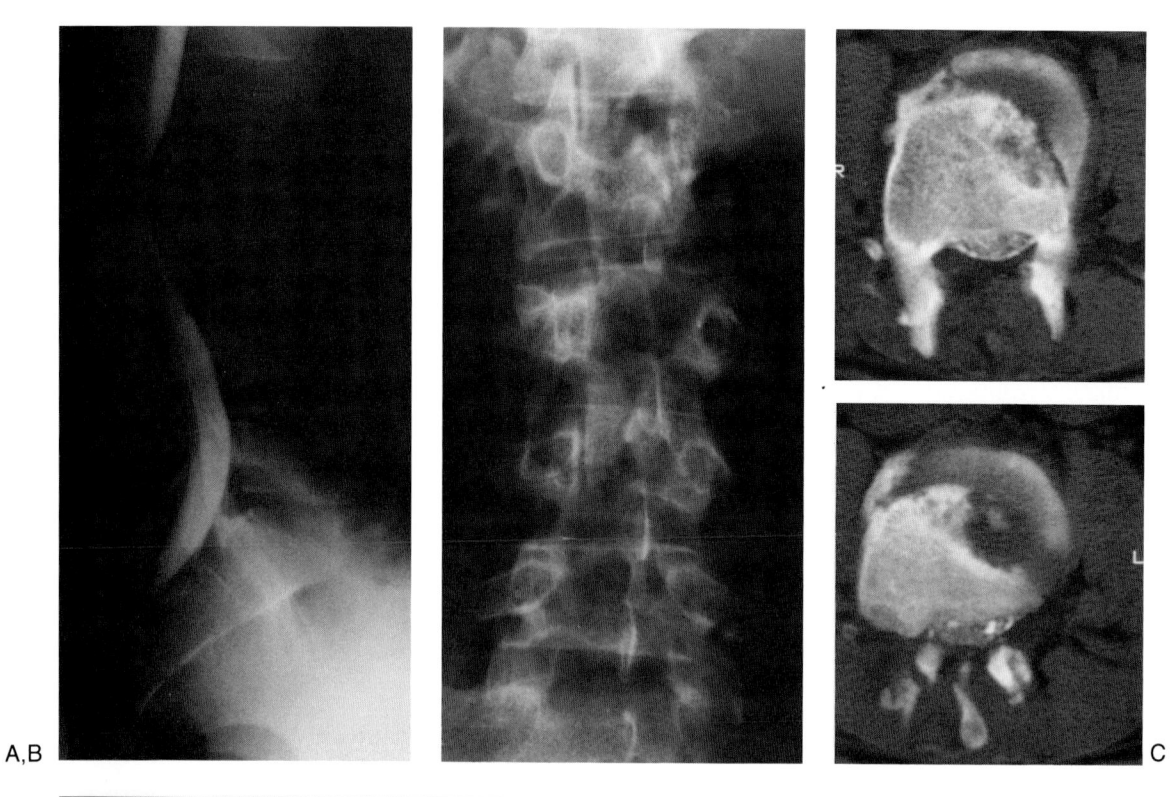

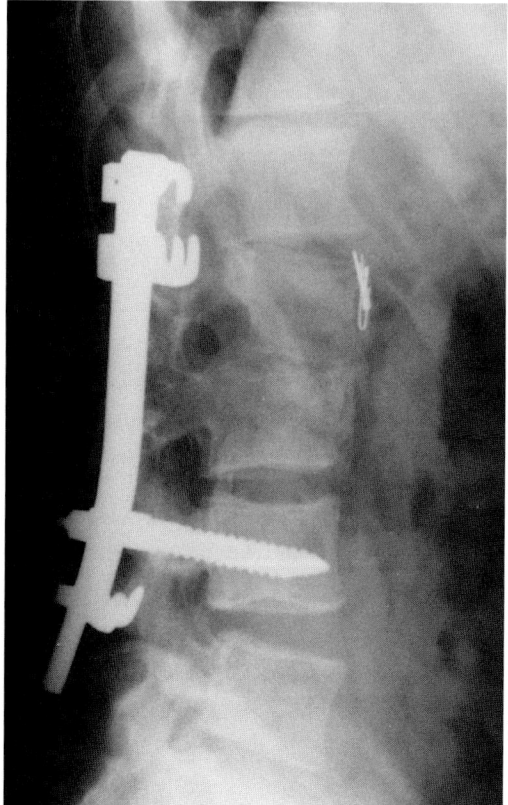

FIG. 4. A: Lateral myelogram view of L2–L3 malunion 1 year following rotation–flexion injury treated with brace alone. **B:** AP view shows right L3 superior articular facet fracture with anterior rotation of L2. **C:** Postmyelogram CT scan at L2–L3 shows severe canal compromise, "double density" sign, and anterior rotation of L2 on L3. **D:** Postoperative lateral view following anterior and posterior osteotomies, realignment, and fusion with instrumentation.

The crucial issues are correction of malalignment and stable restoration of proper three-dimensional contour. As in all intra-articular fractures, failure to reconstruct anatomically results in loss of harmonious function.

SUMMARY

Unilateral or bilateral facet fractures, if left untreated, can set the stage for progressive deformity. In the trauma setting, these injuries are easily overlooked, since attention is focused on more obvious injuries. We stress the need to scrutinize standard radiographs to find the small signs that will trigger appropriate imaging.

Stable, nondisplaced facet fractures without associated segmental deformity that are recognized immediately can be treated closed. Acute displaced facet fractures as well as those with segmental deformity require open reduction and stabilization with internal fixation but without fusion. Reduction, fixation, and fusion of a single-motion segment are required for facet fractures that are unstable, recognized later, or associated with a pars fracture at the same level.

REFERENCES

1. Adams MA, Hutton WC. The effect of posture on the role of the apophyseal joints in resisting intervertebral compression forces. *J Bone Joint Surg* 1980;62B:358.
2. Ahmed AM, Duncan NA, Burke DL. The effect of facet geometry on the axial torque–rotation response of lumbar motion segments. *Spine* 1990;15:391–401.
3. Bedbrook GM. Treatment of thoracolumbar dislocations and fractures with paraplegia. *Clin Orthop* 1975;112:27–43.
4. Berg EE, Gilpin AT. Unilateral jumped thoracic facet dislocation. *Spine* 1991;16:590–592.
5. Boger DC, Chandler RW, Pearce JG, Balciunas A. Unilateral facet dislocation at the lumbosacral junction. *J Bone Joint Surg* 1983;65A:1174–1178.
6. Bradford DS, Lonstein JE, Moe JH, Ogilvie J, Winter RB. *Textbook of scoliosis*, 2nd ed. Philadelphia: Saunders, 1987;7–23.
7. Carl A, Blair B. Unilateral lumbosacral facet fracture–dislocation. *Spine* 1991;16:218–221.
8. Chance GQ. Note on the type of flexion fracture of the spine. *Br J Radiol* 1948;21:452–453.
9. Coessette JW, Farfan HF, Robertson GH, Wells RV. The instantaneous center of rotation of the third lumbar intervertebral joint. *J Biomech* 1971;4:149.
10. DasDe S, McReath SW. Lumbosacral fracture–dislocations. *J Bone Joint Surg* 1981;63B:58–60.
11. Davies WE, Morris JH, Hill V. An analysis of conservative management of thoracolumbar fractures and fracture–dislocations with neural damage. *J Bone Joint Surg* 1980;62A:1324–1328.
12. Denis F. The three column spine and its significance in the classification of acute thoracolumbar spinal injuries. *Spine* 1983;8:817–831.
13. Denis F. Spinal instability as defined by the three-column concept in acute spinal trauma. *Clin Orthop* 1984;189:65–76.
14. Farcy JPC, Weidenbaum M, Glassman SD. The sagittal index in the management of thoracolumbar burst fractures. *Spine* 1990;15:958–965.
15. Frankel HL, Hancock GH, Melzak J, et al. The value of postural reduction in the initial management of closed injuries of the spine with parplegia and tetraplegia. *Paraplegia* 1969;7:179–192.
16. Frymoyer JF, Moskowitz RW. Spinal degeneration pathogenesis and medical management. In: Frymoyer JW, ed. *The adult spine: principles and practice*. New York: Raven Press, 1991;611–634.
17. Garin DM, Leal CV, Granell JB. Fracture–dislocation of L1 through the lower plate of the vertebral body. *Spine* 1991;16:372–373.
18. Gellad FE, Levin AM, Joslyn JN, Edwards CC, Bosse M. Pure thoracolumbar facet dislocation: clinical features in CT appearance. *Radiology* 1986;161:505–508.
19. Gertzbein SD, Court-Brown CM. Rationale for the management of flexion–distraction injuries of the thoracolumbar spine based on a new classification. *J Spinal Disord* 1989;2:176–183.
20. Gumley G, Taylor TKF, Ryan MD. Distraction fractures of the lumbar spine. *J Bone Joint Surg* 1982;64B:520–525.
21. Haher T, Felmly WT, Baruch H. The contribution of the three columns of the spine to rotational stability: a biomechanical model. *Spine* 1989;14:663.
22. Haher TR, Felmly WT, O'Brien M. Thoracic and lumbar fractures: diagnosis and management. In: Bridwell KH, Dewald RL, eds. *Textbook of spinal surgery*. Philadelphia: Lippincott, 1991;858–862.
23. Hedtmann A, Steffan R, Methfessel J. Measurement of human lumbar spine ligaments during loaded and unloaded motion. *Spine* 1989;14:175.
24. Heggeness MH, Esses SI. Translaminar facet joint screw fixation for lumbar and lumbosacral fusion; a clinical and biomechanical study. *Spine* 1991;16:S266–S269.
25. Holdsworth FW. Fractures, dislocations and fracture–dislocations of the spine. *J Bone Joint Surg* 1970;52A:1534.
26. Jacobs RR, Asher MA, Snider RK. Thoracolumbar spinal injuries. *Spine* 1980;5:463–477.
27. King AI, Prasad P, Ewing CL. Mechanism of spinal injury due to caudocephalad acceleration. *Orthop Clin North Am* 1975;6:19.
28. Levine AM, Bosse M, Edwards CC. Bilateral facet dislocations in the thoracolumbar spine. *Spine* 1988;13:630–640.
29. Levine AM, Edwards CC. Lumbar spine trauma. In: Camins M, O'Leary P, eds. *The lumbar spine*. New York: Raven Press, 1987;183–212.
30. Lewis J, McKibbin B. The treatment of unstable fracture dislocation of the thoracolumbar spine accompanied by paraplegia. *J Bone Joint Surg* 1974;56B:603–612.
31. Lorenz M, Pawardian A, Vanderby R. Load bearing characteristics of lumbar facets in normal and surgically altered spinal segments. *Spine* 1983;8:122.
32. Markolf KL. Deformation of the thoracolumbar intervertebral joints in response to external loads: a biomechanical study using autopsy material. *J Bone Joint Surg* 1972;54A:511.
33. McAfee PC, Bohlman HH. Anterior decompression of traumatic thoracolumbar fractures with incomplete neurologic deficit using a retroperitoneal approach. *J Bone Joint Surg* 1985;67A:89–103.
34. McAfee PC, Hansen AV, Fredrickson BE, Lubicky JP. The value of computed tomography in thoracolumbar fractures. *J Bone Joint Surg* 1983;65A:456–473.
35. Miz GS, Engler GL. Unilateral dislocation of a lumbosacral facet. *Spine* 1988;13:956–957.
36. Myklebust JB, Pintar F, Yoganandan N, et al. Strength of spinal ligaments. *Spine* 1988;13:526.
37. Nachemson A. Lumbar intradiscal pressure: experimental studies on post-mortem material. *Acta Orthop Scand* 1960;43(suppl):1–104.
38. Nagel DA, Koogle TA, Piziali RL, Perkash I. Stability of the upper lumbar spine following progressive disruptions and the application of the individual internal and external fixation devices. *J Bone Joint Surg* 1981;63A:62.
39. O'Callaghan JP, Ulrich CG, Yuan HA, Kieffer SA. CT of facet distraction in flexion injuries of the thoracolumbar spine. The "naked" facet. *AJNR* 1980;1:97–102.
40. Panjabi MM, Hausfel JN, White AA. A biomechanical study of

the ligamentous stability of the thoracic spine in man. *Acta Orthop Scand* 1981;52:315.
41. Rissanen P. The surgical anatomy and pathology of the supraspinous and interspinous ligaments of the lumbar spine with special reference to ligament ruptures. *Acta Orthop Scand Suppl* 1960; 46:8–100.
42. Roaf R. A study of the mechanics of spinal injuries. *J Bone Joint Surg* 1960;42B:810.
43. Sullivan JD, Farfan HF. The crumpled neural arch. *Orthop Clin North Am* 1975;6:199.
44. Tencer AF, Mayer TG. Soft tissue strain and facet interaction in the lumbar intervertebral joint. *J Biomech Eng* 1983;105:201.
45. White AA, Hirsch C. The significance of the vertebral posterior elements in the mechanics of the thoracic spine. *Clin Orthop* 1971;81:2.
46. White AA, Panjabi MM. *Clinical biomechanics of the spine.* Philadelphia: Lippincott, 1978;240.
47. Whitesides TE. Traumatic kyphosis of the thoracolumbar spine. *Clin Orthop* 1977;128:78–92.
48. Yang KH, King AI. A mechanism of facet load transmission as a hypothesis for low back pain. *Spine* 1984;9:557–565.
49. Zoltan JD, Gilula LA, Murphy WA. Unilateral facet dislocation between the fifth lumbar and first sacral vertebra. *J Bone Joint Surg* 1979;61A:767–769.

19

Sacral Fractures

Diagnosis and Management

Francis Denis

In spite of pelvic roentgenograms demonstrating a sacral fracture, this condition is frequently ignored and left untreated. The most obvious reason for the oversight is the immediate urgency for management of severe pelvic injuries as a whole. Of course, severe retroperitoneal bleeding is a life-threatening situation and must take precedence over the sacral fracture. However, the latter should be identified from the start, both in terms of stability of the pelvis and in terms of neurological deficits, since they may be improved or cured with the appropriate treatment at the appropriate time.

Richerand (8) appears to be the first to have reported the sacral fracture. Malgaigne (8) did describe vertical shear injuries going through the sacrum. Bonnin (1) gave a classic description of the sacral sciatica, which often remains in conjunction with bladder paralysis the most disabling sequela of sacral fractures. Bonnin also provided us with a most sophisticated classification, demonstrating his very advanced understanding of these injuries. Patterson and Morton (9) described the causal relationship between the level of the lesion and the accompanying neurologic picture.

ROENTGENOGRAPHIC FINDINGS OF SACRAL FRACTURES

An anteroposterior (AP) roentgenogram of the pelvis often gives poor visualization of the sacrum. The Ferguson method produces the best AP view of the upper sacrum and allows visualization of the upper foramina. While a lateral film of the pelvis frequently misses the lower part of the sacrum, a lateral film centered on the sacrum may be of great help in determining a diagnosis, particularly in zone III fractures. AP tomograms are helpful in zones I and II and lateral tomograms are more useful in zone III. Myelography is of limited use in sacral fractures because the dural sac frequently ends at S2 or above and visualization of the root within the foramina is poor, even when metrizamide myelography is performed.

A computerized tomography (CT) scan should be considered whenever neurological damage is present, since the scan will provide better understanding of the traumatic encroachment on sacral roots within the sacral canal. It should involve tilting of the gantry and thin cuts for optimal images in the sagittal plane. MRI shows the nerve roots better than computerized axial tomography, but bone definition is suboptimal.

CLASSIFICATION OF SACRAL FRACTURES

As previously described by the author and co-workers (2), the three-zone classification of sacral fractures is justified by the differences in incidences in quality of neurological symptoms in the three zones (Fig. 1). Zone I, or the alar zone, is rarely accompanied by neurologic deficit (5.9%). In zone II, or the foraminal zone, neurologic deficits are attributable to the sacral fracture in 28.4% of the patients. These are primarily sacral radicular symptoms. Zone III, which is the central canal zone, presents with neurologic damage in 56.7% of the patients. The neurologic deficits involve bowel, bladder, and sexual function in three-quarters of these patients (3,5–7).

F. Denis: Minnesota Spine Center, Minneapolis, MN 55454.

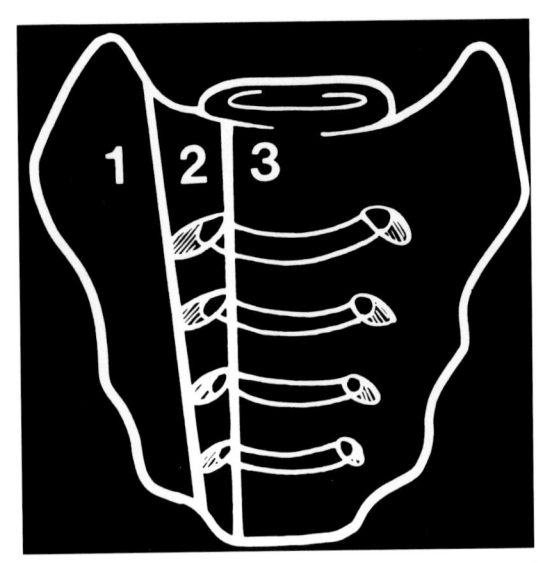

FIG. 1. Classification of sacral fracture; *1*, the region of the ala (zone I); *2*, the region of the foramina (zone II); and *3*, the central sacral canal region (zone III). (With permission from Francis Denis, et al. *Clin Orthop* 227, 67–81, 1988.)

Zone I: Alar Zone

Zone I involves the sacrum lateral to the foraminal line. There are two major types of fractures: alar fractures result from lateral compression injuries; and the other type of fracture involves avulsion of the sacral tuberous ligaments and is responsible for severe pelvic instabilities.

Treatment of the Sacral Fracture in Zone I

Stable alar fractures (Fig. 2) are treated with bed rest and early ambulation, nonweight-bearing on the side of the sacral fracture, or, sometimes, partial weight-bearing with crutches when symptoms permit.

Unstable sacral alar fractures (Fig. 3) are usually accompanied by a significant anterior pelvic instability component. It is difficult to log roll the patient without pain and an anterior fixator may be necessary to stabilize the anterior ring and allow easier nursing. Whatever pubic symphyseal diastasis is present, the likelihood of healing and of maintaining correction is much lower than when a bony injury is encountered. For this reason, one should not hesitate to carry out open reduction and internal fixation of the pubic symphyseal disruption. If a vertical shear injury involving the ala of the sacrum is encountered, examination of the patient should include neurological examination of both lower extremities and, in particular, of the L5 innervated musculature. The L5 root tends to be entrapped as the alar fragment migrates superiorly and posteriorly, which may cause a foot drop (10). Early, powerful traction is then indicated, and posterior open reduction and internal fixation may be the only way to reduce and stabilize this fracture to prevent pressure on the L5 nerve root.

Zone II: the Foraminal Zone

These injuries involve one or several foramina, but they do not involve the central sacral canal (Fig. 4).

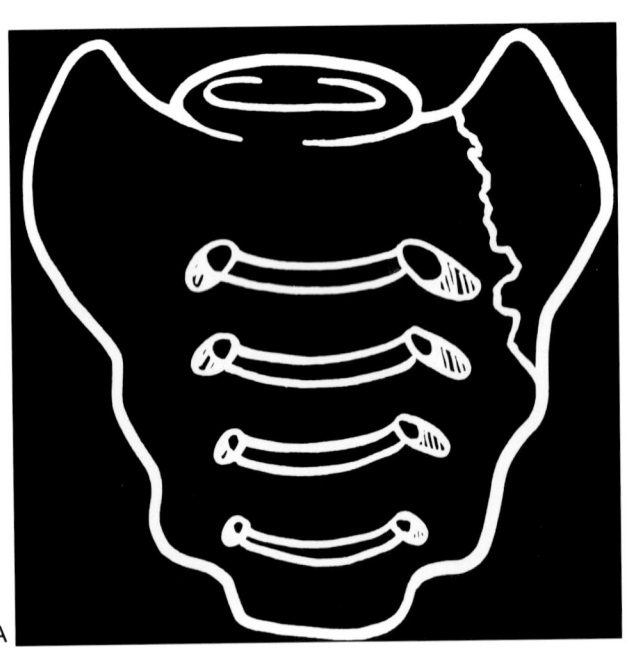

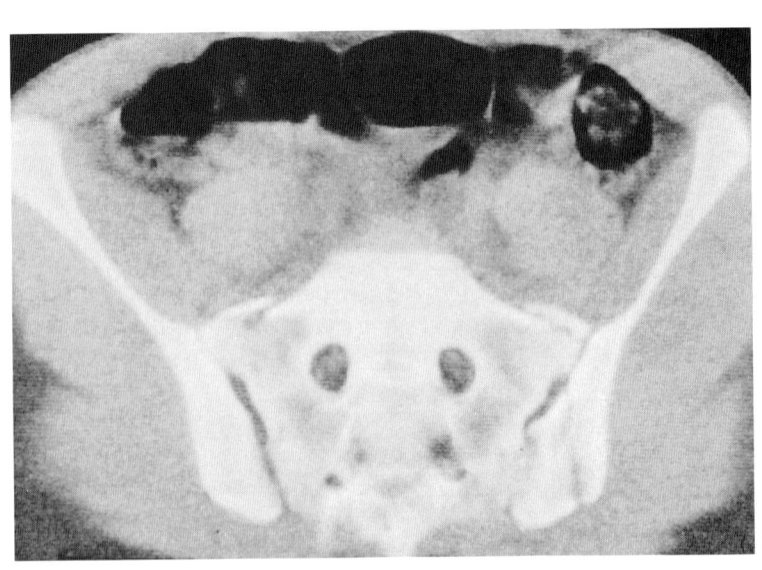

FIG. 2. A: A minor alar fracture (zone I). **B:** CT scan of alar fracture resulting from lateral compression injury to the pelvis. (With permission from Francis Denis, et al. *Clin Orthop* 227, 67–81, 1988.)

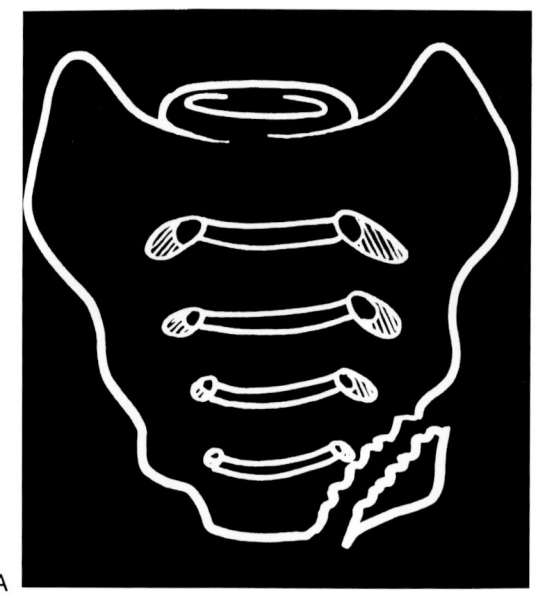

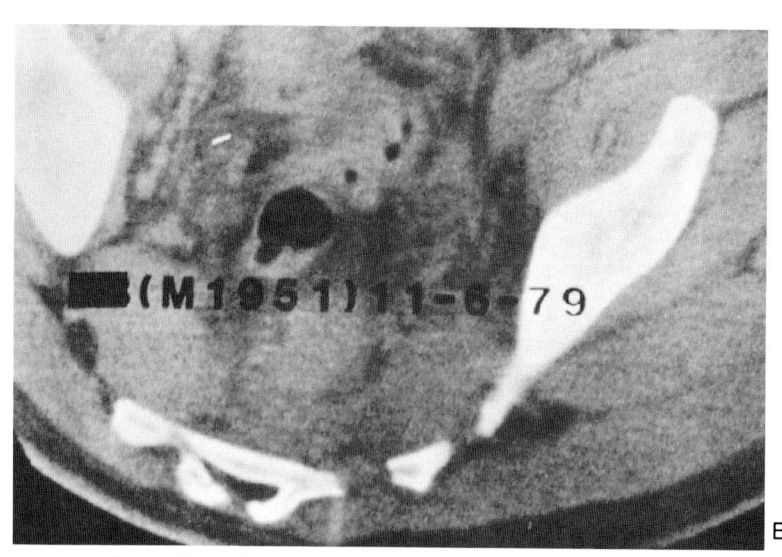

FIG. 3. A: A sacrotuberous ligament avulsion (zone I), indicating a severe pelvic instability. **B:** Sacrotuberous ligament avulsion seen on CT scan. (With permission from Francis Denis, et al. Clin Orthop 227, 67–81, 1988.)

These are typically the patients described by Bonnin with sacral sciatica. The roots involved may be the L5, the S1, or the S2 roots. This type of injury will be seen best on either coronal reconstruction of a CT scan or coronal MRI slices.

Treatment of Stable Foraminal Fractures in Zone II

Patients without sciatica can be turned in bed without major discomfort. The anterior pelvic ring is stable, and they have undisplaced or minimally displaced foraminal fractures. Unless contraindicated, early nonweight-bearing ambulation (on the side of foraminal involvement) with crutches is recommended.

In patients with sciatica, bed rest is the treatment of choice. Ambulation, nonweight-bearing or partial weight-bearing with crutches, may be started on improvement of the sciatica. If the sciatica remains severe after 6 to 8 weeks of rest and a CT scan shows reduction of the first or second sacral foramen size by 50% or more, surgical foraminotomy may be indicated. If both sciatica and foot drop are present, it is probable that both the S1 and S2 roots are involved. An early foraminotomy at both levels is recommended to avoid possible epineural fibrosis with continued sciatica.

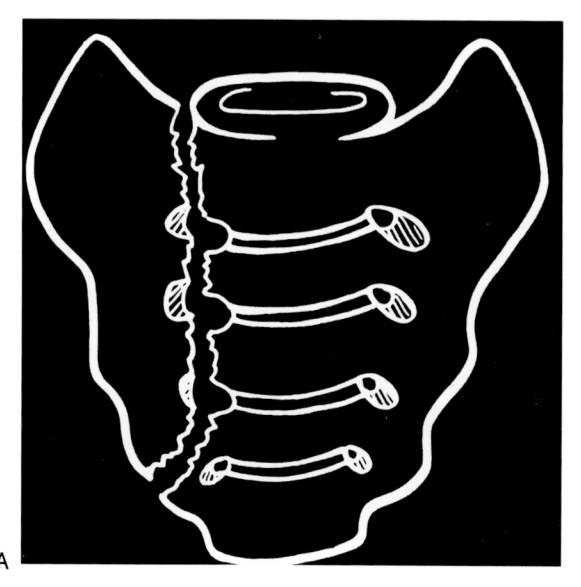

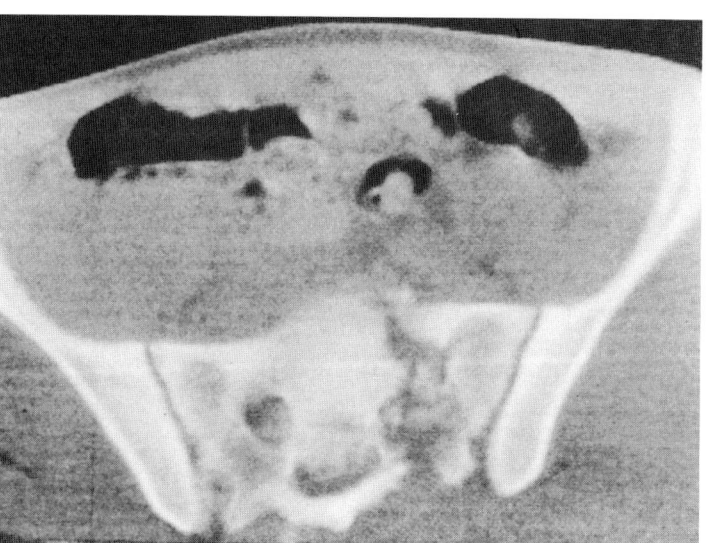

FIG. 4. A: A foraminal fracture (zone II). **B:** Foraminal fracture with significant impingement on the S1 root. (With permission from Francis Denis, et al. Clin Orthop 227, 67–81, 1988.)

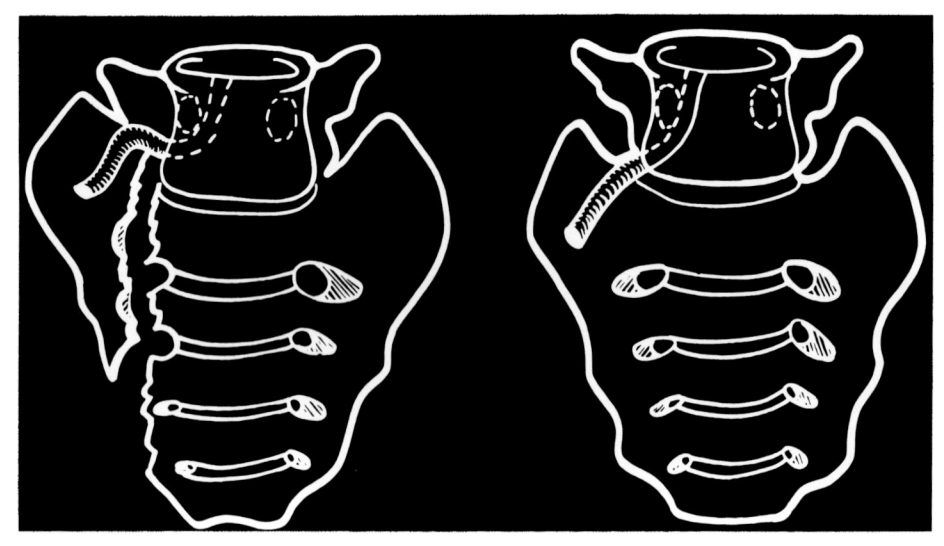

FIG. 5. Mechanism of L5 root damage and/or entrapment in the traumatic "far-out syndrome." The L5 root is caught between the sacral ala and the transverse process of L5 as the alar fragment migrates superiorly and posteriorly. (With permission from Francis Denis, et al. *Clin Orthop* 227, 67–81, 1988.)

Treatment of Unstable Foraminal Fractures in Zone II

In cases with benign-looking foraminal fracture and unstable anterior ring, the patient may benefit from application of an anterior external fixator. Early ambulation, nonweight-bearing or partial weight-bearing may be started when the patient becomes comfortable.

Lateral compression and "open book" pelvic injuries with sacral fractures in zone II are treated much the same as zone I sacral fractures. Neurologic symptoms and deficits are managed as stable foraminal fractures. Anterior stabilization helps healing of the posterior injury.

Vertical shear fractures may involve L5 (Fig. 5), the entire lumbar plexus, and sometimes the sacral plexus. Closed reduction by early traction, with or without manipulation, is recommended. This may decompress the root and maintain the fracture reduced, so that when the patient's general condition permits, delayed internal fixation may be performed. An anterior external fixator alone will stabilize the anterior pelvic ring but will not have much effect on the posterior vertical displacement.

Zone III: Central Sacral Canal Involvement

Zone III fractures primarily involve the central sacral canal, although the fracture line may also go through the other two zones. Neurologic damage occurs frequently and often involves bowel, bladder, and sexual dysfunction (7). The two types of zone III injuries are (a) sacral burst fractures (intact posterior lamina) and (b) fracture/dislocation (horizontal lamina fracture) (Fig. 6).

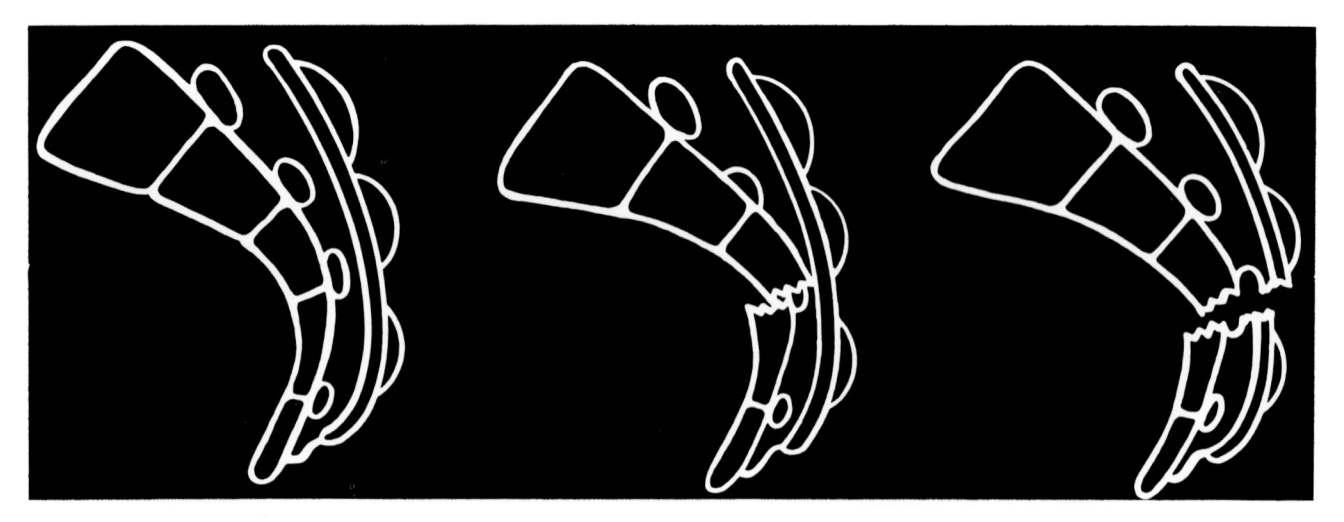

FIG. 6. Zone III injuries. On the **left,** a normal sacrum for comparison. In the **middle,** a sacral burst fracture with higher potential for sacral root compression. On the **right,** a sacral fracture/dislocation with higher potential for sacral root disruption. (With permission from Francis Denis, et al. *Clin Orthop* 227, 67–81, 1988.)

Treatment in Zone III

In the absence of neurologic deficit, treatment is aimed at stabilizing the pelvis and is similar to that for zone I and zone II injuries. However, when neurologic deficits are present, accurate diagnosis of the cause of the deficit is crucial. CT scans with thin cuts, gantry tilting, and reformatting are recommended. Meticulous attention must be given to foraminal encroachment associated with central canal obstruction. In fracture/dislocation, sacral laminectomy and sacral foraminotomy should be considered at least at the level of the transverse fracture, since the foramen is often difficult to visualize on CT scans. Some sacral roots may be torn, or the roots may be intact and compressed. In a sacral burst fracture, a sacral vertebral body may have been retropulsed into the central sacral canal without a horizontal fracture of the sacral lamina posteriorly. Cystometrograms are indicated both before and after the procedure to assess the extent of bladder involvement and postoperative recovery. During the acute phase, decompression of the sacral roots may be relatively uncomplicated. However, after fracture healing, decompression may be more difficult and yield disappointing results. In addition, epineural fibrosis may induce internal strangulation of the nerves, thereby precluding function recovery in spite of a good bony decompression.

CONCLUSION

Cystometrography (CMG) is crucial both in making a diagnosis and providing appropriate follow-up data on neurogenic bladders (4,5). A CMG is systematically recommended in patients with questionable bladder involvement and in all cases involving zone III (5). Recovery of bladder and bowel function in transverse sacral fractures is better with surgical decompression of the central cauda equina than with conservative care. CT scanning and MRI have helped enormously in understanding the pathoanatomy of sacral fractures and, in particular, of their attendant neurologic deficits.

S1 and S2 sacral sciatica improves spontaneously in 75% of patients. Surgical decompression is indicated for the remainder, with about 70% good to excellent results.

Prognosis of foot drop with conservative treatment is poor. Early decompression with anatomic reduction may improve recovery of a foot drop.

REFERENCES

1. Bonnin JG. Sacral fractures and injuries of the cauda equina. *J Bone Joint Surg* 1945;27:113.
2. Denis F, et al. Sacral fractures. *Clin Orthop* 1988;227:67–81.
3. Fallon B, Wendt JC, Hawtrey CE. Urological injury and assessment in patients with fractured pelvis. *J Urol* 1984;131:712.
4. Fardon DF. Displaced transverse fracture of the sacrum with nerve root injury: report of a case with successful operative management. *J Trauma* 1979;19:119.
5. Fountain SS, Hamilton RD, Jameson RM. Transverse fractures of the sacrum. *J Bone Joint Surg* 1977;59A:486.
6. Goodell CL. Neurological deficit associated to pelvic fractures. *J Neurosurg* 1966;24:837.
7. Gunterberg B. Effects of major resection of the sacrum. *Acta Orthop Scand* Suppl 1976;162:1–38.
8. Malgaigne JF. Treatise on fractures. Philadelphia: Lippincott, 1959;523.
9. Patterson FP, Morton KS. Neurologic complications of fractures and dislocations of the pelvis. *Surg Gynecol Obstet* 1961;112:702.
10. Wiltse LL, Guyer RD, Spencer CW, Glenn WV, Porter IS. Alar transverse process impingement of the L5 spinal nerve: the far-out syndrome. *Spine* 1984;9:31.

> # 20

Anterior Techniques of Decompression and Fixation

James C. Bayley, Hansen A. Yuan, and Bruce E. Fredrickson

The anterior surgical approach to the thoracolumbar spine is an important tool in the treatment of spinal fractures. This chapter reviews the history of the development of this approach, discusses the rationale and indications for its use, and describes in detail the techniques involved. The goal will be to familiarize the reader with the potential risks and benefits involved in this approach, with the hope that anterior treatment of thoracolumbar fractures will be facilitated.

HISTORICAL REVIEW

The Treatment of Thoracolumbar Fractures

Spine fractures and the often resulting paralysis have been recognized for centuries. The Edwin Smith papyrus from ancient Egypt states: "thou shouldst say concerning him 'One having a dislocation in a vertebra of his neck while he is unconscious of his two legs and his two arms, and his urine dribbles. An ailment not to be treated'" (12). In more modern times, the relationship between spine fractures and neurologic damage was recognized, but not well understood (38). Through the first half of this century, if the victim survived the initial trauma, the spinal injury was treated with postural reduction and long-term immobilization in bed or on various frames (6,38). The classic work of Holdsworth and Hardy (48) in 1953 was an early attempt at classification of these injuries, both from a neurologic and a structural perspective. They recommended that unstable injuries, which they defined as any fractures with posterior ligamentous injuries, gross displacement, or fractures of the articular processes, should be treated with operative fixation. They noted the disastrous consequences of treating unstable injuries in plaster immobilization, as well as the irreversibility of complete spinal cord lesions. Additionally, these authors were among the first to point out the negative effects of laminectomy, which had previously been widely advocated in the treatment of thoracolumbar fractures. This finding has been confirmed in several later series (9,14).

Perhaps due to increased use of high-speed motor vehicles and certainly due to improved trauma care, survivable fractures of the thoracolumbar spine became increasingly common in the 1960s (66). Treatment continued to be postural reduction and prolonged recumbency, primarily due to the lack of instrumentation available to achieve and maintain adequate reduction of unstable fractures. An early series from 1976 (14) involving the use of neutralization plates and laminectomy in the treatment of unstable fractures condemned the operative approach due to a lower neurologic recovery rate and increased chronic pain in those treated with surgery when compared to nonoperative treatment.

The application of Harrington distraction rods, originally developed to treat scoliosis (43), for fracture treatment, as introduced by Flesch in 1977 (30) and by Dickson in 1978 (20), ushered in the current era of aggressive surgical treatment. Over the past 15 years, there has been a marked increase in the number and complexity of the available spinal implants. The majority of these devices, specifically the A-O Fixateur Interne (19), the Olerud device (71), Edwards rods and

---

J. C. Bayley: Department of Orthopaedic Surgery, Harvard Medical School, and Beth Israel Hospital, Boston, MA 02215.
H. A. Yuan and B. E. Fredrickson: Department of Orthopaedic and Neurological Surgery, State University of New York, Health Science Center at Syracuse, Syracuse, NY 13202-3072.

sleeves (26), and Steffee plates (74), were developed for posterior application to reduce fractures and hold this anatomic position. Recently, several devices, including the Syracuse I-plate (5), the Kaneda device (51), the Dunn device (22), the Kostuik–Harrington device (53), and the Armstrong plate (7), were introduced specifically for anterior fixation of fractures of the thoracolumbar spine following anterior decompression of the spinal cord and/or cauda equina.

The Anterior Approach

Spine fractures have been classified under many different systems (17,60). While minor details and names for the different types of fractures vary between classification schemes, all report that anterior injuries, which occur primarily due to flexion forces, are more common than posterior injuries. Anterior injuries produce more damage to the structures anterior to the spinal canal with the displaced fragments of bone and disc located in that direction. Because the spinal cord may be difficult to mobilize from the posterior direction, especially in the face of anteriorly located compressive lesions, the anterior route for decompression is considered the more direct route.

Traditionally, however, the favored surgical approach to the spine was from the posterior direction for laminectomy or arthrodesis (69). The primary indication for spinal decompression was for surgical drainage and stabilization of tuberculosis of the spine (Pott's disease) (3,44). Von Lackum and Smith (75) described the anterior approach to the lumbar spine for release of scoliotic deformity in 1933. However, perhaps due to unfamiliarity with this approach on the part of orthopaedic surgeons (15) or to fear of catastrophic complications (70), the anterior route was not widely used until resurrected by Hodgson and Stock in 1960 (46), also for the treatment of tuberculous abscesses and arthrodesis. They illustrated the anterior anatomic approach to the thoracolumbar spine in detail and reported excellent results, in marked contrast to previous studies using posterior drainage procedures and/or medical therapy alone (63,67) for treatment of Pott's disease. Harmon (40) advocated anterior fusion for severe lumbosacral spondylolisthesis at approximately the same time. The simultaneous development of effective methods for internal fixation in the anterior spine (see below) expanded the use of this approach so that the anterior approach to the lumbar spine is now the fourth most widely performed procedure in the lumbar spine (77). Thus anterior surgery has become a versatile procedure to be used for many lesions in the thoracolumbar spine, including but not limited to infection (46), tumors (41), spondylolisthesis (11), postlaminectomy instability (34), and fractures with neural compression (55).

Anterior Fixation Devices

Routine application of metallic internal fixation devices to the extremities preceded their use in the spine by many years. Lange (58) first reported a simple plate apparatus for use in the spine in 1910, but these were not widely used. Humphries, Hawk, and Berndt (49) described a plate and screw implant for anterior lumbar interbody fusion in 1959. Surprisingly, the senior author was a vascular, not an orthopaedic, surgeon. In 1964, Dwyer and Schafer (25) invented a cable system for anterior application in scoliosis. By compression across the convex side of the curve, the spine was straightened. Early results, published in 1969 (24), were excellent, but the problem of straightening the lumbar lordosis and increasing strain across the noninstrumented lower lumbar segments was noted by other authors (39). This prompted Zielke (79) to develop a more rigid rod coupled with a derotational device to maintain lumbar lordosis and correct the scoliotic curve and rotation.

Unfortunately, several significant complications were reported associated with the use of the Dwyer and Zielke systems. These include retrograde ejaculation in males (31), ureteral obstruction (50), injury to the spleen (45), and lacerations of a major vessel (23). Fear of these rare but catastrophic complications has limited the application of these bulky devices in the thoracolumbar spine. Additionally, their function in compressing the convex side of a scoliotic curve limited their use in fracture management because of the requirement of distraction to reduce compressed spine fractures.

As noted previously, the application of long Harrington rods to fractures of the thoracolumbar spine, initially summarized by Dickson et al. (20) had been the predominant method of surgical treatment of fractures. Although reduction of displaced spinal fractures and successful arthrodesis were excellent with this apparatus (30), concerns were raised about the length of fusion required for adequate mechanical leverage to produce and maintain fracture reduction (36).

Additionally, the mechanism by which burst fractures cause neural compression and neurologic deficits was clarified with the advent of computed tomography (CT) scanning in the early 1980s (66). It became apparent that the compressive pathology was from the anterior direction (37), and that posterior indirect reduction by Harrington rods was not always successful in alleviating spinal canal compromise (36). Thus approaching the fractured spine from the anterior direction was viewed as more anatomically direct and thus potentially more successful (8). Unfortunately, because 80% of trunk weight is borne by the anterior spinal column, decompression of the spinal canal by debridement of the fractured vertebral body can significantly destabilize the spinal column as a whole if not resupported by an adequate strut. Materials used initially to support the spine following decompression included methyl methacrylate (42) and bone (8) (either autograft or allograft). However, use of these materials unsupported by or unattached to metallic devices resulted in an unacceptable rate of later collapse (64), especially if not reinforced with posterior instrumentation. Thus stable methods for anterior internal fixation in the thoracolumbar spine were sought.

Dunn (22) in 1984 introduced a device for anterior distraction and fusion in the thoracolumbar spine, specifically for treatment of fractures. His system consists of two threaded rods linked by crossbridges attached to the intact vertebral bodies on either side of the fracture by staples and bone screws. Distraction and/or compression as required can be applied to the spine through rotation of the threaded rods. This allows restoration of spinal alignment following anterior decompression of fracture fragments as well as subsequent compression of the bone graft strut spanning the decompressed vertebra. Most importantly, the device is stable enough in vivo to eliminate the need for supplementary posterior instrumentation. Although initial results (22) were excellent and included only three pseudarthroses in 48 patients, the prominence of this instrumentation and its proximity to major vessels led, in inexperienced hands, to several cases of arterial or venous perforation (13). The device is currently not available in the United States.

A similar implant, the Kostuik–Harrington device (54), combines a Harrington distraction rod in front and a compression rod further back clamped to the vertebra by specially modified bone screws. Attachment of these screws to the intact vertebrae adjacent to the fractured level by special staples prevents toggling of the screws. Kostuik's early results (54,55) were excellent: general improvement in partial spinal cord injuries with anterior decompression, no cases of nonunion, few device-related problems, and no early or late vascular complications. The device has not gained any widespread popularity in the United States.

A third dynamic device has recently been introduced by Kaneda et al. (51), who encountered a high failure rate with the Zielke apparatus in lumbar spine fractures. The Kaneda device is similar to the Dunn device and in the largest series reported (51), there was significant neurologic improvement in all partial spinal cord injuries and no loss of fixation. This device is currently under clinical investigation in the United States.

The principal advantage of these three devices is that they allow direct dynamic distraction of the vertebrae to ease exposure of the fracture followed by direct compression of implanted bone graft after decompression of the neural elements. All are extremely rigid once inserted. The principal disadvantage is that the bone screws and connecting rods are prominent, which may increase the danger of early or late injury to the great vessels or peritoneal contents, especially if the device is inadvertently placed anteriorly on the vertebral body. Additionally, the rigidity of the device may promote unwanted stress shielding in instrumented vertebrae and bone graft (65).

In contrast to these bulky dynamic devices, which allow direct compression of the bone graft, two plate systems have been developed for anterior application to the thoracolumbar spine. In 1988, Black, Gardner, and Armstrong (7) introduced a multiholed low-profile plate for lateral placement on the lumbar vertebral bodies. At present, the device has undergone laboratory investigation and is available commercially, but no clinical trials have been published.

The lack of a firm fixation device for anterior stabilization led to the development of a modified A-O dynamic compression plate in 1985 by Yuan et al. (78), called the Syracuse I-plate. Initial experimental data had shown that a standard A-O/ASIF D-C or neutralization plate was not sufficient to resist rotational or translational forces because of the narrowness of the plate and the parallel nature of the vertebral screws applied through the plate.

Thus after several design modifications, the current I-plate was developed, which functions as a neutralization plate following compression of the bone graft (5). The plate is 3 mm thick and angled so that 60° of curvature separates the two adjacent screw holes. The plate is applied with two screws inserted into the intact vertebral body above and below the involved vertebra.

The plate is available in lengths of 70, 80, and 90 mm. The screws are modified A-O/ASIF 6.5-mm cancellous screws consisting of a standard hexagonal head and a 4-mm long nonthreaded 6.5-mm shank for perpendicular fit into the plate. The screws are available in 5-mm increments from 40 to 80 mm. When fully seated, the screws are inset into the surface of the plate. Thus the implant lies flush with the lateral aspect of the vertebrae; the vascular structures are at negligible risk unless the screws disengage or break.

Biomechanically, several of these systems were compared to determine in vitro stability, and for comparison with available posterior instrumentation systems (61,62). These tests, using cadaver spines, showed that the I-plate is as strong as the Kostuik–Harrington and Kaneda devices in all directions tested. However, none of the anterior devices were as stable as the intact spine or the Fixateur Interne when posterior ligamentous disruption or fracture of the posterior elements is present. The authors concluded that the stability of all anterior devices currently available depends on the integrity of the posterior structures, including the facets and capsules, the interspinous and supraspinous ligaments, and the laminae. Any injury involving all three spine columns is a relative contraindication to the use of any currently available anterior device, primarily because posterior instability will allow early loosening and failure of the implant. In these cases, supplemental posterior fixation is generally recommended.

THE ROLE OF ANTERIOR SURGERY IN THE TREATMENT OF THORACOLUMBAR FRACTURES

With this historical discussion as a backdrop, the indications and practices behind the various surgical approaches to fractures of the thoracolumbar spine are discussed.

The vertebral column has two primary purposes: to support the weight of the trunk in the upright or recumbent position and to protect the spinal cord and cauda equina. When failure of the vertebral column occurs through fracture, one or both of these functions may be compromised. Thus there are two issues that must be addressed when planning treatment of any particular spine fracture. The first is the issue of neurologic compromise due to neural injury or compression; the second relates to the stability of the spinal column and its effectiveness in supporting trunk weight, both immediately and long term. These two issues are intimately related, since progressive instability may lead to late neurologic compromise.

In any given spinal injury, the degree of neural damage is closely correlated with the amount of fragment displacement and subsequent spinal canal compromise (16), although the relationship is not directly one to one. Thus a complete dislocation has a higher probability of complete spinal cord injury than does a partial subluxation or minor incongruity in alignment. Various other factors, such as prefracture spinal canal size (27), shape of the spinal canal (59), or age of the patient (66), have an impact on degree of neural injury, but, in general, the degree of displacement of the fragments of the spinal column is the major determinant of neurologic injury (16). Because of this, reversal of spinal canal compromise is a primary goal of fracture treatment. Bohlman and co-workers (8,9) have shown that even late spinal canal decompression can improve neurologic function months after injury.

Reduction of fragments and correction of malalignment causing neural compression can be done in one of three ways. The first is by nonsurgical treatment, commonly referred to as conservative care. Several studies (32,56,76) have documented by sequential CT scanning the gradual improvement of spinal canal compromise with nonoperative treatment of burst fractures. Because of the inherent property of bone to heal and subsequently remodel, minor degrees of spinal canal compromise may correct with time and immobilization. Indeed, Weinstein et al. (76) obtained follow-up of neurologically intact patients with fractures treated conservatively for a mean of more than 20 years. They found that there was no loss of neurologic function and only a moderate degree of kyphosis after this length of time. Pain did not correlate with degree of kyphosis, but instead with socioeconomic factors.

However, because this process of bone remodeling is not always predictable and requires time, even these authors do not advocate conservative treatment if there is any evidence of more than single root neurologic injury. Thus the general consensus (18,53) is that nonoperative treatment is not indicated in fractures with multiple nerve root or partial spinal cord injuries unless the general condition of the patient absolutely precludes operative treatment.

The second method of correction is by indirect operative reduction of the fracture. Much like closed reduction of extremity fractures, this implies that the fracture fragments are not directly visualized, manipulated, or removed. This indirect approach historically is employed in Harrington distraction rods, which can correct both the shortening and excessive kyphosis of thoracolumbar fractures. Fredrickson et al. (33) have clearly shown that distraction, not correction of kyphosis, reduces the intracanal fragments of burst fractures. Recent experimental work by the same authors (4) has shown that the lateral annular attachments of the disc to the fracture fragments, not the posterior longitudinal ligament, are the connections by which the distraction force of indirect reduction is transmitted to the displaced fragments. If these disc attachments are disrupted by the initial injury, reduction will be incomplete. This experimental observation explains the common clinical finding that indirect reduction by distraction does not always lead to relief of spinal canal compression (33,36,54). Thus, although indirect reduction has been utilized successfully for many years, both in the nonoperative postural reduction technique of Guttmann (38) and the operative approach of posterior distraction (1,20,71), it may result in inconsistent reduction and incomplete relief of spinal canal compromise.

The third approach to fracture reduction is by direct removal of displaced spinal column fragments, analogous to ORIF of extremity fractures. Two techniques have been employed. Garfin et al. (35) have advocated a posterolateral approach to the anterior fragments at the time of posterior instrumentation of unstable thoracolumbar fractures. This technique involves resecting the facet joint on the side of greatest spinal canal compromise and removing or directly impacting the displaced vertebral fragments forward out of the spinal canal. The Garfin series reported good results using this approach in a limited number of patients. Problems with this technique include incomplete visualization of some fracture fragments, epidural bleeding anterior to the dural sac where effective control can be difficult, and the difficulty of displacing the fragments if the fracture is more than a few days old. Some authors (72) have advocated the use of ultrasound to verify clearance of fragments from the canal, but this requires cumbersome equipment and an extensive laminectomy.

An alternate method of direct decompression is by the anterior approach to anterior fractures. As noted above, this approach has not been widely used in the past, due both to unfamiliarity with the approach and its attendant risks, and because of inadequate implants to restore spinal stability. Recently, the anterior route has enjoyed more widespread use.

With the anterior approach, the spinal cord is under direct vision. Associated nerve root injuries can be evaluated and/or decompressed. In cases of multiple trauma, retroperitoneal and intraperitoneal injuries can be repaired through the same incision. While significant complications can be associated with the anterior approach, complete decompression of fracture fragments impinging on the dural sac is facilitated due to direct visualization. Bone and soft tissue anterior to the spinal cord and cauda equina can be removed. Thus, all things considered, anterior decompression is the only method that assures complete relief of spinal canal compromise. For this reason, direct anterior decompression and fusion have several advantages over indirect posterior reduction and fusion.

Unfortunately, due both to the fracture and subsequent removal of bone, anterior decompression usually results in spinal column instability, the second major issue involved in the debate on which approach to use. In defining spinal stability, classically the two-column concept of Holdsworth (47) was used. In this scheme, the spinal column is composed of an anterior compression side (the vertebral bodies and intervertebral discs) and a tension side (the posterior elements and attached ligaments). Fractures were considered stable if one column was intact. However, some fractures that should be considered stable according to the Holdsworth scheme, such as flexion–compression injuries or burst fractures, were found to be unstable, leading to late collapse (10). Additionally, widespread use of CT scanning in the evaluation of spinal injuries in the 1980s revealed flaws in this concept, prompting Denis (17) to formulate his three-column concept of the spine. In practice, this mechanistic approach to the evaluation of spine fractures allows classification into stable and unstable injuries depending on whether the middle column (posterior vertebral body, posterior annulus of the disc, and posterior longitudinal ligament) is damaged.

With posterior indirect reduction of fracture fragments via distraction, the integrity of the damaged middle column is not restored. Instead, the posterior instrumentation substitutes a more rigid posterior column for the damaged middle column to restore spinal stability. While this often works successfully, several series have reported late development of kyphosis (36,64) despite intact posterior instrumentation and fusion mass. Additionally, if the hardware fails or becomes disconnected from the spine prior to successful arthrodesis, immediate instability will occur. Thus posterior instrumentation should only be considered as a technique that holds indirect reduction until fracture healing occurs. Occasionally, additional measures such as prolonged recumbency or rigid external orthoses may be required to support the construct in the postoperative period.

The anterior approach, on the other hand, has the advantage of direct repair of the fracture (rarely performed) or reconstruction of the fractured body following decompression, by substitution with other materials at the primary site of instability. Ordinarily, bone graft, either autologous or allograft, has been employed. This bone can serve as a scaffold on which new living host bone can grow, healing the fracture and restoring stability. Other materials such as polymethylmethacrylate (PMMA) have been used but have recently been associated with late failure (64). Synthetic porous materials are in development or use elsewhere (52) but not currently available in the United States. Until these are perfected, bone graft should be considered as the primary material implanted in place of the debrided fracture fragments.

As noted above, the primary difficulty with anterior reconstruction in the past has been to hold the bone graft in position without failure until union occurs. With the recent development of adequate anterior implants that avoid the necessity of subsequent posterior instrumentation, the use of the anterior approach will hopefully become more widespread.

ANTERIOR SURGICAL APPROACHES

There are three different anterior approaches to the fractured thoracolumbar spine: transthoracic, thoracoabdominal, and the lateral retroperitoneal approach. Which one is chosen depends on the location of the fracture. In general, the minimum visualization required is one entire vertebra above and one below the fractured vertebra. Thus the transthoracic approach is used for fractures from T4 to T9, the thoracoabdominal approach for fractures from T10 to L1, and the retroperitoneal approach for fractures from L2 to L5. Fortunately, thoracic injuries requiring the anterior approach above T4 are extremely rare, as this is a very difficult area to expose due to the small ribs and vascular structures (57,68) in the upper mediastinum. The transthoracic approach is ordinarily done through a right thoracotomy because the heart is situated more on the left. The other two approaches are ordinarily performed from the patient's left as the liver may be difficult to mobilize from the right. However, the surgeon's preference and/or the accessibility of fracture fragments from one side or the other may dictate the alternate side of approach.

The Transthoracic Approach

In this approach, a rib is ordinarily removed. Most often, the sixth or seventh rib is chosen because these lie below the scapula when the arm is flexed at the shoulder on an arm holder. This eliminates the necessity of excessive detachment of the muscles from the scapula, required if a higher rib is resected. Additionally, removal of a lower rib frequently limits the exposure of the thoracic vertebra because of the proximity to the dome of the diaphragm. Occasionally, in high thoracic fractures, an approach through the fourth or fifth rib may be required, but this necessitates skeletonizing the scapula. Low intrathoracic fractures can ordinarily be approached through the sixth rib. A Foley catheter is inserted along with large-bore venous catheters. If possible, equipment for collection and retransfusion of blood should be used. Spinal cord monitoring equipment is at the discretion of the surgeon in cases of partial spinal cord injuries or intact patients. However, the authors favor its use to monitor any potential improvement in the case of partial injuries, and to warn of any manipulation-induced neurologic deterioration.

Anesthesia is induced in standard fashion with the exception that a double lumen endotracheal tube must be used. This allows both lungs to be ventilated independently. Failure to do so would result in the right lung inflating during surgery. While the lung can be packed off, any inadvertent tear in the lung tissue would result in an air leak and decreased ventilation of the contralateral lung if a single lumen endotracheal tube were used.

Following intubation, the patient is placed in the left lateral decubitus position with the right arm elevated and flexed forward at the shoulder (Fig. 1). The arm is held suspended in a well padded arm holder or freely across the patient's chest. Draping is such that the midline posteriorly and the midline anteriorly should be prepped and visible. In this position, the first prominent rib below the scapula is ordinarily the fifth. Counting of ribs can be done from the twelfth rib, which explains the need to visualize the midline posteriorly. The skin over the chosen rib is incised from the transverse process of the vertebra, following the rib anteriorly to its ipsilateral costal cartilage. The subcutaneous

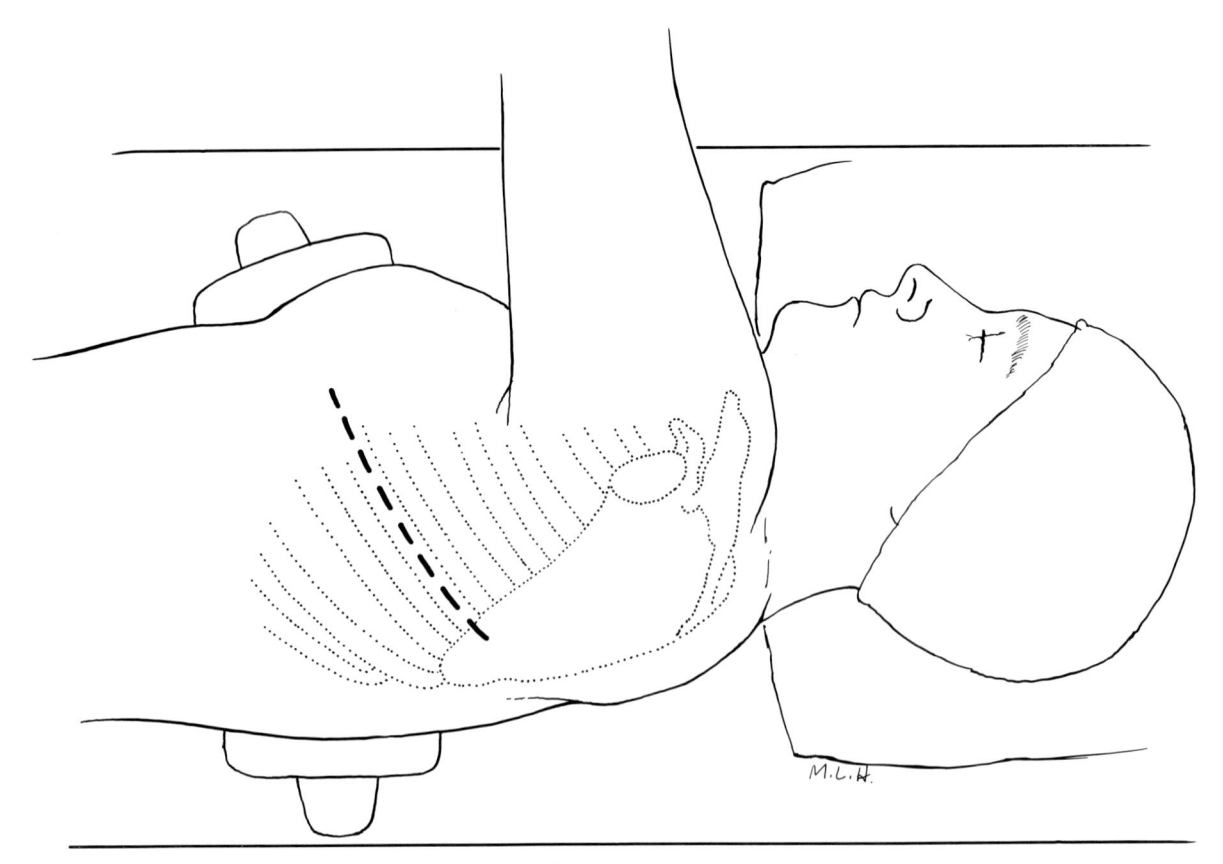

FIG. 1. Positioning of the patient for the transthoracic approach.

tissue is incised with electrocautery down to but not into the superficial muscle layer. Anteriorly, the serratus muscle may be visible attaching to the ribs, but the large muscle encountered posterolaterally is the latissimus dorsi. These muscles are isolated at their free borders and incised over a clamp with electrocautery. The latissimus is incised as far posteriorly as the junction of the rib with the deep surface of the transverse process. With blunt dissection, the chest wall is freed from any attachments to the scapula, and the scapula rotated superiorly and posteriorly to uncover the rib. The periosteum on the rib is sharply incised, and rib elevators are used to strip subperiosteally as far back as the transverse process. At the inferior and superior borders of the rib, Doyon elevators are used to strip the deep periosteum from the rib along with the parietal pleura that is adherent to the periosteum on the undersurface of the rib. Care should be taken at the inferior border of the rib where the neurovascular bundle is located (Fig. 2). If not ligated or cauterized as far posteriorly as possible, the subcostal artery may bleed excessively into the wound or pleural cavity.

After complete elevation of the periosteum from both the superficial and deep surfaces of the rib, the rib is cut as far back as possible with a rib cutter and anteriorly just before the junction with the costal cartilage. A chest spreader is inserted and opened widely over moist sponges, being careful not to fracture adjacent ribs by overdistraction. Occasionally, two ribs may have to be removed to gain adequate exposure in a patient with a stiff chest wall, such as in ankylosing spondylitis. Resection of two adjacent ribs is preferable over multiple rib fractures due to excessive rib spreading; this does not result in any significant chest wall instability unless four or more ribs are removed or fractured. The lung is then deflated and packed off with wet sponges.

Ordinarily, the fractured vertebra is readily identifiable by the paravertebral hematoma and through palpation of the deformity. If not, and frequently for medicolegal reasons in any case, a cross-table AP radiograph can be taken with a large-bore spinal needle in a disc adjacent to the suspected fractured body. The disc spaces are readily apparent as the whitish bulges on the spine. Usually the vena cava and aorta do not interfere with exposure of the spine, as they are well anterior in the mediastinum at this location. However, the azygos vein is frequently located just anterior to the vertebrae. This vein is difficult to mobilize away from the spine, and care must be taken to avoid injury to this vessel with sharp retractors.

Once the fractured vertebra is identified, the segmental vascular bundle overlying the midline of the fractured and two adjacent vertebral bodies should be located. Frequently, these segmental vessels, which are direct branches of the major veins and aorta, are obvious, but occasionally the parietal pleura must be incised and gently teased off the vertebra to identify them. The parietal pleura is incised in an H-shaped fashion from the three vertebral bodies and peeled back without damage to the segmental vessels. These vessels are then carefully isolated over two right-angle clamps, tied off using silk suture, and cut. The vessels should be ligated away from the neural foramina, as they may be important anastomotic channels feeding into the anterior spinal artery. These anastomoses usually are located close to the neural foramina; thus ligation closer to their origin from the aorta will diminish the chance of spinal cord infarction from ischemia in the circulation of the anterior spinal artery. The artery of Adamkiewicz, which supplies a major portion of the blood supply to the spinal cord (21), commonly occurs between T4 and T10, usually on the left side. However, the location is very variable. Theoretically, ligation of this vessel might potentially cause spinal cord infarction. However, several series using the anterior approach in the treatment of fractures have reported no cases of iatrogenic spinal cord infarction (51,54) in large numbers of patients as long as the vessels are ligated away from the neural foramina.

The foramina can then be located by following the nerve root associated with the segmental vessels posteriorly. This localizes the pedicles of the three vertebrae, providing landmarks to define the posterior ex-

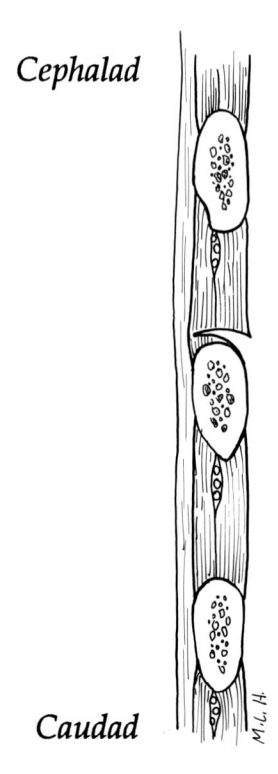

FIG. 2. Entrance into the chest cavity is at the superior border of the rib to avoid injury to the neurovascular bundle on its caudad aspect.

tent of vertebral body resection required for adequate decompression. The techniques of decompression are discussed later.

Following full decompression of the spinal canal, the strut graft is inserted and any required implants applied if indicated. Ordinarily, allograft cortical bone, usually iliac crest, tibia, or femur, is used if the defect is large, as taking such a large piece of autograft iliac crest will leave a sizeable defect. This graft is supplemented with pieces of the resected rib. Frequently, the allograft cortical strut can be hollowed out and packed with pieces of the patient's autograft iliac crest. While this has not been shown to have a higher rate of incorporation compared to allograft alone, it has the theoretical advantages associated with earlier incorporation of autograft compared to allograft (29). The parietal pleura should then be closed if possible. Frequently this is not the case as the bone graft may be too bulky. The pleura will eventually reform and cover the defect, so that closure of the parietal pleura over the vertebra is not absolutely required. The lung should be reinflated and copious amounts of warmed saline poured into the pleural cavity. With serial hyperinflations of the lung, any air leaks due to visceral pleural tearing or lung parenchymal injury will be readily evident. If large, repair or occasionally partial resection of damaged lung may be required. A chest tube is then inserted through a separate stab incision one or two ribs below the resected rib and directed posteriorly and superiorly. A rib approximator is used to place the ribs back in their normal position, and heavy sutures or wire tied around the ribs to hold this position. The bed of the resected rib is then closed in running fashion, as are the incised muscles, subcutaneous tissue, and skin closure as usual.

Postoperatively, the patient should be observed in an intensive care unit, as the potential exists for sudden vascular or neurologic catastrophe. The chest tube is removed when any air leak has ceased and the drainage is minimal. Ordinarily the patient can be placed in a brace or polypropylene body jacket at the discretion of the surgeon and ambulated when stable and comfortable in the thoracolumbosacral orthosis (TLSO).

The Thoracoabdominal Approach

A thoracolumbar retroperitoneal approach is used for fractures from T11 to L2. The spine is usually approached from the patient's left side, since any incidental vascular lacerations are more easily repaired if they occur to the aorta rather than to the thin-walled vena cava. Additionally, the liver may be difficult to mobilize during an approach on the right side. However, either a left or right approach can be used at the discretion of the surgeon. Once again, equipment for collection and retransfusion of any blood lost during surgery should be used except in cases of fractures due to primary or metastatic tumor. Spinal cord monitoring equipment if available should be used to document spinal cord decompression and warn of any impending neurologic injuries during surgery.

The patient should be positioned so that the affected vertebra is over the bend in the table to enhance exposure and provide lateral distraction on the operative side. A double lumen endotracheal tube is helpful to allow deflation of the left lung but is not as necessary as in the transthoracic approach. The patient is placed in the right lateral decubitus position, resting slightly backward on a kidney rest or sandbag (Fig. 3). The

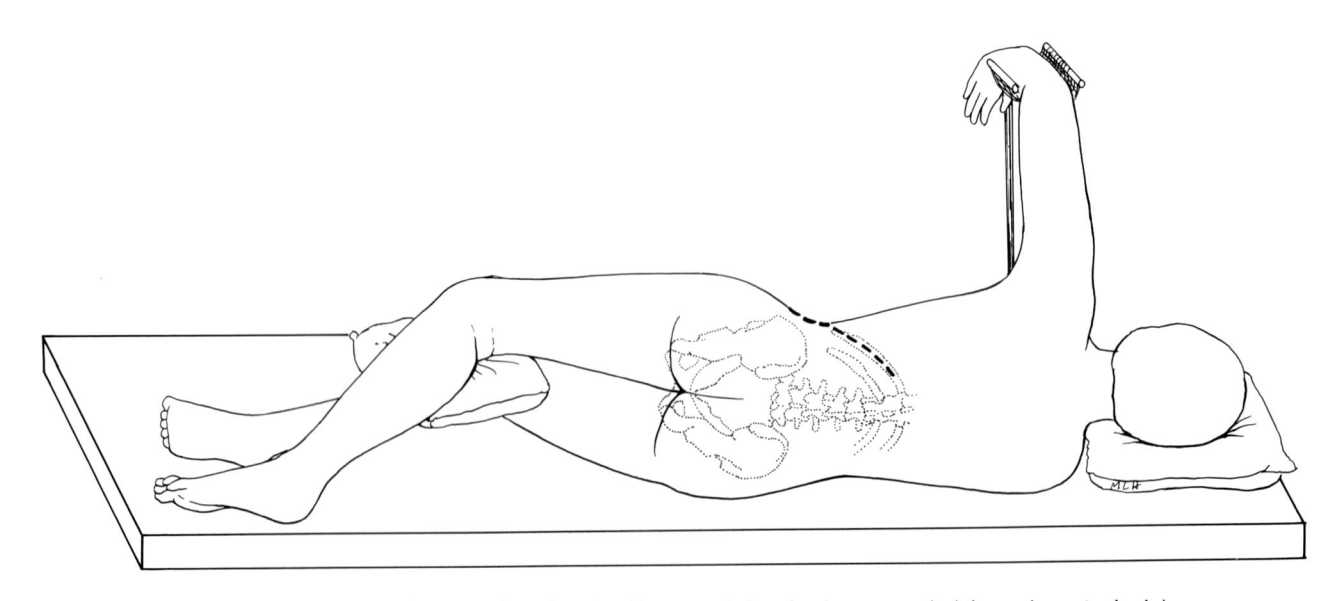

FIG. 3. Positioning of the patient for the thoracoabdominal approach (viewed posteriorly).

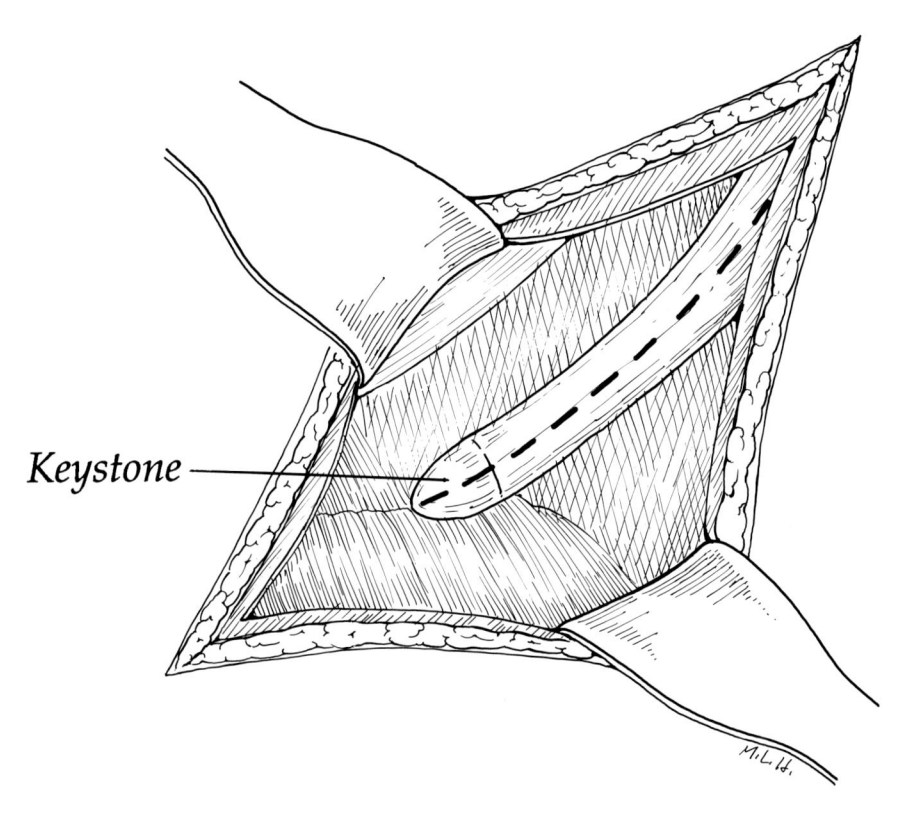

FIG. 4. The rib is exposed after incision of the overlying muscles. The keystone, or cartilaginous tip, is the free end of the floating rib.

entire left side is prepped and draped from axilla to hip including the iliac crest. Autologous or allograft fibula can be used if necessary. An incision is made over the tenth or eleventh rib from the posterior axillary line extending anteriorly and inferiorly to the lateral margin of the rectus sheath. Using electrocautery, the subcutaneous tissue is incised down to the rib through the periosteum. Anteriorly, the external and internal oblique muscles along with the transversus abdominis are incised or split in line with the fibers if possible. The cartilaginous tip of the rib, called the keystone (Fig. 4), is incised sharply and the rib exposed extrapleurally by use of Doyon rib elevators. The rib is osteotomized as far posteriorly as possible, at least as far as the costotransverse junction. The rib is used to provide extra bone graft, or it can be used for a vascularized graft if the vascular pedicle is preserved. The thoracic cavity is entered through the rib bed, and the anterior attachment of the diaphragm to the tip of the tenth rib is identified. By gentle finger dissection, the retroperitoneum is entered through the incised keystone, and by blunt dissection the plane between the diaphragm and the retroperitoneum is developed as far posteriorly as possible. This maneuver isolates the diaphragm from the lung superiorly and the retroperitoneum inferiorly. The diaphragm is then incised at least 1 cm from its peripheral attachment and the central portion is tagged with heavy suture for later reattachment. It is important to leave a peripheral rim of diaphragm for this closure (Fig. 5); the rim, however, is denervated by this maneuver so it should not be overly generous. The retroperitoneum is stripped from the undersurface of the diaphragm back to the crura. Anteriorly, the peritoneum is separated from the retroperitoneum by blunt dissection from the anterior abdominal

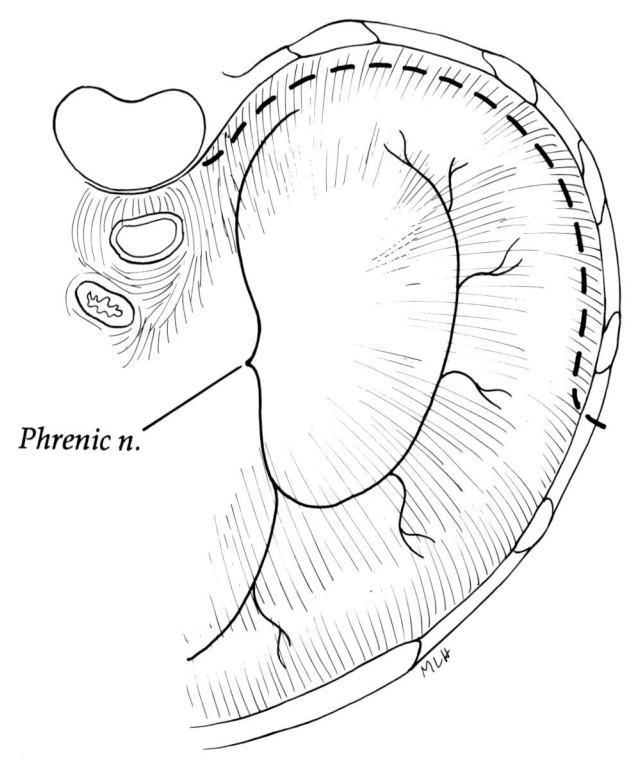

FIG. 5. Incision in the diaphragm (from below). A small peripheral rim must be left for closure. This limits the amount of denervation.

wall as far forward as the rectus sheath. The crura of the diaphragm are then taken down and tagged, leaving a small peripheral portion on the spine for reattachment. This exposes the vertebral bodies from T10 to L2.

The vertebra to be removed is identified. If this is not obvious, a radiograph may be taken with a marker over the suspected body. The lung is deflated and packed off using a soft retractor and a rib spreader is used to widen the space between the ninth and eleventh rib. The peritoneum is gently retracted anteriorly.

The discs are readily identifiable as the glistening white bulges and are safe to incise. The segmental vessels lie on the middle of the vertebral bodies, away from the discs. The vessels are gently elevated from the periosteum using right angle clamps and ligated with sutures or clips. Two ligatures should be tied on the proximal end nearest the aorta. Ligation must be done at least 1 cm from the vertebral foramen to avoid interfering with the anastomotic network of blood supply to the cord as discussed earlier. Ligation of the segmental vessels allows the aorta and vena cava to be mobilized, falling away from the vertebral column. The vertebrae are then stripped subperiosteally back to the neural foramen and pedicles, and forward to the anterior longitudinal ligament. Decompression is described later.

Closure is begun by inserting a #24 chest tube through a separate stab incision. The crura of the diaphragm are repaired using nonabsorbable suture and a running suture is used to close the diaphragm. This may be supplemented with multiple interrupted sutures for added strength. Prior to closure, the lung is checked for air leaks by filling the thoracic cavity with saline and watching for bubbles. The ribs are approximated and sutured together with heavy suture and the muscle layers are closed separately.

Postoperatively, the patient is fitted in a body cast or plastic TLSO. The patient is then allowed progressive ambulation. The chest tube is removed when no air leak is evident and drainage is minimal.

The Retroperitoneal Approach

For exposure of L1 through L5, an extraperitoneal approach through the twelfth rib is used. The patient is anesthetized and positioned as in a thoracoabdominal approach. The eleventh or twelfth rib is palpated and the skin incised over the rib, extending anteriorly and inferiorly to the lateral border of the rectus sheath (Fig. 6). For exposure of the lower lumbar vertebrae, the incision is extended longitudinally toward the pubis just lateral to the rectus sheath. Using electrocautery, the subcutaneous tissue is incised down to the external oblique muscle, which can usually be split by blunt dissection in line with its fibers. The internal oblique and transversus abdominis are cut with electrocautery, being careful not to enter the peritoneum deep to the transversus abdominis muscle. The periosteum of the twelfth rib is incised and the rib is removed as far back as the transverse process of the associated vertebra. Once again, the cartilaginous tip (the keystone) of the twelfth rib is used as a marker to locate the junction of the peritoneum and retroperitoneum. After the key-

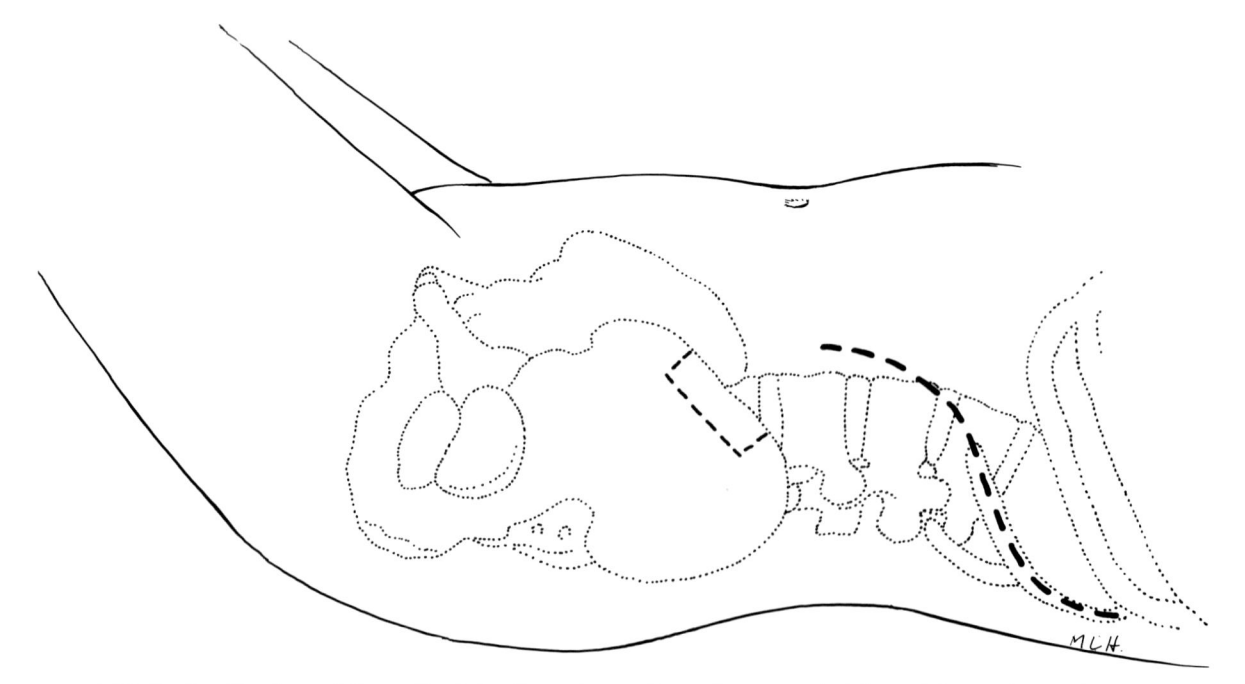

FIG. 6. Positioning of the patient for the retroperitoneal approach (viewed from above the patient).

stone is split with a scalpel, a finger is inserted and swept back and forth, separating the peritoneum and contents anteriorly from the retroperitoneal fat posteriorly. By blunt dissection, the interval between the retroperitoneum and the diaphragm is opened, and the peritoneal contents are retracted anteriorly. Any tears in the peritoneum should be closed with running absorbable suture when identified. For surgery at L2 and below, the diaphragm does not have to be incised.

The psoas muscle is then identified but not entered. The disc spaces are the best landmarks and can be identified as the protruding white bulges. At the anterior border of the psoas muscle, the segmental vessels are located traversing the waist of the vertebral bodies; they are ligated using right angle clamps as in the thoracoabdominal approach. This frees up the aorta and vena cava or their iliac branches, which are retracted anteriorly toward the opposite side. The vertebrae are then stripped subperiosteally as far posteriorly as the vertebral foramen and forward to the anterior longitudinal ligament. This also mobilizes the psoas muscle posteriorly, as well as the sympathetic chain that normally lies in the psoas or on the anterior aspect. Additionally, the segmental nerves that make up the lumbar plexus will be protected if the psoas muscle is left intact and retracted posteriorly. After debridement of the vertebra is performed and any required implants affixed, the wound is closed in separate layers over a drain. Because the thoracic cavity is not entered in this approach, no chest tube is required. Postoperative care is the same as for a thoracoabdominal approach.

Fracture Debridement and Canal Decompression

Following exposure of the fractured and two adjacent vertebral bodies, decompression can proceed. The pedicle attaches to the vertebral body at the anterior margin of the dural sac looking from the anterior direction. Thus the base of the pedicle can serve as a marker to determine the posterior depth for safe decompression. The lateral aspect of the fractured vertebral body on the side of exposure can be removed under direct vision, but the anterior and contralateral cortex should not be routinely removed as these cortical pieces will provide a bed for graft incorporation and may help prevent graft migration or loosening. Large pieces of the fractured vertebra can then be removed with a rongeur, but as the depth of decompression reaches the base of the pedicle, care should be exercised. In a fracture that is more than 24 hr old, the dura may be adherent to the posterior longitudinal ligament and/or fracture fragments. If these are injudiciously torn out with the rongeur, a significant dural tear may result, which can be difficult to close. Unless the base of the pedicle is used as the safe level for initial posterior decompression, inadvertent dural laceration may occur. This is due to the fact that retropulsed fracture fragments will extend to variable distances into the canal, making the exact depth of the dura and contents unpredictable.

The posterior aspect of the vertebral body should be drilled out using a cutting or diamond burr (Fig. 7). At this point, the depth at which the dura is located can frequently be identified. If an edge between the dura and fracture fragments is found, a Penfield elevator or dental pick can be used to separate the two structures, and bone can be removed with a pituitary or Cloward rongeur under direct vision. Dissection should proceed from the contralateral pedicle toward the surgeon, as doing this in the opposite direction allows the dura to bulge into the field of decompression, risking a dural tear. Debridement is performed in a methodical fashion from and including the disc above the fracture to the disc below. The discs are usually adherent to the posterior longitudinal ligament (PLL); a thin posterior rim of disc can be left attached to the PLL if dissection is difficult. The endplates of the adjacent vertebrae should not be damaged, as they will furnish support for the cortical bone graft. Throughout this decompression, bleeding is often excessive due to the vascularity of the vertebra and the fracture. Bone wax and Gelfoam should be packed into areas of bleeding, even if these areas are to be removed later. In this way, overall blood loss will be minimized and the field will not always be obscured by a pool of blood.

Once decompression is complete, bone graft is obtained. Autograft can be taken from the ipsilateral iliac crest through a separate incision or from the ipsilateral fibula. Recently, allograft, which can be femur, tibia, iliac crest, or fibula, has enjoyed more popularity, but concerns about the transmission of blood-borne diseases and a lower rate of graft incorporation (29) may limit the use of allograft. On the other hand, the defect left by decompression of the fracture is frequently quite large, and the available autograft iliac crest may be too weak or too rounded to adequately fit. Thus there is often no choice but to use allograft cortical struts. As noted earlier, there may be a theoretical advantage to packing the center of the allograft cortical strut with autograft cancellous bone from the iliac crest.

Once the graft has been obtained, craters are fashioned in the midportions of the adjacent intact endplates with the cutting burr. The operating table is then flexed as much as possible to provide distraction across the area to be fused. Bone distracting clamps can also be used to distract the intact vertebrae. Occasionally, the A-O femoral distractor can be used across Steinman pins to maximize distraction. The graft is then fashioned with pegs in the ends, which are placed into the craters in the endplates. If necessary, the graft can be impacted posteriorly using the bone impactors.

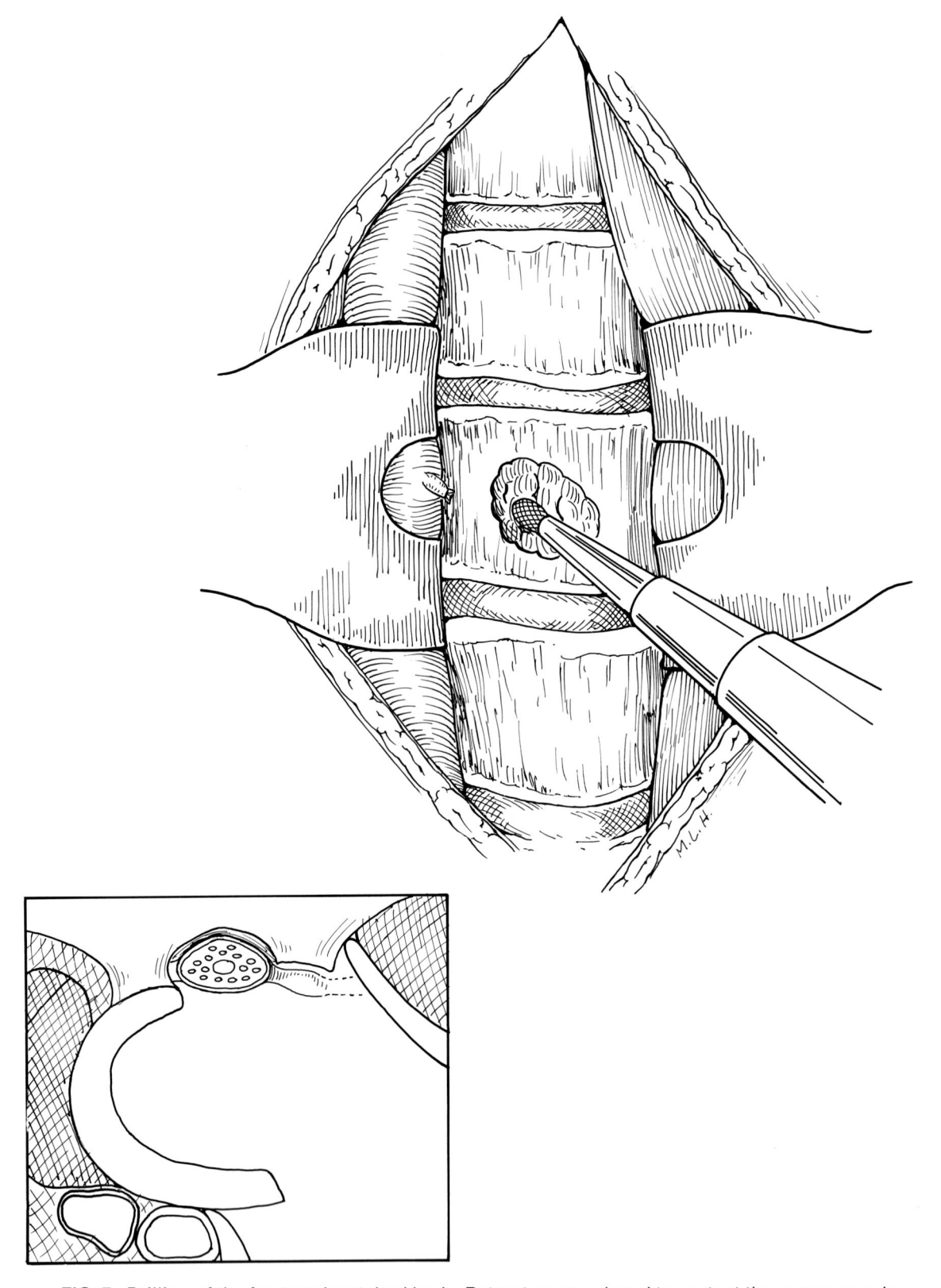

FIG. 7. Drilling of the fractured vertebral body. Retractors are placed to protect the psoas muscle on the ipsilateral side and the major vessels on the opposite side. The extent of decompression is shown in the **inset.**

The distraction is then removed and the table placed back in the neutral position. This locks the graft in place. The internal fixation devices, which are discussed elsewhere in this volume, can then be applied.

RESULTS OF ANTERIOR DECOMPRESSION AND FUSION

Most large series of the surgical treatment of thoracolumbar fractures have consisted primarily of the results of posterior instrumentation. Beginning with the original paper of Flesch et al. (30) in 1977 using long Harrington rods and continuing up to the recent reports of Garfin et al. (35), Aebi et al. (1), and Olerud et al. (71) using more modern instrumentation, most authors report good results from this approach.

When comparing nonoperative treatment of thoracolumbar fractures with posterior surgery, Denis et al. (18) found that all patients treated surgically were able to eventually return to work full time. Seventeen percent of patients treated conservatively developed late neurologic problems, including paraparesis and severe radicular pain. The overall neurologic recovery rates were similar in both groups. They recommended that all thoracolumbar burst fractures be treated with operative reduction and posterior stabilization to minimize postinjury pain and prevent further neurologic deterioration. Similarly, McAfee et al. (66) found that all patients with partial neurologic deficits improved with posterolateral decompression and distraction with Harrington rods. They felt that internal stabilization with Harrington rods reduced the incidence of late kyphosis, neurologic deterioration, and chronic pain, when compared to nonoperative treatment.

Recently, Schlegel et al. (73) have shown that early operative stabilization (within 72 hours of the injury) of thoracolumbar injuries can significantly reduce the rate of serious medical complications. While there were no significant differences in neurologic improvement when comparing early versus late stabilization, pulmonary and skin wound problems were minimized by early surgery, especially in polytrauma patients (those with an Injury Severity Score greater than 17). Thus spinal stabilization appears to minimize both the early and late complications of thoracolumbar fractures, especially if performed within 72 hours of injury.

However, almost all series of posterior stabilization of fractures include failures of this approach, primarily due to inadequate canal decompression, development of late instability, and/or hardware failure. Gertzbein et al. (37) reported on 36 patients in Toronto who underwent posterior Harrington rod instrumentation for thoracolumbar fractures. Over half of those with burst fractures eventually lost reduction, collapsing into more severe kyphosis despite the presence of intact Harrington rods in some. The vast majority of these patients with ongoing pain around the fracture site at last follow-up had unsatisfactory spinal alignment. They concluded that unstable burst injuries, especially those with significant fracture of the anterior vertebral cortex, were prone to late collapse, excessive kyphosis, and chronic pain.

While intrinsically stronger than Harrington rods, pedicle instrumentation systems have also been reported to fail. In the Olerud et al. (71) original series, 20 patients underwent insertion of the PSF device with pedicle screws in the vertebrae on either side of the burst fracture. There were two technical failures due to progressive collapse, and a third patient required subsequent anterior decompression because of ongoing spinal canal compression. Aebi et al. (1) also reviewed the short-term results of the A-O Fixateur Interne in 1987. They noted two cases of instrument loosening in 30 patients, but otherwise reported excellent results at reducing canal compression and restoring lumbar lordosis. In a more comprehensive review, Dick (19) found three instrumentation failures, one screw breakage, two deep infections, and four patients who suffered loss of reduction among 183 patients. Thus, while pedicle fixation systems appear to combine the advantages of short fusions and improved results when compared to Harrington rods, these systems are not problem free and are only now becoming generally available.

In contrast to these problems associated with posterior indirect reduction, whether by long Harrington rods or short pedicle systems, there have been several reports of improved results with anterior decompression and instrumentation. Kostuik (53) described anterior insertion of the Kostuik–Harrington rod system and showed an average improvement of 1.6 Frankel grades in incomplete spinal cord injuries. Failure of the instrumentation occurred in 13 patients, including two nonunions and 11 screw breakages, but this did not appear to affect neurologic recovery or long-term stability. The author did recommend that subsequent posterior instrumentation should be performed in fractures with extensive posterior comminution. In a separate paper, Kostuik (55) also reported a high failure rate when other anterior devices such as Dwyer cables or the A-O D-C plate were used and felt that these devices, which neutralize or compress the anterior column, were inadequate for use in thoracolumbar burst fractures.

Along similar lines, Bohlman et al. (9) found that anterior decompression is more effective than posterior indirect reduction in improving neurologic recovery in partial spinal cord injuries. This was true even with late surgery, in which several patients regained the ability to walk following late decompression. Complications of the anterior procedure included kyphosis of more than 20° in 15%, two fibrous nonunions, and two with transient radiculopathies. Most patients in this series did not have anterior instrumentation placed, instead undergoing later posterior instrumentation to restore spinal stability.

The best series to date comparing anterior with posterior surgery was reported by Esses (28) in 1990. Forty patients with thoracolumbar burst fractures to anterior or posterior decompression and fusion were randomly assigned. At an average follow-up of 20 months, there were no significant differences between the two groups in amount of kyphotic deformity, instrumentation failure rate, or in any preoperative variables. The only significant difference was in degree of canal decompression, with the anterior group having significantly less canal compromise by CT scan. Esses concluded that, in this group of patients, both anterior and posterior instrumentation systems can restore spinal stability, but that the anterior direct approach results in more complete and reliable canal decompression. Whether this improved decompression affects ultimate neurologic recovery is at present unknown.

With the recent development of stronger anterior instrumentation devices, results of the anterior approach continue to improve. Dunn (22) reported on 48 patients who underwent anterior decompression and insertion of the Dunn device. There was neurologic improvement in 40 (83%); complications were limited to three cases of nonunion and three infections, none of which required implant removal. Kaneda's series included 15 patients who underwent insertion of his special anterior device. All partial neurologic deficits improved, there were no hardware failures, and morbidity was limited to the iliac crest bone donor site.

Counterbalancing these excellent results of anterior decompression and fusion is the morbidity of the anterior approach, the risks of catastrophic, although rare, vascular and visceral injury, and the frequent necessity of subsequent posterior instrumentation to restore spinal stability. Clearly, the anterior direct route can assure complete decompression of the spinal canal if done properly. Late stability can be maximized by combining both anterior and posterior instrumentation. Although posterior fusion and stabilization are more familiar to the majority of spinal surgeons, there is a definite role for the anterior route to the spine, especially in cases of ongoing neural compression refractory to posterior indirect reduction.

FUTURE DEVELOPMENTS

Recently, the Morscher plate has been developed for anterior fixation of the cervical spine (2). This plate incorporates titanium inserts placed into the vertebral body, which expand when screws are placed for fixation. This expansion substantially increases the pull-out strength of the plates and significantly lessens the chance of the screw backing out.

Modification of this plate design to one suitable for placement in the thoracolumbar spine may make anterior plating of fractures in this area more successful. Beyond development of a better plate, there are certainly numerous further modifications that can and should be made to the dynamic anterior devices.

Other areas that may facilitate the use of anterior surgery include development of better strut grafts. These involve primarily synthetic materials, which must combine the following properties: biologically inert, strength under compressive loads, ability to adhere to and/or incorporate with intact adjacent vertebrae, and ease of shaping under the conditions of the operating room. While several implants and materials are currently under development, none can yet meet the above criteria. Thus, at the present time, bone graft appears to be the best material available. Unfortunately, bone graft must be supplemented with internal fixation devices, none of which are yet ideal.

CONCLUSIONS

Anterior treatment of thoracolumbar fractures is a crucial method of choice for decompression and stabilization of anterior fractures of the spine. The ideal patient for use of this approach is one with a partial spinal cord or cauda equina injury and extensive anterior compression of the dura. In this case, few would argue with the idea that the anterior approach will guarantee full decompression of the spinal canal, allowing maximal attainable neurologic recovery. A relative indication is in the patient with anterior compression without neurologic deficit, in whom the possibility exists for late development of spinal stenosis due to canal compression or instability. The primary area where the anterior approach is not indicated is in fractures with posterior dural compression or extension–distraction injuries. These are more amenable to posterior decompression and/or stabilization.

Hopefully, the above discussion and description of the anterior approach will allow the reader to become more familiar with its use. It should be considered an integral part of any rational approach to the patient with trauma to the thoracolumbar spine.

REFERENCES

1. Aebi M, Etter C, Kehl T, Thalgott J. Stabilization of the lower thoracic and lumbar spine with the internal spinal skeletal fixation system. Indications, techniques, and first results of treatment. *Spine* 1986;12:544–551.
2. Aebi M, Zuber K, Marchesi D. Treatment of cervical spine inju-

ries with anterior plating: indications, techniques, and results. *Spine* 1991;16:S38–S45.
3. Albee FH. Transplantation of a portion of the tibia into the spine for Pott's disease. A preliminary report. *JAMA* 1911;57: 885–889.
4. Bayley JC, Yuan HA, Donovan DD, et al. Contribution of the posterior annular attachments in the reduction of experimental burst fractures. Orthopaedic Trauma Association Annual Meeting, Nov 7–10, 1990, Toronto, Canada, p. 43.
5. Bayley JC, Yuan HA, Fredrickson BE. The Syracuse I-plate. *Spine* 1991;16:S120–S124.
6. Bedbrook G. Treatment of thoracolumbar dislocation and fractures with paraplegia. *Clin Orthop* 1975;112:27–43.
7. Black RC, Gardner VO, Armstrong GWD, et al. A contoured anterior spinal fixation plate. *Clin Orthop* 1988;227:135–142.
8. Bohlman HH, Eismont FJ. Surgical techniques of anterior decompression and fusion for spinal cord injuries. *Clin Orthop* 1981;154:57–67.
9. Bohlman HH, Freehafer A, Dejak J. Spinal cord injuries and late anterior decompression of spinal cord injuries. *J Bone Joint Surg* 1975;57A:1025–1031.
10. Bohlman HH, Freehafer A, Dejak J. The results of acute injuries of the upper thoracic spine with paralysis. *J Bone Joint Surg* 1985;67A:360–369.
11. Bradford DS, Gotfried Y. Staged salvage reconstruction of grade IV and V spondylolisthesis. *J Bone Joint Surg* 1987;69A: 191–201.
12. Breasted JH. *The Edwin Smith Papyrus*, vol 1. Chicago: University of Chicago Press, 1930;327.
13. Brown LP, Bidwell KH, Holt RJ, Jennings J. Aortic erosions and lacerations associated with the Dunn anterior spinal instrumentation. Presented at the Scoliosis Research Society, 1985.
14. Burke DC, Murray DD. The management of thoracic and thoraco-lumbar injuries of the spine with neurologic involvement. *J Bone Joint Surg* 1976;58B:72–78.
15. Capener N. Spondylolisthesis. *Br J Surg* 1932;19:374–382.
16. Davies WE, Morris JH, Hill V. An analysis of conservative (nonsurgical) management of thoracolumbar fractures and fracture-dislocations with neural damage. *J Bone Joint Surg* 1980;62A: 1324–1328.
17. Denis F. The three column spine and its significance in the classification of acute thoracolumbar spine injuries. *Spine* 1983;8: 817–831.
18. Denis F, Armstrong GWD, Searls K, Matta L. Acute thoracolumbar burst fractures in the absence of neurologic deficit. *Clin Orthop* 1984;189:142–149.
19. Dick W. The "fixateur interne" as a versatile implant for spine surgery. *Spine* 1987;12:882–900.
20. Dickson JH, Harrington PR, Edwin WD. Results of reduction and stabilization in the severely fractured thoracic and lumbar spine. *J Bone Joint Surg* 1978;60A:799–806.
21. Dommisse GF. The blood supply of the spinal cord: a critical vascular zone in spinal surgery. *J Bone Joint Surg* 1974;56B: 225–235.
22. Dunn HK. Anterior stabilization of thoracolumbar injuries. *Clin Orthop* 1984;189:116–124.
23. Dwyer AP. A fatal complication of paravertebral infection and traumatic aneurysm following Dwyer instrumentation. *J Bone Joint Surg* 1979;61B:239–241.
24. Dwyer AF, Newton NC, Sherwood AA. An anterior approach to scoliosis. *Clin Orthop* 1969;62:192–202.
25. Dwyer AF, Schafer MF. Anterior approach to scoliosis: results of treatment in fifty-one cases. *J Bone Joint Surg* 1974;56B: 218–224.
26. Edwards CC, Levine AM, Weigel MC, White JB. Factors affecting neurologic recovery following post-traumatic incomplete paraplegia. *Orthop Trans* 1987;11:453–454.
27. Eismont FJ, Clifford S, Goldberg M, Green B. Cervical sagittal canal size in spine injury. *Spine* 1984;9:663–666.
28. Esses SI. The AO spinal internal fixator. *Spine* 1989;14:373–378.
29. Fernyhough JC, White JI, LaRocca H. Fusion rates in multilevel cervical spondylosis comparing allograft fibula with autograft fibula in 126 patients. *Spine* 1991;16:S561–S564.
30. Flesch JR, Leider LL, Erickson DL, Chou SN, Bradford DS. Harrington instrumentation and spine fusion for unstable fractures and fracture-dislocations of the thoracic and lumbar spine. *J Bone Joint Surg* 1977;59A:143–153.
31. Flynn JC, Price CT. Sexual complications of anterior fusion of the lumbar spine. *Spine* 1984;9:489–492.
32. Fredrickson BE, Yuan HA, Bayley JC. The nonoperative treatment of thoracolumbar injuries. *Semin Spine Surg* 1990;2:70–78.
33. Fredrickson BE, Mann KA, Yuan HA, Lubicky JP. Reduction of the intracanal fragment in experimental burst fractures. *Spine* 1988;13:267–271.
34. Freebody D, Bendall R, Taylor RD. Anterior transperitoneal lumbar fusion. *J Bone Joint Surg* 1971;53B:617–627.
35. Garfin SR, Mowery CA, Guerra J, Marshall LF. Confirmation of the posterolateral technique to decompress and fuse thoracolumbar spine burst fractures. *Spine* 1985;10:218–223.
36. Gertzbein SD, MacMichael D, Tile M. Harrington instrumentation as a method of fixation in fractures of the spine: a critical analysis of deficiencies. *J Bone Joint Surg* 1982;64B:526–529.
37. Gertzbein SD, Court-Brown CM, Marks P, et al. The neurological outcome following surgery for spinal fractures. *Spine* 1988; 13:641–644.
38. Guttmann L. Initial treatment of traumatic paraplegia. *Proc R Soc Med* 1954;47:1103–1121.
39. Hall JE. Current concepts review: Dwyer instrumentation in anterior fusion of the spine. *J Bone Joint Surg* 1981;63A: 1188–1190.
40. Harmon PH. Anterior extraperitoneal lumbar disk excision and vertebral body fusion. *Clin Orthop* 1960;18:169–176.
41. Harrington KD. Anterior cord decompression and spinal stabilization for patients with metastatic lesions of the spine. *J Neurosurg* 1984;61:107–117.
42. Harrington KD. The use of methyl-methacrylate for vertebral body replacement and anterior stabilization of pathological fracture-dislocations of the spine due to metastatic malignant disease. *J Bone Joint Surg* 1981;63A:36–46.
43. Harrington PR. Treatment of scoliosis. *J Bone Joint Surg* 1962; 44A:591–602.
44. Hibbs RA. An operation for progress in spinal deformities. A preliminary report of three cases from the service of the Orthopaedic Hospital. *NY Med J* 1911;93:1013–1016.
45. Hodge WA, Dewald RL. Splenic injury complicating the anterior thoraco-abdominal surgical approach for scoliosis. *J Bone Joint Surg* 1983;65A:396–397.
46. Hodgson AR, Stock FE. Anterior spine fusion for the treatment of tuberculosis of the spine. *J Bone Joint Surg* 1960;42A: 295–310.
47. Holdsworth F. Fractures, dislocations and fracture-dislocations of the spine. *J Bone Joint Surg* 1970;52A:1534–1551.
48. Holdsworth FW, Hardy A. Early treatment of paraplegia from fractures of the thoraco-lumbar spine. *J Bone Joint Surg* 1953; 35B:540–550.
49. Humphries AW, Hawk WA, Berndt KL. Anterior fusion of the lumbar spine using an internal fixation device. *J Bone Joint Surg* 1959;41A:371–376.
50. Johnson RM, McGuire EJ. Urogenital complications of anterior approaches to the lumbar spine. *Clin Orthop* 1981;154:114–118.
51. Kaneda K, Abumi K, Fujiya M. Burst fractures with neurologic deficits of the thoracolumbar spine: results of anterior decompression and stabilization with anterior instrumentation. *Spine* 1984;9:788–795.
52. Kaneda K, Hashimoto T, Abumi K. Anterior decompression and reconstruction with anterior instrumentation for thoracolumbar burst fractures with neurologic deficits. *Orthop Trans* 1990;14:777.
53. Kostuik JP. Anterior fixation for burst fractures of the thoracic and lumbar spine with or without neurological involvement. *Spine* 1988;13:286–293.
54. Kostuik JP. Anterior fixation for fractures of thoracic and lumbar spines with or without neurologic involvement. *Clin Orthop* 1984;189:116–124.
55. Kostuik JP. Anterior spinal cord decompression for lesions of the thoracic and lumbar spine: techniques, new methods of internal fixation and results. *Spine* 1983;8:512–531.
56. Krompinger WJ, Fredrickson BE, Mino DE, Yuan HA. Con-

servative treatment of fractures of the thoracic and lumbar spine. *Orthop Clin North Am* 1986;17:161–170.
57. Kurz LT, Pursel SE, Herkowitz HN. Modified anterior approach to the cervicothoracic junction. *Spine* 1991;16:S543–S547.
58. Lange F. Support for the spondylotic spine by means of buried steel bars, attached to the vertebrae. *Am J Orthop Surg* 1910;8:344–355.
59. Matsuura P, Waters RL, Adkins SH, et al. Comparison of computerized tomography parameters of the cervical spine in normal control subjects and spinal-cord injured patients. *J Bone Joint Surg* 1989;71A:183–188.
60. Magerl F. External spinal skeletal fixation. In: Weber BG, Magerl F, eds. *The external fixator*. Berlin: Springer-Verlag, 1985;291–297.
61. Mann KA, Found EM, Yuan HA, Fredrickson BE, Lubicky J. Biomechanical evaluation of the effectiveness of anterior spinal fixation systems. *Orthop Trans* 1987;11:378.
62. Mann KA, McGowan DP, Fredrickson BE, Falahee M, Yuan HA. A biomechanical investigation of short segment spinal fixation for burst fractures with varying degrees of posterior disruption. *Spine* 1990;15:470–478.
63. Martin NS. Pott's paraplegia: a report in 120 cases. *J Bone Joint Surg* 1971;53B:596–608.
64. McAfee PC, Bohlman HH, Ducker T, Eismont FJ. Failure of stabilization of the spine with methylmethacrylate. *J Bone Joint Surg* 1986;68A:1145–1157.
65. McAfee PC, Farey ID, Shirado O, Sutterlin C, Gurr K, Woodberry K. A quantitative histologic study of stress shielding with transpedicular instrumentation: a canine model. *Orthop Trans* 1990;14:37–38.
66. McAfee PC, Yuan HA, Lasda N. The unstable burst fracture. *Spine* 1982;7:365–373.
67. Medical Resource Council Working Party on Tuberculosis of the Spine. Five year assessments of controlled trials of ambulatory treatment, debridement and anterior spinal fusion in the management of tuberculosis of the spine: studies in Bulawayo (Rhodesia) and in Hong Kong. *J Bone Joint Surg* 1978;60B:163–177.
68. Micheli LJ, Hood RW. Anterior exposure of the cervicothoracic spine using a combined cervical and thoracic approach. *J Bone Joint Surg* 1983;65A:992–997.
69. Mixter WJ, Barr JS. Rupture of the intervertebral disc with involvement of the spinal canal. *N Engl J Med* 1934;211:210–215.
70. Newman PH. Editorial: lumbo-sacral arthrodesis. *J Bone Joint Surg* 1965;47B:209–210.
71. Olerud S, Karlstrom G, Sjostrom L. Transpedicular fixation of thoracolumbar vertebral fractures. *Clin Orthop* 1988;227:44–51.
72. Quencer RM, Montalvo BM, Eismont FJ, et al. Intraoperative spinal sonography in thoracic and lumbar fractures: evaluation of Harrington rod instrumentation. *Am J Neuroradiol* 1985;6:353–359.
73. Schlegel J, Yuan HA, Fredrickson BE, Bayley JC. Timing of operative intervention in the management of acute spinal injuries. *Orthop Trans* 1991;15:257.
74. Steffee AD, Biscup RS, Sitkowski DJ. Segmental spine plates with pedicle screw fixation. A new internal fixation device for disorders of the lumbar and thoracolumbar spine. *Clin Orthop* 1986;203:45–53.
75. von Lackum HL, Smith AF. Removal of vertebral bodies in the treatment of scoliosis. *Surg Gynecol Obstet* 1933;57:250–256.
76. Weinstein JN, Collalto P, Lehmann TR. Thoracolumbar "burst" fractures treated conservatively: a long-term follow-up. *Spine* 1988;13:33–38.
77. White AA. Editorial comment on anterior interbody fusion. In: *Lumbar spine surgery*. St Louis, MO: CV Mosby, 1990;432.
78. Yuan HA, Mann KA, Found EM, et al. Early clinical experience with the Syracuse I-plate: an anterior spinal fixation device. *Spine* 1988;13:278–285.
79. Zielke K. Derotation and fusion: anterior spinal instrumentation. Presented at the Twelfth Annual Meeting of the Scoliosis Research Society, Hong Kong, 1977.

21

Anterior Decompression and Instrumentation in the Management of Thoracolumbar Injuries, with Special Reference to Burst Fractures

Yizhar Floman

Failure to achieve canal clearance by posterior instrumentation techniques employing ligamentotaxis and/or posterior decompression may necessitate a more direct approach for decompression—the anterior approach. This is especially true in burst injuries. According to Yuan et al. (40), anterior approach to the spine was described as early as 1750 by Geraud, and in 1852 by Maisonneuve. In 1928, Royle (36) was the first to describe hemivertebra excision by the anterior approach. The technique did not gain much popularity until Hodgson and Stock (17) reported on anterior decompression techniques in the management of tuberculous spondylitis associated with neurologic damage almost 30 years later.

The technique of anterior decompression has been employed since then in a variety of pathological conditions, such as osteomyelitis, both pyogenic and tuberculous; rigid angular kyphotic deformities; and, more recently, in both burst injuries of the spine and metastatic cord compression.

Most of the earlier reports described the method of anterior cord decompression without instrumentation. The first anterior device designed for anterior spine fixation was described by Milgram in New York City in 1953. Unfortunately, this device used for kyphosis correction was not successful (24).

In the late 1960s Dwyer (7), in Australia, was the first to devise and popularize an anterior spinal fixation system for scoliosis surgery. The system consisted of vertebral body screws connected to each other by a braided titanium cable. One of the shortcomings of the Dwyer device was the inadvertent creation of iatrogenic lumbar kyphosis. In Boston, Hall further popularized the technique and introduced some modifications to the Dwyer instrumentation, including a rod to connect the vertebral screws (15). Zielke (42) further modified the Dwyer system by replacing the cable of the instrumentation with a solid rod, enabling the induction of lordosing forces. Later on, Slot (38) modified the Zielke apparatus and described a distractor and fixator for anterior use in management of kyphotic deformities.

Dunn (5) developed an anterior distraction fixation device for the management of lumbar burst injuries. This was a biomechanically sound device that was able to withstand both axial and rotational loading. A number of fatal aortic and common iliac aneurysms as a result of the bulkiness of the device and its proximity to great vessels led to the removal of the implant from the market. In the meantime, in Japan, Kaneda devised a similar anterior fixation device (18) with a lower profile, and hence a safer implant, that has gained general popularity and is being used with increasing frequency (Fig. 1).

In Canada, Kostuik (20) adapted the Harrington system for anterior use. Dwyer screws were modified to accept the Harrington distraction or compression rods. In the Kostuik-Harrington system, a standard Har-

---

Y. Floman: Department of Orthopaedic Surgery and Spine Surgery Unit, Hebrew University–Hadassah Medical School, Hadassah University Hospital, Jerusalem 91120, Israel.

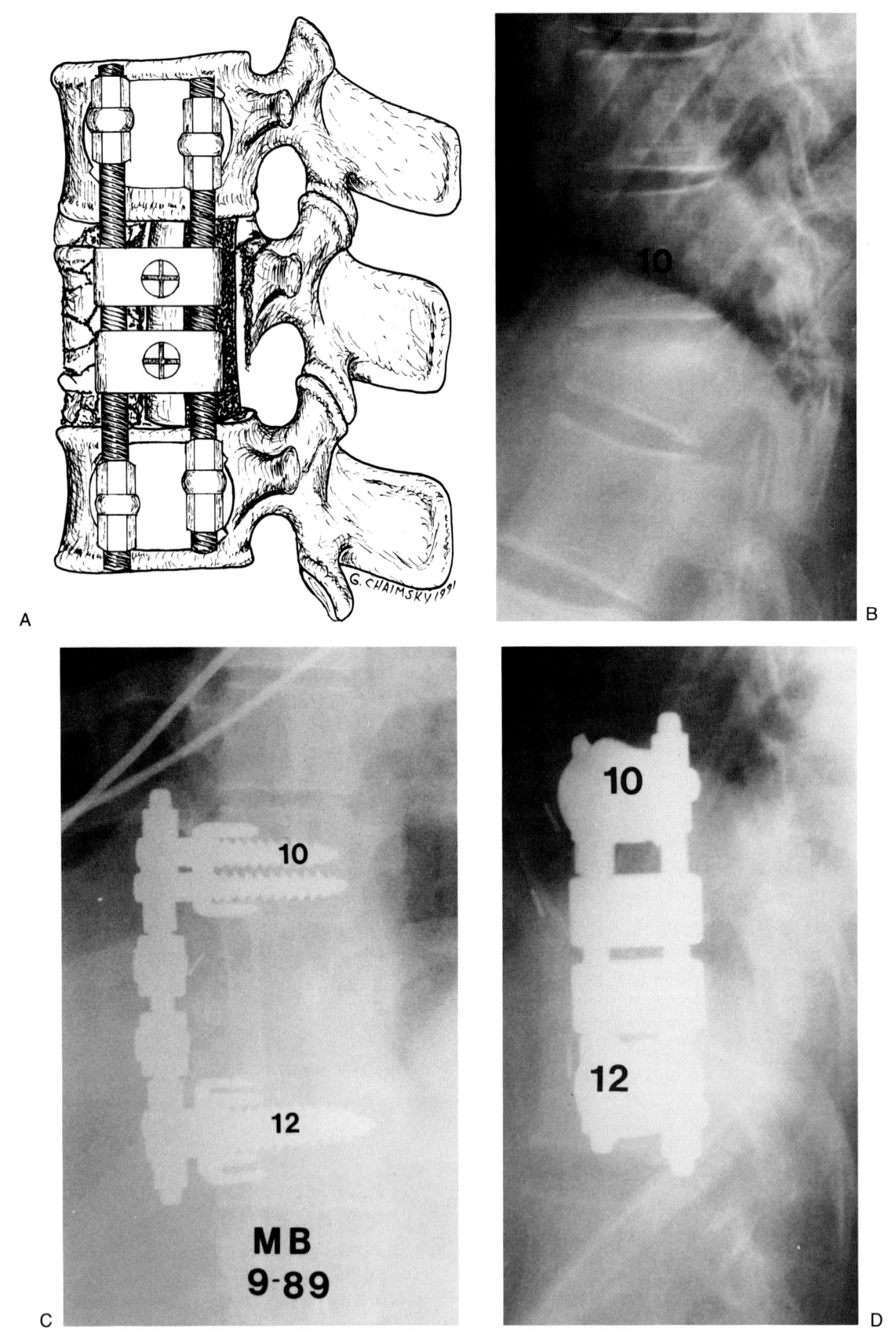

FIG. 1. A: The Kaneda anterior spinal device. It consists of vertebral plates, vertebral screws that fix the plates to the vertebral body, rigid threaded rods that connect the vertebral screws, nuts, and transverse fixators connecting the rods. This is a depiction of the use of the Kaneda device in a lumbar burst fracture following anterolateral decompression and iliac crest bone graft. **B–D:** Application of the Kaneda device in a burst fracture of T9 after anterior decompression and bone grafting. (Case courtesy of R. Geoffrey Wilber, M.D., Cleveland, OH.)

rington round-ended rod is used with a larger-holed screw for the ratchet end of the distraction rod. A smaller-holed (collar) screw is used for the collar end of the distraction rod or a heavy compression rod. Washers are used between the screw head and the vertebral body.

Kostuik has used this modified system in over 350 cases (22). The indications for the application of the Kostuik–Harrington system are correction of angular kyphosis, Scheuermann's kyphosis, anterior fixation of burst fractures, and anterior fixation of posterior pseudarthrosis.

All anterior implants described so far raise concern for possible vascular erosion over the prominent metal rods or cables. Therefore attempts have been made to utilize spinal plates. The Syracuse (Yuan) I-plate was developed to allow firm fixation without the danger of vascular injury by virtue of its flat, nonprominent profile (40). The system was developed in 1985, initially by modifying an A-O/ASIF dynamic compression plate into an I-configuration by broadening the upper and lower ends. The plate was curved to allow it to wrap around the vertebral body, and the plate's middle holes were eliminated. The fixating screws are modified 6.5-mm cancellous A-O screws. The current plate is 3 mm thick. Fixation is realized by fixing the plate to the vertebral bodies above and below the resected, injured, or pathologic vertebral corpus (Fig. 2).

Other types of instrumentation available for anterior use are the Armstrong plate (26), the A-O plate (14) (Fig. 3), and several other plates including the Senegas plate (37). Although plates are reasonably good fixation devices, they do not provide the ability to apply distraction forces, feasible in the various rod systems.

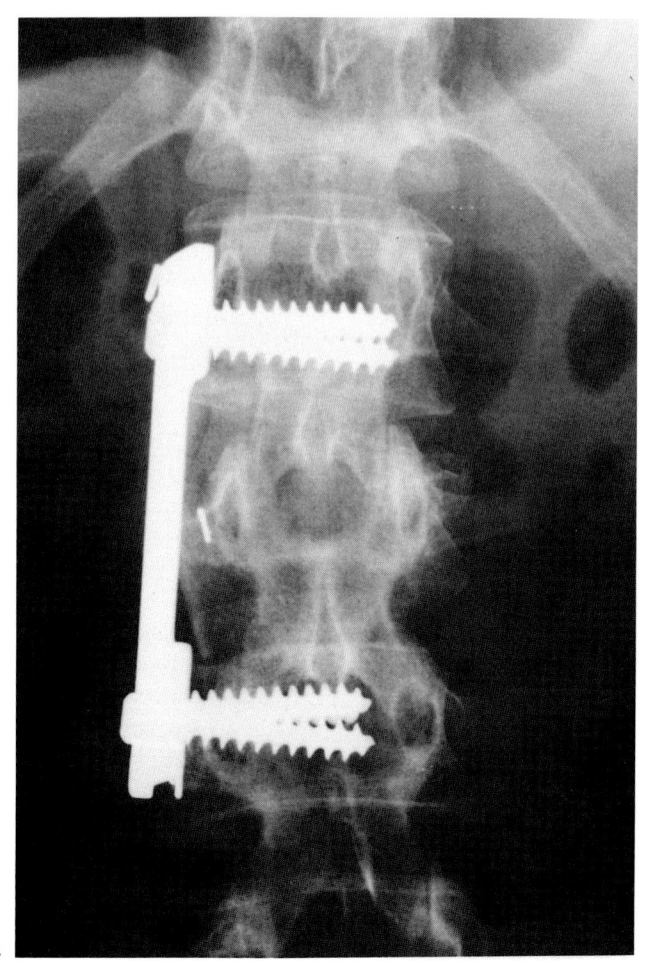

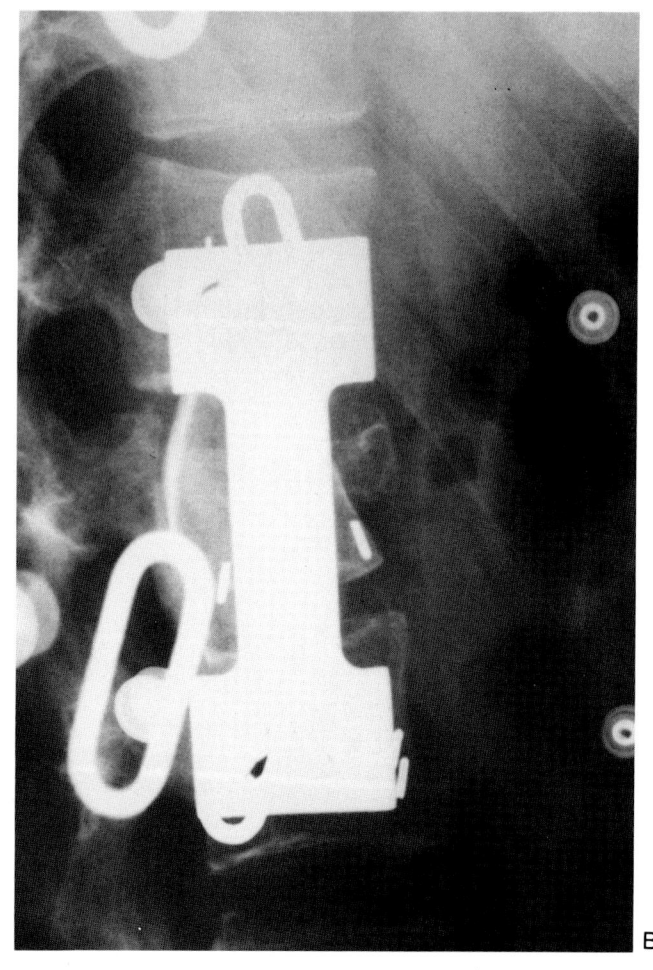

FIG. 2. Anteroposterior **(A)** and lateral **(B)** radiographs of the lumbar spine in a patient with an L2 burst fracture, who underwent anterior decompression, strut grafting, and stabilization with the Syracuse I-plate. (Case courtesy of Dr. B. Fredericksen; from ref. 27.)

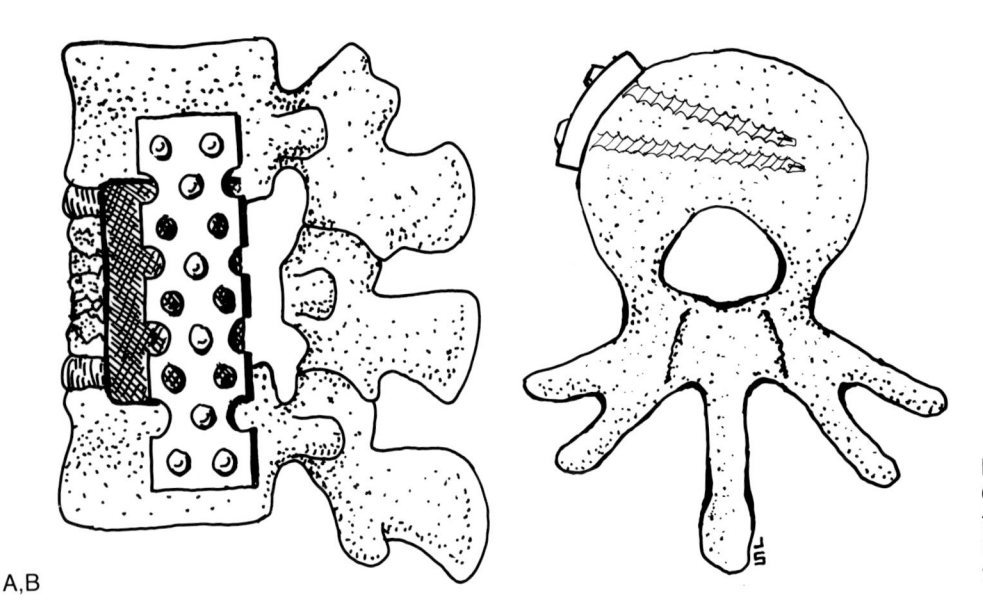

FIG. 3. A: Specially contoured A-O spinal plate. **B:** It allows more than two screws to be inserted into the vertebral body. (Modified from ref. 14.)

In general, anterior spinal devices fall into three major categories: plates, rods, and interbody devices. Existing plates are the A-O plate (14), Armstrong plate (26), Yuan plate (40), and Senegas plate (37). Anterior rod systems include the Dunn (5), Kaneda (18), Slot (38), Zielke (42), and Kostuik–Harrington (20). Interbody devices include the Rezaian device, the Harms interbody "cage" that may be fixed to a posterior or anterior Harms–Zielke instrumentation by pedicle screws (3) (Fig. 4), and temporary distraction devices such as the Pinto distractor.

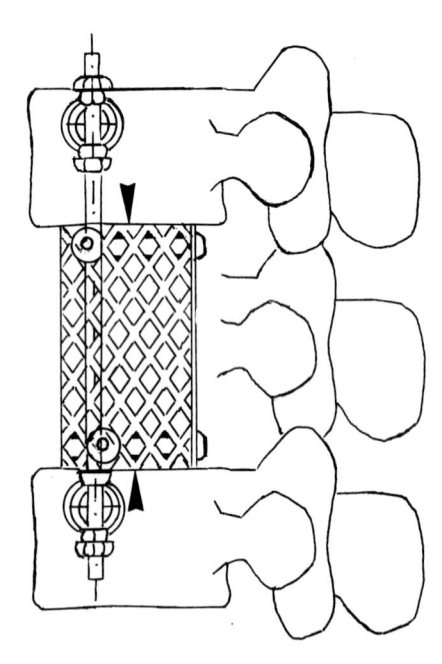

FIG. 4. The Harms "cage" is a titanium mesh cylinder with metallic vertebral endplates used for replacement of the vertebral body. Fixation can be supplemented by the modular segmented spine instrumentation of Harms–Zielke anteriorly or posteriorly.

BIOMECHANICAL EVALUATION OF ANTERIOR DEVICES

Gurr, McAfee, and Shih (12) studied the biomechanical stability of three anterior fixation techniques and four posterior instrumentation systems in a calf "corpectomy" model. The anterior systems were the iliac strut graft, Kaneda device, and methyl methacrylate with Harrington rod and hooks placed anteriorly. The posterior constructs were Harrington distraction rods, Luque rectangle, Cotrel–Dubousset pedicular fixation, and Steffee pedicle plate fixation. The least rigid constructs in torsion were the iliac graft, followed by the Harrington rod, and Luque rectangle. The most rigid constructs were the Kaneda device, Cotrel–Dubousset pedicular screw system, and Steffee pedicle screws and plates. The clinical relevance of this study is that, following vertebral corpectomy (as in burst fracture), spinal stability can be regained by implanting a Kaneda device one level cephalad and one level caudad to the lesion. An alternative would be an iliac crest bone graft with posterior, two-level cephalad and two-level caudad Cotrel–Dubousset or Steffee pedicular system. A recent study by the same group (41) showed that anterior instrumentation with anterior grafting provided a higher percentage of bony fusion with more rigidity than did fixation with posterior devices.

The rigidity of the I-plate was tested and compared to the Kostuik–Harrington construct and the Kaneda device in a burst fracture model (30). All but the Kostuik–Harrington system, which was less stable in flexion, improved the stability of the uninstrumented burst fracture model, and all constructs, including the Kostuik–Harrington device, were more stable than the intact spine in extension. In further biomechanical testing comparing the I-plate to the Dick device, a posterior pedicular system, Mann et al. (31) found that the I-plate was more stable in axial rotation than the Dick device when the posterior elements were intact. Similarly, both systems were more stable than the intact spine in flexion, extension, and lateral bending. However, when the posterior vertebral complex was compromised, the I-plate was less stable than the intact spine.

Mann et al. (31) concluded that the Syracuse I-plate was inadequate to stabilize a burst fracture model with posterior disruption. However, for burst fracture with intact posterior elements, the I-plate provided significant increase in stability over the intact spine in flexion, extension, and lateral bend loading.

INDICATIONS FOR ANTERIOR SURGERY IN THORACOLUMBAR FRACTURES

In general, the advantages of anterior surgery in the management of thoracolumbar fractures are several. Since in many instances the pathological process is anterior, the anterolateral approach provides direct access to the pathology and allows adequate decompression and placement of graft material directly at the site of the deformity and instability (Fig. 5). Similarly, direct reconstruction of the deformity is feasible. The anterior approach allows a short fixation, saving as many intact levels as possible.

There are several indications for anterior spine surgery in patients with thoracolumbar fractures, specifically burst injuries:

1. In patients with burst fracture, accompanied by conus, or cauda equina injury, in which there is canal occlusion of more than 70% by the retropulsed bone fragments.

2. In patients on whom posterior decompression, posterior instrumentation, and fusion were already performed and follow-up CT examination revealed a significant residual canal occlusion.
3. When surgery was delayed for 10 days or more after injury (25). In these three instances, anterolateral decompression of the spinal canal with bone grafting and eventual anterior instrumentation are performed.
4. In a burst injury in which there is deficient anterior bone stock, such as in the case of "eggshell or empty" vertebra. In this instance, anterior grafting and, occasionally, instrumentation are performed after posterior instrumentation.
5. In patients who present with late progression of a sagittal plane deformity with Sagittal Index exceeding 25° (9,35). Simultaneous anterior and posterior approaches may be dictated.
6. In patients with instability following laminectomy, anterior bone grafting and instrumentation are performed.

Bone graft material for anterior bone grafting following a vertebral corpectomy is usually harvested from the iliac crest. A tricortical bone graft will best sustain axial loads. However, there may be donor site problems from harvesting this kind of bone graft. Therefore some surgeons obtain bicortical graft from under the iliac crest. J. P. C. Farcy (*personal communication*) obtains his grafts from the posterior part of the ilium and claims to have no donor site problems. Others use bone allografts (33) augmented with vascularized rib grafts in the thoracic spine or morsalized autologous cancellous bone.

The surgical approach is described by Bayley et al. in Chapter 20. Note also the extracavity approach described by McCormick and Stein in Chapter 13.

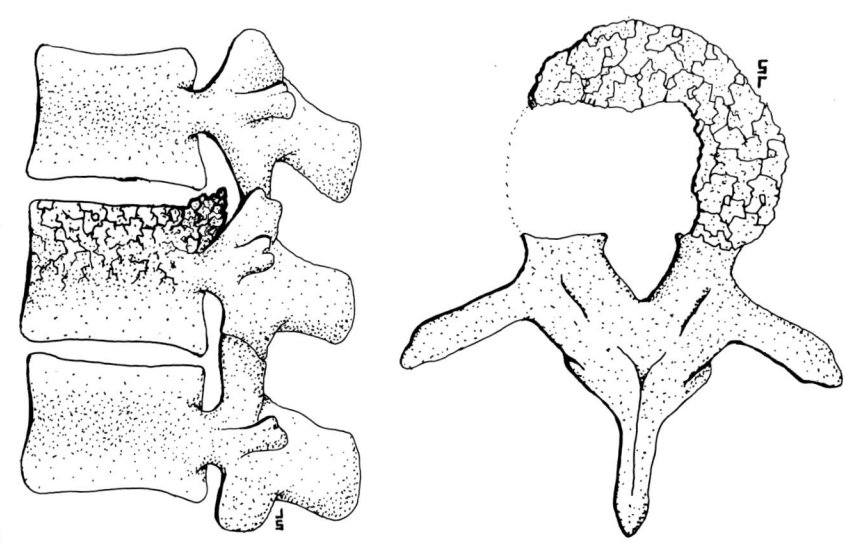

FIG. 5. Anterolateral decompression following a typical burst fracture. **A:** The burst vertebra. **B:** Following spinal canal decompression.

RATIONALE FOR DECOMPRESSION

The role of anterior decompression in thoracolumbar injuries is still undetermined. In selected cases with incomplete neurologic deficit, anterior decompression is effective in improving the neurologic outcome (8,20,21). It is logical to assume that excision of the offending bone fragments that compress and distort the neural elements may bring about recovery of neural function. Although this clinical concept is valid and may be beneficial, this is "not the whole story." Despite demonstration of retropulsed bone fragments in the spinal canal, no direct correlation exists between the percentage of canal occlusion and signs of neural compromise (19). This is at odds with the opinion of others, who have stated a contrary opinion (16,39). In addition, the spinal cord or cauda equina has been contused at the moment of impact or with momentary translation during the injury and this may be the main reason for the neurologic sequelae. Moreover, hematoma, edema, and vascular ischemia perpetuated by various neurotrophic and vasoactive agents may sustain the neurologic damage; and decompression may add little to the desired neural recovery, since the mere presence of bone fragments in the canal does not equate with a neural lesion.

In order to assess the role of decompressive surgery, we have to be reminded that about 60% of patients with injuries below T12 will recover with nonoperative measures (13). This probably represents the natural history of such lesions.

There is, however, ample evidence to suggest that late decompression, even several years following the original injury, may enhance neural recovery both at the cord level (2), conus, and cauda equina (4,32).

Therefore it would appear that anterior decompression is warranted and, in concert with fracture deformity reconstruction and spinal stabilization, will ensure the proper environment for maximal neural recovery.

Dunn (6) concluded that neurologic recovery is more certain with anterior decompression, especially when compared with published series of patients managed by either posterior instrumentation or nonoperative treatment. This was particularly true in lesions at L2 or lower.

CLINICAL RESULTS WITH THE VARIOUS ANTERIOR FIXATION SYSTEMS

Kostuik et al. (25) studied 80 patients with burst injuries that were managed by early anterior decompression, grafting, and anterior stabilization by the Kostuik–Harrington device. Some of the patients underwent a second stage posterior instrumentation. Fifty-seven of the 80 patients had a neurologic lesion. Most improved their neurologic status. With prompt surgical intervention, there was a tendency to greater improvement of neurologic status as measured by the Frankel scale. The nonunion rate was 4%. Thirteen patients had screw breakage. There were no vascular complications, either early or late.

Kostuik described his technique of anterior instrumentation in burst fractures of the lumbar spine (21–23). He found this technique of particular importance in burst fractures of L3 or lower (Fig. 6), where anterior decompression and fusion involved only two disc levels. His technique entails a lateral decubitus approach, preferably through the left side if possible. The burst vertebra is resected while the anterior one-quarter of the vertebral body is preserved (Fig. 6B). The dura is then fully decompressed, and the Kostuik screws are inserted (Fig. 6C). Distraction is performed, and the C-clamp is applied. An iliac crest bone graft is added, followed by implantation of the heavy compression Harrington rod with the collar-ended Kostuik screws (Fig. 6D,E). Finally, the screw heads are crimped.

Kostuik used this technique in 100 fractures (22). Twenty-three screws and one rod broke in the follow-up period. There were no early or late vascular complications. Average neurologic improvement was 1.6 grades on the Frankel scale.

Yuan recommends the Syracuse I-plate for management of the unstable burst fracture with partial neurologic deficit (40). In these patients, anterior decompression, grafting, and supplemental I-plate fixation are indicated. If posterior ligamentous injury is present, the addition of posterior instrumentation is also recommended. In a recent report on the clinical use of I-plate as well as a 4-year follow-up (1), there were four instances of plate loosening in a group of 28 burst fractures managed by this method. In two of the four cases, osteoporosis was the cause of plate loosening and, in the other two, a significant posterior ligamentous disruption was present before surgery. The implants failed in translation-induced screw loosening (1).

Haas et al. (14) reviewed their experience with use of anterior A-O plates in 39 patients with thoracolumbar injuries. No plate fractured or loosened, but four screws broke during the follow-up period.

A different mechanical solution was adopted by Rao and colleagues (34) in China. They employed a dual blade plate as an anterior fixation device (intervertebral body fixator, or IVBF). They reported its use in 88 cases with a variety of pathologic conditions including thoracolumbar fractures. In three cases, the dual blade plate failed. No biomechanical testing of the device was provided.

A,B

C

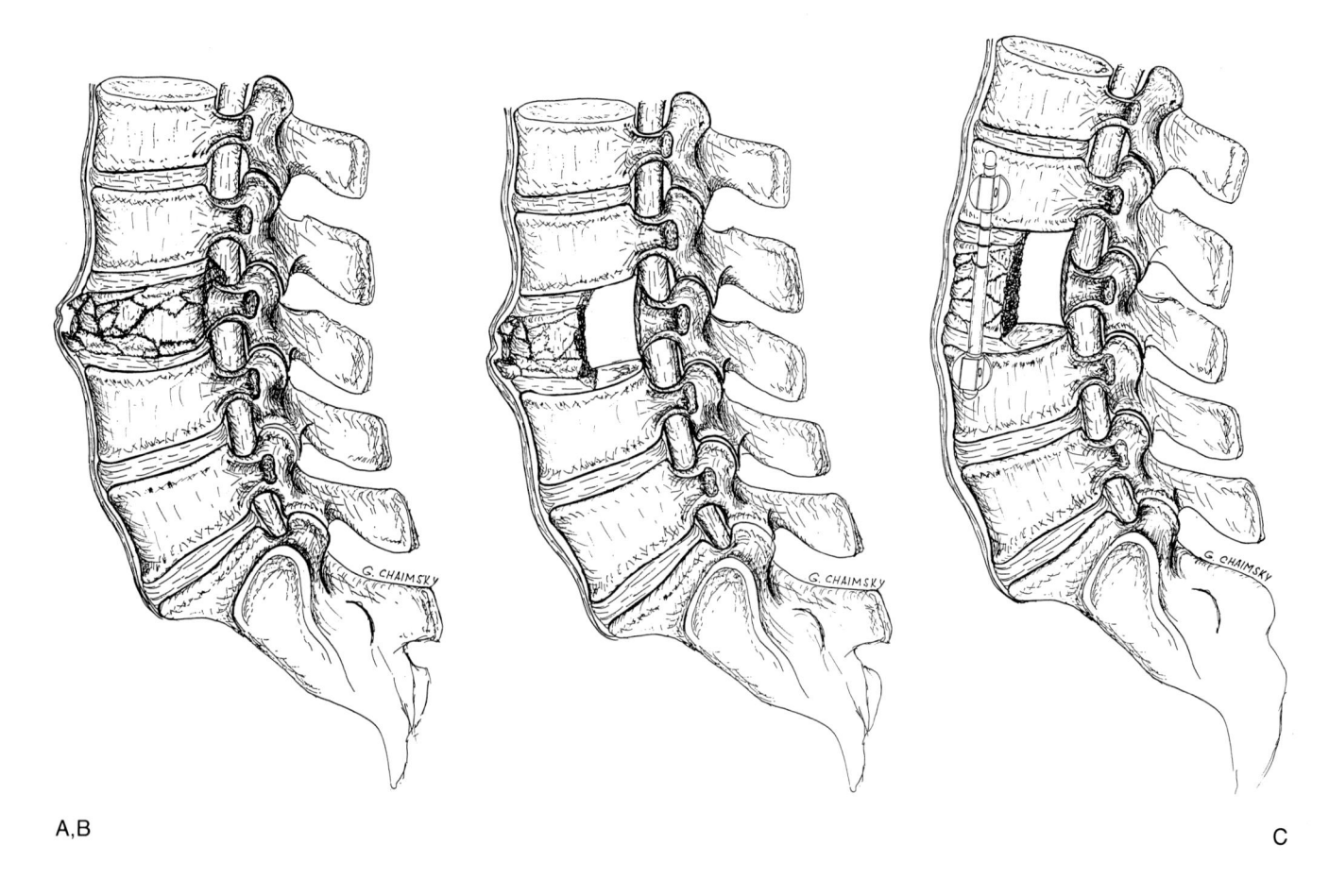

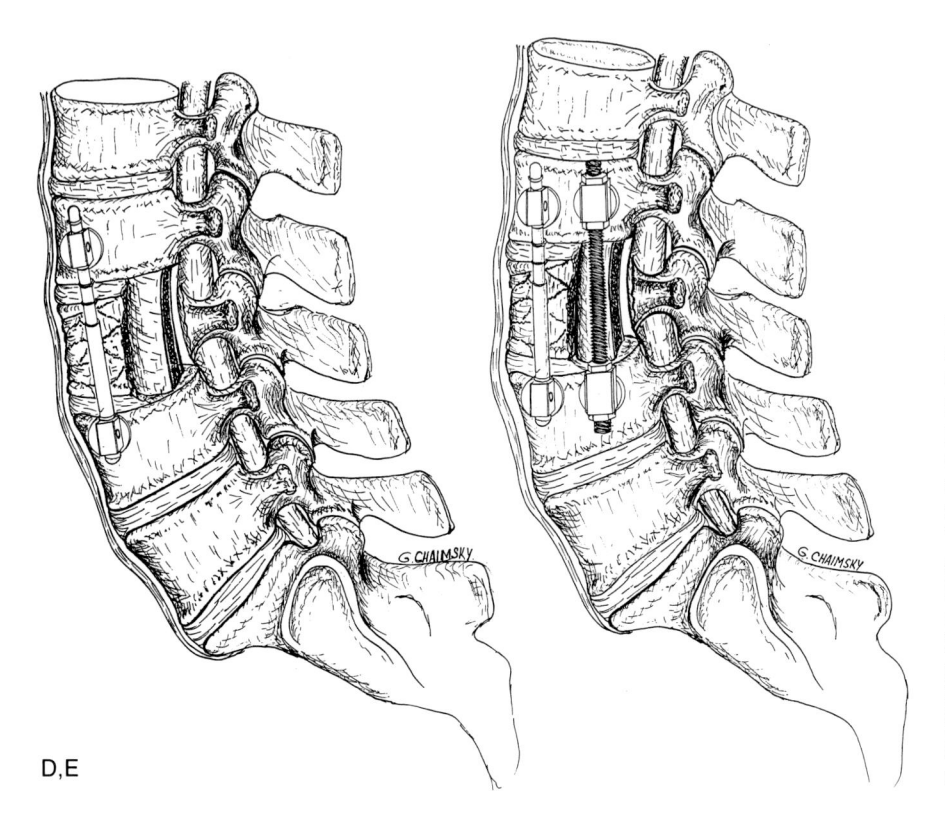

D,E

FIG. 6. A: The Kostuik technique for anterior decompression and fixation of burst fractures. His technique entails a lateral decubitus approach, preferably through the left side if possible. **B:** The burst vertebra is resected while the anterior one-quarter of the vertebral body is preserved. **C:** The dura is then fully decompressed, and the Kostuik screws are inserted. Distraction is performed, and the C-clamp is applied. **D, E:** An iliac crest bone graft is added, followed by implantation of the heavy compression Harrington rod with the collar-ended Kostuik screws. Finally, the screw heads are crimped. (Modified from ref. 24.)

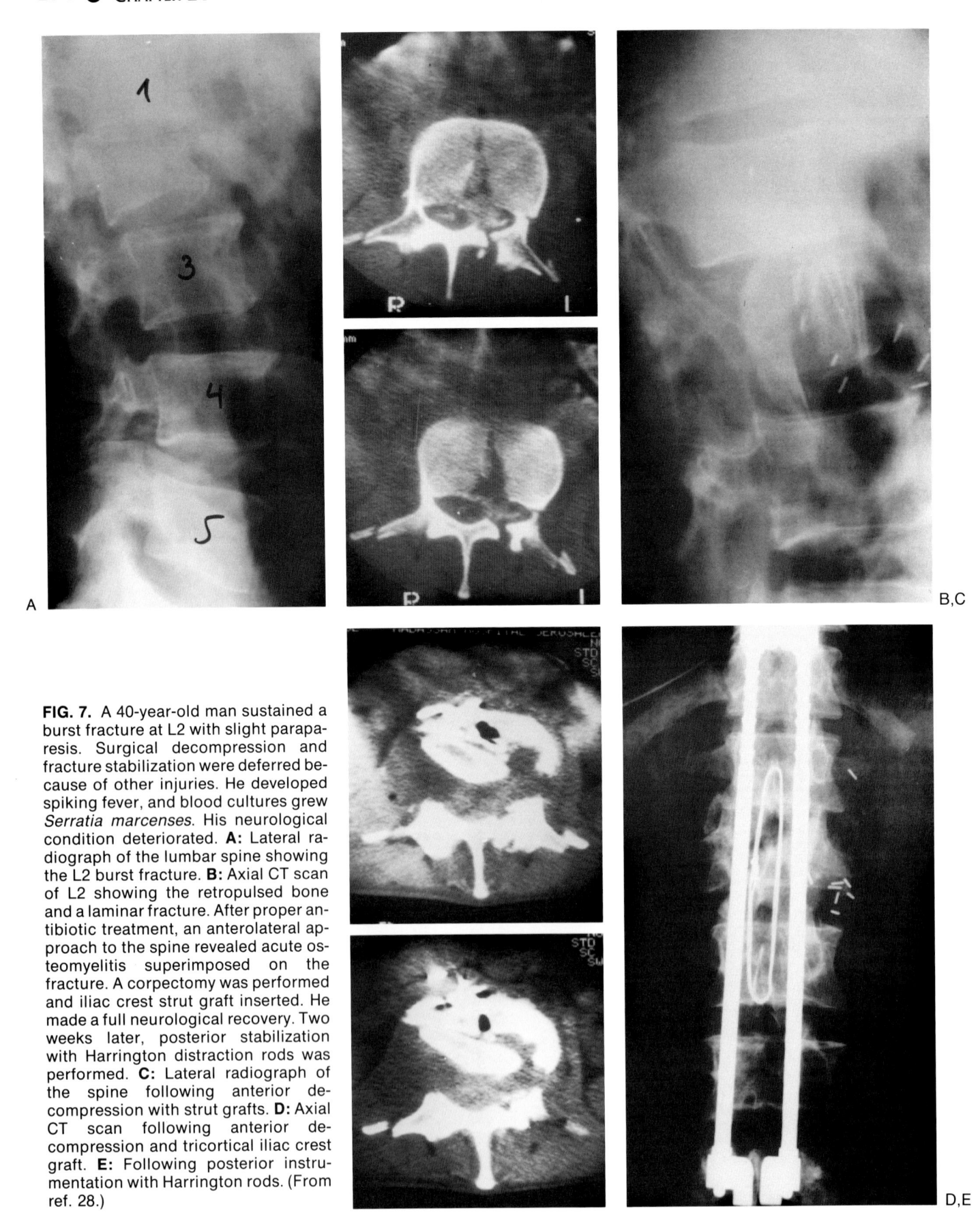

FIG. 7. A 40-year-old man sustained a burst fracture at L2 with slight paraparesis. Surgical decompression and fracture stabilization were deferred because of other injuries. He developed spiking fever, and blood cultures grew *Serratia marcenses*. His neurological condition deteriorated. **A:** Lateral radiograph of the lumbar spine showing the L2 burst fracture. **B:** Axial CT scan of L2 showing the retropulsed bone and a laminar fracture. After proper antibiotic treatment, an anterolateral approach to the spine revealed acute osteomyelitis superimposed on the fracture. A corpectomy was performed and iliac crest strut graft inserted. He made a full neurological recovery. Two weeks later, posterior stabilization with Harrington distraction rods was performed. **C:** Lateral radiograph of the spine following anterior decompression with strut grafts. **D:** Axial CT scan following anterior decompression and tricortical iliac crest graft. **E:** Following posterior instrumentation with Harrington rods. (From ref. 28.)

ANTERIOR VERSUS POSTERIOR SURGERY

Bradford and McBride (4) compared the results of anterior approach versus posterior approach in managing patients with thoracolumbar fractures accompanied by neurologic deficit. The neurologic recovery was greater with anterior decompression (88% versus 64%). This was even more evident with regard to bladder and bowel control (69% versus 33%). In addition, Bradford and McBride reported on patients with inadequate posterior decompression and neural deficits who recovered following an anterior decompression.

Gertzbein et al. (11) combined anterior and posterior approaches in 18 patients with canal compromise greater than 50%. Eighty-one percent of the patients with incomplete lesions demonstrated neurologic improvement. Local kyphosis was corrected from 21.8° to 17.1°. Kostuik et al. (25) are currently comparing posterior decompression and pedicle fixation with anterior decompression and stabilization. So far, the same results have been achieved in both groups, but canal clearance is greater after anterior decompression (100% versus 80%).

Kaneda et al. (18) reported 92% neurologic improvement in patients with incomplete paraplegia who underwent anterior decompression and stabilization with the anterior Kaneda device. Similar results were reported by Kostuik (21), and almost similar results were reported by McAfee et al. (32). Since anterior instrumentation is not always available, anterior decompression followed by posterior instrumentation may be indicated (Figs. 7 and 8).

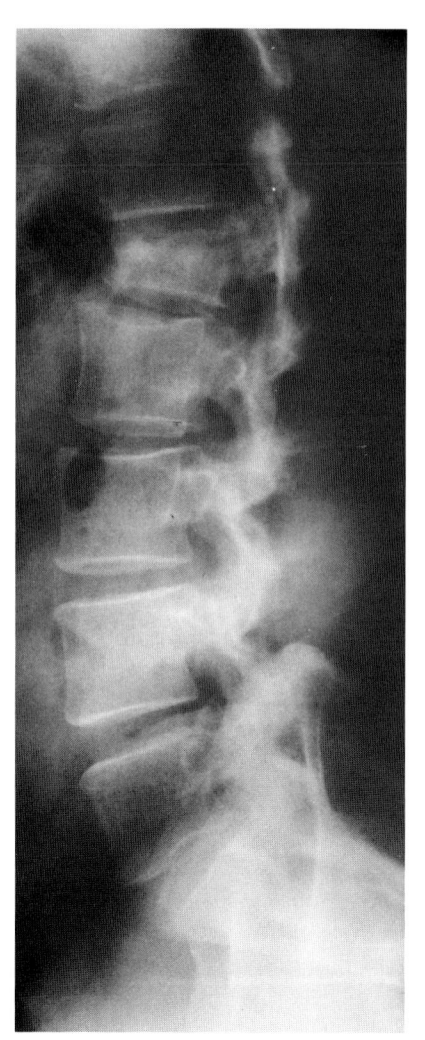

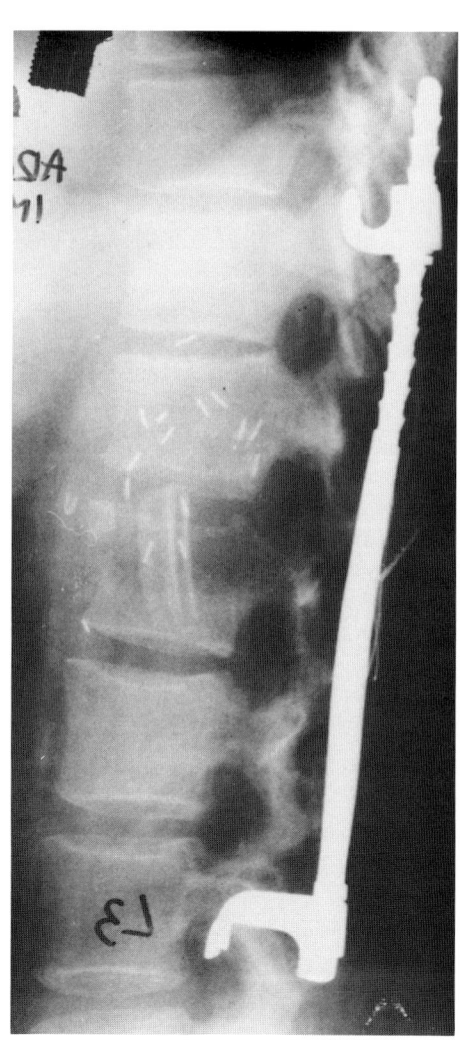

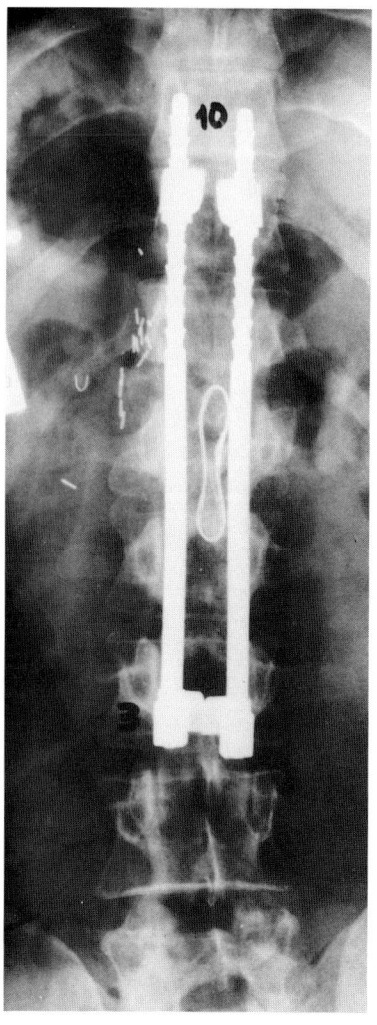

FIG. 8. A 30-year-old man sustained a burst fracture of L1 in a road accident with mild neurologic deficit. He underwent anterolateral decompression with rib strut grafts and posterior Harrington instrumentation from T10 to L3. He made a full neurologic recovery. **A:** Lateral radiograph of the lumbar spine with localized kyphosis and a typical burst fracture at L1. **B,C:** Following anterior decompression and posterior spine fusion, sagittal alignment is restored. Shown are a lateral radiograph (B) and an anteroposterior radiograph (C).

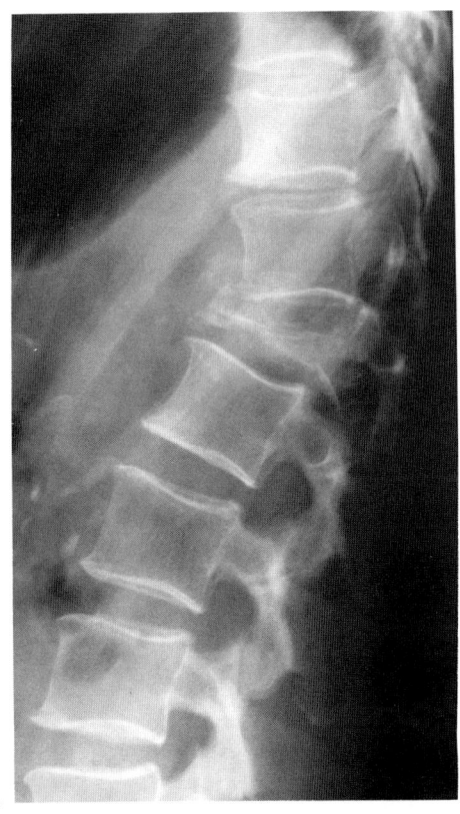

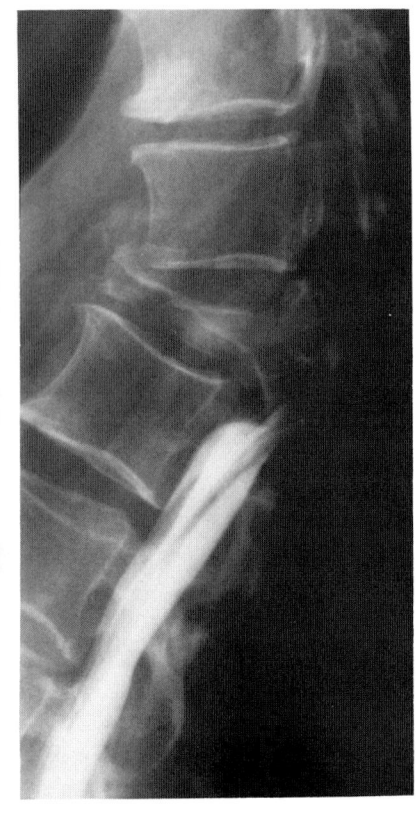

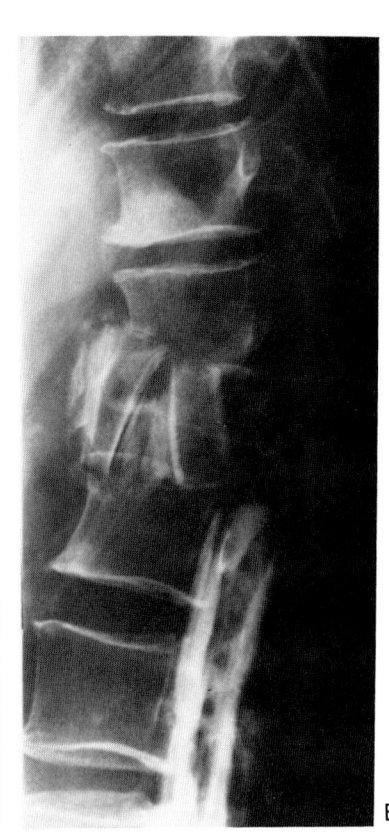

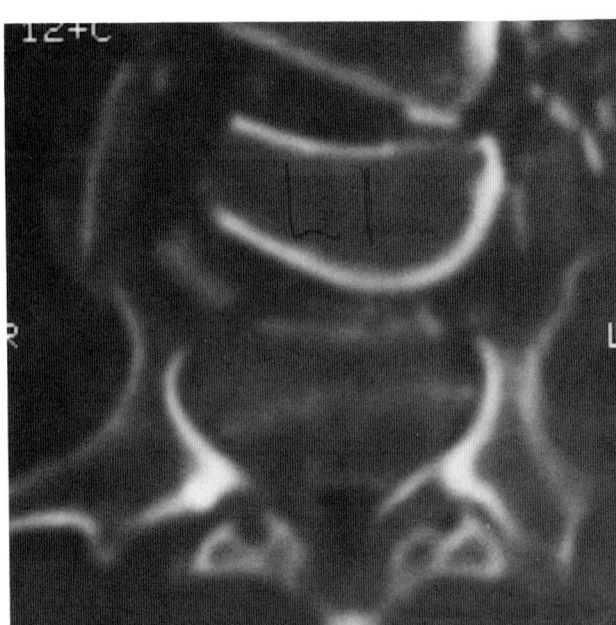

FIG. 9. A: Lateral radiograph of a 57-year-old woman who sustained an L1 burst fracture with bilateral leg weakness (Frankel C) following a fall in an archeological excavation in a third world country. Note also the marked local kyphosis. **B:** Myelogram showing a partial block. The patient underwent "anterior decompression" and bone grafting. Neurological deterioration to Frankel B was noted postoperatively, and the patient was transferred to New York. **C:** A repeat myelogram showed a complete block at the L1 level. Note also the anterior bone graft and uncorrected local kyphosis. **D:** CT scan demonstrated complete canal occlusion from retropulsed bone of the burst fracture. Note also the bone graft that was laid down without prior canal decompression.

Gertzbein et al. (10) studied 60 consecutive patients with spinal injuries and greater than 20% encroachment of the spinal canal with regard to neurologic outcome. They evaluated the outcome of posterior surgery versus anterior surgery. There was no significant change in whether posterior or anterior surgery was performed with regard to neurologic improvement (the rates of improvement were 85% and 88%, respectively). There was no apparent difference between the degree of canal encroachment and the initial Frankel grade. As a result of this study, Gertzbein and his colleagues concluded that (a) fracture/dislocation should be stabilized by posterior instrumentation; (b) burst fractures with canal occlusion greater than 50% should be decompressed anteriorly; and (c) burst dislocation should be posteriorly stabilized. If, at follow-up, the CT scan at the burst level still reveals canal encroachment greater than 50%, anterior decompression should be per-

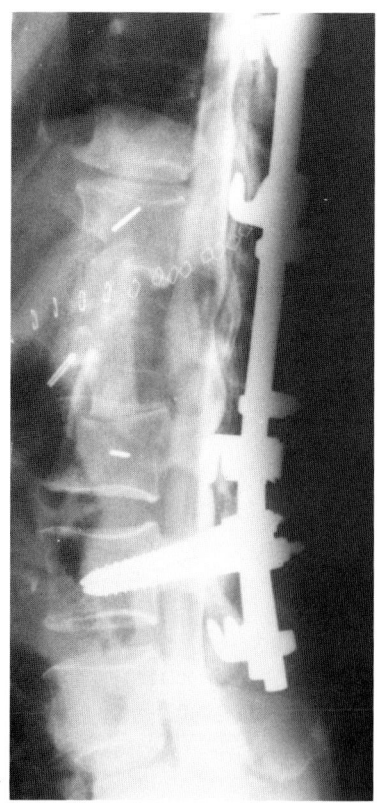

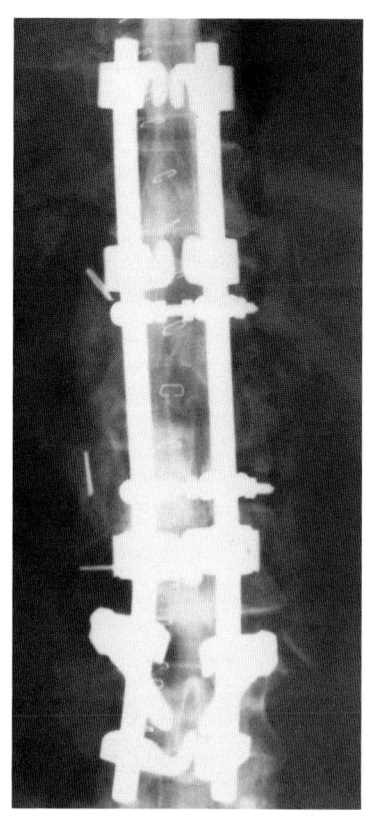

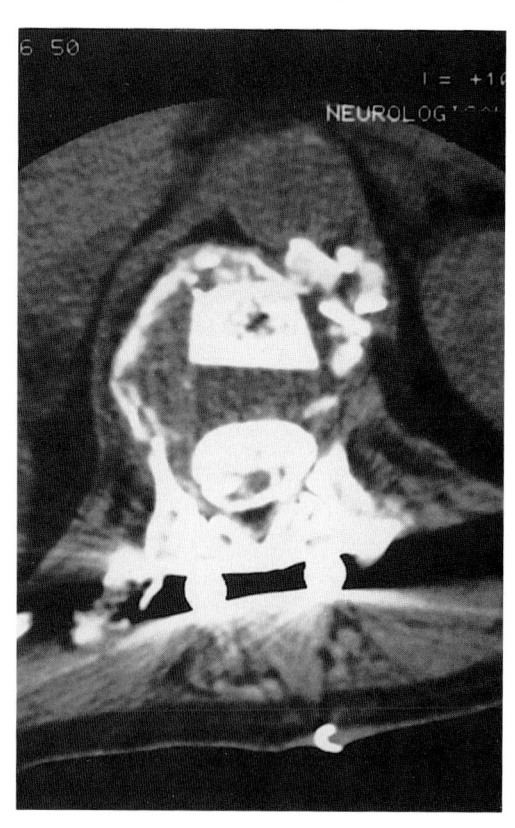

FIG. 9. *Continued.* **E,F:** Lateral and AP myelogram following simultaneous combined anterior decompression and posterior Cotrel–Dubousset instrumentation from T11 to L3. Note the uninterrupted flow of the dye column, indicating complete canal decompression. Note also the restoration of the Sagittal Index to its normal value. **G:** Postoperative CT-myelography showing complete canal decompression. The patient made a full neurological recovery. (Case courtesy of Dr. J.-P. C. Farcy.)

formed as well. In the latter instance, or in cases of late malunion, it is perhaps better to perform a simultaneous posterior stabilization and anterior decompression (Fig. 9).

Esses, Botsford, and Kostuik (8) conducted a prospective randomized protocol in which patients with burst fractures were treated either by posterior distraction instrumentation with the A-O fixateur or anterior decompression with Kostuik–Harrington fixation and bone grafting. Anterior decompression and instrumentation enabled better canal clearance than was afforded by application of a posterior pedicular system; residual canal occlusion was 4% versus 16.5% ($p < 0.0001$). In most cases, however, canal decompression was adequately managed by a posterior pedicular system. Kyphosis correction was similar in both treatment groups. Blood loss was higher with the anterior surgery.

Esses et al. (8) concluded that burst fractures with major neurologic compromise or injuries older than 72 hr with neurologic deficit should undergo anterior decompression. In other modes of presentation of burst fractures, posterior surgery with pedicle screw fixation is the treatment of choice.

In kyphotic deformities, as in late post-traumatic kyphosis, attempts at anterior fusion without either anterior or posterior instrumentation may result in a pseudarthrosis rate as high as 50% (29), and use of supplementary posterior fixation is recommended. It must be remembered that a single, anteriorly placed rod cannot withstand rotational or lateral bending loads. Therefore insertion of an additional rod, a posterior fixation system, or an external orthosis is recommended. According to Kostuik et al. (25), if the posterior elements are intact, there is no need for posterior instrumentation. However, if more than one vertebral body has been resected or the posterior elements are deficient, posterior instrumentation is mandatory.

Kostuik and Matsusaki (23) reported their experience in 27 patients who underwent surgery for late post-traumatic kyphosis with anterior surgery and fixation with the Kostuik–Harrington system. Indications for surgery were increasing deformity, pain, spinal stenosis, and persistent neurologic deficit. Stable arthrodesis with correction of the kyphosis occurred in 36 of the 37 patients. Pain was reduced in 78% of the patients, and six of eight paraparetic patients had neurologic improvement. (See also Chapter 31 by Glassman and Farcy.)

SUMMARY

Anterior approach to the spine is useful in achieving a thorough decompression of the neural elements. This may enhance neural recovery in patients who have plateaued after posterior fixation and decompression, or in patients presenting later after injury. In addition, patients with a significant bone deficiency of the anterior column require anterior buttressing by bone grafting and, probably, anterior instrumentation. Finally, combined anterior and posterior procedures may be indicated in late progressing sagittal plane deformities.

Anterior instrumentation in conjunction with tricortical iliac crest bone graft is sufficient to sustain physiologic loads when the posterior column is intact. With disruption of the posterior complex, posterior stabilization is recommended as well.

REFERENCES

1. Bayley JC, Yuan HA, Fredrickson BE. The Syracuse I-plate. *Spine* 1991;16(3S):S120–S124.
2. Bohlman HH, Freehater A, Dejak J. Late anterior decompression of spinal cord injuries: a report of 36 cases. *J Bone Joint Surg* 1975;52A:1025.
3. Bohm H, Harms J, Donk R, Zielke K. Correction and stabilization of angular kyphosis. *Clin Orthop* 1990;258:56–61.
4. Bradford DS, McBride G. Surgical management of thoracolumbar spine fractures with incomplete neurological deficits. *Clin Orthop* 1987;218:201–216.
5. Dunn HK. Anterior stabilization of thoracolumbar injuries. *Clin Orthop* 1984;180:116–124.
6. Dunn HK. Anterior spine stabilization and decompression for thoracolumbar injuries. *Orthop Clin North Am* 1986;17:113–119.
7. Dwyer AP. Experience of anterior correction of scoliosis. *Clin Orthop* 1973;93:191–206.
8. Esses SI, Botsford DJ, Kostuik JP. Evaluation of surgical treatment of burst fractures. *Spine* 1990;15:667–673.
9. Farcy JPC, Weidenbaum M, Glassman SD. Sagittal index in management of thoracolumbar fractures. *Spine* 1990;15:598–965.
10. Gertzbein SD, Court-Brown CM, Marks P, Martin C, Fazl M, Schwartz M, Jacobs RR. The neurological outcome following surgery for spinal fractures. *Spine* 1988;13:641–644.
11. Gertzbein SD, Court-Brown CM, Jacobs RR, et al. Decompression and circumferential stabilization of unstable spinal fractures. *Spine* 1988;13:892–895.
12. Gurr KR, McAfee PC, Shih CM. Biomechanical analysis of anterior and posterior instrumentation systems after corpectomy. *J Bone Joint Surg* 1988;70A:1182–1191.
13. Guttmann L. *Spinal cord injuries: comprehensive management and research.* Oxford: Blackwell Scientific Publishing, 1957.
14. Haas N, Blauth M, Tscherne H. Anterior plating in thoracolumbar spine injuries. *Spine* 1991;16(3S):S100–S111.
15. Hall JE, Micheli LJ. The use of modified Dwyer instrumentation in anterior stabilization of the spine. Presented at the Scoliosis Research Society, Hong Kong, 1977.
16. Hashimoto T, Kaneda K, Abumi K. Relationship between traumatic spinal canal stenosis and neurologic deficits in thoracolumbar burst fractures. *Spine* 1988;13:1268–1272.
17. Hodgson AR, Stock FE. Anterior spinal fusion: a preliminary communication on radical treatment of Pott's disease and Pott's paraplegia. *Br J Surg* 1956;44:266–275.
18. Kaneda K, Abumi K, Fujiya M. Burst fractures with neurologic deficits of the thoracolumbar–lumbar spine. Results of anterior decompression and stabilization with anterior instrumentation. *Spine* 1984;9:788–795.
19. Keene TS, Fischer SP, Vanderleg R, Drummond DS, Tursk PA. Significance of acute post-traumatic bony encroachment of the neural canal. *Spine* 1989;14:789–802.
20. Kostuik JP. Anterior spinal cord decompression for lesions of the thoracic and lumbar spine, techniques, new methods of internal fixation and results. *Spine* 1983;8:512–531.
21. Kostuik JP. Anterior fixation for burst fractures of the thoracic and lumbar spine with or without neurologic involvement. *Spine* 1988;13:286–293.
22. Kostuik JP. Anterior Kostuik–Harrington distraction systems in the treatment of kyphotic deformities. *Spine* 1990;15:169–180.
23. Kostuik JP, Matsusaki H. Anterior stabilization instrumentation and decompression for post traumatic kyphosis. *Spine* 1989;14:379–386.
24. Kostuik JP. Anterior techniques of stabilization in thoracic and lumbar trauma. In: Errico JJ, Bauer RD, Waugh T, eds. *Spinal trauma.* Philadelphia: Lippincott, 1991;282.
25. Kostuik JP, Huler RJ, Esses SI, Stauffer ES. Thoracolumbar spine fracture. In: Frymoyer JW, ed. *The adult spine.* New York: Raven Press, 1991;1307.
26. Kostuik JP, Huler RJ, Esses SI, Stauffer ES. Thoracolumbar spine fracture. In: Frymoyer JW, ed. *The adult spine.* New York: Raven Press, 1991;1309.
27. Levine AM. New trends in instrumentation of the lumbar spine. In: Floman Y, ed. *Disorders of the lumbar spine.* Gaithersburg, MD: Aspen Publishers, 1990;690.
28. Lowe J, Kaplan L, Liebergall M, Floman Y. Serratia osteomyelitis causing neurological deterioration after spine fracture. A report of 2 cases. *J Bone Joint Surg* 1989;71B:256–258.
29. Malcolm BW, Bradford DS, Winter RB, Chow SN. Post traumatic kyphosis. *J Bone Joint Surg* 1981;63A:891.
30. Mann KA, Found EM, Yuan HA, Fredrickson BE, Lubicky J. Biomechanical evaluation of the effectiveness of anterior spinal fixation systems. Presented at the Orthopaedic Research Society, San Francisco, January 1987.
31. Mann KA, McGowan DP, Fredrickson BE, Falahee M, Yuan HA. A biomechanical investigation of short segment spinal fixation for burst fracture with varying degrees of posterior disruption. *Spine* 1990;15:470–473.
32. McAfee PC, Bohlman HH, Yuan HA. Anterior decompression of traumatic thoracolumbar fractures with incomplete neurological deficit using a retroperitoneal approach. *J Bone Joint Surg* 1985;67A:89–104.
33. McBride GC, Bradford DS. Vertebral body replacement with femoral meek allografts and vascularized rib strut graft. A technique for treating post-traumatic kyphosis with neurologic deficit. *Spine* 1983;8:405.
34. Rao SC, Mou ZS, Hu YZ, Shen H. The IVBF dual-blade plate and its applications. *Spine* 1991;16(3S):S112–S119.
35. Rawlins BA, Weidenbaum M, Glassman SD, Farcy J-PC. Simultaneous anterior and posterior procedures for short segment spine pathology. European Spinal Deformity Society, Lyon, June 17–29, 1992, p 93.
36. Royle ND. The operative removal of an accessory vertebra. *Aust Med J* 1928;1:467.
37. Senegas J, Vidal JM, Banling D, Gernier F. L'osteosynthese du rachis dorso-lombaire par plaque vissee anterolateral. *Rev Chir Orthop Supp* 1987;II:157–160.
38. Slot GH. A new distraction system for the correction of kyphosis using the anterior approach. Presented at the Scoliosis Research Society, Montreal, Quebec, Canada, September 1981.
39. Trafton PG, Boyd CA. Computed tomography of thoracic and lumbar spine injuries. *J Trauma* 1984;24:508–515.
40. Yuan HA, Mann KA, Found EM, et al. Early clinical experience with the Syracuse I-plate: an anterior spinal fixation device. *Spine* 1988;13:278–285.
41. Zdeblick TA, Shirado O, McAfee PC, deGroot H, Warden K. Anterior spinal fixation after lumbar corpectomy. *J Bone Joint Surg* 1991;73A:527–534.
42. Zielke K. Ventral derotation spondylodese: Behandlungsergebnisse bein idiopathischen lumbar skoliosen. *Orthopade* 1982;120:320–329.

22

Posterior Instrumentation in the Management of Thoracolumbar Injuries

Yizhar Floman

The goals of surgical management of spine injuries are to provide stability to the axial skeleton, regain sagittal and frontal alignment, and create a stable environment for enhancing neurologic recovery and function. When spinal architecture has been violated or destroyed, the maintenance of proper spinal alignment and stability often depends on internal fixation. Such fixation must maintain reduction and stability without jeopardizing neural structures until bony union occurs.

Internal fixation of spine fractures is a legitimate and valid management option, as is internal fixation of long bone fractures. However, this is a relatively new avenue of treatment that replaced the nonoperative management advocated by Guttmann (63). He was a strong proponent of postural nonoperative reduction of spine fractures. At the time, the alternative to this treatment modality was "decompressive" laminectomy that proved to be futile and destabilized the spine even further. Guttmann's approach was echoed by Watson-Jones (124) and Bedbrook (12), who emphasized the beneficial role of postural nonoperative spine fracture reduction. Later, Holdsworth (67) was one of the first to advocate operative stabilization of spine fractures.

There are numerous advantages to surgical management of thoracolumbar fractures. Operative fixation of spine fractures enables reduction of the fracture/deformity, allows decompression, either direct or indirect, of the neural canal, and provides stabilization. It also enhances the chances of neural recovery and allows early mobilization, better nursing, and shortens hospitalization. Surgery may prevent occurrence of late deformity.

It is well known that, in most cases, laminectomy does not decompress the neural elements, since often the offending structures are anterior to the cord or cauda equina (120). Laminectomy increases the instability of the fracture, which may lead to further neurologic deterioration, but decompression as deemed necessary in conjunction with stabilization may enhance neurologic recovery (30,68).

Decompression can be achieved by anatomic realignment of the fracture and by bony decompression via posterior, posterolateral, or anterolateral approach. Decompression was found to be effective in models of spinal cord compression in experimental animals (34). Although 60% of patients with fractures below T12 accompanied by neurologic deficit improve with conservative management (63), late decompression performed up to 2 years postinjury can bring about further neurologic recovery, long after the natural improvement has plateaued (15,30,122). There is ample evidence to suggest that decompression of the cord, conus, or cauda equina in thoracolumbar fractures does change the natural history of neurologic recovery (15,91,97,122). Recently, Anderson et al. (4) reported on better neurologic recovery in patients with thoracic fractures managed by decompression and stabilization: 91% recovery in operated patients versus 61% in patients managed by postural reduction. To enhance neural recovery, a stable, anatomically reduced spinal column and spinal canal are necessary. This is best achieved with various forms of internal spinal fixation.

AVAILABLE POSTERIOR INSTRUMENTATION

The earliest spinal implants were reported by Hadra (64) in 1891 and Lange (82) in 1910. These implants

---

Y. Floman: Department of Orthopaedic Surgery and Spine Surgery Unit, Hebrew University–Hadassah Medical School, Hadassah University Hospital, Jerusalem 91120, Israel.

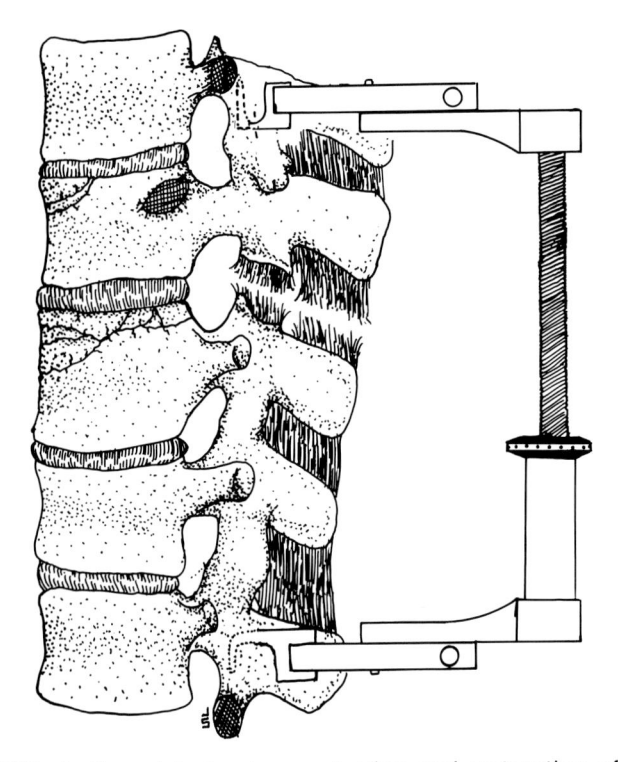

FIG. 1. Complete fracture reduction and restoration of vertebral height can be achieved with the Harrington outrigger. Hooks are inserted two levels above and below the fracture site and are connected to the outrigger. The outrigger is then distracted to allow for fracture reduction and vertebral body height restoration by ligamentotaxis.

were either a suture tied around the spinous processes or a wire that anchored a metal rod to the spinous processes. Although these constructs most probably were able to resist tensile loads, apparently they were unable to sustain flexion or anterior shear forces (80). The next spinous process implants to be developed were plates (119,129); internal fixation of the spine was performed by double spinous process plating (108,109). The spinous process plate fixation and spinous process wires were the only spinal fixation systems available until the middle of the 20th century. Kaufer and Hayes (74) reported 21 patients managed by open reduction with interspinous wiring and plaster cast immobilization and claimed to have good clinical results. They performed a short segment fusion and emphasized the advantage of their technique over the spinous process plates.

Spinous process plates were fixed to the spinous process with a 3-mm diameter bolt. Theoretical biomechanical analysis reveals that, although spinous process plates were able to withstand tensile, compression, and shear loads, they failed in flexion, creating a kyphotic deformity (80). Their use resulted in a high percentage of failure, with the implant cutting out of the spinous process and causing recurrent fracture-deformity (108). Lewis and McKibbin (86) reported on 27 patients with spine fractures managed with the Meurig–Williams spinous process plates, which achieved superior results to those obtained by

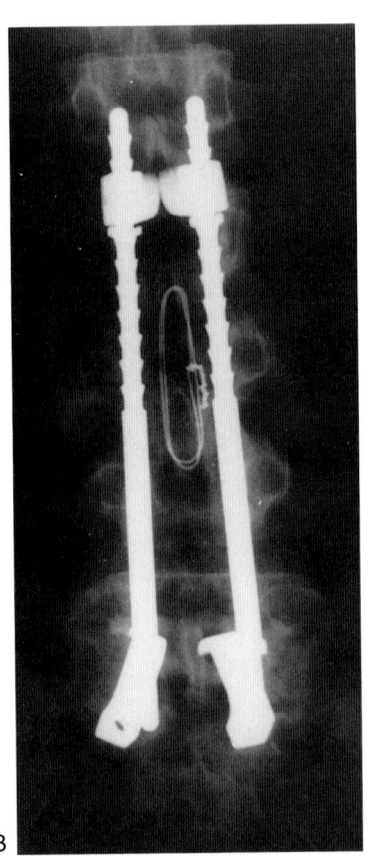

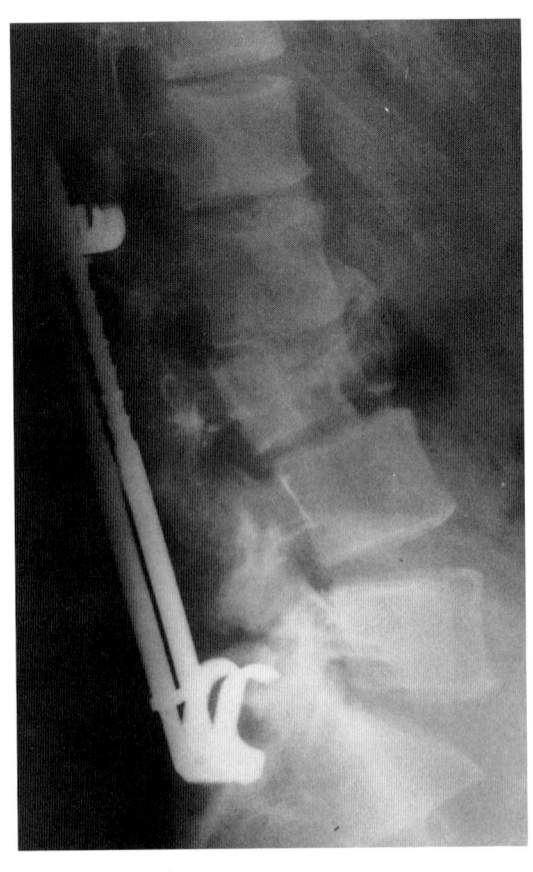

FIG. 2. Burst fracture of L3 instrumented with Harrington distraction rods from L1 to S1. Both lower hooks and rods are dislodged, with recurrent local kyphosis. **A:** AP view. **B:** Lateral view.

A,B

postural reduction. There was, however, a high percentage of instrumentation failure; implant loosening necessitated plate removal in nine of 27 patients. Today, none of the spinous process-anchored plates are in use; this includes the Meurig–Williams plate, the Williams plate, and the Crawford–Adams plate.

Paul Harrington, a pioneer in the field of spine fixation, developed an instrumentation system for surgical management of scoliosis and other spinal deformities in the late 1950s (66). It was soon modified for use as an internal fixation device for stabilization of thoracic and lumbar spine fractures (33). Dickson et al. (33) used dual Harrington distraction rods to stabilize and fuse unstable thoracic and lumbar spine injuries. The introduction of the Harrington system allowed, for the first time, effective stabilization of the unstable injured spine, as well as full restoration of vertebral body height (51,65,68). Reduction was achieved by application of the Harrington outrigger inserted into hooks placed at equal distances above and below the injury level (Fig. 1). Gradual, progressive distraction was applied and fracture reduction was verified by radiographic control. The advantages of the Harrington instrumentation were readily recognized and, to a large extent, the system remains in worldwide use. Despite the numerous modifications that have been introduced over the years, it certainly remains the standard of surgical management for thoracolumbar spine fractures.

Nevertheless, shortcomings of the system were soon recognized. Although originally Harrington planned his system to be used as a segmental fixation device, its application in the fractured spine was not segmental, and postoperative external immobilization was necessary until consolidation of the spinal arthrodesis occurred. Hook or rod dislodgements were common, with loss of operative correction (132) (Fig. 2). Another problem with the Harrington system was its failure to control or preserve sagittal plane curves. This is crucial at the thoracolumbar junction and lumbar spine, where the Harrington system tends to eliminate the natural lumbar lordosis. The "flatback" syndrome due to this iatrogenic induction of lumbar kyphosis (78,99) was, and still is, a serious complication of the Harrington instrumentation that may necessitate surgical revision to restore lumbar sagittal alignment (76).

The latter problem was addressed by Moe, who introduced square-ended Harrington rods, bent into lordosis, and square-ended Harrington hooks (29,99). Nevertheless, this modified Harrington system was unable to sufficiently preserve lumbar lordosis (20). A different modification, aimed at preservation of lumbar lordosis, was the use of Harrington compression rods either as a replacement for one of the distraction rods, or as a midline supplement between the two distracting rods (75). An additional modification was the introduction of the interspinous compression wire technique to counteract the Harrington distraction rods (51) (Fig. 3). Other shortcomings of the Harrington system were the need to instrument long motion segments, the lack of proper segmental fixation, and the late loss of correction that had been obtained at surgery.

In order for the posteriorly applied distraction forces to be mechanically effective, a long lever arm (long rod) is needed. The standard recommended rod length in fracture management is a length that spans three motion segments above and three motion segments below the lesion (106). Later, this was modified to three segments above and two segments below the lesion (51). The sacrifice of five or six motion segments for a single-level injury is a serious disadvantage of the Harrington system. This is of paramount significance when the injury level is at L3 or below, since use of the Harrington system will necessitate spine fusion either to L5 or the sacrum.

This particular problem has led to the adoption of the "instrument long, fuse short" strategy (68,69), which

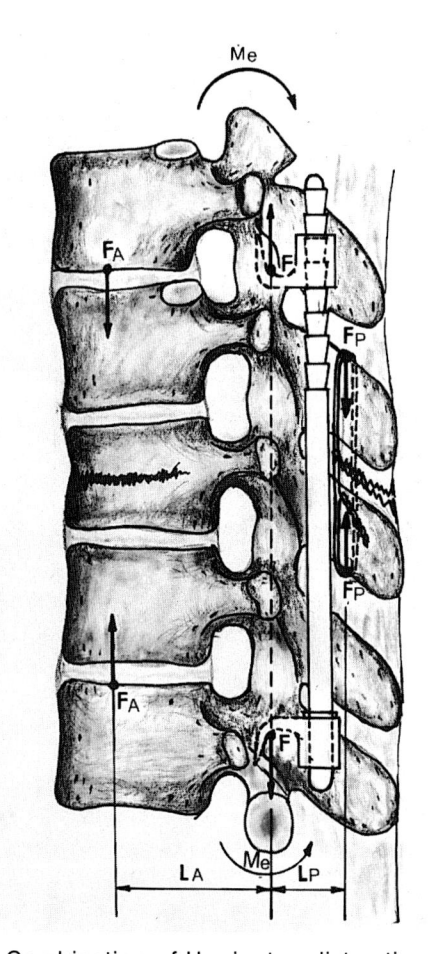

FIG. 3. Combination of Harrington distraction rods and an interspinous compressive wire. Overdistraction is resisted by FA (intact anterior elements) and FP provided by the wire. Because the wire is stiffer than the anterior longitudinal ligament, an extension moment (Me) develops in the defined direction, correcting the local kyphosis. (From ref. 51.)

requires removal of the instrumentation after fracture union. The latter technique is somewhat controversial, as it is thought that the immobilized, nonfused, facet joints may later develop painful osteoarthrosis after rod removal (72,73). Kahanovitz and co-workers (72,73) have demonstrated both in experimental models and in humans managed by this technique that an irreversible osteoarthrosis develops in the immobilized facet joints. Similarly, Urban et al. (123) showed that immobilization of normal discs induced degenerative changes, manifested by disc desiccation and decreased metabolic activity of the disc. Thus it is argued that, even after rod removal, the instrumented spinal segments may be plagued by disc degeneration and facet joint arthrosis, leading to postoperative back pain. Lately, Gardner and Armstrong (53) have found little clinical and radiologic evidence of facet osteoarthritis in long-term follow-up of patients managed by the technique of "rod long, fuse short." In addition, the majority of their patients did not have back pain and were able to return to their prefracture jobs.

The problem of instrumentation length is now better addressed by the use of pedicle screws. This technique will be discussed later in the chapter.

Weiss springs modified from implants used in scoliosis surgery were used as an internal fixation device in thoracolumbar injuries (126). These springs were first developed by Gruca in 1956 for the correction of scoliosis. In 1975, Weiss modified the springs for stabilization of lumbar spine fractures. The system consists of two springs with hooks for attachment at both ends of the spine. One spring is attached to each side of the spine, and the springs are attached under tension, spanning the injured segment. The hooks at the end of the spring are attached either to the laminae or transverse processes. The springs exert a large bending moment to correct the angular deformity and a compressive moment posteriorly. Theoretically, flexion/distraction injuries may be managed by modified Weiss springs (92). While the original Weiss springs had poor resistance to rotational and laterally applied forces, the modified Weiss springs, which contain steel rods, provide better resistance against such forces (13). The resistance to these forces can be increased further by fixing the rods to the spinous processes with Parham bands (83). Larson (83) reported on 127 patients instrumented with the modified Weiss springs; only four had to be removed because of pain associated with spring

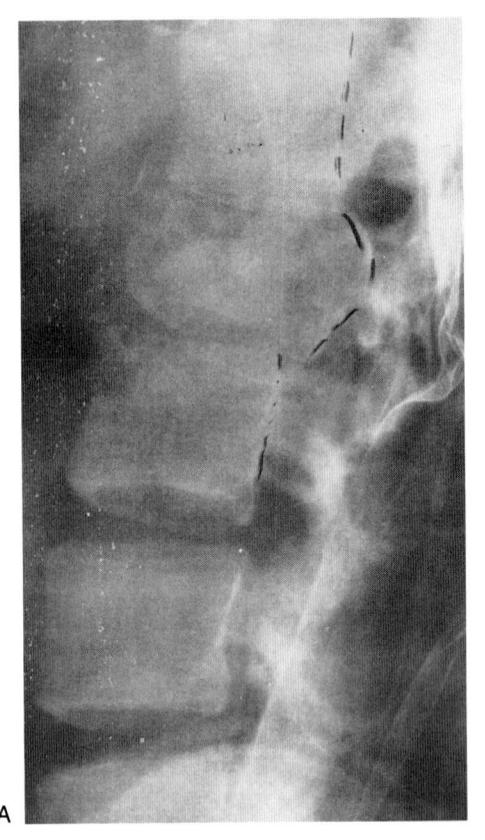

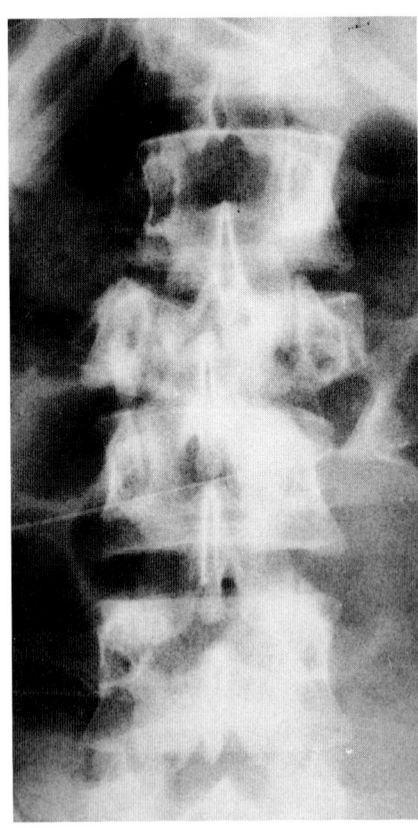

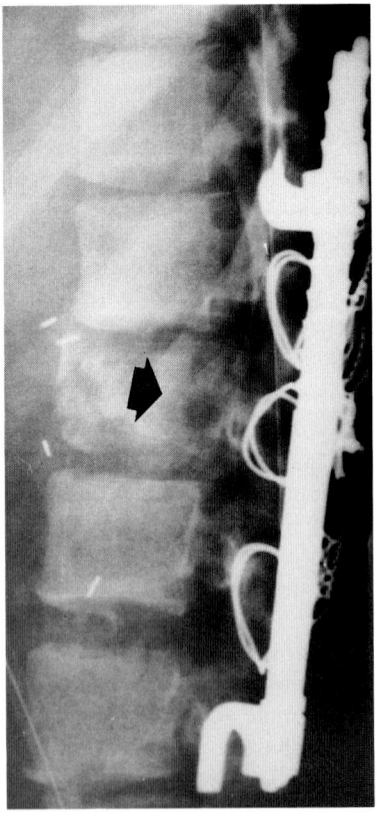

FIG. 4. A 19-year-old man sustained complete paraplegia due to a burst fracture of L2. Restoration of vertebral height and sagittal alignment was achieved by bilateral Harrington distraction rods with sublaminar wires (T12–L5). **A,B:** Lateral and AP radiographs of the lumbar spine showing the L2 burst fracture. Note the retropulsed bone fragment and the increased interpedicular distance at L2. **C:** Lateral radiograph of the lumbar spine following instrumentation with the "Harri–Luque" system.

breakage. Weiss springs are no longer in use because the system is nonrigid. Its use may be indicated only in a few, uncommon spine fractures (13).

The lack of proper segmental fixation dictates the use of postoperative external immobilization in either a cast or a "plastic jacket" for at least 3 months with all the systems we have mentioned so far. Because of the viscoelastic properties of the spine and the lack of segmental fixation, loss of correction in the sagittal plane may occur in the postoperative course (56,132). An additional, significant problem is related to bone loss at the fractured vertebral body, especially in severe vertebral body comminution, such as in burst injury ("eggshell" or "empty vertebra"). This may lead to late postoperative vertebral body collapse with progression of kyphosis at the injury site despite the presence of posterior instrumentation (128). This is a greater problem if the spinal instrumentation is removed later, as in the "instrument long, fuse short" technique.

Some of these problems were prevented by the use of the Luque technique that employed sublaminar segmental wires. Eduardo Luque, an orthopaedic surgeon from Mexico, developed his system for the treatment of spine deformities. As with the Harrington system, the Luque instrumentation was adopted for use in management of spine fractures (89). The Luque system allows application of transverse forces that, in some cases, enable better correction of the deformity (127). The Luque instrumentation is a rigid system because of its segmental application, but the system cannot apply or maintain compression or distraction forces. The two major advantages of the system are the elimination of postoperative external support and the ability to extend the instrumentation and fusion either to the cervical spine or the sacrum. Unlike the Harrington system, Luque instrumentation is stable in rotation. Sagittal curves can easily be contoured to the Luque rods to maintain normal sagittal alignment, especially in the cervical and lumbar spine.

The recommended length of a Luque construct is at least two levels above and below the unstable motion segment. The Luque system is contraindicated in fractures that exhibit comminution of the "middle column" because of the danger of pushing fragments from this unstable column into the spinal canal. A major disadvantage of the Luque system is the need to pass sublaminar wires in the epidural space, with potential for neurologic injury. The system may be safely used in patients with complete cord lesions.

The disadvantages of Luque rods have led to the development of the "Harri–Luque" system, a combination of Harrington distraction rods and sublaminar wires (127) (Fig. 4). This has improved the axial load resistance of the system and enables better rotational control (100). To reduce the incidence of hook or rod dislodgement, sublaminar wiring is performed around the Harrington rod one level below the proximal hooks and one level above the distal hooks (18). Caution should be exercised with this technique; the sublaminar wire may push the rod against bone, which may push the hook into the spinal canal.

Because of the danger of passing sublaminar wires into the epidural space, spinous process wire fixation was developed by Drummond et al. (35). This is a useful technique that provides a segmental fixation system without danger of encroachment on the spinal canal. Noel et al. (102) reported that use of the Wisconsin interspinous process segmental spine instrumentation in patients with thoracolumbar fractures shortened hospitalization and brace time when compared to use of the Harrington system without segmental fixation. Similar conclusions were drawn by Phillips et al. (105).

A further refinement of the Harrington technique was the development of rod sleeves by Edwards (37). Rod sleeves provide better mechanical stability and better control of the natural sagittal alignment (i.e., lordosis). These high-density polyethylene rod sleeves enable better three-point fixation and add an active, anteriorly directed, corrective force to combat angular kyphosis at the fracture site (Fig. 5).

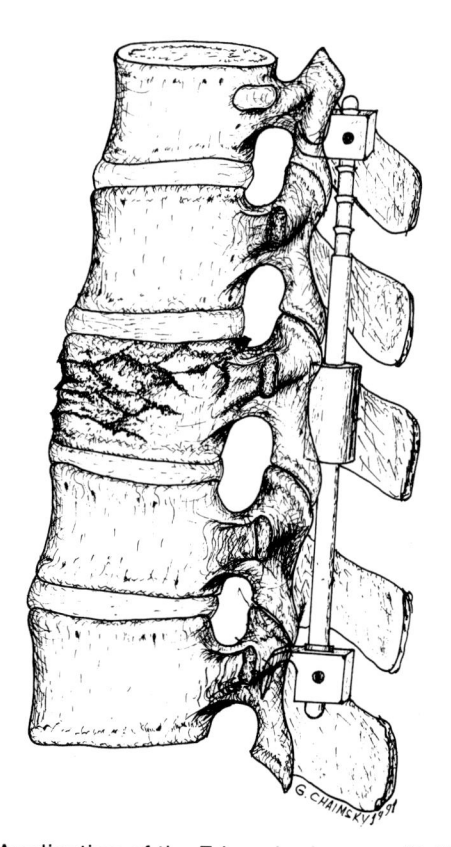

FIG. 5. Application of the Edwards sleeves with Harrington distraction rods in the lumbar spine. The rod sleeves exert an anteriorly directed force that will correct localized kyphosis and help to restore lumbar lordosis.

To eliminate some of the problems with the Harrington instrumentation and its modifications, Jacobs et al. (71) devised the locking hook spinal rod system (Fig. 6). The system provides partial segmental fixation and, most important, allows application of lordosing forces by prebending the rods. It is three times stronger than the classic Harrington construct and does not require postoperative external immobilization.

The technique of insertion of the Jacobs rod entails insertion of the lower hook two levels below the fracture. A trial hook is inserted to ensure proper seating of the lower hook. Next, the superior hook, which spans three intact lamina above the fracture, is inserted. The rod is introduced after appropriate sagittal contouring, and the superior hook is locked to the rod. The system is removed after fracture healing, implementing the philosophy of the "rod long, fuse short" technique.

Based on experience with 110 patients, Gertzbein et al. (59) found that kyphosis correction at the fracture site was from 21° preoperatively to 13° following surgery. If anterior surgery also was performed, the efficacy of kyphosis correction was markedly reduced. In 12 patients, the rods loosened. There was a 5° loss of kyphotic reduction due to late settling, especially in burst fractures. Complications occurred in 13.7% of the patients. These results are better than those achieved with Harrington rods in fracture management; complications may occur in up to 45% of cases (33,56,94,132). Jacobs and Ghista (69) stressed the importance of accurate rod contouring to the expected sagittal alignment so that the rod will resist bending moments. In addition, a longer rod decreased by 50% the force transmitted to the bone–hook interface by the rod.

A further departure from the original Harrington technique was the development of the Cotrel–Dubousset (C-D) system by Cotrel and Dubousset (23,24). The system employs segmental fixation with hooks or screws and allows the hooks to be placed on the same rod simultaneously, in distraction or compression mode. The addition of transverse connecting rods (cross-linkage) converts the construct to a very rigid frame (24) (Fig. 7). In fracture management, the C-D system can be applied with the usual three-point fixation technique to enable fracture reduction (44), or by the rotation maneuver as advocated for correction of scoliosis (39). The main advantages of the C-D system are elimination of postoperative external immobilization and the ability to correct and preserve sagittal alignment. A relative disadvantage is its high cost. Numerous reports (3,6,7,44,45) attest to its effectiveness in the management of thoracolumbar fractures.

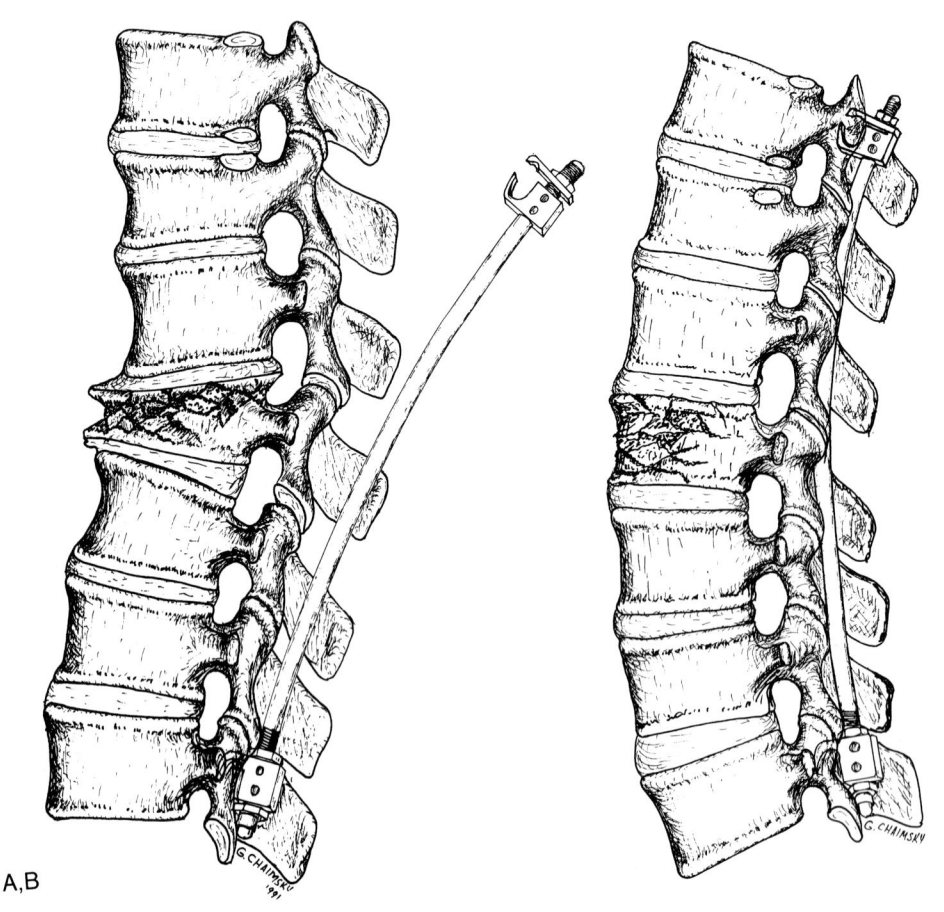

FIG. 6. The locking hook spinal rod system device of Jacobs and co-workers. Fracture reduction is achieved by approximating a pre-contoured rod to the spine, allowing fracture reduction and a correction of sagittal plane alignment. This technique necessitates a long instrumentation with adoption of "rod long, fuse short" technique, requiring later removal of the "hardware." **A:** The lower hook is inserted first two to three levels below the injury site. **B:** Next, the superior hook is approximated to the spine and inserted three levels above the lesion. The superior hook is locked around the superior lamina.

A,B

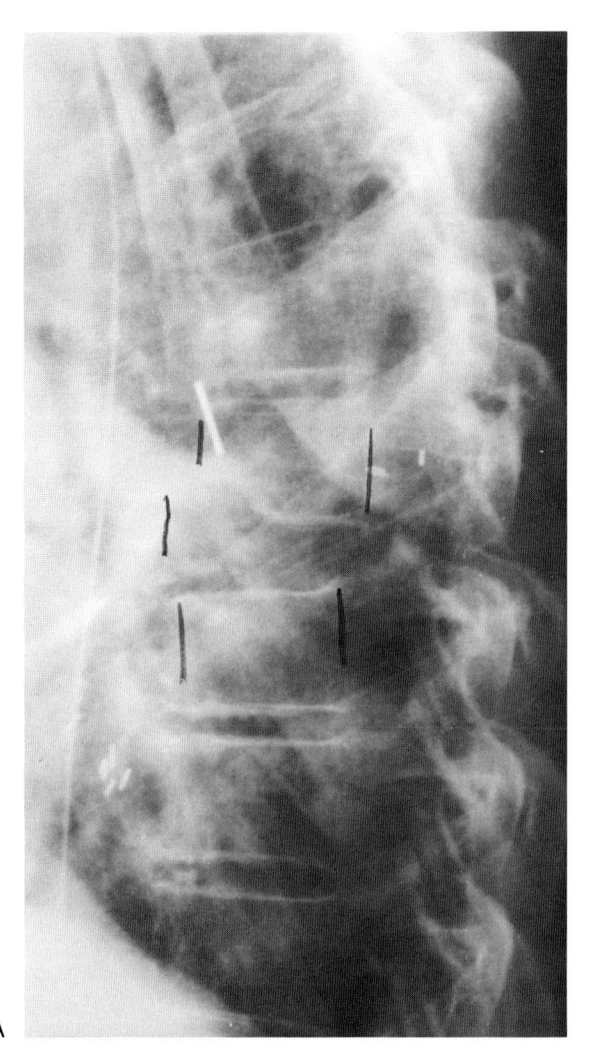

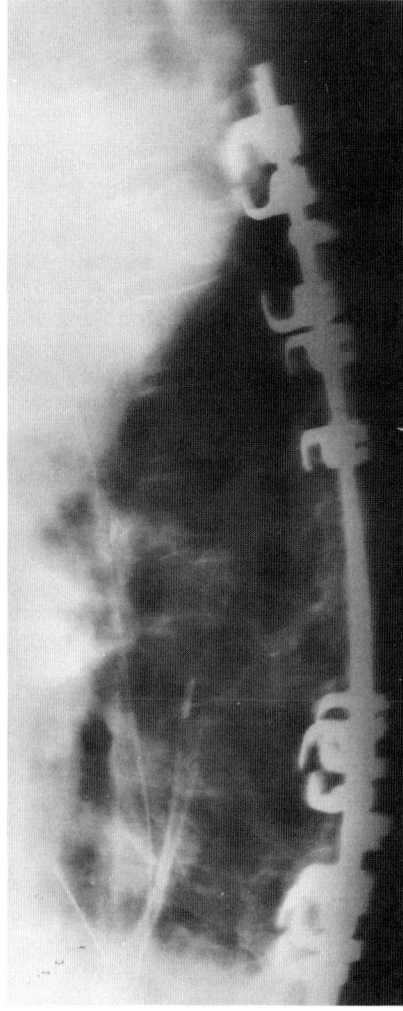

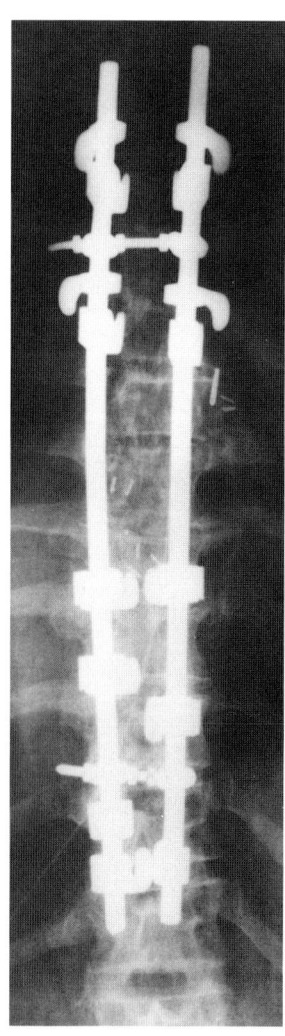

FIG. 7. A 60-year-old woman sustained fracture dislocation of the midthoracic spine with complete paraplegia. The fracture was stabilized with a C-D instrumentation to allow easier nursing and early rehabilitation. **A:** Lateral radiograph of the thoracic spine, showing the fracture dislocation. **B,C:** Lateral and AP radiographs after application of the C-D instrumentation. Note the double-level grips above and below the fracture.

Newer systems are the TSRH (Texas Scottish Rite Hospital) system (11), similar to the C-D system, and the Isola system (9), which combines many innovations of the Harrington, Luque, Drummond, and C-D techniques (Fig. 8).

Pedicle screws should serve as firm anchorage sites to the spine. Pedicle screw fixation directly controls the three columns of the spine with use of a posterior insertion, provides four-point fixation, and allows short constructs that "save" uninjured spinal motion segments. Pedicle screw fixation was introduced in 1959 by Boucher (16) and popularized in the 1960s and 1970s by Roy-Camille et al. (110), who developed a system of spinal plates and pedicle screws. Magerl (90) developed the external fixator for stabilization of spine fractures and employed Schantz pedicular screws. This system was modified by Dick (31), who developed the internal fixator as a fully implantable system.

The advantages of pedicle screw fixation are numerous. It provides a strong anchor to the spine, resulting in shorter constructs in fracture fixation. A three vertebrae, two motion segment "montage" is feasible and avoids unnecessary sacrifice of uninjured motion segments. This is especially important in the lumbar spine when fixing fractures at or below L3. Since pedicle screw fixation is firmly anchored to the spine, it allows application of stronger corrective forces, especially in the case of a burst fracture. The major disadvantage of pedicle screw fixation is the danger of root injury if the screw is malplaced (i.e., out of the confines of the pedicle). In addition, the potential injury to structures anterior to the spine (i.e., major blood vessels) must also be recognized (42,54).

A thorough knowledge of pedicular dimensions and size is crucial for the safe application of pedicle fixation. Saillant (112) provided mean values of thoracic

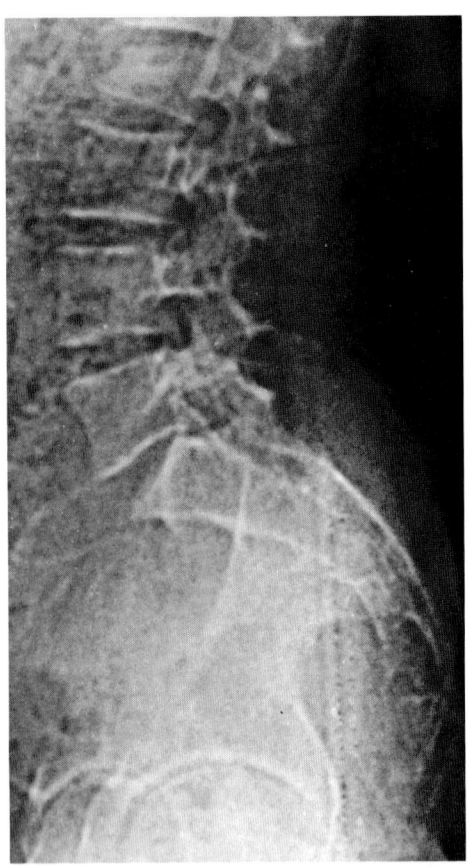

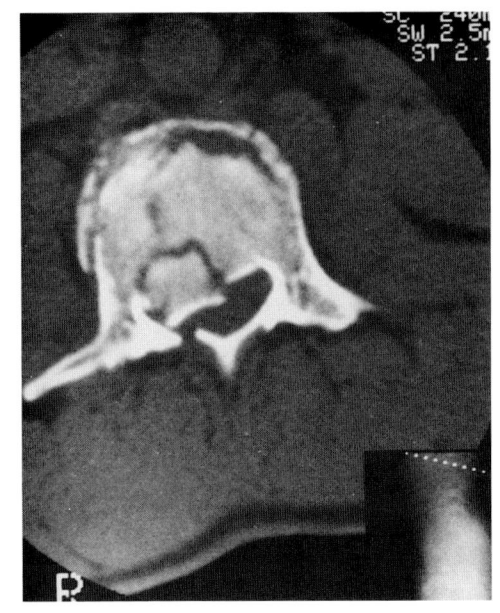

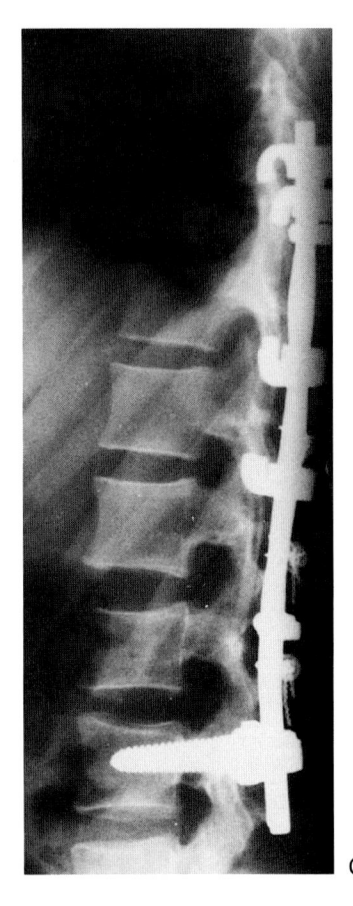

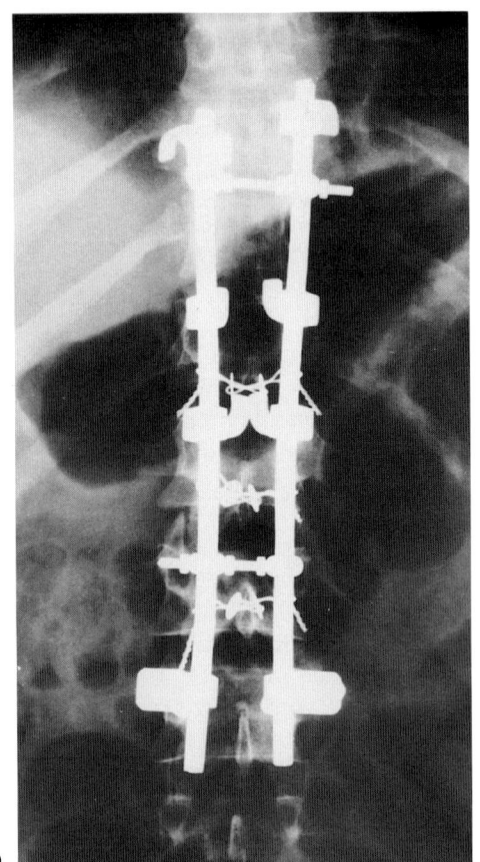

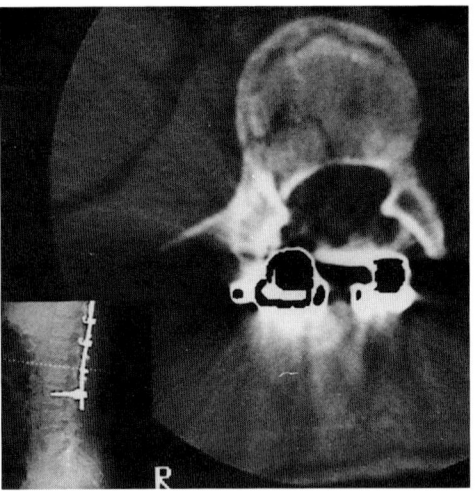

FIG. 8. A 30-year-old construction worker sustained a burst fracture at L2 and a compression fracture at T11 (not shown). He was neurologically intact. **A:** Lateral radiograph of the lumbar spine, showing the L2 burst. **B:** Axial CT scan shows a significant canal occlusion by the retropulsed posterior wall. There is also a laminar fracture. **C,D:** Lateral and AP radiographs following fixation with Steffee screws at L3, hooks at T9, T11, and T12, with two rods (Isola), as well as spinous process wires (Drummond). **E:** Axial CT scan. Note the complete clearance of the bony fragments from the spinal canal by ligamentotaxis.

and lumbar pedicle dimensions, but the most extensive study on pedicular anatomy was provided by Zindrick et al. (134). The oval-shaped pedicle is narrowest in the transverse plane and widest in the sagittal plane. The transverse plane pedicle angle is medial in the lumbar spine, becomes gradually neutral at L1, and angles laterally at T12. Further cephalad, the angle will again angulate medially. In the sagittal plane, the higher the vertebra, the greater the pedicle angle will be. Exceptions to the rule are L4, which is neutral, and L5, which angles caudally. The distance to the anterior cortex is significantly greater along the axis of the pedicle at most levels, except for T11 and T12. The pedicle is widest at L5 and narrowest at T5.

While Zindrick et al. (134) and Saillant (112) studied the morphometry of thoracic and lumbar pedicles, Gertzbein and Robbins (60) studied pedicular placement in vivo. They analyzed 167 pedicular screws inserted with the Dick device, by measuring postoperative CT scans. Eighty-one percent of screw insertions were within 2 mm or less of encroachment into the epidural space, beyond the medial border of the pedicle. Fifteen percent were inserted 2 to 8 mm into the spinal canal. Two of eight patients in whom the canal was encroached from 4.1 to 8.0 mm developed transient neurological symptoms. Four percent of the screws were placed lateral to the pedicle. Transverse pedicular screw angles measured according to Zindrick et al. (134) revealed that angles greater than 15° were associated with an increased incidence of unacceptable canal encroachment. However, a change in the port of entry, with a more lateral insertion of the screws, may avoid significant canal encroachment even though the angle exceeds 15°.

Improvement in screw placement was noted by Gertzbein and Robbins (60) in the last 25% of their cases, reflecting a "learning curve" associated with the technique of pedicular fixation. Canal intrusion of 4 mm or less was considered by these investigators to be safe, since there is a 2-mm epidural space and 2 mm of subarachnoid space (60). Another important parameter is the width of the pedicular isthmus. This is particularly important in the lower thoracic spine, where T7 can accommodate a 5.0 screw (133,134). Indeed, three of the five screws inserted at the level of T8 by Gertzbein and Robbins were out of the confines of the pedicle (60). (For further details on the anatomy of the pedicle and the techniques of screw insertion, see Chapter 2 by de Peretti and Argenson.)

The external fixator of Magerl (90) allows fracture reduction while immobilizing one level above and one level below the injured vertebra. Since it is a temporary external device, it was modified by Dick (31) to an "internal fixator," which is an implant, not an external device. It consists of a 5-mm Schantz screw placed into the pedicle and 7.0-mm flattened stainless steel rods that are connected to the pedicle screws. The connecting unit of the Schantz screws to the rod is mobile and allows introduction of kyphosis or lordosis to facilitate fracture reduction. Distraction or compression forces can also be applied. The Schantz screws are long and provide a strong lever arm that helps during fracture reduction (Fig. 9). After application of the appropriate corrective forces, the Schantz screws are cut (Fig. 9).

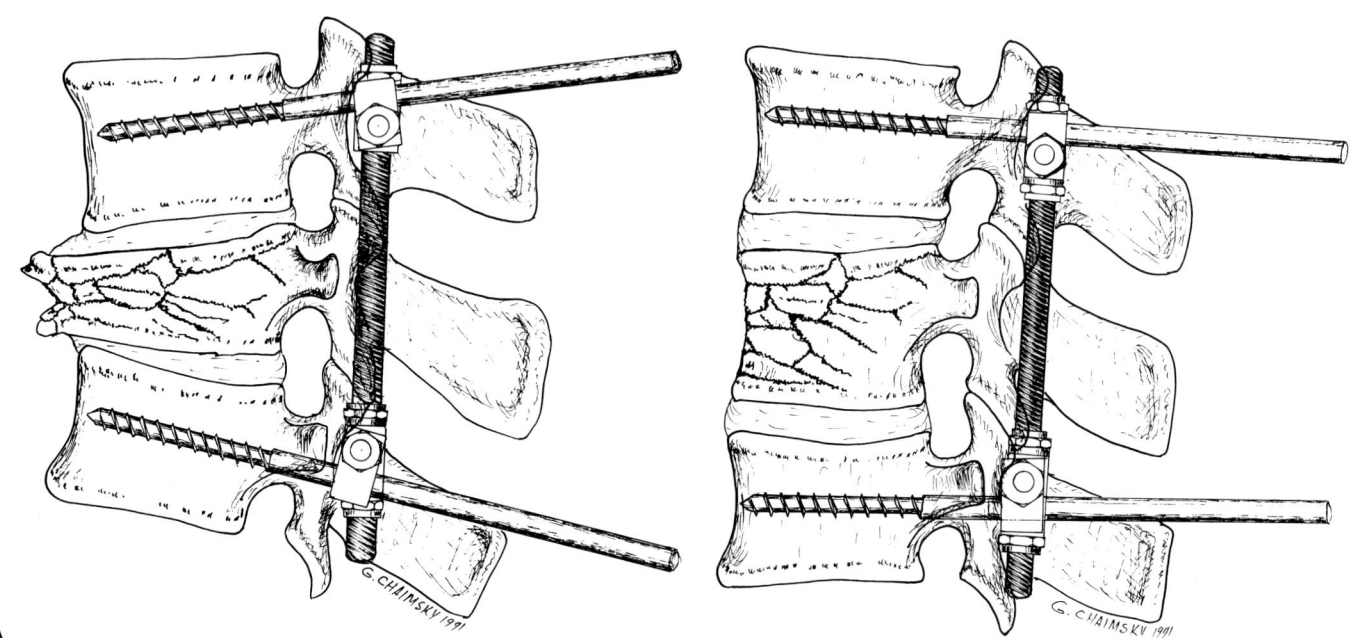

FIG. 9. The Dick (A-O) internal fixator. The system consists of 5-mm Schantz screws and 7.0-mm rods. **A:** The system *in situ*. **B:** Following application of corrective forces with restoration of vertebral architecture and sagittal alignment.

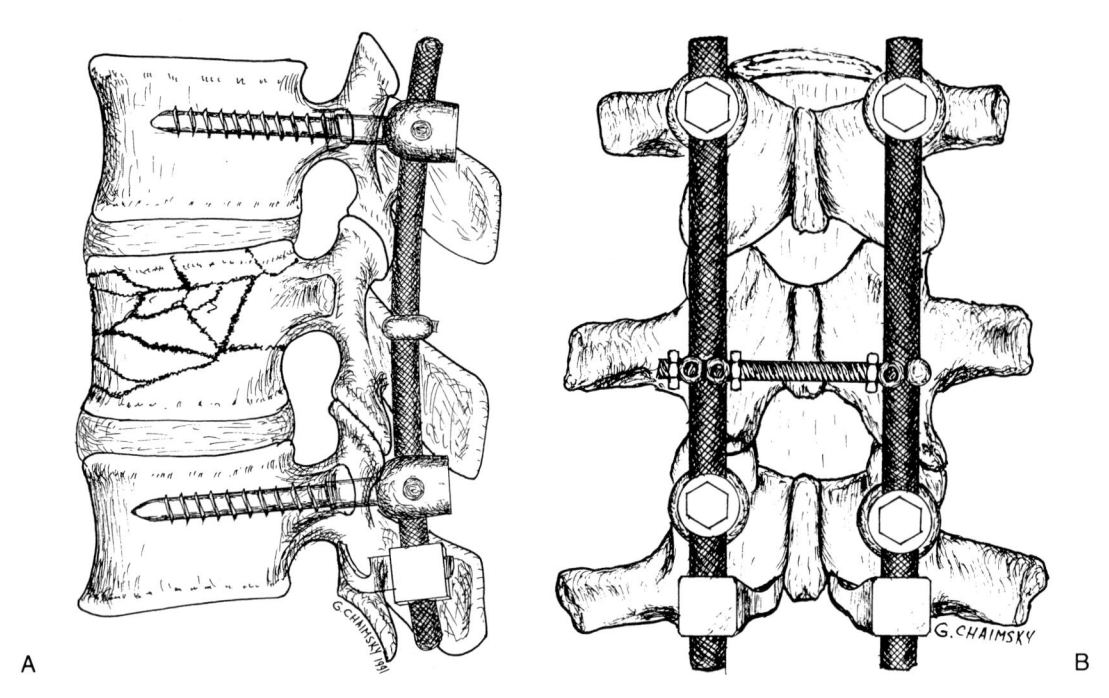

FIG. 10. The C-D pedicular system for fracture fixation in the lumbar spine. **A:** Lateral view. **B:** AP view. Note the "Tulip" screw with locking mechanism for the Cotrel rod, the "DTT" transverse connector, and the "protecting" hooks below the lower screws.

The Dick device has been used successfully in thoracolumbar fractures (32,40).

Esses et al. (41) reported on 120 patients with a variety of thoracolumbar fractures who were managed with the Dick device. There was a 32% improvement in canal clearance and an average kyphosis reduction of 14°. There was a 4.3% incidence of screw malplacement and two cases of neurologic injury after surgery.

In a prospective study, Lindsey and Dick reported on the use of the A-O fixateur in 80 consecutive patients with thoracolumbar fractures (87). Kyphosis was corrected from 17° to 8°. There was a 5° loss of correction after removal of the device due to collapse of the superior disc. They recommended interbody fusion of this injured disc.

Another available pedicular instrumentation is the C-D system, which employs pedicle screws of various designs that connect to standard C-D rods. C-D pedicle screws are available with "closed bodies" or as posterior open screws (Tulip) to accept C-D rods. In the latter instance, the rod is locked onto the open screw with a screw-top mechanism (22) (Fig. 10). Similarly, Steffee screws can be connected to the smooth, stainless steel rods of the Isola system, which is suitable for both fracture and deformity fixation (9) (Fig. 8).

Pedicle screw systems with plate fixation are also available. The classic design is that of Roy-Camille et al. (110), which has been used, mainly in France, since the early 1960s. The plates, perforated by holes at 13-mm intervals for screw placement, are precontoured and designed for use in the thoracic and lumbar spines. The screws are 3.5 to 4.5 mm in diameter; lengths range from 32 to 46 mm. The system is a four-point fixation device, immobilizing normal motion segments above and below the lesion.

Roy-Camille et al. (110) reported a 75% rate of acceptable fracture reduction. There was a 25% incidence of screw breakage, either at the proximal or distal end of the plate. This system should be protected by postoperative external immobilization for 3 to 6 months.

The Steffee pedicular screw–plate system is also a four-point fixation device (117,118). The Steffee screw, a modified cancellous bone screw, ranges in diameter from 5.5 to 7.0 mm and comes in various lengths. It is connected to a nested, slotted plate (VSP plates, or variable screw placement) with specialized nuts.

Other available pedicular systems are the notched A-O spinal plates, Luque plates, Rene Louis plates, Zielke posterior pedicular system, and the Hartshill rectangle system.

BIOMECHANICAL TESTING OF THE POSTERIOR DEVICES

In in vitro trials, Fidler (48) studied 14 different patterns of posterior instrumentation strategies in an anterior spine model, grossly destabilized after removal of a vertebral body. To eliminate individual variation in the anatomic and mechanical properties of human cadaveric spines, Fidler used a plastic spine model. The various constructs were tested with compression forces necessary to produce a deformity of 3 mm, and axial torque necessary to produce 27° torsion. Among the constructs tested, the most rigid was a steel rectangle fastened to the vertebrae with sublaminar wires. The addition of bone cement significantly increased the construct's rigidity. Harrington distraction rods were less rigid than double Luque rods. Double distraction Harrington rods incorporating three vertebrae above and below the lesion were stronger than similar constructs spanning only two levels above and below the lesion. Similarly, a one-level Harrington construct above and below the lesion was weaker than a two-level Harrington construct. Addition of sublaminar wires increased the construct's rigidity.

Panjabi et al. (103) created an injured spine model in fresh cadaveric human spines. They studied the comparative multidirectional stability provided by devices spanning five vertebrae. Among other measurements, they also observed translatory motions at the injury site for the first time. Luque rods and Luque rectangle provided the most stability in flexion, extension, and lateral bending, but stability in axial rotation was deficient. The next most stable devices were the Harrington distraction compression assembly and the Harrington distraction rods with Edwards sleeves. Constructs spanning five vertebrae were significantly stronger than shorter, three vertebrae constructs such as a short Luque rectangle or the anterior Dunn device (103).

In another study from the same group, Abumi et al. (2) studied the stability of shorter constructs in a fresh human cadaveric spine injury model. They studied translatory and rotatory multidirectional stability at the fracture site. None of the constructs restored stability to the values of the intact spine. Under physiologic flexion load, the most stable device was the Magerl external fixator. Other stable constructs were Harrington rods with reversed ratchets, Luque rectangle, and the Kaneda device. Almost identical results were obtained in extension. In lateral bending, the most stable device was the Kaneda anterior instrumentation. Axial rotation was the most difficult direction in which to obtain stability. Another important finding of the Abumi et al. (2) study was that it was easier to restore rotatory stability than translatory stability at the fracture site for all constructs evaluated.

Jacobs and associates (70) compared Weiss springs, Roy-Camille plates, vertebral body plates, Harrington compression rods, and Harrington distraction rods fixed to cadaveric spines. They compared the stability of these systems in simulated posterior ligamentous injury, vertebral body injury, and a combined injury. In the posterior ligamentous injury model, Harrington compression rods were as stable as the intact spine. In the anterior body defect model, Harrington distraction rods (three levels above and below the lesion) were as stable as the intact spine. In the combined injury, the Harrington distraction system again was the most stable system. However, in the latter instance, the overall stability achieved was lower than in single anterior or posterior lesions.

Wittenberg and associates (130) studied fatigue of four posterior implants in a burst fracture model of a calf spine. They tested the Dick fixator, Steffee plates, Harrington distraction rods with Drummond's spinous process fixation, and Luque pedicle screws and plates. Simulation of the posterior muscle tone and the physiologic axial preload was added to the experimental system during cyclic loading and compression testing. The Dick system was less stiff than the Luque plate. The Harrington–Drummond system allowed for less posterior distraction than the Steffee or the Dick systems.

Nasca et al. (101) studied fatigue of various spinal devices and found that Harrington rods were superior to Luque rods. Nasca and coinvestigators studied various posterior instrumentation designs in nondestructive cyclic testing (101). They studied Harrington–Moe distraction rods, paired Luque rods, and the "Harri–Luque"–Drummond system, with each system attached to porcine spines in vitro. Each spine was cycled 28,000 times. Displacement of the Harrington hooks was seen during off-axis compression/torsion testing. There was no evidence of loosening of either the Drummond or Luque implants or fatigue failure of any component. Throughout torsion testing, none of the implants showed statistically meaningful rotational stability. The Luque and Drummond constructs displaced less in axial compression, off-axis compression, and off-axis compression/torsion.

Thus clinical considerations in choosing the right implant should include not only a spinal construct's rigidity but also the length of its fatigue life. If a fatigue fracture occurs in a Harrington rod, it will usually occur at the shaft–rachet junction, as expected in an area of stress concentration.

Ferguson et al. (47) evaluated the stiffness of motion segments in the intact spine, two spine fracture models (partially and totally destabilized), and after the application of five posterior instrumentation systems. The systems studied were Jacobs rods two levels above and below the lesion; Harrington distraction rods with Moe hooks and sublaminar wires two levels above and below the lesion; compression Harrington rods ($3/16$ in.) with sublaminar wires; Roy-Camille plates with six screw fixation two levels above and below the fracture; and the Vermont fixator, fixed to the pedicles above and below the lesion. Combined compression/flexion, compression/extension, and compression/lateral bending loads were tested. Axial torque and cyclic loading were tested, as well. Three independent relative displacements between the two vertebrae adjacent to the simulated fracture were measured. In torsion, the posterior fixation devices had the least effect on stiffness compared to the normal spine. The Roy-Camille plates were the stiffest system in angular and shear measurements in all tested planes of motion. The segmentally wired Harrington distraction rods were the second stiffest. Cyclic loading resulted in loss of stiffness in torsion in the Harrington rods, Roy-Camille plates, and the Vermont fixator. Lateral bending stiffness was maintained in the pedicular systems but was lost in both wired systems. Asher and associates (8) found that a rigid cross-link between two spine rods was better than wires in achieving greater axial torsional resistance.

Farcy and associates (43) performed a biomechanical study comparing the stiffness and stability of Cotrel–Dubousset instrumentation to that of segmentally wired Harrington distraction rods with Moe hooks and segmentally wired Luque rods. A single-level instability (corpectomy) was created in bovine spine specimens, and the various instrumentations were mounted. Cotrel–Dubousset instrumentation provided 50% more torsional stability than double-level, segmentally wired Luque rods. Cotrel–Dubousset instrumentation fixed one level above and below the lesion was rotationally more stable than the same instrumentation fixed two levels above and below the lesion. Axial load stability with second-level Cotrel–Dubousset instrumentation was 400% that of double-level wired Harrington rods. Farcy et al. concluded that single-level Cotrel–Dubousset instrumentation may be suitable in management of rotational instability, while double-level Cotrel–Dubousset constructs are more appropriate for management of axial load injuries (i.e., burst fractures). Gepstein et al. (55) found that a C-D construct two levels cephalad to the lesion and one level caudad to the fracture was more stable and rigid than Harrington distraction rods three levels above and two levels below the fracture, or a similar construct with the Luque system.

McAfee et al. (95) developed an animal model for anterior and posterior column instability to allow in vivo observation on bone remodeling and arthrodesis after posterior spinal instrumentation and fusion. They studied Harrington distraction rods, Luque rectangle, and Cotrel–Dubousset pedicular fixation. There was a significant improved probability of achieving spinal fusion if spinal instrumentation had been used. Fusions performed in conjunction with instrumentation were found to be more rigid. They did find a device-related osteoporosis, especially with the Harrington or Cotrel–Dubousset instrumentations, but the improved mechanical properties of the fusion mass with use of spinal instrumentation compensated for the occurrence of device-related osteoporosis. In a later study by the same investigators, device-related osteoporosis was found to be more pronounced in pedicle screw fixation systems (96). However, the benefits of achieving a mature, solid fusion with instrumentation outweighed the influence of osteoporosis.

Krag (79) developed the Vermont spinal fixator and showed that there is ample room for safe pedicle fixation and, furthermore, that 80% screw penetration is accompanied by a 30% gain in resistance to screw pullout, as compared to 50% screw penetration. The major advantages of pedicle fixation according to Krag (79,80) are (a) only two to three vertebrae are incorporated in the construct, as opposed to five to seven vertebrae with the Harrington system; (b) three-dimensional fixation is achieved, resulting in prevention of hook or rod dislocation and allowing force application in more than one plane; (c) elimination of deliberate (as opposed to inadvertent) spinal canal encroachment by wires or hooks; and (d) the ability to instrument segments that had undergone laminectomy.

Skinner et al. (114) studied pullout strength, displacement, and energy absorption before failure of several pedicle screw designs in human cadaveric vertebrae. The best ranking screws were the 6.5-mm Steffee and 6.5-mm A-O screws. The greater the screw diameter, the greater the pull-out strength. They also found that placement of pedicle screws into the vertebral endplate increased pull-out strength. Conversely, penetration of the anterior cortex was not associated with increased pull-out strength. An exception to this is the sacrum, where anterior penetration of the S1 cortex is important for firm fixation of the pedicular screw (6,36).

Magerl (90) found the external fixator to be more stiff and stable than dorsal plate fixation, Jacobs rods, and Harrington rods.

Zindrick et al. (133) found that sacral pedicle screws directed 45° medially or laterally had the greatest pull-out strength. They also found that osteoporosis was important in decreasing pull-out strength, and that methyl methacrylate could restore this deficiency. A similar conclusion regarding bone mineral density of vertebrae was found by Wittenberg and associates (131). Interestingly, these investigators did not find a difference in pull-out strength whether screw placement was started with probing or drilling. Coe and his coinvestigators (21) found that hook fixation was superior to pedicle or spinous process fixation in osteoporotic vertebra. A different approach to overcome the negative effects of osteoporosis on pedicle screw fixation was proposed by Ruland et al. (111). They found that triangulated constructs with pedicle screws and transverse plates provided better fixation than conventional pedicle screws or laminar hooks.

Gillet et al. (61) studied short segment internal fixation versus longer segment fusion in thoracolumbar fractures. They created an unstable burst fracture at L1 in human and calf cadaveric spines and compared the stability of Harrington rods (T10 to L3), Harrington–Moe rods (T10 to L3), Roy-Camille plates both long and short (T11–T12 to L2–L3 and T12 to L2), extended hook–pedicle screw Cotrel–Dubousset instrumentation (T11 to L2), and a short pedicular Cotrel–Dubousset construct (T12 to L2). Under pure axial load, short C-D instrumentation was as stable as long Roy-Camille plates. Short Roy-Camille plates were less stable, but better than Harrington or Harrington–Moe rods. Under anterior bending tests, short C-D instrumentation was less stable than long Roy-Camille plates. However, long hook–pedicle screw C-D constructs were as stable as long Roy-Camille plates. They therefore recommended that short C-D constructs should be protected postoperatively by a Jewett brace.

Although pedicle screw fixation provides significant stability of the instrumented segment, fatigue fractures of the screws have been noted clinically. Ashman and coinvestigators (10) studied five different pedicle screw systems, examining the relative stiffness of each construct and the stresses generated within the implant in a corpectomy model that used "one level above and one level below" constructs. The systems evaluated were the Zielke system, Steffee plate system, Dick device, Luque pedicle–plate system, and notched A-O plates. Axial and torsional stresses were comparable in all systems tested. Stresses at the root of the pedicle screws were found to exceed the endurance limit of stainless steel in systems with rigid screw plate attachments (i.e., the Steffee plate and the Dick device). Devices with a flexible screw–plate attachment load the screws in tension, while the constrained systems load the screws in cantilevered bending. However, since screws can pivot in the nonconstrained systems, screw pull-out strength becomes a more important issue in these devices.

Finally, if bony fusion is incomplete, any system will eventually show fatigue failure. Therefore the techniques for arthrodesis are no less important than the implants themselves.

RECOMMENDED FIXATION FOR SPECIFIC INJURIES

Flexion injuries of the thoracolumbar spine result in compression of the anterior spinal column and tension at the posterior column, while the middle column serves as a hinge. Injuries that result in less than 50% reduction in the anterior column height, less than 30° of local kyphosis, and without evidence of posterior ligamentous disruption are managed nonoperatively. Indeed, many years ago, Bohler (14) advocated closed reduction of compression fractures of the thoracolumbar spine. He obtained reduction by hyperextension, raising the upper trunk and extending the lower extremities in the prone position. The reduction was maintained by external immobilization usually with three-point fixation by plaster of Paris. Louis et al. (88) described a similar technique under general anesthesia with longitudinal traction of 50% of the patient's weight.

More severe eccentric flexion injuries with involvement of the posterior ligamentous complex (46) necessitate surgical stabilization. Fixation may be achieved by a compression assembly that will restore anterior vertebral height and close the posterior disruption (75,93). It should be noted that these injuries also can be managed by Harrington distraction rods with a compressive interspinous wire. Flexion/compression injuries that involve all three columns of the spine can be managed by Harrington distraction rods.

Lateral flexion injuries, if severe enough to initiate a lateral spine curvature, are best treated by a distraction device on the concave side and a compression device on the convex side of the spine. A combination of Harrington distraction and compression rods or the C-D system with one rod in distraction and the other in compression will achieve the goal of vertebral body realignment with correction of the acute scoliotic deformity.

Flexion/distraction injuries are a result of a tension failure of the three spinal columns that starts posteriorly and progresses anteriorly. The lower thoracic spine and upper lumbar spine are usually involved. These injuries may occur with the use of lap seat belts and are accompanied by visceral trauma in a high percentage of the cases (58,107). The injury may be a pure bony injury (Chance fracture), a pure ligamentous injury, or a combination of both (58).

These lesions can be stabilized by Harrington compression rods acting as a tension band (Fig. 11). Harrington threaded compression rods are either $\frac{1}{8}$ or $\frac{3}{16}$ in. in diameter. In vitro testing shows that heavy Harrington compression rods are stronger than Harrington distraction rods. In vivo, they also have less tendency to loosen with time when compared to Harrington distraction rods (69). Their best use is in posterior ligamentous disruption injuries, when the posterior part of the vertebral body is intact. A compressive apparatus two levels above and two levels below the lesion is recommended with localized fusion and removal of the rods at 1 year postsurgery to preserve lumbar spine motion (58). Alternatively, a compression assembly one level above and below the lesion can be used as depicted in Fig. 11 or C-D compression assembly can also be used. Pure, bony Chance-type injuries may be managed conservatively with a brace or cast for 2 to 3 months.

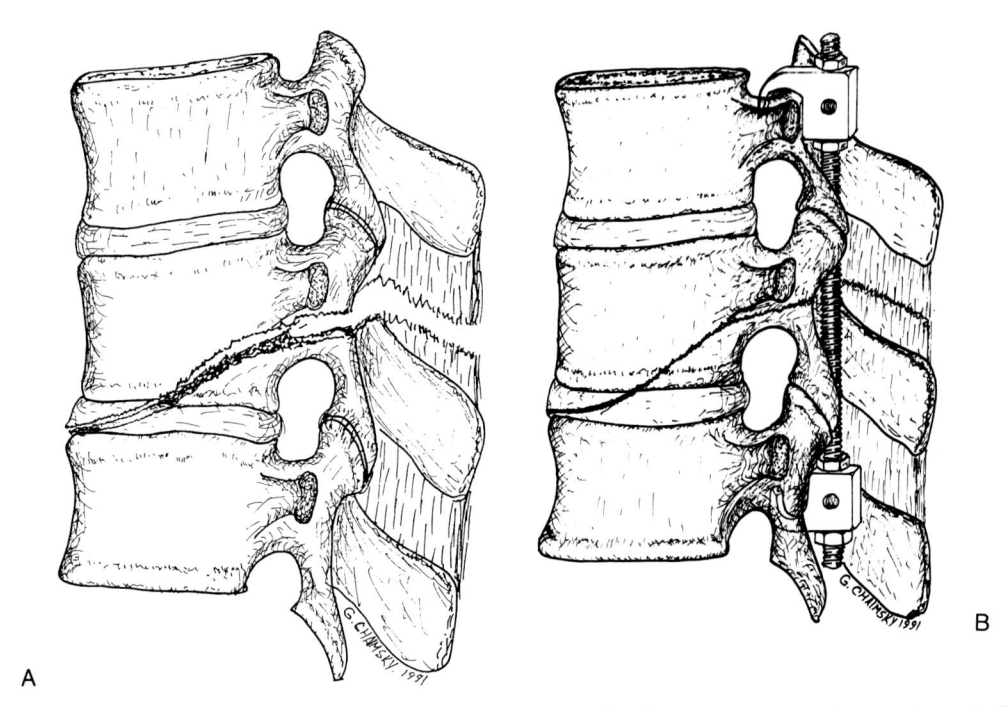

FIG. 11. Fixation of a flexion distraction injury with the Harrington compression system. **A:** The injury. **B:** After application of the Harrington system.

Fracture/dislocations of the thoracolumbar spine are highly unstable injuries and require spinal instrumentation and fusion to prevent deformity and neurologic damage (17). Flesch et al. (50) reported their experience in management of spine fractures with the Harrington system, using the Harrington outrigger. Jacobs disagreed with the use of this technique in fracture fixation, since the scoliosis outrigger applies distraction to the posterior structures without the three-point fixation principle (69). This may cause overdistraction, increased angular deformity, and possible injury to the neural elements. Stauffer and Neil (116) emphasized that the principle of three-point fixation is essential to proper use of the Harrington distraction system.

In fracture/dislocation managed with Harrington distraction rods, the rods function as a beam-column, loaded by end compressive forces and end flexion moments that are caused by the eccentric load of the torso's weight above the level of injury (69). The rod pushes anteriorly on the laminae immediately above and below the fracture site. For proper reduction, the rods should be contoured to the proper sagittal contour of the spine.

The application of distraction instrumentation per se may be dangerous in this setting (51). Because the normal constraints to distraction are ruptured, use of the Harrington outrigger may overdistract the spine at the injury level, leading to distraction of the spinal cord itself, with increased neurologic damage the result (Fig. 12A,B). To overcome this problem, a simultaneous application of compressive and distractive forces is recommended (51). Initially, the Harrington outrigger is mounted and progressively distracted without full correction. A double 18-gauge wire is then applied across the fracture/dislocation. When the wire is tightened, a compressive moment is applied, and further distraction can be exerted by the outrigger (51). After reduction of the fracture and restoration of the vertebral body height are verified by intraoperative radiographs, Harrington distraction rods replace the outrigger (Fig. 12C).

Similarly, a C-D system can be used. Application of a C-D compressive assembly is followed by a C-D distraction assembly. Alternatively, two Harrington distraction rods can be applied with the addition of a single midline compression Harrington rod.

Akbarnia et al. (3) reviewed the experience with thoracic fracture managed with the C-D system in 41 patients. Various hook arrangements were used in each case. At least one pediculo-transverse grip and one lamino-laminar grip were realized at the ends of the instrumentation. They concluded that the technique was safe and effective in treatment of unstable thoracic spine fractures. Argenson et al. (5) arrived at the same conclusion.

Levine et al. (85) studied bilateral facet dislocations in the thoracolumbar spine and reported on 30 patients. On pure biomechanical grounds, compression mode instrumentation is the treatment of choice. However, compression instrumentation was recommended by these authors only for patients with complete cord lesions; they recommended distraction instrumentation

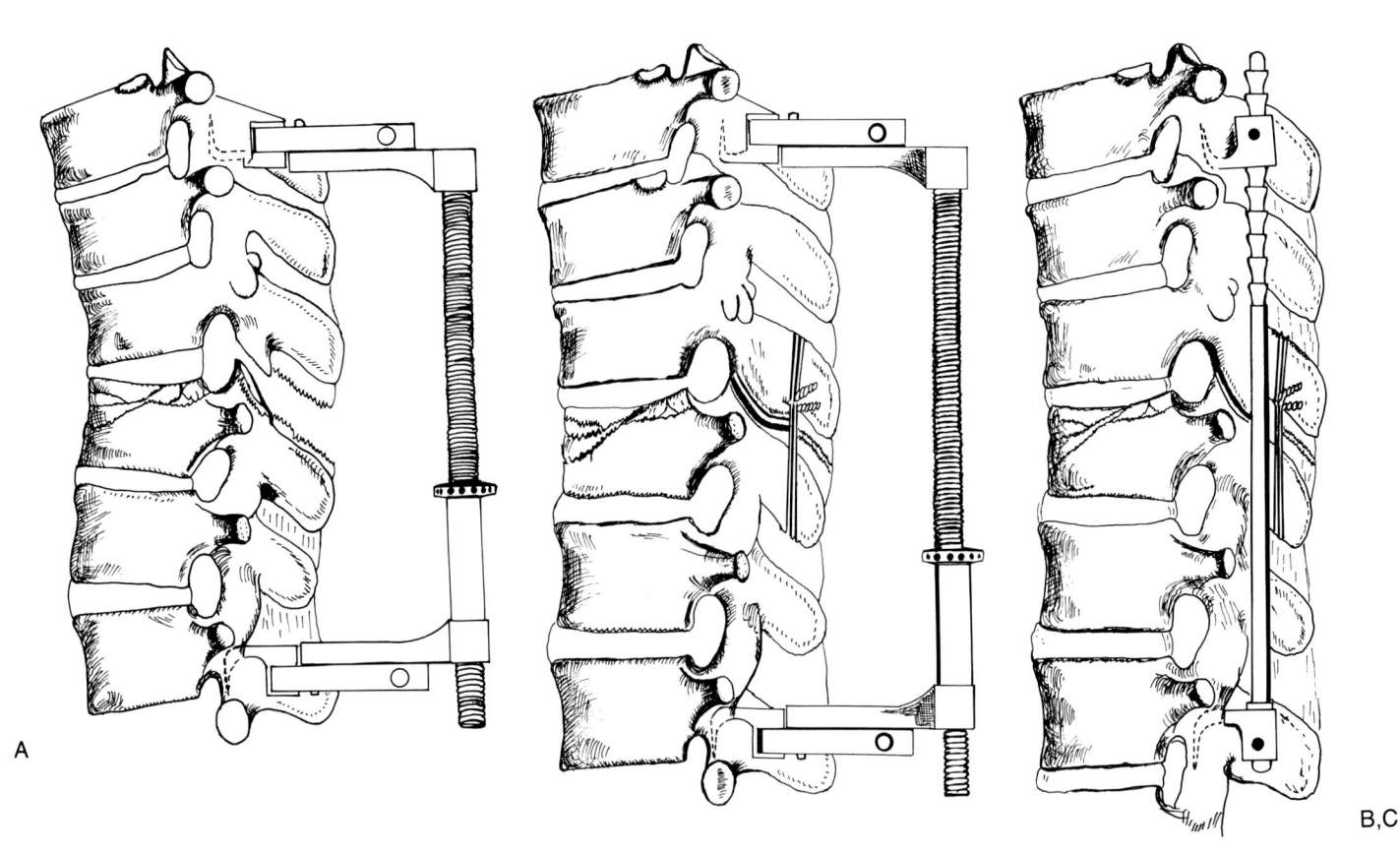

FIG. 12. Because the normal constraints to distraction are ruptured, use of the Harrington outrigger may overdistract the spine at the injury level, leading to distraction of the spinal cord itself, with increased neurologic damage the result. **A,B:** To overcome this problem, a simultaneous application of compressive and distractive forces is recommended (51). Initially, the Harrington outrigger is mounted and progressively distracted without full correction. A double 18-gauge wire is then applied across the fracture dislocation. When the wire is tightened, a compressive moment is applied, and further distraction can be exerted by the outrigger. **C:** After reduction of the fracture and restoration of the vertebral body height are verified by intraoperative radiographs, Harrington distraction rods replace the outrigger.

for partial neurologic deficits or neurologically intact patients. The reason for use of distraction mode instrumentation was to avoid posterior bulging of the injured disc that may occur with application of compression forces. If this lesion occurs in the lumbar spine, where distraction is to be avoided, discectomy of the injured disc should precede the application of a compression system (84,85). Likewise, compression rods should not be used in burst injuries for fear of pushing the bony fragment posteriorly, causing further encroachment on the neural elements.

Torsional flexion dislocations are usually reduced by anchoring a prebent rod to the spine proximal to the fracture. The rod is lowered to the distal hooks below the fracture, considering the Sagittal Index as the final goal. This allows correction of the deformity and reduction of the dislocation. Reduction can be obtained by either the Harrington or the C-D system.

Burst fractures account for 15% of all thoracolumbar injuries (28). Although some authors have recommended conservative management of burst fracture, others recommend surgical treatment. Surgical approaches themselves are controversial, and both anterior and posterior surgery have been advocated, sometimes even in combination.

Conservative care of burst fractures consists of short bed rest, followed by reduction with a brace or cast, and physical therapy mobilization (125). Weinstein et al. (125) reported excellent long-term results in patients managed conservatively, the majority of whom returned to work. There was no correlation between residual kyphosis and back pain and, most importantly, canal remodeling occurred with resorption of the bone fragments (125).

There is no doubt that this avenue of therapy is indicated for neurologically intact patients with "stable" burst injuries. However, problems with prolonged bed rest and immobilization as well as evolving late pain and deformity may lead to suboptimal results. Denis (28) contended that patients with spine fractures managed nonoperatively had more back pain. In addition, 17% of Denis' patients developed late neurological symptoms. Krompinger et al. (81) also reported that a significant percentage of patients managed nonoperatively had back pain.

We would recommend nonoperative treatment to neurologically intact patients with mild sagittal plane deformities of up to 15° on the Sagittal Index (62,81). (See discussion below and Chapter 31 by Glassman and Farcy.)

Posterior surgery is the most frequent mode of operative management of burst fractures. The mainstay of operative intervention was, and still is, the application of Harrington distraction instrumentation (Figs. 13 and 14). Although preliminary results with the Harrington instrumentation were encouraging, Gertzbein et al. (56) found that the results of Harrington instrumentation in burst fractures were inferior to its results in other types of vertebral fractures. If canal decompression by ligamentotaxis is the goal, then the instrumentation must exert a powerful distraction force.

Traditionally, burst injuries were managed by Harrington distraction rods. The mechanism of ligamentotaxis usually allows the full restoration of vertebral body height and partial clearance of bony fragments from the spinal canal. Tencer and associates (120,121) studied an experimental model of a burst fracture with 35% spinal canal occlusion. Laminectomy did not decrease spinal cord compression. They recommended avoiding overdistraction (more than 5.2 mm), compression of more than 3.2 mm, and flexion of more than 20°. Fredrickson et al. (52) found that the major force that provides clearance of bony fragments from the spinal canal is the distraction force. Effective canal clearance may be achieved only if the operative correction is carried out within the first 96 hr (25,38).

In general, posterior distraction techniques may enlarge the canal by reduction of the retropulsed fragment. Canal enlargement is usually from 40% to 75% (1,57). Crutcher et al. (26) found that Harrington distraction instrumentation was able to achieve canal decompression in burst fractures of the thoracolumbar spine. Canal decompression by indirect distraction ligamentotaxis was at least 50% of the initial canal occlusion. In Denis type A burst fractures, canal encroachment decreased from 62.5% to 19.2%; in type B burst fractures, canal decompression was less successful and was reduced only from 66.3% to 38.9%. Distraction is more effective in type A fractures in clearing the spinal canal, possibly because this fracture has a high degree of comminution. In Denis type B burst fractures, the bony fragments in the canal are usually one or two large pieces of bone locked between the two halves of the fractured vertebral body.

Even if canal clearance is not complete, bony fragments may resorb with time due to spinal canal remodeling (38,49,125). In addition, the presence of retropulsed bone in the canal in a neurologically intact patient is usually not associated with late neurologic deterioration (81,128).

If the retropulsed fragment is rotated, or canal occlusion is greater than 50%, ligamentotaxis is not efficient and posterior decompression should be performed as well. If canal clearance is inadequate following posterior instrumentation or after posterior or posterolateral decompression, anterior decompression is indicated (15,77). Also, if more than 75% of canal occlusion is noted preoperatively, anterior decompression should be performed first, followed by posterior fixation, preferably with pedicle screws. If CT examination suggests that a laminar fracture is present, it is better to first approach the spine from the back, since the dura may be torn and the cauda equina roots may be trapped in the fracture (19) (Fig. 15).

Using a posterior rod–hook system raises the issue of the rod length as well as the extent of arthrodesis. Dickson et al. (33) recommended two levels above and two levels below the injury site, with fusion along the length of the rods. Conversely, Peterson and Armstrong (104) recommended instrumentation of three levels above and below the lesion with full length fusion. Jacobs and Ghista (69) reported better anatomic reduction with the latter method, although without full length fusion.

There are two biomechanical explanations as to why longer rods are preferable. Contouring of longer rods to the preferred sagittal alignment of the spine is better because it allows better contact with the laminae, creating a better three-point fixation. In the "three above, three below" construct, the lever arm is almost twice that of "two above and below," resulting in a 50% decrease in force applied to the bone by the fixation device (69).

Despite the development of newer fixation systems, the Harrington spinal instrumentation is still the mainstay of vertebral fracture fixation because of its simplicity, surgeons' familiarity with the system, and its relatively low cost. Figures 13 and 14 depict the application of the Harrington system in burst fractures.

However, the Harrington system is plagued by many shortcomings that are especially significant when managing lumbar burst fractures. Hook dislodgement and late collapse are frequently encountered. Flattening of the lumbar lordosis and fusion of long segments are the most important drawbacks of this system. Rod sleeves, locking rods and hooks, Moe rods and hooks (square ended), and contoured Harrington rods with sublaminar wires represent the many attempts to circumvent these complications.

Luque instrumentation is not appropriate in the management of burst fractures, since it does not provide the axial resistance necessary to avoid further retropulsion of bony fragments into the spinal canal.

Pedicle screw fixation is certainly a better solution

POSTERIOR INSTRUMENTATION • 295

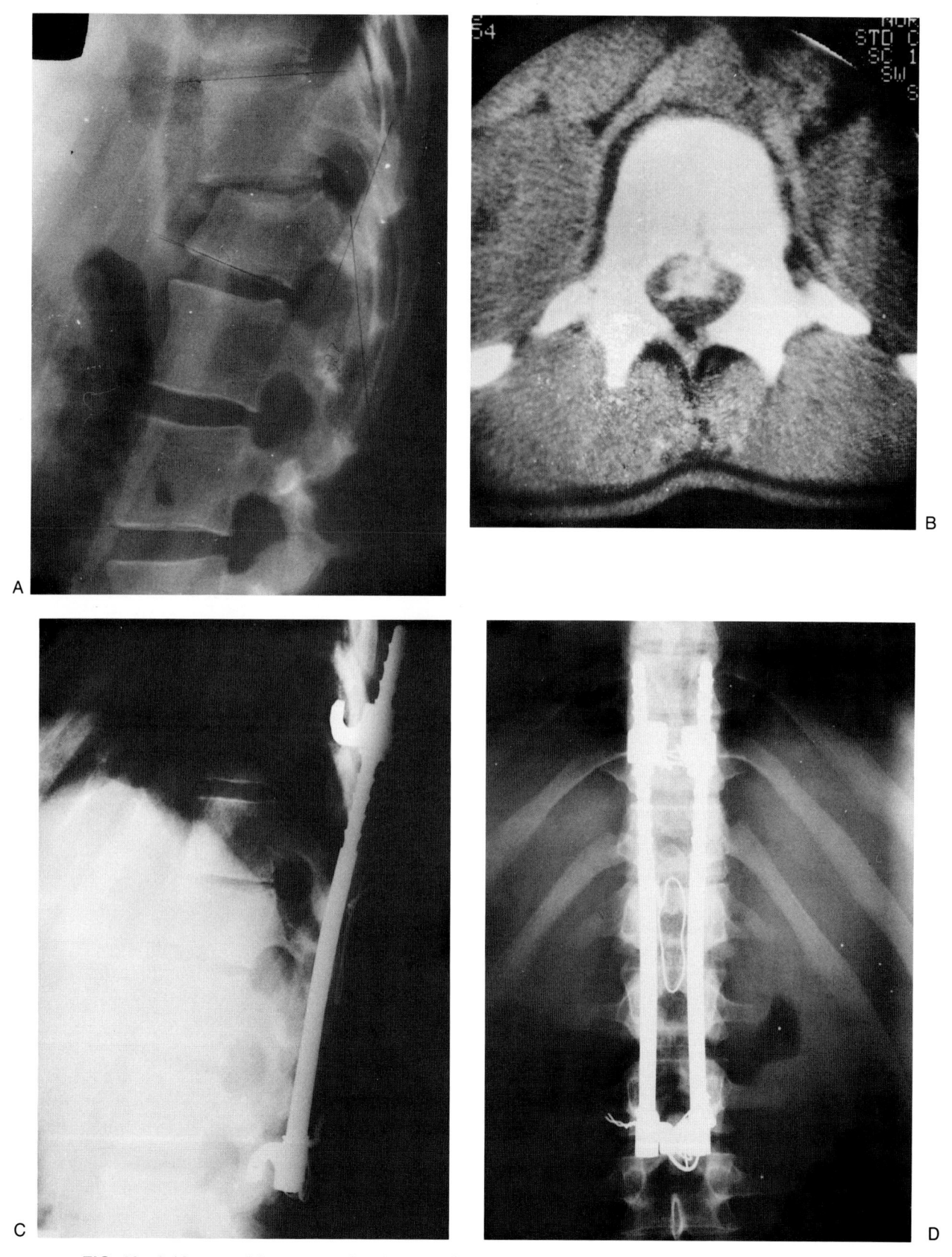

FIG. 13. A 19-year-old man sustained a burst fracture of L1 with localized kyphosis of 26° degrees **(A)** and retropulsed bone in the canal **(B)**. He was neurologically intact. **C,D:** Lateral and AP radiographs following instrumentation with two Harrington distraction rods and spinous process wires from T10 to L3.

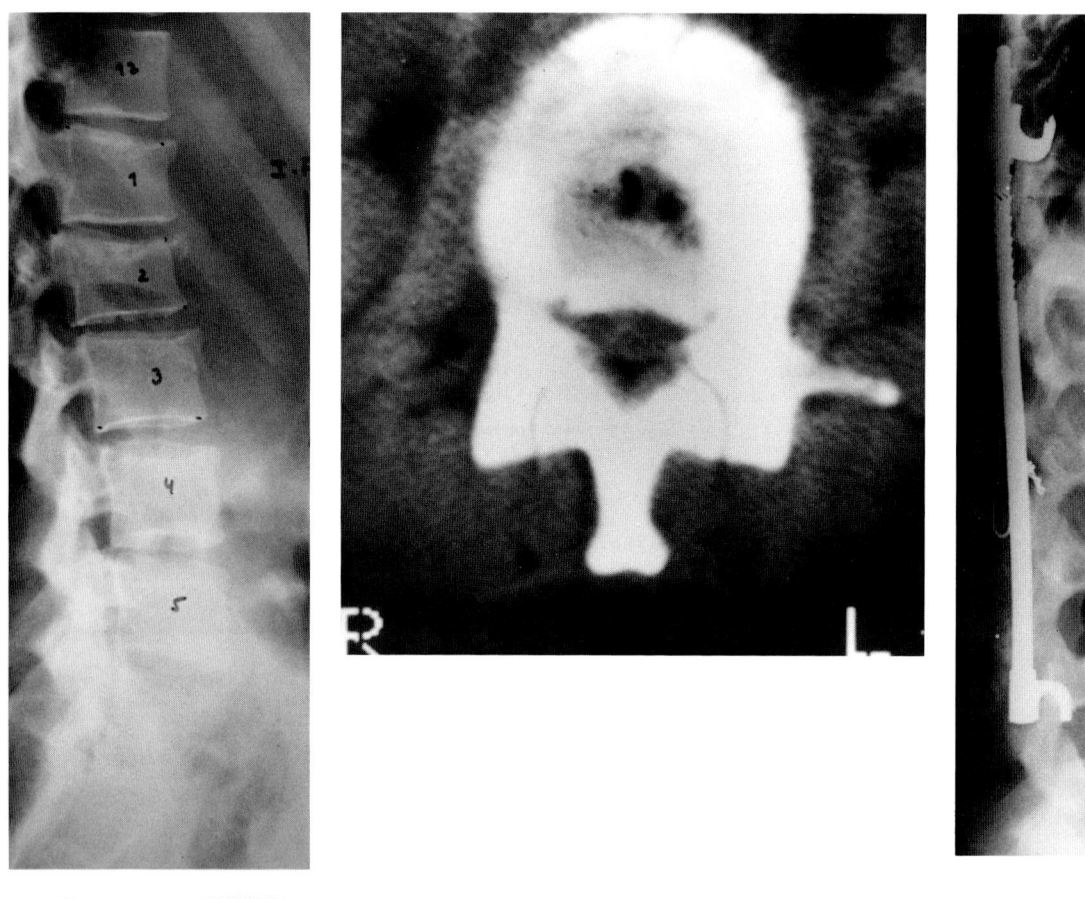

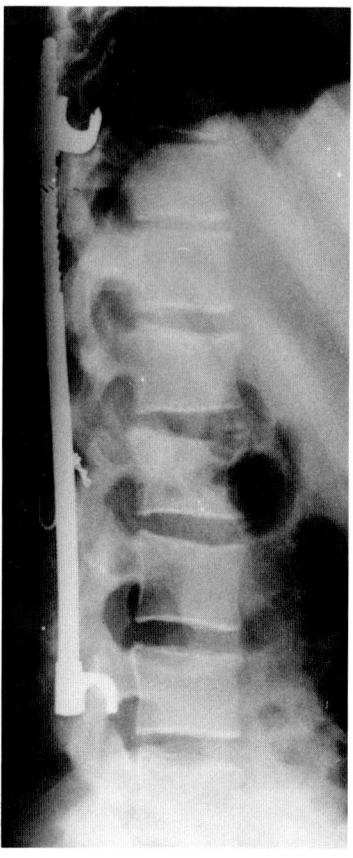

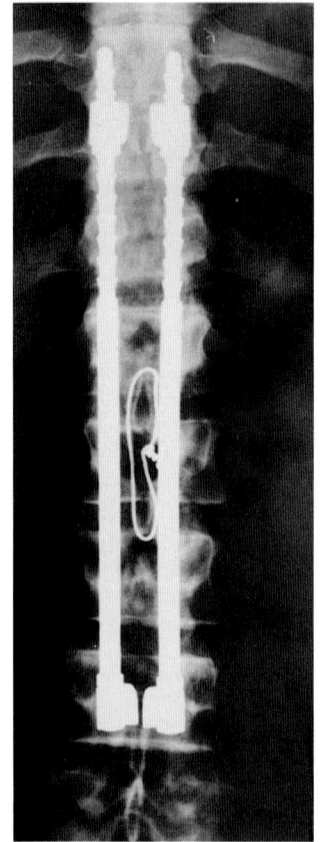

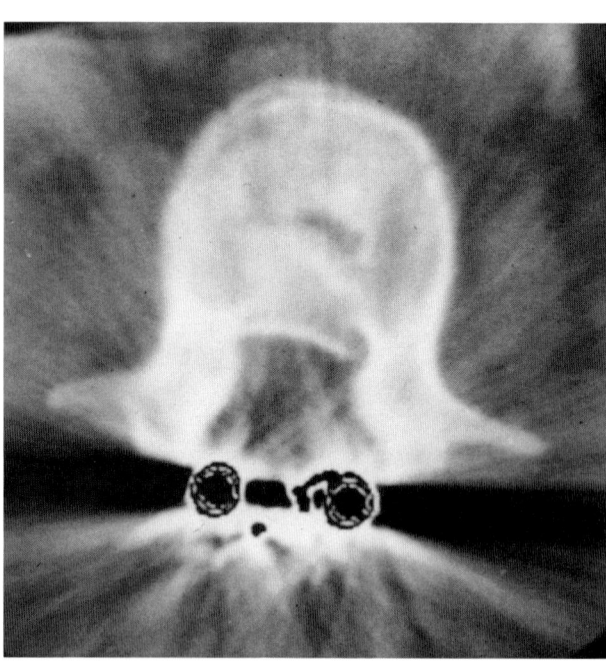

FIG. 14. An 18-year-old psychotic woman was injured in a suicidal attempt sustaining a burst fracture of L2 with Frankel D paraparesis. **A:** Lateral radiograph. **B:** CT scan showing the retropulsed bony fragment. **C,D:** Lateral and AP radiographs following instrumentation with Harrington distraction rods from T10 to L4 with an interspinous compressive wire between L1 and L2. **E:** CT scan showing canal clearance by ligamentotaxis.

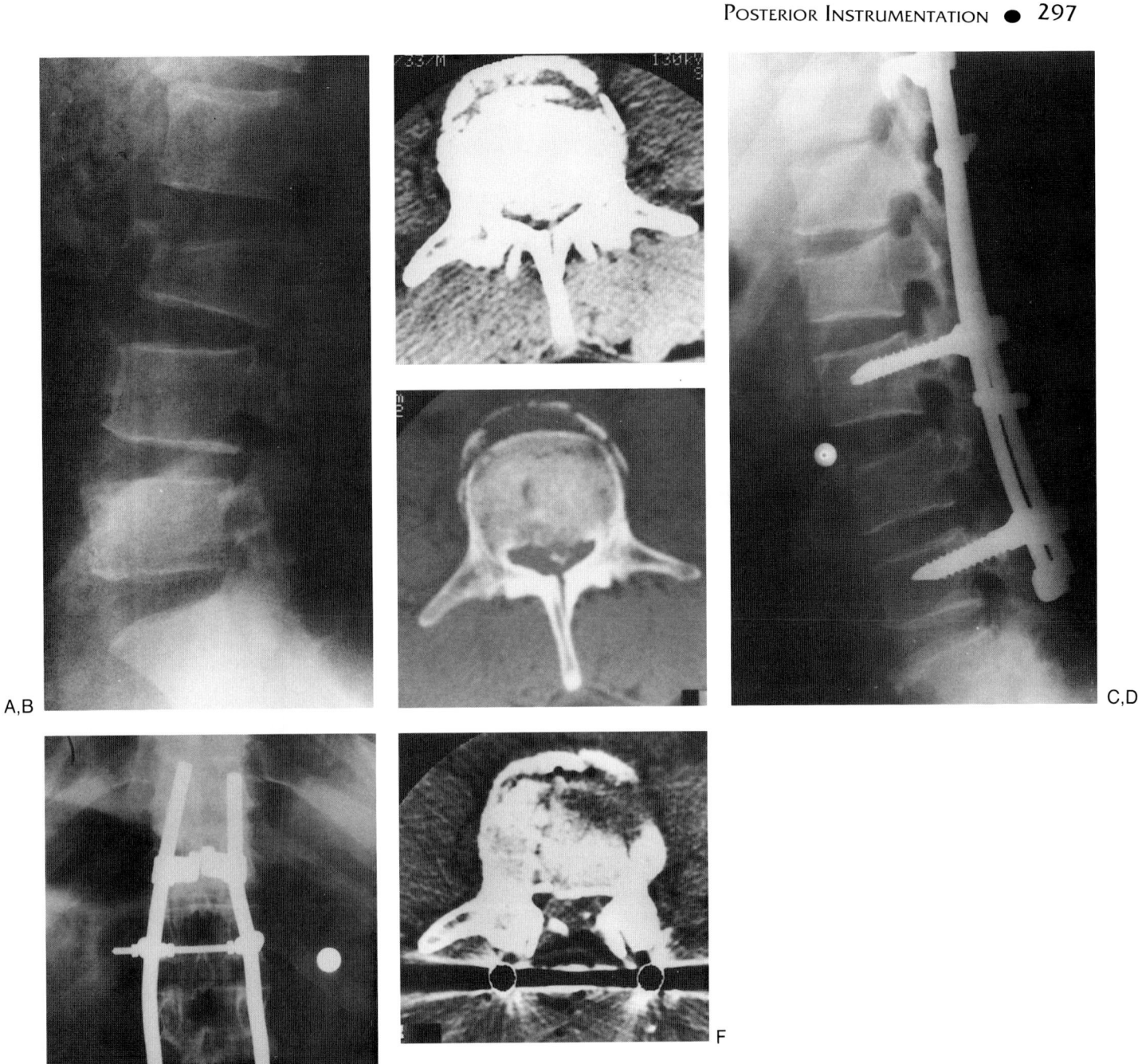

FIG. 15. A 34-year-old construction worker fell from 4 meters and sustained an L3 burst fracture with severe weakness of both legs and loss of sphincteric control. He also sustained compression fractures of T12 and L1. Lateral view **(A)**. CT showed more than 90% canal occlusion **(B)** as well as a laminar fracture **(C)**. Following pedicle screw fixation at L4 and L2 with instrumentation to T10 to bypass the compression fractures **(D,E)**, a laminectomy of L3 was performed. There was a complete tear of the dura with cauda roots entrapped in the laminar fracture. Following repair of the dura and impaction of the bone fragments back to the vertebral body, the patient made a partial but significant neural recovery. Note the significant canal reconstruction **(F)**.

to these problems, as it is possible to restore lumbar lordosis and yet perform a short fusion (three vertebrae, two motion segments) (Fig. 16).

A combination of pedicle screws below the lesion and hooks above the lesion also is a useful and easy construct to apply, especially in a multilevel spine injury (Figs. 17 and 18). It may have the theoretical advantage of preventing late collapse at the fracture site.

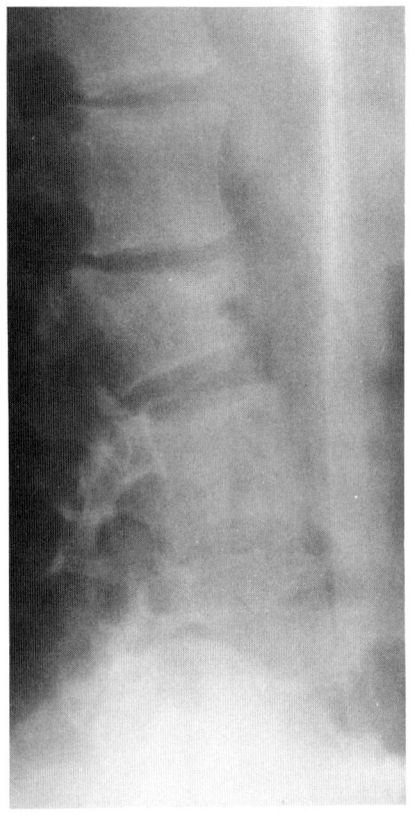

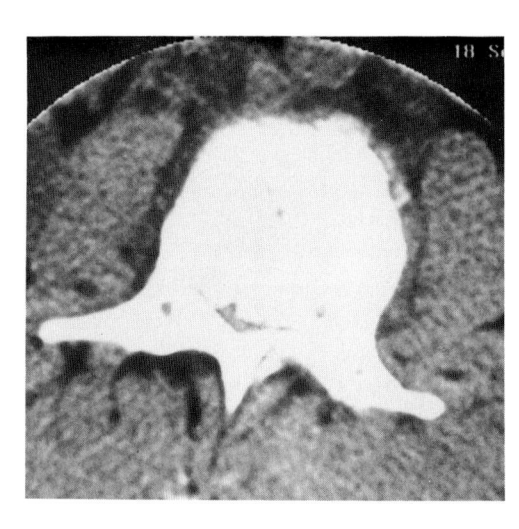

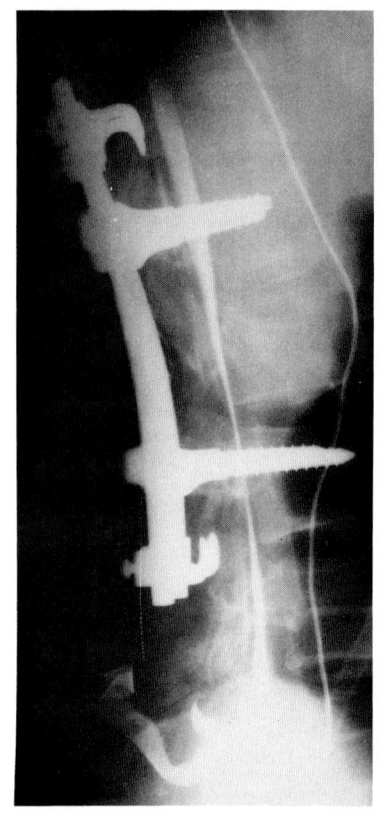

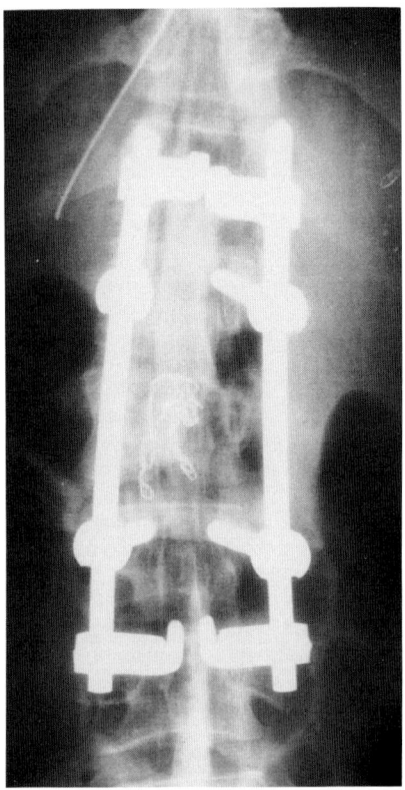

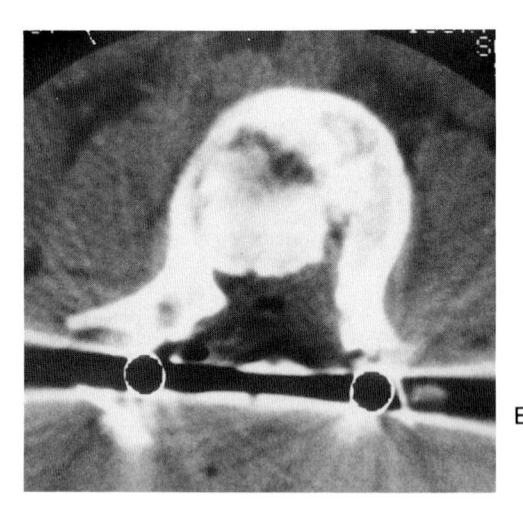

FIG. 16. An 18-year-old man fell 6 meters and sustained a burst fracture of L2 with severe weakness of both legs (left more than the right). **A:** Lateral radiograph showing the localized kyphosis and the retropulsion of the upper part of L2 posteriorly. **B:** CT scan shows more than 90% canal occlusion. **C,D:** Following pedicle screw insertion at L3 and L1 with rod contouring, sagittal alignment was regained. Laminectomy with impaction of the retropulsed bone back to the vertebral body was performed as well. Intraoperative myelogram shows free passage of the contrast. **E:** CT scan shows restoration of the canal.

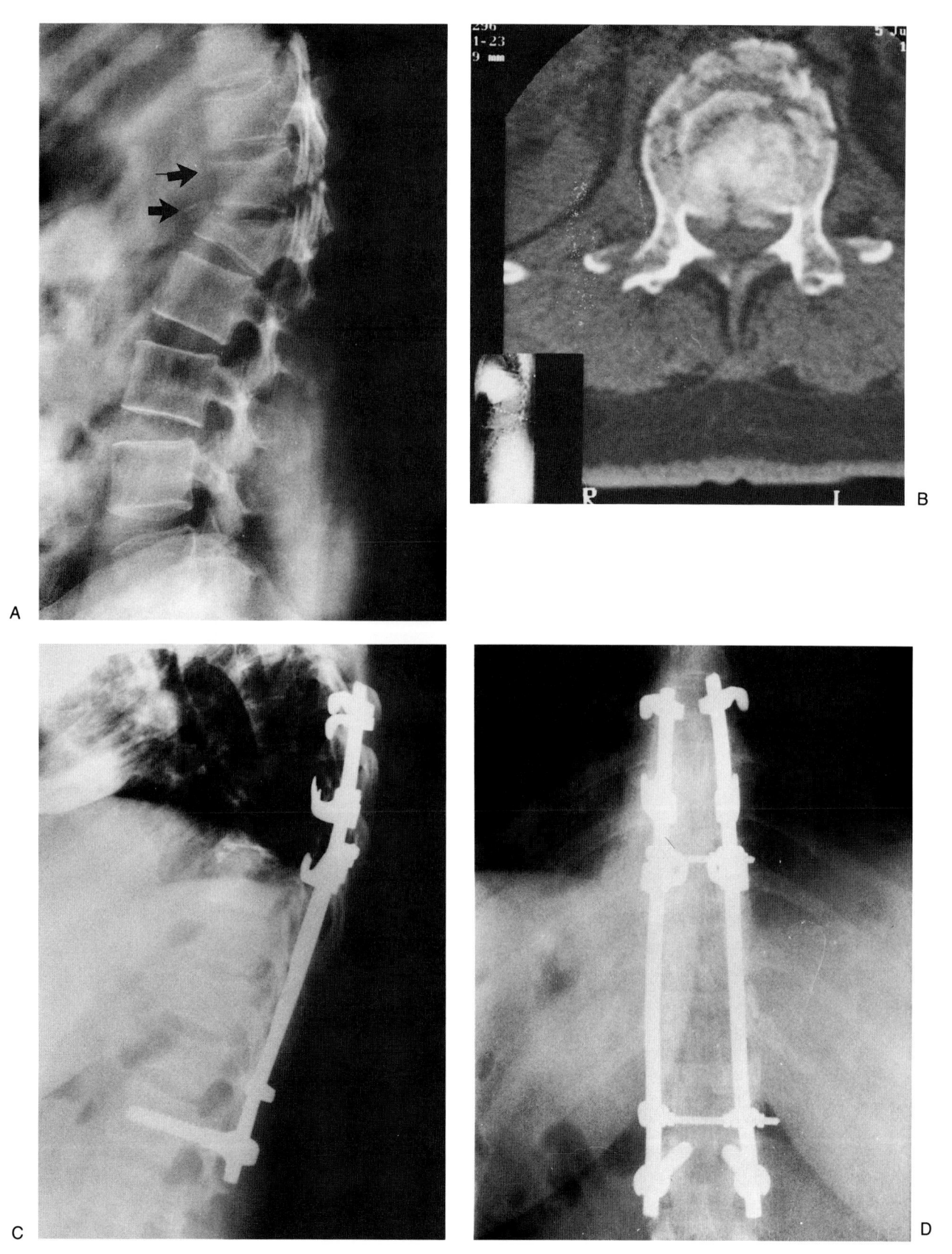

FIG. 17. A 50-year-old woman was involved in a road accident and sustained burst fractures of T12 and L1 and compression fracture of T11. There was no neurological deficit. **A:** Lateral radiograph. **B:** CT scan showing the retropulsed bone. **C,D:** Lateral and AP radiographs following instrumentation with C-D screws at L2 and hooks at T6–T7 and T8.

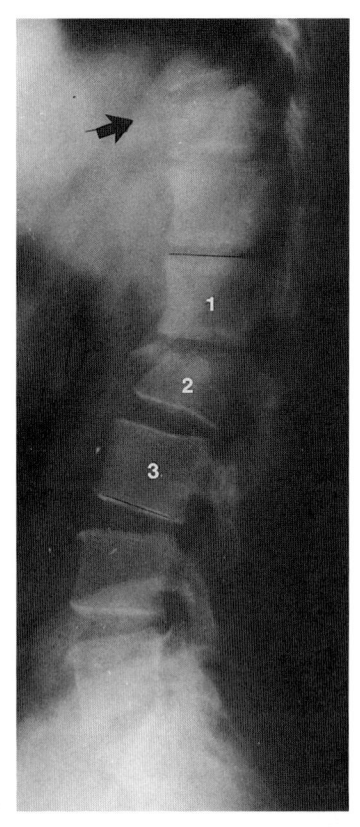

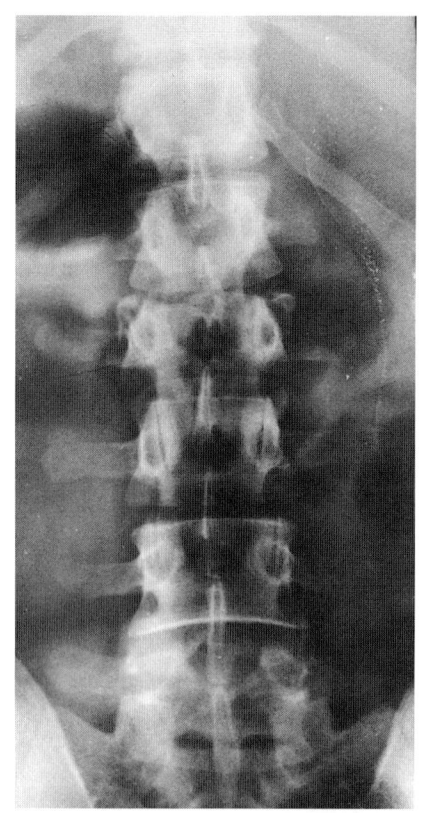

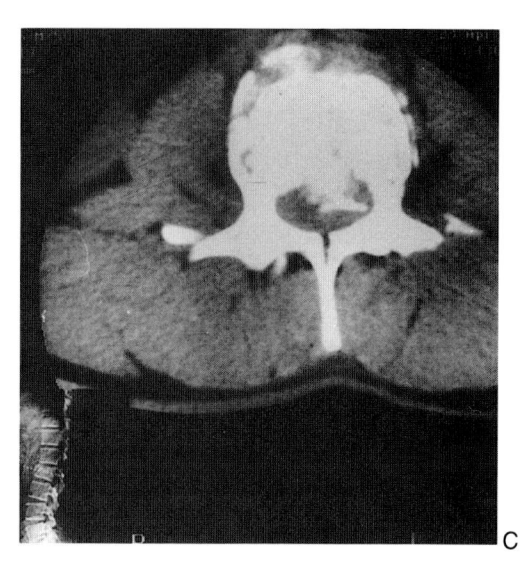

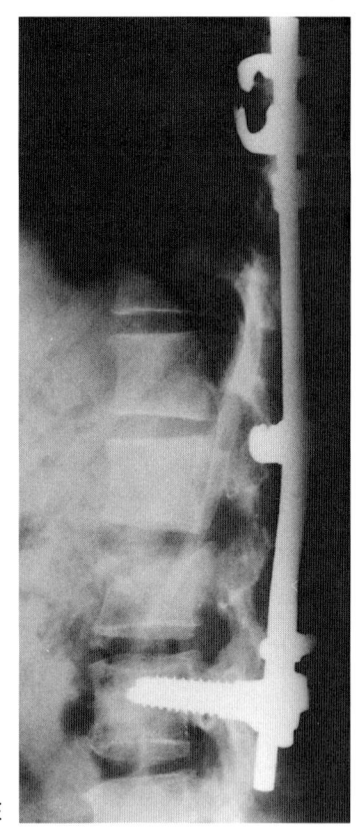

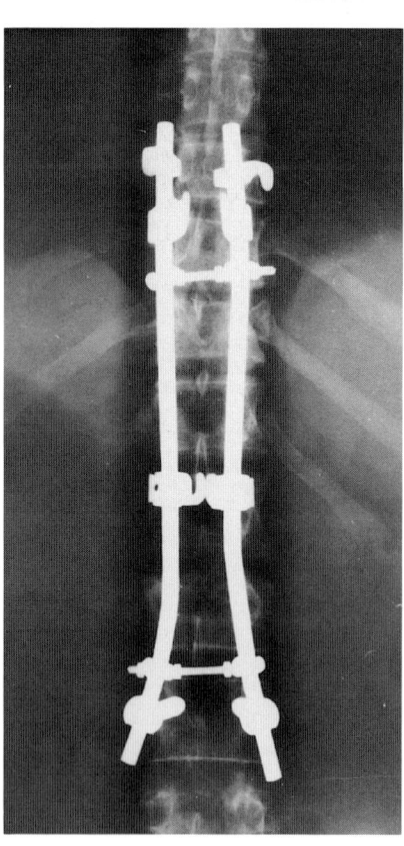

FIG. 18. A 30-year-old man sustained a burst fracture of L2 and compression fracture at T11 after falling 10 meters. **A:** Lateral radiograph. **B:** AP radiograph. **C:** Bony retropulsion of the posterior wall of L2. **D,E:** Following C-D instrumentation with pedicle screws at L3 and hooks at T12 and T8.

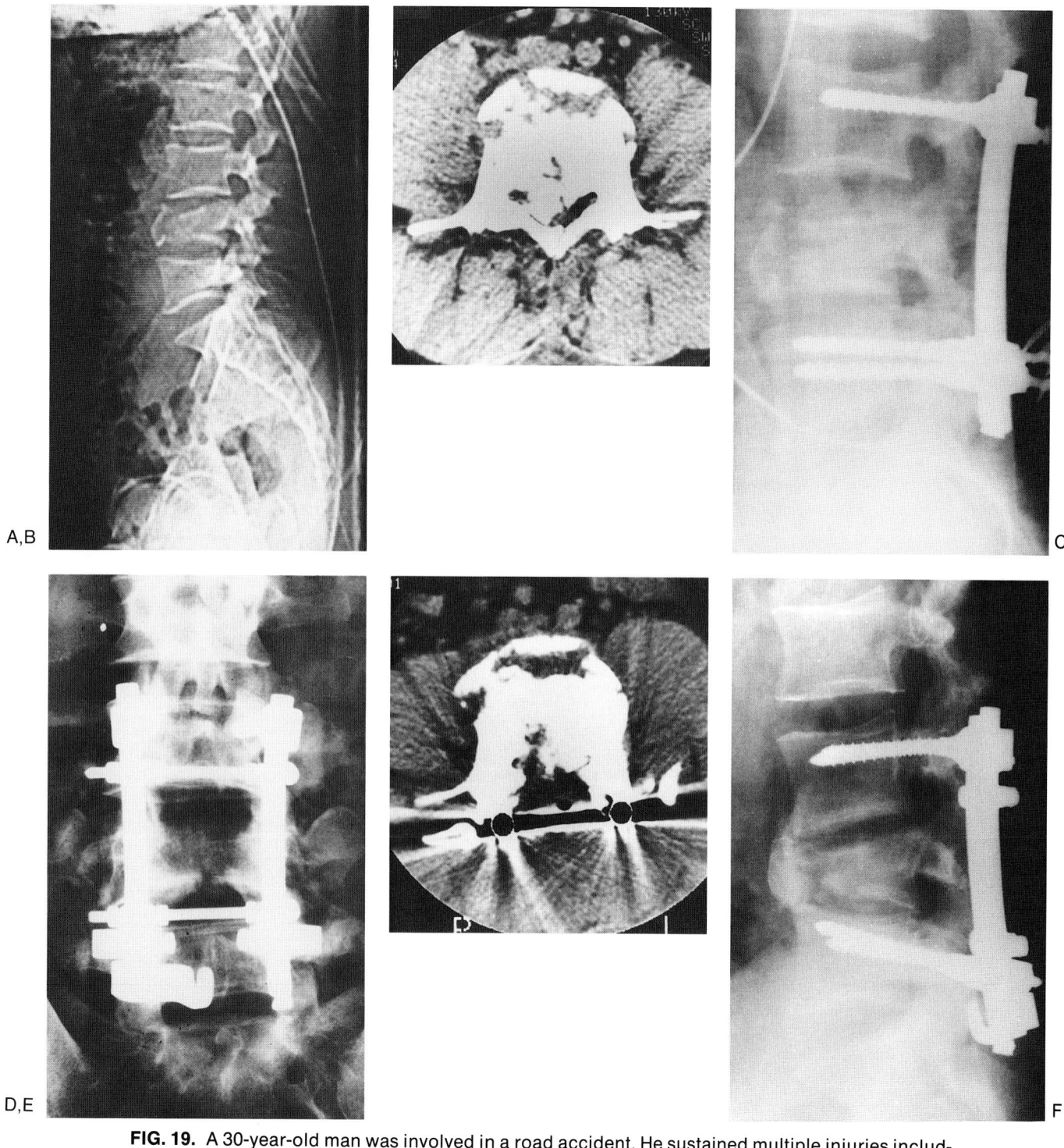

FIG. 19. A 30-year-old man was involved in a road accident. He sustained multiple injuries including a burst fracture of L4 with bilateral leg weakness. **A:** Lateral radiograph of the lumbar spine showing a burst fracture of L4, with marked kyphosis. **B:** CT scan showing a typical burst fracture. Following instrumentation with pedicle screws at L3 and L5 (C-D) and connection to Cotrel rods. A laminectomy with decompression and removal of the bony fragments was performed as well. He had a full neural recovery. **C,D:** Lateral and AP radiographs following instrumentation. **E:** Note canal clearance following decompression. **F:** Despite a part time use of a postoperative corset, there was vertebral body collapse with screw bending.

Because there always is loss of bone as a result of the burst vertebral body, with formation of an eggshell, or empty vertebra, late collapse at the fracture site is quite common. The A-O group recommends transpedicular bone grafting to account for the bony loss. Nevertheless, it is quite common to have vertebral collapse at the fracture site with a three vertebra, two motion segments, and four pedicle screw construct.

Argenson et al. (6) presented their experience with the C-D system in managing 87 thoracolumbar fractures. For a thoracolumbar junction fracture (T11–L2), short constructs with pedicle screws with "protecting" hooks above and below the screws were found to be the most efficient in preventing late collapse. A later report from the same group (7) described their experience in managing 63 patients of thoracolumbar burst injury with the C-D pedicular system. The C-D construct consisted of one screw below the lesion and one screw above it. A buttress hook was placed below the caudal screw at the same vertebral level, as well as a protecting hook cephalad to the upper screw, one vertebral level higher. (See Argenson, *this volume*.) Twenty-five of the patients had a neural deficit, and all improved at least one Frankel grade. Local kyphosis was corrected to an average of 3°. However, at final follow-up the kyphosis increased to 5.7° due to disc disruption above the burst. These authors also stressed the importance of contouring the rods to accomplish sagittal contour restoration.

Thus late sagittal collapse may partially be avoided by addition of hooks above and below the pedicle screws or by using longer constructs proximally. The addition of two or three motion segments proximally is usually not associated with significant motion loss or late, unwarranted sequelae.

McKinley et al. (98) also reported that, in lumbar burst injuries managed by a short C-D pedicular construct, late collapse will occur, with recurrent localized kyphosis (Fig. 19). They therefore advocated that in cases with loss of structural integrity of the anterior column, massive bone grafting via an anterior approach should be performed and prolonged postoperative bracing instituted.

Daniaux et al. (27) proposed a somewhat different approach. According to these authors, late vertebral collapse may occur not only because of bone loss but also due to damage of the upper disc space (above the fractured body). Therefore, in these instances, they recommend disc excision and interbody fusion and devised a special technique of accomplishing this via a posterior approach that also combines plate and pedicle screw fixation.

A novel approach to the sagittal contour malalignment was developed by Farcy. Farcy et al. (45) described the Sagittal Index as an indicator in management of burst fractures at the thoracolumbar junction.

The Sagittal Index was defined as measurement of segmental kyphosis at the level of a given segment (one disc plus one vertebra) adjusted to the baseline "normal" sagittal curvature at that level. The baseline sagittal values are derived from the studies by Stagnara et al. (115).

Farcy et al. (45) incorporated the Sagittal Index into their operative technique. The correct Sagittal Index is contoured into a C-D rod and, following connection of the rod to a proximal hook claw, the rod is lowered and anchored two levels below the kyphotic angle to a pair of pedicular screws. Following radiographic verification of deformity reduction, decompression and strut grafts are performed via an anterior approach.

Farcy et al. reported their experience with 35 patients managed according to the Sagittal Index (45). They also assessed the risk of late deformity progression (kyphosis) by the Sagittal Index. Burst fractures with a Sagittal Index greater than 15° were destined to progress (45). While patients with a Sagittal Index of 15° to 25° required only posterior instrumentation and arthrodesis, patients with a Sagittal Index greater than 25° at injury or later required anterior and posterior arthrodesis in addition to posterior instrumentation. (See Chapter 31 by Glassman and Farcy.)

SUMMARY

The Harrington system, including its various modifications, is still the main spinal fixation device employed around the world for fracture fixation. Its main advantages are its availability (especially in "developing" countries), surgeons' familiarity with the device, ease and speed of insertion of the system, and its low cost. As new segmental fixation devices combining hooks and pedicle screws have developed in the last decade, better fixation systems that enable a better deformity reduction, better canal decompression (direct and indirect), and greater patient comfort and well-being, with shorter arthrodesis length and, perhaps, better long-term results are available.

There is no "best" instrumentation system, and each device has its merits and disadvantages. The surgeon embarking on a new spinal fixation system should choose the fixation device prudently. Surgeons should use a system with which they have gained familiarity and with which they feel comfortable while dealing with complex injuries and deformities.

Eccentric flexion injuries, if unstable (50% loss of vertebral height or 30° local kyphosis), should be managed by a segmental instrumentation in compression mode, two levels above and below the injury level.

Ligamentous flexion/distraction injuries should be managed in the same manner if at the thoracolumbar junction, but should be immobilized by pedicle screw fixation "one above, one below" with transverse connection of the rods or plates in the lumbar spine. A Harrington compression assembly is also a legitimate alternative.

Fracture/dislocation of the thoracic spine and the thoracolumbar junction should be managed by segmental fixation two to three levels above and two levels below, with transverse-laminar claws proximally and lamino-laminar or pedicle screw–laminar claws distally. A more "old fashioned" contoured Harrington distraction assembly with sublaminar wire may be the only system needed in patients with complete cord lesions.

Lumbar burst fractures should be managed nonoperatively if the patient is neurologically intact and the Sagittal Index at the fracture site does not exceed 15°, even in the presence of significant canal encroachment.

Neurologically intact patients with Sagittal Index greater than 15° but less than 25° should undergo instrumentation and indirect decompression either by a short pedicle screw construct with protective hooks above and below, or with a distal screw and proximal hooks two levels above the injury (61). In addition, patients with neurologic involvement should undergo posterior and posterolateral decompression. Patients with Sagittal Index greater than 25° should undergo anterior decompression and grafting followed by posterior instrumentation as outlined earlier. Patients with neurologic signs and canal occlusion of more than 70% should undergo initial anterior decompression.

REFERENCES

1. Aebi M, Etter C, Kehl T, Thalgott J. Stabilization of the lower thoracic and lumbar spine with internal spinal skeletal fixation system. Indication, techniques and first results of treatment. *Spine* 1987;12:544–551.
2. Abumi K, Panjabi MM, Duranceau J. Biomechanical evaluation of spinal fixation devices. Part III: Stability provided by six spinal fixation devices and interbody bone graft. *Spine* 1989; 14:1249.
3. Akbarnia BA, Moskowitz A, Merenda JT, Carl A, Niemann PF, Measeck B. Surgical treatment of thoracic spine fractures using Cotrel–Dubousset instrumentation. In: *Proceedings of the 6th International Congress on Cotrel–Dubousset instrumentation*. Montpellier: Sauramps Medical, 1989;25–30.
4. Anderson PA, Krengel WF, Hanley MB. Neurologic recovery in patients with incomplete paraplegia due to thoracic level cord injury. AAOS 57th Annual Meeting, New Orleans, February 8–13, 1990.
5. Argenson C, Boileau P, de Peretti F, Lovet J, Diazotto H. Fractures of the thoracic spine (T1–T10). *Fr J Orthop Surg* 1989;3:238–254.
6. Argenson C, Lovett J, de Peretti F, Cambas PM, Griffet J, Boileau P. Treatment of spinal fractures with Cotrel–Dubousset instrumentation. Results of the first 85 cases. European Spinal Deformities Society and the Scoliosis Research Society, combined meeting, Amsterdam, The Netherlands, Paper 144, pp 586–587, 1989.
7. Argenson C, Peretti A, Pernaud M, Lacour C, Puch JM. C-D instrumentation for thoracolumbar burst fractures. Scoliosis Research Society, Minneapolis, September 1991.
8. Asher M, Carson W, Heining C, Strippgen W, Arendt M, Lark R, Hartley M. A modified spinal rod linkage system to provide rotational stability. *Spine* 1988;13:272.
9. Asher M. An improved technique for the correction of adolescent idiopathic scoliosis: thoracolumbar and lumbar deformities. 6th Annual Meeting of North American Spine Society, Keystone, CO, July 31–August 3, 1991, p 298.
10. Ashman RB, Galpin RD, Corin JD, Johnston CE. Biomechanical analysis of pedicle screw instrumentation systems in a corpectomy model. *Spine* 1989;14:1388.
11. Ashman RB, Herring JA, Johnston CE. Texas Scottish Rite Hospital Instrumentation System. In: Bridwell KH, DeWald RL, eds. *The textbook of spinal surgery*. Philadelphia: Lippincott 1991;219–248.
12. Bedbrook GM. Stability of spinal fractures and fracture dislocations. *Paraplegia* 1971;9:23.
13. Benzel EC, Larsen SJ. Operative stabilization of post-traumatic thoracic and lumbar spine: a comparative analysis of the Harrington distraction rod and the modified Weiss spring. *Neurosurgery* 1986;19:378.
14. Bohler L. General consideration in the treatment of spinal fracture. In: *Treatment of fractures*. New York: Grune & Stratton, 1956;328–387.
15. Bohlman HH, Eismont FJ. Surgical techniques of anterior decompression and fusion for spinal cord injuries. *Clin Orthop* 1981;154:57–67.
16. Boucher HH. A method of spinal fusion. *J Bone Joint Surg* 1959;41B:248.
17. Bradford DS, Akbarnia BA, Winter RB, Seljeskog EL. Surgical stabilization of fracture and fracture dislocations of the thoracic spine. *Spine* 1977;2:185–196.
18. Bryant CE, Sullivan JA. Management of thoracic and lumbar spine fractures with Harrington distraction rods supplemented with segmental wiring. *Spine* 1983;8:532–537.
19. Cammisa FP, Eismont FJ, Green BA. Dural laceration occurring with burst fractures and associated laminar fractures. *J Bone Joint Surg* 1989;71A:1044–1052.
20. Casey MP, Asher MA, Jacobs RR, Orrik JM. The effect of Harrington rod contouring on lumbar lordosis. *Spine* 1987;12:750–753.
21. Coe JD, Warden KE, Herzig MA, McAfee PC. Influence of bone mineral density on the fixation of thoracolumbar implants. A comparative study of transpedicular screws, laminar hooks and spinous process wires. *Spine* 1990;15:902–907.
22. Cotrel Y. CDI 1989. In: *Proceeding of the 6th International Congress on Cotrel–Dubousset instrumentation*. Montpellier: Sauramps Medical, 1990;99–111.
23. Cotrel Y, Dubousset J. A new technique of spine fixation by a posterior approach in the treatment of scoliosis. *Rev Chir Orthop* 1987;70:489–494.
24. Cotrel Y, Dubousset J, Guillaumat M. New universal instrumentation in spinal surgery. *Clin Orthop* 1988;227:10–23.
25. Crowe P, Gertzbein SD. Spinal canal clearance in burst fractures using the A-O internal fixator. Scoliosis Research Society, Amsterdam, September 1988.
26. Crutcher JP, Anderson PA, King HA, Montesano PY. Indirect spinal canal decompression in patients with thoracolumbar burst fractures treated by posterior distraction rods. *J Spinal Disord* 1991;4:39–48.
27. Daniaux H, Seykora P, Genelin A, Lang T, Kathrein A. Application of posterior plating and modifications in thoracolumbar spine injuries: indications, techniques and results. *Spine* 1991; 16(3S):S125–S133.
28. Denis F. The three column spine and its significance in the classification of acute thoracolumbar spinal injuries. *Spine* 1983;8:817–831.
29. Denis F, Ruiz H, Scarls K. Comparison between square ended distraction rods and standard round ended distraction rods in the treatment of thoracolumbar spinal injuries. *Clin Orthop* 1984;189:162–167.
30. DeWald RL. Burst fractures of the thoracic and lumbar spine. *Clin Orthop* 1984;189:150–161.
31. Dick W. The "fixator interne" as a versatile implant for spine surgery. *Spine* 1987;12:882–900.
32. Dick W. *Internal fixation of thoracic and lumbar spine fractures*. Toronto: Hans Hauber Publishers, 1989.

33. Dickson JH, Harrington PR, Erwin WD. Harrington instrumentation in the fractured unstable thoracic and lumbar spine. *Tex Med* 1973;69:91–98.
34. Dolan EJ, Tator CM, Endrenyi L. The value of decompression for acute experimental spinal cord compression injury. *J Neurosurg* 1980;53:749–755.
35. Drummond D, Guadagni J, Keene JS, et al. Interspinous process segmental spinal instrumentation. *J Pediatr Orthop* 1984;4:397–404.
36. Edwards CC. Sacral fixation device: design and preliminary results. Proceedings of 19th Annual Meeting of the Scoliosis Research Society, 1989.
37. Edwards CC, Levine AM. Early rod–sleeve stabilization of the injured thoracic and lumbar spine. *Orthop Clin North Am* 1986;17:121–145.
38. Edwards CC, Rosenthal MS, Levin AM, Gellad F. The fate of retropulsed bone following thoracolumbar burst fractures. Late stenosis or resorption? *Orthop Trans* 1988;13:32–33.
39. Engler G. Cotrel–Dubousset instrumentation for reduction of fracture dislocation of the spine. *J Spinal Disord* 1990;3:62–66.
40. Esses SI. Spinal internal fixator: review of fifty cases. *Orthop Trans* 1989;13:38.
41. Esses SI, Botsford DJ, Wright T, Bendar D, Bailey S. Operative treatment of spinal fractures with the A-O internal fixator. *Spine* 1991;16(3S):S146–S150.
42. Esses SI, Botsford DJ, Huler RJ, Rauschning W. Surgical anatomy of the sacrum: a guide for rational screw fixation. *Spine* 1991;16(3S):S283–S288.
43. Farcy JPC, Weidenbaum M, Michelsen CB, Hoeltzel DA, Athranasion KA. A comparative biomechanical study of spinal fixation using Cotrel–Dubousset instrumentation. *Spine* 1987;12:877–881.
44. Farcy JPC, Weidenbaum M. Pitfalls in fracture fixation with Cotrel–Dubousset instrumentation. In: *Proceedings of the 5th International Conference on Cotrel–Dubousset instrumentation*. Montpellier: Sauramps Medical, 1989;103–110.
45. Farcy JPC, Weidenbaum M, Glassman SD. Sagittal index in management of thoracolumbar fractures. *Spine* 1990;15:958–965.
46. Fergusen RL, Allen BL. A mechanistic classification of thoracolumbar spine fractures. *Clin Orthop* 1984;189:77–88.
47. Ferguson RL, Tencer AF, Woodward P, Allen BL. Biomechanical comparisons of spinal fracture models and the stabilizing effect of posterior instrumentations. *Spine* 1988;13:453–460.
48. Fidler MW. Posterior instrumentation of the spine. An experimental comparison of various possible techniques. *Spine* 1986;11:367–372.
49. Fidler MW. Remodelling of the spinal canal after burst fracture. A prospective study of two cases. *J Bone Joint Surg* 1988;70B:730–732.
50. Flesch JR, Lieder LL, Erickson DL. Harrington instrumentation and spine fusion for unstable fractures and fracture dislocations of the thoracic and lumbar spine. *J Bone Joint Surg* 1977;59A:143–153.
51. Floman Y, Fast A, et al. The simultaneous application of an interspinous compressive wire and Harrington distraction rods in the treatment of fracture-dislocation of the thoracic and lumbar spine. *Clin Orthop* 1986;205:207–215.
52. Fredrickson BE, Mann KA, Yuan HA, Lubicky JP. Reduction of the intracanal fragments in experimental burst fractures. *Spine* 1988;13:267.
53. Gardner VO, Armstrong GWD. Long term lumbar facet joint changes in spinal fracture patients treated with Harrington rods. *Spine* 1990;15:479–484.
54. Georgis T, Rydevik B, Weinstein JN, Garfin SR. Complications of pedicle screw fixation. In: Garfin SR, ed. *Complications of spine surgery*. Baltimore: Williams & Wilkins, 1989;200–210.
55. Gepstein R, Latta L, Shufflebarger HL. Cotrel–Dubousset instrumentation for lumbar fractures. A biomechanical study. In: *Proceedings of the 4th International Congress on Cotrel–Dubousset instrumentation*. Montpellier: Sauramps Medical, 1988;91.
56. Gertzbein SD, MacMichael D, Tile M. Harrington instrumentation as a method of fixation in fractures of the spine. A critical analysis of deficiencies. *J Bone Joint Surg* 1982;64B:526–529.
57. Gertzbein SD, Court-Brown CM, Jacobs RR, et al. Decompression and circumferential stabilization of unstable spinal fractures. *Spine* 1988;13:892–895.
58. Gertzbein SD, Court-Brown CM. Fractures of the lumbar spine. In: Floman Y, ed. *Disorders of the lumbar spine*. Gaithersburg, MD: Aspen Publishers, 1990;615–662.
59. Gertzbein SD, Jacobs RR, Stoll J, Martin C. Results of the locking-hook spine rod for fractures of the thoracic and lumbar spine. *Spine* 1990;15:275–280.
60. Gertzbein SD, Robbins SE. Accuracy of pedicular screw placement *in vivo*. *Spine* 1990;15:11–14.
61. Gillet PH, Meyer R, Fatemi F, Lemaire R. Short segmental internal fixation using CD instrumentation with pedicular screws versus Roy-Camille plates or Harrington rods in the treatment of the thoracolumbar spine. Biomechanical testing. In: *Proceedings of the 6th International Congress on Cotrel–Dubousset instrumentation*. Montpellier: Sauramps Medical, 1990;19–24.
62. Goutallier D, Hernigon P, Piat C. Le traitement orthopedique des fractures du rachis dorsolombaire et lombaire avec recul du mur corporeal posterieur sans ou avec troubles neurologiques mineurs. *Rev Chir Orthop* 1988;74:77.
63. Guttmann L. *Spinal cord injuries: comprehensive management and research*. Oxford: Blackwell Scientific Publications, 1957.
64. Hadra BE. Wiring of the spinous process in injury and Pott's disease. *Trans Am Orthop Assoc* 1891;4:206.
65. Hannon KM. Harrington instrumentation in fractures and dislocations of the thoracic and lumbar spine. *South Med J* 1976;69:1269–1273.
66. Harrington PR. Treatment of scoliosis. Correction and internal fixation by spine instrumentation. *J Bone Joint Surg* 1962;44A:591–602.
67. Holdsworth F. Fracture, dislocations and fracture/dislocations of the spine. *J Bone Joint Surg* 1970;52A:1534–1551.
68. Jacobs RR, Asher MA, Snider RK. Thoracolumbar spine injuries. A comparative study of recumbent and operative treatment in 100 patients. *Spine* 1980;5:463–477.
69. Jacobs RR, Ghista DN. A biomechanical basis for the treatment of injuries of the dorsolumbar spine. In: Ghista DN, ed. *Osteoarthromechanics*. New York: McGraw-Hill, 1982;435–471.
70. Jacobs RR, Nordwall A, Nachemson A. Reduction stability and strength provided by internal fixation systems for thoracolumbar spinal injuries. *Clin Orthop* 1982;171:300.
71. Jacobs RR, Schlaepfer F, Mathys R, Nachemson A, Perren S. A locking hook spinal rod system for stabilization of fracture dislocations and correction of deformities of the dorsolumbar spine. A biomechanical evaluation. *Clin Orthop* 1984;189:168–177.
72. Kahanovitz N, Arnoczky SP, Levine DB, Otis JP. The effects of internal fixation on the articular cartilage of unfused canine facet joint cartilage. *Spine* 1984;9:268–272.
73. Kahanovitz N, Bullough P, Jacobs RR. The effect of internal fixation without arthrodesis on human facet joint cartilage. *Clin Orthop* 1984;189:204–208.
74. Kaufer H, Hayes JT. Lumbar fracture dislocation. *J Bone Joint Surg* 1966;48A:712.
75. Keene JS, Wackwitz DL, Drummond DS, Breed AL. Compression–distraction instrumentation of unstable thoracolumbar fractures: anatomic results obtained with each type of injury and method of instrumentation. *Spine* 1986;11:895–902.
76. Kostuik JP, Gross M. Correction of iatrogenic lumbar kyphosis–flat back syndrome. *Orthop Trans* 1982;6:27.
77. Kostuik JP. Anterior fixation for fractures of the thoracic and lumbar spine with and without neurologic involvement. *Clin Orthop* 1984;189:103–115.
78. Kostuik JP, Errico TJ, Gleason TF. Techniques for internal fixation for degenerative conditions of the lumbar spine. *Clin Orthop* 1986;203:219–231.
79. Krag MH. An internal fixation for posterior application to short segments of the thoracic, lumbar or lumbosacral spine. *Clin Orthop* 1986;203:75–98.

80. Krag MH. Biomechanics of thoracolumbar spinal fixation. A review. *Spine* 1991;16(3S):S84–S98.
81. Krompinger WJ, Fredrickson BE, Mino DE, Yuan HA. Conservative treatment of fractures of the thoracic and lumbar spine. *Orthop Clin North Am* 1986;17:161–169.
82. Lange F. Support for the spondylitic spine by means of buried steel bars attached to the vertebrae. *Am J Orthop Surg* 1910;8:344–361.
83. Larson SJ. The thoracolumbar junction. In: Dunsker SB, Schmidek HH, Frymoyer J, Kahn A, eds. *The unstable spine.* New York: Grune & Stratton, 1986;127–152.
84. Levine A, Edwards CC. Lumbar spine trauma. In: Camins M, O'Leary PF, eds. *The lumbar spine.* New York: Raven Press, 1987;183–212.
85. Levine AM, Bosse M, Edwards CC. Bilateral facet dislocation in the thoracolumbar spine. *Spine* 1988;13:630–640.
86. Lewis J, McKibbin B. The treatment of unstable fracture dislocations of the thoracolumbar spine accompanied by paraplegia. *J Bone Joint Surg* 1974;56B:603–612.
87. Lindsey RW, Dick W. The fixateur interne in the reduction and stabilization of thoracolumbar spine fractures in patients with neurologic deficit. *Spine* 1991;16(3S):S140–S145.
88. Louis R, Maresea C, Bel P. Fractures instables du rachis. La reduction orthopedique. *Rev Chir Orthop* 1977;63:449–451.
89. Luque ER, Cassis N, Ramirez-Wiella G. Segmental spinal instrumentation in the treatment of fractures of the thoracolumbar spine. *Spine* 1982;7:312–317.
90. Magerl FP. Stabilization of the lower thoracic and lumbar spine with external fixation. *Clin Orthop* 1984;189:125–141.
91. Maiman DJ, Larson SJ, Benzel EC. Neurological improvement associated with late decompression of the thoracolumbar spinal cord. *Neurosurgery* 1984;14:302–307.
92. Maiman DJ, Sances A, Myklebust J, Larson SJ, Flately T, Neseman S. Comparison of the failure biomechanics of spinal fixation devices. *Neurosurgery* 1985;17:574–580.
93. McAfee PC, Yuan HA, Fredrickson BE, Lubicky JP. The value of computed tomography in thoracolumbar fractures: an analysis of one hundred consecutive cases and a new classification. *J Bone Joint Surg* 1983;65A:461–473.
94. McAfee PC, Bohlman HH. Complications following Harrington instrumentation for fractures of the thoracolumbar spine. *J Bone Joint Surg* 1985;64A:672–686.
95. McAfee PC, Farey ID, Sutterlin CE, Gurr KR, Warden KE, Cunningham BW. Device related osteoporosis with spinal instrumentation. *Spine* 1989;14:919–926.
96. McAfee PC, Farey ID, Sutterlin CE, Gurr KR, Warden KE, Cunningham BW. The effect of spinal implant rigidity on vertebral bone density. A canine model. *Spine* 1991;16(3S):S190–S197.
97. McBride GG, Bradford DS. Vertebral body replacement with femoral neck allograft and vascularized rib strut graft: a technique for treating post traumatic kyphosis with neurologic deficit. *Spine* 1983;8:406.
98. McKinley LM, Obenchain TG, Roth KR. Late kyphosis in short segment pedicle fixation in cases of posterior transpedicular decompression. In: *Proceedings of the 6th International Congress on Cotrel-Dubousset instrumentation.* Montpellier: Sauramps Medical, 1989;37–39.
99. Moe JH, Denis F. Iatrogenic loss of lumbar lordosis. *Orthop Trans* 1977;1:131.
100. Munson G, Satterlee C, Hammond S, et al. Experimental evaluation of Harrington rod fixation supplemented with sublaminar wires in stabilizing thoracolumbar fracture dislocations. *Clin Orthop* 1984;189:97–102.
101. Nasca RJ, Hollis JM, Lemons JE, Cool TA. Cyclic axial loading of spinal implants. *Spine* 1985;10:792.
102. Noel SH, Keene JS, Rice WC. Improved postoperative course after spinous process segmental instrumentation of thoracolumbar fractures. *Spine* 1991;16:132–136.
103. Panjabi MM, Abumi K, Duranceau J, Crisco JJ. Biomechanical evaluation of spinal fixation devices. Part II: Stability provided by eight internal fixation devices. *Spine* 1988;13:1135.
104. Peterson EW, Armstrong WD. Immediate reduction and fixation of major spinal fractures and dislocations as an aid to the recovery of function. American Association of Neurological Surgery, Annual Meeting, San Francisco, 1976.
105. Phillips DL, Brick GW, Spengler DM. A comparison of Harrington rod fixation with and without segmental wires for unstable thoracolumbar injuries. *J Spinal Disord* 1988;1:151–161.
106. Purcell GA, Markolf KL, Dawson EG. Twelfth thoracic–first lumbar vertebral mechanical stability of fractures after Harrington rod instrumentation. *J Bone Joint Surg* 1981;63A:71–78.
107. Ritchie W. Combined visceral and vertebral injuries from lap type seat belts. *Surg Gynecol Obstet* 1970;131:431.
108. Roberts PH. Internal metallic splintage in the treatment of traumatic paraplegia. *Injury* 1969;1:4–11.
109. Roberts JR, Curtiss PH. Stability of the thoracic and lumbar spine in traumatic paraplegia following fracture and fracture dislocation. *J Bone Joint Surg* 1970;52A:1115–1130.
110. Roy-Camille R, Saillant G, Mazel C. Internal fixation of the lumbar spine with pedicle screw plating. *Clin Orthop* 1986;203:7–17.
111. Ruland CM, McAfee PC, Warden KE, Cunningham BW. Triangulation of pedicle instrumentation. A biomechanical analysis. *Spine* 1991;16(3S):S270–S276.
112. Saillant G. Etudes anatomique de pedicules vertebraux. Application chirurgicale. *Rev Chir Orthop* 1976;62:151–160.
113. Senegas J, Baulny D, Gerrier F, Vital JW. L'osteosynthese du rachis dorsolombaire per plaque vissee anterolateral. *Rev Chir Orthop Supp* 1987;II:157–160.
114. Skinner R, Transfeldt EE, Maybee J, Venter R, Chalmas W. Experimental pullout testing and comparison of variables in transpedicular screw fixation: a biomechanical study. *Spine* 1990;15:195–201.
115. Stagnara P, DeMauroy JC, Dran G, Gonan GP, Contanzo G, Dimnet J, Parquet A. Reciprocal angulation of vertebral bodies in a sagittal plane: approach to references for the evaluation of kyphosis and lordosis. *Spine* 1982;7:335–342.
116. Stauffer ES, Neil JL. Biomechanical analysis of structural stability of internal fixation in fractures of the thoracolumbar spine. *Clin Orthop* 1975;112:159.
117. Steffee AD, Biscup RS, Sitkowski DJ. Segmental spine plates with pedicle screw fixation: a new internal fixation device for disorders of the lumbar and thoracolumbar spine. *Clin Orthop* 1986;203:45–53.
118. Steffee AD, Sitkowski DJ. Posterior lumbar interbody fusion and plates. *Clin Orthop* 1988;227:99–102.
119. Straub LR. Lumbosacral fusion by metallic fixation and grafts. *J Bone Joint Surg* 1949;31B:478.
120. Tencer AF, Allen BL, Ferguson RL. A biomechanical study of thoracolumbar spinal fractures with bone in the canal. I: The effect of laminectomy. *Spine* 1985;10:580–585.
121. Tencer AF, Ferguson RL, Allen BL. A biomechanical study of thoracolumbar spinal fractures with bone in the canal. II: The effect of flexion, angulation distraction and shortening of the motion segments. *Spine* 1985;10:586–589.
122. Transfeldt E, White D, Bradford DS, Ogilivie J, Kahman R, Cohen M, Roche B. Delayed anterior decompression in patients with spinal cord and cauda equina injuries of the thoracolumbar spine. Scoliosis Research Society, Amsterdam, September 1989.
123. Urban JP, Holm S, Maroudas A, Nachemson A. Nutrition of the intervertebral disc: effect of fluid flows on solute transport. *Clin Orthop* 1982;170:296–302.
124. Watson-Jones R. *Fractures and joint injuries.* Edinburgh: Livingstone, 1962;957–965.
125. Weinstein JN, Collalto P, Lehman TR. Thoracolumbar "burst" fractures treated conservatively: a long-term follow up. *Spine* 1988;13:33–38.
126. Weiss M. Dynamic spine alloplasty (spring loading corrective devices) after fracture and spinal cord injury. *Clin Orthop* 1975;112:150–158.
127. Wenger DR, Carollo JJ. The mechanics of thoracolumbar fractures stabilized by segmental fixation. *Clin Orthop* 1984;189:89–96.

128. Willen J, Lindahl S, Nordwall A. Unstable thoracolumbar fractures. A comparative clinical study of conservative treatment and Harrington instrumentation. *Spine* 1985;10:111–112.
129. Williams EWM. Traumatic paraplegia. In: Mathews DN, ed. *Recent advances in surgery in trauma*. New York: Churchill Livingstone, 1963;171–186.
130. Wittenberg RA, Coffee MS, Swatz DE, Edwards WT, White AA, Hayes WC. Fatigue properties of lumbar spine traction devices. 7th Meeting of European Society of Biomechanics, Aarhus, Denmark, 1990.
131. Wittenberg RH, Lee KS, Coffee M, White AA, Hayes WC. The effects of screw design and fixation in human and calf vertebral bodies. 7th meeting of the European Society of Biomechanics, Aarhus, Denmark, 1990.
132. Yosipovitch Z, Robin GC, Makin M. Open reduction of unstable thoracolumbar injuries and fixation with Harrington rods. *J Bone Joint Surg* 1977;59A:1003–1015.
133. Zindrick MR, Wiltse LL, Widell EH, Thomas JC, Holland WR, Feld BT, Spencer CW. A biomechanical study of intrapedicular screw fixation in the lumbosacral spine. *Clin Orthop* 1986;203:99–112.
134. Zindrick MR, Wiltse LL, Doornick A. Analysis of the morphometric characteristics of the thoracic and lumbar spine. *Spine* 1987;12:160–166.

23

Thoracic and Lumbar Spine Injuries in Children

Gerard Bollini

Spine injuries are less frequent in children than in adults, but their consequences are more grave as they affect the growing spine. Spine injuries in children will cause deformities at the level of injury; when there is a cord injury, deformities may develop below the level of the injury.

Spine injuries are not as well known in children as in adults, and our knowledge of adult spinal injury is not applicable to children. Children with spine injuries must be treated with a more conservative approach than adults, since some surgical indications are questionable, and quite a few are dangerous. This category includes laminectomies, which are responsible for many late deformities.

In children, injuries at the level of the growth cartilage are difficult to recognize and can be overlooked in the presence of multiple associated lesions/multiple trauma. Therefore we must stress the high incidence of multiple level spinal injuries. Also, "spinal cord injuries without radiographic abnormalities" (SCIWORA) are found more frequently in children than in adults.

REVIEW OF LITERATURE

Children rarely sustain spine injuries, although they account for 1% to 10% of all spine injuries regardless of age (38). Spine injuries represent a small percentage of overall injuries to children—0.34%, according to Hubbard (21).

A review of the literature pertinent to children's spine injuries is noteworthy in two respects. First, there is a prevalence of cervical spine injuries as indicated by percentages: 76% according to Ruge et al. (38); 42% for Hadley et al. (19); 29% for Hubbard (22); 70% for Anderson and Schutt (2); 50% for McPhee (29); and 35% of our 118 cases (6).

The second aspect relative to the incidence of spine injuries in children is the variation in the range of ages selected by each author. Ruge et al. (38) and others chose a range from 0 to 12 years of age. The age range was increased by Hubbard (22) and others to include 0 to 17 years of age. Including patients aged 14 to 17 years increased the incidence of spine injuries to children.

Skeletal maturation is an accepted landmark in the classification of musculoskeletal injury in the "pediatric" group, but no criterion exists to define the completion of skeletal maturation. Fusion between the growth plate and vertebral body, which is the usual radiologic criterion for skeletal maturation, can occur long after the age of 17.

The literature shows discrepancies in evaluation of the prevalence of cervical involvement when compared to thoracic and lumbar injuries, which varies from one series to another, statistically as well as clinically. Due to these discrepancies, spine injuries in children are not so well addressed as in adults; our knowledge of adult spinal injury is not applicable to children.

Among the most important series are: 156 cases from Anderson and Schutt (2); 122 cases from Hadley et al. (19); 118 cases from Bollini et al. (6); 47 cases from Ruge et al. (38); and 42 cases in the separate series of Hubbard (21) and McPhee (29). The series of two groups, Pouliquen et al. (35) (64 cases) and Lesoin et al. (27) (67 cases), excluded cervical spine injuries. The prevalence of spine injury in boys as opposed to girls shows consistency, with 61% to 66% (2,19–21,27,38), in spite of two series that showed only 29% (6) and 54% (35). The incidence of complete or partial spinal cord injury (SCI) varies from 14% to 50% (2,6,19,21,27,29,35,38).

Traffic accidents are the dominant cause of chil-

G. Bollini: Department of Orthopaedic Surgery, Hôpital Timone Enfants, 13385 Marseille Cedex 5, France.

dren's spine injuries: 59% from Hadley et al. (19); 37% from Bollini et al. (6); 36% from Hubbard (21); and 25% from Anderson and Schutt (2). The child is more often injured as a passenger in an auto than as a pedestrian hit by a car and is injured even less frequently when riding a bicycle.

Falls are the second most frequent cause of children's spine injuries: 15% in the Hadley et al. (19) series, 33% in the Hubbard series (21), 18% in the Anderson and Schutt (2) series, and 29% in the Bollini et al. (6) series. In two series, injuries caused by falls outnumbered those caused by traffic accidents: in the Ruge et al. (38) series, falls caused 38% of the injuries; in the series of McPhee (29), they accounted for 40%.

Sports injuries hold third place as a causative factor in children's spine injuries: diving into shallow water accounts for a fair number of cervical spine injuries.

In some studies, in which thoracic, thoracolumbar, and lumbar injuries are separated from each other and from cervical injuries, the rate of involvement of each spine segment varies by author, respectively, from 46%, 20%, and 34% in Hubbard's (21) series to 70%, 21%, and 9% in the Horal et al. (20) series, 49%, 9%, and 42% in the Bollini et al. (6) series, and 52%, 21%, and 27% in the series of McPhee (29).

EPIDEMIOLOGY

Spinal Cord Injuries and Fractures

The incidence of cord injury after spinal trauma is far less in children than in adults. Studies over a 25-year period by Melzac (32) reported SCI in 93 children; of these, only 29 were caused by trauma. This can be compared to the 44% rate of spine injuries in adult trauma that was recorded in the same hospital during the same period of time. In a 5-year study of 328 SCIs, Cheshire (9) found only four SCIs in children under 13 years of age, which accounted for only 1.2% of all SCIs.

Kewalramani and co-workers (23,24) made a 2-year epidemiologic survey of 18 counties in California. Fifty-eight of 619 victims of SCI were children between 1 and 15 years of age. They accounted for 9.4% of SCIs. Another study (24) of 733 SCIs over a 7-year period at the Texas Institute for Rehabilitation and Research included 97 children between 1 and 15 years of age who accounted for 13.2% of SCIs. Reviewing 2698 SCIs over 14 years, Ruge et al. (38) found 71 children below the age of 12, or 2.7% of these injuries.

Depending on the referral conditions of each medical center, the data vary, and the proportion of children's SCIs ranges from 1.2% to 13.2% of the adult population with SCI. This low incidence of SCI in children parallels the low incidence of spinal injury in children when compared to the adult population.

Anderson and Schutt (2) found 44 SCIs, or 28%, among 156 young victims of spinal injury who were less than 14 years of age. Hadley et al. (19) counted 61 SCIs (50%) among 122 children 16 years of age or younger who suffered spinal injuries. In 1974, Hubbard's study (21) of 42 children below age 17 included six SCIs, or 14%, and McPhee (29) found six SCIs (14%) in a group of 42 children, age 15 and younger, with spinal cord injury. Lesoin et al. (27) found 28% SCIs, or 19 of 67 children with spinal injury who were younger than age 15. Among 118 children younger than age 16 with spinal injuries, Bollini et al. (6) found 28 SCIs, or 14%.

The incidence of SCI among spinal injuries in children varies from 14% to 28% with the exception of Hadley et al. (19), whose series reflects a 50% occurrence. Other isolated series reported children's SCI statistics that correlated neither with adult nor children's SCI.

Audic and Maury (4) had 15 cases and Lancourt et al. (25) 50 cases of SCI over a period of 17 years in children less than 14 years of age. Hachen (18) studied 18 children younger than 15 years of age over 12 years, Burke (8) had 25 patients younger than 13, and Ruge et al. (38) saw 25 patients under 12 years of age over a period of 14 years.

Analysis of these reports shows that one to two new cases of SCI in children are directed to a specialized center each year. In conducting a comparison of complete versus incomplete SCI, the authors found variable statistics, as seen in Table 1.

Complete SCIs do not recover (2,6,8,23,29), however, Hubbard (22) described some neurologic recoveries. SCI recuperation is usually incomplete, although partial recovery is routinely expected.

SCI associated with other injuries frequently causes death, as reported by Kewalramani et al. (23). Seventy-six percent represents 34 deceased of 58 patients; 13

TABLE 1. *Comparison of complete versus incomplete SCI*

Study	Complete SCI	Incomplete SCI	Percentage complete
Anderson and Schutt (2)	16	28	36
Ruge et al. (38)	9	11	45
Hadley et al. (19)	21	40	34
Hubbard (21)	4	2	66
McPhee (29)	3	3	50
Burke (8)			86
Lesoin et al. (27)	12	3	80
Kewalramani et al. (24)			69
Bollini et al. (6)	21	7	76

of these patients died within the initial 20 min at the hospital.

Burke (8) reported two deaths in his study of 29 SCIs. Anderson and Schutt (2) reported 11 deaths of 16 patients with complete SCI, but the death of only two of 28 patients with incomplete SCI. McPhee (29) reported the death of two of six patients. Discrepancies can be ascribed to data accounting for death at the scene, upon arrival, or after admission. The victim of complete SCI with associated injuries usually dies shortly after hospital admission.

Motor vehicle accidents were responsible for most of the injuries in the practice of Kewalramani et al. (23): 43% in their practice, and 65.5% in a survey of 18 counties in California (23). Other percentages were: Hachen (18), 39%; Hubbard (22), 36%; and Bollini et al. (6), 39%.

According to decreasing occurrence, children sustained injury (a) as passengers in a motor vehicle accident (MVA), (b) as pedestrians run over by a motor vehicle, and (c) by falls from height [25% for Bollini et al. (6)]. Ruge et al. (38) reported more occurrences from falls than from MVA. Diving into shallow water occurred less often.

Most of the SCI publications do not always report the level of injury, which could be cervical in addition to thoracic and/or lumbar. Kewalramani et al. (23) reported 62 cervical injuries of 97 patients with SCI. This distribution appears to be usual.

SCIWORA in children is reported in the literature either in association with SCI due to vertebral injuries or as an isolated syndrome (Table 2).

Incidence of SCIWORA

Except for Anderson, the incidence of SCIWORA in the SCI population varies from 20% according to Andrews and Jung (3) to 66% according to Pang and Wilberger (34). SCIWORA as an isolated syndrome was described by Ahmann et al. (1), two cases; Choi et al. (10), eight cases; Walsh et al. (42), eight cases; Leblanc and Nadell (26), three cases; and Pollack et al. (36), 54 cases.

Eight series with a total of 65 patients indicated the level of the cord lesion (1,6,9,10,18,26,34,42). The lesions were 46% cervical, 27% high thoracic, 20% low thoracic, and 7% lumbar.

In summary, the incidence of SCI in a spine-injured population is far smaller in children than adults. It varies from 1.2% to 13% (9,23,24,32,38) depending on the referral patterns of each medical center. This low incidence parallels the low incidence of spinal injury in children compared to the incidence in the spine-injured adult population. The incidence of SCI in the population of spine-injured children varies from 14% to 28% (2,6,19,21,27,29), with a peak at 50% in one series (19).

SCI can present as complete (2,6,8,19,21,23,27,38) (34–86%), showing no recovery (2,6,8,23,29), or incomplete, with potential for recovery.

VERTEBRAL GROWTH

The growth plates determine the specific patterns of injury in children. At birth, a large bony nucleus occupies almost the entire vertebra, from front to back. A cartilaginous endplate separates the nucleus from adjacent discs (Fig. 1). Growth cartilage connects the cartilaginous endplate to the bony nucleus; this growth cartilage will finally disappear at the age of 20. The cartilaginous endplate becomes thicker at its periphery as the child gets older. During this process, the bony nucleus is surrounded by a ring that creates a step-off in front of the vertebral body.

As early as age 5, calcium deposits appear in the cartilaginous endplate and will progress in the dorsoventral direction. Simultaneously, the edges of the cartilaginous endplates begin to ossify. The ossified zones

TABLE 2. *Reports on SCIWORA*

Study	SCIWORA	SCI (including SCIWORA)
Burke (8)	17	29
Kewalramani et al. (23)	5	25
Hachen (18)	9	18
Andrews and Jung (3)	7	15
Pang and Wilberger (34)	24	36
Melzac (32)	16	29
Lesoin et al. (27)	5	19
Ruge et al. (38)	10	27
Anderson and Schutt (2)	2	44
Bollini et al. (6)	8	28

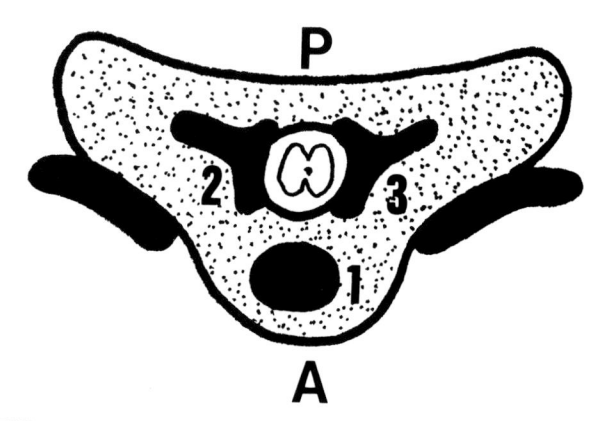

FIG. 1. Anteroposterior view of an embryo. Number 1 is the primary enchondral ossification nucleus for the vertebral body. Number 2 indicates the primary perichondral ossification nucleus for the pedicles and posterior arch.

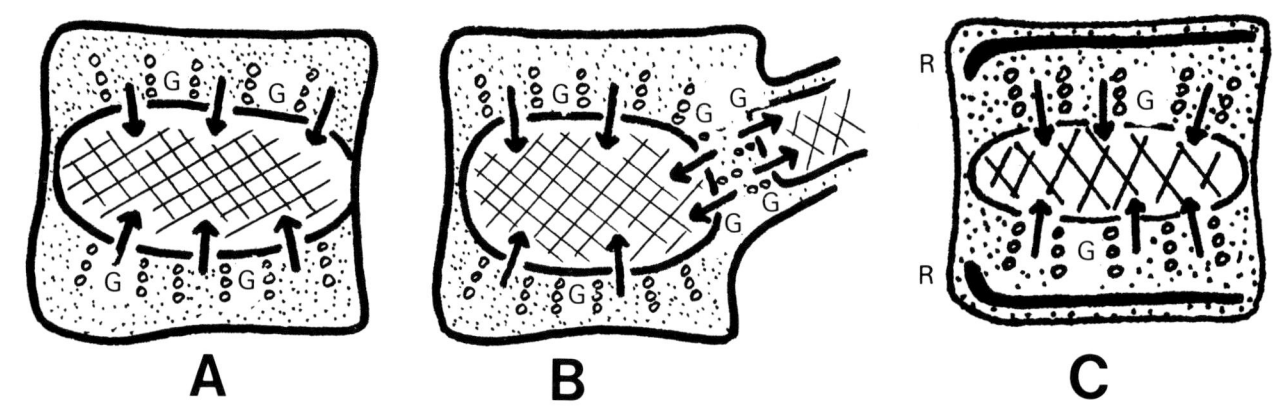

FIG. 2. Sagittal view of a vertebral body. **A:** Sagittal midline slice at age 2 years. Growth cartilage columns (G) induce growth in height of the vertebral body. **B:** Sagittal paramedian slice of the same vertebra shows two cartilages of the neurocentral cartilage, which allow pedicle growth (GG). **C:** Rims (R) do not participate in the growth in height of the vertebral body.

will fuse in the ventrodorsal direction, creating a marginal ossified circular ring at the age of 12 according to Tondury (41), and at the age of 15 according to Mallet et al. (30) (Fig. 2).

The marginal ring is the beginning of a process of fusion with the vertebral body at age 14 or 15; the process is completed only at age 24 or 25 (Fig. 3). The stratified growth plate between the endplate and the vertebral body induces growth in height. The neurocentral cartilage induces growth in the horizontal plane.

T7 grows an average of 16 mm between birth and adulthood, that is, 8 mm from each stratified cartilage at each growth plate. T7 averages 6 mm at birth, 11 mm at age 2, 13 mm at age 4, 16 mm at age 10, and ceases growth at approximately 22 mm.

L2 grows an average of 25 mm between birth and adulthood, which means an average of 12.5 mm from each stratified cartilage at each growth plate. L3 is 8 mm at birth, 16 mm at age 2, 20 mm at age 4, 24 mm at age 10, and 33 mm at age 18 (13). The size of a vertebral body at age 3 is one-half its adult size.

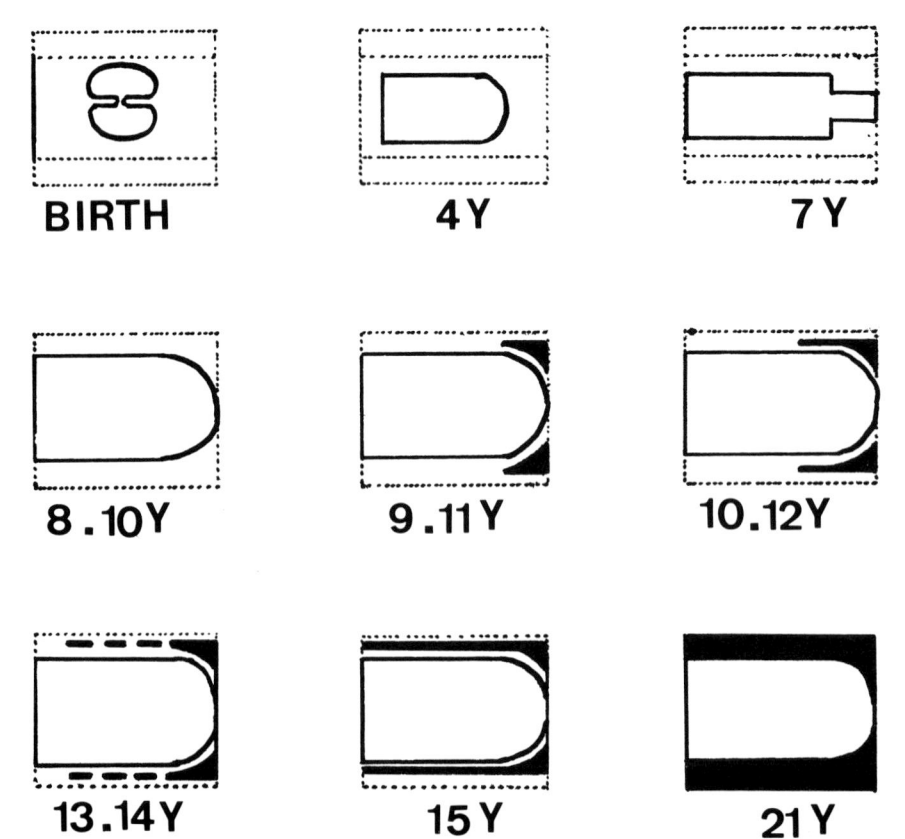

FIG. 3. Vertebral body bony nucleus shape at sequential ages (30).

PATHOANATOMY

Aufdermaur (5) reported autopsy results of 100 spines of which 12 were children younger than 18 years of age; only one fracture had been diagnosed before the patient's death. There were seven cervical injuries, four thoracic, and one lumbar. Death was recorded 24 to 36 hr postinjury.

Histologically, the fracture lines involved the layers of the growth zone almost exclusively. These layers were split in irregular, wavy lines. There were four patients with multiple cartilage plate injuries. The proximal growth plate was injured in 12 patients, the caudal plate in six patients. Histologic findings were similar for cervical, thoracic, and lumbar vertebrae. In two of the cases, the anterior longitudinal ligament was also ruptured. In three cases, the supraspinous and infraspinous ligaments, the ligamentum flavum, and the capsules of the posterolateral joints were ruptured in addition to ruptures of the endplate and the anterior longitudinal ligament. Similar lesions were noted when 20 intact spines from juveniles of similar age groups who had died were subjected to mechanical stresses.

According to this study, the incidence of spine injuries in children is likely to be underestimated (5).

CLASSIFICATION

With some modifications, Denis' classification (12) for adult thoracolumbar fractures can be extended to children's fractures.

Compression Fractures

According to Denis' three-column concept, compression fractures represent a failure of the anterior column under compression; only the anterior column is injured. Type D (Figs. 4 and 5) is more often found with compression of the midvertebral body and endplates intact and preserved. Anterior compression creates a kyphotic deformity, lateral compression a scoliotic deformity, and combined anterior and lateral compression create a kyphoscoliosis. Discs and growth plates remain intact. These fractures are stable, and late deformities are unlikely.

Type B fractures compress the cranial endplate (Fig. 5); in type C fractures, there is compression of the caudal endplate. In both of these fractures, the endplate and growth cartilage are fragmented and damaged in children. An example is type A fractures, in which a

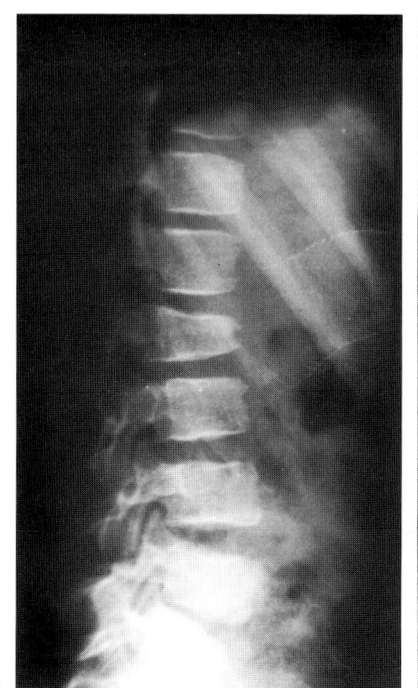

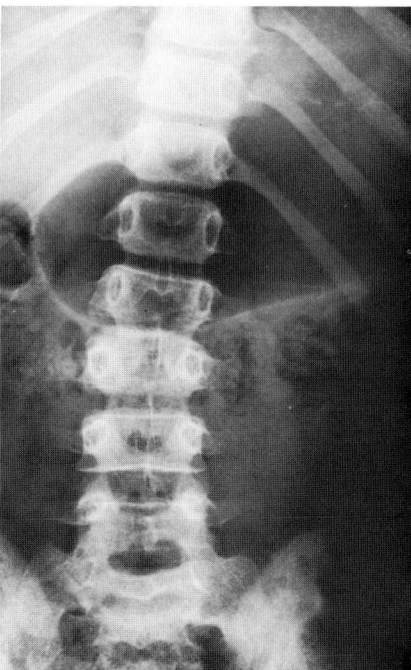

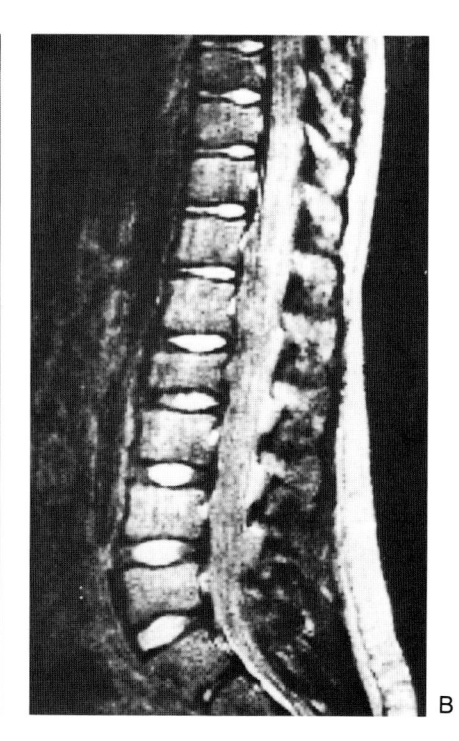

FIG. 4. A: L2 compression fracture responsible for an acute kyphosis. **B:** Discs are preserved, as shown on MRI scan.

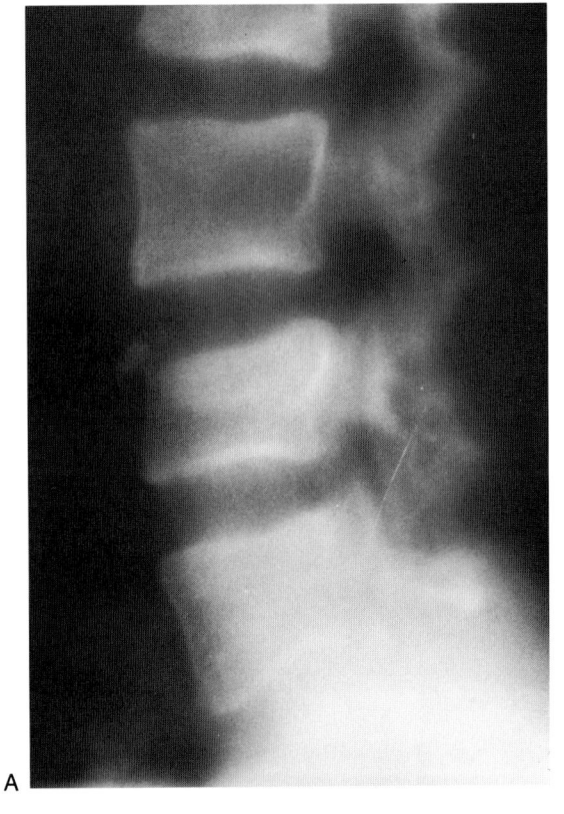

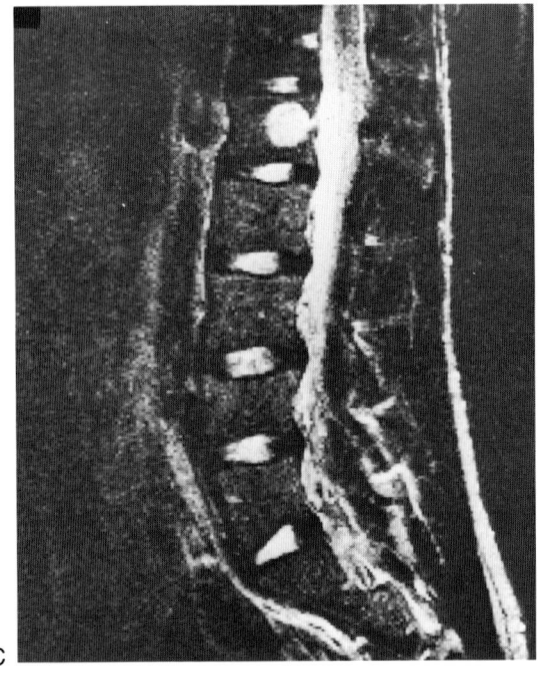

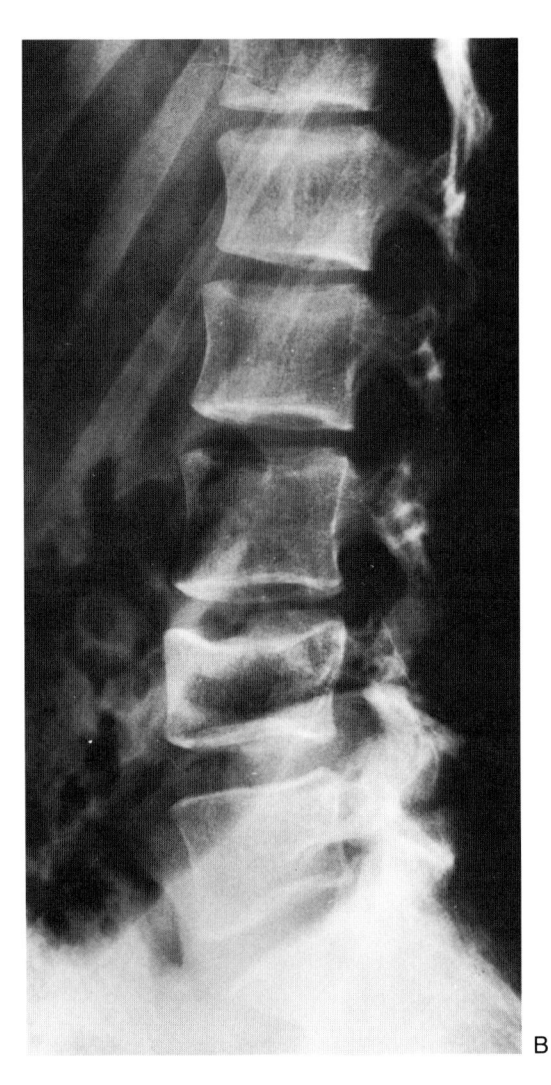

FIG. 5. A: L5 compression fracture at age 15 years. **B:** The same patient, 2 years later. **C:** MRI scan at the 2-year follow-up visit.

fracture line divides the vertebral body in the frontal plane (Fig. 6).

It is important to understand that, after injury to the growth plate and cartilaginous endplate, epiphysiodesis is unlikely. The epiphysis is reduced to a margin that ossifies later as a ring and may not slow the growth of a vertebra. Destruction of the growth plate, comparable to a Salter–Harris type V, represents the major risk. The evolution of the fractures (Figs. 5 and 6) shows that vertebral growth and vertebral spine balance are not always correlated.

Spinal contours depend on the ratio of anterior to posterior vertebral body height in the sagittal plane and the ratio of lateral vertebral body height in the frontal plane. Figure 5 shows that the sagittal spine contour can remain satisfactory over a period of 2 years even though the growth in height of L4 is delayed in the center of the vertebral body.

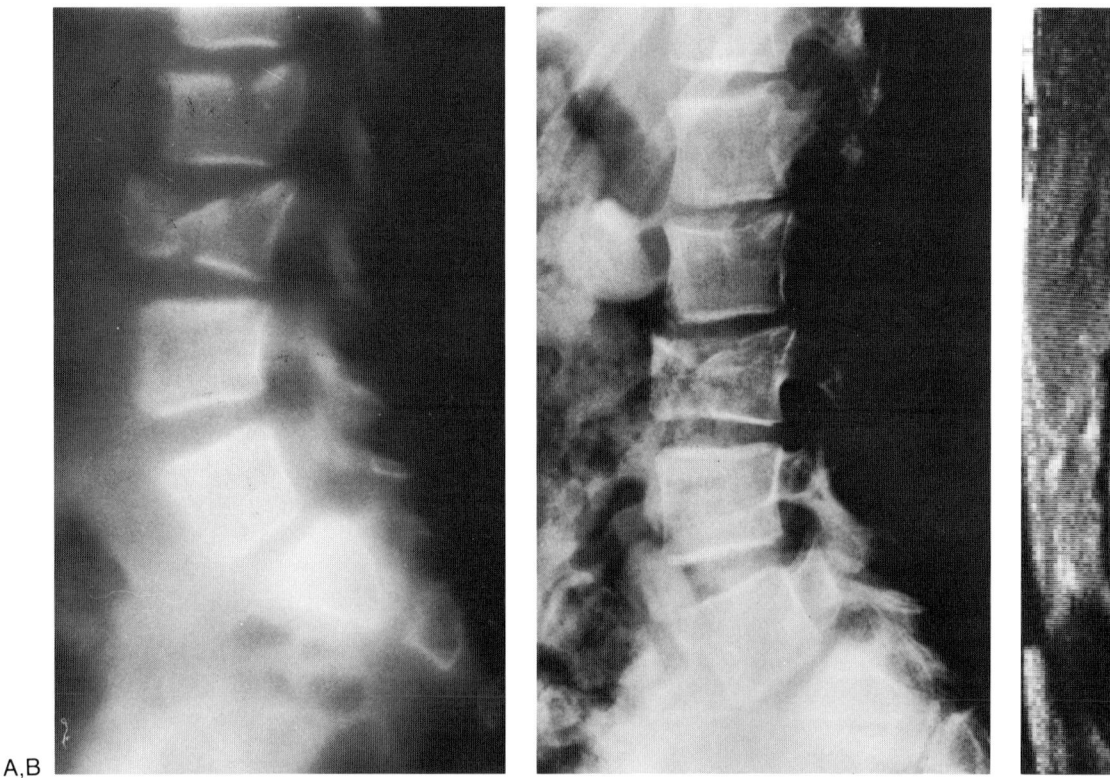

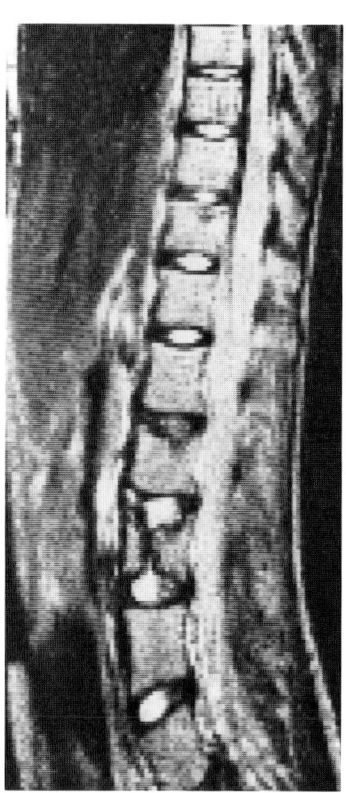

FIG. 6. A: L2 compression fracture (Denis type IA) and L3 compression fracture (Denis type IB) in a 9-year-old girl. **B:** One year follow-up radiograph. **C:** Three-year follow-up MRI scan.

Figure 6 is even more conclusive. The MRI scan shows vertebral body pseudarthrosis at 3-year follow-up. The sagittal contour is normal, since the anterior and posterior parts of the vertebral body have grown simultaneously.

In contrast, Fig. 7 shows vertebral growth and contour derangement following Denis type I fractures. Figure 7 shows an angular kyphosis caused by growth interruption due to anterior fracture disruption of a thoracic vertebra. MRI casts a different light on disc

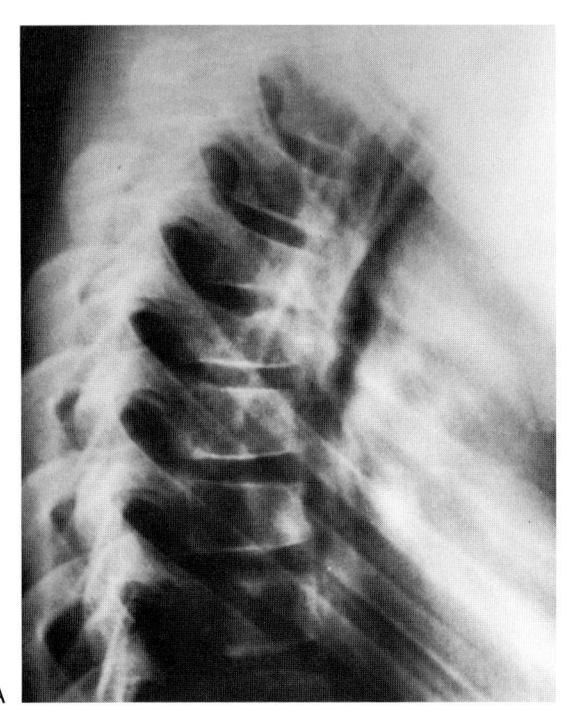

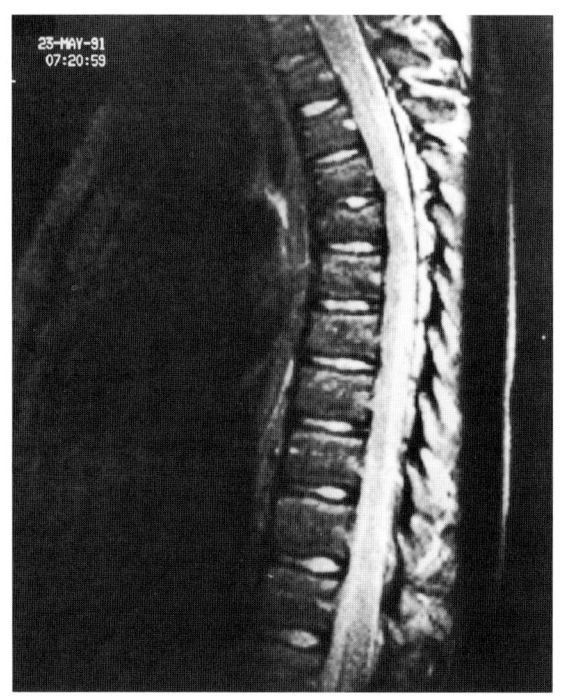

FIG. 7. A: T5–T6 compression fracture in a 13-year-old girl. **B:** Segmental kyphosis at 1-year follow-up.

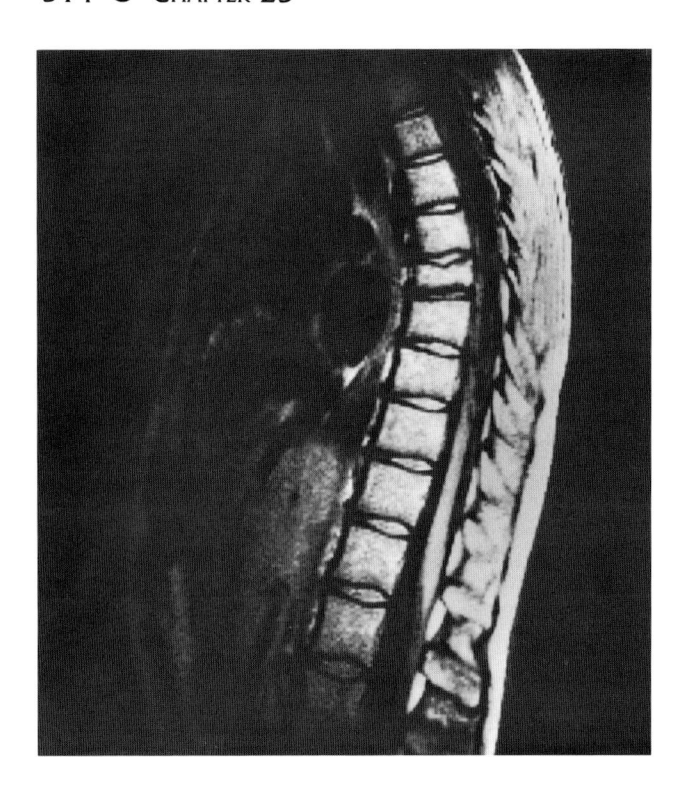

FIG. 8. MRI scan of a thoracic burst fracture treated by a brace at seven-year follow-up.

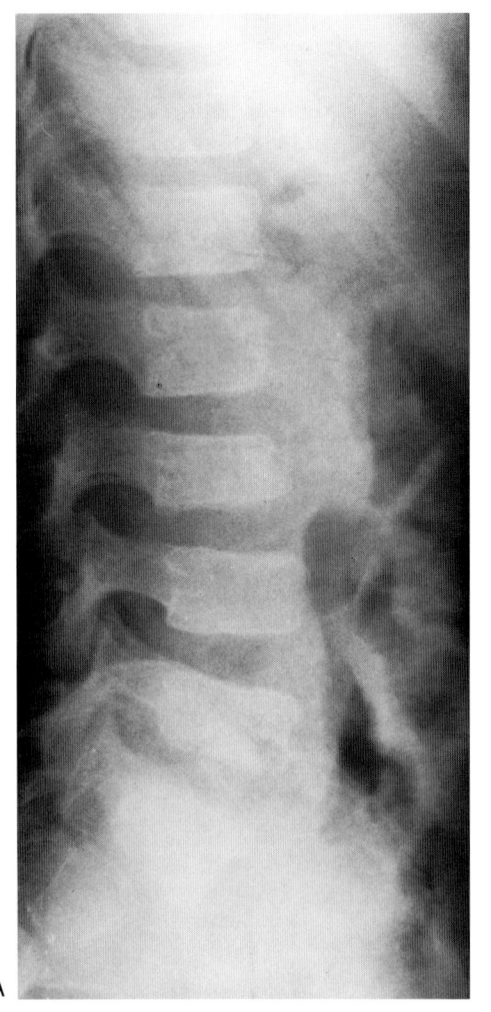

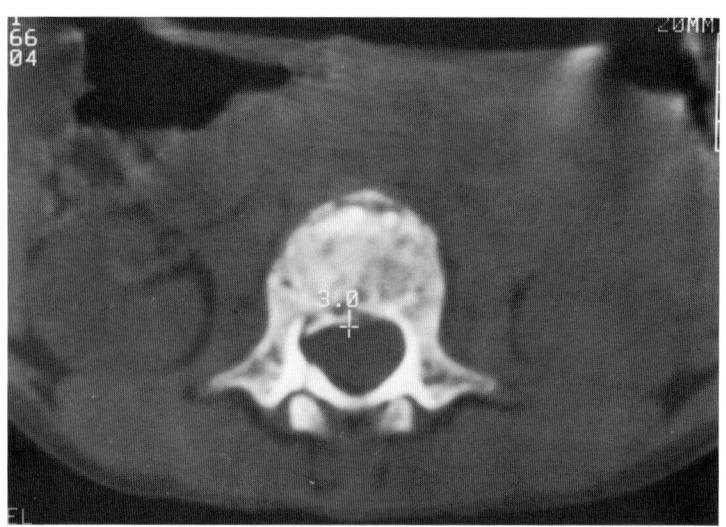

FIG. 9. L3 burst in a 5-year-old girl, neurologically intact, following a fall from a third floor. **A:** Lateral radiograph. **B:** CT scan.

integrity in compression fractures in children. Even though the patients in Figs. 4 and 5 do not show disc injuries, they are different from other cases that show different patterns.

In Fig. 6, there is a change in the MRI disc signal for the L1–L2 disc; L2 sustained a type IB fracture, and L3 sustained a type IA fracture. Figure 7 shows that the MRI disc signal is perceived less at this level in front than at the other levels. Change in MRI disc signal is likely to be related to the magnitude of the injury and may indicate possible vertebral growth problems.

Burst Fractures

Burst fractures result from failure of the anterior and middle columns, both from compression due to axial load with tilting and retropulsion of a bone fragment into the canal. Not often encountered in young children, burst fractures in adolescents have almost the same incidence as in adults. When a burst fracture occurs, the retropulsed bony fragment is small, and the canal diameter is merely reduced. In our series, canal decompression was never indicated.

Figure 8 shows an MRI scan of a 21-year-old woman, 7 years after a burst fracture. At age 14, when the burst fracture occurred, growth was unlikely to resume, and remodeling was not able to prevent a mild kyphotic deformity and reduced vertebral height.

Figure 9 shows an L3 burst fracture; a 5-year-old child fell from a fifth story window. The criteria for burst fracture were not easy to find on the spine roentgenograms (Fig. 9A). Diagnosis was made after a CT scan (Fig. 9B).

CT scans routinely performed for all compression fractures may show small, retropulsed bony fragments from the middle column protruding into the spinal canal. Therefore these fractures, Denis group I (12), must be reclassified as burst fractures.

Ultimate spine contours obey the same growth laws. The same guidelines for treatment apply to compression and burst fractures.

Seat Belt Injuries

A child seated in a vehicle's front seat and wearing a seat belt is unusual, so just a few seat belt fractures are encountered in children. Wearing a seat belt while seated on the auto's rear seat is more likely to increase the number of children's seat belt injuries (Fig. 10).

The "Chance-like" fracture with a posterior fracture line, well shown with MRI (Fig. 10A) will result in a contour deformity after 2 years. The patient was a 14-year-old girl who was treated in a body cast for 2 months.

In adults, Chance fractures become stable when the fracture line through bone has healed. They fail to sta-

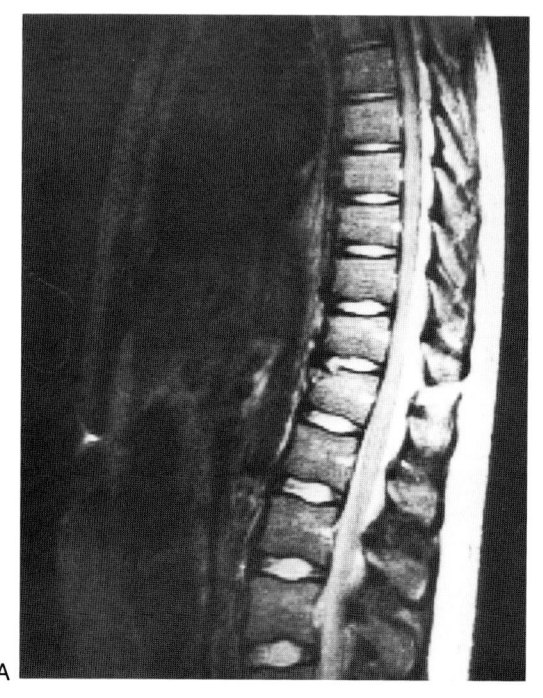

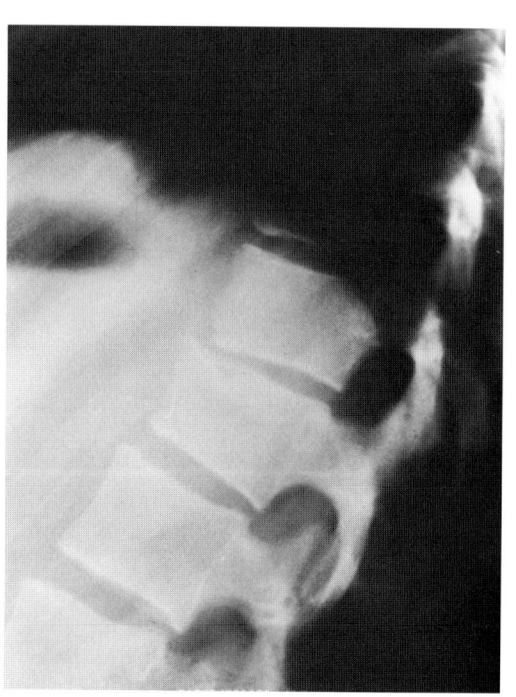

FIG. 10. Chance-like fracture. **A:** Emergency MRI scan. **B:** Radiograph at 2-year follow-up.

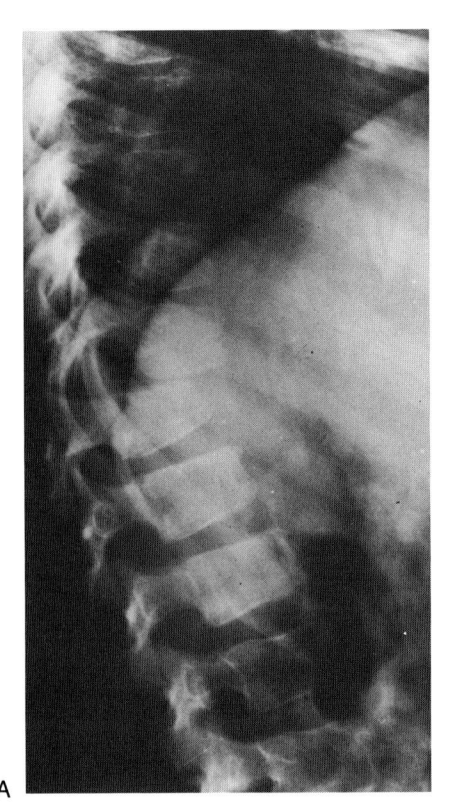

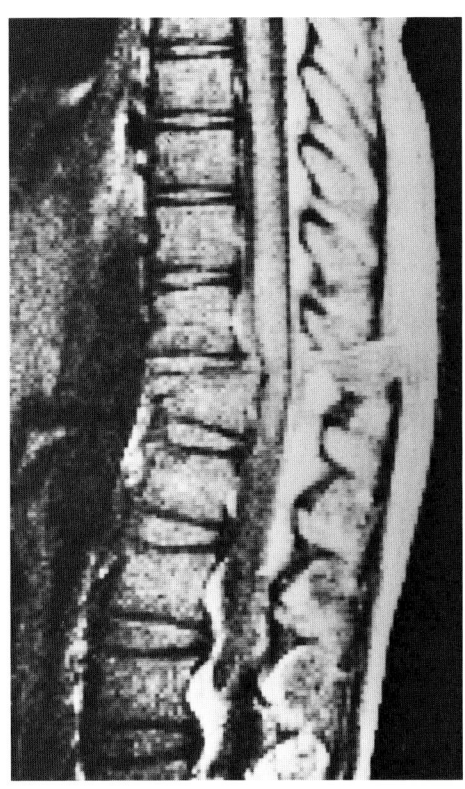

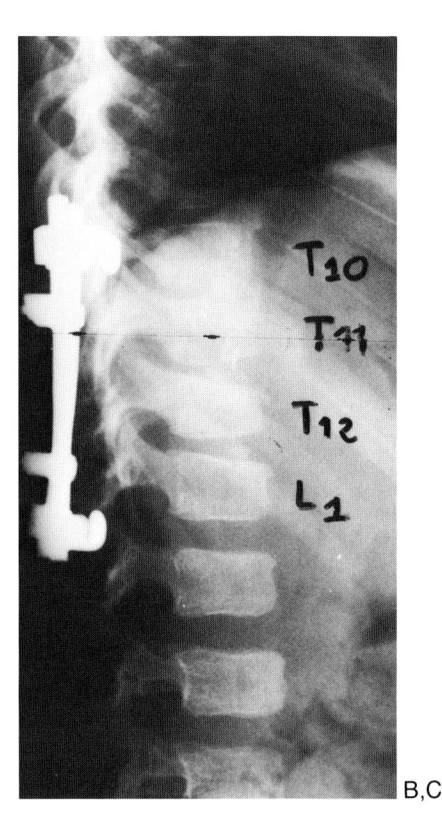

FIG. 11. A: Roentgenogram of neurologically intact 6-year-old boy showing a T11–T12 fracture/dislocation. **B:** MRI scan in emergency. **C:** Reduction, instrumentation, and circumferential arthrodesis.

bilize when the fracture line is through the disc. In children, the fracture line can be an epiphysiolysis and may heal, preserving late stability.

Fracture/Dislocation

The dislocations observed in our series resulted from shear and flexion/distraction. Most of the cord injuries were found in the cases of fracture/dislocation. Figure 11A shows T11–T12 flexion/distraction dislocation with facet joint dislocation. In Fig. 11B, the MRI scan documents the fracture line and tissue disruption from the subcutaneous tissues. Reduction, internal fixation, and posterior arthrodesis were followed by anterior arthrodesis that was indicated by the age (7 years) of the patient, who was neurologically intact. Bone and cord lesions in fracture/dislocation due to shear injury are well documented with MRI, as evidenced by Fig. 12.

Immediate and late stability in this type fracture are compromised, and surgical reduction and stabilization are indicated. Other injuries may be found in children, in addition to those fractures already included in the Denis classification (12).

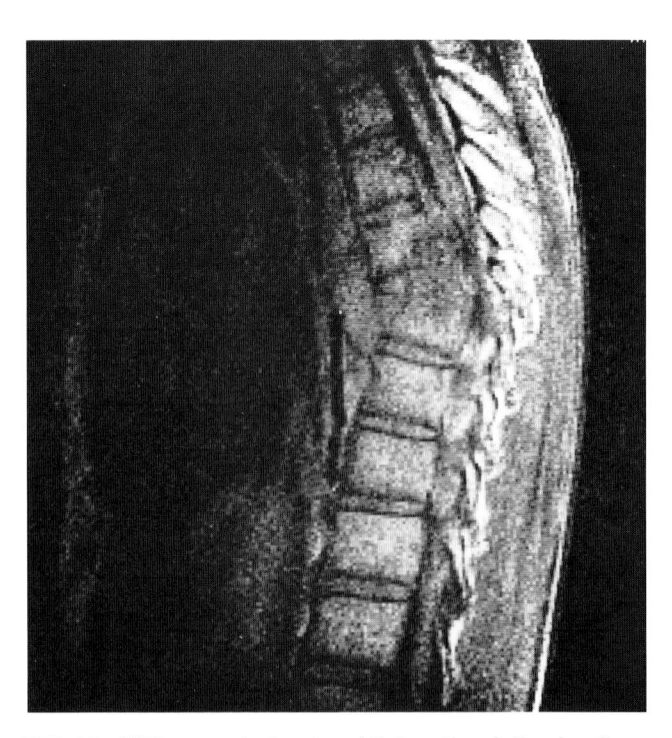

FIG. 12. MRI scan of a fracture/dislocation following flexion/distraction. Patient presented a complete paraplegia.

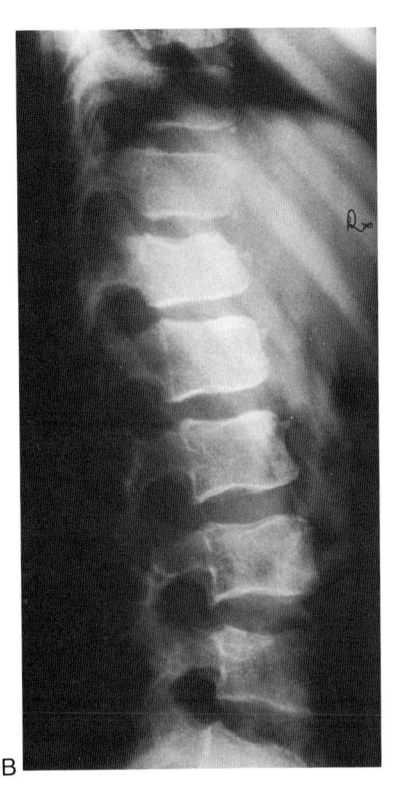

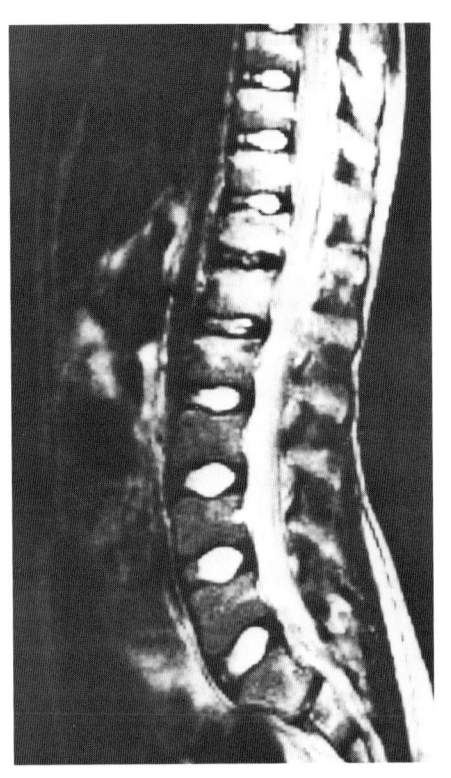

FIG. 13. **A:** Pull-out of the marginal anterior rim by extension fracture. **B:** MRI scan showing signal modifications in the vertebral body.

Anterior Ring Epiphysis Avulsion Due to Extension/Distraction Injury

The anterior longitudinal ligament may be pulled from its annulus fibrosus insertions with the anterior part of the ring margin epiphysis (Fig. 13).

Posterior Avulsion of the Ring Margin Epiphysis (Rim Fracture)

The ring margin, or rim, can become detached and extruded into the canal (Fig. 14). In 1988, Takata et al. (40) described three types of rim fractures (Fig. 15):

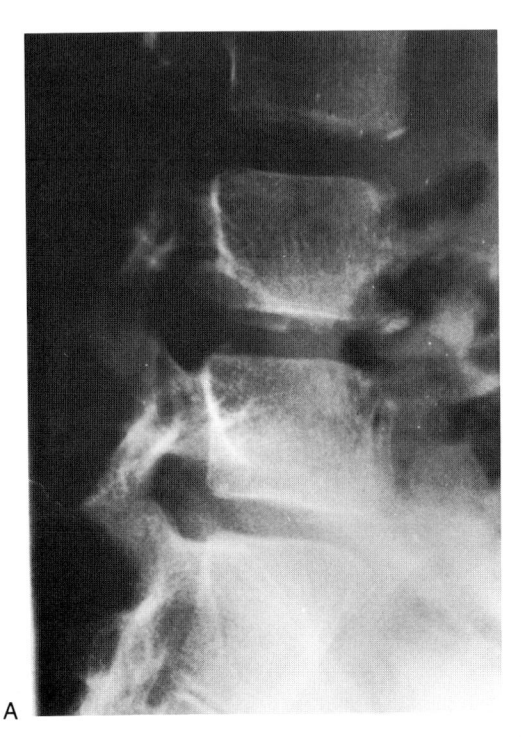

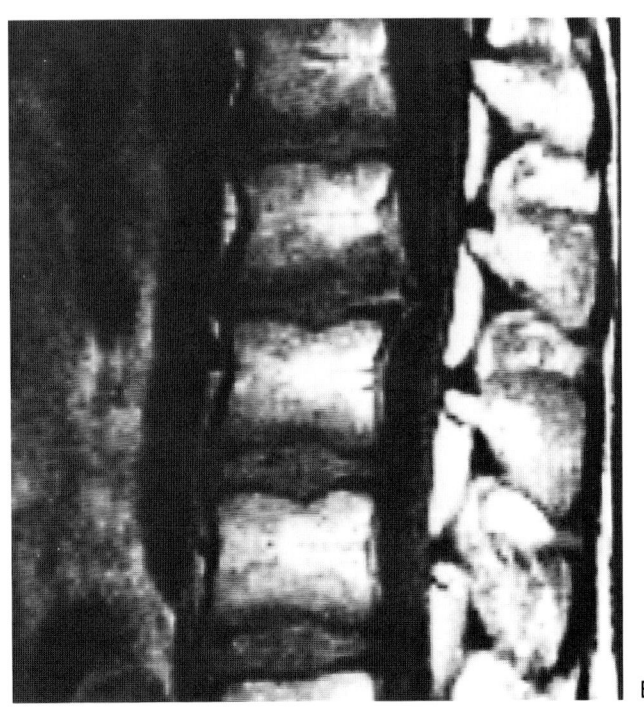

FIG. 14. **A:** Rim fracture of the inferior L4 endplate. **B:** MRI scan showing L2–L3 rim fracture on a different patient.

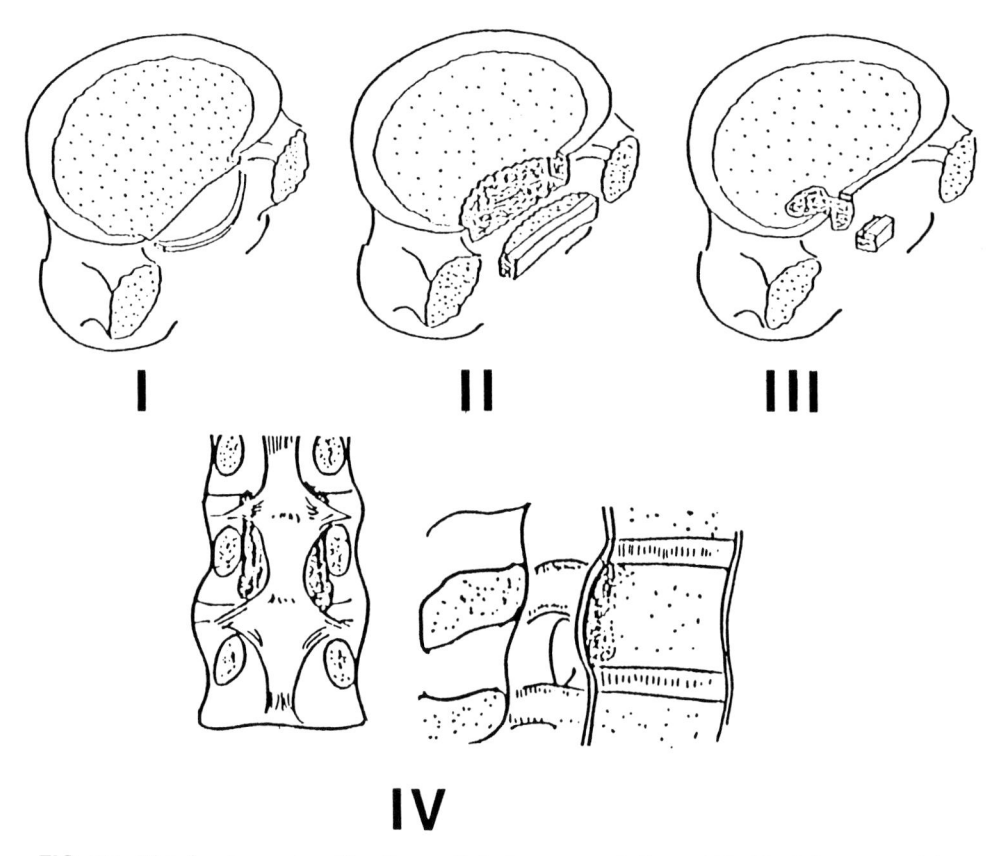

FIG. 15. Rim fracture classifications: Takata groups I, II, and III; Epstein group IV.

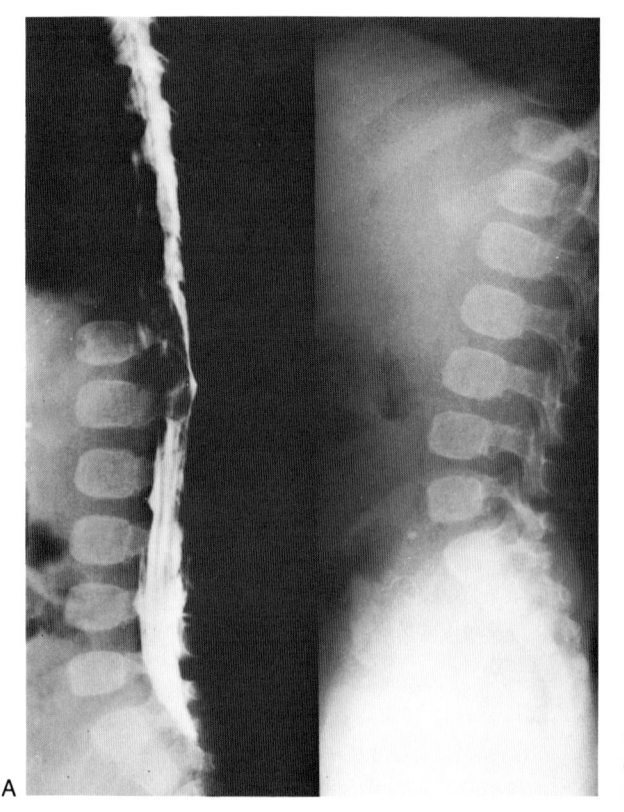

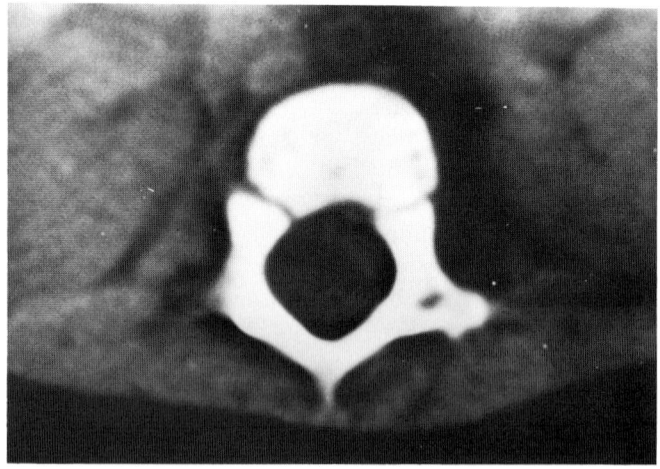

FIG. 16. A: Roentgenogram and myelogram of a 9-month-old paraplegic baby after spinal injury. **B:** Unilateral enlargement of the neurocentral cartilage on CT scan.

Type I   Simple separation of the entire posterior margin
Type II   Avulsion fracture of some of the substance of the vertebral body, including the margin
Type III More localized, lateral fracture of the posterior margin of the vertebral body

Epstein et al. (15) added a fourth type to the three types described by Takata et al. (40): this fracture extends between the endplates, beyond the margins of both the disc and the full length of the vertebral body. If the injury is undiagnosed, this fracture (type IV) effectively displaces bone posteriorly. In the absence of treatment, the spinal canal will be filled anteriorly by a combination of reconstituted cortical and cancellous bone, accompanied, in part, by scar formation.

Neurocentral Cartilage Separation

Only CT scan can document this fracture; when the injury extends bilaterally, it is similar to a fracture of both pedicles that is quite often found in children at the cervical spine level (hangman fracture) after a motor vehicle accident (Fig. 16). A 9-month-old child held in its mother's arms on the front seat sustained a paraplegia without obvious bone and ligamentous lesions. CT/myelogram showed a block on myelography with unilateral enlargement of the neurocentral cartilage on CT scan, which documented the separation (Fig. 16).

Pars Interarticularis Fractures

Repeated microtraumatic injuries can be the cause of isthmic spondylolysis. Direct, high-energy injury may cause isthmic fractures that should heal with 3 months immobilization. Documentation of intact pars interarticularis before injury, fracture after injury, and healing after immobilization should be available for comparison. Since it is unrealistic to expect to obtain this documentation at once, the above hypothesis remains controversial.

CLINICAL DIAGNOSIS OF SPINE FRACTURES

Clinical evaluation of spine injuries in children is dominated by two major concerns: finding associated lesions and finding nerve compromise. Spinal shock and the resultant loss of sympathetic vasomotor tone may complicate the general evaluation and mimic the symptoms of shock from internal bleeding.

The clinical evaluation must be performed without spine mobilization after stabilizing the blood pressure. Abdominal reflexes may be absent, and guarding or complaints of abdominal pain may not be present in a patient with a high cord lesion. History and physical examination of a neurologically intact patient may reveal skin lesions, which can aid the clinician to understand the mechanism of injury. It is unlikely that acute deformities will be found. Pain may be found with light percussion and palpation. Complete loss of muscle function and reflexes accompanying complete loss of all modes of sensitivity at the same level indicate a complete cord injury. There is a larger incidence of complete cord injury in the juvenile population than in the adult population, in which 50% to 60% of the cord injuries are incomplete.

When in pain, children in a coma may show facial grimacing in the absence of a withdrawing of extremities and loss of deep tendon reflexes that suggest cord injury. In the thoracolumbar region, as many as 11 spinal segments can lie between the spinous processes of T10 and L1 (33).

The clinical neurologic examination is similar to that for the adult. However, there are different neurologic patterns of compromise.

Spinal shock remains a misunderstood phenomenon. There is a flaccid paralysis, and deep tendon reflexes cannot be elicited. Urinary retention is usual; the sphincter tone is merely disturbed. There are patchy zones in which pin prick and deep pain sensation may be preserved. When recovery of neural function occurs, it may begin very early, within a few hours, or be delayed for a few days, according to the magnitude of the injury. In babies, reflex activity of the isolated cord may be almost indistinguishable from normal motor function.

Medullary infarction frequently accounts for the number of quadriplegics who will remain flaccid.

Cord injuries with a short spinal shock and early return (within hours) of sacral reflexes are likely to become spastic.

Brown–Sequard is defined as a loss of touch and proprioception that occurs on the same side as the motor loss. Analgesia occurs on the contralateral side and may be two or three levels below the motor level. In the case of anterior spinal artery insult, the syndrome is defined as a loss of all long tract functions with preservation of touch and proprioception.

Central cord injury, which very rarely occurs in children, may present with a preserved sacral sensitivity.

Radiculopathy:

Isolated radicular pain may indicate a rim fracture, which can occur in adolescents and young adults. Epstein et al. (15) reviewed the literature and analyzed a 10-patient series, which showed that, in adolescents, fractures of the vertebral rim typically involve the L4–L5 level (L4 caudally), whereas both L4–L5 and L5–S1 are more commonly affected in young adults.

Takata et al. (40) did not confirm this localization and instead found most of the lesions at the posterior cephalad rim of S1. This may relate more to the type of fracture than to the location of the fracture, which is typical of the adolescent. Takata types I and II (40) are almost always found in adolescents, in contrast to Takata type III (40) and Epstein type IV (15), which are almost always found in adults, as shown in Fig. 15.

The tethered chain concept (14) as well as mild idiopathic dysplasia of the vertebral ring (37) are hypotheses that may explain the pathophysiology of unconfirmed rim fractures.

There are three important clinical aspects of SCI which are typical of a children's population and, because they may be misleading, must be described separately. It is important to know the characteristics of each in order to avoid errors.

SCIWORA

Spinal cord injury without radiographic abnormalities (SCIWORA) must be considered in children who present with clinical myelopathy as a result of injury. Their plain radiograph, myelogram, CT scan, and MRI scan may show no evidence of skeletal injury or subluxation.

SCIWORA syndrome can affect children of all ages and occurs in conditions similar to the rest of SCI. There is an analogy to a birth injury that occurs with cervical hyperextension in breech delivery. Inasmuch as the patient is younger, the SCIWORA is more serious. According to Pang and Wilberger the age of eight years is the landmark that divides SCIWORA syndrome.

SCIWORA does not always appear immediately after injury; delay of the onset of symptoms can be up to 4 days. Retrospective analysis frequently found transient neurologic deficit that was overlooked. Patients were discharged home, with delayed development of SCIWORA related to a new, minor injury (1,8, 9,34).

Spine instability was considered a possible cause, but documentation by stress radiograph failed because of muscle contractures. Late instability was never found, and this hypothesis is unproved.

The second hypothesis is related to the original cord injury, which could have started the slow but progressive destruction of neural tissues. The insult may be ischemic, as documented twice by Ahmann et al. (1).

Pathophysiology of Medullary Lesions in SCIWORA

Leventhal's (28) cadaver study of the longitudinal compliance of the neonatal spine is most revealing, showing that the elastic spinal column of the neonate can be stretched 2 in. without signs of structural disruption. But the spinal cord, devoid of elastic elements, can stretch only ¼ in. before rupturing.

Hyperextension, hyperflexion, distraction, and repeated flexion/extension of battered children can cause SCIWORA (17,34). The discrepancy between the elasticity of the cord and the *bony* spine is enough to relate any of these mechanisms of injury to SCI. Cord ischemia, often increased by severe general hypotension upon admission, is also responsible for SCI (34). Ischemia with large cord infarction is responsible for cord destruction, which occurs frequently in the upper thoracic level and causes flaccid paralysis.

Among SCIWORA syndromes, it is possible that growth plate fractures with large displacement on injury can be reduced by positioning and maintained reduced by muscle contracture after cord damage. Early healing of the chondrocartilage does not allow documentation.

As reported by Pollack et al. (36), transient forms of SCIWORA may be recognized. Children younger than 8 years of age who sustain hyperflexion injuries are candidates for a transient SCIWORA, and the family must be advised of possible nerve deficit, which will require attention in the coming days after discharge.

Lesions with Minimal Injury

Finding a spine fracture with a history of minimal injury must alert the clinician to a pathologic fracture. Eosinophilic granuloma or neuroblastoma metastasis will be evident earliest on a young patient. Aneurysmal bone cyst or osteoblastoma may be suspected in an older child, rather than the infrequent Ewing tumor. Systemic diseases, such as the hemoglobinopathies (thalassemia, drepanocytosis, sicklemia, or leukemia), steroid treatment, or bone diseases, such as osteogenesis imperfecta, may be responsible for fractures.

Injury Not Reported

The battered child and battered baby syndromes (11) should not be overlooked. Cullen (11) and Swischuk (39) reported 12 cases, with age range 2 to 24 months at the time of diagnosis, which led Cullen (11) to discuss battered babies rather than battered children.

With the exception of one T3 lesion, the other 11 fractures were distributed between T11 and L3. Three patterns usually were found:

- Compression.
- Subluxation or fracture dislocation.
- Narrowing of intervertebral disc space and anterior notching of a vertebral body.

As Swischuk (39) noted, a neurologically intact baby is merely symptomatic. The clinician cannot exclude the consideration that some vertebral notching, otherwise possibly considered a variant of the "normal," is related to the battered baby syndrome.

Scheuermann's disease can also raise discussion of diagnosis. Its classic symptoms are:

- Wedge-shaped vertebral body, predominantly symmetrical.
- Irregular endplates and intracorporeal disc protrusions.
- Repetition of findings at three adjacent levels.

Signal modification in the MRI image of the vertebral body is diagnostic for fracture.

IMAGING IN CHILDREN'S SPINAL INJURIES

Radiographs

AP and lateral radiographs are still the standard. The cervicothoracic junction is notable for its poor radiographic imaging. Lateral asymmetrical compression is responsible for late scoliosis and can be well documented on AP views, as can increased interpedicular distance, which suggests a burst fracture. Sagittal deformity of the vertebra, disc space integrity, and enlargement of the interspinous process space are well documented on lateral radiographs.

The entire spine must be seen, keeping in mind the possible involvement of multiple levels (Fig. 17). An average of two vertebrae were involved in a thoracic compression fracture series (6). As many as five vertebrae can be involved; both T5 and T6 were injured 13 times, and T11 and T12 were injured 11 times, although noncontiguous as well as contiguous vertebrae can be affected. Anterior and posterior margins must be recognized on lateral radiographs to identify either forward or backward displacement to diagnose a rim fracture.

Tomograms

AP tomograms can be useful to find a sagittal fracture line, and lateral tomograms may help to eliminate bony lesions in spinal cord injuries without radiologic abnormalities.

Myelogram may be indicated, followed by CT scan.

MRI, which can document compression fractures that are not visible on standard roentgenograms, has legal implications. MRI signals also may help to evaluate the integrity of the intervertebral discs, cord, and spinal canal relationships.

Thirty-seven patients with spinal injuries underwent MRI evaluation (7). Eight patients with normal MRI scans were neurologically intact, but the 29 patients who presented with neurologic involvement were distributed within three groups.

Group I consisted of 10 patients who demonstrated a decreased signal intensity, consistent with acute intraspinal hemorrhage. Group II was comprised of 16 patients who demonstrated a bright signal intensity, consistent with acute cord edema. The three patients in group III demonstrated a mixed signal of central hypointensity and peripheral hyperintensity consistent with contusion.

All patients were reevaluated after 1 year. Group I remained at the same Frankel level/score, but groups II and III improved at least one level in the Frankel classification (16).

CT scan is the best imaging to evaluate the bony lesion. Rim fracture can be diagnosed and classified into one of the four groups only after viewing CT images.

SPINE STABILITY

Long-term evolution of spine balance following spinal injury in children is the main concern. Kyphosis, scoliosis, or kyphoscoliosis is likely to develop at the level of a compression fracture such as Denis type I. However, the neurologically intact patient is unlikely to develop increasing late deformities, since deformities at the level of the injury are not likely to become symptomatic even after long follow-up (6,20,22,35).

Compression fractures of thoracic or lumbar vertebrae do not carry a long-term morbidity as regard to back pain and late deformities, even though kyphosis

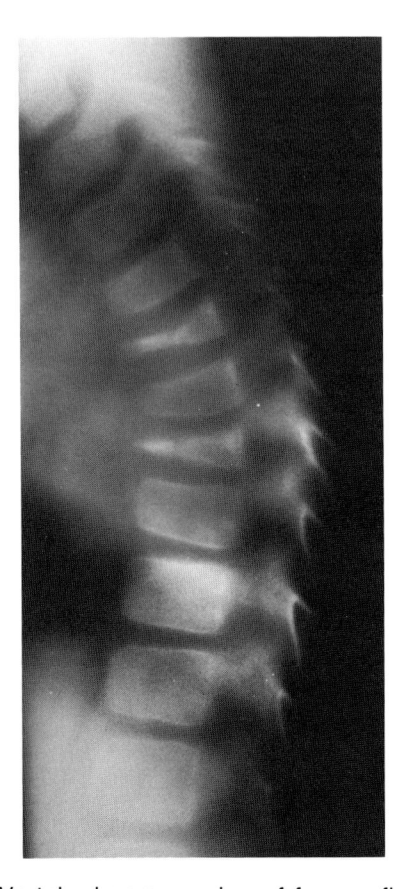

FIG. 17. Vertebral compression of four or five thoracic vertebrae.

and lordosis are of concern. However, poor evaluation of the injury may lead to shortcomings, as in Fig. 6, which shows a patient whose lesion did not require surgery. This is contrasted to the patient in Fig. 10, who required late surgical stabilization.

Late deformities depend on the neurologic status after injury. Deformity is a different issue at the level of the fracture in a neurologically intact patient and at the level of the spine below the lesion in a paralyzed patient.

Locally, on a neurologically intact patient, it is rare to find a late deformity that develops at the same level as a compression fracture. No segmental kyphosis exceeds 10°, and some hyperlordoses are found (20,22). Reduction, correction, and fusion are almost never indicated (6) (Fig. 18). Scoliosis can be expected when a

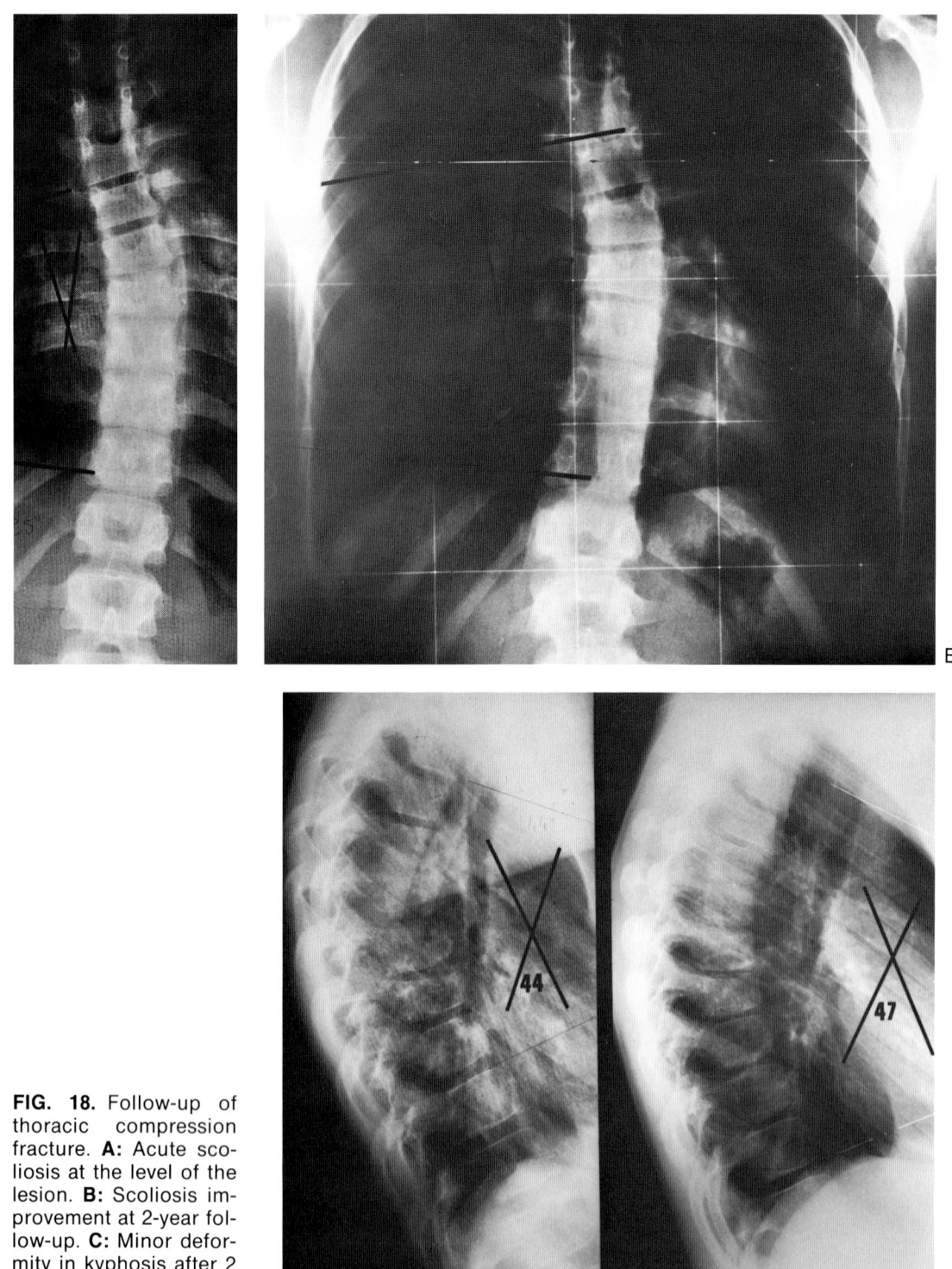

FIG. 18. Follow-up of thoracic compression fracture. **A:** Acute scoliosis at the level of the lesion. **B:** Scoliosis improvement at 2-year follow-up. **C:** Minor deformity in kyphosis after 2 years.

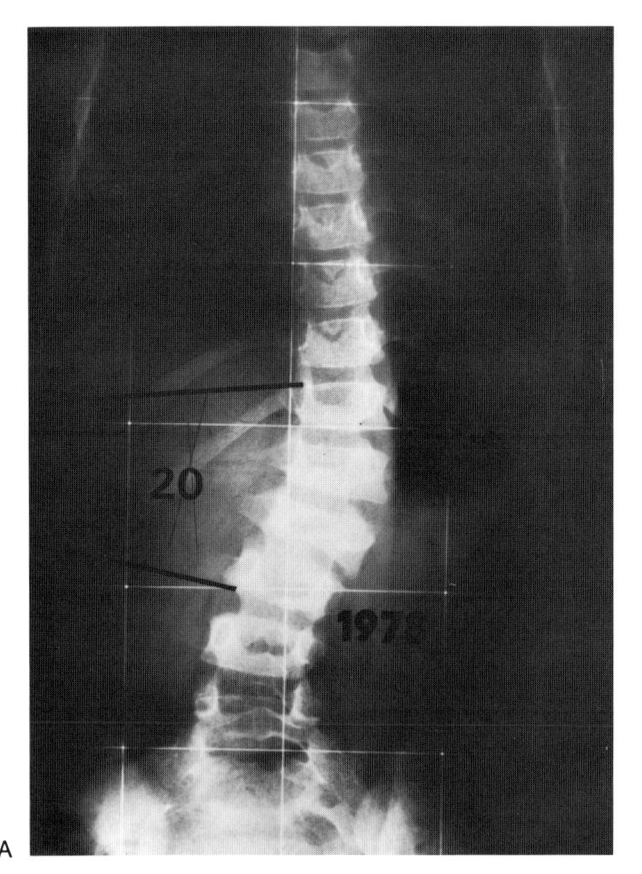

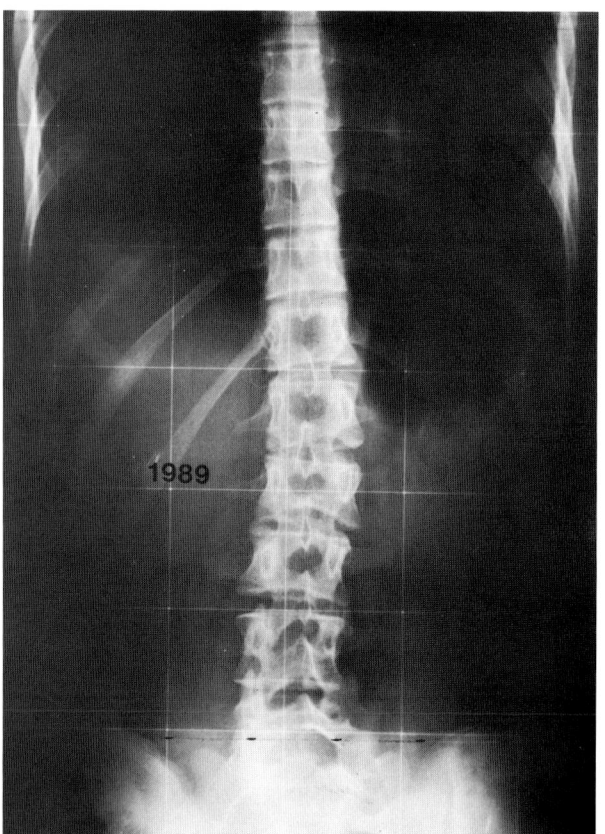

FIG. 19. A: A 20° left lumbar scoliosis following an asymmetric compression fracture in a 5-year-old girl. **B:** Same patient at 11-year follow-up.

lateral compression is found, but there is no report of a scoliosis with late angulation exceeding 20°. Figure 19 shows treatment by 3 months in a cast followed by 1 year in a brace. The deformity at 11-years follow-up does not impair spine balance.

Laminectomy performed for decompression may not prevent neural compression, but does create instability. Thus patients who undergo laminectomy may show progression with important late deformity (35).

Fracture/dislocation, if not treated, carries a high risk of late deformity. However, these fractures are almost always treated by open reduction and internal fixation with fusion.

Burst fractures can be responsible for variable deformity, according to the patient's age at the time of injury. However, the potential late deformity is theoretical because just a few have been reported. Seat belt fractures are likely to cause late deformities when posterior ligament injury is present and associated with anterior disc injury. They must be treated by fusion.

Seat belt and Chance fractures, lesions mainly in bone or the growth plate, routinely healed well in a cast, without risk of late deformities. Late deformities are addressed in detail by Dubousset in Chapter 24.

TREATMENT GUIDELINES

In Neurologically Intact Patients

Compression Fractures

Even with a serious compression fracture, there is no indication for early surgery. When there is a moderate compression fracture, even at multiple levels, which does not compromise spine balance, treatment is always conservative. Three weeks in bed are enough, and the pain disappears rapidly if strict bed rest is respected.

When the compression fracture is significant (more than one-third of the vertebral body height) with kyphotic deformity, closed reduction is indicated. Reduction is performed on a Cotrel or Risser table according to Boehler's principles, without general anesthesia.

Twenty-four to 48 hr are necessary to observe relief of pain and monitor the vital signs to diagnose associated injuries without the inconvenience of a body cast. On a patient who is stable, sedated, and awake, a three-point body cast is applied with a large anterior window. The body cast will be extended cranially by a Minerva for high thoracic fractures. As soon as the cast is dry, the patient can get out of bed and may ambulate. Early discharge home with physical therapy is indicated. The cast is left in place for 3 months. After 3 months, if there is still a deformity, a body jacket is indicated. The length of time in the brace varies according to the deformity and the age of the patient. Since progression of deformities in this type of fracture is unlikely, wearing of the brace should not exceed 1 year.

Burst Fractures

Cast immobilization as first treatment is always indicated in children. In young children, decompression is exceptionally indicated. However, reduction must be extremely prudent, and any maneuver to forcefully reduce the deformity is contraindicated. The patient must be stable and awake without positioning in hypercorrection. The patient will stay in bed for 1 month without being allowed out of bed. A CT scan is performed after the cast application. After 1 month in bed, treatment is continued as if it were a compression fracture.

In older children and mature adolescents, indications for decompression are the same as for adults.

Seat Belt Fractures

Surgery is not indicated in children younger than 8 years of age, even in the presence of a discoligamentous injury. In our experience, the treatment of compression fracture can be extended to 3 months in a cast, followed by stress radiographs. If late instability is documented on stress radiographs, surgical stabilization may be indicated. In this case, a circumferential arthrodesis must be performed to avoid further growth-induced deformities. In children older than 8 years of age, a posterior arthrodesis with segmental instrumentation must be performed for late instability.

A neurocentral cartilage disruption does not require reduction. It requires 1 month in a cast to heal.
Hyperextension fractures must be casted in a neutral position for 3 months. It is not necessary to apply a brace after cast removal.
Rim fractures require surgical decompression.

Acute rim fractures with a mobile bony fragment require only a flavectomy to provide access for elective removal of the fragment. A discectomy is not necessary.

In lumbar rim fractures seen late, a laminectomy is necessary to remove the bony fragment. Dissection of a disc protruding into the canal is extremely difficult, and a discectomy must be performed in these cases.

In Patients with Neurologic Lesions

The patient is admitted, treated, and monitored in the ICU, as are all cord injury patients. The guidelines for orthopaedic treatment vary with age and diagnosis.

Fracture/Dislocation

The patient with a fracture/dislocation who is neurologically intact is an exception but will, nevertheless, be treated in a similar manner. Posterior reduction with instrumentation and arthrodesis is indicated. It must be performed early, almost as an emergency if the neurological lesions are incomplete.

On a paraplegic child younger than 8 years of age, one must recognize that late deformities below the lesion are inevitable. A long posterior segmental arthrodesis extended caudally must be performed.

Anterior arthrodesis can be performed as a second stage to prevent hyperlordosis induced by further anterior growth. This second stage will be performed when the patient is stable, after a delay to allow recovery. Laminectomy must be avoided at any cost.

SCIWORA

Preventing transient SCIWORA from getting worse is the primary concern. When diagnosed, a transient SCIWORA must be immobilized in a body jacket for a 3-month period. Early physical therapy is indicated, and ambulation is allowed. SCIWORA with paralysis will require treatment of late deformities as indicated for any paralytic spine.

Late deformities are addressed in Chapter 24 by Dubousset.

CONCLUSION

It must be remembered that the child's spine is a structure in transformation. Growth is a reality that must be kept in mind when treating spine fractures during childhood. The post-traumatic result with regard to stability is far better in a child than in an adult. A child's SCI has no more potential for recovery than does an adult's SCI. The spine of the paralyzed child with SCI will, unfortunately, continue to deform with growth.

REFERENCES

1. Ahmann PA, Smith SA, Schwartz JF, et al. Spinal cord infarction due to minor trauma in children. *Neurology* 1975;25: 301–307.
2. Anderson JM, Schutt AH. Spinal injury in children. A review of

156 cases seen from 1950 through 1978. *Mayo Clin Proc* 1980; 55:499–504.
3. Andrews LG, Jung SK. Spinal cord injuries in children in British Columbia. *Paraplegia* 1979;17:442–451.
4. Audic B, Maury M. Les deformations du tronc apres paraplegie chez les enfants et les adolescents. *Rev Chir Orthop* 1970;56: 139–153.
5. Aufdermaur M. Spinal injuries in juveniles. *J Bone Joint Surg* 1974;56B:513–519.
6. Bollini G, Jouve JL, Cottalorda J. Spinal trauma in children. Eighth Annual Stonwin Medical Conference, New York, July 15–17, 1991.
7. Bondurant FJ, Cotler HB, Kulkarni MV, et al. Acute spinal cord injury. A study using physical examination and magnetic resonance imaging. *Spine* 1990;15:161–168.
8. Burke DC. Traumatic spinal paralysis in children. *Paraplegia* 1974;11:268–276.
9. Cheshire DJE. The paediatric syndrome of traumatic myelopathy without demonstrable vertebral injury. *Paraplegia* 1977;15: 74–85.
10. Choi JU, Hoffman HJ, Hendrick EB, et al. Traumatic infarction of the spinal cord in children. *J Neurosurg* 1986;65:608–610.
11. Cullen JC. Spinal lesions in battered babies. *J Bone Joint Surg* 1975;57B:364–366.
12. Denis F. The three column spine and its significance in the classification of acute thoracolumbar spinal injuries. *Spine* 1983;8: 817–831.
13. Dimeglio A, Bonnel F. *Le rachis en croissance.* Paris: Springer-Verlag, 1990.
14. Ehni G, Schneider SJ. Posterior lumbar vertebral rim fracture and associated disc protrusion in adolescence. *J Neurosurg* 1988;68:912–916.
15. Epstein NE, Epstein JA, Mauri T. Treatment of fractures of the vertebral limbus and spinal stenosis in five adolescents and five adults. *Neurosurgery* 1989;24:595–604.
16. Frankel HL, Hancock DO, Hyslop G, et al. The value of postural reduction in the initial management of closed injuries of the spine with paraplegia and tetraplegia. *Paraplegia* 1969;7: 179–182.
17. Glasauer FE, Cares HL. Biomechanical features of traumatic paraplegia in infancy. *J Trauma* 1973;13:166–170.
18. Hachen HJ. Spinal cord injury in children and adolescents. *Paraplegia* 1977;15:55–64.
19. Hadley MN, Zabramski JM, Browner CM et al. Pediatric spinal trauma. *J Neurosurg* 1988;68:18–24.
20. Horal J, Nachemson A, Scheller S. Clinical and radiological long term follow up of vertebral fractures in children. *Acta Orthop Scand* 1972;43:491–503.
21. Hubbard DD. Injuries of the spine in children and adolescents. *Clin Orthop* 1974;100:56–65.
22. Hubbard DD. Fractures of the dorsal and lumbar spine. *Orthop Clin North Am* 1976;7:605–614.
23. Kewalramani LS, Kraus JF, Sterling HM. Acute spinal cord lesions in a pediatric population: epidemiological and clinical features. *Paraplegia* 1980;18:206–219.
24. Kewalramani LS, Tori JA. Spinal cord trauma in children. Neurologic patterns, radiologic features and pathomechanics of injury. *Spine* 1980;5:11–18.
25. Lancourt GE, Dickson TH, Carter ME. Paralytic spinal deformity following traumatic spinal cord injury in children and adolescents. *J Bone Joint Surg* 1981;63A:47–53.
26. Leblanc HJ, Nadell J. Spinal cord injuries in children. *Surg Neurol* 1974;2:411–414.
27. Lesoin F, Kabbaj K, Dhellemmes P, et al. Fractures du rachis chez l'enfant. Problemes diagnostics et therapeutiques. *Neurochirurgie* 1984;30:289–294.
28. Leventhal HR. Birth injuries of the spinal cord. *J Pediatr* 1960; 56:447–453.
29. McPhee IB. Spinal fractures and dislocations in children and adolescents. *Spine* 1981;6:533–537.
30. Mallet J, Rey JC, Raimbeau G. Dystrophie rachidienne de croissance. *Ann Orthop Ouest* 1975;7:95–116.
31. Mayfield JK, Erkkila JC, Winter RB. Spine deformity subsequent to acquired childhood spinal cord injury. *J Bone Joint Surg* 1981;63A:1401–1411.
32. Melzac J. Paraplegia among children. *Lancet* 1969;2:45–48.
33. Ogden JA. *Skeletal injury in the child.* Philadelphia: Lea & Febiger, 1982;385–422.
34. Pang D, Wilberger JE Jr. Spinal cord injury without radiographic abnormalities in children. *J Neurosurg* 1982;57:114–129.
35. Pouliquen JC, Beneux J, Pennecot GF. Le risque de deviation rachidienne evolutive dans les fractures et luxations du rachis chez l'enfant. *Rev Chir Orthop* 1978;64:487–498.
36. Pollack IF, Pang D, Sclabassi R. Recurrent spinal cord injury without radiographic abnormalities in children. *J Neurosurg* 1988;69:177–182.
37. Reigel DH. Slipped lumbar apophyseal ring. In: *Concepts of pediatric neurosurgery*, vol 5. Basel: Karger, 1984;34–40.
38. Ruge JR, Sinson GP, McLone DG, Cerullo LJ. Pediatric spinal injury: the very young. *J Neurosurg* 1988;68:25–30.
39. Swischuk LE. Spine and spinal cord trauma in the battered child syndrome. *Radiology* 1969;92:733–738.
40. Takata K, Inoue SI, Takahashi K, Ohtsuha Y. Fractures of the posterior margin of a lumbar vertebral body. *J Bone Joint Surg* 1988;70A:589–594.
41. Tondury G. *Entwicklungsgeschichte und fehl bildungen Der Wirbersaule.* Stuttgart: Hippokrates-Verlag, 1958.
42. Walsh JW, Stevens DB, Young AB. Traumatic paraplegia in children without contiguous spinal fracture or dislocation. *Neurosurgery* 1983;12:439–445.

24

Spinal Deformities Secondary to Traumatic Lesions Involving the Spine and Spinal Cord in Children

Jean Dubousset

Late spinal deformities are typical in a child who has sustained both spinal and cord injuries. The mode of development of the deformity and its incidence rate are different in children and adults who sustain the same type of injury. Addressing these differences was my rationale for writing this chapter.

Late end results of spine injuries in children can be, more or less, studied at two levels: at the level of the lesion with all possible derangements—instability, alignment, gross and subsequent spinal cord lesions; and below the level with all the aftermath of residual paralysis—scoliosis, kyphosis, lordosis, balance and imbalance, pelvic obliquity, lower limb functions and contractures, and the inability to stand, walk, and sit. In addition, collapsing factors that oppose growth, trophic problems, and urinary impairment are also cause for concern.

To understand the multiple possible outcomes, we must remember the normal growth pattern at the level of the "functional unit," as well as the normal active and passive balance that are compatible with harmonious, normal growth.

GROWTH AND BALANCE OF THE NORMAL AND PATHOLOGICAL SPINES

At the Level of the Vertebra and the Functional Unit

Growth is accomplished by three groups of growing cartilage, which allow three-dimensional growth of the vertebra (Fig. 1). The cartilage of the vertebral endplate is like the growth plate of a long bone, providing for growth in height through the same mechanism. When subjected to trauma, the shear between bone and cartilage occurs more often at the lower endplate than at the upper endplate. The neurocentral cartilage is unique, vertical, and located between the body and posterior arch. It is a bipolar cartilage that induces growth of the body and pedicles in the horizontal plane. Connection between the horizontal cartilage of the endplate and the bipolar cartilage provides for a true three-dimensional expansion. Commonly, the cartilage ossifies between 9 and 11 years of age. Specimens have demonstrated some remnants of the cartilage as late as age 13.

Finally, growing cartilage is also present in the posterior arches, facet joints, and spinous and transverse processes. In addition, resorption apposition at the level of the periosteum occurs. This induces spinal canal remodeling and body remodeling. The ring apophysis fuses with the vertebral body at an age that varies between 15 and 24 years. In height, the mean growth of each vertebra has been estimated to be 0.7 mm per vertebra, per year.

The growth and maturation of each vertebra are regulated not only by general hormonal factors but also by the proper, special balance that is contributed by the function of muscles and ligaments surrounding the vertebrae. For example, a localized paralysis can occur at the level of the paravertebral muscles, as demonstrated after removal of a neuroblastoma and resection of one or two intercostal bundles close to or even inside

---

J. Dubousset: University of René Descartes, and Department of Pediatric Orthopaedic Surgery, St. Vincent de Paul Hospital, 75014 Paris Cedex 14, France.

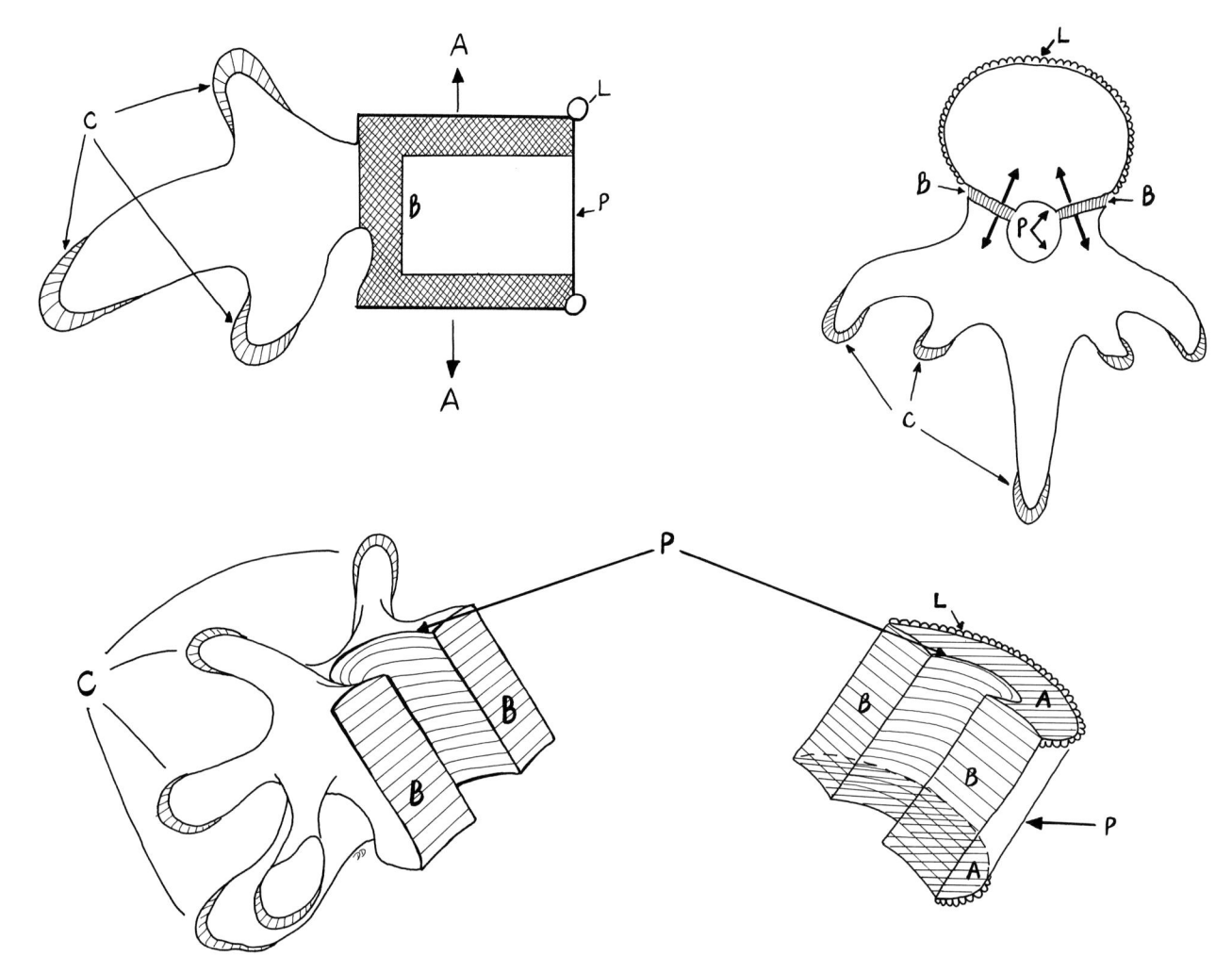

FIG. 1. Growing cartilage of the vertebra. *A,* Vertebral endplate; *B,* neurocentral cartilage (bipolar) closes between 8 and 13 years; *C,* facet: transverse and spinous processes cartilage (apophyseal type); *L,* ring apophysis—fusion obtained between ages 15 and 24; *P,* periosteum (apposition–resorption).

the foramen. This procedure results in localized paralysis and imbalance, hyperpressure on the opposite side due to the remaining, normal muscle function, and deformity in the coronal plane with convexity on the side of the paralysis.

Vertebral growth is controlled by evenly distributed, even weight-bearing that guarantees a proper sagittal contour of the spine. Tetraplegia, when it happens to a young child, modifies weight-bearing and disturbs natural growth. Vertebral height increases more in proportion than vertebral width, and the endplate becomes biconvex with reduction of the disc space (2). Similarly, following laminectomy, instability and anterior overload will slow the anterior growth, inducing kyphosis.

At the Level of the Entire Spine

Harmonious growth and its impact on the final sagittal contour are closely related to the development of proper standing posture. Starting with a global kyphosis at birth, a lumbar lordosis appears when the infant sits and stands. The lordosis becomes temporarily excessive before postural muscle balance has been completed. At this stage, genetically induced variations control the orientation of the L5–S1 inclination as well as the amount of thoracic kyphosis and cervical lordosis. The rate of growth plays an important role, mainly at puberty, when it reaches a peak.

Development of muscle balance, which shapes the spine of a child when he/she stands spontaneously, is missing in a paralyzed child, even when the child uses a brace parapodium. Impaired muscle function will always lead to spinal deformity, and hormonal factors at the time of puberty will cause the deformity to worsen.

SECONDARY DEFORMITIES

At the Level of the Lesion

Pathophysiology

The pathophysiology will depend on two factors: the first factor originates from the evolution of the bony and ligamentous lesions; the second factor evolves from the neural injury (spinal cord and roots), with or without progressive syringomyelia.

Evolution of Bony, Cartilaginous, and Ligamentous Lesions

Direct damage to bone, cartilage, and ligaments at the time of injury causes one aspect of the deformities. The initial lesion may involve only ligaments and soft tissues. In neonates or infants, these lesions cannot be detected on plain films, which may look normal.

The lesions occur more frequently at the cervical and upper cervical levels. Dislocation can happen with ligament, capsule, and/or disc injury but without fracture. Division of the cartilage and fracture of the growth plate can also appear, and coexist, with fragment rupture. Both bone and ligaments can be ruptured, presenting indeed as an obvious fracture with some dislocation, including a crushed and collapsed vertebral body. When plain radiographs fail to demonstrate the lesion and instability, stress radiographs (flexion and extension) may provide a decisive answer.

Each of these bone lesions has a specific evolution.

1. Complete healing with fusion of the damaged part of the spine occurs with good alignment or malalignment. If the initial injury has damaged the growth potential of the growth cartilage, deformity will progress.
2. The outcome is doubtful when ligaments and discs have "healed." Healing can be stable or unstable and, in many cases, will be insufficient, leading to chronic instability. This is most likely to happen after disc injury, which often never heals. This reality justifies careful evaluation of a local injury, even years after it occurred. The evaluation requires good quality plain and dynamic radiographs in all pertinent planes of the spine. CT and MRI scans will provide additional information regarding the spinal canal and neural content.

Plain radiographs may suggest the presence of spine instability if malalignment exists, the bone fragments are not in continuity, or healing is not homogeneous, that is, showing a mixture of bone and soft tissue healing. Dynamic radiographs may demonstrate abnormal motion. If the dynamic radiographs are normal, a hyperextension test done very slowly in the supine position may demonstrate real, abnormal motion. In some cases, the dynamic radiographs will be normal, but the other features, such as acute malalignment and nonhomogeneous healing at the injury site as well as severe deficiency of the posterior interlocking elements, may lead to the diagnosis of potential or chronic instability.

We can summarize the physiopathology at the level of the spine in four categories that are isolated but may be mixed.

1. Immediate instability will be demonstrated by dynamic radiographs that show real, abnormal motion that presents danger to the spinal cord. Typically, this case is represented by pseudarthrosis of the odontoid process.
2. Chronic or potential instability may present with negative dynamic radiographs, but there will be malalignment and nonpure bony fusion with a progressive deformity, mainly in the sagittal plane. The deformity is rarely in the frontal plane. It more often presents as a rotatory dislocation, especially at the junction of two spine segments that rotate in opposite directions, as happens in post traumatic kyphoscoliosis. A typical case of traumatic kyphoscoliosis is one in which an old fracture/dislocation occurred. But alignment was not reestablished, the disc was injured, and the posterior ligaments remained elongated or were destroyed. In such a case, minor or repetitive trauma due to microscopic pathological movements will increase the deformity until the instability becomes evident.
3. The initial injury disturbed the proper relationship of the growing cartilage and bone, or when only the growing cartilage was damaged. In the latter case, the deformity will continue to progress without instability and will create progressive compression of the spinal cord.
4. It is not infrequent to observe, in patients with permanent neurologic damage, a local, bony dystrophy that leads to the so-called "Charcot spine." In this instance, the three spinal columns may be involved in the dystrophic process, creating a genuine pseudarthrosis of the spine.

The second part of the spinal deformity at the local level of injury results from the local treatment, that is, laminectomy.

Laminectomy creates problems in children. In a child, a wide laminectomy with removal of facet joints, ligamentum flavum, and interspinous ligament at the same level will lead to progressive kyphotic deformity in 100% of cases. The laminectomy can augment the instability due to injury that is already present and that leads to a major, progressive deformity.

Very often, anterior decompression will address the anterior encroachment on the spinal cord better than a laminectomy can. When a posterior approach is necessary, reconstruction of posterior stability is mandatory. This can be accomplished by a laminotomy or by precise reconstruction, sometimes with instrumentation and fixation. Adequate external immobilization is also a possibility.

Evolution of the Spinal Cord and Nervous System Lesions

Nerve root lesions can be partial or complete, as in nerve root avulsion. If the root is stretched, elongated, or compressed, it can recover, and this recovery also may influence the "sublesional" pathology. Root recovery is of the utmost importance in the cervical spine, where recovery of the C4 root may allow diaphragmatic function and prevent permanent tracheostomy. Involvement of the bulbomedullary junction may cause development of major cardiac, respiratory, and autonomous reflex problems, leading to the need for permanent or quasipermanent respiratory assistance. In the thoracolumbar region, it is quite different if an L3 or S1 root recovers; the L3 root will provide quadriceps function and the S1 will provide gluteal function. Lesions of the meninges, such as dural ectasia or arachnoiditis, may cause more problems for neurologic recovery.

Similarly, lesions of the spinal cord can be partial or complete. In addition, syringomyelia may develop and increase neurologic deficit. The consequences of such nervous and spinal cord lesions are respiratory but may include cardiac complications: primary if there is involvement of the bulbomedullary junction, secondary if the complications are related to respiratory failure. Urinary and trophic changes also are of the utmost importance, so that orthopaedic management in conjunction with other medical specialties in a multidisciplinary approach are of the utmost importance.

Treatment at the Level of Injury

Treatment priorities are as follows.

1. Decompression of the spinal cord or cauda equina is essential, even at a late stage, especially if the lesion is partial. Following decompressive surgery, we have observed some recovery as late as 2 years after initial injury. The decompression should be realized according to the level and anatomy of the compression (i.e., anterior, posterior, lateral). MRI and CT scans can be more effective than myelogram in localizing the site of compression and will dictate whether decompression should be anterior, anterolateral, or with the combined anterior and posterior approaches.

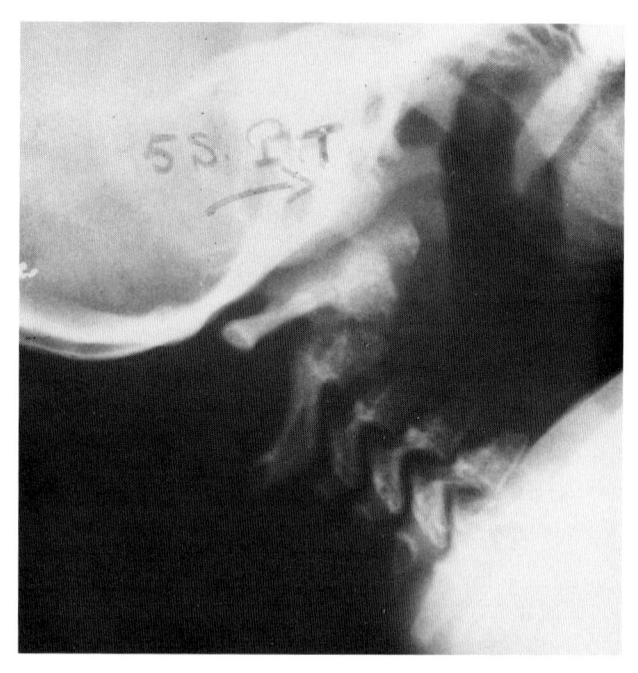

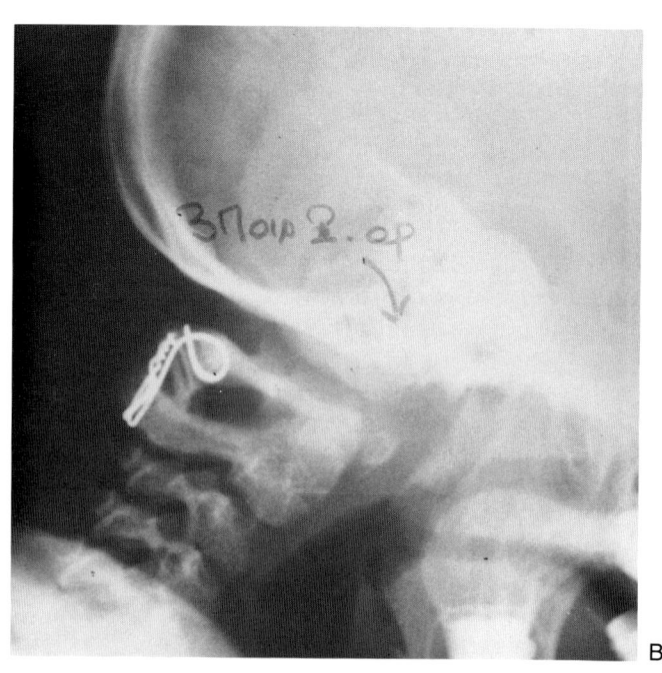

FIG. 2. A: Fracture dislocation of C1–C2 with post-traumatic hemiplegia seen 5 weeks after injury. **B:** Instability is cured by C1–C2 instrumentation and fusion. Perfect stabilization but no neurologic improvement.

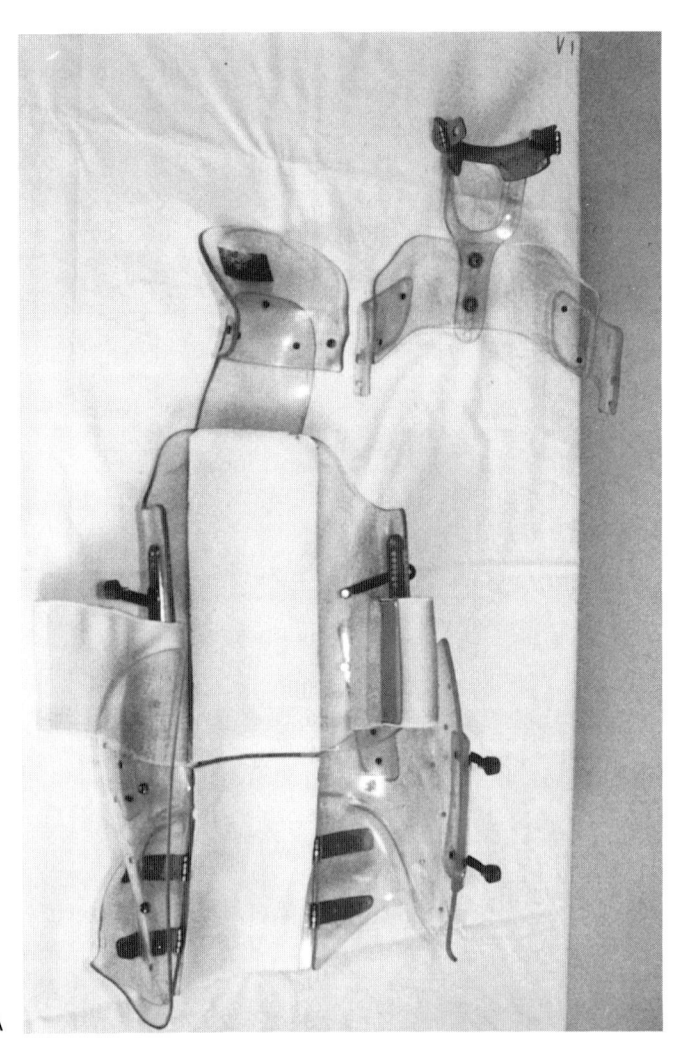

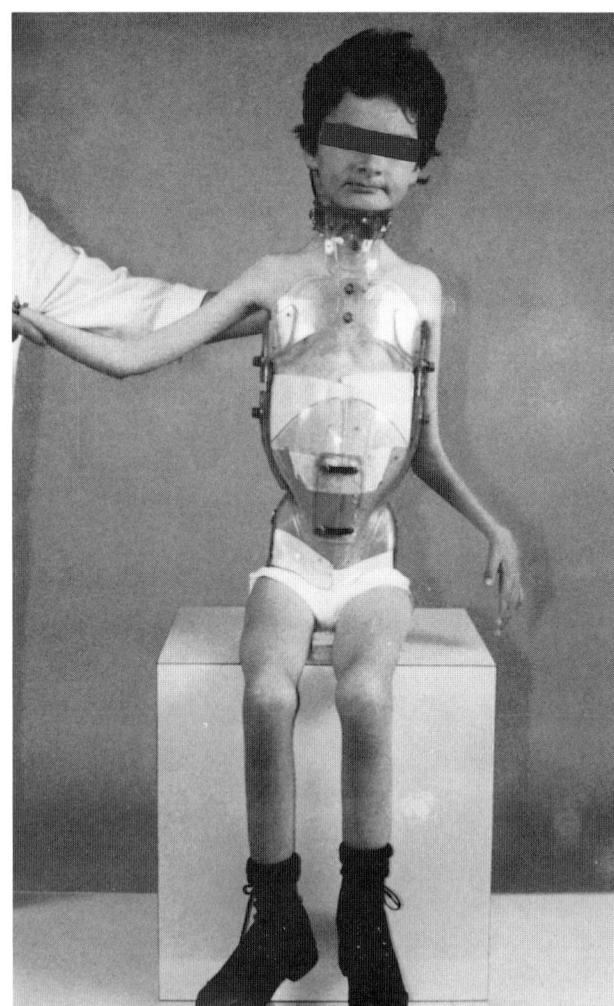

FIG. 3. A,B: The Garchois brace closed and open. In our department, it was found to be the best brace for a paralytic spine in a growing child.

2. Stabilization (Fig. 2) must be achieved at the time of decompression, or alone if decompression is deemed unnecessary because of use of instrumentation and fusion. In the case of an older child, strong spinal instrumentation is suggested. Cotrel–Dubousset (C-D) instrumentation is used for an adolescent of adult size; the pediatric size is used if the child is more than 4 years of age. In very young children wiring with fusion is the only possibility. In such cases, in which stability is not provided by the instrumentation, or when there is no instrumentation, we must use external stabilization with cast or halo cast/vest.

3. Fusion is the only way to achieve permanent stability. Fusion should be accomplished with autograft (iliac or tibial) and good decortication and should be done from the back and front in cases in which the lesion involves both sides of the spine.

In fact, anterior spine instability (disc, bone, cartilage) must be managed from the front of the spine, always trying to recover proper alignment (i.e., correction of kyphosis) and locking the fusion mass in concordance with the gravity axes. On the other hand, posterior instability must be addressed from the back, rebuilding the posterior elements with good posterior fusion. If the posterior elements are missing after laminectomy, bone for fusion can always be found at the lateral part of the spine (transverse processes or the lateral part of the remaining facets) to achieve the best possible circumferential fusion. This is also mandatory in the case of a Charcot spine in which both the front and back of the spine are damaged.

4. Prevention by proper reduction and management of the initial trauma during the stage of acute treatment is a priority. Prevention includes realignment of the spine and reduction; decompression of the cord if necessary, choosing laminotomy as often as possible instead of the classic laminectomy; and adequate immobilization with or without instrumentation and fusion.

5. Bracing difficulties and problems are major, especially when there is neurologic involvement. The difficulties stem from two sources: lost skin sensation leads to skin sores; and the collapse of the paralytic spine is

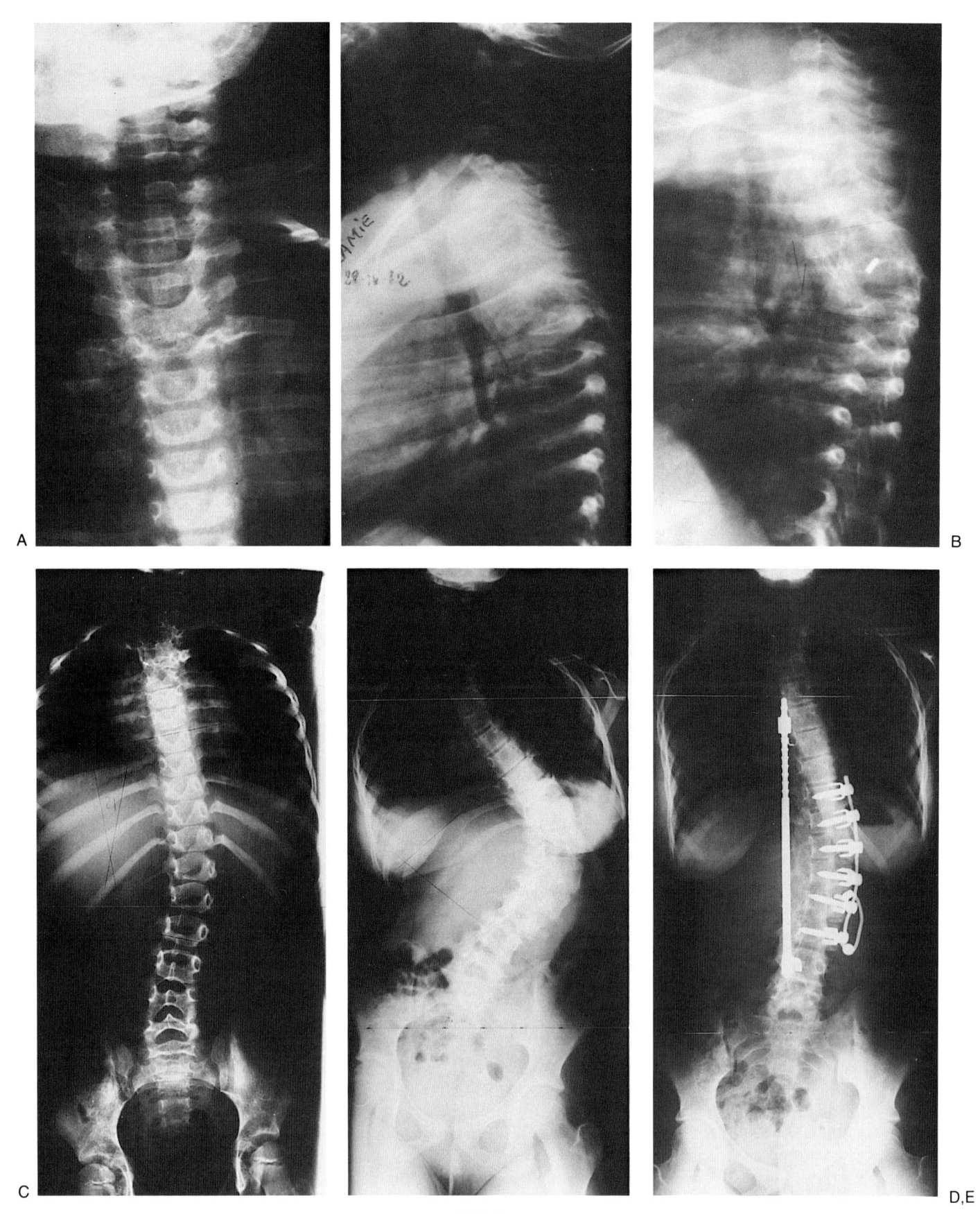

FIG. 4.

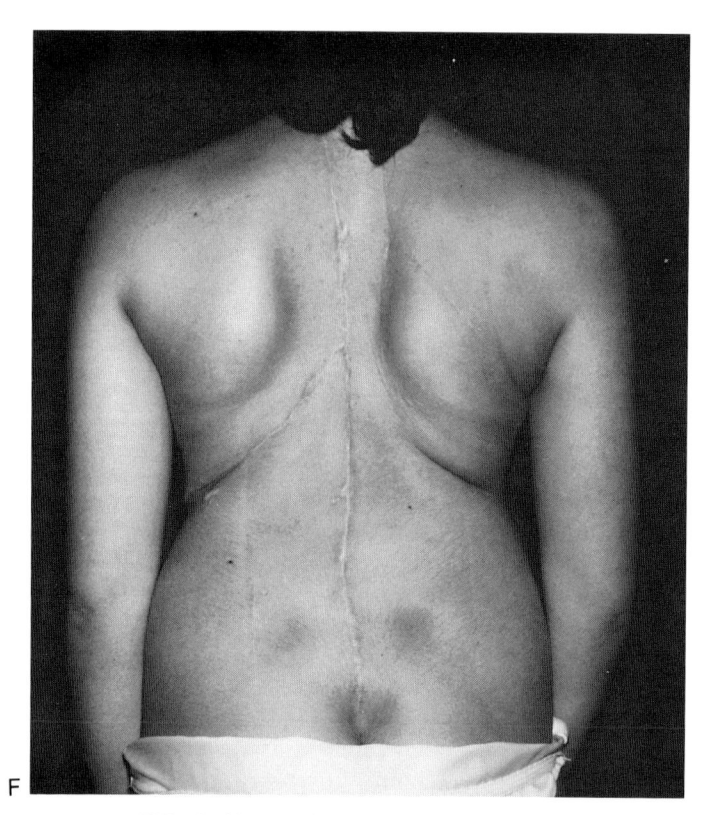

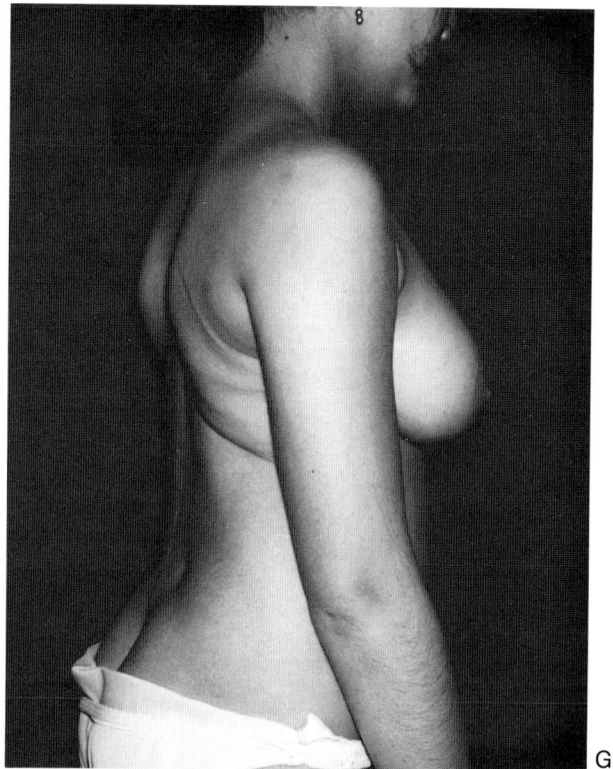

FIG. 4. Upper thoracic lesion at birth, with progressive paraplegia at age 5 months. **A:** Acute kyphosis, AP and lateral. **B:** Local treatment: anterior decompression and fusion, and posterior fusion. **C:** Sublesional paralytic spine: progression between the ages of 5 months and 6 years. **D:** Bracing: progression until 12 years of age. **E:** Final treatment: fusion and instrumentation at age 12; results at age 15. **F,G:** Clinical result at age 15.

pronounced when the lesion is located at a high level of the spine.

The Milwaukee brace has proved to be inefficient in these cases because the area of skin contact with the brace is too small. The thoracolumbosacral orthosis (TLSO) seems to be better, but it is difficult for parents to apply because of the elasticity required for correct brace fit; the paralytic child must be twisted when only one person takes care of him/her. In our experience, we have found the Garchois brace to be good. This brace opens like a book, allowing a perfect fit to be achieved by one caretaker. In addition, the volume and the rigidity of the material used to build the brace allow the best possible ventilatory and respiratory function (Fig. 3).

6. Finally, even with perfect local treatment at the injury level, we cannot avoid secondary progression of the deformity because of the growth of the spine.

SPINAL LEVELS BELOW THE LESION

The consequence of tetraplegia or paraplegia is a paralyzed spine below the level of injury.

Physiopathology

The paralytic spine may develop a deformity that is mainly scoliotic, kyphotic, or lordotic. This is caused by a mixture of paralysis, contractures, and collapsing factors at the level of the trunk (thoracic, thoracolumbar, lumbar, abdominal) muscles. As a consequence of gravity, we must recognize the importance of pelvic and hip contractures or paralysis, symmetrical or asymmetrical.

The prognostic factors for these deformities are as follows:

1. Relationship to age. The younger the patient, the worse the deformity. Deformities arose in more than 90% of the cases in which spinal and spinal cord trauma occurred before puberty, and in almost 100% when trauma happened at the neonate or infant period. Of course, we know the constant influence of the pubertal growth spurt; sometimes it may relieve the deformity but, more often, deformity increases (Fig. 4).

This problem should be taken into consideration in the planned course of management since, if the treatment of paralytic spines takes place before the end of growth, it is mandatory to perform anterior and posterior fusions. Otherwise, secondary deterioration due to the crankshaft phenomenon will occur with growth.

2. Relationship to the level of the cord lesion. Particular danger exists with cervical lesions, where tetraplegia above the diaphragm (C4) involving bulbomedullary function adds to paralytic problems of trunk, upper and lower limbs, and respiratory muscles such as the diaphragm. Other consequences are possible reflex and direct impairment of cardiorespiratory and temperature regulatory functions that, in turn, can cause major functional instability (tetraplegia, tracheostomy).

Specific danger also exists for lower cord lesions, where urinary problems are important considerations. Of course, fewer pulmonary and respiratory problems are present at this level. There are fewer functional problems with wheelchair management, which may actually improve. Walking ability will be variable, with or without callipers and braces, dictated by the level of injury and the number of the roots that remain functional.

3. Relationship to the type of neurologic disorder. Some cases are flaccid with hypermobility, leading to greater collapse of the spine, hip dislocation from time to time, and, according to orientation, either a significant lordosis or kyphosis. The consequences may be respiratory but more often will involve pelvic and urinary problems.

Many patients are spastic when asymmetry of the lesion and contractures lead to deformities in any plane. The most difficult is the associated asymmetry of the spine, pelvis, and hips, the so-called wind-swept deformity.

The majority have a mixed neurologic pattern: flaccid, spastic, and with dystrophic, bony or cutaneous problems.

4. Relationship to pelvic and trunk asymmetry and balance. The pelvic vertebra concept considers the entire pelvis as one unique vertebra, moving between the lower limbs and the spine. This concept is important in understanding pelvic obliquity, which may be due to:

a. Infrapelvic pathology related to the lower limbs, mainly hip joint asymmetry. We have to remember that, when we are seated, the sitting frame of the body is represented not only by both ischial tuberosities but also by the posterior aspect of both thighs. Therefore it is important to consider mobility, balance, flexion contractures, paralysis of the lower limbs, and, especially, knee and hip joints.
b. Suprapelvic pathology, which is represented by three-dimensional deformities of the spine, especially in the thoracolumbar, lumbar, and lumbosacral regions.
c. Finally, within the pelvis itself, deformity is represented by the progressive twist and structural deformity of the pelvis, conceptualized as one unique vertebra. The asymmetry of the pull of the muscle strength is able not only to displace the entire pelvis in three dimensions but also to distort the bone structure according to the various strengths and orientations of the deforming forces.

This leads to classification of pelvic obliquities, emphasizing the relationship and function of this pelvic vertebra between the spine and the lower limbs.

Sometimes the pelvis and the spine may displace in the same direction; this is called "regular pelvic obliquity." Other times they displace in opposite directions; this is called "opposite pelvic obliquity." The above considerations will determine the necessity for, and technique of, spine fusion to the pelvis.

Pathophysiology Summary

All these conditions produce three-dimensional deformities of the spine in which the lesional level must always be included.

A three-dimensional deformity develops at the level of the lesion, which may correct or increase the deformity below the level of the lesion.

Finally, the deformity always exists in three dimensions but is dominant in one plane:

1. Mainly frontal, with cervicothoracic or thoracolumbar scoliosis for spinal cord lesion below T4. In this plane, the pelvic obliquity is more important for patients not ambulating and for patients living in a wheelchair without a brace; and is increased by the asymmetry of the hip joint contractures and mobility and, without prevention, leads to considerable deformities with no possible sitting position.
2. For other patients, the major deformity is found mainly in the sagittal plane. The thoracolumbar or lumbar lordosis can arise from asymmetry between anterior and posterior muscles, weak abdominal muscles, active or spastic paraspinal muscles, weak glutei, and spastic or contracted hip flexors. The progression of the lordosis creates incorrect sitting balance, abdominal and pelvic pressure with urethral and urinary compression, loss of vital capacity and decrease of pulmonary function, and increased risk of sores on the sacrum. To compensate, the cervical spine becomes kyphotic.

This situation progresses through childhood and, when it becomes fixed, necessitates large, complicated, and dangerous surgery, potentially complicated by generally poor pulmonary function.

Finally, in other patients, lumbar or thoracolumbar kyphosis occurs mainly in a sitting position when hip flexion is limited partially by contracture of the glutei or hamstring muscles, but the deformity occurs mainly by the collapse of the spine. When established at this level, a compensatory thoracic lordosis also may occur, with consequences of worsening pulmonary function.

These collapsing kyphotic deformities can be corrected only by posture and bracing over a long period of time. However, usually they slowly become more fixed and require extensive surgery, both front and back.

To reiterate, sagittal deformity increases abdominal and thoracoabdominal compression and initiates pressure sores on the sacrum and even on the lumbar spinous processes. Sagittal deformity thereby impairs pulmonary function and the functional mobility of wheelchair-bound patients.

This evolution during childhood demonstrates the absolute necessity for *prevention* of the deformity.

Treatment

As we have seen, the first goal is early detection, prevention of evolution and the resulting progression of deformity.

Prevention and Early Treatment During Growth

Prevention addresses all elements responsible for the deformity.

The first goal is to preserve mobility, balance, and complete motion of the lower limbs if paralyzed. Prevention of asymmetrical contracture may be accomplished by stretching, manipulation, bracing, night splints, and weight-bearing, with or without braces. *Asymmetrical contractures* of the hip in all planes *must be prevented.*

Correction can be done with tenotomies, sometimes with osteotomies, to keep the femoral head centered inside the acetabulum. The goal is to retain as much symmetry and mobility as possible. Weight-bearing, with or without ambulation, is good for prevention of trophic disorders of bone and soft tissue.

It is most important to detect beginning asymmetry of the spine muscles and the concomitant beginning of scoliosis to prevent collapse of the spine. This situation must be prevented with appropriate bracing; we prefer the Garchois brace, with or without chin piece (Fig. 5). Simultaneously, care must be taken to control or

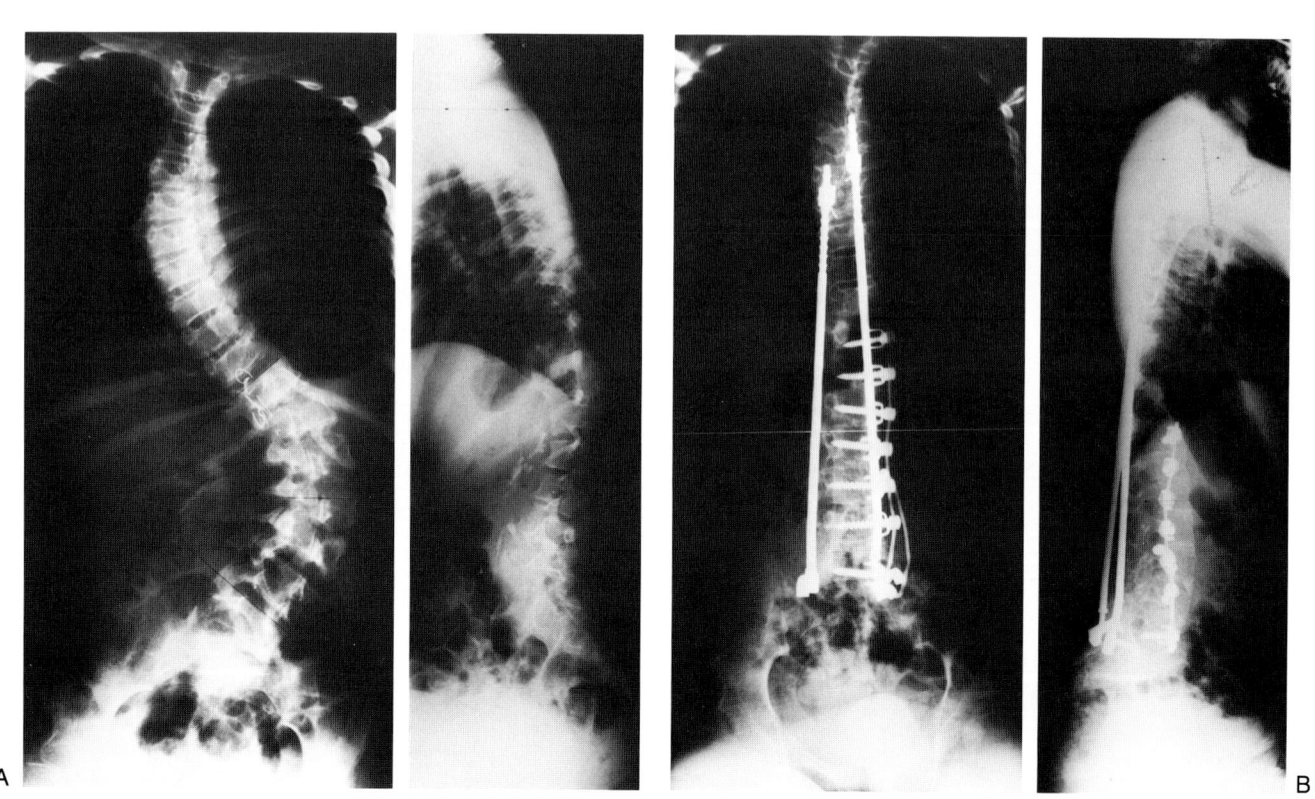

FIG. 5. A: Post-traumatic paraplegia occurred at age 5. T8–T9 fracture/dislocation with CSF fistula. Neurosurgical repair and wiring of the broken lamina. Bracing, with progression of paralytic scoliosis until age 12. **B:** Correction with Dwyer anterior and Harrington posterior instrumentation and fusion. Postoperative casting for 6 months. Roentgenographic result with 5-year follow-up.

correct any respiratory problems, with the aid of a breathing machine, such as a Bird if necessary.

It is very important to take precise care of the posture of the patient whether standing, sitting, or supine. If the sitting position is asymmetrical, the patient should be placed in a molded sitting brace. Prevention of contractures and asymmetry with physical therapy and treatment of spasticity (e.g., with local injection of alcohol at the neuromuscular junction) are necessary.

Control of the spine deformity may necessitate a surgical procedure, since nonoperative treatment may delay progression of deformity without stopping it completely. When the deformity is still progressing, we use subcutaneous rods without fusion in order to assist bracing. When rotation at the apex of the curve is too big and the deformity continues to progress, an apical anterior hemiepiphysiodesis may be indicated in conjunction with posterior subcutaneous rods and bracing.

Every 6 months to 1 year, a small surgery will allow distraction of the instrumentation to help guard against further collapse of the spine in any plane. The best method is realized with upper and lower claws composed of hooks, with a smooth rod between the claws to prevent too much soft tissue sclerosis.

This treatment often allows the patient to reach the pubertal growth spurt before the definitive spinal fusion is performed, with the patient in the best possible respiratory, nutritional, and functional condition.

Final Treatment: Indications and Techniques for Correction and Stabilization of the Paralytic Spine

After correction of possible deformities, contractures, and dislocation of the lower limbs, the goal is to maintain good hip joint congruency and mobility

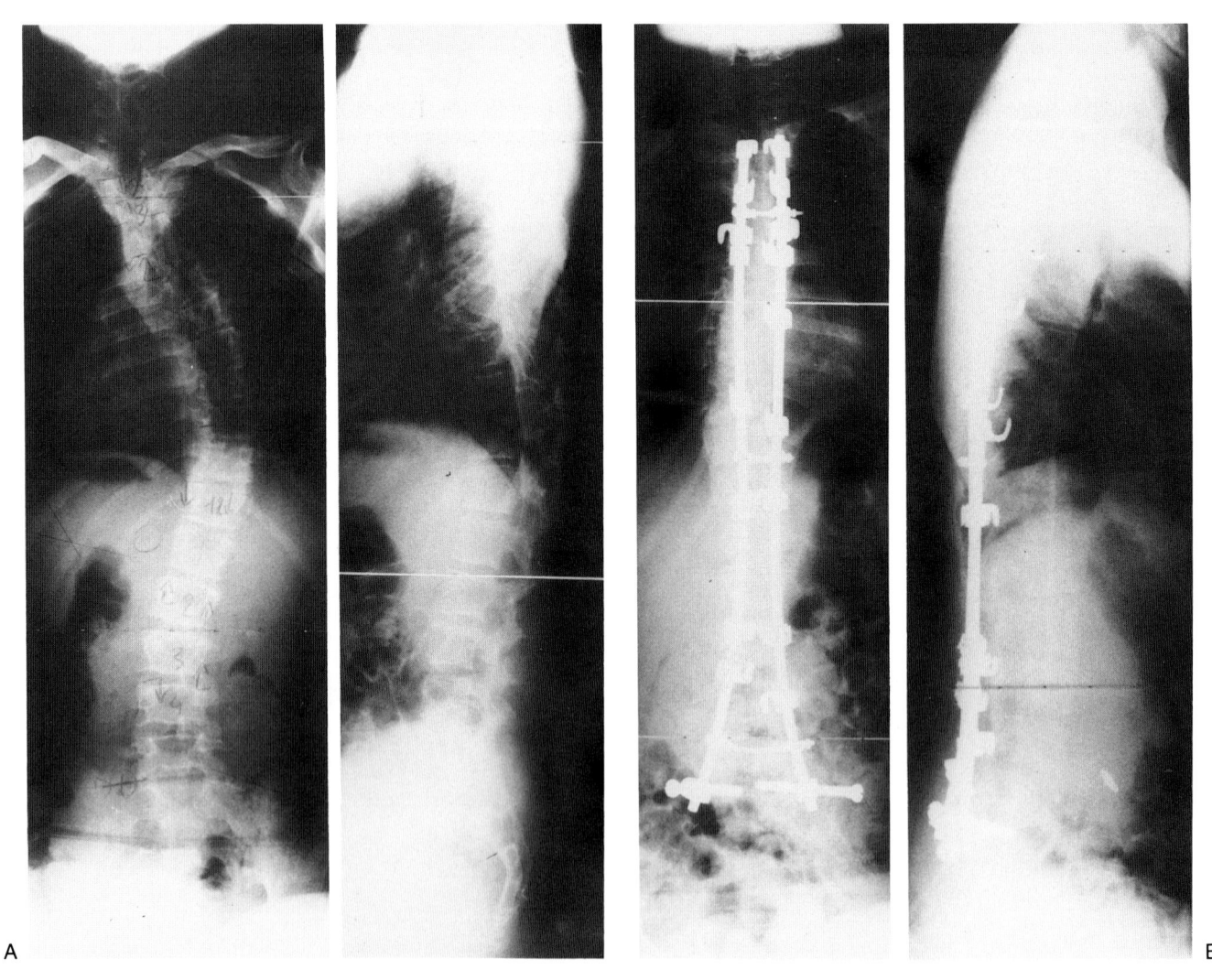

FIG. 6. A: Post-traumatic T4 paraplegia with kyphoscoliosis and collapse of the spine. **B:** Posterior reduction, stabilization, and fusion with C-D instrumentation. Anterior interbody fusion with tibial strut graft at the apex of the kyphosis.

without too much asymmetry, while the correction and stabilization of the spinal deformities attempt three goals:

1. Prevention of collapse and progression of deformity, which may continue even into adulthood. This requires a good spine fusion with sufficient extension to the proximal spine (thoracic or, sometimes, upper thoracic level).
2. Good position of the trunk to allow the best possible function in standing, if possible, or sitting position, most frequent. Good comprehension of the problem and a strategy to correct the pelvic obliquity are necessary.
3. Prevention of decrease in vital capacity and pulmonary function requires good cardiorespiratory pre- and postoperative management with a good, specialized medical team.

To reach these goals, the techniques must combine anterior and posterior surgery with fusion. As much as possible, postoperative immobilization, casting, and bracing should be avoided (Fig. 5).

Anterior surgery is mandatory when kyphosis remains after conservative treatment. If the kyphosis is angular, the anterior "palisade" with strut bone grafts is a good technique. If there is a predominant rotatory scoliosis, anterior convex apical releases and fusion are useful to prevent the "crankshaft" phenomenon in an immature spine. This is also a valid option for an adolescent (Fig. 5).

The posterior instrumentation is done with C-D instrumentation (Fig. 6), almost always with bone graft from the iliac crest or tibia. The fusion and instrumentation to the sacrum depend on the type of pelvic obliquity. The only case in which the pelvis is not included in the fusion and not instrumented is when, after correction of deformities below the pelvis and correction of the spinal deformity, the pelvic vertebra remains stable, mobile, and balanced in three dimensions both at rest and during motion. For all other cases, fusion to the sacrum is required.

In our hands, the best pelvic fixation for pelvic obliquity is achieved by the iliosacral screw with cylindrical Beurrier or "Cardan" hooks. The strategy for correction will depend on three-dimensional analysis of the relationship between the spine and pelvis. The goal is to rebuild the thoracic kyphosis and lumbar lordosis to provide height for the trunk, prevent collapse, balance the spine in three dimensions, and place the pressure point of the body in the best possible balance when the patient is in a sitting frame.

In planning such correction, one must address the deformity at the level of the lesion, which must be included in the overall spinal balance.

The final point of treatment must include care of the other parts of the body. For example, it must be remembered that spine instrumentation and fusion will give height to the trunk of a tetraplegic patient; this means that the distance from the hand to the mouth is increased. If the strength of the upper limbs is bad, the correction of the spine changes the use of these weak upper limbs, sometimes requiring external power to help the weak upper limbs function. Further rehabilitation may be required (e.g., after correction of thoracolumbar spine deformity) for urinary problems.

The final goal of all this treatment is to attain better function and social integration. This stage of treatment underscores the reason why treatment, from its earliest stages in the infant or child, must be addressed not only by one person but by a coordinated, multidisciplinary team that includes a neurosurgeon, cardiorespiratory, acute and chronic care physicians, an orthopaedic surgeon, a urologic surgeon, rehabilitation medicine personnel, a physical therapist, a brace maker, a general medical practitioner, and a social worker.

BIBLIOGRAPHY

1. Audic B, Maury M. Secondary vertebral deformities in childhood and adolescence. *Paraplegia* 1969;7:10–16.
2. Brandner ME. Normal values of the vertebral body and intervertebral disc index during growth. *Am J Roentgenol* 1970;110:618.
3. Campbell J, Bonnett C. Spinal cord injury in children. *Clin Orthop* 1975;112:114–123.
4. Hadley MN, Zabramski JM, Browner CM, Rekate H, Sonntag VKH. Pediatric spinal trauma: review of 122 cases of spinal cord and vertebral column injuries. *J Neurosurg* 1988;68(1):18–24.
5. Kewalramani LS, Tori JA. Spinal cord trauma in children: neurologic patterns, radiologic features and pathomechanics of injury. *Spine* 1980;5:11–18.
6. Lancourt JE, Dickson JH, Carter RE. Paralytic spinal deformities following traumatic spinal cord injury in children. *J Bone Joint Surg* 1981;63A:47–53.

# Thoracolumbar Fractures in Osteoporosis

Felicia Cosman and Robert Lindsay

Osteoporosis is a disease in which there is a reduction in bone mass accompanied by aberrations in microarchitecture that result in an increase in the risk of fracture.

It has been recognized over the past several years that osteoporosis is a major public health problem involving many countries. The disorder affects primarily postmenopausal women with increasing prevalence and incidence as age advances (141). As the society ages, the number of individuals at risk increases. For this reason, the magnitude of the osteoporotic problem can be expected to increase over the next 50 years.

Osteoporosis is only important clinically after fracture occurs with minimal or no antecedent trauma. The principal fractures that result from osteoporotic change within the skeleton are fractures of the vertebrae, femoral neck, and distal radius (Colles' fractures) although fractures at other sites also occur (26,58,115). While hip fractures are the most serious from a public health standpoint, vertebral fractures are the most frequent and most feared of the osteoporotic fractures. Postmenopausal patients attending specialty clinics for evaluation of their risk of osteoporosis cite vertebral fractures, with accompanying morbidity and changes in body configuration, over hip fracture when asked their particular concerns about osteoporosis.

EPIDEMIOLOGY

Reliable data about the epidemiology of osteoporotic fractures have been difficult to obtain. Only recently have epidemiologists become interested in the consequences of osteoporosis. Since hip fracture requires hospital admission in almost all instances, those fractures have been subject to study more than any other and considerable data are now available about hip fracture epidemiology. Approximately 250,000 hip fractures occur annually in the United States (26,58,115), associated with a high morbidity and a 5% to 20% excess mortality over age-matched individuals during the year after the occurrence of the fracture (28). Both morbidity and mortality increase with age at fracture. Since hip fracture almost always requires hospital admission and surgical intervention, it is a major acute health care expense in the elderly ($5–10 billion in 1985 dollars) (27). Hip fracture is also a common precipitant of admission to a nursing home or other chronic care facility, further increasing the cost of osteoporosis to society. As the population ages, the total number of hip fractures can be expected to increase, doubling by early next century. In addition, some considerable data, mostly of European origin, suggest that there is also an increase in the age-specific incidence of hip fractures. Health care costs for hip fracture alone have been predicted at $16 billion by the year 2040 (27).

In contrast, there are only limited epidemiological data concerning osteoporotic vertebral fractures. In part, this is due to the lack of agreement on the precise definition of vertebral fracture. Additionally, the asymptomatic nature of many radiological abnormalities detected on routine spinal radiographs contributes to the lack of epidemiological data (61,119,140). Finally, even symptomatic vertebral fractures often cause modest morbidity and no mortality, rarely require hospital admission, and therefore are difficult to detect and track in the population. Estimates of prevalence of vertebral fractures, not surprisingly therefore, vary markedly, ranging from 5% to 70% depending on the population studied and method of evaluation, among other factors (62,80,117). Vertebral fractures are undoubtedly the most common of the osteoporotic fractures. Falls do not play a major role in vertebral

---

F. Cosman and R. Lindsay: Department of Medicine, Regional Bone Center, Helen Hayes Hospital, West Haverstraw, NY 10993; and Columbia University College of Physicians and Surgeons, New York, NY 10032.

fracture occurrence, and specific traumatic incidents are often not elucidated by the patients. Normal everyday repetitive stresses, which exert compressive loads on the vertebral bodies, can produce fracture (96,151).

It has been suggested that younger patients (5–15 years postmenopausal) are more likely to present with marked vertebral compression and severe pain (141). Older patients are often found to have apparently relatively painless, multiple wedge deformities that may affect as many as 80% of the population (62,80,117). This makes the assessment of true incidence difficult. The most recent data utilizing the unique record linkage system in Rochester, Minnesota, indicate that vertebral fracture incidence increases from 84:100,000 person years at age 50 to 1452:100,000 person years at age 85 and older (22). Curiously, the estimated overall sex ratio in that study suggested a female to male predominance of only 2:1, similar to that seen for the femoral neck. This differs substantially from other reported estimates where female to male ratios are cited as 8–10:1 (62,80,117).

Vertebral fracture prevalence varies in different geographical locations. In North Dakota, regions where water fluoride content is naturally high have shown a lower rate of vertebral fracture than low fluoride regions in the same state (10).

Extrapolation from prevalence data reveals that around 60% of vertebral fractures remain undiagnosed during the year of occurrence. In fact, the data from Rochester, Minnesota suggest that approximately 5 million women in the United States will have vertebral fractures each year, but only 83,000 will seek medical attention (22). Few data have carefully evaluated differences in distribution of vertebral fractures by race, although in clinic populations, vertebral fractures are rare among black women.

Colles' fractures are also more common than hip fractures and may cause considerable morbidity for some individuals but have a negligible mortality and, because hospitalization is rarely required, have a low financial cost to society (26).

INTERRELATIONSHIPS AMONG FRACTURES

It is well known that patients presenting with one type of osteoporotic fracture often have another. Vertebral fractures are several times (perhaps as much as 10 times) more common among patients presenting with hip fracture compared with the general population. Moreover, additional vertebral fractures are much more common in those presenting with pre-existing vertebral fractures (144a). Patients presenting with vertebral fractures also have a similarly high risk (five times greater) for hip fracture (62,80,117). Despite this relationship, *most* patients do not present with new fractures at other sites and it is therefore inadequate to use a history of fracture (e.g., Colles' fracture, which occurs on average 10–20 or more years earlier than hip fractures) to predict a future hip fracture. Bone mass measurement can be used to predict overall risk of future fracture for these patients (*vide infra*).

PATHOPHYSIOLOGY

Bone mass at any point in adult life is the algebraic sum of the skeletal mass accumulated during growth and the mass of skeletal tissue subsequently lost during aging. The accumulation of skeletal mass is dependent primarily on genetic factors (37,51,105,131,152,159), but the capacity to reach that potential is dependent on a variety of extrinsic factors (Table 1). These include nutrition, especially calcium and caloric intake (83,108,109), life-style, especially physical activity (2,5,29,83,123), and intercurrent illnesses, especially those resulting in prolonged immobility and paralysis (70,120,175). Peak skeletal mass is achieved at around 20 to 30 years of age, and bone mass subsequently changes only modestly if at all prior to the gradual decline in ovarian function that precedes the overt menopause. The menopause, the failure of ovarian function that occurs ubiquitously among women at the average age of 51 years, is the single major event of public health importance, causing loss of skeletal tissue among aging women (101). The effect of menopause is compounded by a wide variety of proposed risk factors, each of which can increase the rate or duration of bone loss (Table 2). These include premature hypogonadism (prior to menopause), endocrine disorders, certain chronic medical disorders, drugs, and life-style factors, most importantly smoking and alcohol ingestion (4,7,12,25,26,31,33,38–42,45,50,52,64,67,71,79,81,88,106,110,116,127,138,149,153,154,159,163,169). In addition, since most nonvertebral osteoporotic fractures also require some degree of trauma as a precipitant (26,58,77,115), falls (Table 3) (6,17,66,132,135,168), which also increase with age (6,17,66), add to the risk of osteoporotic fracture.

TABLE 1. *Factors controlling peak bone mass*

Genetic: Sex
　　　　　Race
　　　　　Familial factors
　　　　　Disorders such as Turner's syndrome or Klinefelter's syndrome
Calcium intake during youth
Physical activity or inactivity during youth
Gonadal function or dysfunction
Other life-style factors (e.g., smoking, alcohol intake)

TABLE 2. *Factors causing increased bone loss*

Premature hypogonadism
  Early age of menopause
    Oligomenorrhea/amenorrhea
      Exercise induced
      Anorexia nervosa
      Hyperprolactinemia
  Low testosterone in men
    Hyperprolactinemia
    Idiopathic
    Anorexia nervosa
Other endocrine disorders
  Cushing's syndrome
  Thyrotoxicosis
  Insulin-dependent diabetes mellitus
  Primary hyperparathyroidism
Lifestyle
  Smoking
  Alcohol consumption
  Thin body habitus
  Immobilization/inactivity
  Dietary
    Low calcium
    High protein, caffeine, sodium, fiber
Drugs
  Glucocorticoids
  Excessive thyroid hormone
  Antiepileptics
  Chemotherapy
  Heparin (prolonged use)
Systemic diseases
  Gastrectomy
  Malabsorption
  Chronic liver disease
  Chronic renal disease
  Chronic obstructive pulmonary disease
  Some hematologic/neoplastic diseases
    (lymphoma/leukemia/multiple myeloma
    mastocytosis/hemochromatosis)
  Radiotherapy (localized)

Bone Remodeling

Bone is a vital tissue that undergoes a continuous remodeling process that is necessary preventive maintenance (126). Although the control of bone remodeling is as yet inadequately understood, the process itself has been well defined from a variety of histological studies (126,128). The remodeling sequence is discrete in both time and space and is performed by a team of cells often termed a basic multicellular unit (BMU). The surface of bone at rest is covered by a thin layer of unmineralized tissue, which in turn is covered by a layer of cells thought to be resting osteoblasts, or surface osteocytes. In the *activation* of remodeling (171), these cells appear to contract, exposing the surface underneath to the adjacent bone marrow in cancellous and endocortical bone. These cells may also be responsible for preliminary digestion of the unmineralized lining tissue. The control of this activation step is unknown. Mineralized bone, the underlying remaining surface, appears to be chemotactic for osteoclasts, the multinucleated giant cells of the monocyte–macrophage series responsible for bone resorption. A team of osteoclasts (often called pre-osteoclasts before fusion occurs to convert them to mature osteoclasts) is recruited to the remodeling site. These cells adhere closely to the surface of bone creating a microenvironment between the cell and bone interface. The osteoclasts secrete hydrogen ion and a variety of enzymes into this space, creating an acid environment with the capacity to digest collagen. Thus both mineral and organic matrix are removed by these cells. Each team of osteoclasts appears to remove a predetermined amount of bone, creating a Howship's lacuna in cancellous bone and a cutting cone in cortical bone. The *resorption* phase lasts approximately 2 months and bone is removed to an average depth of 31 μm in cancellous bone (137).

At the end of the resorption period, the osteoclasts disappear from the bone surface (their fate is unknown) and are replaced by mononuclear cells whose function appears to be to prepare the surface for bone formation, including perhaps the secretion of a substance that becomes the cement line seen in biopsy speci-

TABLE 3. *Factors altering risk of falling*

Intrinsic	Extrinsic
Acute illness	Lighting
Postural hypotension	Glare
Neurologic disease	Excessive shadows
Parkinson's disease	Floors
Hemiparesis	Rug
Alzheimer-type	Trailing cords
dementia	Small objects (litter)
Cognitive disorders	Waxed surfaces
Vision	Stairs
Hearing	Lighting
Vestibular function	Rails
Proprioception	Contrasting steps
Musculoskeletal disorders	Adequate repair
Muscle weakness	Kitchen
Slow gait (senile gait)	Cupboards within
Medications	reach, etc.
Sedatives, tranquilizers	Bathroom
Hypotensive agents	Grab bars: showers,
Diuretics	toilets, baths
Anticonvulsants	Nonskid floor on
Alcohol	shower
Hypoglycemic agents	Shower chair
	Footwear
	Form-fitting shoes
	Nonskid
	Outdoors
	Ice, snow
	Terrain uneven
	Tools, etc.
	Lighting

mens. This process, in which resorption reverses to formation, is known as the *reversal* phase. Active osteoblasts are recruited to the surface and proceed to synthesize collagen, which is organized extracellularly into fibrils. Other noncollagenous proteins are also synthesized by these cells including osteocalcin, osteonectin, and osteopontin (14). The matrix is subsequently mineralized extracellularly in a poorly understood process. The phase of *formation* and mineralization takes about 200 days but varies in normal individuals from 70 to 600 days (171).

Osteoblasts synthesize a variety of potential local regulators of cell function including IGFs, TGF-β, prostaglandins, and interleukins (134). Osteoblasts have receptors for hormones responsible for calcium homeostasis including PTH and $1,25(OH)_2D$ (134) and probably also sex steroids (48,90). Thus osteoblasts have the capability to be the controlling influence over the bone remodeling system. Osteoclasts have receptors for calcitonin and perhaps also for estrogen but no demonstrable physiological response has as yet been observed to hormones other than calcitonin (171). Interleukins, prostaglandins and TGF-β may all be local modulators of osteoclast activity. Factors that control the amount of bone resorbed, the linkage of formation to resorption, and the amount of bone formed at each remodeling site are not understood.

Role of Menopause

Prior to menopause, at each remodeling site, the amount of new bone formed is approximately equal to the amount of bone that is resorbed (126). That is, there is a balance in each remodeling unit and bone mass remains essentially stable. Following menopause, at each remodeling site more bone is removed than is subsequently formed (164). Thus there is net loss of bone

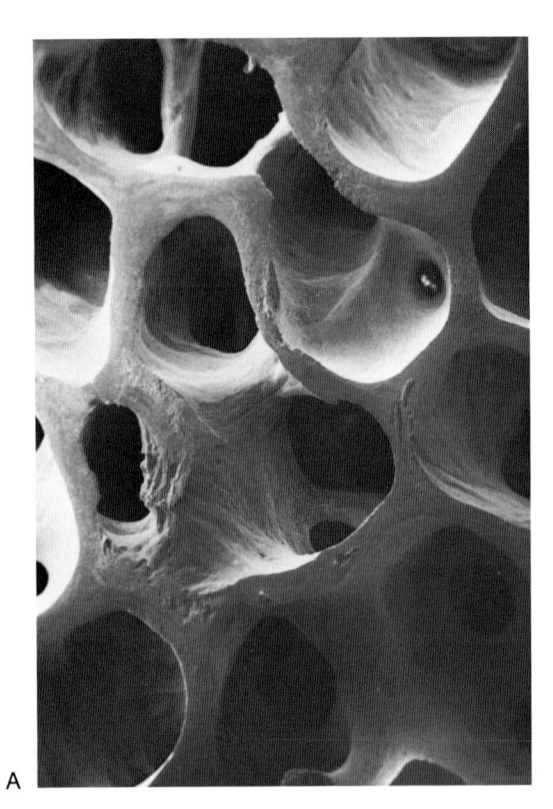

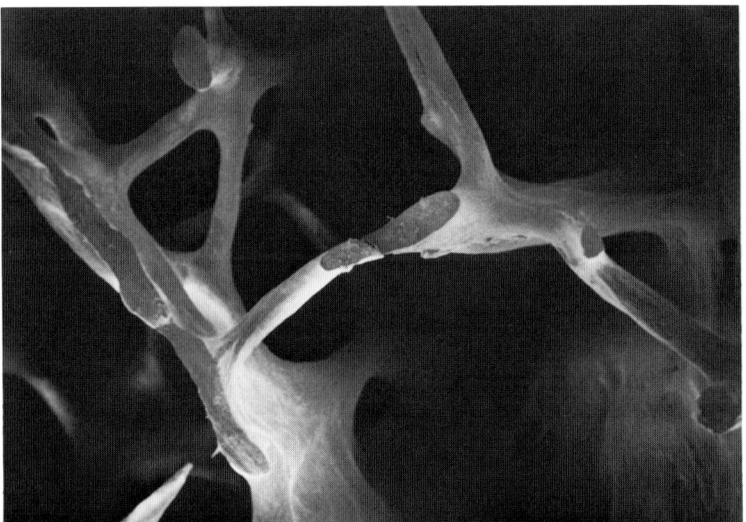

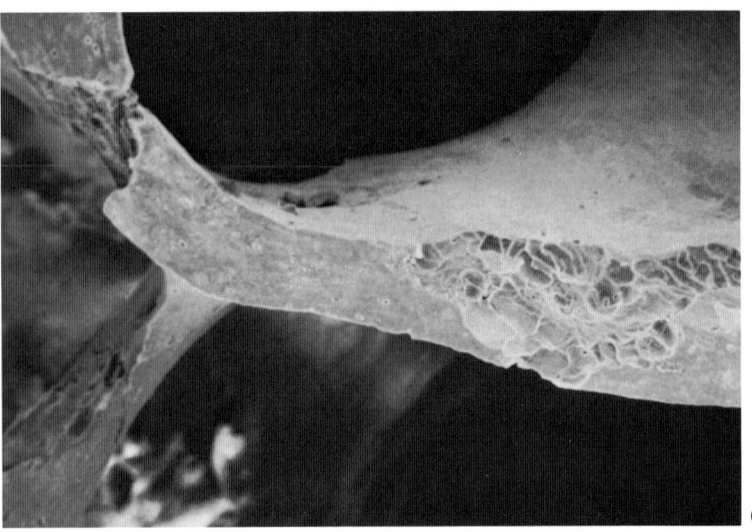

FIG. 1. Electron micrographs of trabecular bone taken from iliac crest biopsy specimens in normal **(A)** and osteoporotic **(B)** individuals. (From ref. 36.) **C:** A trabecular plate perforated in two areas by intense osteoclastic bone resorption. (From ref. 35.)

at each remodeling site. In addition, there is increased activation of new remodeling sites with an overall increase in bone turnover, resulting in a potentially rapid phase of bone loss (164). Increases in biochemical indices of bone turnover, including urine calcium and hydroxyproline, and serum calcium, alkaline phosphatase, and osteocalcin (101,165), confirm the increased remodeling rate. Kinetic studies show an increase in calcium movement into and out of the skeleton at menopause, but the transmenopausal increment in movement of calcium from the skeleton is greater, confirming the net loss of bone tissue (73,74).

The changes in skeletal homeostasis that occur at menopause are likely to be intrinsic alterations in skeletal homeostasis caused by the decline in estrogen secretion by the ovary, perhaps in part mediated by increased sensitivity of the skeleton to the effects of parathyroid hormone (PTH) (24,69). At the same time, there appears to be a decline in renal sensitivity to PTH with reduced production of $1,25(OH)_2D$ (57,170). The consequence of the latter is a well-documented decline in intestinal calcium absorption (57). Increased bone turnover and imbalance within individual remodeling units lead to a net loss of bone mass. The rate of loss is greatest in the first few years after cessation of ovarian function (111,122,143).

Sudden cessation of ovarian function such as premenopausal ovariectomy or use of GnRH superagonists might result in an even more dramatic loss of bone (165). Loss of ovarian function, irrespective of cause, including amenorrhea secondary to excessive exercise (42,95,104,106,145), anorexia nervosa (13,142), or hyperprolactinemia (89,91,125,148), results in loss of skeletal tissue. Bone mass is also reduced in Turner's syndrome (8) (ovarian agenesis), where ovarian function is absent or deficient.

Since bone remodeling occurs primarily on bone surfaces, the rate of bone loss is greatest in cancellous bone, which has a higher surface to volume ratio than cortical bone. Using quantitated computed tomography (QCT), average annual rates of loss are about 5% in the cancellous bone of the vertebral body (59). Annual rates of loss are somewhat lower (2–3%) when measurements of entire vertebrae (including posterior, predominantly cortical elements) are made using dual photon absorptiometry (DPA) or its derivative, dual energy x-ray absorptiometry (DXA) (1,62,122,143).

At menopause, increased remodeling activation frequency appears to be accompanied by an increase in the activity of each osteoclast team, resulting in larger resorption cavities and therefore a greater chance that the osteoclast team can perforate through individual trabeculae (126). Puncturing a trabecula in this fashion (Fig. 1) (35,36) destroys the template on which new bone can be formed. Consequently, since formation cannot follow resorption in that perforated area, there is acceleration in net loss of bone tissue as well as permanent changes in trabecular architecture. Once trabeculae are fenestrated in this fashion, further action of osteoclast teams creates rods from trabecular plates, and eventually eliminates these rods. In vertebral bodies, there is preferential loss of horizontal trabeculae and relative maintenance of vertical trabeculae, as shown in Fig. 2. The reason for this is not entirely clear, but it is presumed to be related to the greater axial stress on the latter units. The same imbalance of remodeling in the endocortical surface results in erosion of the cortex, a process often referred to as trabecularization of the cortex (Fig. 3) (34).

Age-Related Bone Loss

In addition to the effect of the menopause, bone loss also appears to occur as a phenomenon of increasing

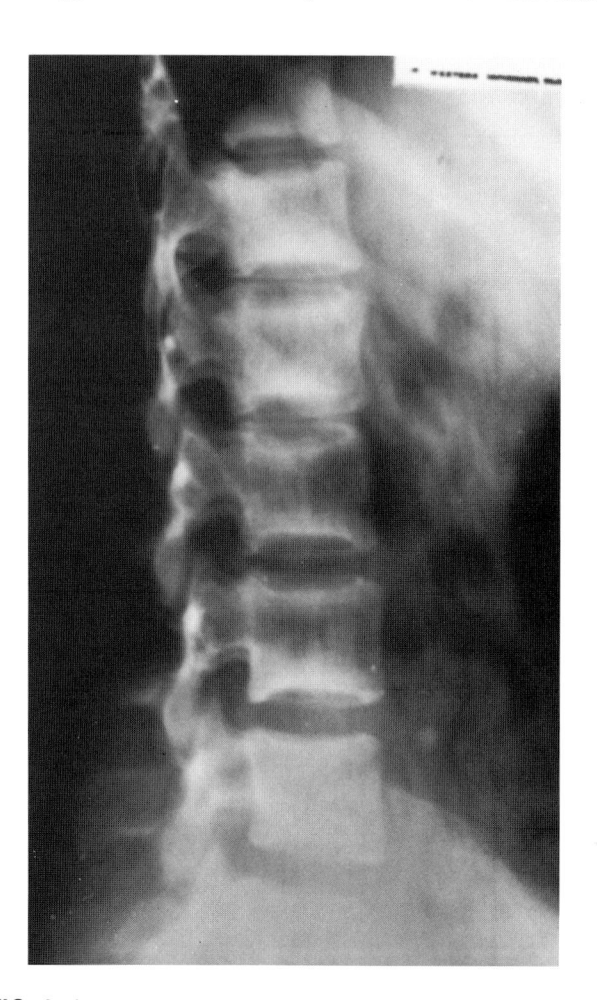

FIG. 2. Lumbar radiograph of a patient with osteopenia but no compression fractures. Note the prominent longitudinal markings representing vertical trabeculae, caused by a loss of reinforcing horizontal trabeculae, which commonly occurs early in vertebral osteoporosis. Note also the prominent vertebral endplates, a sign seen frequently in steroid-treated patients and other metabolic bone diseases such as renal osteodystrophy.

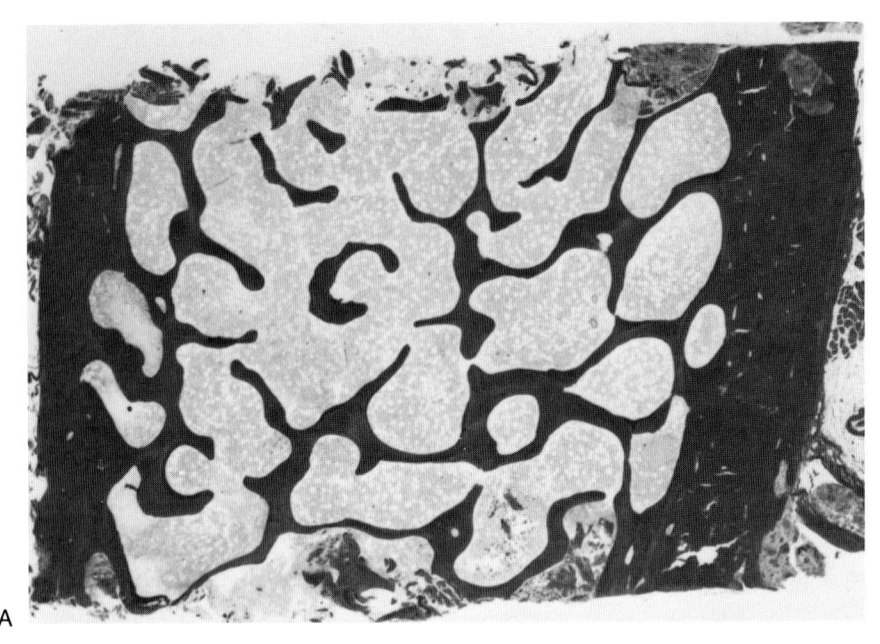

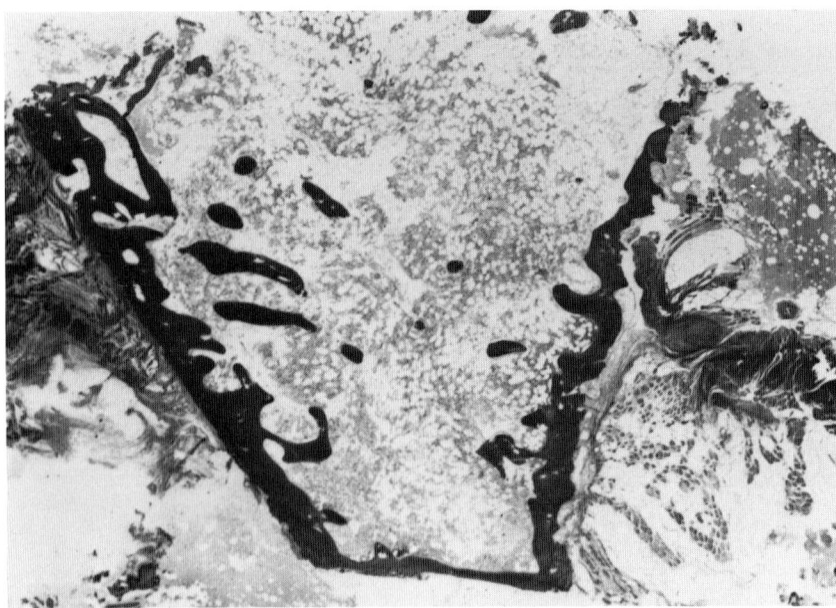

FIG. 3. Iliac crest biopsy specimens showing normal cortical structure in normal **(A)** but thinned **(B)**, eroded, perforated cortex, known as trabecularization, in an osteoporotic patient. Also note the marked reduction in cancellous bone volume. (From ref. 34.)

age and affects both sexes (111). In this case, the rate of loss is slower than that affecting women in the early years after menopause. The mechanism also seems to be different. In age-related bone loss, there appears to be a reduction in the amount of bone synthesized by teams of osteoblasts at each remodeling site but probably not enhanced activity of osteoclastic bone resorption (126). There is thus a small negative balance at each site with gradual thinning of trabeculae and cortex. The cause of this alteration in osteoblast function is not clear. It may be related to declining physical activity with age, increased frequency of nutritional calcium deficiency, or secondary hyperparathyroidism as the kidney fails to produce adequate amounts of $1,25(OH)_2D$ with increasing age and diminution in renal mass and function (44,118).

CLINICAL FEATURES

Clinically, osteoporosis often becomes apparent when a fracture occurs on minimal trauma and vertebral crush fracture is considered the hallmark of postmenopausal osteoporosis. Vertebral fractures occurring in this way are often discovered on routine radiographs. The percentage of patients who actually present with an acute fracture as stated above is not known but could range from 1% to 40%. In some patients there is sudden acute severe pain at the time of fracture, localized to the approximate site of fracture, sometimes with lateral radiation (55). The incident precipitating the pain can be extremely trivial, such as bending, stretching, lifting, or stumbling (55,94). Paravertebral muscle spasm is common and may be severe. In some patients distension of the capsule leads to a paralytic ileus with associated nausea, anorexia, abdominal pain, and constipation. The pain gradually subsides, persisting only for a few days or up to 8 weeks. Tenderness can often be elicited at the site of fracture. Neurological signs are rarely, if ever, seen in an uncomplicated osteoporotic fracture. It is possible that the pain is related to the suddenness of the episode and in those whose fractures develop more gradually, symptoms are often less severe. After the acute episode, pain may disappear completely or be replaced by a dull ache. This secondary pain is related to abnormal stretching of the posterior ligaments and paraspinal muscles and is less well localized. The pain is aggravated by the erect posture and relieved by rest. The symptoms become gradually worse as the day progresses with some patients complaining that their back feels "tired" and that they find it difficult to maintain the erect posture.

Patients experiencing gradual compression of multiple vertebrae, particularly of the wedge variety, may present with significant height loss or an exaggerated thoracic kyphosis or "dowager's hump" (Fig. 4). These patients may complain of lower back pain incited by an exaggeration of the normal lumbar lordosis, which occurs to compensate for the anterior displacement of the center of gravity caused by the exaggerated thoracic kyphosis (55). When multiple fractures have occurred, patients may exhibit pain in the lower chest area or, more specifically, in the lower ribs or flanks bilaterally. This is usually caused by pressure and irritation induced by the close contact between lower ribs and iliac crests occurring as a result of the loss of vertebral height, which maintains a physical space between these structures. This discomfort, like the muscular pain associated with the changes in body configuration,

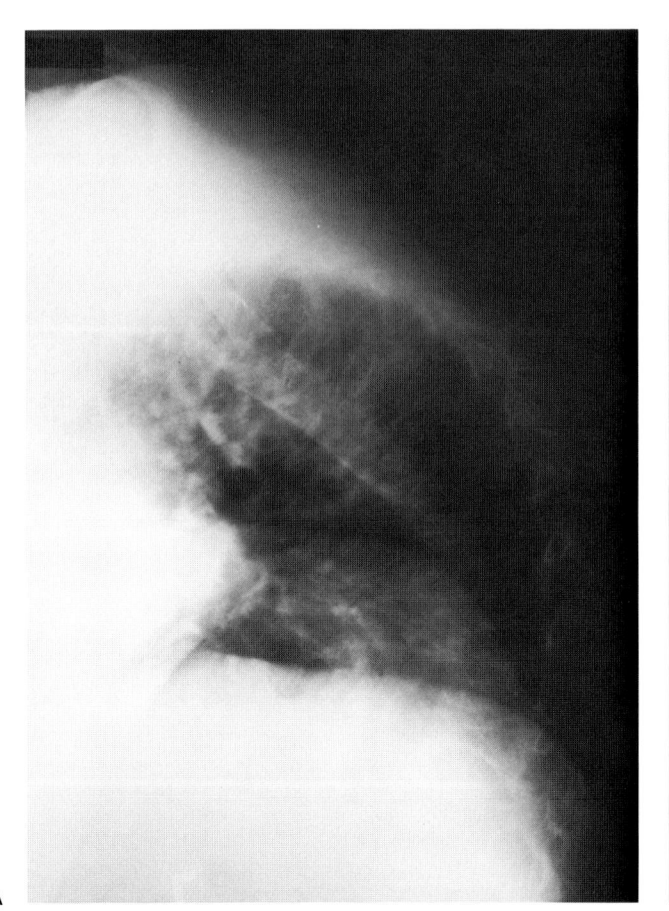

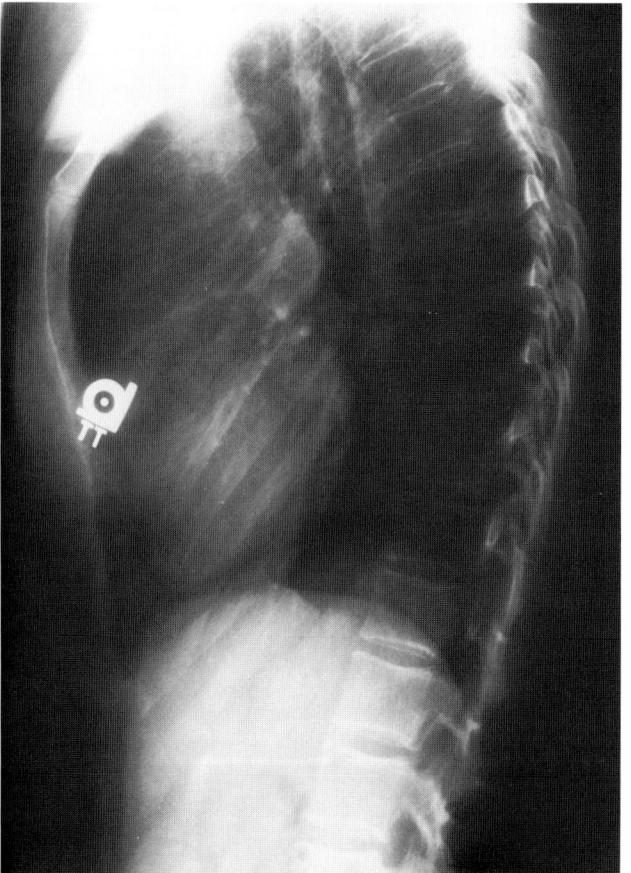

FIG. 4. A: Multiple thoracic vertebral deformities and an extremely exaggerated kyphosis in this man with severe osteoporosis. This patient lost 18 in. of height over an 18-month period. **B:** Normal thoracic spine.

is often worse after standing during the day and improves when the pressure between the structures decreases, in the supine position.

RADIOLOGY

Vertebral deformities are often detected in asymptomatic patients on routine radiographs. An inexact definition of the normal features of vertebral geometry results in confusion and disagreement about the definition of vertebral fractures (43,76,121,158). Vertebral bodies vary in size, being related both to overall height and the position of the vertebral body in the spinal column (32,56). The shape of each vertebral body also depends on its position in the chain. The normal thoracic kyphosis results in vertebral bodies that have anterior heights less than their posterior heights, particularly in the upper and middle thoracic regions. At the lumbar level, anterior and posterior heights are approximately equal. The shape of thoracic vertebrae may be a consequence of modeling of the bone in response to greater pressure exerted on the anterior surface of vertebral bodies in the erect posture. Consistent with this hypothesis is the finding that in quadrupeds, anterior and posterior vertebral heights appear equal throughout the thoracolumbar spine. In humans, an increase in this natural wedging might be expected with age and may contribute to the high prevalence of such findings on routine radiographs of the elderly, but insufficient data have been published to confirm this. There is, however, clearly an increase in what most would call vertebral "deformity" with age and it is possible that at least some of these deformities are produced by gradual shape changes as vertebral bodies model their shape in response to stress and therefore are not true fractures.

The simplest and most widely used method of determining the presence of vertebral fracture is assessment of a true lateral radiograph (centered on midthoracic or midlumbar vertebrae to reduce problems created by parallax; see Fig. 5). Qualitative assessment may result in significant disagreement among readers (43,76, 121,158). Semiquantitative assessments have been used to obtain a spinal fracture (or deformity) score (124,147), which has been used to assess the severity of osteoporosis. The more quantitative evaluation of vertebral shape has been applied by some groups mainly to classify patients for entry into clinical re-

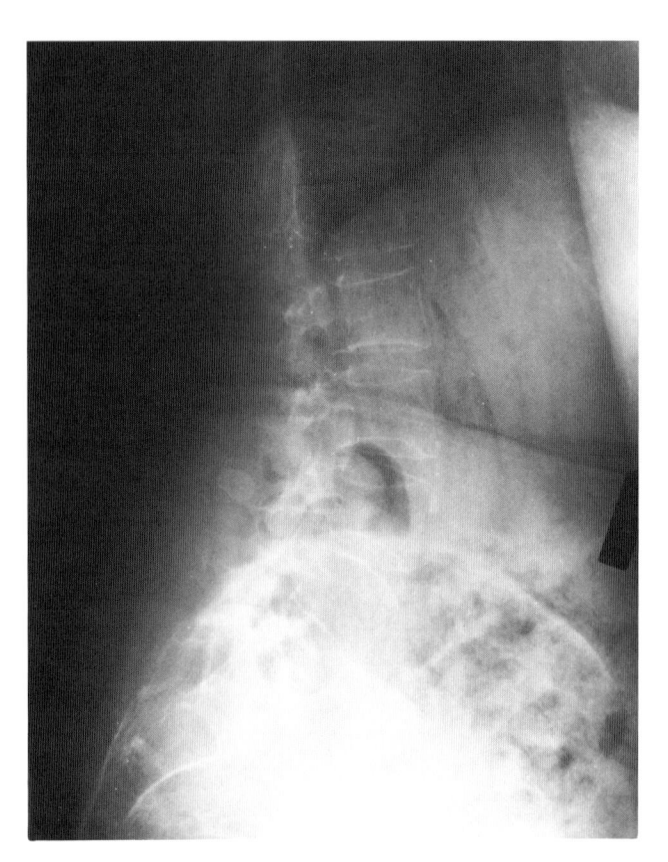

FIG. 5. Osteopenia and moderate wedge type abnormality of T12. Note apparent biconcavity of lumbar vertebrae caused by parallax of x-ray beam most prominent at L3–L5. These vertebrae are actually normally shaped.

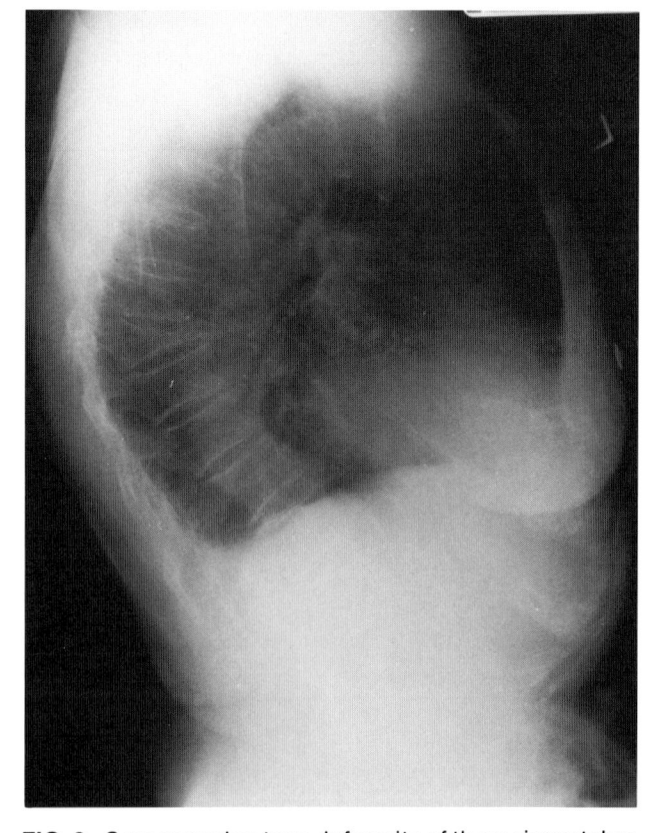

FIG. 6. Severe wedge type deformity of thoracic vertebra, nearly flat at the anterior surface. Also seen is some hypertrophic lipping anteriorly, confirming the existence of both osteoporosis and spinal osteoarthritis in this patient.

search studies, and to record "fracture" frequency as patients progress through clinical trials. Such techniques can also be used to evaluate individual patients in routine practice and are briefly described here.

Most techniques for classification of vertebral deformity use measurements of anterior height, posterior height, and the height of the central portion of the vertebral body, either as absolute measures or in a variety of calculated ratios related to each other or to measurements of neighboring vertebrae (32,43,56,76,121,124, 147,158). Where normative data are available, these have usually been obtained for radiographs of similar populations as the study population but in people without the presence of overt crush fractures as defined by an experienced radiologist (32,56). This may not be the most appropriate method of defining normality. Examination of radiographs using an age-matched population might underestimate the alterations in vertebral geometry due to osteoporosis as subjects with anterior vertebral body modeling would be included in the "normal population." Evaluation of vertebral bodies from lateral radiographs of young adults would provide normal vertebral morphometry at a point prior to the onset of age-associated modeling and thus provide what could be considered the closest to perfection for each vertebral body. This would by necessity, however, result in higher estimates of vertebral deformation in any older population.

In general, wedge fractures refer to vertebrae where the anterior height is substantially reduced with normal posterior height (Fig. 6), crush fracture refers to a reduction in both anterior and posterior height (Fig. 7), and biconcave fractures (Fig. 8) show a reduction in the central vertebral height with normal anterior and posterior dimensions.

Although there is variation in the location and prevalence of fractures depending on the population studied, with increasing numbers of fractures, there is a greater likelihood of fractures involving both anterior and posterior heights (75). Crush fractures are most common in the lumbar region and wedge fractures most common in the midthoracic to lower thoracic regions (75).

Schmorl's nodes, which are sometimes thought to be pathognomonic for osteoporosis, are cartilaginous intervertebral disc herniations into the substance of the vertebral body (Fig. 9). This can be caused by any abnormality of the vertebral endplate or weakness of the subchondral bone and thus can be seen in various metabolic bone diseases in addition to osteoporosis and can also be seen in infection or malignancy.

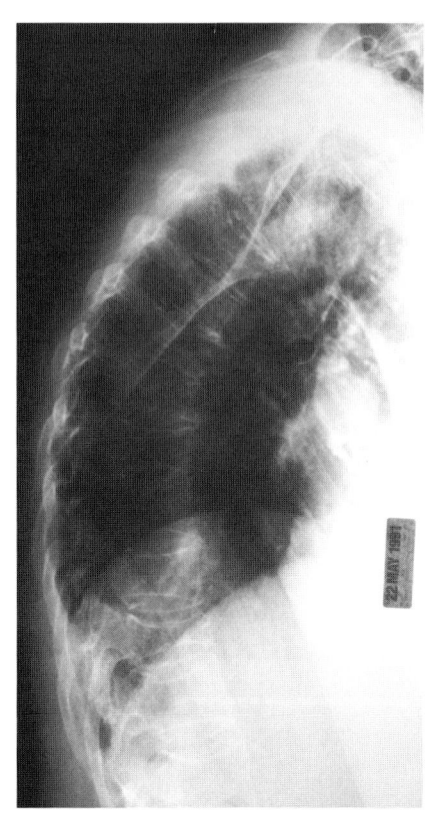

FIG. 7. Multiple thoracic vertebral deformities are visible with crush type deformity of T12 in this 65-year-old woman with postmenopausal osteoporosis.

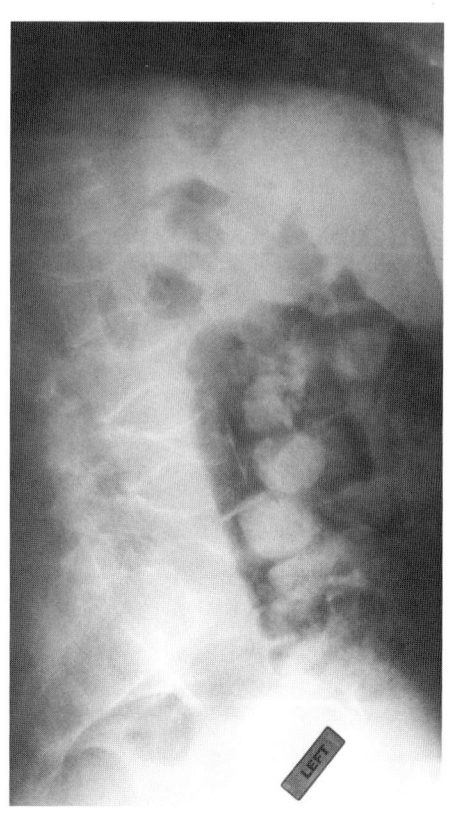

FIG. 8. Multiple severe biconcave deformities of the lumbar spine.

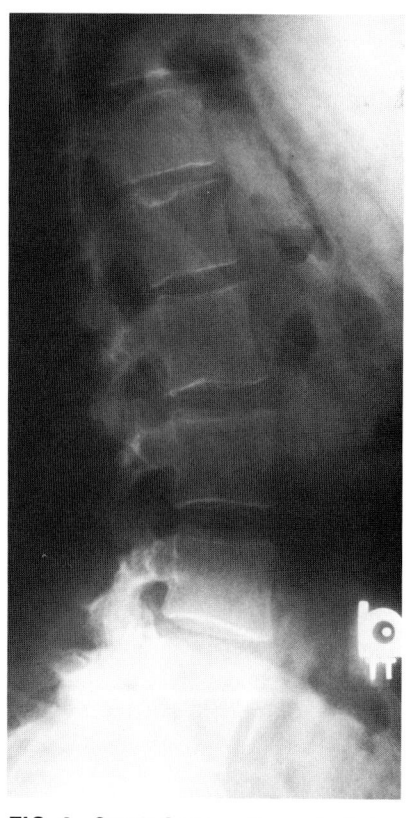

FIG. 9. Small Schmorl's node (intervertebral disc herniation into vertebral body) into posterior superior aspect of L1.

DIFFERENTIAL DIAGNOSIS

The most common cause of vertebral fractures is osteoporosis but other conditions including old trauma, malignancy, and other metabolic bone diseases can also cause vertebral fractures and must be distinguished from osteoporosis since treatment and prognosis depend on the correct primary diagnosis.

Occasionally, an apparently asymptomatic fracture is seen in a postmenopausal female who by bone density criteria does not have osteoporosis. Often such a fracture may be the consequence of long forgotten trauma, often in childhood or young adolescence. In such patients, a radionuclide bone scan will be negative, since scans remain positive only for 1 to 2 years after the incident.

Metastatic disease can produce a fracture that can be mistaken for an osteoporotic fracture, especially among elderly individuals. The inclusion of the posterior aspect of the vertebral body, especially when involved to a greater extent than the anterior, the extension of the lesion to the pedicles, or neurological compromise necessitates an evaluation to rule out malignancy. Occasionally, hematologic malignancies can present as general rarefaction and vertebral collapse. This is especially true of multiple myeloma, which must be considered in every patient presenting with vertebral crush fracture.

Osteomalacia only rarely in the United States presents as vertebral crush fracture. The radiological findings when present are distinctive but may mimic osteoporosis. The cortical and trabecular surfaces have indistinct surfaces, and other evidence of excessive resorption due to secondary hyperparathyroidism may be present. Incomplete fractures (Looser's zones or Milkman's fractures) are common in osteomalacia but are not pathognomonic for this condition (18,46,107), as they can also be found in Paget's disease, renal osteodystrophy, and osteoporosis. In osteomalacia, the vertebrae may be biconcave, but they are often uniformly biconcave unlike in osteoporosis. Intracortical tunneling resorption classically occurs in secondary hyperparathyroidism associated with osteomalacia and renal osteodystrophy and may best be appreciated by a hand radiograph. The most common form of osteomalacia is that associated with nutritional vitamin D deficiency, to which the elderly, the infirm, and the institutionalized are particularly susceptible. The biochemical findings are distinctive, with low serum phosphorus, low normal serum calcium, high alkaline phosphatase, and low serum 25-hydroxyvitamin D level. The presence of a mild nutritional vitamin D deficiency may coexist with osteoporosis, since both are relatively common in the elderly age group. Whether the existence of such vitamin D insufficiency exaggerates the problem of osteoporosis is not clear as yet.

Renal osteodystrophy (84,144) occasionally presents with vertebral crush fractures. The radiological findings are distinctive with a classical pattern of sclerosis and lucency in the vertebral bodies to which the term "rugger jersey" spine has been attached. Secondary hyperparathyroidism is often extreme in this condition, and the other traditional radiological and biochemical signs are present. Renal osteodystrophy is associated with extremely high levels of PTH particularly when C-terminal assays are used, since those larger peptides are retained in the circulation in renal failure. Circulating $1,25(OH)_2D$ levels are usually low or undetectable.

Crush fractures are occasionally seen in patients with Paget's disease (11). The classical radiological and bone scan appearances of Pagetic lesions usually differentiate the disorders (Fig. 10). The classic radionuclide scan may not be differentiating, however, since increased uptake can be found in recently fractured vertebrae from any cause or Paget's disease without compression (Fig. 11).

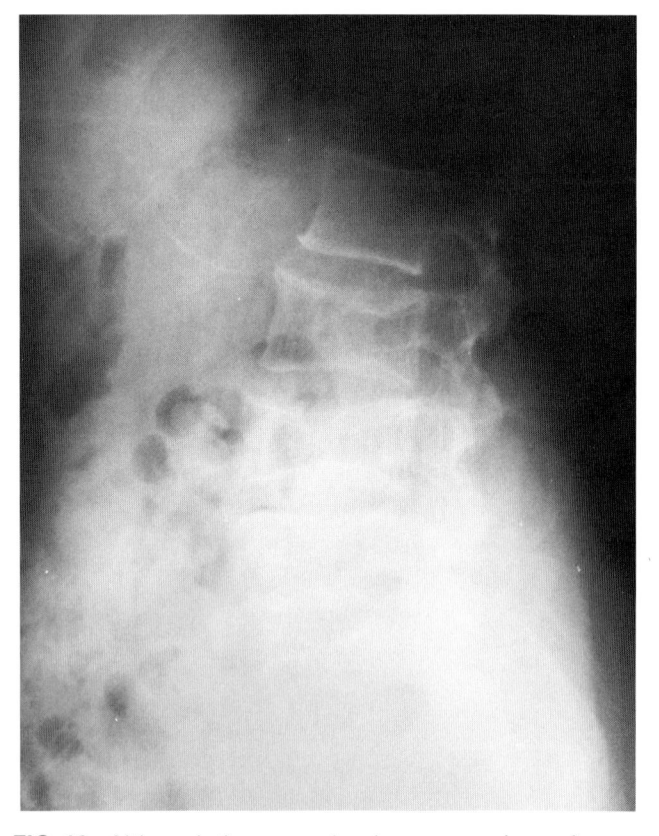

FIG. 10. Although there are clearly compressions of varying degrees in L3–L5, note the expanded anteroposterior diameter in these vertebrae. This patient has Paget's disease, not osteoporosis.

THORACOLUMBAR FRACTURES IN OSTEOPOROSIS • 349

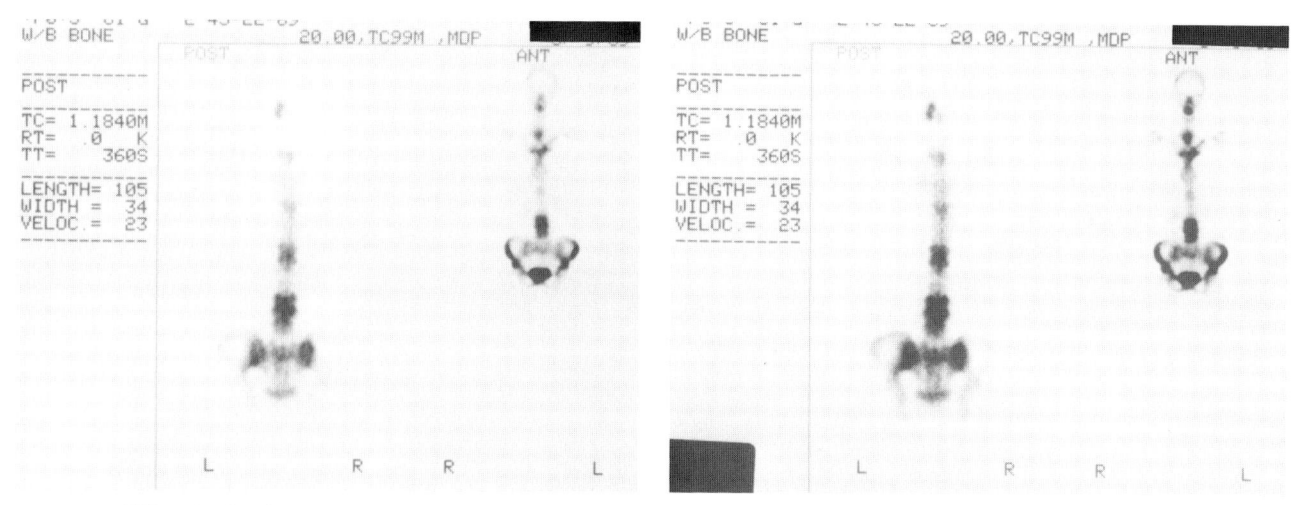

FIG. 11. Radionuclide bone scan showing multiple areas of increased uptake in both the lumbar and thoracic spine representing recent osteoporotic compression fractures. Increased uptake can be present up to 12 months after a fracture so precise dating of the incidents cannot be determined.

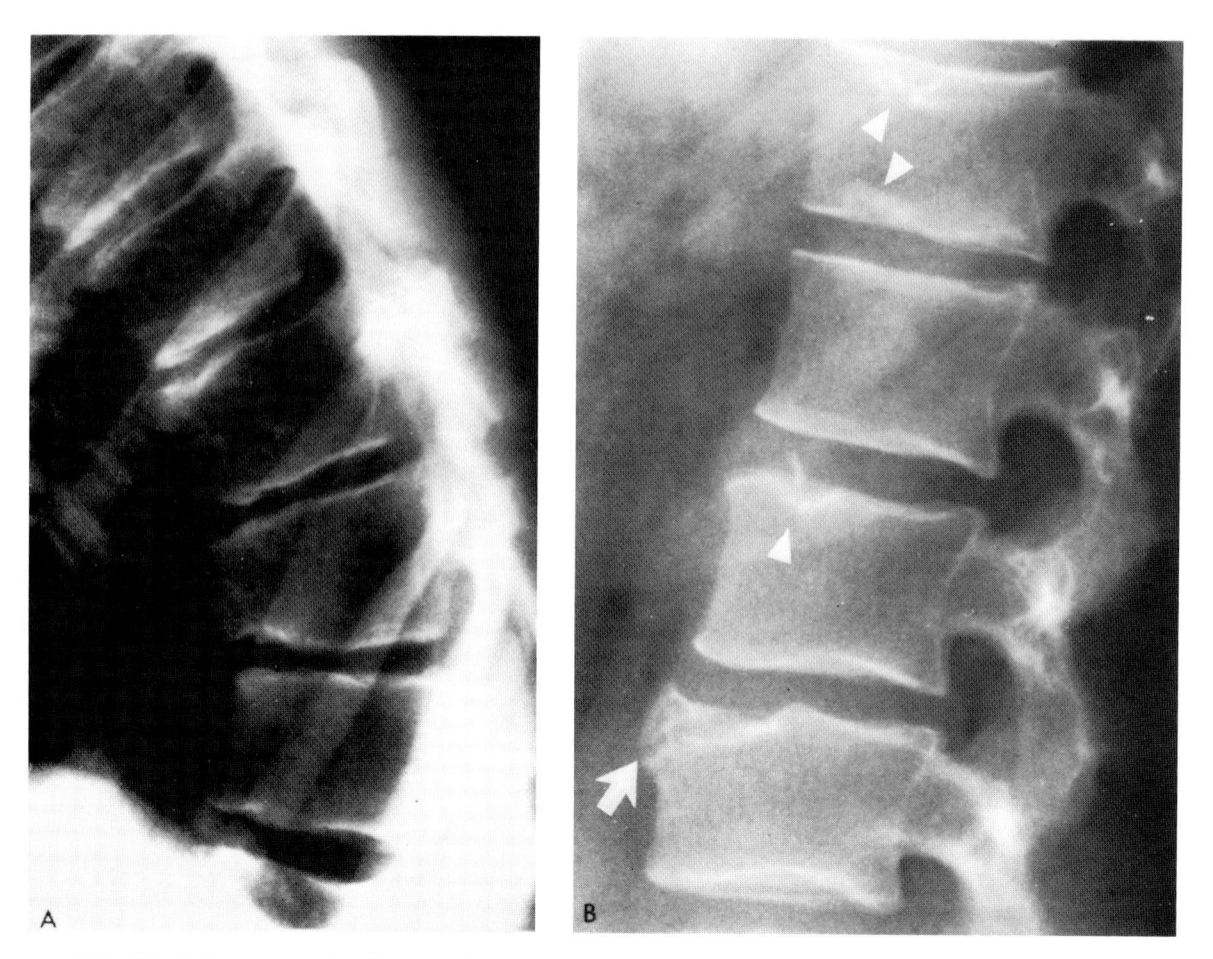

FIG. 12. Scheuermann's disease. **A:** Irregular vertebral contour with some reactive sclerosis, intervertebral disc space narrowing, and anterior vertebral wedging in thoracic spine. **B:** Lumbar spine showing several lucent cartilaginous nodes with resultant surface irregularity. An anterior discal herniation of the lowest vertebra shown has produced an irregular anterosuperior corner. (From ref. 139.)

In primary hyperparathyroidism, as it presents today, crush fractures are uncommon (129). This disorder is now seen as a relatively mild biochemical disease, readily cured by surgery or estrogen therapy and without significant morbidity in many cases even if not treated at all. In addition, the relatively small increments in circulating PTH do not appear to have the same detrimental effects on cancellous bone and there is little if any loss of vertebral substance (130,176).

Osteogenesis imperfecta (21,155) may present with vertebral fractures but often other fractures, affecting parts of the skeleton with large cortical components, are more common in this disease. A mild adult form of osteogenesis imperfecta may be difficult to diagnose except by fibroblast collagen assay, as many of the classic phenotypic characteristics such as blue sclerae and deafness may be absent. Osteogenesis imperfecta, when present in women, predisposes to osteoporosis since bone mass is compromised.

Patients with Scheuermann's disease or juvenile kyphosis (Fig. 12) (139) may have clinical and radiologic appearances suggestive of osteoporosis but this disease occurs most commonly during the teenage years and the abnormalities when patients are seen as adults have been longstanding. Schmorl's nodes and decreased intervertebral disc space are often seen in this disease secondary to an abnormality causing weakness of the vertebral endplate. Abnormal vertebral shape is also often seen due to dysfunction of the endplate as well as abnormal vertebral growth induced by cartilaginous node herniation within the vertebral body (139).

Osteoporosis itself occurs as both primary and secondary types. Primary osteoporosis is considered to be that associated with ovarian failure at the time of menopause or advancing age. The former is the most common type of osteoporosis and was described best by Albright some 50 years ago (101). Bone loss occurring with increasing age is the second most common form. Secondary osteoporosis is that which occurs with some clear insult other than menopause or age, the most common being the exogenous administration of glucocorticoids. Other medications such as excessive doses of thyroid hormone, immunosuppressants, and cytotoxic agents are also known to exacerbate osteoporosis. Various chronic medical conditions in which vertebral fractures can be seen as part of generalized osteoporosis are listed in Table 2 (4,7,12,25,26, 31,33,38–42,45,50,52,64,67,71,79,81,88,106,110,116, 127,138,149,153,159,163,169).

THE USE OF BONE MASS MEASUREMENT

The development of noninvasive techniques for the estimation of bone mass has improved the evaluation of patients thought to be at risk for osteoporotic fracture and the management of patients with known vertebral abnormalities (82). Several techniques are available for estimation of bone mass including dual and single energy absorptiometric techniques and computed tomography (CT). The commonly used techniques are listed in Table 4, together with some of their characteristics (59,82,112). All methods essentially rely on the differential absorption of radiation by bone in comparison to soft tissue. This allows calculation of the amount of skeletal tissue present in the path of radiation transmitted through the region. Currently, most techniques use monochromatic sources of x-rays, but isotope techniques have also been used with some considerable success.

The original technique described was single energy photon absorptiometry (SPA), a technique that uses an isotope source, usually iodine, to provide a stream of photons that are allowed to pass through a segment of the body. The energy of the photons, and the fact that only a single energy is released by iodine (112), allows measurement only of the appendicular skeleton, which has only modest soft tissue covering. The region of interest must be immersed in a soft tissue equivalent material (usually water) to provide a constant path

TABLE 4. Bone mass measurement techniques

Type	Site measured	Exposure to radiation	Precision error	Accuracy error	Time required
Single photon absorptiometry	Radius Os calcis	<15 mrem	1–2%	4–5%	10–15 min
Dual photon absorptiometry	Lumbar spine Hip Total body	<5 mrem	2–4%	3–6%	30 min 20 min 45 min
Dual x-ray absorptiometry	Lumbar spine Hip Total body Wrist	2–4 mrem	1%	3–6%	9 min 8 min 20 min 10 min
Quantitative computed tomography	Spine—vertebral body only	100–300 mrem	1–3%	5–10%	15 min

length of simulated soft tissue. Consequently, SPA has been used primarily to measure the radius, but other bones such as the metacarpal, calcaneus, and humerus have been measured. The technique is precise, involves a low radiation dose, and can be used repeatedly in the same individual. The major problem is that the standard site of measurement, consists of a high proportion of cortical bone (112). Under most clinical conditions, the changes that occur in primarily cortical bone are too slow to allow calculation of rates of loss of bone tissue within a useful time frame (154).

Dual photon absorptiometry (DPA) is a similar technique that uses gadolinium as the source of photons. Gadolinium emits a spectrum of radiation, which can be separated into two specific energies. The presence of two energies allows corrections to be made for alterations in the amount of soft tissue in the energy path since the two energies are differentially absorbed by bone and soft tissue. The technique can therefore be used to measure regions of the skeleton that are inaccessible to the single photon technology. The development of DPA therefore allows for the first time bone density measurement of the sites of major importance in osteoporotic fracture, principally the spine and femoral neck (112). The technique is relatively accurate and precise although errors occur with alteration in isotope activity and purity. Again, radiation dose is modest, allowing multiple measurements, but the precision is insufficient to allow calculation of rates of change over short periods of time.

A more recent adaptation of the dual photon technique is dual energy x-ray absorptiometry (DXA). This technique is to all intents and purposes identical to DPA but uses an x-ray tube as the source of photons. The results for spine and femoral neck are similar to those obtained with DPA but the stability of the radiation source and the elimination of the purity problems of isotopes have resulted in a significant improvement in precision. The higher photon flux obtained from the x-ray source reduces the patient contact time and radiation exposure.

Quantitative computed tomography also allows measurement of the lumbar spine. It has been suggested that the value of this technique is that it measures purely cancellous bone in the center of a vertebral body. This method is less precise and accurate than DXA, however, particularly in a commercial radiology department, and results in a significantly higher radiation dose to the patient. Finally, there is no clear understanding about the value of measurement of purely cancellous bone. Consequently, DXA has become the technique used most commonly for estimation of bone mass.

The measurement of bone mass by any technique is available in only a modest number of institutions at present. For those practitioners who wish a measurement where the technology is not readily available, measurement of mass can be made using standard x-ray equipment and an aluminum alloy reference wedge. A hand radiograph is obtained in the standard radiology department and specialized computer-aided analysis of the radiograph is performed at a specialized center subsequently. This technique (radiographic absorptiometry) provides an estimate of bone mass in the phalanges, which correlates relatively well with measurements at other skeletal sites using either DPA or DXA (23).

The National Osteoporosis Foundation has provided some guidelines for the clinical use of bone mass measurement (82). First, bone mass is a good predictor of future risk of fracture. This prediction is actually better than the prediction of risk of myocardial infarction using cholesterol level, or other lipoprotein measurements. For each standard deviation below the mean normal bone mass in young individuals, fracture risk doubles. For those who feel they might be at risk of fracture, usually at time of menopause, a bone mass measurement will give an indication of risk and allow for evaluation for preventive therapy (Fig. 13) (103). The first recommendation from the National Osteoporosis Foundation is the use of bone mass in estrogen-deficient women to evaluate the requirement for estrogen replacement therapy.

For those who present with vertebral abnormalities on radiograph, a bone mass measurement is useful in determining the presence of low bone mass and its severity. Thus, for example, for the individual with a vertebral fracture on radiograph, but no recent history of sudden back pain, a measurement of bone mass can determine the presence or absence of osteoporosis, and the necessity of intervention designed to prevent further loss of skeletal tissue. Often, the determination of the severity of the problem can be used to improve compliance with the regimen of intervention.

The advent of DXA with improved precision has raised the possibility that the technique can be used to monitor the response to intervention. While this is done in clinical trial settings, it has yet to be demonstrated to be a useful tool in clinical practice. Certainly, in this situation also, the capability to demonstrate a response to treatment is likely to improve compliance.

For all patients in whom glucocorticoid therapy is being initiated, bone mass measurement is a tool that allows evaluation of the skeleton at the start of treatment and during the early phase of therapy when the most rapid bone loss occurs. Use of the technique allows more critical evaluation of the requirement for therapy with steroids, adjustment of the dose downward where possible, and assessment of the patient for other intervention designed to protect the skeleton from the ravages of steroids, where necessary. The information obtained from bone mass measurements

Vertebral BMD: __.68__ g/cm²

Femoral Neck BMD: __.50__ g/cm²

Vertebral BMD: __.86__ g/cm²

Femoral Neck BMD: __.84__ g/cm²

Vertebral BMD: __1.25__ g/cm²

Femoral Neck BMD: __.96__ g/cm²

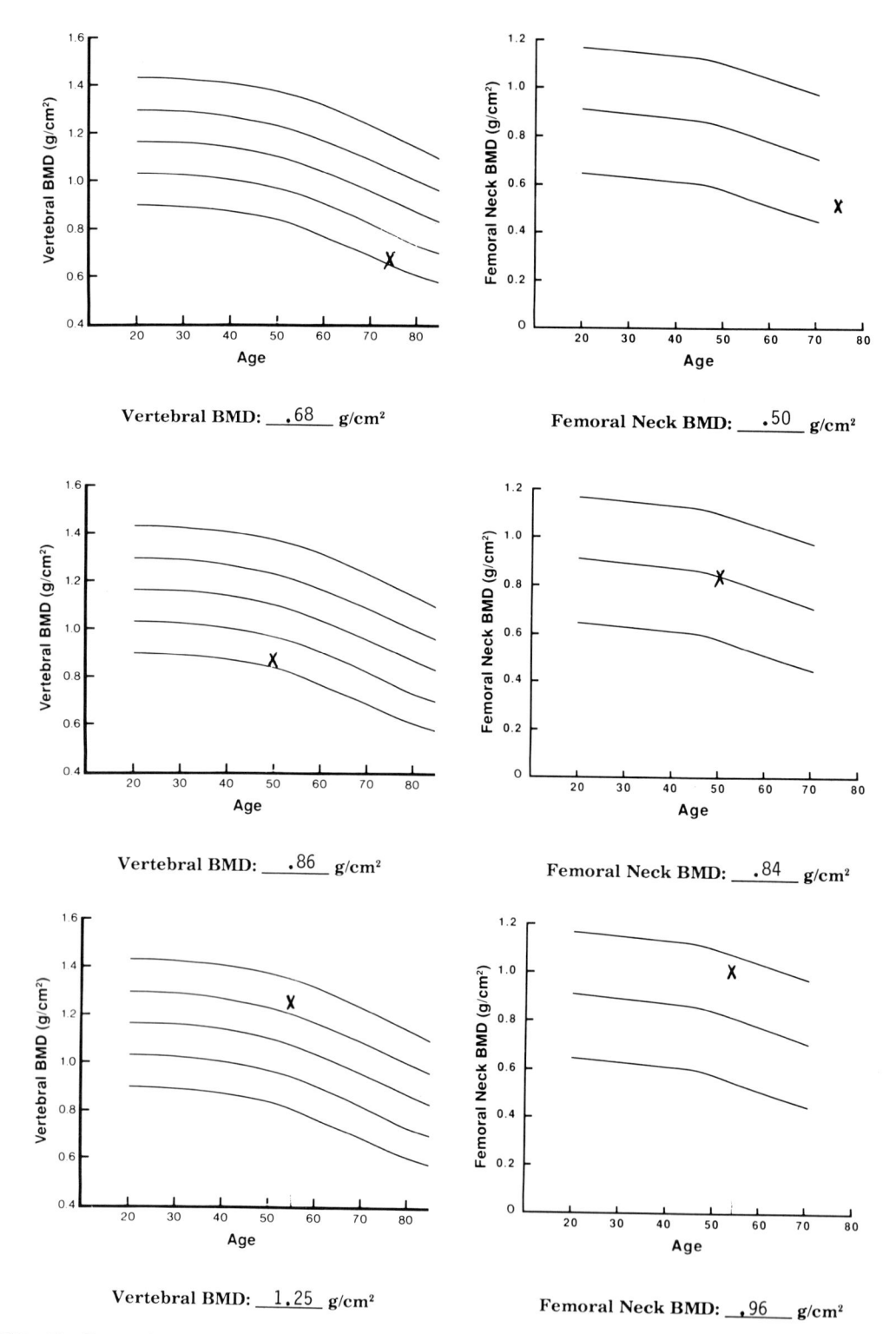

FIG. 13. Bone density measurements plotted by (X) on graphs of normal women measured at ages 20–85 (103). For spine, middle line is mean BMD with 1 and 2 standard deviation lines above and below mean. For femoral neck, mean ± 2 SD are shown. **Top panel:** A 74-year-old woman with known osteoporosis and low bone density in both the spine and femoral neck. Intervention might be advised to prevent any further loss of bone and attendant increase in future fracture risk. **Middle panel:** A 50-year-old woman just 3 years after menopause. Note a low vertebral density indicating an elevated risk of future fractures. Her femoral neck density is higher proportionately than her spine, a common pattern seen in early postmenopausal bone loss where cancellous bone of the spine is lost prominently first, followed later by bone loss in sites with larger amounts of cortical bone (e.g., femoral neck). This woman would benefit by pharmacologic inter-

cannot be obtained by other methods. The use of clinical markers for osteoporosis risk does not allow prediction of bone mass (87,172). There is no demonstrated clinical method for determining bone mass, just as there is no group of risk factors for hypertension that takes the place of blood pressure measurement.

We recommend therefore that all patients who present with a fracture thought to be osteoporotic in origin or who wish to assess their risk of osteoporosis be offered bone mass measurement as part of their clinical assessment. Should bone mass be low (i.e., more than 1.5–2 standard deviations below the mean for young normal individuals), the patient should be evaluated further and treated. If bone mass is below the mean, but not more than 1.5 standard deviations below, the patient should be given advice regarding behavior modification to prevent further loss of bone but may be observed without pharmacologic intervention. Patients with bone mass measurements above the mean do not have osteoporosis and at least in the near future are not likely to develop osteoporosis. Further intervention in this group is usually unnecessary unless there is a change in the medical condition.

TREATMENT OF VERTEBRAL FRACTURES

Acute Management

Pain from vertebral fractures may be sufficiently severe to require bed rest and occasionally admission to a hospital for analgesia and for help in day-to-day functioning during the acute period. This acute stage usually lasts 1 to 5 days with pain gradually settling. No data delineate the best method for remobilization of the patient and in particular it is not clear if early or late mobilization influences the final outcome. Generally, we use pain as a guide and encourage early weight-bearing (within 72 hr) when possible. Shorter periods of bed rest avoid any potential influence of immobilization aggravating bone loss in a patient who already suffers from low bone mass.

The use of a therapeutic pool allows activity in a comfortable gravity-free environment and is often useful in assisting early mobilization. Moist heat may also help alleviate the muscle spasm often associated with an acute fracture and responsible for a large part of the initial discomfort. Many patients also get temporary relief from hot packs, which should be applied under supervision to avoid skin damage. Selecting the most comfortable position in bed is important and the use of multiple pillows to provide support to the upper back and under the knees can be helpful. The diet should be light to avoid approbating an ileus.

The use of a nonsteroidal anti-inflammatory drug is often of benefit in reducing pain from vertebral fractures. Potent analgesics, including narcotics, may be required during the first few days after fracture. Antispasmodic agents such as diazepam or flexeril may be required if paraspinal muscle spasms are a problem. The use of salmon calcitonin at this stage may be helpful in some patients. Calcitonin is a specific inhibitor of osteoclast action and in the long term can be used to stabilize bone mass. In the short term, however, considerable data support the concept that calcitonin has analgesic activity and its use immediately after a fracture can reduce the requirement for a narcotic analgesic. Doses of up to 400 units administered subcutaneously have been recommended. Calcitonin administered subcutaneously, however, is associated with dose-related nausea, vomiting, and flushing and care must be taken to avoid making a miserable patient more unhappy by adding iatrogenic symptoms. In practice, we begin by injecting 25 units subcutaneously, increasing the dose by 25 units every 12 hr if side effects are not a problem. When these appear, reducing the dose by 25 units is often sufficient to reduce or eliminate them.

Returning to a standing posture is often painful especially in the first weeks after a fracture. The use of a soft spinal support is often helpful and improves mobility especially, but not only, for fractures in the lumbar area. Rigid supports are often uncomfortable to the patient and should not be used; we commonly experience patients coming to clinic carrying the support in a shopping bag, which they tell us is more comfortable than wearing it. Recommendations by some physicians that patients wear a rigid support whenever they are out of bed often result in patients who are relegated to far more bed rest than required for pain management, and there is no evidence to suggest that this will aid healing.

Occasionally, patients have a more prolonged course with staggered improvements and pain exacerbations, perhaps in part related to further settling of a fractured vertebral body before a final stable position is reached. Often these patients are those who have had multiple fractures and in whom the muscles and ligaments are already strained into abnormal positions. In this subgroup of patients, further nonnarcotic attempts to

---

vention to prevent further bone loss. **Lower panel:** A 55-year-old woman 5 years postmenopause with normal BMD in both spine and femoral neck. This screening measurement shows the patient to be at low risk of future fractures and pharmacologic intervention would probably not be recommended for the purpose of osteoporosis prevention.

reduce pain are warranted and work in some patients. These include ultrasound massage and transcutaneous nerve stimulation. Usually the pain does subside and patients can return for the most part to their previous life-style.

Chronic Treatment

Certain movements including heavy lifting, reaching far forward, jarring the body, and rapidly twisting increase compressive forces on the spine and should be avoided to prevent further episodes of fractures. Attempts should be made to improve life-style factors known to accelerate bone loss, including discontinuing smoking and reducing or eliminating excessive alcohol ingestion. Iatrogenic factors such as excessive thyroid hormone replacement or excessive glucocorticoid use should be eliminated.

Role of Calcium

Assessment of total dietary calcium intake should be made. Although the U.S. RDA for calcium is only 800 mg/day, patients should be advised to increase dietary calcium or take a calcium supplement to reach a total daily intake of 1000 mg if estrogen replete or 1500 mg if estrogen deficient. Primarily, this is to ensure that there is no exacerbation of bone loss by providing sufficient dietary calcium so that skeletal calcium is not liberated to maintain calcium homeostasis. Although most people would not need 1500 mg/day to maintain homeostasis, because there is such a large variability in calcium absorption, this intake assures that all people will maintain calcium balance (72–74). Calcium carbonate is well absorbed and well tolerated but other preparations can be used (47), provided they dissolve normally in weak acid (such as vinegar, where tablets should dissolve within 30 min). Patients must be instructed to look for the contribution of elemental calcium from the calcium preparation rather than the total mass of the calcium plus congener. Calcium supplements should be taken in divided doses with food.

Exercise Prescription

Almost all patients can benefit from an exercise program (68). Most exercise studies in both normal and osteoporotic individuals have suggested that reduction in the rate of bone loss can be attained through some combination of aerobic exercise (such as rapid walking or jogging on a free surface or treadmill, step climbing, aerobic dancing) and a muscle strengthening calisthenic program (3,19,30,68,93,146,150,156, 157,160–162). We recommend low-impact aerobic exercise to avoid excessive compression on the spine. For walkers, we advocate adding light weights to the wrists and ankles to add to the benefit. Exercises designed particularly to build strength in the paraspinal musculature are beneficial in helping to avoid muscular laxity, which increases the thoracic kyphosis by the end of the day and puts increased chronic compressive force on the anterior vertebral bodies.

Pharmacologic Therapy

For those patients with vertebral fractures as well as those patients with low bone mass (>1.5 or 2 SD below mean young normal), antiresorptive therapy may be warranted. Estrogen and calcitonin are the only two drugs approved so far by the FDA for this purpose. Estrogen has been shown in numerous trials to maintain bone mass at all important sites of fracture (1,20, 49,78,97,99,100,102,133,136). Epidemiologic data indicate that women treated with estrogen for at least 5 years in the immediate postmenopausal period will have a 50% reduction in hip fracture and 75% reduction in vertebral fracture risk (49,54,63,85,92,174). Estrogen is usually given in the form of Premarin 0.625 mg/day (conjugated equine estrogen) or its equivalent (98). Estrogens in any form (transdermal, subcutaneous, percutaneous) all reduce bone loss (166). For women with an intact uterus, cyclic (5–10 mg/day, 12–14 days each month) or continuous medroxyprogesterone (2.5 mg/day) are recommended to prevent chronic endometrial hyperstimulation. All patients should undergo mammography before beginning estrogen therapy and annually thereafter. Regular gynecologic follow-up is also recommended. Estrogen has powerful potential benefits for the cardiovascular system (possibly reducing ischemic heart disease by 50%) (9,15,16) in addition to its ability to decrease bone loss and reduce the risk of fracture. This additional potential benefit far outweighs the combined risk of uterine, breast, and ovarian cancer in women.

For patients who have had breast cancer or uterine cancer or have a close family history of breast cancer (mother or sister), estrogen is usually contraindicated and injectable salmon calcitonin may be an effective alternative. Calcitonin has been shown to prevent bone loss at least for up to 3 years in postmenopausal women (53,60,65,113,114), but no large scale studies have yet shown prevention of fractures by calcitonin. Injectable calcitonin may be associated with nausea and flushing but these symptoms are usually short-lived and avoided by increasing the dose slowly. As stated earlier, calcitonin may have an analgesic effect on bone pain. Intranasal calcitonin spray, currently undergoing clinical testing, will be a much easier alternative if it proves to be efficacious and may avoid the side effects associated with the injectable form.

Intermittent etidronate therapy may be effective at decreasing bone loss over a 2- to 3-year period and preliminary data suggest that it may decrease the number of spinal fractures (167,173); however, its long-term efficacy and long-term complications have not yet been fully assessed. Continuous etidronate administration may cause a mineralization abnormality and thus a detrimental effect on skeletal integrity.

Sodium fluoride has been shown in multiple studies to increase bone mass but its efficacy in reducing fracture frequency is not well documented in controlled studies and it has too many adverse effects, including a possible increase in nonvertebral fractures, the painful limb syndrome (possibly due to small stress fractures), and gastrointestinal irritation, to warrant its use currently (86,140). Clinical trials of intermittent dosing, reduced doses, and other forms of fluoride may be warranted before rejecting this agent completely.

Numerous agents are currently being investigated for potential treatment of osteoporosis, including growth factors, growth hormone, parathyroid hormone, anabolic steroids, newer diphosphonates, and regimens involving combinations of agents. For now and the near future, it is clear that osteoporosis is a disease that is much more easily prevented than treated.

REFERENCES

1. Al-Azzawi F, Hart DM, Lindsay R. Long-term effect of oestrogen replacement therapy on bone mass as measured by dual photon absorptiometry. *Br Med J* 1987;294:1261–1262.
2. Aloia JF, Cohn SH, Babu T, et al. Skeletal mass and body composition in marathon runners. *Metabolism* 1978;27:104–107.
3. Aloia JF, Cohn SH, Ostuni JA, et al. Prevention of involutional bone loss by exercise. *Ann Intern Med* 1979;89:356–358.
4. Aloia JF, Cohn SH, Vaswani A, et al. Risk factors for postmenopausal osteoporosis. *Am J Med* 1985;78:95–100.
5. Aloia JF, Vaswanit AN, Yeh JK, et al. Premenopausal bone mass is related to physical activity. *Arch Intern Med* 1988;148:121–123.
6. Baker SP, Harvey AH. Fall injuries in the elderly. Symposium on falls and the elderly. Biological and behavioral aspects. *Clin Geriatr Med* 1985;1:501–508.
7. Bardin T, Lequesne M. The osteoporosis of heparinotherapy and systemic mastocytosis. *Clin Rheumatol* 1989;8:119–123.
8. Barr DG. Bone deficiency in Turner's syndrome measured by metacarpal dimensions. *Arch Dis Child* 1974;49:821–822.
9. Barrett-Connor E, Brown WV, Turner J, Austin M, Criqui MH. Heart disease risk factors and hormone use in postmenopausal women. *JAMA* 1979;241:2167–2169.
10. Bernstein DS, Sadowsky N, Hegsted DM, et al. Prevalence of osteoporosis in high-/low-fluoride areas in North Dakota. *JAMA* 1966;198:499–504.
11. Bijvoet OLM, Vellenga CJLR, Harinck HIJ. Paget's disease of bones: assessment, therapy, and secondary prevention. In: Kleerekoper M, Krane SM, eds. *Clinical disorders of bone and mineral metabolism.* New York: Mary Ann Liebert, 1989; 525–542.
12. Biller BMK, Saxe V, Herzog DB, et al. Mechanisms of osteoporosis in adult and adolescent women with anorexia nervosa. *J Clin Endocrinol Metab* 1987;64:1021–1026.
13. Biller BMK, Saxe V, Herzog DB, et al. Mechanisms of osteoporosis in adult and adolescent women with anorexia nervosa. *J Clin Endocrinol Metab* 1989;68:548–554.
14. Boskey AL. Noncollagenous matrix proteins and their role in mineralization. *Bone Miner* 1989;6:111–123.
15. Bush TL, Barrett-Connor E, Cowan LD. Cardiovascular mortality and noncontraceptive use of estrogen in women. Results from the Lipid Research Clinics Program Follow-Up Study. *Circulation* 1987;75:1102–1109.
16. Bush TL, Barrett-Connor E. Non-contraceptive estrogen use and cardiovascular disease. *Epidemiol Rev* 1985;7:80–104.
17. Campbell AJ, Reinken J, Allan BC, et al. Falls in old age: a study of frequency and related clinical factors. *Age Ageing* 1981;10:264–270.
18. Campbell GA. Osteomalacia: diagnosis and management. *Br J Hosp Med* 1990;44:332–338.
19. Chow R, Harrison JE, Notarius C: Effect of two randomised exercise programmes on bone mass of healthy postmenopausal women. *Br Med J* 1987;295:1441–1444.
20. Christiansen C, Rodbro P. Does postmenopausal bone loss respond to estrogen replacement therapy independent of bone loss rate. *Calcif Tissue Int* 1983;35:720–722.
21. Cole WG. Osteogenesis imperfecta. In: Martin TJ, ed. *Clinical endocrinology and metabolism: international practice and research.* London: Bailliere Tindall, 1988;243–265.
22. Cooper C, Atkinson E, O'Fallon WM, et al. The epidemiology of vertebral fractures in Rochester, Minnesota, 1985–1989. *J Bone Miner Res* 1991;6(suppl 1):S300.
23. Cosman F, Herrington B, Himmelstein S, Lindsay R. Radiographic absorptiometry: a simple method for determination of bone mass. *Osteoporosis Int* 1991;2(1):34–38.
24. Cosman F, Shen V, Xie F, et al. A mechanism of estrogen action on the skeleton: protection against the resorbing effects of (1–34)hPTH infusion as assessed by biochemical markers. *Ann Intern Med* 1992;118:337–343.
25. Crilly RG, Anderson C, Hogan D, et al. Bone histomorphometry, bone mass, and related parameters in alcoholic males. *Calcif Tissue Int* 1988;43:269–276.
26. Cummings SR, Kelsey JL, Nevitt MC, et al. Epidemiology of osteoporosis and osteoporotic fractures. *Epidemiol Rev* 1985;7:178.
27. Cummings SR, Rubin SM, Black D. The future of hip fractures in the United States. *Clin Orthop* 1990;252:163–166.
28. Cummings SR. Osteoporotic fractures: the magnitude of the problem. In: Christiansen C, Johansen JS, Riis BJ, eds. *Osteoporosis.* Copenhagen: Osteopress, 1987;1193–1196.
29. Dalen N, Olsson KE. Bone mineral content and physical activity. *Acta Orthop Scand* 1974;45:170–174.
30. Dalsky GP, Stocke KS, Ehsani AA, et al. Weight-bearing exercise training and lumbar bone mineral content in postmenopausal women. *Ann Intern Med* 1988;108:824–828.
31. Daniell HW. Osteoporosis of the slender smoker. *Arch Intern Med* 1976;136:298–304.
32. Davies KM, Recker RR, Heaney RP. Normal vertebral dimensions and normal variation in serial measurements of vertebrae. *J Bone Miner Res* 1989;4:341–349.
33. Dempster DW. Bone histomorphometry in glucocorticoid-induced osteoporosis. *J Bone Miner Res* 1989;4:137–141.
34. Dempster DW. Bone quantification and dynamics of turnover. In: *Principles and practice of endocrinology and metabolism.* Philadelphia: Lippincott, 1990;247–252.
35. Dempster DW. Bone remodeling. In: Coe FL, Favus MJ, eds. *Disorders of bone and mineral metabolism.* New York: Raven Press, 1992.
36. Dempster DW, Shane E, Horbert W, Lindsay R. A simple method for correlative light and scanning electron microscopy of human iliac crest bone biopsies: quantitative observations in normal and osteoporotic subjects. *J Bone Miner Res* 1986;1:15–21.
37. Dequeker J, Nijs J, Verstraeten A, et al. Genetic determinants of bone mineral content at the spine and radius: a twin study. *Bone* 1987;8:207–209.
38. DeVernejoul MC, Bielakoh T, Heire M, et al. Evidence for defective osteoblastic function: a role for alcohol and tobacco

consumption in osteoporosis in middle-aged men. *Clin Orthop* 1983;179:107–115.
39. Devogelaer JP, Crabbe J, DeDeuxchaisnes CN. Bone mineral density in Addison's disease: evidence for an effect of adrenal androgens on bone mass. *Br Med J* 1987;294:798–850.
40. Diamond T, Stiel D, Lunzer M, et al. Thanol reduces bone formation and may cause osteoporosis. *Am J Med* 1989;86: 282–288.
41. Diamond T, Stiel D, Posen S. Osteoporosis in hemochromatosis: iron excess, gonadal deficiency, or other factors. *Ann Intern Med* 1989;110:430–436.
42. Drinkwater BD, Nilson KL, Chesnut CH III. Bone mineral content of amenorrheic and eumenorrheic athletes. *N Engl J Med* 1984;311:277–281.
43. Eastell R, Cedel SL, Wahner HW, et al. Classification of vertebral fractures. *J Bone Miner Res* 1991;6:207–215.
44. Eastell R, Heath HH III, Kumar R, et al. Hormonal factors: PTH, vitamin D, and calcitonin. In: Riggs BL, Melton LJ III, eds. *Osteoporosis: etiology, diagnosis, and management.* New York: Raven Press, 1988;373–388.
45. Eastall R, Riggs BL. Diagnostic evaluation of osteoporosis. *Endocrinol Metab Clin North Am* 1988;17:547–571.
46. Eisman JA. Osteomalacia. In: Martin TJ, ed. *Clinical endocrinology and metabolism: international practice and research.* London: Bailliere Tindall, 1988;125–155.
47. Ekman M, Reizenstein P, Teigen SW, Ronnenberg R. Comparative absorption of calcium from carbonate tablets, lactogluconate/carbonate effervescent tablet, and chloride solution. *Bone* 1991;12:93–97.
48. Erikssen EF, Colvard DS, Berg NJ. Evidence of estrogen receptors in normal human osteoblast-like cells. *Science* 1988; 241:84–86.
49. Ettinger B, Genant HK, Cann CE. Long-term estrogen therapy prevents bone loss and fracture. *Ann Intern Med* 1985;102: 319–324.
50. Ettinger B, Winger J. Thyroid supplements: effect on bone mass. *West J Med* 1982;136:472–476.
51. Evans R, Marel GM, Lancaster EK, et al. Bone mass is low in relatives of osteoporotic patients. *Ann Intern Med* 1988;1: 870–873.
52. Fallon MD, Perry HM III, Bergfeld M, et al. Exogenous hyperthyroidism with osteoporosis. *Arch Intern Med* 1983;143: 442–444.
53. Fatourechi V, Heath HH III. Salmon calcitonin in the treatment of postmenopausal osteoporosis. *Ann Intern Med* 1987; 107:923–925.
54. Finn-Jensen M, Christiansen C, Transbol I. Fracture frequency and bone prevention in postmenopausal women treated with estrogen. *Obstet Gynecol* 1982;60:493–496.
55. Frost HM. Clinical management of the symptomatic osteoporotic patient. *Orthop Clin North Am* 1981;12:671–681.
56. Gallagher JC, Hedlund LR, Stoner S, et al. Vertebral morphometry: normative data. *Bone Miner* 1988;4:189–196.
57. Gallagher JC, Riggs BL, Eisman JA, et al. Intestinal calcium absorption and serum vitamin D metabolites in normal subjects and osteoporotic patients. *J Clin Invest* 1979;64:729–736.
58. Garraway WM, Stauffer RN, Kurland LT, et al. Limb fractures in a defined population. *Mayo Clin Proc* 1979;54:701–707.
59. Genant HK, Ettinger B, Harris ST, et al. Quantitative computed tomography in assessment of osteoporosis. In: Riggs BL, Melton LJ III, eds. *Osteoporosis: etiology, diagnosis and management.* New York: Raven Press, 1988;221–249.
60. Gennari C, Chierichetti SM, Bigazzi S, et al. Comparative effects on bone mineral content of calcium and calcium plus salmon calcitonin given in two different regimens in postmenopausal osteoporosis. *Curr Ther Res* 1985;38:455–464.
61. Gershon-Cohen J, Rechtman AM, Schrarer H, et al. Asymptomatic fractures in osteoporotic spines of the aged. *JAMA* 1953;153:625–627.
62. Geusens P, Dequeker J, Verstraeten A, Nijs J. Age-, sex-, and menopause-related changes of vertebral and peripheral bone: population study using dual and single photon absorptiometry and radiogrammetry. *J Nucl Med* 1986;27:1540–1549.
63. Gordan GS, Picchi J, Roof BS. Antifracture efficacy of long-term estrogens for osteoporosis. *Trans Assoc Am Physicians* 1973;86:326–332.
64. Greenspan SL, Neer RM, Ridgway EC, et al. Osteoporosis in men with hyperprolactinemic hypogonadism. *Ann Intern Med* 1986;104:777–782.
65. Gruber HE, Ivey JL, Baylink DJ, et al. Long-term calcitonin therapy in postmenopausal osteoporosis. *Metabolism* 1984;33: 295–303.
66. Gryfe CI, Amies A, Ashley MJ. A longitudinal study of falls in an elderly population: 1. Incidence and morbidity. *Age Ageing* 1977;6:201–210.
67. Hahn TJ. Drug induced disorders of vitamin D and mineral metabolism. *J Clin Endocrinol Metab* 1980;9:107–129.
68. Harris SS, Caspersen CJ, DeFriese GH, et al. Physical activity counseling for healthy adults as a primary preventive intervention in the clinical setting. Report for the US Preventive Services Task Force. *JAMA* 1989;261:3590–3598.
69. Heaney RP. A unified concept of osteoporosis. *Am J Med* 1965; 39:377–380.
70. Heaney RP. Radiocalcium metabolism in disuse osteoporosis in man. *Am J Med* 1962;33:188–200.
71. Heaney RP, Recker RR. Effects of nitrogen phosphorus and caffeine on calcium balance in women. *J Lab Clin Med* 1982; 99:46–55.
72. Heaney RP, Recker RR, Saville PD. Calcium balance and calcium requirements in middle-aged women. *Am J Clin Nutr* 1990;30:1603–1611.
73. Heaney RP, Recker RR, Saville PD. Menopausal changes in bone remodeling. *J Lab Clin Med* 1978;92:964–970.
74. Heaney RP, Recker RR, Saville PD. Menopausal changes in calcium balance performance. *J Lab Clin Med* 1978;92: 953–963.
75. Hedlund LR, Gallagher JC, Meeger C, et al. Change in vertebral shape in osteoporosis. *Calcif Tissue Int* 1989;44:168–172.
76. Hedlund LR, Gallagher JC. Vertebral morphometry in diagnosis in spinal fractures. *Bone Miner* 1988;5:59–67.
77. Holbrook TL, Grazier K, Kelsey JL, et al. The frequency of occurrence, impact, and cost of musculoskeletal conditions in the United States. *Am Acad Orthop Surg* 1984;163–166.
78. Horsman A, Gallagher JC, Simpson M, et al. Prospective trial of estrogen and calcium in postmenopausal women. *Br Med J* 1977;2:789–792.
79. Jackson JA, Kleerekoper M, Parfitt AM, et al. Bone histomorphometry in hypogonadal and eugonadal men with spinal osteoporosis. *J Clin Endocrinol Metab* 1987;65:53–58.
80. Jensen GF, Christiansen C, Boesen J, et al. Epidemiology of postmenopausal spinal and long bone fractures. *Clin Orthop* 1982;166:75–81.
81. Johnell O, Nilsson BE. Lifestyle and bone mineral mass in perimenopausal women. *Calcif Tissue Int* 1984;36:354–356.
82. Johnston CC, Melton LJ III, Lindsay R, et al. Clinical indications for bone mass measurement. *J Bone Miner Res* 1989;4: 1–28.
83. Kanders B, Dempster DW, Lindsay R. Interaction of calcium nutrition and physical activity on bone mass in young women. *J Bone Miner Res* 1988;3:145–149.
84. Kanis JA, Cundy TF, Hamdy NAT. Renal osteodystrophy. In: Martin TJ, ed. *Clinical endocrinology and metabolism: international practice and research.* London: Bailliere Tindall, 1988; 193–241.
85. Kiel DP, Felson DT, Anderson JJ. Hip fracture and the use of estrogens in postmenopausal women. *N Engl J Med* 1987;317: 1169–1174.
86. Kleerekoper M, Peterson EL, Nelson DA, et al. A randomized trial of sodium fluoride as a treatment for postmenopausal osteoporosis. *Osteoporosis Int* 1991;1:155–161.
87. Kleerekoper M, Peterson E, Nelson D, et al. Identification of women at risk for developing postmenopausal osteoporosis with vertebral fractures: role of history and single photon absorptiometry. *Bone Miner* 1989;7:171–186.
88. Klibanski A, Greenspan SL. Increase in bone mass after treatment of hyperprolactinemic amenorrhea. *N Engl J Med* 1986; 315:542–546.

89. Klibanski A, Neer RM, Beitins IZ, et al. Decreased bone density in hyperprolactinemic women. *N Engl J Med* 1980;303: 1511–1514.
90. Komm BS, Terpening CM, Benz DJ. Estrogen binding, receptor mRNA, and biologic response in osteoblast-like osteosarcoma cells. *Science* 1988;241:81–84.
91. Koppelman MCS, Kurz DW, Morrish KA, et al. Vertebral body bone mineral in hyperprolactinemic women. *J Clin Endocrinol Metab* 1984;59:1050–1053.
92. Kreiger N, Kelsey JL, Holford TR. An epidemiological study of hip fracture in postmenopausal women. *Am J Epidemiol* 1982;116:141–148.
93. Krolner B, Toft B, Pors Nielsen S, et al. Physical exercise as prophylaxis against involutional vertebral bone loss: a controlled trial. *Clin Sci* 1983;64:541–546.
94. Lane JM, Cornell CN, Healey JH. Orthopaedic consequences of osteoporosis. In: Riggs BL, Melton LJ III, eds. *Osteoporosis: etiology, diagnosis, and management*. New York: Raven Press, 1988;433–455.
95. Lindberg JS, Fears WB, Hunt MM. Exercise-induced amenorrhea and bone density. *Ann Intern Med* 1984;101:647–648.
96. Lindhe M. Biomechanics of the lumbar spine. In: Frankel VH, Nordin M, eds. *Basic biomechanics of the skeletal system*. Philadelphia: Lea & Febiger, 1980;255–290.
97. Lindsay R, Aitken JM, Anderson JB, et al. Long-term prevention of postmenopausal osteoporosis by oestrogen. *Lancet* 1976;1:1038–1041.
98. Lindsay R, Hart DM, Clark DM. The minimum effective dose of estrogen for prevention of postmenopausal bone loss. *Obstet Gynecol* 1984;63:759–763.
99. Lindsay R, Hart DM, Forrest C, et al. Prevention of spinal osteoporosis in oophorectomized women. *Lancet* 1980;2: 1151–1154.
100. Lindsay R, Hart DM, Purdie P, et al. Comparative effects of oestrogen and a progestogen on bone loss in postmenopausal women. *Clin Sci* 1978;54:193–195.
101. Lindsay R. Sex steroids in the pathogenesis and prevention of osteoporosis. In: Riggs BL, Melton LJ III, eds. *Osteoporosis: etiology, diagnosis and management*. New York: Raven Press, 1988;333–358.
102. Lindsay R, Tohme J. Estrogen treatment of patients with established postmenopausal osteoporosis. *Obstet Gynecol* 1990;76: 1–6.
103. Lindsay R, Williams S, Dempster DW, et al. Bone mineral density changes with age, body size and crush fractures. *J Bone Miner Res* 1985;1:121.
104. Linnel SL, Stager MM, Blue PW. Bone mineral content and menstrual regularity in female runners. *Med Sci Sports Exec* 1989;16:343–348.
105. Maller M, Horsman A, Harvald B, et al. Metacarpal morphometry in monozygotic and dizygotic elderly twins. *Calcif Tissue Res* 1975;25:197–201.
106. Marcus R, Cann C, Madvig D. Menstrual function and bone mass in elite women distance runners. *Ann Intern Med* 1985; 102:158–163.
107. Marel GM, McKenna JM, Frame B. Osteomalacia. In: Peck WA, ed. *Bone and mineral research*. New York: Elsevier, 1991;335–412.
108. Matkovic V, Kostial K, Simonovic I, et al. Bone status and fracture rates in two regions of Yugoslavia. *Am J Clin Nutr* 1979;32:540–549.
109. Matkovic V, Tominac C, Fontana D, Chesnut C. Influence of calcium on peak bone mass: a 24-month follow-up. *J Bone Miner Res* 1988;3(suppl 1):S85.
110. Mazanec DJ, Grisanti JM. Drug-induced osteoporosis. *Cleve Clin J Med* 1989;56:297–303.
111. Mazess RB. On aging bone loss. *Clin Orthop* 1982;165:237–252.
112. Mazess RB, Wahner HM. Nuclear medicine in densitometry. In: Riggs BL, Melton LJ III, eds. *Osteoporosis: etiology, diagnosis, and management*. New York: Raven Press, 1988; 251–295.
113. Mazzouli GF, Passeri M, Gennari C, et al. Effects of salmon calcitonin in postmenopausal osteoporosis: a controlled double-blind clinical study. *Calcif Tissue Int* 1986;38:3–8.
114. McDermott MT, Kidd GS. The role of calcitonin in the development and treatment of osteoporosis. *Endocrinol Rev* 1987;8: 377–390.
115. Melton LJ III. Epidemiology of fractures. In: Riggs BL, Melton LJ III, eds. *Osteoporosis: etiology, diagnosis, and management*. New York: Raven Press, 1988;133–154.
116. Melton LJ III. Epidemiology of fractures. In: Riggs BL, Melton LJ III, eds. *Osteoporosis: etiology, diagnosis, and management*. New York: Raven Press, 1988;155–179.
117. Melton LJ III, Kan SH, Frye MA, et al. Epidemiology of vertebral fractures in women. *Am J Epidemiol* 1989;129:1000–1011.
118. Melton LJ III, Riggs BL. Clinical spectrum. In: Riggs BL, Melton LJ III, eds. *Osteoporosis: etiology, diagnosis, and management*. New York: Raven Press, 1988;155–180.
119. Melton LJ III, Riggs BL. Epidemiology of age-related fractures. In: Avioli LV, ed. *The osteoporotic syndrome*. New York: Grune & Stratton, 1983;45–72.
120. Minare P, Meunier P, Edouard C, et al. Quantitative histological data on disuse osteoporosis. Comparison with biological data. *Calcif Tissue Res* 1974;17:57–63.
121. Nelson D, Peterson E, Tilley B, et al. Measurement of vertebral area on spine x-rays in osteoporosis: reliability of digitizing techniques. *J Bone Miner Res* 1990;5:707–716.
122. Nilas L, Christiansen C. Bone mass and its relationship to age and the menopause. *J Clin Endocrinol Metab* 1987;65:697–701.
123. Nilsson BE, Westlin NE. Bone density in athletes. *Clin Orthop* 1971;77:179–182.
124. Nischelsky JE, Harms HM, Sylvester S, et al. Vertebral deformity index (Kleerekoper) in osteoporosis: data of an outpatient clinic. *Osteoporosis* 1990;2:909–913.
125. Nystrome E, Leman J, Lundberg PA, et al. Bone mineral content in normally menstruating women with hyperprolactinemia. *Horm Res* 1988;29:214–217.
126. Parfitt AM. Bone remodeling: relationship to the amount and structure of bone, and the pathogenesis and prevention of fractures. In: Riggs BL, Melton LJ III, eds. *Osteoporosis: etiology, diagnosis, and management*. New York: Raven Press, 1988; 45–93.
127. Parfitt AM. Dietary risk factors for age-related bone loss and fractures. *Lancet* 1983;2:1181–1185.
128. Parfitt AM. The cellular basis of bone remodeling: the quantum concept reexamined in light of recent advances in the cell biology of bone. *Calcif Tissue Int* 1984;36:37–45.
129. Parisien M, Silverberg SJ, Shane E, et al. Bone disease in primary hyperparathyroidism. *Endocrinol Metab Clin North Am* 1990;19:19–34.
130. Parisien M, Silverberg SJ, Shane E, et al. The histomorphometry of bone in primary hyperparathyroidism: preservation of cancellous bone structure. *J Clin Endocrinol Metab* 1990;70: 930–938.
131. Pocock NA, Eisman JA, Hopper JL, et al. Genetic determinants of bone mass in adults. *J Clin Invest* 1987;80:706–710.
132. Prudham D, Evans JG. Factors associated with falls in the elderly: a community study. *Age Ageing* 1981;10:141–146.
133. Quigley MET, Martin BL, Burnier AM, et al. Estrogen therapy arrests bone loss in elderly women. *Am J Obstet Gynecol* 1987; 156:1516–1523.
134. Raisz LG, Kream BE. Regulation of bone formation. *N Engl J Med* 1983;309:29–35.
135. Ray WA, Griffin MR, Schaffner W, et al. Psychotropic drug use and the risk of hip fracture. *N Engl J Med* 1987;316:363–369.
136. Recker RR, Saville PD, Heaney RP. The effect of estrogens and calcium carbonate on bone loss in postmenopausal women. *Ann Intern Med* 1977;87:649–655.
137. Recker RR, Kimmel DB, Parfitt AM. Static and tetracycline-based bone histomorphometric data from 34 normal postmenopausal females. *J Bone Miner Res* 1988;3:133–144.
138. Reid IR. Pathogenesis and treatment of steroid osteoporosis. *Clin Endocrinol (Oxf)* 1989;30:83–103.
139. Resnick D. The osteochondroses. In: Resnick D, Niwayama G, eds. *Diagnoses of bone and joint disorders*. Philadelphia: Saunders, 1981;2874–2912.
140. Riggs BL, Hodgson SF, O'Fallon WM, et al. Effect of fluoride

140. treatment on the fracture rate in postmenopausal women with osteoporosis. *N Engl J Med* 1990;322:802–809.
141. Riggs BL, Melton LJ III. Involutional osteoporosis. *N Engl J Med* 1986;314:1676–1686.
142. Rigotti NA, Nussbaum SR, Herzog DB, et al. Osteoporosis in women with anorexia nervosa. *N Engl J Med* 1984;311:1601–1606.
143. Riis BJ, Christiansen C. Measurement of spinal or peripheral bone mass to estimate early postmenopausal bone loss. *Am J Med* 1988;84:646–653.
144. Ritz E, Drueke T, Merke J, Lucas PA. Genesis of bone disease in uremia. In: Peck WA, ed. *Bone and mineral research.* New York: Elsevier, 1991;309–374.
144a. Ross PD, Davis JW, Epstein RS, Wasnich RD. Pre-existing fractures and bone mass predict vertebral fracture incidence in women. *Ann Intern Med* 1991;114:919–923.
145. Sanborn CF, Martin BJ, Wagner WW. Is athletic amenorrhea specific to runners. *Am J Obstet Gynecol* 1982;143:859–861.
146. Sandler RK, Cauley JA, Hom DL, et al. The effects of walking on the cross-sectional dimensions of the radius in postmenopausal women. *Calcif Tissue Int* 1987;41:65–69.
147. Sauer P, Leidig G, Minne HW, et al. Spinal deformity index versus other objective procedures of vertebral fracture identification in patients with osteoporosis: a comparative study. *J Bone Miner Res* 1991;6:227–238.
148. Schlechte JA, Sherman B, Martin R. Bone density in amenorrheic women with and without hyperprolactinemia. *J Clin Endocrinol Metab* 1983;56:1120–1123.
149. Schlechte J, El-Khoury G, Kathol M, et al. Forearm and vertebral bone mineral in treated and untreated hypoprolactinemic amenorrhea. *J Clin Endocrinol Metab* 1987;64:1021–1026.
150. Schoutens A, Laurent E, Poortsmans JR. Effects of inactivity and exercise on bone. *Sports Med* 1989;7:71–81.
151. Schultz AB, Anderson GBJ, Haderspeck K, et al. Analysis and measurement of lumbar trunk loads in tasks involving bends and twists. *J Biomech* 1991;15:669–675.
152. Seeman E, Hopper JL, Bach LA, et al. Reduced bone mass in daughters of women with osteoporosis. *N Engl J Med* 1989;320:554–558.
153. Seeman E, Melton LJ III, O'Fallon WM, et al. Risk factors for spinal osteoporosis in men. *Am J Med* 1983;85:977–983.
154. Seeman E, Wahner HW, Offord KP, et al. Differential effects of endocrine dysfunction on the axial and the appendicular skeleton. *J Clin Invest* 1982;69:1302–1309.
155. Sillence D. Osteogenesis imperfecta: an expanding panorama of variants. *Clin Orthop* 1981;159:11–25.
156. Simkin A, Ayalon J, Leichter I. Increased trabecular bone density due to bone-loading exercises in postmenopausal osteoporotic women. *Calcif Tissue Int* 1987;40:59–63.
157. Sinaki M, Mikkelsen BA. Postmenopausal spinal osteoporosis: flexion versus extension exercises. *Arch Phys Med Rehabil* 1984;65:593–596.
158. Smith-Bindman R, Cummings SR, Steiger P, et al. A comparison of morphometric definitions of vertebral fracture. *J Bone Miner Res* 1991;6:25–34.
159. Smith DM, Nance WE, Kang K, et al. Genetic factors in determining bone mass. *J Clin Invest* 1973;52:2800–2811.
160. Smith EL, Gilligan C, McAdam M, et al. Deterring bone loss by exercise intervention in premenopausal and postmenopausal women. *Calcif Tissue Int* 1989;44:312–321.
161. Smith EL, Reddan W. Physical activity: a modality for bone accretion in the aged. *Am J Radiol* 1976;126:1297.
162. Smith EL, Reddan W, Smith PE. Physical activity and calcium modalities for bone mineral increase in aged women. *Med Sci Sports Exec* 1981;13:60–64.
163. Stall GM, Harris S, Sokoll LJ, et al. Accelerated bone loss in hypothyroid patients overtreated with L-thyroxine. *Ann Intern Med* 1990;113:265–269.
164. Steiniche T, Hasling C, Charles P, et al. A randomized study of the effects of estrogen/gestagen or high dose oral calcium on trabecular bone remodeling in postmenopausal osteoporosis. *Bone* 1989;10:313–320.
165. Stepan JJ, Pospichal J, Presl J, et al. Bone loss and biochemical indices of bone remodeling in surgically induced postmenopausal women. *Bone* 1987;8:279–284.
166. Stevenson JC, Cust MP, Gangar KF, et al. Effects of transdermal versus oral hormone replacement therapy on bone density in spine and proximal femur in postmenopausal women. *Lancet* 1990;336:265–269.
167. Storm T, Thamsborg G, Steiniche T, et al. Effects of intermittent cyclical etidronate therapy on bone mass and fracture rate in women with postmenopausal osteoporosis. *N Engl J Med* 1990;322:1265–1271.
168. Tinetti ME, Speechley M, Ginter SF. Risk factors for falls among elderly persons living in the community. *N Engl J Med* 1988;319:1701–1707.
169. Travis WD, Chin-Yang L, Bergstralh EJ, et al. Systemic mast cell disease. Analysis of 58 cases and literature review. *Medicine (Baltimore)* 1988;67:345–368.
170. Tsai K, Heath HH III, Kumar R, et al. Impaired vitamin D metabolism with aging in women: possible role in pathogenesis of senile osteoporosis. *J Clin Invest* 1984;73:1668–1672.
171. Vaes G. Cellular biology and biochemical mechanism of bone resorption. *Clin Orthop* 1988;231:239–271.
172. van Hemert AM, Vandenbroucke JP, Birkenhager JC, et al. Prediction of osteoporotic fractures in the general population by a fracture risk score. *Am J Endocrinol* 1990;132:123–135.
173. Watts NB, Harris ST, Genant HK, et al. Intermittent cyclical etidronate treatment of postmenopausal osteoporosis. *N Engl J Med* 1990;323:73–79.
174. Weiss NS, Ure CL, Ballard JH. Decreased risk of fractures of the hip and lower forearm with postmenopausal use of oestrogen. *N Engl J Med* 1980;303:1195–1198.
175. Whedon GD. The influence of activity on calcium metabolism. *J Nutr Sci Vitaminol* 1991;31:41–44.
176. Wilson RJ, Rao DS, Ellis B, et al. Mild asymptomatic primary hyperparathyroidism is not a risk factor for vertebral fractures. *Ann Intern Med* 1988;109:959–962.

26

Surgical Management of Primary and Secondary Bone Tumors of the Thoracolumbar Spine

Joseph Y. Margulies, Yizhar Floman, and Michael G. Neuwirth

Neoplastic involvement of the spine is frequently encountered by spine surgeons, especially if they practice in a medical center with a busy oncology service. While the number of primary bone tumors of the spine is relatively small and most likely constant, the number of patients with spinal metastases is growing steadily. This is due both to longer life expectancy in the Western world and better treatment protocols of primary tumors, leading to longer survival. The increased longevity of cancer patients leads, however, to an increased incidence of spine metastases. The various advances in imaging studies, oncologic protocols, improved anesthetic techniques as well as sound biomechanical spinal instrumentation enable today a better, more efficient management of these various tumors. This, in turn, has yielded a better quality of life for patients with primary or secondary spine tumors and, in many cases, even enabled achieving a cure.

The spine surgeon, when confronted with a spine tumor patient, should address four basic issues: (a) What is the tissue diagnosis (is the tumor benign or malignant, primary or secondary)? (b) Is the tumor causing neurologic embarrassment? (c) Is the tumor jeopardizing spinal stability, or will surgical resection create spinal instability? (d) Is surgical cure feasible or is palliation the main aim?

The objectives of this chapter are to outline the clinical approach and the decision-making process when managing spine tumors. One has to be reminded that surgical care of malignant spine tumors is only one part of the process. These patients are managed by a multidisciplinary team of professionals of various specialties. The spine surgeon is part of the team.

INCIDENCE

The incidence of spinal tumors varies according to the underlying pathology. The two main groups encountered are primary and secondary bone tumors.

The incidence of primary bone tumors in general is 0.4% of all tumors; less than 10% of these are found in the spine (22). Ten percent of osteoid osteomas (which comprise 3% of all spine tumors) appear in the spine (51). Osteoblastomas comprise about 1% of all bone tumors; however, 40% of osteoblastomata appear in the spine (61). Osteochondromas of the spine comprise 1% of all bone tumors (40). Giant cell tumors comprise about 3% of all vertebral tumors (84). Less than 3% of osteosarcomas (23) and 10% of chondrosarcomas (50) appear in the spine. Chordoma, which arises predominantly in the spine, consists of between 1% and 4% malignant bone tumors (93).

While primary bone tumors of the spine are rare, metastatic secondary spine tumors are much more frequent. Of approximately one million new cases of cancer that are discovered every year in the United States, about 60% eventually develop distant metastases (3).

J. Y. Margulies and M. G. Neuwirth: Orthopaedic Department/Spine Service, Hospital for Joint Disease/Orthopaedic Institute, New York, NY 10003.

Y. Floman: Department of Orthopaedic Surgery and Spine Surgery Unit, Hebrew University–Hadassah Medical School, Hadassah University Hospital, Jerusalem 91120, Israel.

The skeletal system is the third most common site for metastasis, after the lungs and liver (10). Breast and prostate tumors metastasize to bone in 84% of the cases, thyroid tumors in 50%, lung neoplasms in 44%, and kidney tumors in 37% (8,32). Among skeletal metastases, the vertebral column has been found to be the most common site (10,33,64). Vertebral metastases were noted in large autopsy series in about 15% to 40% of patients dying of cancer (13). The thoracic spine and thoracolumbar spine are the most common sites of spinal metastases (6,39,73). There are predilections of certain tumors to specific regions in the spine (12,69). Breast and lung cancer have a predilection to the thoracic spine, while prostatic carcinoma has a predilection to the lumbar spine (39). Of the secondary spinal lesions, 12.5% appear without a known primary site (12).

ANATOMICAL CONSIDERATIONS

Benign tumors of the spine are usually located in the posterior elements of the vertebrae. Conversely, primary malignant tumors arise mainly from the vertebral body. Vertebral metastases usually spread through the venous system, as hypothesized many years ago by Batson (7) and others (21). Spinal metastases usually start within Denis' "middle" column, that is, the posterior part of the vertebral body. Thus it is possible to have a relatively early spread of the metastatic tumor into the epidural space. Indeed, Barron et al. (6) found, in autopsies of patients who died of carcinoma, that 5% had evidence of metastatic cord compression. The tumor may also spread to the vertebral pedicle, giving rise to the well-known radiologic sign of the "winking owl" (Fig. 1). The local invasion of the vertebral body and spinal canal may cause a pathological compression fracture and further contribute to pain and neurological compromise. Occasionally, the tumor may spread by direct extension to the spine, for example, in renal cell carcinoma or lung cancer presenting as a Pancoast tumor. Lymphoma is also known to invade the spinal canal from its paravertebral location, via the intervertebral foramina (72). Rarely, direct epidural metastasis may occur (13).

Pain, which is the most common symptom of primary or secondary spine tumors, arises from involvement of specific anatomical structures. It may be due to expansion of the tumor cells within the bone, periosteal irritation, or from a pathologic vertebral fracture. In addition, the pain may arise from compression of the dura, a nerve root, or invasion of a neural plexus. Back pain due to neoplastic involvement may be localized or diffuse and at times will have a radicular component.

Signs of neurologic compromise depend on the biology of the tumor, location of the lesion in the vertebral column, and the structural integrity of the axial skeleton. Gradual progressive paresis can be noted, associated with a high-grade myelographic block (39). Rapid onset of paralysis may appear suddenly within 24 hr (59,90). The slower the development of the weakness, the better the prognosis following surgical decompression. Occasionally, weakness without pain can be noted and may be confused with general debilitation of the patient. Bowel and bladder symptoms may also have an indolent or acute presentation. Involvement of the thoracic spine is more likely to result in neurologic deficit. The thoracic spinal canal is relatively narrow, and the vascular supply to the thoracic cord is relatively scarce. A tumor, in the thoracic spine, may therefore interfere with the blood supply of the cord or may cause an early cord compression. Due to the kyphotic posture of the thoracic spine, the cord at this site is even more vulnerable to compression. Thus a thoracic pathologic compression fracture will further augment the natural kyphosis and increase the likelihood of neural compromise (69). Spinal cord compression usually occurs at the anterior aspect of the cord, due to involvement of the posterior part of the vertebral body (the middle column) (Fig. 2).

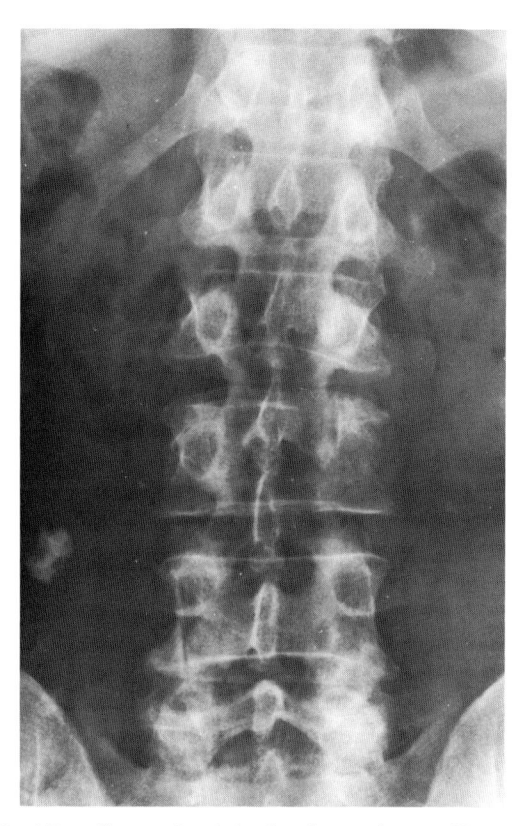

FIG. 1. AP radiograph of the lumbar spine: a 60-year-old patient with malignant fibrosarcoma involving the body of L3. Note the "missing" left pedicle, giving rise to the "winking owl" sign.

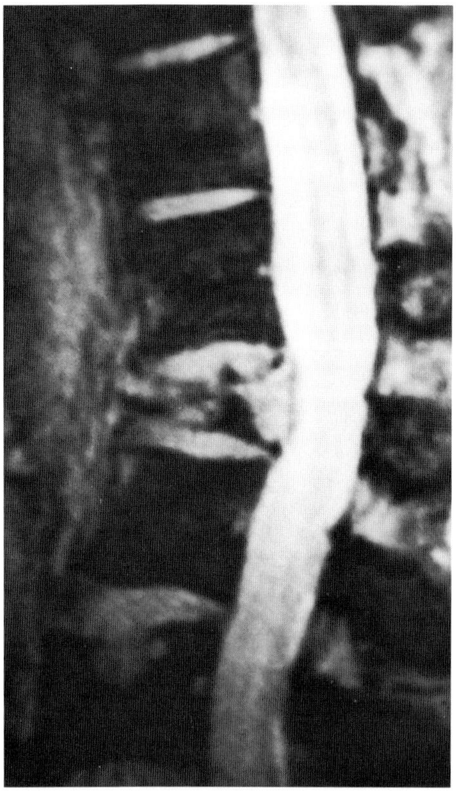

FIG. 2. MRI scan of the thoracic spine showing a pathological fracture (breast carcinoma) of a midthoracic vertebra with compression of the thecal sac from tumor located in the posterior part of the vertebral body.

The discs are not invaded by most tumors, yet discal damage occurs secondary to collapse of the invaded vertebral endplates or due to blockage of blood supply to the disc by the tumor (103).

A comprehensive model of spinal tumors relying on functional anatomy has been proposed by Weinstein (99). His classification uses the three-column model of the spine proposed by Denis (26) and Enneking's compartmental approach to tumors (28). Weinstein's approach is based on the anatomic location of a tumor within the vertebrae and whether the tumor is confined to bone or has expanded outside the body borders. The classification includes three grades:

A   Intraosseous lesion
B   Extraosseous lesion
C   Metastatic spread

Each of these grades is further defined by the exact anatomic location of the tumor within the vertebrae:

I   Laminae, inferior articular processes, spinous process
II Transverse processes, pars interarticularis, superior articular processes
III Anterior two-thirds of the vertebral body
IV Posterior one-third of the vertebral body

In addition to providing a logical framework for operative planning, it provides a comprehensive model for interinstitutional databases and statistics.

Asdourian et al. (5) presented data on the natural history of spinal deformity secondary to metastatic breast cancer. Their data relate the spinal deformity to the anatomic location of the secondary tumor deposition. Their observations and classification seem applicable to all metastatic vertebral lesions.

MODES OF PRESENTATION OF PATIENTS

Treatment Decisions

Pain is the most common presenting symptom of a spine tumor, whether primary or secondary (39,57,100). Certain features should alert the managing physician to the possible diagnosis of an axial skeleton neoplasm. Back pain when resting and nocturnal pain that may be relentless and progressive in nature are common symptoms of a spine tumor. Sometimes a nerve root is involved, leading to radicular pain. Radiculitis of the upper or lower extremity is easy to diagnose; however, one has to be alert to the presence of girdle-type radicular pain, typical for neoplastic involvement of the thoracic spine. In the series of Weinstein and McLain (100), 84% of the patients presented with pain, while weakness, solitary or in combination with other neurologic symptoms, was present in 41.5%. Spinal pain may be attributed to one or more of the following origins: mechanical instability, including pathologic fractures; pressure on neural structures; or marrow infiltration by the tumor. Pain can appear up to 6 months before a neurologic deficit can be detected (13,71).

Neurologic compromise secondary to a spinal tumor is the most important factor influencing therapeutic decision-making. Neurologic compromise means that the disease is advanced and treatment should be pursued immediately; procrastination may lead to permanent neural deficit. Paralysis is associated with bad prognosis and shortens the life expectancy of the cancer patient (91). Paralysis precedes sensory changes due to the proximity of the tumor cells in the posterior aspect of the vertebral body to the motor nerve cells in the anterior aspect of the spinal cord. Compression of the cauda equina will result in a lower motor neuron lesion. Isolated sphincter dysfunction is rarely a presenting symptom and occurs only if the lesion is in the conus region (18,39).

Patients may be referred to the radiologist or surgeon for a spinal biopsy for tissue diagnosis. Basically, a

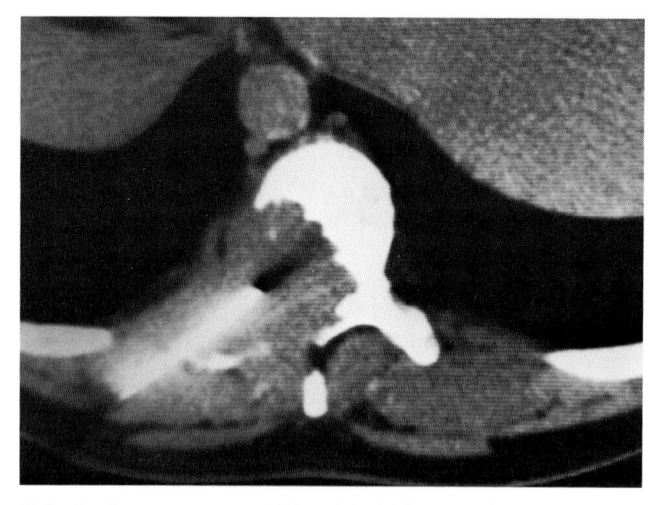

FIG. 3. Percutaneous CT-guided biopsy of a lesion in a thoracic vertebra. Note the large tumor mass invading the right lamina, pedicle and the vertebral body.

biopsy is performed in two clinical situations. Either the patient may have a known primary tumor elsewhere and a spine biopsy is needed for confirmation that the spinal lesion is a metastatic one, or the patient may present with a primary spinal neoplasm or a metastasis without a known primary. Indeed, 9% to 12% of patients with metastatic cord compression present without a known primary site (12,39). A closed biopsy, either under fluoroscopy control or with a CT-guided needle, can provide a tissue diagnosis most of the time (20,37,53,70) (Fig. 3). If a closed biopsy fails to establish the diagnosis, an open "limited" biopsy can be obtained via a costotransversectomy or via a transpedicular approach. The accurate tissue diagnosis especially in a case of epidural cord compression is essential for prescribing the most effective treatment.

Once the tissue diagnosis is established, a treatment protocol may be developed. Surgery is almost always

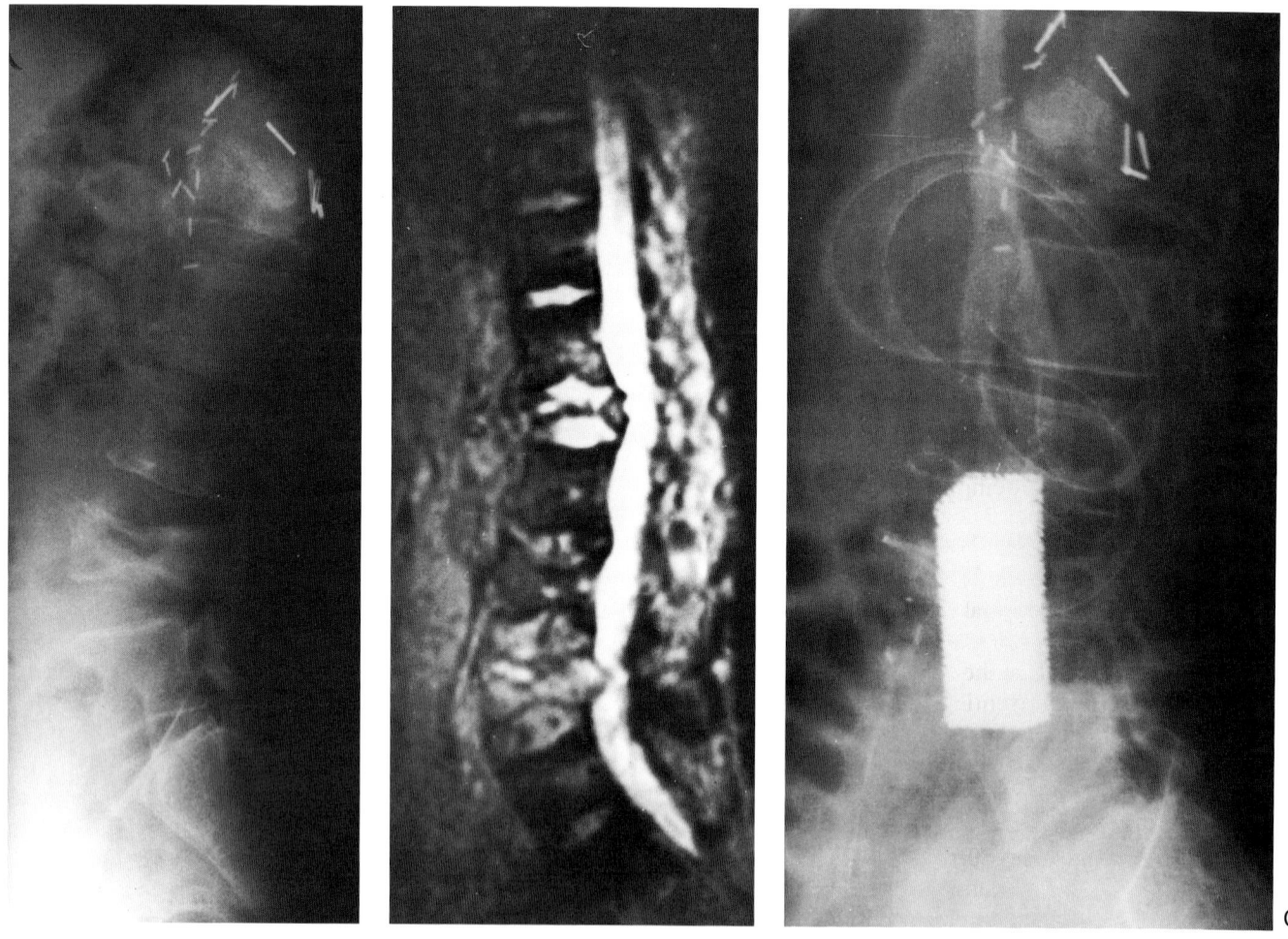

FIG. 4. A 40-year-old man with Gaucher's disease with clinical symptoms of cauda equina compression. He was previously operated on at the T12–L1 level for similar symptoms. **A:** Plain lateral radiograph of the lumbar spine showing an L4 "burst-like" fracture. Note the "vascular" clips at T12–L1. **B:** MRI scan of the same patient showing the fracture of L4 with compression of the dural sac, and also a mild compression at T12–L1. **C:** Following anterior retroperitoneal resection of the body of L4 with decompression of the cauda equina and vertebral replacement with a titanium block.

TABLE 1. *Indications for surgical treatment of metastatic cord compression*

Primary unknown
Relapse after previous radiation therapy
Radioresistant tumor
Neurologic deterioration during radiotherapy
Mechanical instability
Pathological fracture—bone compression of the neural elements

---

contemplated in primary spine tumors. Surgical treatment is also indicated when the tumor is known to be resistant to other modes of treatment, or when the mechanical or neurological functions of the spine and the cord are compromised (17). The majority of spine metastases and metastatic cord compressions can be managed by chemotherapy and/or radiation therapy. Surgery is indicated only if these measures fail to control pain or deformity or preserve neural function. Surgery is almost always indicated in a case of metastatic cord compression, without a known primary. Likewise, if mechanical stability is at stake or neurological deterioration is evolving rapidly, then primary surgery is the treatment of choice.

In summary, surgery is indicated when the diagnosis is in doubt, if there is a relapse of neurological symptoms after previous radiation therapy, or if there is a significant spinal instability or when the compressing tissue is bone (Table 1). Recently, Sundaresan et al. (97) found in a prospective study that de novo surgery is the treatment of choice in selected patients with neoplastic spinal cord compression. Surgery de novo was superior to radiotherapy or surgery performed after radiation therapy in achieving long-term preservation of walking ability (97).

Differential Diagnosis

Several nontumor, pathological lesions need to be considered in the differential diagnosis. The most important is the common osteoporotic fracture, which may sometimes pose a diagnostic dilemma. While most osteoporotic fractures are compression type fractures, occasionally these may be of the burst type, leading to neurologic compromise (80). Tuberculosis, osteomyelitis, and pseudoinfectious diseases such as eosinophilic granuloma must be considered as well. Gaucher's disease can also lead to a pathological fracture and cord compression (Fig. 4A). The degree of aggressiveness of these lesions varies, but the spinal problems that these conditions create usually justify surgical resection and a spinal reconstruction similar to solutions adopted in tumor surgery (Fig. 4).

NEUROLOGIC DEFICITS: CONSIDERATIONS

Overall, the goal of managing patients with spine tumors is to have a neurologically intact pain-free patient with a stable spine.

Neurologic deterioration is the most important indication for aggressive treatment. Fourteen percent of patients with spinal metastasis will present with a neurological deficit (88,89). Several factors that may influence the extent of the neurologic damage are to be considered.

Location

In order to inflict neurologic damage, it is not enough for the tumor to be located in the spine, but it has to produce pressure on neural tissue. This usually occurs by invasion of the tumor cells into the epidural space of the spinal canal, leading to encroachment of the available space for the neural tissue. Neural damage can also be inflicted by structural damage to the vertebrae leading to direct mechanical pressure on the neural tissue by the affected bone.

The Rate of Development of the Neural Deficit

The pathophysiology of the neural damage is based not only on the effect of direct mechanical pressure, but also on the relative ischemia of the neural tissue induced by local edema formation and decreased blood flow (90). Vascular changes can influence the rate of the developing neural deficit.

Abrupt onset of neurologic deficit, especially paraplegia, is a bad prognostic sign for the patient and for the neurological function. This has to do most probably with the cell biology of the specific tumor. On the other hand, the prognosis for an insidious neurologic compromise is more favorable with proper surgical decompression (46). The sooner the decompression is accomplished, the better are the odds for neural function improvement.

Pathological Fractures

Pathologic fractures of the thoracolumbar spine due to neoplastic infiltration of the vertebrae, with and without neural compromise, usually differ from traumatic injuries of the axial skeleton. While pathological fractures usually occur in middle aged or elderly, relatively sick individuals, traumatic injuries of the spine characteristically occur in young, otherwise healthy persons. Fracture patterns also differ in both conditions, and specific patterns may be recognized in each type (5,26).

A pathologic fracture may produce clinical symptoms due to mechanical instability and/or compression of neural tissue (see Fig. 2). Tumors cause vertebral fractures by interfering with the mechanical integrity of the bone; that is, the normal bone is replaced by the neoplasm. The tumor-infiltrated bone is less competent mechanically; this leads to mechanical insufficiency and collapse of the vertebra, irrespective of whether the tumor is osteoblastic or osteolytic. Tumors that cause fractures are usually moderately slow growing. Rapidly growing, malignant tumors usually cause severe pain or neural compression before fracture occurs.

Whether the neurologic deficit is caused by direct tumor cell invasion of the epidural space or by a pathologic fracture, surgical decompression should address the problem in its actual anatomical site (i.e., anterior, posterior, etc.). A general "decompression" by laminectomy, a once common practice, seldom addresses the problem and is no longer adequate.

IMAGING STUDIES

Modern imaging technologies make diagnosis of spine lesions relatively simple. The most important issue in the diagnosis of spinal tumors is therefore clinical awareness or a "high index" of suspicion. In most cases, plain radiographs may establish the diagnosis of a spinal bone tumor. However, bone scans, CT scans, MRI scans, and other investigative modalities are indicated to stage the lesion for an appropriate treatment plan.

The first efforts should be aimed toward locating the exact spinal level of the lesion.

Bone scans are frequently used as a screening examination. It is the best tool for detecting vertebral tumors including metastasis, with an accuracy of 95% to 97% (9,16). Morishita et al. (67) found that routine performance of technetium bone scans detected "hot spots" in the spine in 25%, 29.5%, 24.3%, and 47%, respectively, of patients with breast, lung, uterine/cervix, and prostatic cancer. These "hot spots" represent metastatic deposition (Fig. 5). Although bone scans are more sensitive than plain radiographs in detecting bony metastasis (34), they are inadequate for predicting the level of cord compression. Moreover, a ^{99m}Tc bone scan may sometimes yield false-negative results when the tumor produces pure bone lysis, such as in the case of multiple myeloma. Recently, MRI was found to be more sensitive than Tc bone scan in detecting vertebral metastasis (2,81).

Plain radiographs from at least two angles often indicate the nature of a lesion and the bone quality. Pathologic fractures and spinal deformity can easily be diagnosed on plain films. Once the lesion is confirmed by

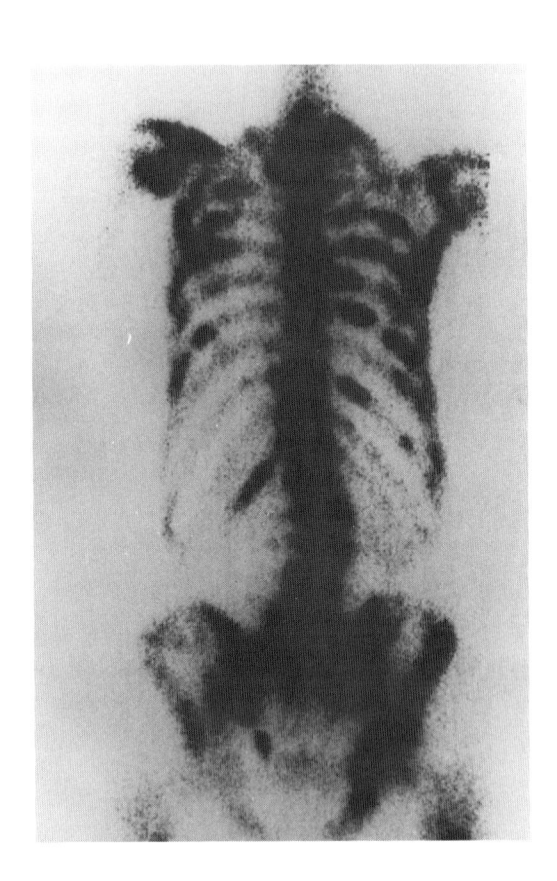

FIG. 5. ^{99m}Tc bone scan of a 70-year-old man showing multiple "hot spots" in spine, pelvis, and ribs representing metastatic prostatic cancer.

radiographs, the next step is to gain further anatomic information about the lesion. CT or MRI scans with dye enhancement, such as intra-arachnoid metrizamide or i.v. gadolinium, should be performed. Computed tomography is excellent in both diagnosing the extent of tumor deposition and planning the surgical approach. In addition, it may provide data on the stability of the spine, and whether there is neural encroachment. A traditional tomogram may be useful in some cases.

In patients with neurologic compromise, the next important information to obtain is the identification of the upper and lower ends of the compromised cord with myelography (6). This may necessitate a cisternal puncture in addition to a lumbar puncture. Identification of skip lesions with myelography is also important. The routine use of CT-myelography in cancer patients with complaints of back pain may provide the possibility for earlier detection of cord compression (101) and will increase the likelihood that these patients will retain their ambulatory status with proper management (78). MRI may soon replace myelography in many of these diagnostic situations.

Angiography should be performed prior to surgery if it is suspected that the tumor is hypervascular. If so, embolization of the tumor can be accomplished during the angiography, as a means of cutting down on intraoperative bleeding (11).

After the lesion has been anatomically defined, evaluation of the patient's general condition and the magnitude of the disease spread is of utmost importance for further decision-making regarding treatment. The immune status of the patient must also be included in the preoperative considerations. The immunologically compromised patient represents a poor surgical risk.

If a patient presents with a progressive neurologic problem, especially if it is of recent onset, then immediate surgical decompression is indicated. A complete diagnostic work-up is impossible in these circumstances. Nevertheless, the spine level should be confirmed by CT-myelography or MRI before surgery. Prior to radiation, chemotherapy or surgical intervention, systemic high-dose steroids are administered (44,98).

TREATMENT: THE ROLE OF THE SPINE SURGEON

Management of spine tumors is usually pursued by a team of specialists. The spine surgeon is involved either in obtaining a tissue diagnosis or, in other instances, in providing definitive treatment of the affected spine. However, one must remember that surgery is only part of the overall management of the spine tumor patient. One must consider the life expectancy of the patient, the operative risk, the magnitude of the proposed procedure, and the patient's physical and mental ability to participate in the plan of management. Alternative methods of treatment must also be considered. For example, it has been found that only 11% of patients with breast metastasis required surgery, the rest responded well to radiation therapy (17). On the other hand, renal cell carcinoma, multiple myeloma, and lung carcinoma do not respond well to these conservative measures. In these cases, surgery is dictated by the appearance of signs of cord compression.

The ideal objectives of any treatment, including operative treatment, are to radically *excise the tumor*, leaving a *stable, pain-free* spine, *without neurologic impairment*.

The first goal has to do with radical tumor excision. However, not infrequently marginal or intralesional resection are the only realistic possibilities.

The second goal of treatment is to restore stability (30,55,95). Instability due to tumor deposition differs from traumatic instability. A motion segment with tumor involvement in two of the three spinal columns may still retain a reasonable mechanical stability. Ligaments are usually spared by the neoplastic process, although ligamentous attachments may be jeopardized. In these circumstances, spine instability may be related to continued tumor growth. However, if the specific tumor that caused the spinal instability responds to conservative measures, such as radiation, the spine may restabilize, as, for example, in breast carcinoma (54). Conversely, extensive infiltration of two spinal columns, by a tumor that is not responsive to oncologic treatment (radiotherapy and chemotherapy), requires surgical stabilization. Radiologic evidence of involvement of *all* three spinal columns usually warrants stabilization.

Kostuik et al. (55) devised their own system for evaluating spinal stability in neoplastic involvement; they divided the spine into anterior and posterior columns. The anterior column, consisting of the vertebral body, was divided into right and left anterior and posterior quadrants. The posterior column, which is comprised of the pedicle and the posterior arch, was also divided into right and left parts (55). Kostuik et al. stated that tumor deposition in more than three to four subcolumns should be considered mechanically unstable.

The technique and principles of spine stabilization are somewhat different from those employed in traumatic fracture surgery. Tumor surgery requires "filling in" of zones of bone loss, frequently not encountered in trauma surgery. For patients with life expectancy of more than 2 years, regular bone grafting techniques are appropriate. Sometimes a mixture of cement in the anterior and middle columns of the spine and bone

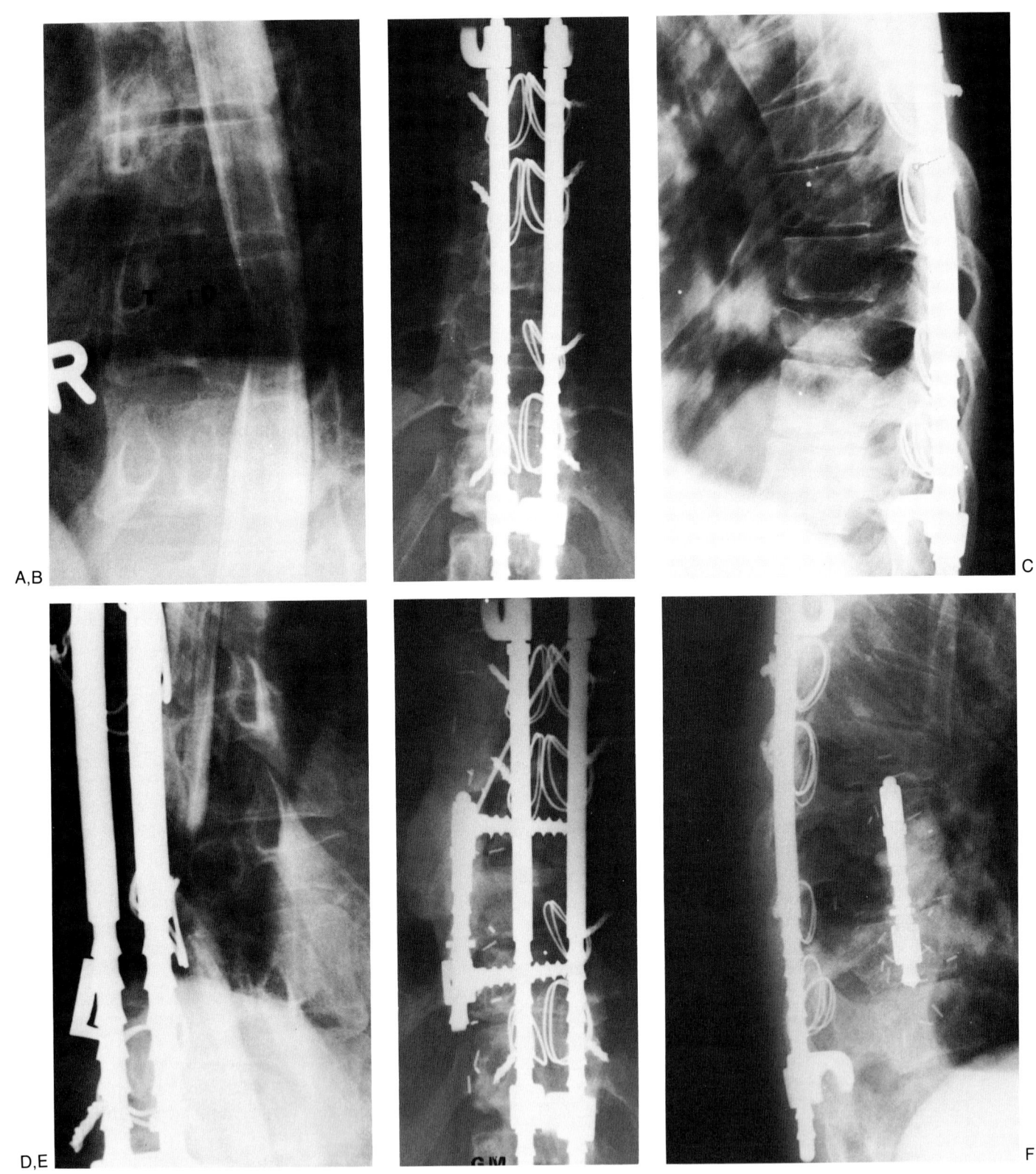

FIG. 6. A 35-year-old woman with metastatic malignant melanoma of the thoracic spine (T10) with clinical signs of cord compression. **A:** A myelogram showing the involvement of the right pedicle of T10 with compression on the dye column. **B,C:** AP and lateral views of the spine. The patient underwent a laminectomy and right pediculectomy to decompress the cord. The spine was stabilized with Harrington distraction rods and sublaminar wires from T6 to L12. **D:** Myelogram. The tumor recurred 9 months later. Note compression on the dye column from tumor invading the vertebral body. **E,F:** AP and lateral views of the spine. Patient underwent a right thoracotomy with resection of the vertebral body with "filling in" of the gap with bone cement and stabilization with Kostuik–Harrington instrumentation.

grafting in the posterior column is the proper course for the destabilized, tumor-ridden spine (Fig. 6). Bone cement alone is appropriate in patients with short life expectancy. Estimated life expectancy can be provided by the managing oncologist. For example, only 19% of the lung cancer patients stay alive for more than 1 year if metastases are diagnosed, while more than 74% of breast, prostate, and uterine/cervix carcinoma patients stay alive more than 1 year after metastasis detection (67). It must be remembered that there are numerous complications with the use of bone cement, including leakage of the cement into the spinal canal (27).

Preservation of the neural function is the most important goal of treatment. It is well known that laminectomy or radiation therapy, or a combination of both, has resulted in limited success in ensuring neurological recovery (63,66,104). Livingston and Perrin (57) reported that only 40% of patients undergoing "decompressive" laminectomy for neoplastic spinal cord compression showed satisfactory neural recovery. The percentage of nonambulatory patients regaining their ability to walk was even lower (11%). The overall success rate in restoring neural function with radiation therapy and laminectomy is between 20% and 40%. Gilbert and Kagan (38) found that radiation therapy alone was as effective as a combination of laminectomy and radiotherapy (49% versus 46%). As neural compression occurs usually in the anterior aspect of the canal, laminectomy is usually contraindicated because it does not relieve the pressure on the neural elements and may increase spinal instability. Moreover, laminectomy may even increase the neurologic deficit, especially if performed in a case of a pathological fracture with a kyphotic deformity (29). From a historical point of view, laminectomy was the main mode of decompression, mainly because it was the only procedure mastered by surgeons at that time. Its efficiency in clinical situations other than posterior cord compression is, however, very limited and is most often hazardous.

Employment of a more direct surgical approach to the site of cord compression (i.e., the anterior approach) facilitated better and more efficient tumor excision and neural decompression (47,55,88,89,95). Accordingly, the results achieved were significantly better. Harrington (47) reported 84% return of neural function following anterior decompression. The findings of Sundaresan et al. (95) were similar. It can be expected that 70% of patients who are nonambulatory may improve with surgery; this percentage of improvement is twice that achieved by radiotherapy (55,58,95).

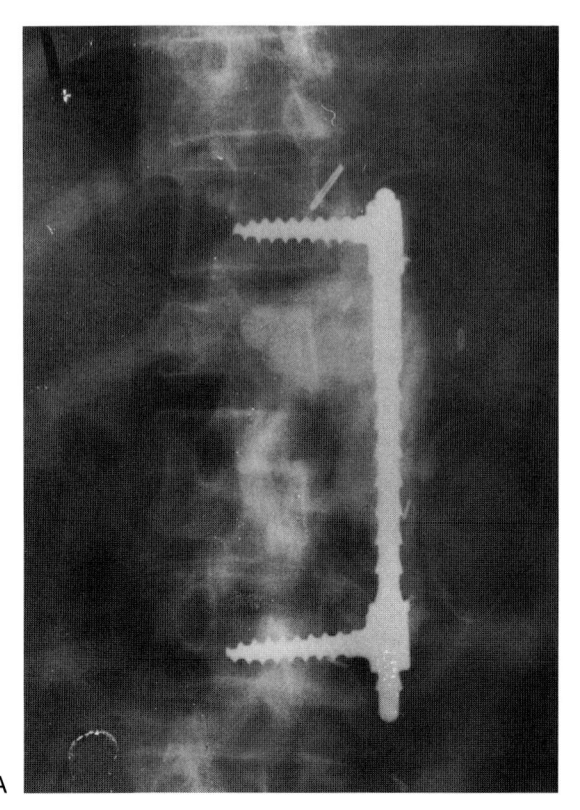

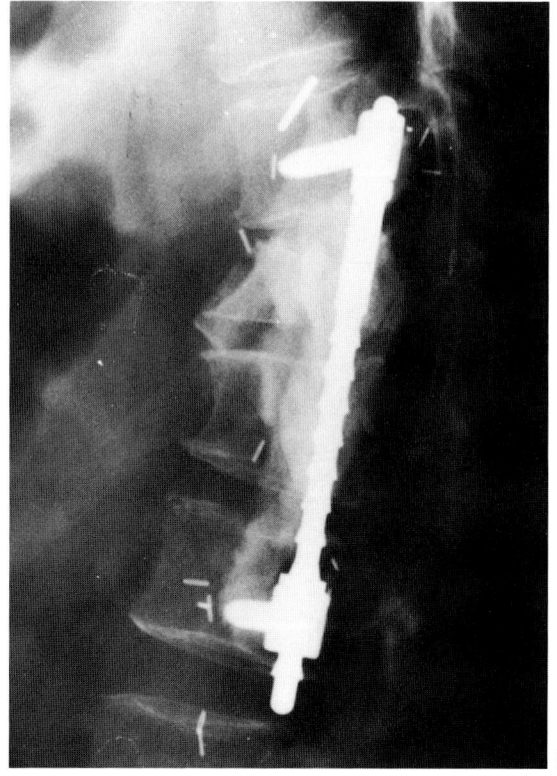

FIG. 7. AP **(A)** and lateral **(B)** views of the spine. Metastatic thyroid carcinoma in a 44-year-old man. Following anterior excision of the lesion, the spine was stabilized with a Kostuik–Harrington device augmented with bone cement.

Siegal and Siegal (88,89) found that radiation therapy was effective in 30% of patients with cord compression, laminectomy in 40%, while anterior decompression achieved 80% neural recovery. It has to be stressed that patients with pathological fractures and cord compression are not candidates for radiotherapy and will necessitate surgery.

The nature of the tumor and its anatomical location dictate whether radical tumor excision or only intralesional resection is possible. Next, the mechanical status of the spine after tumor excision must be considered. Obviously, removal of the tumor involves decompression of the neural tissue, if indicated. After excision of the tumor, the next objective is to leave the patient with a stable spine. This is achieved by reconstruction of two stable continuous columns, the anterior and the posterior. The continuity of the anterior column must be based preferably on bone grafting and bony healing, or by a metal spacer or bone cement, rather than relying only on metal rods or plates. In general, the role of spinal implants is to support and augment immediate stability until biologic healing takes place.

As stated earlier, if the patient's projected survival is short term, instrumentation with mechanical augmentation with methyl methacrylate is the only procedure performed (Fig. 7). If the projected time of survival is more than 1 year, stabilization procedures, accompanied by biologic arthrodesis, as employed in surgery for trauma or for degenerative diseases should be accomplished.

In certain circumstances, the radiated vertebra with secondary tumor deposition is not excised, but spinal stability is addressed by "bypassing" the lesion with instrumentation and fusion. This procedure is beneficial to many patients with vertebral metastasis, by eliminating most of their axial pain, thus improving their life quality (Figs. 8 and 9) (35). All these procedures can be followed, if indicated, by adjunct radiotherapy and chemotherapy.

The two objectives—tumor excision and spine stabilization—dictate the operative approach. In some cases, either the anterior or posterior approach will suffice and, at other times, a combined approach must be utilized.

While neurologic function is never sacrificed for

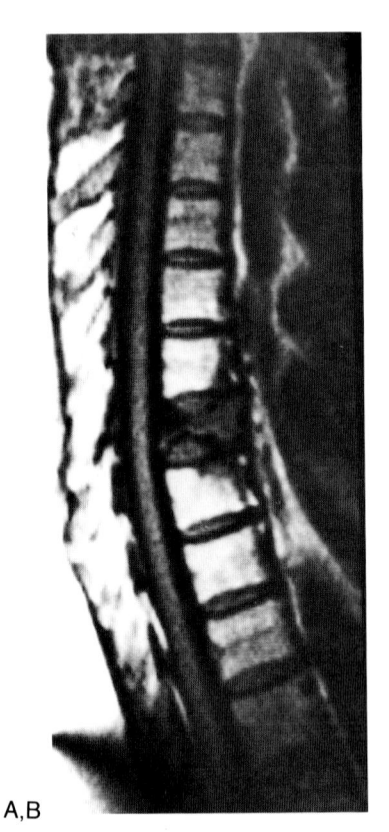

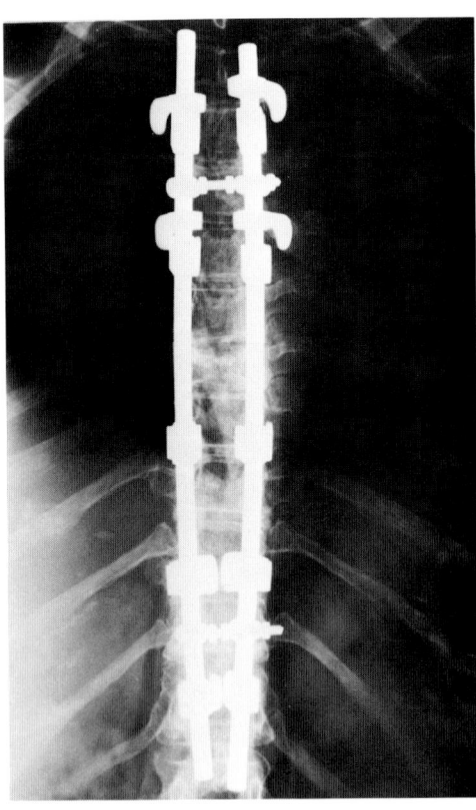

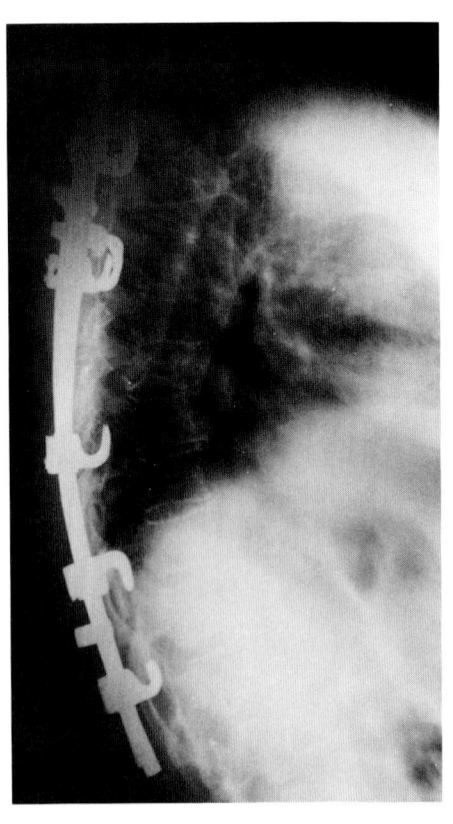

FIG. 8. A 50-year-old woman with metastatic breast cancer to the thoracic spine. She had incapacitating back pain due to mechanical instability. No signs of cord compression were evident. **A:** MRI scan showing tumor invasion of T7. **B,C:** AP and lateral views of the spine: following stabilization with C-D instrumentation. The patient had complete relief of her back pain until her death 2 years later.

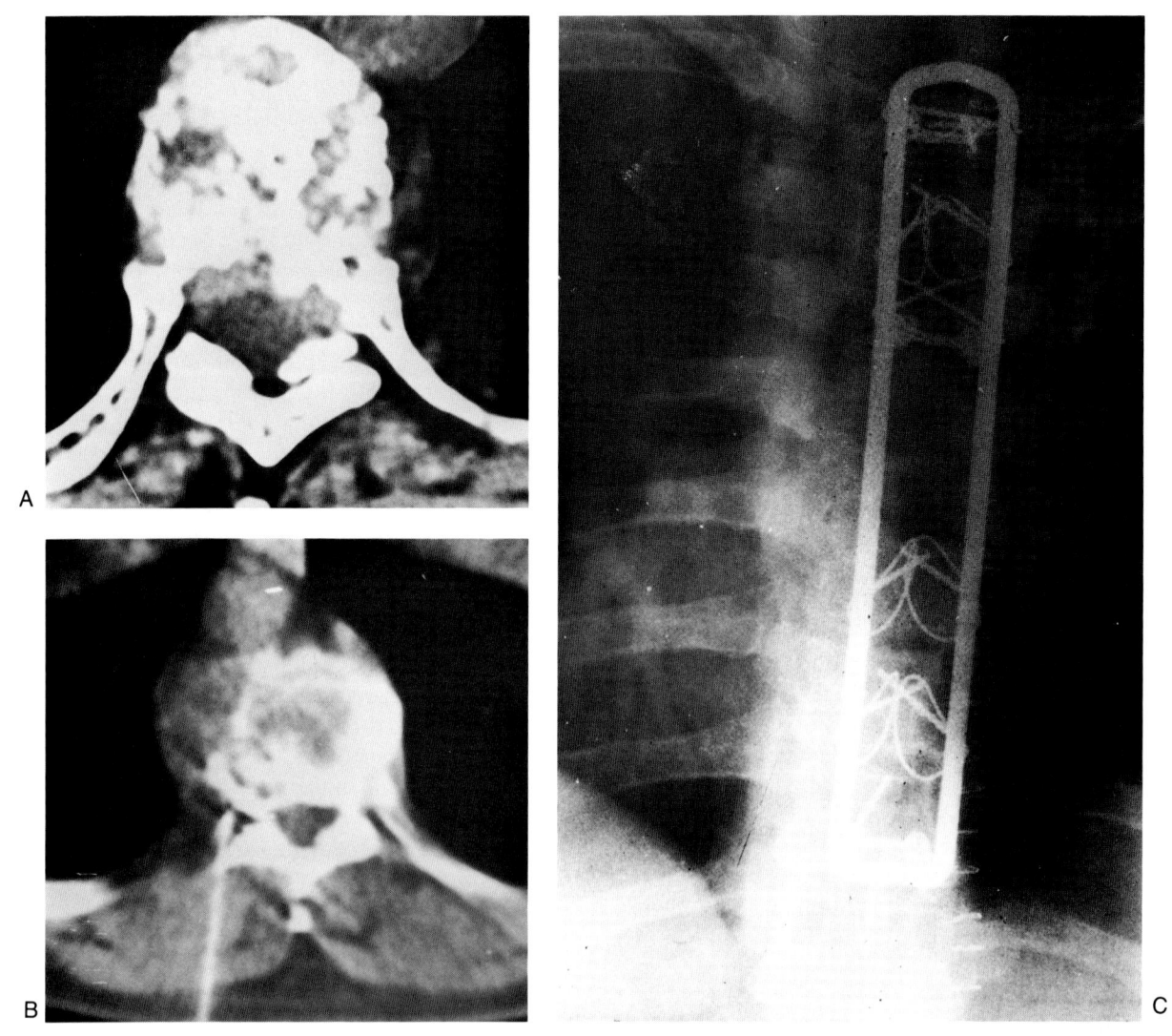

FIG. 9. Kimura's tumor involving the T8 body. The patient, a 45-year-old man, had mechanical thoracic spine pain. **A:** CT scan showing involvement of the T8 body. **B:** Needle biopsy establishing the histological diagnosis. **C:** The spine was stabilized with a Hartshill frame, and the patient was referred for radiotherapy.

spinal stability, neurologic integrity may occasionally be sacrificed to achieve a radical tumor excision (i.e., in sacral tumors).

SURGICAL APPROACHES

The appropriate surgical approach has to be chosen to meet the most important surgical objectives, which are removal of the tumor and decompression of the neural tissue. Another consideration in choosing the surgical approach is spinal stability. The name of the game is a proper exposure, which will enable accomplishment of all objectives without the need to compromise.

Many patients undergo radiation therapy prior to surgery; these patients present an increased risk for postoperative skin necrosis and/or infection. This factor may sometimes modify the surgical approach.

Anterior Approaches and Instrumentation

The anterior approach is used to solve problems caused by tumors that are located in the vertebral body. Every anterior operation of this type has four main objectives to fulfill:

1. Adequate exposure.
2. The possibility of radically excising the tumor.
3. Adequate neural decompression.
4. The ability to stabilize the spine.

The dorsal spine may be accessed by two anterior routes, either extrapleural or intrapleural, through a thoracotomy. The extrapleural approach carries less morbidity to the patient but is technically more difficult. Usually the transpleural approach is preferred. Both usually require a rib resection and, in higher thoracic levels, also necessitate mobilization of the scapula. The anterior approach above T4 is technically difficult, since the area of exposure is limited by the small ribs and adjacent vascular structures in the upper mediastinum. A costotransversectomy might yield a slightly better exposure of the upper thoracic spine. However, a modified anterior approach to the cervicothoracic junction is preferred. A T-shaped incision over the clavicle and upper sternum with midsternotomy and resection of the medial third of the clavicle allow for good exposure of the upper thoracic spine (56).

The two main anterior exposures of the lumbar spine are retroperitoneal and transperitoneal. Each of these exposures gives access to the various aspects of the vertebrae, according to the anatomy. The retroperitoneal approach is adequate for lesions of the upper lumbar spine. A better access to the fourth and fifth lumbar vertebrae is the transperitoneal route. (For more details on the anterior approach, see Chapter 20 by Bayley, et al.)

Excision of the tumor, usually the first goal of surgery, is done according to the principles of tumor excision in general: preferably extracompartmental or through disease-free borders (i.e., "en bloc" resection). It is, however, hard to discuss extracompartmental excisions in the spine, because the compartments are not well defined and the cord may hinder attempts at radical excision. Therefore a "piecemeal" debulking may sometimes be the only surgical alternative. Even in these circumstances, one should arrive at tumor-free tissue.

The extent of the required excision dictates the need for spinal stabilization and "hardware" implantation. A stabilizing construct consists of two components, a spacer to fill the bony gap created by the tumor excision (Fig. 6) and a construct that will preserve the spinal contour until bony healing has taken place. Technically, the fewer motion segments fused, the more favorable the outcome for the patient (Fig. 10).

Traditionally, anterior stabilization was achieved by a bony strut graft. This technique was associated with a high percentage of strut graft dislocation and/or loosening and difficulty in preserving spinal stability until bony union occurred. In the past 10 years, stable anterior instrumentation has been introduced, yielding better clinical results. (For more details, see Chapter 21 by Floman). Kostuik–Harrington (Figs. 6, 7, and 10), Kaneda, Zielke, and Slot instrumentations are all longitudinal member (rod) systems. Plate systems include the Yuan, Armstrong, Senegas, and other systems (Fig. 11). The Kaneda device seems to be more stable than the other implants and in conjunction with anterior strut grafting provides higher fusion rates and a more rigid spinal segment (105). A newly introduced system is the Harms cylinder for vertebral body replacement (see Fig. 17).

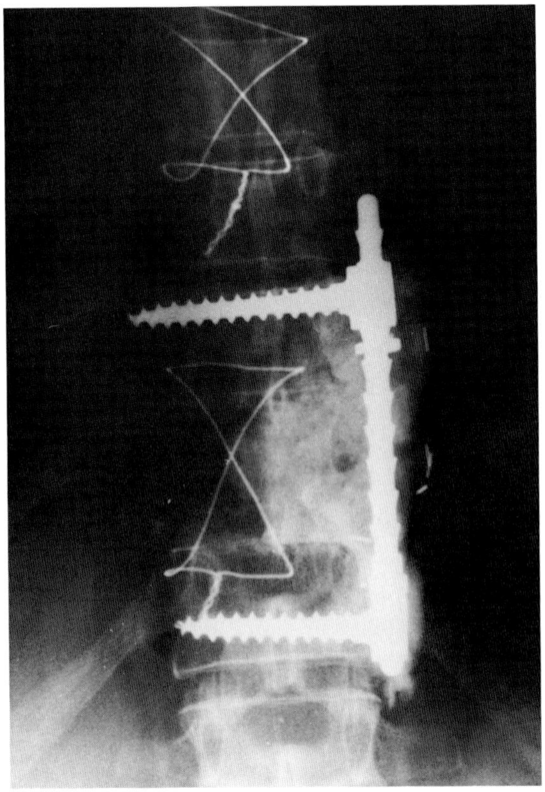

FIG. 10. Metastatic carcinoma of the colon managed by vertebral body resection with fixation by bone cement and Kostuik–Harrington distraction rod.

FIG. 11. Metastatic cord compression in a 79-year-old man with prostatic carcinoma. **A:** Lateral view showing a "compression" fracture of T8. **B:** Sagittal MRI scan showing anterior cord compression at the T7 level. **C,D:** AP and lateral views following vertebrectomy of T7, strut grafting T6–T8, and femoral shaft allograft, as well as stabilization with an Armstrong plate. (Case courtesy of Dr. E. H. Simmons, Jr., Buffalo, NY.)

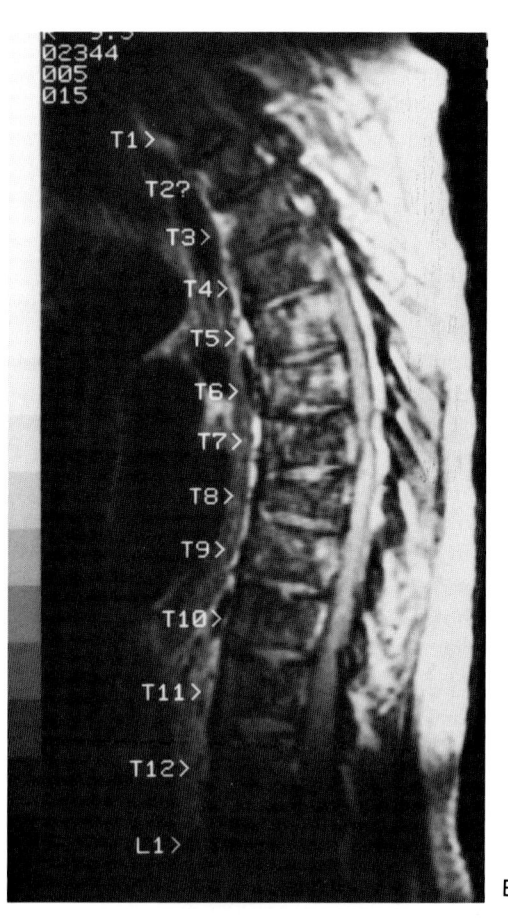

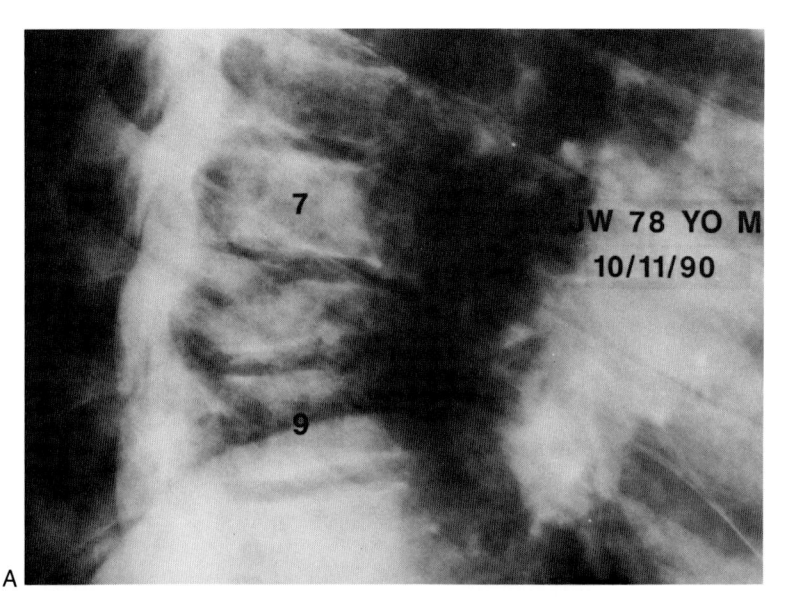

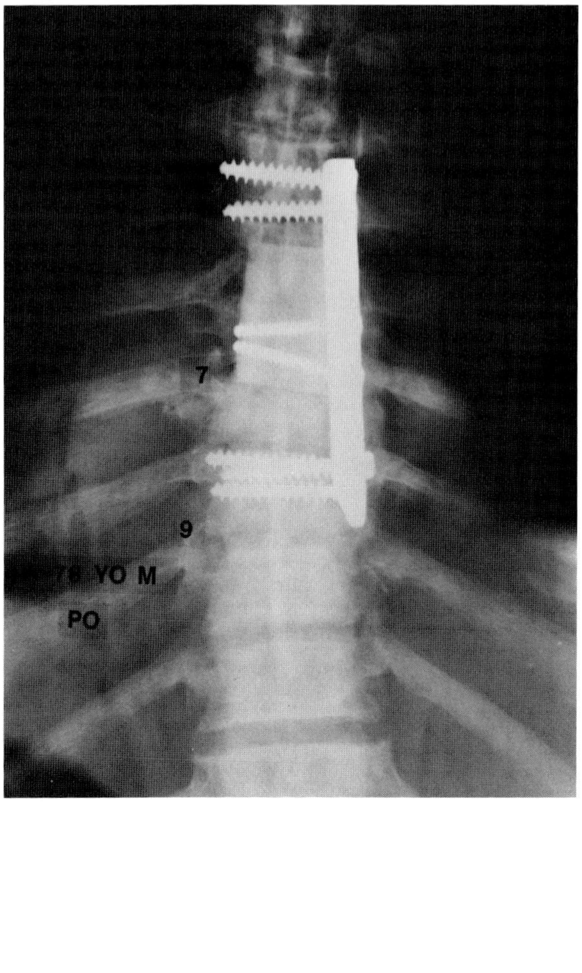

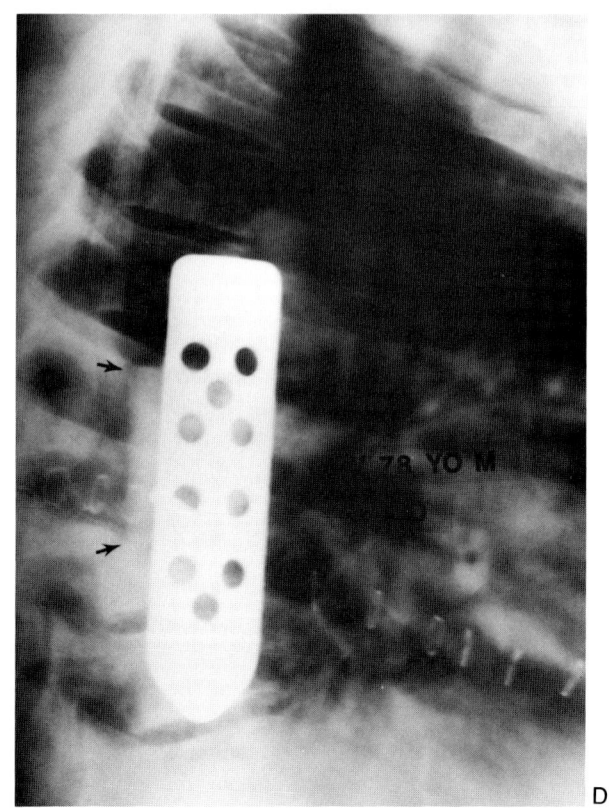

Posterior Approaches and Instrumentation

The posterior approach can solve problems caused by tumors located in the posterior elements of the spine. Because most of the metastatic lesions arise from the middle column, and the pressure on the neural tissues is anterior, laminectomy has had limited success in restoring neural function. Occasionally, the spinal cord can be decompressed through a posterior approach via the pedicle with excision of the posterior vertebral body; however, decompression and tumor resection are quite limited. Similarly, a costotransversectomy can be employed again, with limited exposure. The latter approach is practical for biopsy or drainage but is not suitable for proper neural decompression. Total corporectomy through a posterior approach has been reported by Roy-Camille (79); however, most spine surgeons do not master this complex technique.

The posterior approach can provide stability for problems caused by the excision of tumors in either site of the vertebral column. The modern posterior fixation systems are based on a strong purchase of the posterior elements, in conjunction with segmental fixation. In addition, insertion of pedicular screws provides a direct and more rigid fixation of all three spinal columns, even in osteopenic patients. Some of the available posteriorly installed systems are the Cotrel–Dubousset, Isola, TSRH, and the A-O internal fixator (see Fig. 8). All these systems include rods with hook and pedicle screw connections. In addition, plate systems with pedicle screw fixation, such as the Steffee or Roy-Camille, are also available. (For more details see Chapter 22 by Floman.)

Combined Approaches

A combined or circumferential approach may be needed when the tumor is located in all three columns of the spine (i.e., the body and posterior elements) or when stability was lost as a result of the tumor removal. Gurr et al. (45) utilized a corpectomy model and showed that solid stabilization required implantation of posterior and anterior devices with a strong purchase and a spacer. Figures 6E and 6F are examples of such constructs.

SPECIFIC TUMORS

Primary Bone Tumors of the Spine

In contrast to metastatic spinal tumors, primary bone tumors of the axial skeleton are rare. When detected in children or young adults, these primary tumors are usually benign, while in older individuals they may be malignant. The presenting symptoms of these primary bone tumors are usually nonspecific. Not all tumors present as pathological fractures or cause neurologic deficit. The very small, benign tumors do not produce a serious neurologic or mechanical problem. These benign spinal bone tumors tend to appear in the posterior element and may cause, in addition to pain, a reactive scoliosis. Tumor excision will usually result in regression of the scoliotic deformity. Yet the surgical excision of such tumors may sometimes hinder the mechanical stability.

Certain tumors have a characteristic radiological picture and a preoperative histological diagnosis is unnecessary (i.e., osteoid osteoma). In other primary bone tumors of the spine, needle biopsy of the lesion should be obtained, for better planning of the operative procedure. If necessary, even an open biopsy should be performed.

Primary Benign Tumors of the Spine

Hemangioma

This is the most common benign tumor of the spine. Schmorl and Junghans (85) reported that 10% of spines examined postmortem showed evidence of vertebral hemangioma. Indeed, this tumor (or perhaps a hamartoma) can be detected incidentally on spinal radiographs taken for a variety of reasons. Vertebral hemangioma has a predilection for the thoracic spine. The

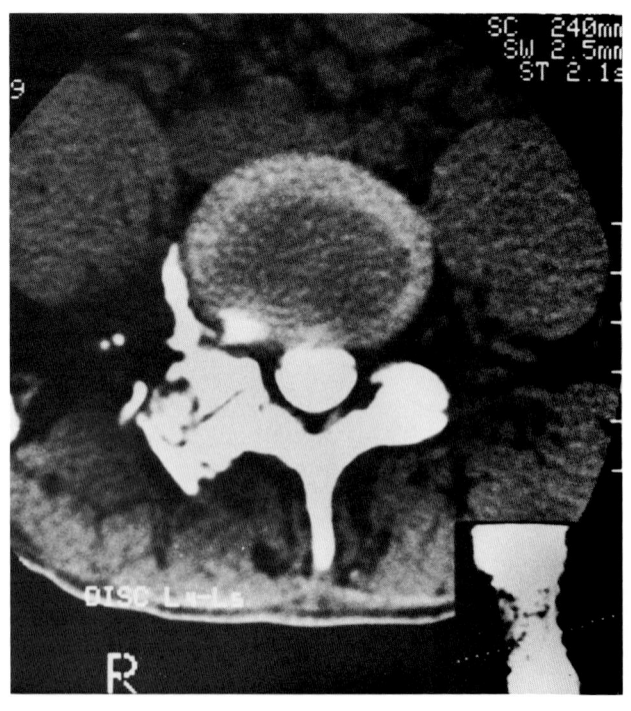

FIG. 12. Axial CT scan showing a typical osteoid osteoma of the right facet joint at L4–L5. This 25-year-old man had persistent low back pain and referred right leg pain.

radiological picture has a characteristic appearance of thick vertical sclerotic strands of bone trabeculae located in the vertebral body (48). On CT examination, the hemangioma appears as dense white dots spread in the vertebral corpus. The lesion is in most cases asymptomatic. Rarely, a pathologic fracture may result in a neurologic compromise (42). This may necessitate surgical excision and spinal reconstruction.

Osteochondroma

This benign lesion arises usually from the spinous process or the facet joint and has a distinct radiological appearance of a broad or pedunculated bony projection covered with a cartilaginous cap. One can easily distinguish the continuity of the bony cortex, as well as the spongiosa between the intact posterior elements and the lesion.

Osteochondromas are usually silent but occasionally, because of their large size, can give rise to local symptoms. Rarely, neurologic compromise can occur as well (52).

Osteoid Osteoma

In the spine, this small, bone-forming tumor involves almost invariably the posterior elements, facet joints, pedicle, and transverse processes (31,76). Rarely, it can be found in the vertebral body itself.

The tumor presents with localized pain, often nocturnal in nature, and may be accompanied by a reactive scoliotic deformity. Typically, the pain is relieved by aspirin and other NSAIDs. Spinal motion is usually severely restricted.

This benign tumor is most often encountered in children, adolescents, and young adults and is not found in elderly people. Radiologically, the size of the lesion is less than 2 cm in diameter. It is a bone-forming tumor with a central radiolucent zone surrounded by thick sclerotic reactive bone. Focal increased isotope uptake is seen on Tc bone scan, and the lesion can easily be identified (without the need for histological confirmation) on tomograms or CT scan (Fig. 12). Treatment is by surgical resection or by complete curettage, otherwise the pain may recur. Excision of the tumor usually leads to the regression of the scoliotic deformity and seldom results in spinal instability.

Benign Osteoblastoma

Osteoid osteoma and benign osteoblastoma are members of the same family of benign bone-forming tumors and may be histologically indistinguishable (61). Despite the similarity of the histological picture,

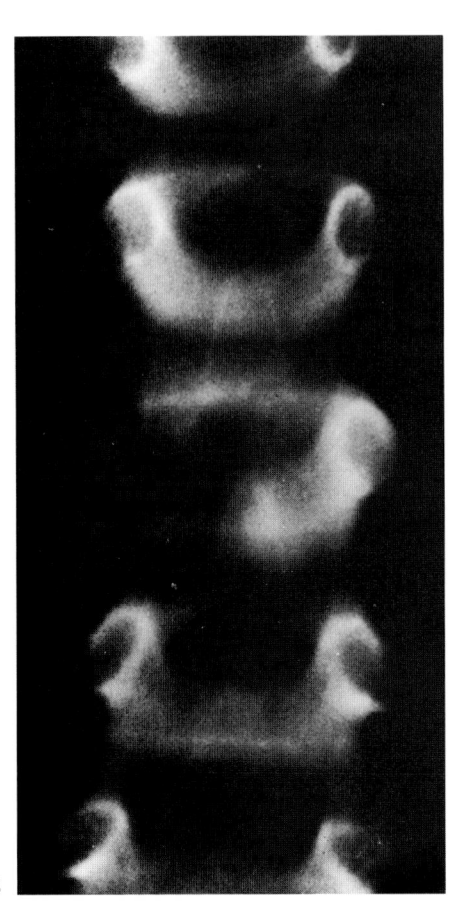

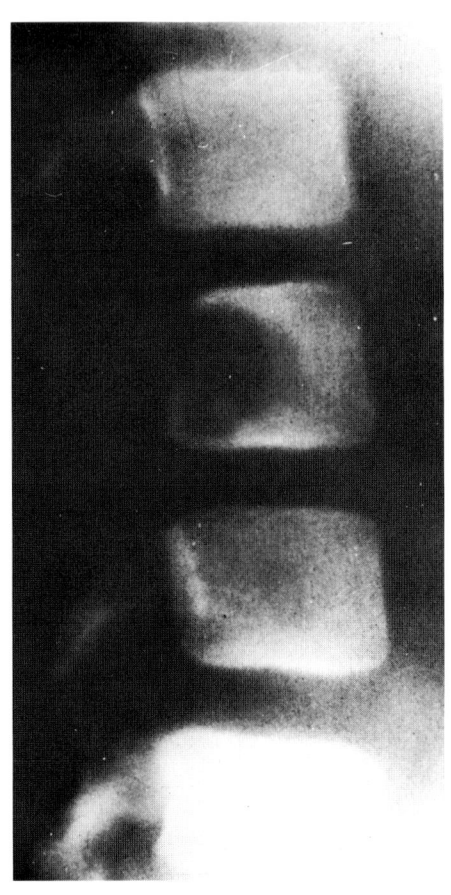

FIG. 13. A 6-year-old boy with persistent low back pain. Pedicular destruction is noted on the AP view **(A)**. The lateral view **(B)** shows a large osteolytic lesion in the posterior half of the vertebral body. After surgical excision, the lesion was found to be an osteoblastoma. (From ref. 77.)

these tumors have a different radiological appearance and biological behavior. This difference is probably the result of the different locations of these benign tumors; whereas osteoid osteoma arises in cortical bone, osteoblastoma originates in spongy bone. This may explain the limited growth potential of osteoid osteoma, and the more locally aggressive growth of osteoblastoma.

The spine is the most common site for benign osteoblastoma (31). Osteoblastoma arises most often in the posterior elements of the spine but occasionally may appear in the ribs. Spinal osteoblastoma is found in the second or third decades of life and causes local spinal pain, reactive scoliosis, and not infrequently neurological symptoms (Fig. 13).

Radiologically, osteoblastoma appears as a well circumscribed lesion of a large osteolytic nidus surrounded by a thin radiodense shell. It has the tendency to invade the soft tissues or encroach the spinal canal, giving rise to neurologic symptoms.

Surgical treatment is accomplished by "en bloc" resection and usually necessitates some form of surgical stabilization and spine fusion. In some instances, local recurrence appears, especially after piecemeal excision (31). Rarely, the lesion may become malignant, with pulmonary spread (36). It is then indistinguishable from osteosarcoma.

Aneurysmal Bone Cyst

This tumor of the spine is characterized by aneurysmal dilation of the bony structure. It may involve the posterior elements or the vertebral body (1,15,25,49). It usually occurs in the second or third decade of life. Its etiology is unclear, and it has been proposed that the lesion represents a vascular anomaly secondary to altered bone hemodynamics (1,77). It is a hypervascular lesion that may reach a very large size. It has been reported that in about one-third of the cases the aneurysmal lesion is secondary to another primary bone tumor such as osteoblastoma or giant cell tumor of bone (1). The tumor may invade more than one vertebral level.

Radiologically, there is an aneurysmal dilation of the bone with a surrounding eggshell thin cortex. It may invade the soft tissues or the spinal canal, with a significant encroachment of the neural elements (Fig. 14). The lesion may cause collapse of the vertebral body with the appearance of a vertebra plana or localized kyphosis leading to a neurological catastrophe.

Management of these tumors includes complete resection, with occasional bone grafting and internal fixation.

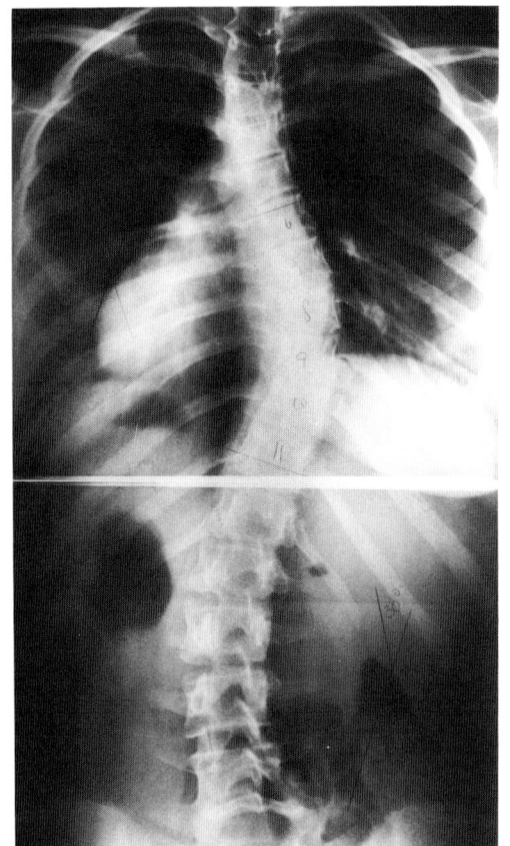

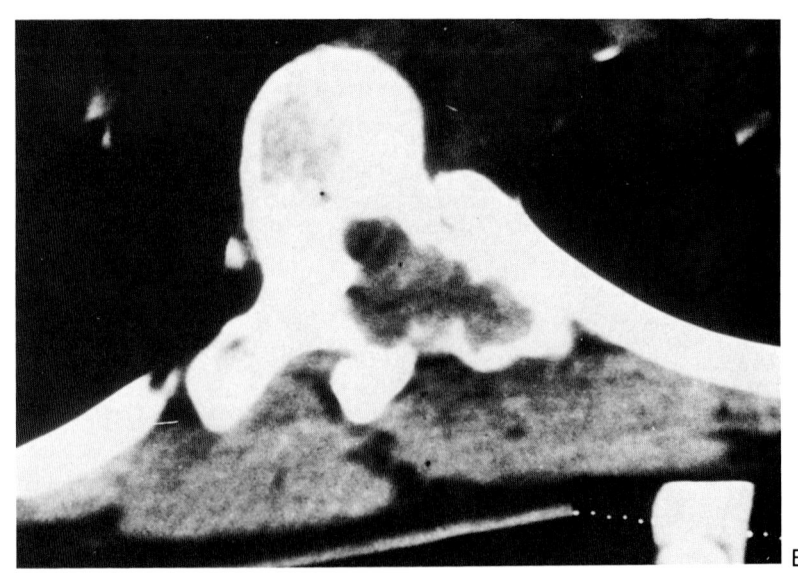

FIG. 14. This 15-year-old girl had persistent nocturnal thoracic spine pain. On examination, there was a stiff right thoracic scoliosis **(A)**. A bone scan showed an increased focal uptake at the apex of the curve on the concave side. Axial CT scan **(B)** revealed an aneurysmal bone cyst of T9 causing impingement of the dural sac. The tumor was resected with complete pain relief. The scoliotic deformity was managed by a Milwaukee brace.

Giant Cell Tumor of Bone

This is an osteolytic tumor that affects young adults. It usually involves the vertebral body. It has a predilection to the sacrum. It is a slow growing, locally aggressive tumor with a tendency to local recurrences, and occasionally to distant metastases (24,82,100). It can lead to a pathological fracture with a severe neurological compromise. Surgical treatment is indicated with wide excision (not always possible without sacrificing the neural elements) and some form of internal fixation and bone grafting (Fig. 15).

Other Benign Tumors

Other benign tumors of bone may be encountered in the spine, such as chondromyxoid fibroma or desmoplastic fibroma.

Tumor-like Lesions Affecting the Spine

Eosinophilic granuloma and histiocytosis-X may affect the spine (68). The typical radiological picture is that of vertebra plana, although atypical radiological presentation is not rare. Clinical symptoms include pain without neural embarrassment in most cases. Rarely, spinal eosinophilic granuloma can cause neurologic compromise (43).

Gaucher's Disease

Gaucher's disease may involve the spine, leading to pathological fractures and cord compression (see Fig. 4).

Malignant Primary Bone Tumors of the Spine

Solitary Plasmacytoma and Multiple Myeloma

Solitary plasmacytoma and multiple myeloma are distinct manifestations of B cell lymphoproliferative disease. These are the most common primary malignant bone tumors in adults. The tumor, which originates from plasma cells in the hematopoietic marrow, is more common in men than women and occurs in middle aged and elderly people. It appears as either a solitary bone destructive lesion or as a systemic condition affecting numerous bones such as the spine, skull, and pelvis (19). The prognosis of solitary plasmacytoma is far better than that of multiple myeloma.

Pain is the most common presenting symptom. Occasionally, neurologic involvement may occur as a result of invasion of tumor cells into the spinal canal or as a result of a pathological compression fracture. Roentgenograms reveal a pure lytic lesion involving the vertebral body. In the case of a solitary plasmacytoma, there may be evidence of expansion of the lesion to the soft tissues and spinal canal. In the case of multiple myeloma, punched-out lesions without sclerosis and generalized osteopenia are characteristic. These plasma cell neoplasms are unique because in the vast majority, Tc bone scan may be negative, as a result of the pure bone reabsorbing process.

In the case of multiple myeloma, blood tests may be helpful in establishing the diagnosis. Typically, elevated erythrocyte sedimentation rate and abnormal proteins are present in the serum and urine.

The tumor is sensitive to radiotherapy and chemotherapy. Surgery may be indicated when tissue diagnosis is not available, especially when the presenting signs are neurologic and when vertebral reconstruction is indicated (60,62) (Fig. 16). Surgery is always followed by radiation and chemotherapy.

Lymphoma

This malignant tumor may rarely affect primarily the bone and present in a similar fashion to myeloma and plasmacytoma (75,77). Radiologically, there are radiolucent lesions, occasionally accompanied by reactive sclerosis. When the bone is affected secondarily, wide-

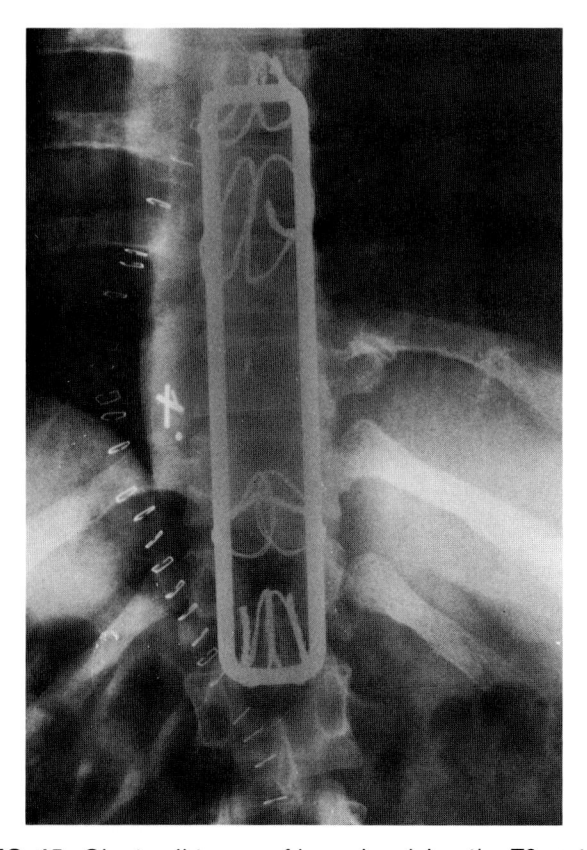

FIG. 15. Giant cell tumor of bone involving the T9 vertebra. Following decompression through a right costotransversectomy, the spine was stabilized with a Hartshill frame and sublaminar wires.

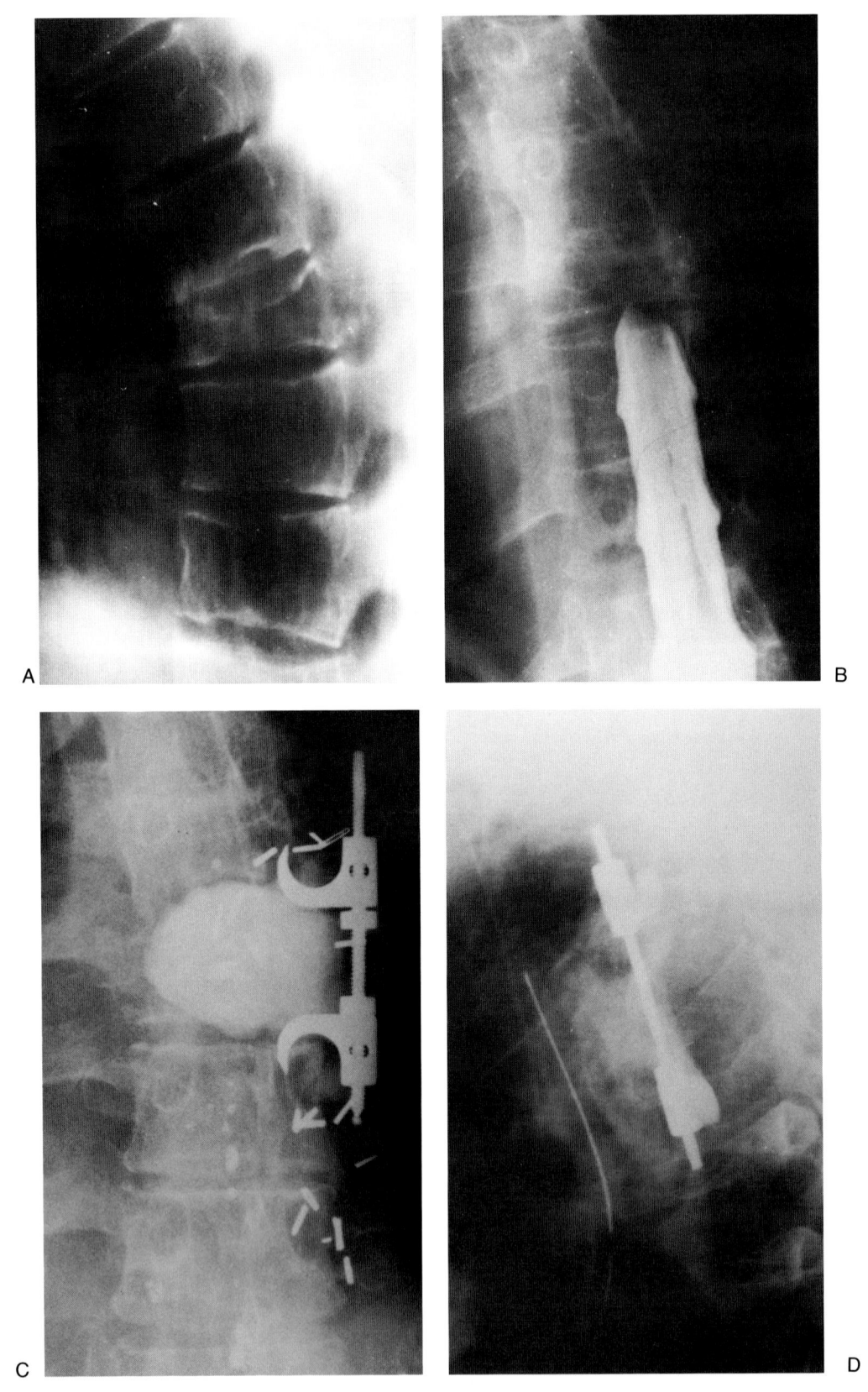

FIG. 16. A 65-year-old man with solitary plasmacytoma of T9. His main complaint was thoracic and girdle-type pain. The histological diagnosis was established after surgery. **A:** Plain radiograph showing the compression fracture of T9. **B:** A "full stop" is noted on myelography. **C,D:** AP and lateral views of the spine. Following vertebral body resection with stabilization with bone cement and Harrington compression rods incorporated in the methyl methacrylate.

spread spinal involvement may be found, leading to the "typical" osteoblastic spinal lesions. Occasionally, lymphoma can invade the spinal canal via the intervertebral foramina, causing extradural cord or cauda equina compression.

Surgery (or biopsy) may be indicated when tissue diagnosis of the lesion is not known or when the patient presents with acute paralysis (Fig. 17). In most cases, the treatments of choice are radiation therapy and chemotherapy.

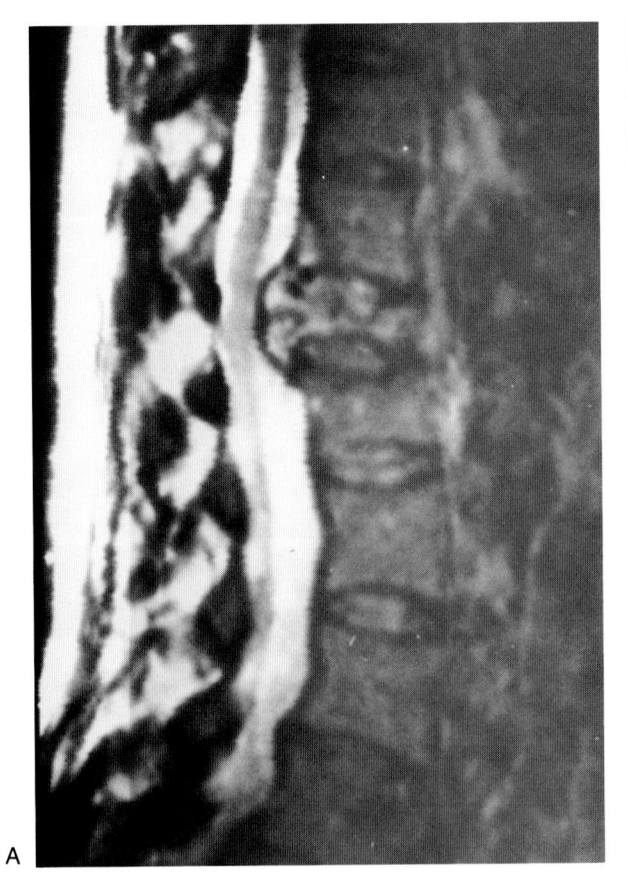

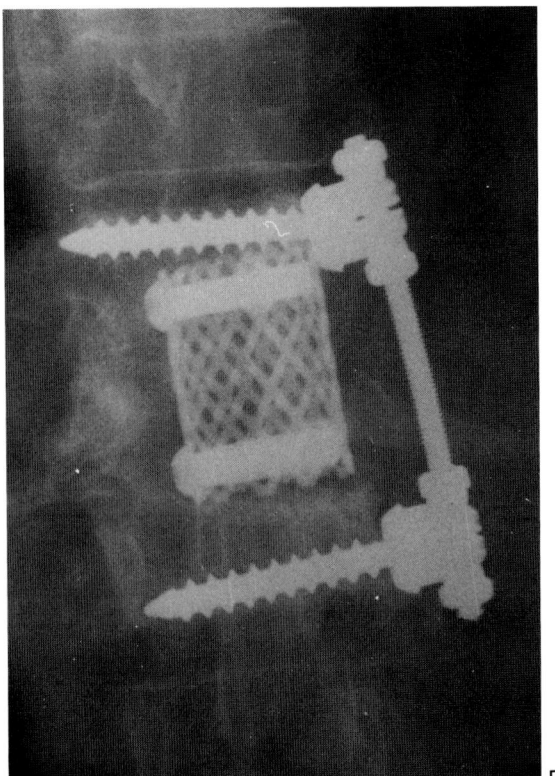

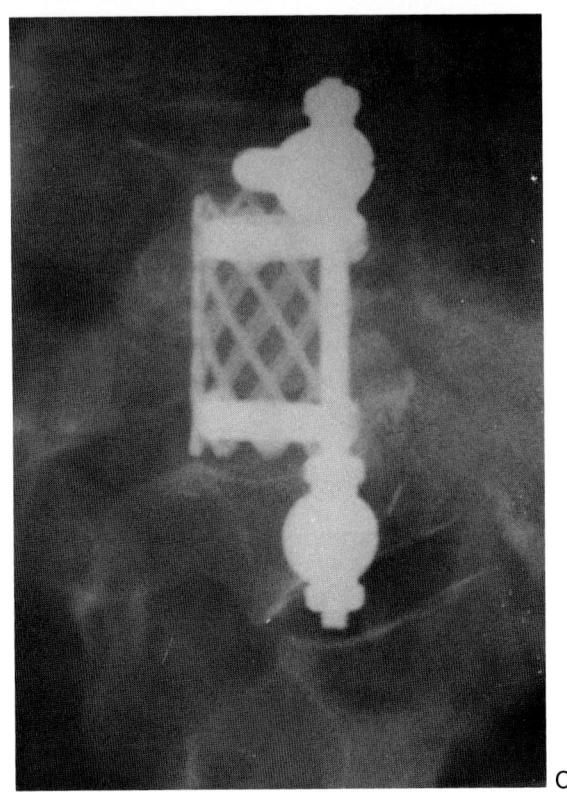

FIG. 17. A 65-year-old woman presented with persistent incapacitating thoracic spine and girdle pain, accompanied by paresthesias in both legs. She was diagnosed elsewhere to suffer from "chondrosarcoma" of T12. **A:** MRI scan showed a collapsed T12 body with significant impingement of the thecal sac. **B,C:** AP and lateral radiographs of the spine. The T12 body was resected through a left thoracoabdominal approach. A paravertebral mass was found to involve the left psoas muscle. The spine was stabilized with a Harms titanium cage and pedicle screws at T11 and L1 connected with a short rod. The histopathologic diagnosis was lymphoma.

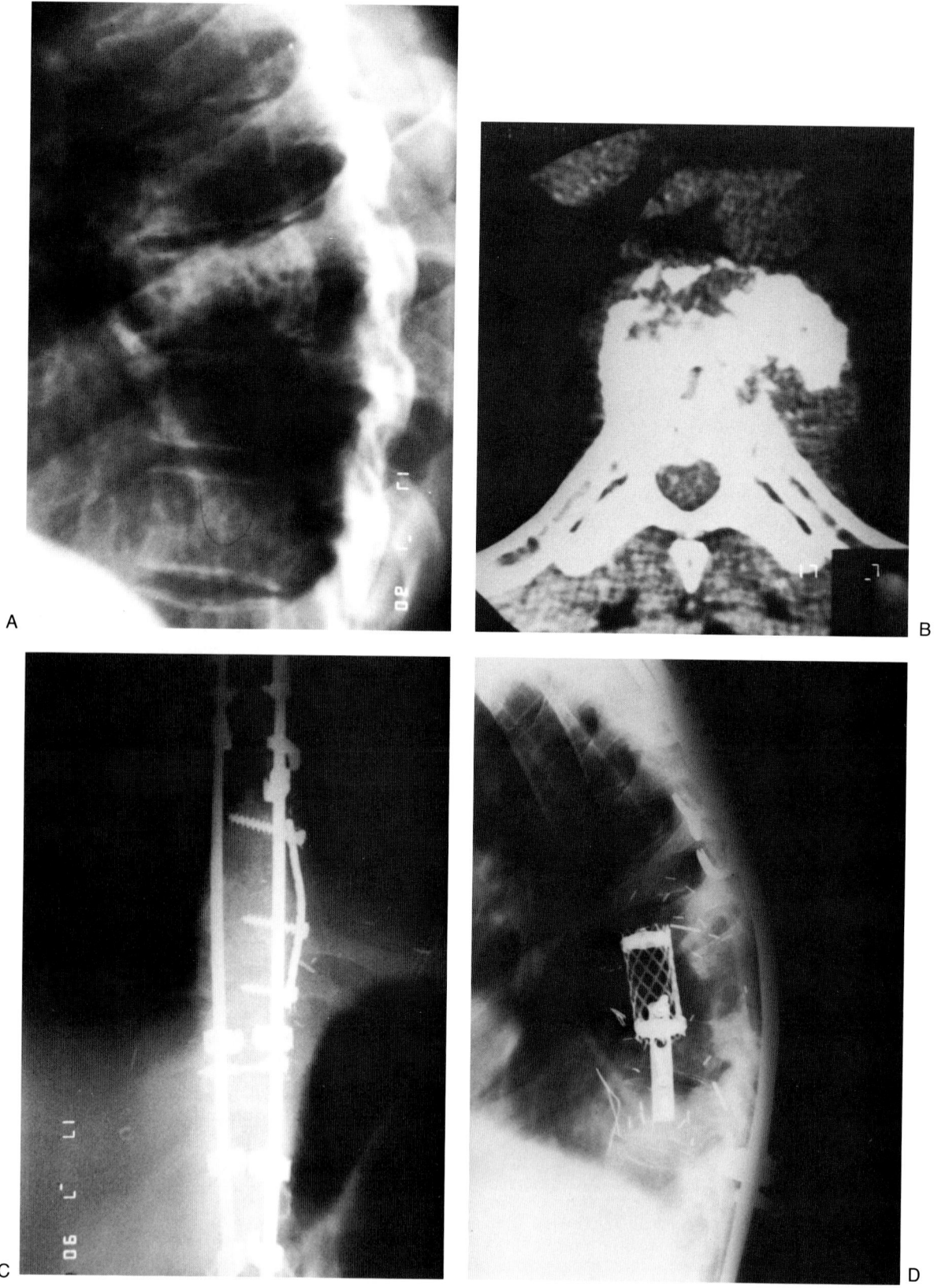

FIG. 18. A 44-year-old man with chondrosarcoma of T9. Presenting symptoms were protracted mild back pain. A CT-guided Craig needle biopsy established the diagnosis of a low-grade chondrosarcoma. **A:** Plain lateral radiograph of the thoracic spine shows a compression fracture of T9 with areas of bone stippling. **B:** Axial CT scan showing a lytic lesion of T9 with intralesional

Chondrosarcoma

This is an uncommon primary malignant bone tumor of the spine (14,87). It is much more common in the long bones and pelvis. It occurs in middle aged adults and is most often found in the lumbar spine and sacrum. Radiologically, a lytic lesion with calcific mottling and variable soft tissue involvement are typical. Pain is the most common presenting symptom and may be of long duration. Radical excision, whenever feasible, is the treatment of choice, accompanied by spinal column reconstruction (Fig. 18). Radiotherapy may be utilized as an adjunct to incomplete resection. A low histological grading may be associated with a better prognosis, although local recurrences will eventually lead to paralysis. Late distant metastasis may also occur.

Osteosarcoma

This is a very rare primary bone tumor of the spine (86). It involves the body or neural arch and may present as an osteolytic or osteoblastic lesion or both. Occasionally, it arises as a result of malignant degeneration of Paget's disease or after radiation therapy. Occasionally, it is difficult to distinguish histologically between aggressive osteoblastoma, malignant osteoblastoma, and osteosarcoma.

Total ablation of the lesion is impossible in the spine. The prognosis is therefore very poor.

Chordoma

This malignant bone tumor is a specific tumor of the spine as it is derived from notochordal remnants (65,77,92,93). Its most common locations are the base of the skull and sacrum, but occasionally it may involve the lumbar spine. Radiographs reveal an asymmetric bone destruction of the vertebral body, usually the sacrum. This is a slow growing tumor and symptoms arise after the tumor has gained a considerable size. The only treatment available is surgical. Total extirpation of the tumor is feasible if the tumor is located in the sacrococcygeal region. Local recurrences are typical and may necessitate multiple local resections. Radiotherapy is seldom of any help.

Ewing's Sarcoma

Ewing's sarcoma rarely occurs in the spine (74,77). It affects teenagers or young adults, most often in the sacrum and lumbar spine. It usually presents with pain and not infrequently with neural signs. Surgery may be indicated in establishing the diagnosis for decompression and rarely for stabilization. The treatment of choice is radiotherapy and chemotherapy.

Other Malignant Tumors

These may include fibrosarcoma, malignant fibrohistiocytoma, and malignant ganglioneuroma.

Specific Metastatic Tumors

Patients with metastatic breast, prostate, and lung cancer are those most frequently encountered by spine surgeons. It should be stressed again that the spine surgeon is part of a team managing the patients. The team has to make the therapeutic decision about specific patients, and surgery is usually not the first step in the management of these patients. New drugs and other modes of therapy are being developed and the team approach is highly important to achieve the most updated treatment protocol and hence better results.

Lung Cancer Metastasis

Lung cancer, with its four different histological types, is a most aggressive tumor. Pulmonary cancer accounts for 22% of all cancer in men and less frequently in women (94). Spinal metastasis may be the only site of hematogenous spread and may lead to paraplegia and early death. Likewise, the patient may present with signs of cord compression without a known primary site. Sundaresan et al. (94) reported that with aggressive surgical treatment by anterolateral decompression and stabilization, 24 out of 25 patients

---

calcifications and a left paravertebral mass. **C:** AP view of the spine. Surgery was carried out employing combined consequential posterior and anterior approaches. Initially, a posterior approach with resection of the lamina of T9 and bilateral pedicle resection and Cotrel–Dubousset instrumentation from T4 to L1 were accomplished. This was followed by a left thoracotomy with T9 vertebral body resection with replacement of the body by a femoral head allograft and stabilization with an acetabular reconstruction plate. **D:** Sixteen months later, the tumor recurred, invading the femoral head allograft. After tumor excision the gap was filled with the Harms titanium cylinder. The prosthesis was anchored by a small A-O plate.

regained ambulation and 90% had significant pain relief. Despite the general poor prognosis and the projected short life expectancy, surgical decompression should be contemplated.

Breast Cancer Metastasis

About 10% of American women will develop breast carcinoma sometime in life (3). Although this tumor is responsible for the highest number of deaths in young women, its prognosis is improving constantly as new avenues of therapy are developed. Breast metastases are usually insidious and slow growing. In autopsy studies, 85% of women with breast cancer had skeletal involvement (102). Spinal involvement, which leads to both mechanical and neurological compromise, is also very common (Fig. 19) (83). As bone metastases are relatively sensitive to radiotherapy, chemotherapy, and even hormonal treatment, the surgical management is limited to cases of instability, neurological deficit, or intractable pain resistant to the above-mentioned measures.

Radiologically, breast cancer metastases are either lytic in nature, osteoblastic, or sometimes a mixture of both. Involvement of several noncontiguous vertebrae is typical.

The yield of treatment of any of the types mentioned is high. Patients who improve neurologically following spine surgery doubled their life expectancy (21.4 months with no intervention to 42 months following surgery) (64). Conversely, those not improving by surgery died after several months. The general long survival of these patients justifies an aggressive surgical approach to spinal metastasis, including repeated surgical interventions.

Prostate Cancer Metastasis

The spine is the most common site involved in metastatic prostatic cancer. This is a common cancer that is found in almost half the autopsies of men older than 50 years. In some of them, the prostatic cancer was clinically unnoticed.

Bone metastases may often be the presenting symptoms of prostatic carcinoma (see Fig. 11) (41). Their radiological appearance is osteoblastic in a very high percentage and the acid phosphatase blood levels are elevated.

Treatment consists of hormonal therapy followed by chemotherapy and radiotherapy. Surgery is indicated for neural compression, instability, and for intractable pain. The general life expectancy of patients with prostate cancer justifies an aggressive approach to the metastatic disease. Prostate metastases tend to involve more often the posterior elements rather than the vertebral body. Decompressive laminectomy is therefore adequate in many cases.

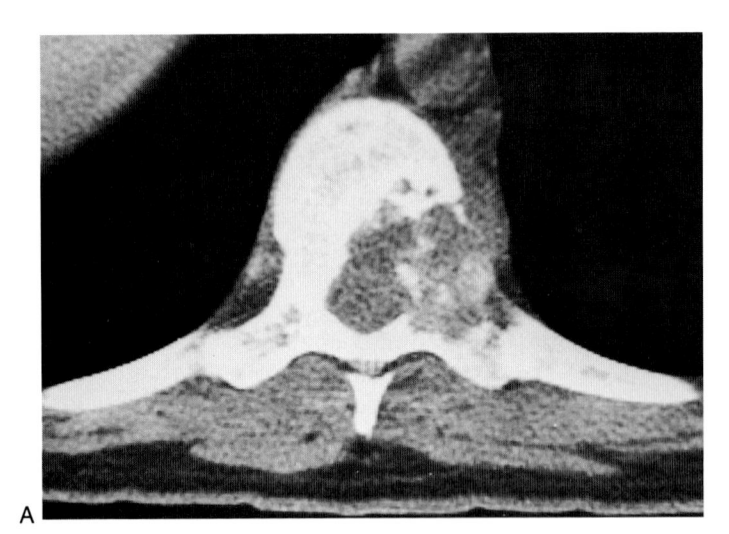

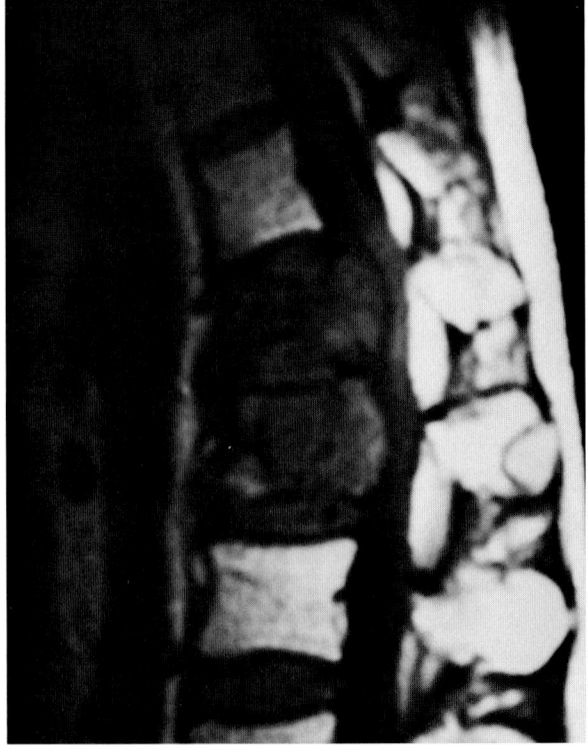

FIG. 19. A: Breast carcinoma involving the left pedicle of T7. **B:** Breast carcinoma involving two adjacent thoracic vertebrae with marked cord compression.

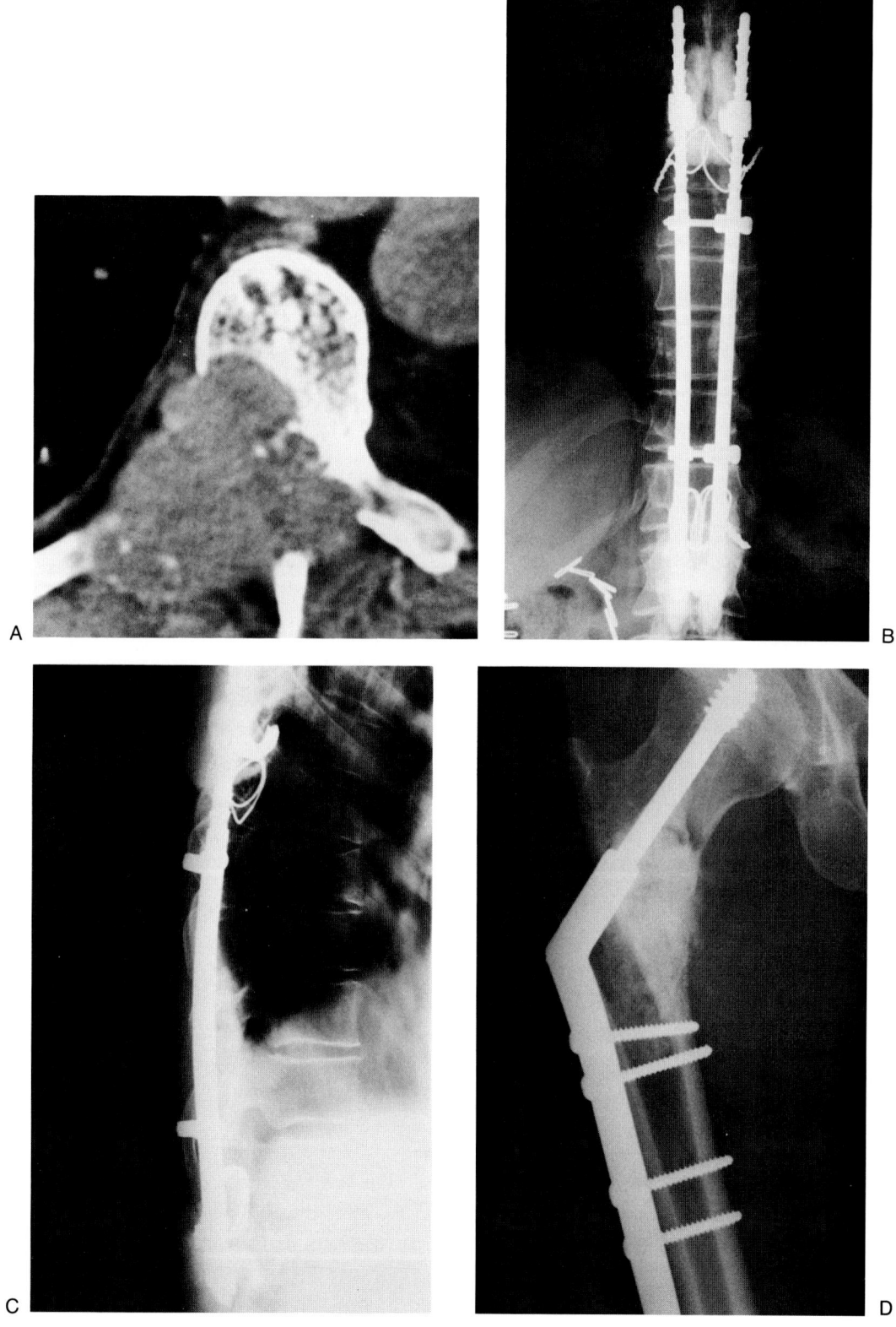

FIG. 20. A 65-year-old man with metastatic renal cell carcinoma presented with signs of cord compression at the T8 level. There was also a lytic lesion of the right proximal femur. **A:** Axial CT scan showing a lytic lesion involving both laminae, the right pedicle, and the right side of the posterior T8 body with tumor invading the epidural space and encroaching on the cord. **B,C:** AP and lateral views of the spine. The patient underwent decompressive laminectomy, pediculectomy, and partial corpectomy with cord decompression and Harrington rod instrumentation from T6 to L1 augmented with sublaminar wires and methyl methacrylate. **D:** The right femur was fixed with a Richard's compression hip screw and the lytic lesion was filled with bone cement.

Renal Cancer Metastasis

Although this cancer is less common, it has certain characteristics worth mentioning especially for its hypervascular nature, causing extensive bleeding during surgery. The aggressive tumor also has characteristic bone metastatic behavior: about 2% of the patients suffer from bone metastases that are so aggressive that they do not appear even in a bone scan. Ribs and the thoracic and lumbar spine are each involved in more than 30% of the cases (4).

The tumor is radioresistant and also not sensitive to chemotherapy and, in the case of cord compression, surgery should be considered (Fig. 20). Sundaresan et al. (96) reported that patients with metastatic spinal renal cell carcinoma had a 13-month median survival following surgical decompression and stabilization as opposed to 3 months if managed only by radiation therapy. Surgery can be complicated by extensive hemorrhage, and angiography with catheter embolization of the feeding vessel is recommended (11). Embolization of vessels may cause ischemia of the cord by itself.

REFERENCES

1. Akbarnia BA. Aneurysmal bone cyst of the spine. *Spine: State of Art Rev* 1988;2:265.
2. Algra PR, Bloem JC, Tissing H, Falke TH, Arndt JW, Verboom LJ. Detection of vertebral metastasis: comparison between MR imaging and bone scintigraphy. *Radiographics* 1991;11:219–232.
3. American Cancer Society. *Cancer facts and figures*. New York: American Cancer Society, 1982.
4. Arkless R. Renal carcinoma: how it metastasizes. *Radiology* 1965;84:496.
5. Asdourian PL, Mardjetko S, Rauschning W, et al. An evaluation of spinal deformity in metastatic breast cancer. *J Spinal Disord* 1990;3:119.
6. Barron KD, Hirano A, Arak S, Terry RD. Experience with metastatic neoplasm involving the spine. *Neurology* 1959;9:91.
7. Batson OV. The function of the vertebral veins and their role in the spread of metastasis. *Am Surg* 1940;112:138–149.
8. Bhardwaj S, Holland JF. Chemotherapy of metastatic cancer in bone. *Clin Orthop* 1984;169:28–37.
9. Blair RJ, McAfee JB. Radiological detection of skeletal metastases: radiography vs. scans. *Int J Oncol* 1976;1:1201.
10. Boland PJ, Lane JM, Sundaresan N. Metastatic disease of the spine. *Clin Orthop* 1982;169:95–102.
11. Bowers TA, Murray JA, Charnsangavej C, et al. Bone metastases from renal carcinoma. The preoperative use of transcatheter arterial occlusion. *J Bone Joint Surg* 1982;64A:749.
12. Brihaye J, Ectors P, Lemort M, Van Houtte P. The management of spinal epidural metastases. *Adv Tech Stand Neurosurg* 1988;16:121.
13. Byrne TN, Waxaman SG. *Spinal cord compression*. Philadelphia: FA Davis, 1990;146–178.
14. Camins MB, Duncan AW, Smith J, Marcove RC. Chondrosarcoma of the spine. *Spine* 1978;3:202.
15. Capanna R, Albisini U, Picci P, Calderon P, Campanacci M, Springfield DS. Aneurysmal bone cyst of the spine. *J Bone Joint Surg* 1985;67A:527.
16. Citrin DL, Bessent RG, Craig WR. A comparison of the sensitivity and accuracy of the 99 Tcm phosphate bone scan and skeletal radiograph in the diagnosis of bone metastases. *Clin Radiol* 1972;28:107.
17. Cobb DC, Leavens ME, Eckles N. Indications for nonoperative treatment of spinal cord compression due to breast cancer. *J Neurosurg* 1977;47:613–618.
18. Constans JP, De Divitis E, Donzelli R, et al. Spinal metastases with neurological manifestations. Review of 600 cases. *J Neurosurg* 1983;59:111.
19. Corwin J, Lindberg RD. Solitary plasmacytoma of bone vs. extramedullary plasmacytoma and their relationship to multiple myeloma. *Cancer* 1979;43:1007.
20. Craig FS. Vertebral body biopsy. *J Bone Joint Surg* 1956;38A:93.
21. Crock HV, Yoshizawa H, Kame SK. Observations on the venous drainage of the human vertebral body. *J Bone Joint Surg* 1973;55B:528.
22. Dahlin DC. *Bone tumors, general aspects and data on 6221 cases*. Springfield, IL: Charles C Thomas, 1986.
23. Dahlin DC, Coventry MG. Osteogenic sarcoma: a study of 600 cases. *J Bone Joint Surg* 1967;49(A):101–110.
24. Dahlin DC. Giant cell tumor of vertebrae above the sacrum. A review of 31 cases. *Cancer* 1977;39:1350.
25. Dahlin DC, McLeod RA. Aneurysmal bone cyst and other non-neoplastic conditions. *Skeletal Radiol* 1982;8:243.
26. Denis F. Spinal instability as defined by the three-column spine concept in acute spinal trauma. *Clin Orthop* 1984;189:65–76.
27. Dolin MG. Acute massive dural compression secondary to methyl methacrylate replacement of a tumorous lumbar vertebral body. *Spine* 1989;14:109–110.
28. Enneking WF. *Musculoskeletal tumor surgery*. New York: Churchill Livingstone, 1983.
29. Findlay GF. The role of vertebral body collapse in the management of malignant spinal cord compression. *J Neurol Neurosurg Psychiatry* 1987;50:151.
30. Flately TJ, Anderson MH, Anast GT. Spinal instability due to malignant disease. Treatment by segmental spinal stabilization. *J Bone Joint Surg* 1984;66A:47.
31. Floman Y, Milgrom C, Kenan S, Sabato S, Robin GC. Spongious and cortical osteoblastomata of the axial skeleton. *Orthopaedics* 1985;8:1478.
32. Fournasier VL, Horne JG. Metastases to the vertebral column. *Cancer* 1975;36:590–594.
33. Galasko CSB. The anatomy and pathways of skeletal metastases. In: Weiss L, Gilbert HA, eds. *Bone metastasis*. Boston: GK Hall, 1981;49–63.
34. Galasko CSB. The development of skeletal metastases. In: Weiss L, Gilbert HA, eds. *Bone metastasis*. Boston: GK Hall, 1981;83–113.
35. Galasko CSB. Spinal instability secondary to metastatic cancer. *J Bone Joint Surg* 1991;73B:104–108.
36. Gertzbein SD, Cruickshank B, Hoffman H, et al. Recurrent benign osteoblastoma of the second thoracic vertebra. A case report. *J Bone Joint Surg* 1973;55B:841.
37. Ghelman B, Lospinuso MF, Levine DB, O'Leary PF, Burke SW. Percutaneous computed tomography-guided biopsy of the thoracic and lumbar spine. *Spine* 1991;10:736.
38. Gilbert HA, Kagan R. Evaluation of radiation therapy for bone metastases: pain relief and quality of life. *Am J Radiol* 1977;129:1095.
39. Gilbert RW, Kim JH, Posner JB. Epidural spinal cord compression from metastatic tumor: diagnosis and treatment. *Ann Neurol* 1978;3:40–51.
40. Glasser DB, Cammisa FP, Lane JM. Benign cartilage tumors of the spine. In: Sundaresan N, ed. *Tumors of the spine*. Philadelphia: Saunders, 1990;146.
41. Goris MC, Bretille J. Skeletal scintigraphy for the diagnosis of malignant metastatic disease of bone. *Radiother Oncol* 1985;4:319.
42. Graham JJ, Uang WC. Vertebral hemangioma with compression fracture and paraparesis treated with preoperative embolization and vertebral resection. *Spine* 1984;9:97.
43. Green VE, Robertson J, Kirlow AW. Eosinophilic granuloma of the spine with associated neural defect. *J Bone Joint Surg* 1980;62A:1198.
44. Greenberg HS, Kim JH, Posner JB. Epidural spinal cord compression from metastatic tumor: results with a new treatment protocol. *Ann Neurol* 1980;8:361–366.

45. Gurr KR, McAfee PC, Shih CM. Biomechanical analysis of anterior and posterior instrumentation systems after corpectomy. A calf-spine model. *J Bone Joint Surg* 1988;70(A):1182–1191.
46. Harrington KD. Metastatic disease of the spine. *J Bone Joint Surg* 1986;68A:1110.
47. Harrington DK. Anterior decompression and stabilization of the spine as a treatment for vertebral collapse and spinal cord compression from metastatic malignancy. *Clin Orthop* 1988;233:177.
48. Haughton VM, Williams AL. *Computed tomography of the spine*. St. Louis: CV Mosby, 1982.
49. Hay MC, Paterson D, Taylor TKF. Aneurysmal bone cyst of the spine. *J Bone Joint Surg* 1978;60B:406.
50. Huvos AG. *Bone tumors: diagnosis, treatment and prognosis*. Philadelphia: Saunders, 1979;206–237.
51. Jackson IG. Osteoid osteoma of the lamina and its treatment. *Am Surg* 1953;19:17–23.
52. Kak UK, Prabhakar S, Khosla VK, Banerjee AK. Solitary osteochrondroma of the spine causing spinal cord compression. *Clin Neurol Neurosurg* 1985;87:135.
53. Kattapuram SV, Khurana JS, Rosenthal D. Percutaneous needle biopsy of the spine. *Spine* 1982;17:561–564.
54. Kostuik JP. Diagnosis and treatment of pathologic spinal fractures secondary to metastatic disease. In: Errico TJ, Bauer D, Waugh T, eds. *Spinal trauma*. Philadelphia: Lippincott, 1991;499.
55. Kostuik JP, Errico TJ, Gleeson TF, Errico CC. Spinal stabilization of vertebral column tumors. *Spine* 1988;13:250.
56. Kurz LT, Pursel SE, Herkowitz HN. Modified anterior approach to the cervicothoracic junction. *Spine* 1991;16:542–547.
57. Livingston KE, Perrin RG. The neurological management of spinal metastases causing cord and cauda equina compression. *J Neurosurg* 1978;49:839.
58. Manabe S, Tateishi A, Abe M, Ohno T. Surgical treatment of metastatic tumors of the spine. *Spine* 1989;14:41–47.
59. Manabe S, Tanaka H, Hibo Y, Park P, Ohno T, Tateishi X. Experimental analysis of the spinal cord compressed by spinal metastasis. *Spine* 1989;14:1308–1315.
60. Margulies JY, Kenan S, Michowitz SD, Okon E, Peretz T, Matzner Y, Floman Y. Cord compression as the presenting symptom of extradural malignant lymphoma. *Arch Orthop Trauma Surg* 1987;106:291–296.
61. Marsh BW, Bonfiglio M, Brady LP, Enneking WF. Benign osteoblastoma: range of manifestations. *J Bone Joint Surg* 1975;57A:1–9.
62. McLain RF, Weinstein JN. Solitary plasmocytomas of the spine: a review of 84 cases. *J Spinal Disord* 1989;2:69–74.
63. Millburn L, Hibbs GG, Hendrickson FR. Treatment of spinal cord compression from metastatic carcinoma: review of the literature and presentation of a new method of treatment. *Cancer* 1968;21:447.
64. Miller F, Whitehill R. Carcinoma of breast metastatic to the skeleton. *Clin Orthop* 1984;184:121–127.
65. Mindell EP. Chordoma. *J Bone Joint Surg* 1981;63A:501.
66. Mones FJ, Dozier D, Berret A. Analysis of medical treatment of malignant extradural spinal cord tumors. *Cancer* 1966;19:1842.
67. Morishita S, Onomura T, Inoue T, Maeda H, Akagi H. Bone scintigraphy in patients with breast cancer, pulmonary cancer, uterine cervix cancer and prostatic cancer. *Spine* 1989;14:784–789.
68. Nesbit ME, Keiffer S, D'Angio GI. Reconstitution of vertebral height in histiocytosis X: a long term follow-up. *J Bone Joint Surg* 1969;51A:1360.
69. Nottebaert M, von Hochstetter AR, Exner GU, Schreiber A. Metastatic carcinoma of the spine: a study of 92 cases. *Int Orthop* 1987;11:345.
70. Ottolenghi CE. Aspiration biopsy of the spine: techniques and results in 1078 cases. *J Bone Joint Surg* 1967;49A:1479.
71. Paillas JE, Alliez B, Pellet W. Primary and secondary tumors of the spine. In: Vinken PJ, Bruyn GW, eds. *Handbook of clinical neurology*, vol 20. Amsterdam: North-Holland, 1976;19–54.
72. Posner JB. Spinal metastases: diagnosis and treatment. In: Posner JB, ed. *Neuro-oncology*. Course at Memorial Sloan–Kettering Cancer Center, New York, 1981;42–54.
73. Posner JB. Back pain and epidural spinal cord compression. *Med Clin North Am* 1987;71:185–204.
74. Pritchard DJ, Dahlin DC, Dauphone RT, Taylor WF, Beabont KW. Ewing's sarcoma: a clinicopathological and statistical analysis of patients surviving 5 years or longer. *J Bone Joint Surg* 1975;57A:10.
75. Pui CH, Dahl GV, Huston HO, Murphy SB. Epidural spinal cord compression as the initial finding in childhood acute leukemia and non-Hodgkin's lymphoma. *J Pediatr* 1985;106:788.
76. Ransford AO, Pozo JL, Hutton PAN, Kirwam EOG. The behavior pattern of the scoliosis associated with osteoid osteoma or osteoblastoma of the spine. *J Bone Joint Surg* 1984;66B:16.
77. Robin GC. Tumors of the lumbar spine and sacrum. In: Floman Y, ed. *Disorders of the lumbar spine*. Gaithersburg, MD: Aspen Publishers, 1990;823.
78. Rodichok LD, Ruckdeschal JC, Haper GR, et al. Early detection and treatment of spinal epidural metastases: the role of myelography. *Ann Neurol* 1986;20:696–702.
79. Roy-Camille R, Mazel C. Vertebrectomy through an enlarged posterior approach for tumors and malunions. In: Bridwell KH, DeWald RL, eds. *The textbook of spinal surgery*. Philadelphia: Lippincott, 1991;1243.
80. Salomon C, Chopin D, Benoist M. Spinal cord compression, and exceptional complication of spinal osteoporosis. *Spine* 1988;13:222–224.
81. Sarpel S, Sarpel G, Yu E, et al. Early diagnosis of spinal epidural metastasis by magnetic resonance imaging. *Cancer* 1987;59:1112–1116.
82. Savini R, Gherlinzoni F, Morandi M, Neff JR, Picci P. Surgical treatment of giant cell tumor of the spine. The experience at the Institute Orthopaedico Rizzoli. *J Bone Joint Surg* 1983;65A:1283.
83. Schaberg JC, Gainor BJ. A profile of metastatic carcinoma of the spine. *Spine* 1985;10:19.
84. Schajowicz F. *Tumors and tumor-like lesions of bone and joints*. New York: Springer-Verlag, 1981.
85. Schmorl G, Junghans H. *The human spine in health and disease*, 2nd ed. New York: Grune & Stratton, 1971.
86. Shives TC, Dahlin DC, Sim FH, Pritchard DJ, Earle JP. Osteosarcoma of the spine. *J Bone Joint Surg* 1986;68A:660.
87. Shives TC, McLeod RA, Unni KK, Schray MF. Chondrosarcoma of the spine. *J Bone Joint Surg* 1989;71A:1158.
88. Siegal TZ, Siegal T. Vertebral body resection for epidural compression by malignant tumors. *J Bone Joint Surg* 1985;67A:375.
89. Siegal TZ, Siegal T. Surgical decompression of anterior and posterior malignant epidural tumors compressing the spinal cord. *Neurosurgery* 1985;17:424.
90. Siegal TZ, Siegal T. Current consideration in the management of neoplastic spinal cord compression. *Spine* 1989;14:223–228.
91. Siegal TZ, Siegal T. Neurologic compromise due to spinal tumors. In: Sundaresan N, ed. *Tumors of the spine*. Philadelphia: Saunders, 1990;272.
92. Stener B, Gunterberg B. High amputation of the sacrum for extirpation of tumors: principles and techniques. *Spine* 1978;3:351.
93. Sundaresan N. Chordomas. *Clin Orthop* 1986;204:135–142.
94. Sundaresan N, Mains M, McCormick P. Surgical treatment of spinal cord compression in patients with lung cancer. *Neurosurgery* 1985;16:350.
95. Sundaresan N, Galicich JH, Lane JE, et al. Treatment of neoplastic epidural cord compression by vertebral body resection and stabilization. *J Neurosurg* 1985;63:676.
96. Sundaresan N, Scher H, DiGiacinto GV, Yagoda A, Whitmore W, Choi IS. Surgical treatment of spinal cord compression in kidney cancer. *J Clin Oncol* 1986;4:1851.
97. Sundaresan N, DiGiacimto GV, Hughes JEO, Cafferty M, Vallejo A. Treatment of neoplastic spinal cord compression. Results of a prospective study. *Neurosurgery* 1991;29:645–650.
98. Vecht CJ, Haaxma-Reichett H, Van Putten WLJ, et al. Initial bolus of conventional versus high-dose dexamethasone in metastatic spinal cord compression. *Neurology* 1989;39:1255–1257.

99. Weinstein JN. Spinal tumors. In: Weinstein JN, Wiesel GW, eds. *The lumbar spine*. Philadelphia: Saunders, 1990;741–759.
100. Weinstein JN, McLain R. Primary tumors of the spine. *Spine* 1987;12:843–851.
101. Weissman DE, Gilberg M, Wang H, et al. The use of computed tomography of the spine to identify patients at high risk for epidural metastases. *J Clin Oncol* 1985;3:1541–1544.
102. Willis RA. Secondary tumors of bones. In: *The spread of tumors in the human body,* 3rd ed. London: Butterworth, 1973; 229.
103. Yasuma T, Yamauchi Y, Arai K, Makino E. Histopathologic study of tumor infiltration into the intervertebral disc. *Spine* 1989;14:1245–1248.
104. Young RF, Post EM, King GA. Treatment of spinal epidural metastases: randomized prospective comparison of laminectomy and radiotherapy. *J Neurosurg* 1980;53:741.
105. Zdeblick TA, Shirado O, McAfee PC, deGroot H, Warden K. Anterior spinal fixation after lumbar corpectomy. *J Bone Joint Surg* 1991;73A:527–534.

27

Fractures of the Spine in Ankylosing Spondylitis

Edward H. Simmons and Avi J. Bernstein

Ankylosing spondylitis, Marie–Strümpell disease or Bechterew's disease (4), has been incorrectly referred to as "rheumatoid" spondylitis. Clearly, it is a different disease from rheumatoid arthritis (22,31,39). Ankylosing spondylitis is more common in men, with a predilection for affecting the spine and major joints. Rheumatoid arthritis is more common in women, with a predilection for smaller joints of the appendicular skeleton. Ankylosing spondylitis has a different serology. There is a significant incidence of the disease, which, on a clinically active basis, is two to three patients per 1000 population.

In ankylosing spondylitis, the spine becomes inflamed, painful, osteopenic, and later ossified (8). If the spine ossifies in normal alignment, the affliction is not too severe but, all too frequently, the spine may become ossified in a deformed position (41). Superimposed on these issues is the extreme susceptibility of the ankylosed spine to fracture.

The main clinical problems related to the spine presenting with ankylosing spondylitis are gross, fixed deformities (40,41). In rheumatoid arthritis, the main problems of the spine are local destruction and instability (42). Fractures of the spine in ankylosing spondylitis embody completely different principles than fractures of the normal spine.

SPINAL FRACTURE

In ankylosing spondylitis, the spine is extremely susceptible to fracture from minor trauma for a number of reasons. First, the process of ankylosing spondylitis turns a mobile, multisegmented organ into a stiff rod. This causes the bending moments to become magnified in even minor trauma. Second, the process of ankylosis in an osteopenic structure makes the structure more susceptible to fracture. This is well supported in the literature. Statistically, the majority of spinal fractures in ankylosing spondylitis occur following minor or trivial trauma (10,24–26,32,52).

Spinal fracture in ankylosing spondylitis carries grave implications. Neurologic impairment is extremely high when compared to the non-ankylosing spondylitis fracture group. Mortality and permanent neurologic loss are about twice the rate reported for non-ankylosing spondylitis spinal trauma patients: 30% to 50% and 60% to 80%, respectively (16,17,24,25,29, 32–34,51,53).

Fractures of the spine in ankylosing spondylitis are similar to fractures of an osteoporotic tubular long bone, with a transverse shear pattern (5). The fracture may occur at any level, although 75% of fractures in ankylosing spondylitis occur in the cervical spine (10,25,30). The site of injury is usually at the base of the neck at the cervicothoracic junction (38) from C6 to T2, most commonly in the area of C7 or T1. This is probably because the cervicothoracic region is the point of greatest stress, even in minor falls.

The mechanism frequently is extension of the cervicothoracic junction (2,10,21,32,52). The scenario in which a patient falls forward and the head strikes the ground first because of the patient's inability to extend the neck in a defensive manner produces an extension

---

E. H. Simmons: Department of Orthopaedic Surgery, State University of New York at Buffalo, Buffalo, NY 14203; and University Orthopaedic Spine Service, Orthopaedic Department, Buffalo General Hospital, Buffalo, NY.

A. J. Bernstein: Department of Orthopaedic Surgery, University of Chicago, The Pritzker School of Medicine; and the Lutheran General Hospital, Park Ridge, IL 60068-1145.

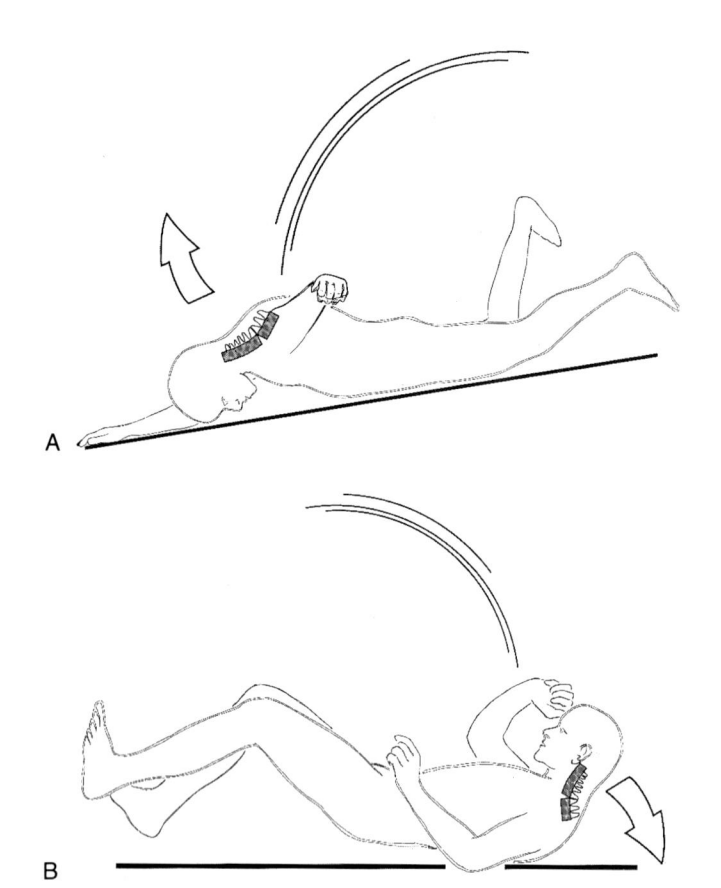

FIG. 1. A: Diagrammatic outline demonstrating patient with kyphotic deformity falling forward and striking head against the ground. The cervicothoracic junction is the point of greatest stress with an extension moment being applied. **B:** Diagrammatic view demonstrating patient with kyphotic deformity falling backward and landing on apex of kyphos. Significant extension forces are experienced at the point of greatest stress, the cervicothoracic junction.

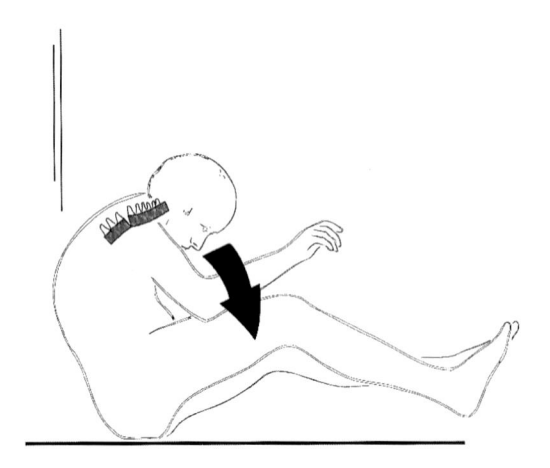

FIG. 2. Diagram of patient with flexion deformity falling onto buttocks. The anterior position of the head relative to the body results in a significant flexion moment at the cervicothoracic junction.

injury at the point of greatest stress, the cervicothoracic junction. In another situation, the patient falls backward and strikes the kyphotic upper thoracic spine against the ground exerting a hyperextension moment at the cervicothoracic junction that results in a hyperextension injury (Fig. 1).

Flexion type fracture mechanisms also play a prominent role in these patients. Many patients have mild to moderate kyphotic deformity prior to injury, with the head aligned anterior to the center of gravity of the body. With the weight of the head at one end of the rigid cervical spine, which is fixed to the thorax, any vertical drop or forward trajectory will result in a significant flexion moment. In a simple fall onto the buttocks, significant flexion injury can occur because of the anterior position of the center of gravity of the head relative to the body (Fig. 2). Front end automobile collisions in which the passenger either is restrained by a seat belt or the chest collides with the steering wheel result in flexion injury as the head projects forward, unrestrained. This mechanism of injury creates a significant flexion moment. This scenario in these at risk patients supports the use of airbag safety restraint systems. A rear end collision results in an extension moment as the trunk is restrained by the car seat (Fig. 3). The extent of fracture and displacement depends on the rigidity of the cervical spine, the amount of preexisting deformity, the extent of osteoporosis (strength of the spine), and the mechanism and force of injury.

Thoracolumbar fractures in ankylosing spondylitis are high risk injuries and account for a minority of the injuries seen (15,38). Diagnosis of these fractures can be difficult because of low suspicion and difficult visualization caused by osteoporosis and superimposition of the shoulders. The slice or shear fracture is the most unstable, with serious neurological risk, and can lead to devastating consequences including hemothorax (27) and aortic laceration (29). Missed, the fracture may go on to pseudarthrosis. A shear crack may be missed on initial presentation, later going on to erosive collapse and deformity. Fracture pseudarthrosis should be distinguished from spondylodiscitis, which is an inflammatory manifestation of ankylosing spondylitis. The basic tenets of treatment outlined for cervicothoracic fracture should be adopted in the rest of the spine (50).

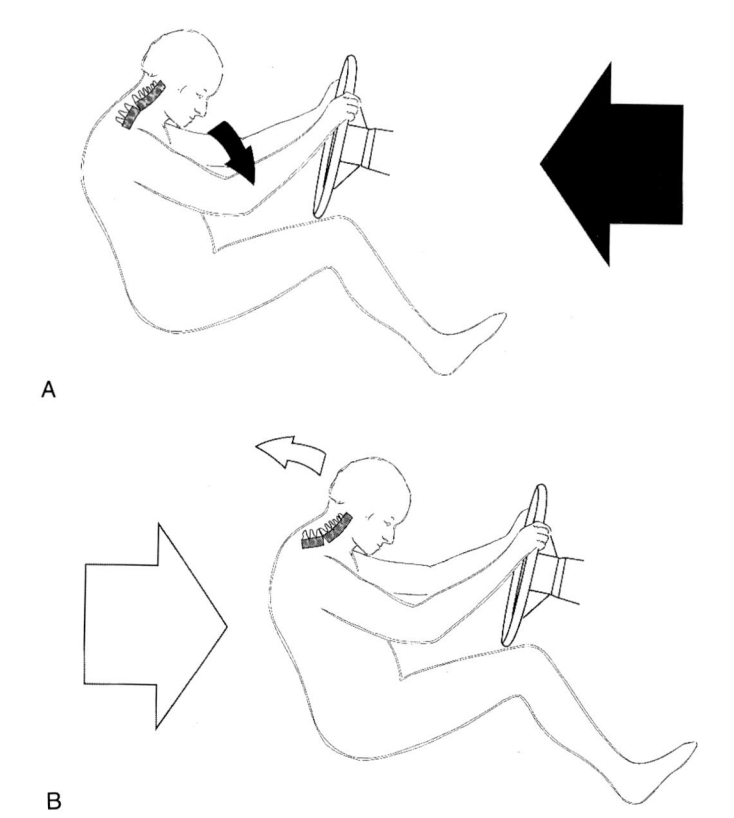

FIG. 3. A: Diagram showing front end collision (*dark arrows*). Even a minor "fender bender" can result in serious injury as the head is thrown forward. **B:** Diagram of rear end collision. Minor impact can result in serious extension injury as the head is thrown backward and the body is restrained by the seat.

The patient with ankylosing spondylitis whose trunk alignment has been relatively unchanged and relatively pain-free over a significant interval who then sustains minimal or even insignificant trauma with subsequent painful progressive flexion deformity of the neck should be considered to have a fracture of the spine until proved otherwise (41,43). The increased pain is often mistakenly attributed to the patient's disease. The fracture undergoes gradual erosion with compression collapse anteriorly, allowing the chin to approach the chest. The patient notices that the position of the head varies during the day. It will be more elevated on awakening in the morning and will approach the chest during the day as the attempt is made to maintain upright position of the trunk. On presentation, the patient may hold his/her head with the hands to ease the distress.

These patients do not require cervical osteotomy for correction of deformity. A cervical halo should be applied, with initial traction along the line of the neck to slowly restore normal alignment. With careful neurologic assessment, the head is restored to its normal

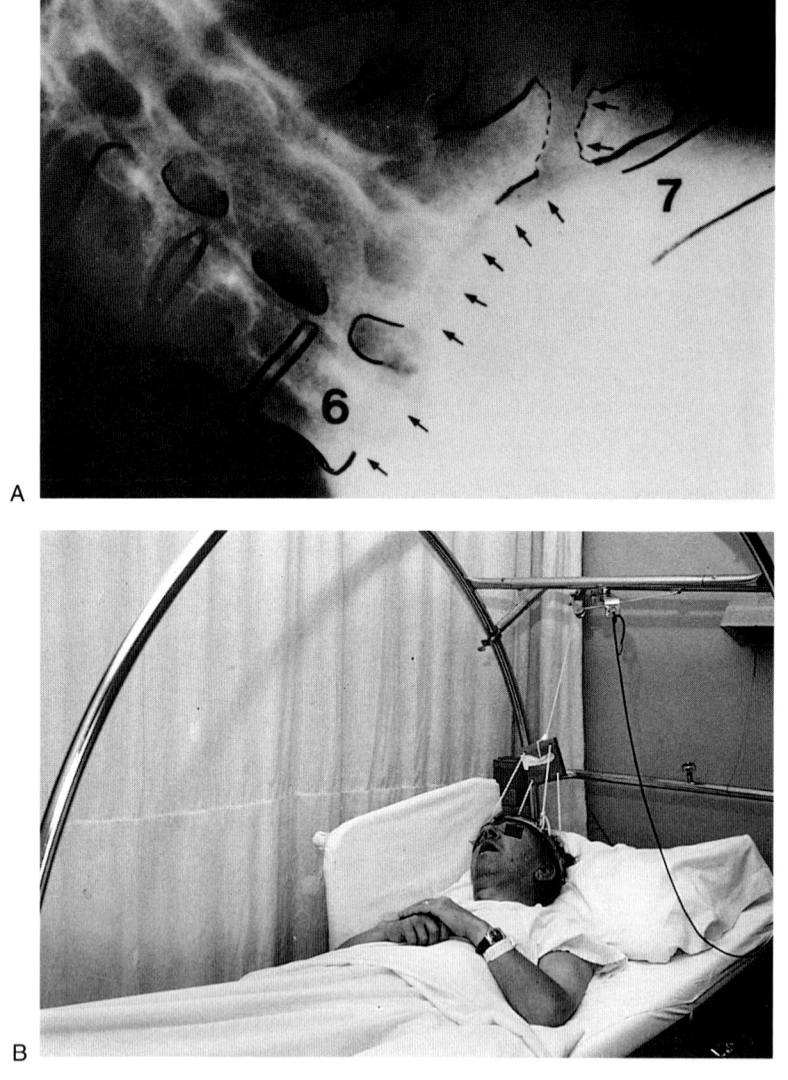

FIG. 4. A: Lateral radiograph demonstrating C6–C7 shear fracture in a 55-year-old man following trauma. Fractures at this level may be difficult to see due to superimposition of the shoulders. **B:** Photograph of 55-year-old man with cervical fracture in halo traction being nursed in a circ-o-electric bed. Initial traction is in line with the neck in both sagittal and coronal planes, gradually restoring alignment to the preinjury position. Improvement in the preinjury chin–brow to vertical angle is considered a bonus.

functional position (Fig. 4). This is most efficiently accomplished with the patient supported on a circ-o-electric bed. A fairly normal chin–brow to vertical angle can usually be obtained with the alignment restored to at least the preinjury state. A standard halo vest will not supply adequate immobilization and a cast is essential, so the patient should be immobilized in a well molded halo cast for 4 months. In our experience, union occurs almost consistently over this interval, which is followed by a shorter period of bracing (Fig. 5). If in a rare or unusual instance spontaneous healing does not occur, anterior cervical fusion using a keystone graft or posterior fusion–fixation will be required. Unrecognized fractures at the base of the cervical spine, if untreated, ultimately heal as the chin approaches the chest, at which time the pain disap-

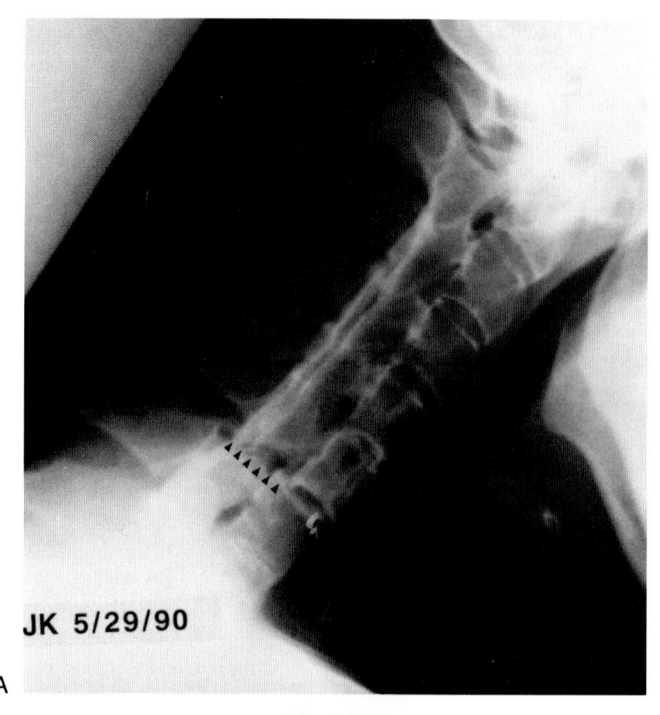

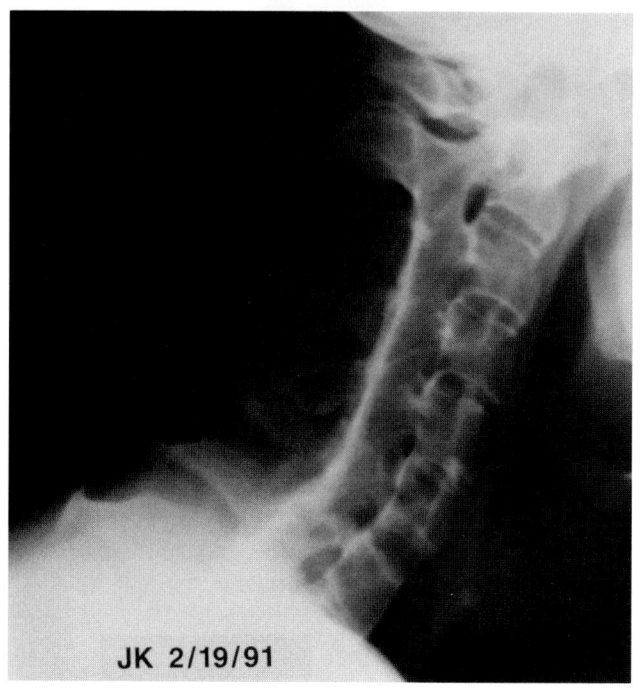

FIG. 5. A: Lateral radiograph of a 36-year-old man with ankylosing spondylitis following injury from a fall. The patient noted immediate neck pain and paresthesias in the index finger. A transverse shear fracture with 25% displacement is seen at C6–C7. **B:** Lateral radiograph demonstrating healing of the fracture anteriorly after treatment. The patient was treated with halo traction for 9 days with careful monitoring of neurologic status and had improvement of chin–brow to vertical angle from 40° to 5°.

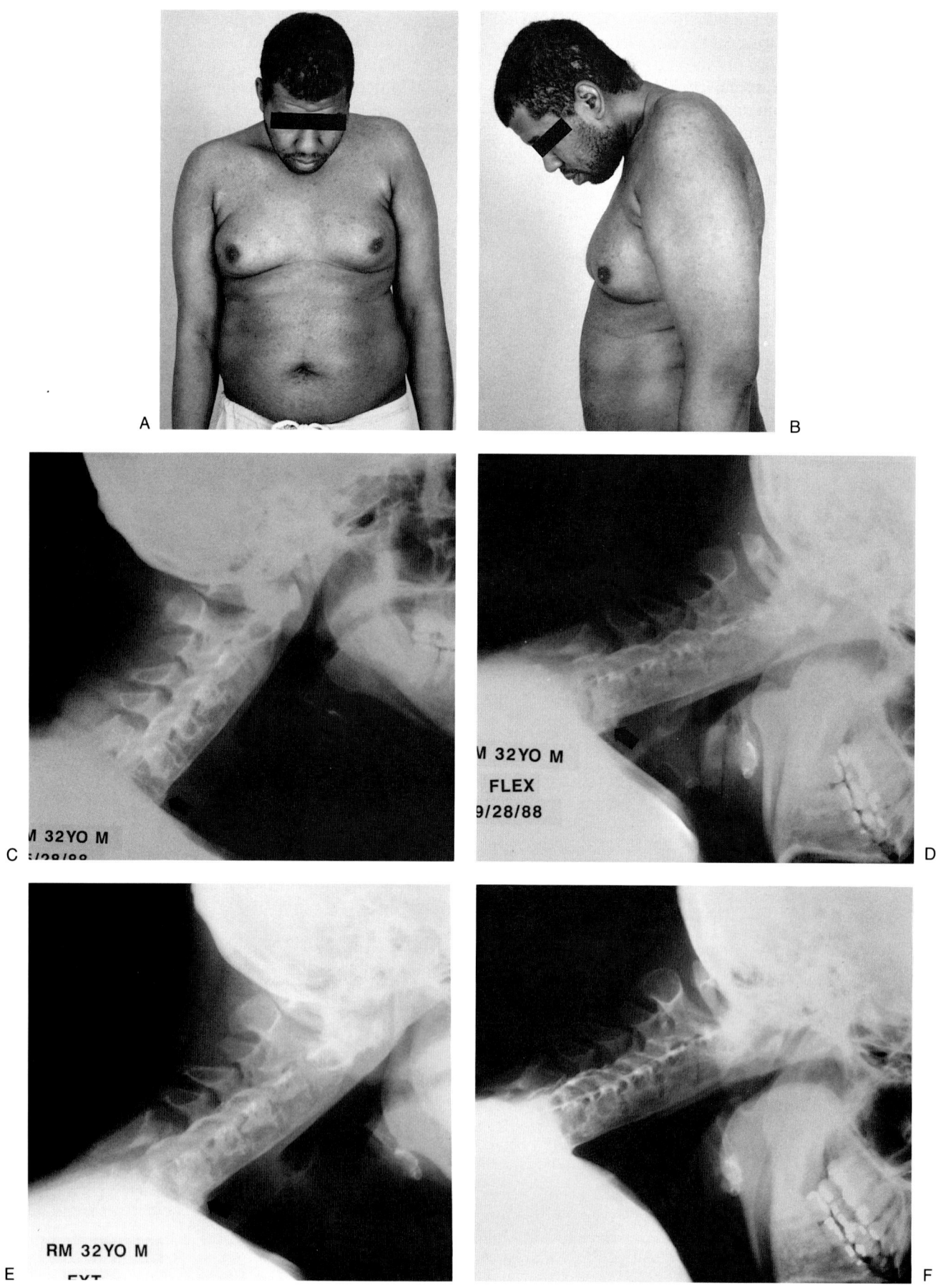

FIG. 6.

pears, leaving the patient with a painless, fixed flexion deformity. At this stage, osteotomy is required for correction (39,41,42) (Fig. 6).

When incomplete spinal cord injury with residual fracture displacement has occurred, open reduction and internal fixation may be required to protect the cord, since further injury may be caused by motion induced from the solid segments above and below. Decompression of the cord is accomplished by the accuracy of the reduction (10).

It is important to recognize the dangers of attempting operative reduction under general anesthesia (37). The movement of the neck required for intubation can cause further major spinal cord injury to a rigid upper

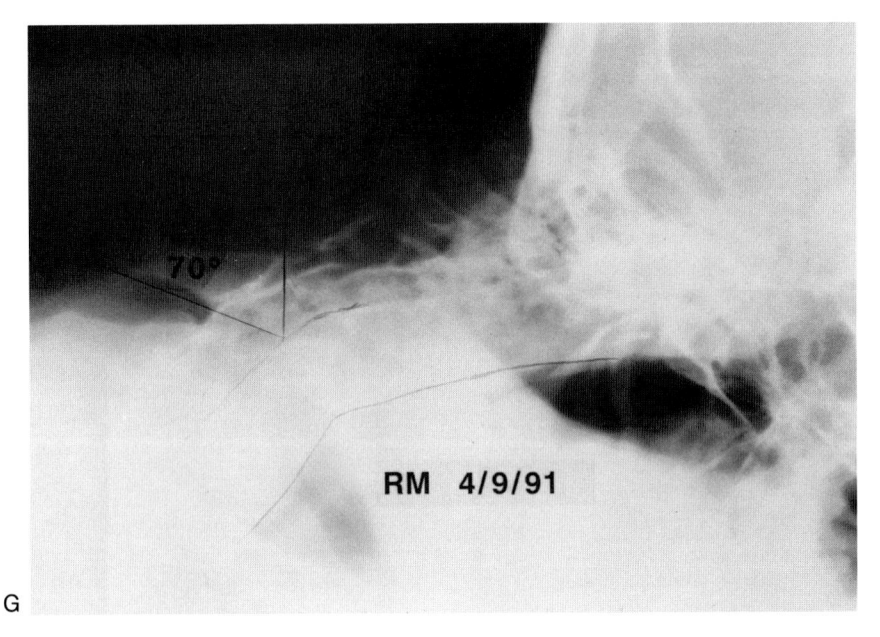

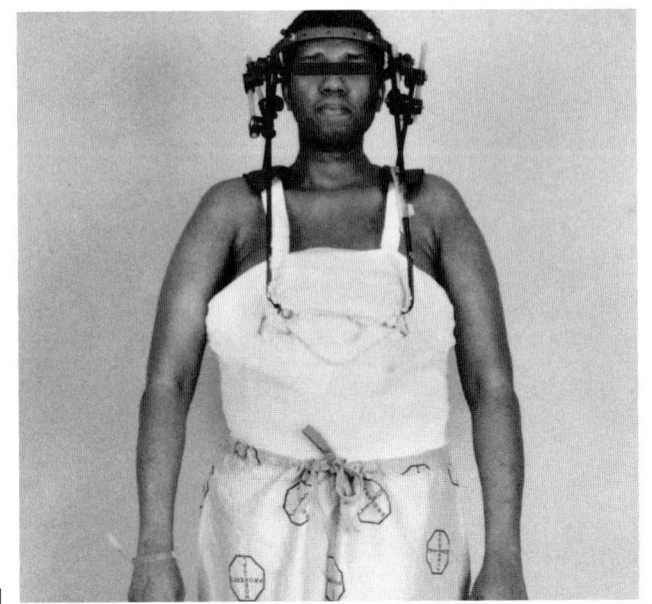

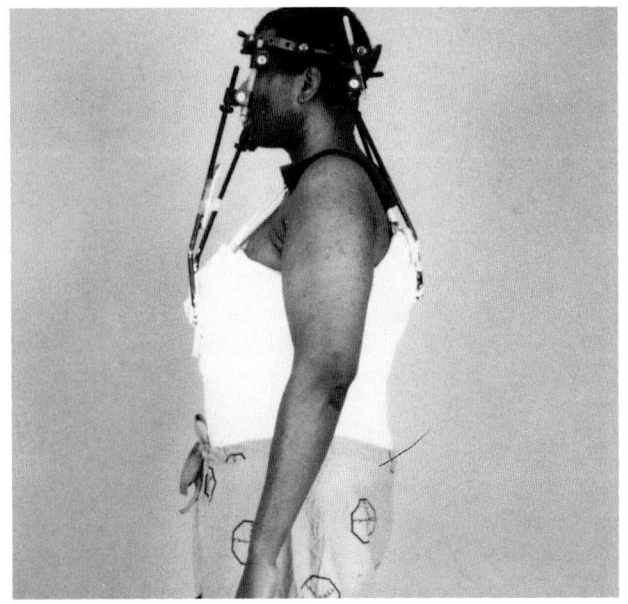

FIG. 6. A,B: Anterior and lateral views of 34-year-old man with ankylosing spondylitis and severe flexion deformity causing difficulty eating, shaving, and walking due to restricted field of view. C: Lateral radiograph demonstrating fracture at C7, which was missed at initial assessment following injury. The diagnosis of associated ankylosing spondylitis was not made for 5 months after injury. D,E: Lateral flexion and extension radiograph showing development of flexion deformity 4 months after injury. F: Preoperative lateral radiograph 1 year after injury with fixed painless flexion deformity following healing of fracture with chin-on-chest deformity. G: Lateral preoperative tomogram shows 70° wedge required to perform resection–extension cervical osteotomy. H,I: Anterior and lateral views of patient following cervical osteotomy with immobilization in halo cast. A normal chin–brow to vertical angle is restored.

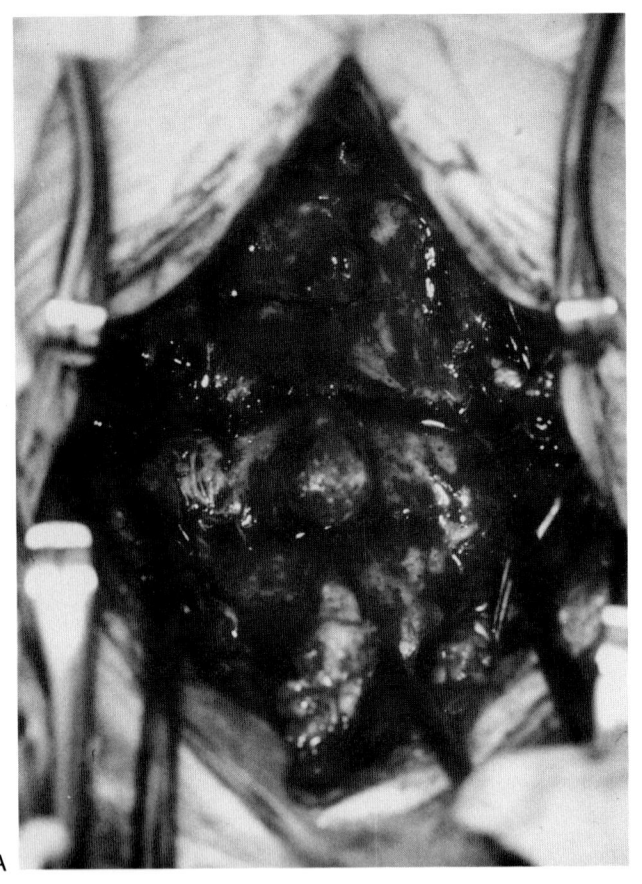

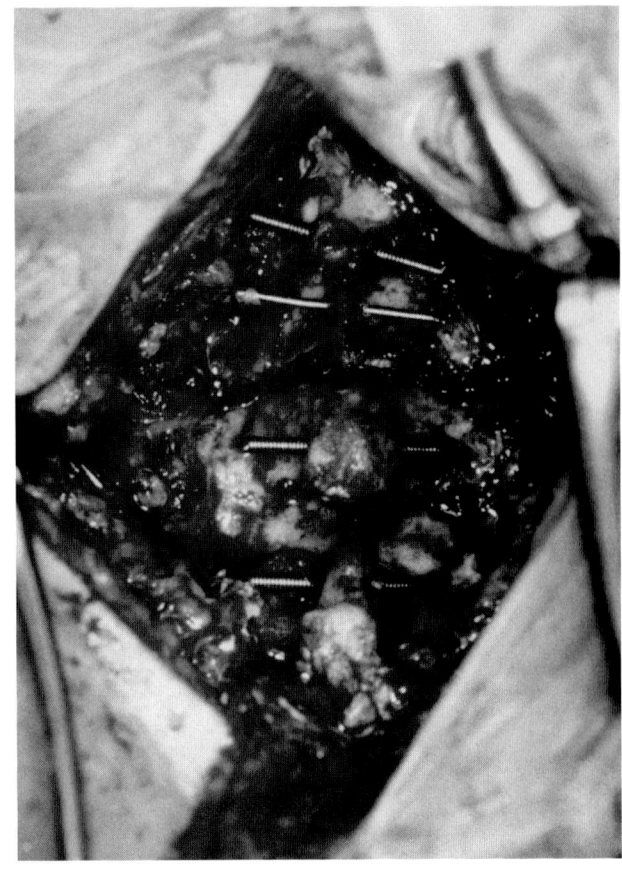

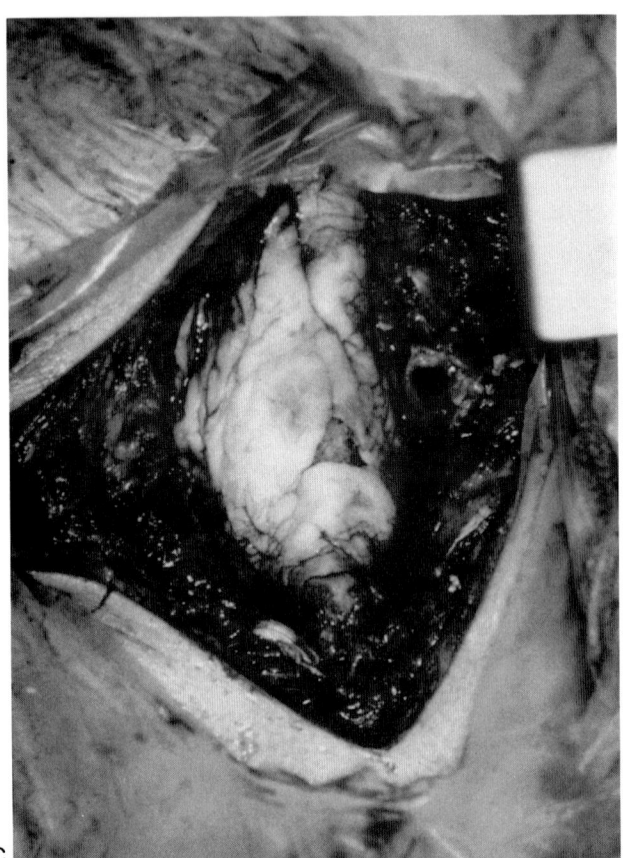

FIG. 7. A: Posterior operative view of the cervical spine of a 32-year-old spondylitic man suffering fracture/dislocation of C6–C7 with partial quadriplegia following an automobile accident. The patient was placed in a halo vest with some displacement persisting. The displacement and instability in this type of patient are magnified by the solid column of bone above and below. Operation was performed under local anesthesia with the patient in the sitting position. The halo was suspended along the normal line of the neck to add to the immobilization of the halo vest. The fracture has been reduced with the C5 and C6 spinous processes exposed above, and the spinous processes of C7 and T1 below. **B:** Operative posterior view showing reduction of shear fracture-dislocation, with threaded Compere wires in position through the posterior arches of C5, C6, C7, and T1. The wires were inserted percutaneously from the left lateral aspect of the neck, transfixing the bases of the spinous processes. The wires were then cut lateral to the spine. **C:** Posterior operative view showing methyl methacrylate incorporating the Compere wires and spinous processes, maintaining reduction with instant fixation of the unstable shear fracture. The procedure provides normal alignment of the canal and prevents the deleterious effect of continuing motion on the neural elements until bony healing occurs. If midline decompression is necessary, bridges of methylmethacrylate may be placed laterally on each side, leaving the midline free.

cervical spine. Transferring to an operating table and positioning for surgery presents significant risks if the patient is not awake. The patient is most safely operated on while awake and in the sitting position.

After the neck has been stabilized with a halo jacket, which has been firmly applied, surgery can be performed in the sitting position. Traction applied along the line of the neck assists with immobilization. The posterior cervical spine can be exposed under local anesthesia and the fracture accurately reduced and fixed internally with methyl methacrylate. This may be accomplished by passing threaded Compere pins percutaneously through the bases of the spinous processes above and below with an encircling stainless steel wire. Methyl methacrylate is then used to fix the spine, incorporating the threaded wires. This provides instant fixation, relieves the patient's pain, and maintains accurate alignment until healing occurs anteriorly (Fig. 7).

Following the surgery, the halo vest should be changed to a well molded halo cast that will supply more rigid and accurate immobilization. The cast must be molded below the costal cage and over the iliac crests to prevent any up or down motion. This is worn for 4 months. The restoration of accurate alignment of the spinal canal is the main factor in decompression. In more longstanding cases with residual displacement or in the presence of a small spinal canal, additional decompression can be accomplished by removing the adjacent arches at the fracture site. Mobilization is then accomplished by placing methyl methacrylate laterally on each side as a bridge from the segments above to below (45,47).

The other area where lesions of the cervical spine may occur, causing the patients to present with painful flexion deformity, is the craniocervical junction. Erosive fractures through the posterior arch of C1 and subluxation at C1–C2 may present with painful neck flexion with or without neurologic symptoms (13). Destructive arthritis at the atlanto-occipital joints may cause the patient to flex the neck, with the chin held downward, at these joints.

A lateral radiograph of the cervical spine is a clue to the recognition of these possibilities. It will show a relatively normal cervical lordosis with flexion deformity at the craniocervical junction. The lesions should be recognized and the deformity corrected by graduated halo traction. This is initially applied along the line of the neck to restore a normal chin–brow to vertical angle and is followed by posterior stabilization. When reduction is obtained for a C1–C2 dislocation, then posterior atlantoaxial arthrodesis, using the Gallie technique, may be all that is required. For occipitocervical destructive change and erosive fractures of the arch of C1, occipitocervical fusion is required with, when necessary, excision of the posterior fragmented arch of C1 (45,47) (Fig. 8).

Ankylosing spondylitic patients with stiffened, brittle spines are subject to the higher forces of modern, mechanized society and may experience complex traumatic forces with fractures occurring in other regions. Once the fracture has occurred, the segment is typically more unstable due to a rigid column of bone above and below. The spinal canal, which is a rigid tube, typically shears through both the anterior and posterior elements, much like a Chance fracture. This injury is inherently unstable. The fracture is at the junction of two long, ankylosed tubes, and any movement of the trunk translates all the force or motion to the fracture. This fracture is more like a long bone fracture than a typical spinal fracture.

It should be recognized that patients with this ankylosing spondylitis are at major risk and are prone to disastrous results with the conventional methods of treatment used for fracture/dislocation in patients without ankylosing spondylitis. Numerous reports of patients with fractures in ankylosing spondylitis who had neurologic decline in the immediate or the early hospital period are available (7,33). The incidence of neurologic deterioration reported in the normal patient with spine fracture has improved with the advent of greater care and expertise in the field and emergency room prior to definitive treatment.

The same maneuvers, however, may prove hazardous to the ankylosing spondylitic patient (35). In an ankylosing spondylitic patient with a previous flexion deformity of the neck, taping or strapping the head to a baseboard in the field can prove disastrous. The neutral position for a normal patient may be an excessively hyperextended position in the spondylitic patient. A common observation by relatives of a patient with a fracture of the cervical spine, when the patient is first seen after admission to the emergency department, is that "the neck is straight" when, prior to the injury, the patient had a well-known forward flexion alignment. It is important to get a history of previous flexion deformity in these patients so that this complication can be avoided.

In a review of 300 traumatic spine fractures, eight patients were found to have ankylosing spondylitis (6). This group did poorly compared to the nonspondylitic patients. In four of the eight patients the diagnosis of cervical spine injury was not made initially in the emergency room, and the patients were not admitted to hospital for inpatient care. Three of these four patients subsequently developed increasing quadriparesis that required return to hospital. Only one of the eight patients did not have paralysis. Of the seven patients with neural deficit, five had an anterior cord syndrome and two had complete quadriplegia. Only three of the eight

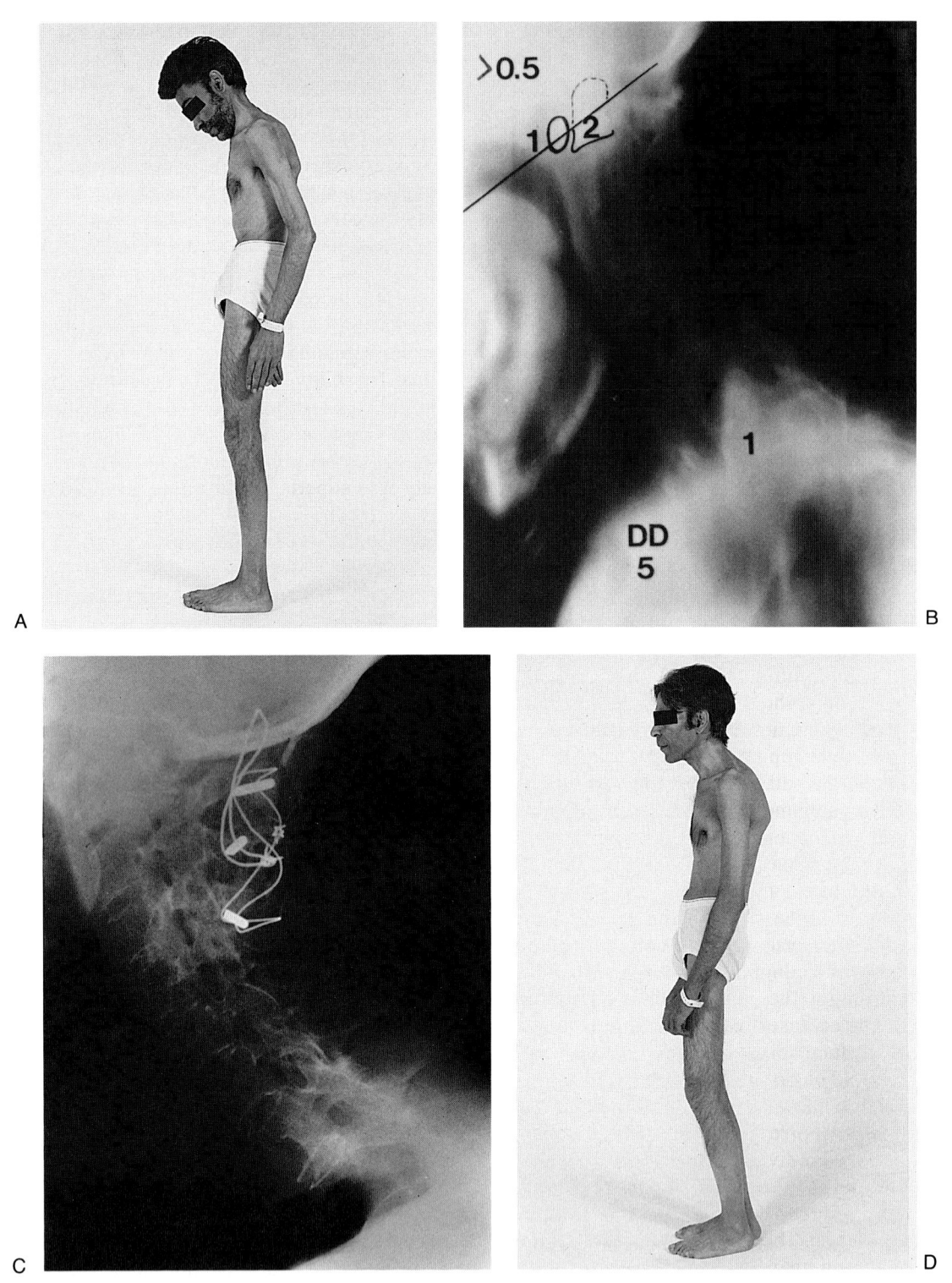

FIG. 8. A: Lateral view of physicist with painful chin-on-chest deformity. The patient held his head with his hands when sitting to control his pain. **B:** Lateral tomogram of the cervical spine showing normal lordosis and normal alignment at the cervicothoracic junction. The C1–C2 relationships are normal. The mandible approaches the cervical spine, indicating the deformity is at the occipitoatlantal junction. The dense posterior arch of C1 was eroded and loose, likely causing dural irritation and neck flexion. There were destructive changes at the occipitoatlantal joints. **C:** Lateral postoperative radiograph following reduction of the deformity with halo traction, excision of the loose posterior arch of C1, and solid posterior occipitocervical fusion. Double onlay iliac grafts were used, fixed to the skull and upper cervical spine, augmented with cancellous grafts. **D:** Lateral postoperative view showing correction of chin-on-chest deformity with restoration of normal chin–brow to vertical angle.

patients survived. This small group of patients illustrates a number of the problems in treating patients with ankylosing spondylitis and fracture.

The difficulty in making the diagnosis of neck fracture in these patients is documented in the medical literature. The typical location of the fracture in the lower cervical spine or at the cervicothoracic junction makes radiographic visualization difficult. Visualization also is obscured because of severe osteoporosis. In any patient who presents with neck pain following even trivial trauma, the presence of a fracture must be assumed until proved otherwise.

In Bohlman's series, four of his eight ankylosing spondylitis patients developed significant epidural hematomas (6). This represented 50% of the eight spondylitic patients, while none of the other 292 patients in the series had a diagnosis of epidural hematoma. The susceptibility of these patients to epidural hematoma must be considered in the presence of a worsening neurologic examination (10,14,17). The exaggerated motion at the fracture site, predisposed by the solid column of bone above and below, probably aggravates the tendency to hematoma formation. This development of an epidural hematoma is a definite indication for surgical intervention with reduction, decompression, and rigid stabilization of the fracture and, if significant, laminectomy and evacuation of the hematoma.

Many authors have reported on the rapid rate of union in patients with ankylosing spondylitis (19,20,32). This phenomenon may be the only fortunate mechanism in these patients with spinal fracture. In series comparing operative versus nonoperative treatment of these fractures, little benefit can be gained from surgery except in the case of the declining neurologic deficit (32,51). These patients should be placed in halo traction with reduction of the fracture to the preinjury position. Injudicious extension of the fracture in an effort to decrease the patient's fixed kyphotic deformity can produce spinal cord injury. Any extension obtained should be on a careful, gradual basis with the patient awake to allow careful monitoring of neurological function. Any correction of preinjury deformity should be considered a dividend (23). It should not be the primary goal and should not supplant the basic principles of fracture reduction (47) (Fig. 9).

Once reduction has been achieved, the patient should be placed in a halo cast. Neurologic deterioration has occurred with patients in halo traction when the patient has turned in bed or during radiographic procedures. A lateral tomogram with routine radiographic studies is the most valuable aid determining the alignment at the fracture site.

Fractures of the cervical spine in ankylosing spondylitis appear to have a significant influence on the severe deformity that often presents for spinal osteotomy. Simmons and Duncan (48) reviewed 39 patients who had undergone surgical correction of severe flexion deformity of the cervical spine associated with ankylosing spondylitis. Fourteen patients (36%) had evidence of preexisting fracture. In 12 (31%), the fracture had caused significant superimposed deformity and functional disability. When compared to the uninjured group, those with injury were found to have suffered an episode of sudden increase, followed by relentless progression of the deformity. This phenomenon typically was superimposed on a moderate, fixed flexion deformity that had previously been considered quiescent or only mildly progressive.

Patient education and physician education may help prevent some of these serious injuries and complications (17,50,53). Patients should be informed about the fragile nature of their spines and their susceptibility to injury. Patients should report all incidences of head and neck trauma to their physicians, who should always suspect fracture. Simple precautions may make grave differences in the lives of these patients. Night lights, hand rails, avoidance of alcohol, and use of automobile seat belts should be strongly encouraged. Physician education should result in a higher percentage of fracture diagnosis at initial presentation.

A halo vest is suitable for emergency stabilization. However, for prolonged rigid immobilization to allow healing with minimal motion at the fracture site, the halo cast has proved to be the most efficient and reliable. New orthoses, including the Lev-Tec unit and inflatable vests, may prove adequate, but they cause problems of skin pressure and adjustment and have not been evaluated adequately in patients with ankylosing spondylitis.

All patients with neck pain following head or neck trauma should be assumed to have a cervical fracture until proved otherwise. All fractures must be assumed to be highly unstable with a high potential for neurologic complications. All fractures should be rigidly immobilized using halo head control, and all fractures should be reduced to the preinjury position.

Text continues on page 397.

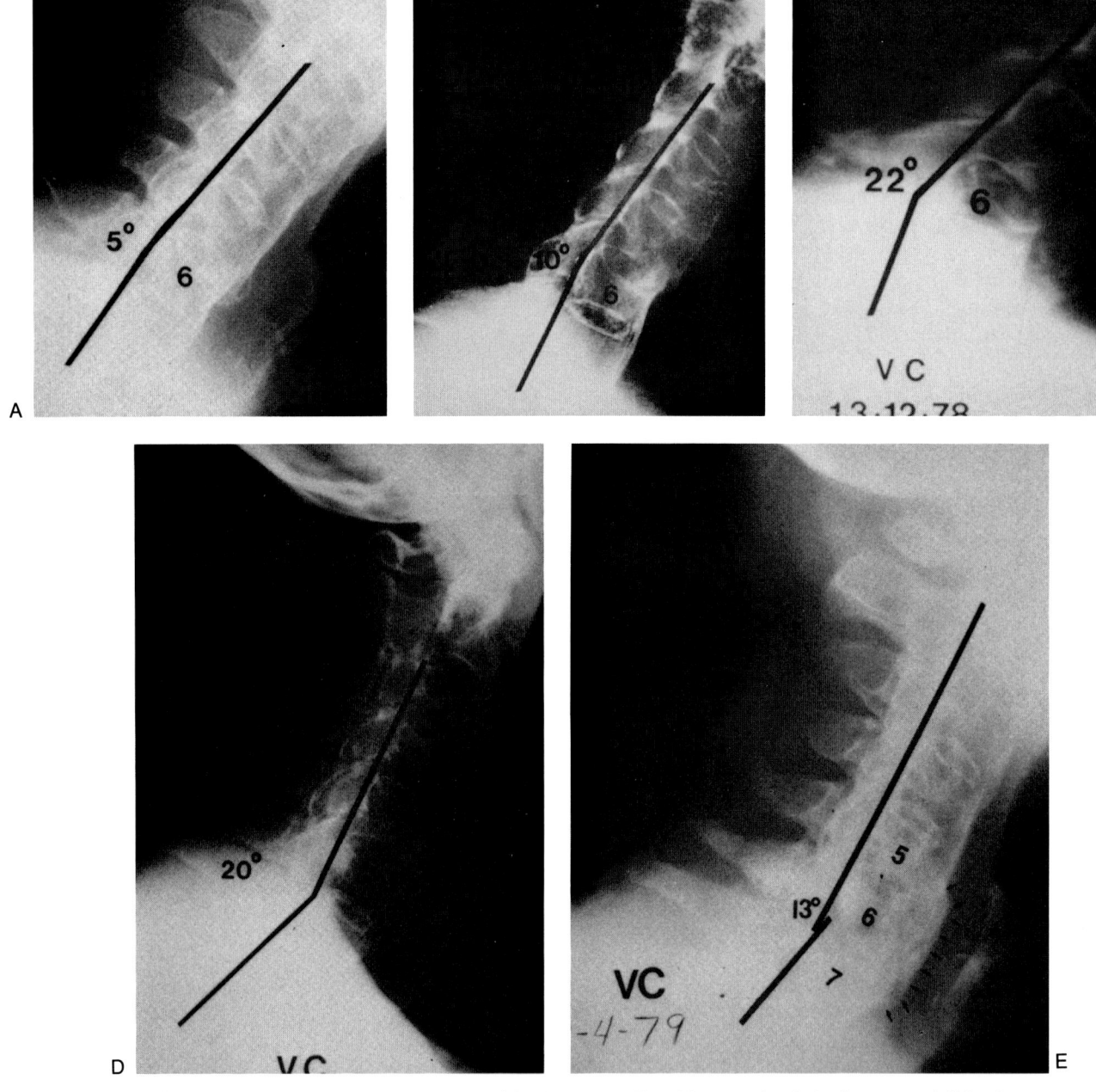

FIG. 9. A: Lateral radiograph of man with a longstanding history of ankylosing spondylitis showing recent shear fracture at C5–C6. **B:** A further lateral view of the cervical spine 13 days later shows increasing flexion deformity. At that time, the patient had increasing pain in the C7 distribution. **C:** A further lateral radiograph 36 days following injury. The patient now had gross triceps weakness with severe pain on movement and 22° fracture flexion deformity. **D:** Lateral radiograph of the cervical spine following graduated halo traction reduction. The patient was symptom-free with return of normal neurologic function. **E:** Lateral radiograph of the cervical spine showing solid healing 4 months following treatment. The patient's spinal alignment has been improved over the preinjury state.

DIFFERENTIATION OF FRACTURE PSEUDARTHROSIS FROM SPONDYLODISCITIS

A radiographic characteristic of ankylosing spondylitis is erosion and sclerosis of bone adjacent to the sacroiliac joint (18). Occasionally, the erosive sclerotic process extends into the intervertebral discs and adjacent bone. It is then called "spondylodiscitis." These erosive lesions of the vertebral bodies were first reported by Andersson (1) in 1937.

Speculation on the nature of the lesions is resolved into two opposing views. The first is that spondylodiscitis is an expression of the inflammatory process affecting the intervertebral disc and the surrounding bone (49). Detailed assessment and biopsy specimens support this view. The second, less commonly held view is that spondylodiscitis is due to trauma, with excessive forces localized at one intervertebral segment, resulting in mechanical destruction and a functional pseudarthrosis (12,28).

The inflammatory mechanism appears to arise from, and is part of, the spondylitic process. This inflammatory process is seen in other areas where ligaments attach to the skeleton and is often referred to as spondylitic enthesopathy (3,8). Erosion of bone surfaces such as the iliac crest, the greater trochanter, the tips of the vertebral spinous processes, the symphysis pubis, and the sternomanubrial joints has been reported. Biopsy specimens of the lesions reveal a primary inflammatory process.

A similar process leads to the characteristic changes of ankylosing spondylitis seen in the vertebral bodies; vertebral squaring and "shining corners" (18). This mechanism of primary inflammation is also supported by destructive intervertebral lesions in the spine with intact posterior elements. This is in contrast to the presumed pseudarthrosis following trauma in which the posterior elements are also involved in the lesion. Lesions have also been reported in thoracic spines that were neither rigid nor deformed, supporting a primary inflammatory process (3,9).

The impression of "spinal pseudarthrosis" at a disc space is believed to occur when forces, which would tend to bend the spine, are concentrated on an unstable diseased space. This weakness predisposes to disruption of the posterior spinal elements. Fang et al. (12) evaluated 40 destructive vertebral lesions in 35 patients and found fractures through the ankylosed posterior elements in line with the anterior lesion in 31 disc lesions in 26 patients. The histopathology in 18 lesions that underwent anterior spinal fusion was considered pseudarthrosis.

It is a consistent observation at surgery that, in a completely ossified spine, the ossified ligamentum flavum, ligaments, and discs are much stronger and harder than the vertebral bony elements, which are often osteoporotic. Force applied to this type of spine will produce disruption through the weaker bone, rather than through the ossified intervertebral ligamentous connections, including the ossified disc. True fracture pseudarthroses will be seen in nonunions of slice fractures through the true bony elements (Fig. 10) in contradistinction to inflammatory spondylodiscitis, which is always at the disc space (44,47,48) (Fig. 11).

The radiographic appearance of spondylodiscitis is fairly typical, with a reported incidence of 5% to 6% (49). The erosive process widens the disc space, with destruction of the subchondral bony plates. The surrounding bone becomes sclerotic and radiodense (47,48) (Fig. 12). Either erosion or sclerosis may appear more prominent. The majority of the lesions develop in the thoracic spine. About one-half of the cases present with back pain, and a little over 50% are discovered on routine radiological review, since they are asymptomatic. It appears that the lesion generally follows a benign course and will usually respond to conservative management. Occasionally, surgical stabilization may be required for intractable pain, particularly where there is an associated fracture or disruption of the posterior fused spine at the same level.

The lesion of spondylodiscitis can easily be confused with infection. The differential diagnosis of the destructive intervertebral disc lesion includes infection, neoplasia, and axial neuroarthropathy (Charcot arthropathy). With a single lesion neoplasia is unlikely, but it should not be completely discounted (Fig. 13). The major concern is distinguishing these lesions from infection. The absence of fever, leukocytosis, increased erythrocyte sedimentation rate, a history of recent infection, or intravenous drug abuse make infection unlikely. Biopsy specimens and culture may be required to make this diagnosis.

The incidence of spondylodiscitis may be greater than what the literature would suggest. Undoubtedly, its recognition requires an awareness of its presence. Of 157 cases of ankylosing spondylitis referred for evaluation and surgical correction of spinal deformity, 133 still had available radiographs of the entire spine available for study (49). Of these, 31, or 23%, were found to have spondylodiscitis. The high incidence may be partly attributable to the severity of the deformities analyzed.

The chief complaint was progressive kyphotic deformity in 26 cases. Nine of the 26 patients described a traumatic episode that produced increasing pain and deformity in the area of spondylodiscitis. There were no neurologic deficits secondary to the lesion. The site of spondylodiscitis ranged from T7 to L5. Most commonly, it was found at T11, T12, or L1. There were seven cases of multiple level involvement.

Text continues on page 406.

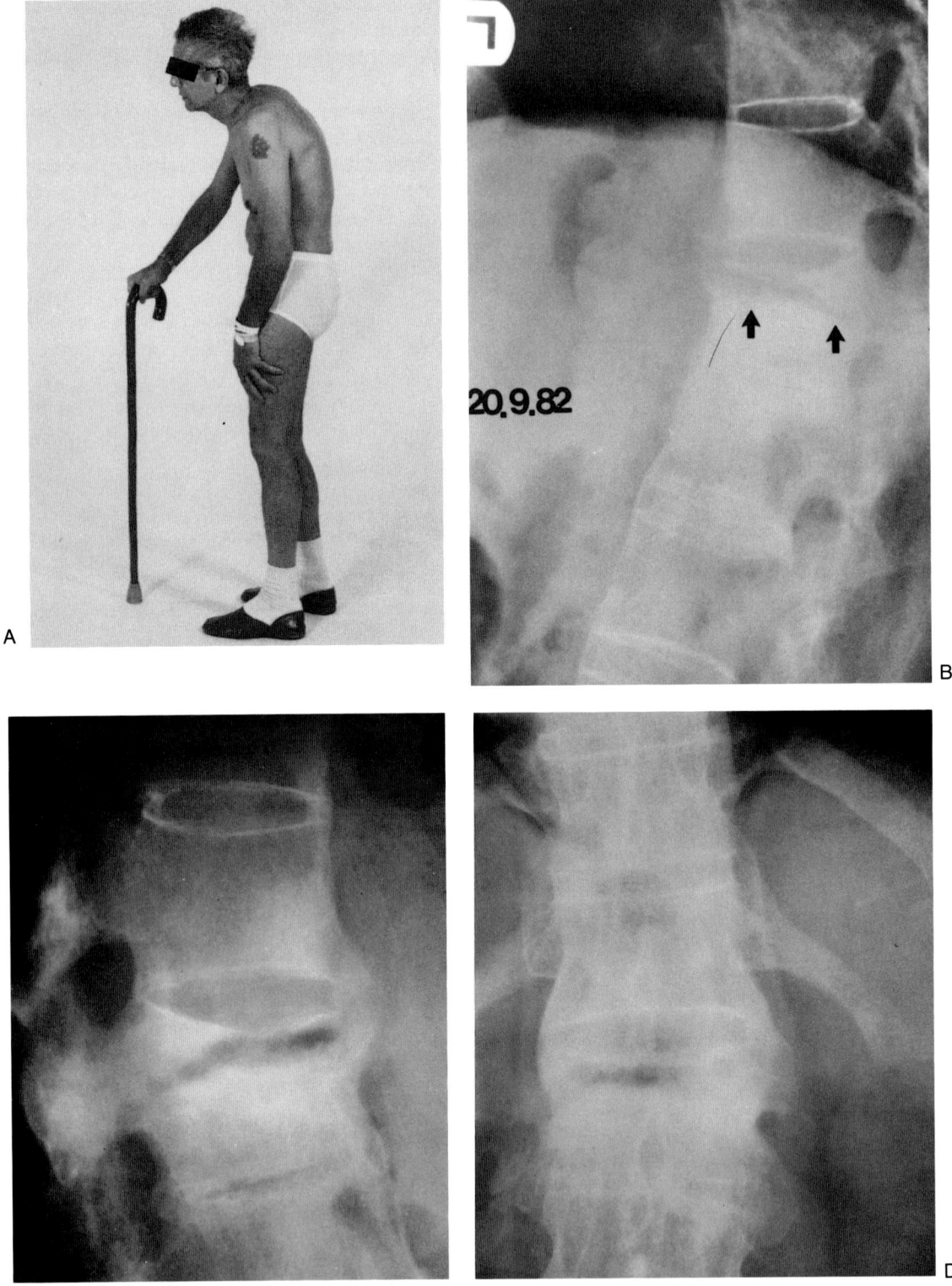

FIG. 10. A: Lateral view of a 56-year-old man with painful thoracolumbar flexion deformity following significant injury to the spine. His pain was in keeping with a fracture pseudarthrosis. **B:** Lateral radiograph showing nonunion of a transverse shear fracture through the upper body of L1 going through the posterior elements. **C:** Close-up view showing a typical pseudarthrosis in the vertebral body of L1 not involving the disc space. **D:** Anterior view showing typical appearance of fracture pseudarthrosis without gross bone destruction. **E:** Lateral standing 3-ft radiograph of spine showing the lesion under shear stress with the weight-bearing line of the body anterior to the fracture site. **F:** Postoperative standing lateral 3-ft radiograph showing correction of the spinal deformity by lumbar extension osteotomy, with the weight-bearing line shifted posteriorly and the area of pseudarthrosis under compression with spontaneous healing.

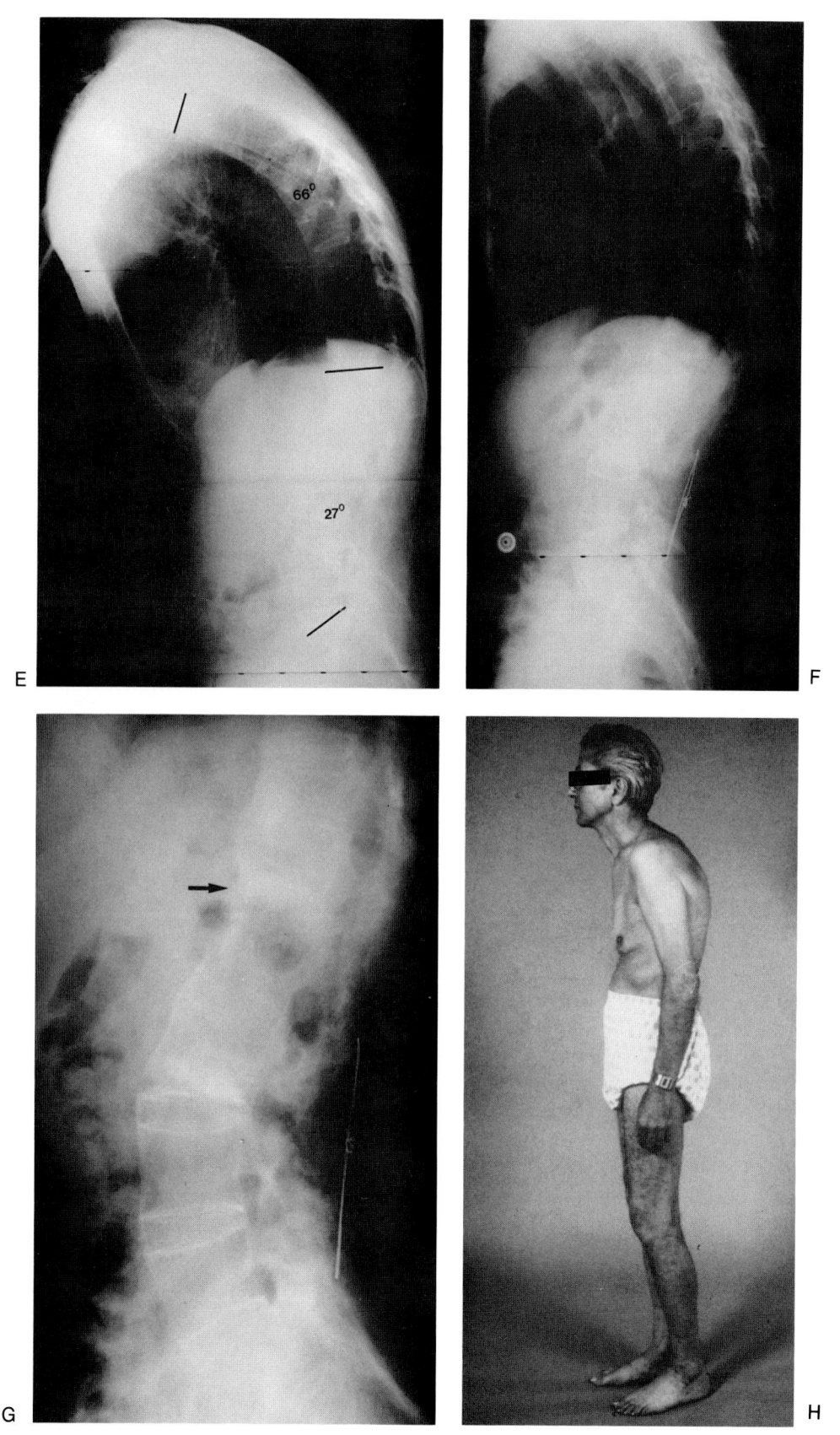

FIG. 10. (*Continued.*) **G:** Lateral postoperative radiograph of the lumbar spine showing extension osteotomy, with spontaneous healing of the pseudarthrosis of the L1 vertebra after the lesion had been placed under compression by correction of the deformity. **H:** Postoperative standing lateral view of patient showing correction of spinal deformity with normal spinal alignment.

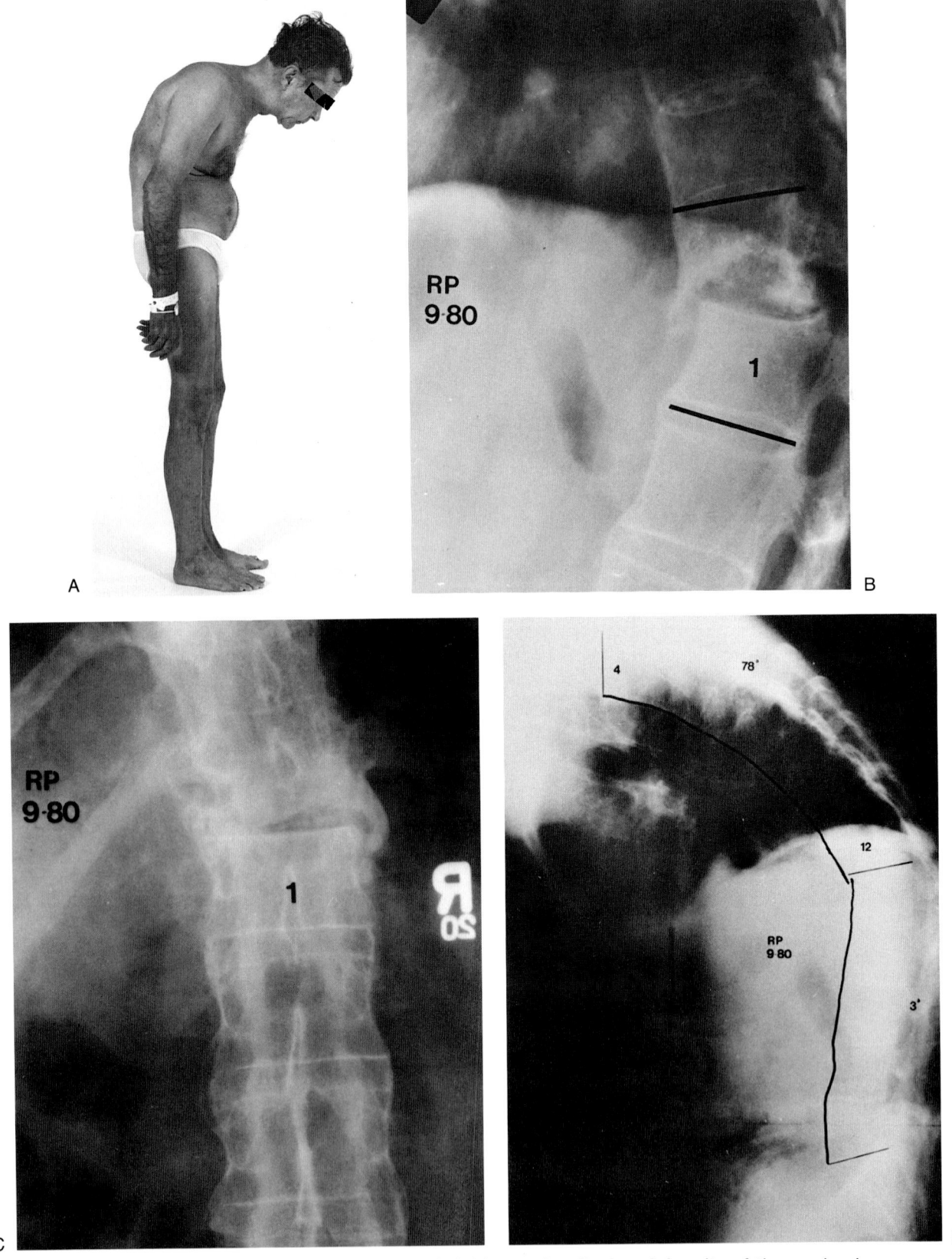

FIG. 11. A: Lateral view of patient with painful increasing flexion deformity of thoracolumbar spine associated with spondylodiscitis. Note thoracolumbar apex. **B:** Lateral radiograph showing gross destructive spondylodiscitis at T12–L1 with endplate destruction and bone absorption. **C:** AP radiograph showing changes of T12–L1 disc space. **D:** Standing lateral 3-ft radiograph of spine showing weight-bearing line well anterior to the area of destructive spondylodiscitis.

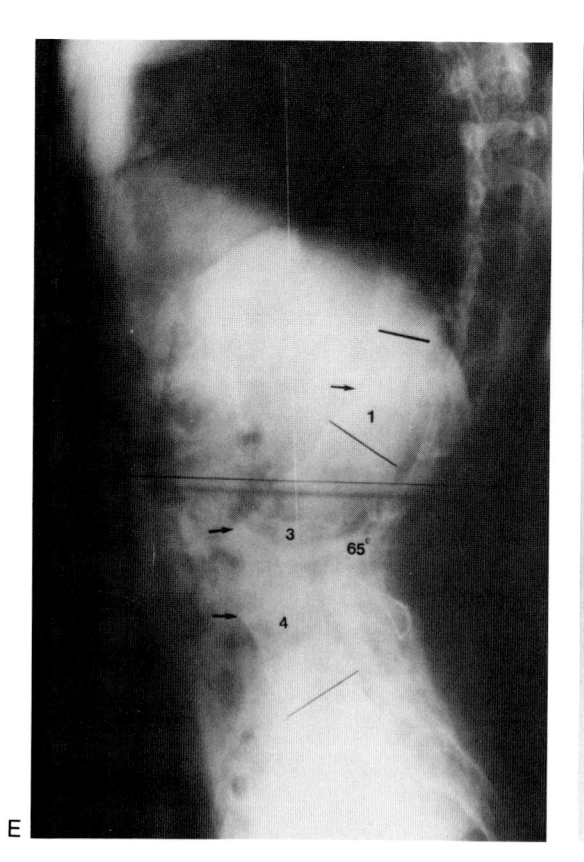

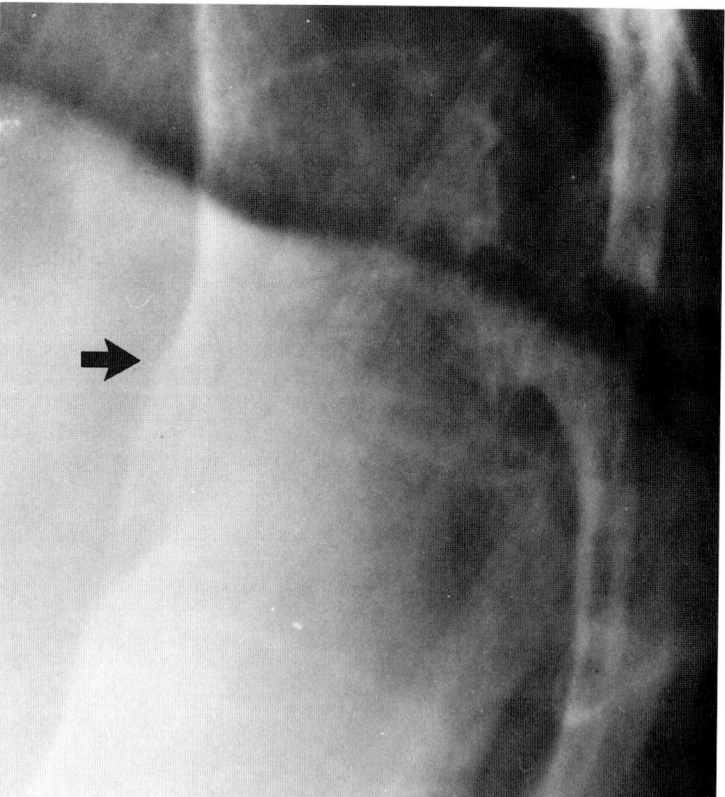

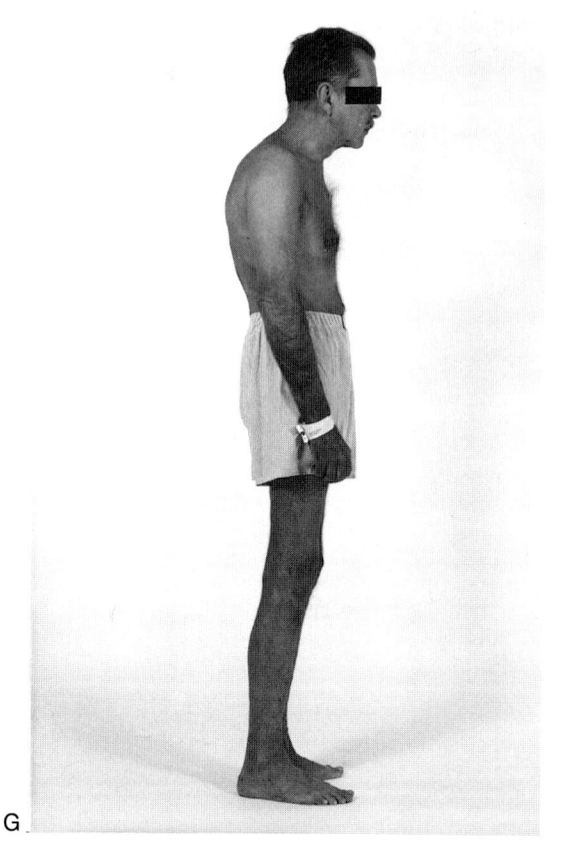

FIG. 11. (*Continued.*) **E:** Postoperative standing lateral 3-ft radiograph showing resection–extension osteotomy of midlumbar spine shifting the weight-bearing line posteriorly, converting shear force at the site of the spondylodiscitis to compression. **F:** Lateral radiograph of T12–L1 obtained 4 months postoperatively showing spontaneous healing of the area of spondylodiscitis as a result of conversion of shear stress to compression by lumbar osteotomy. **G:** Lateral view of patient following union of osteotomy and area of spondylodiscitis, showing correction of deformity.

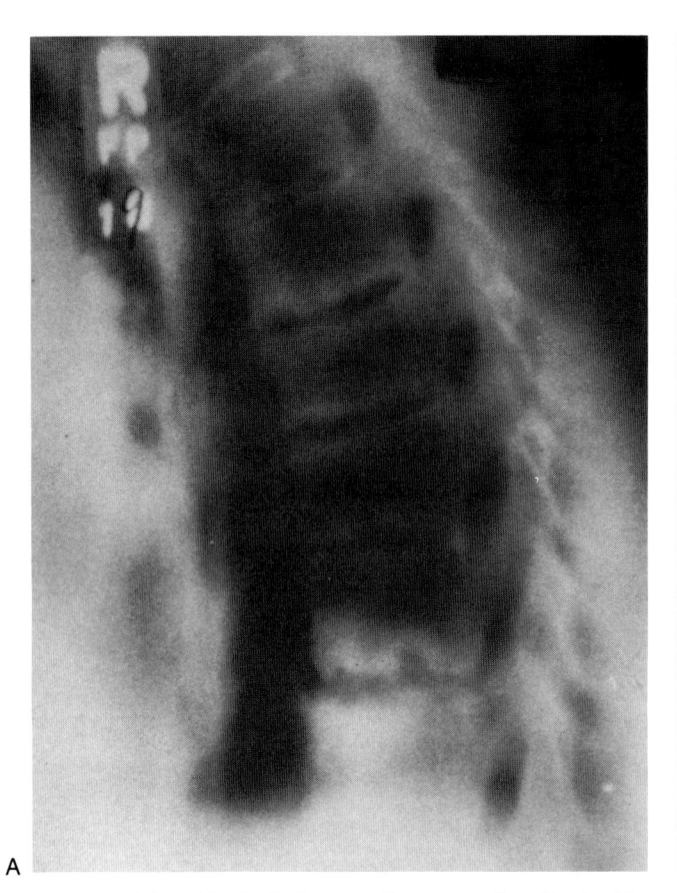

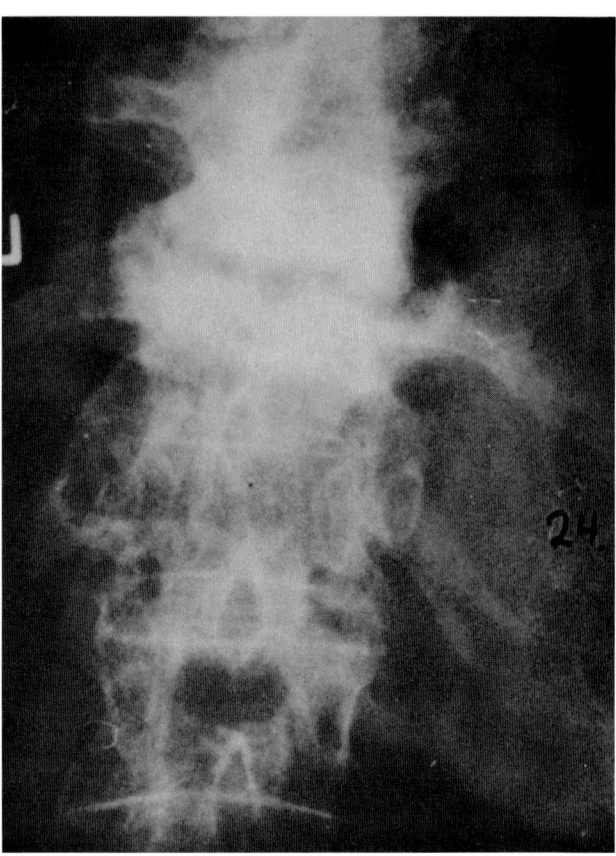

FIG. 12. A: Lateral radiograph of patient with ankylosing spondylitis showing areas of spondylodiscitis. The typical main lesion is in the lower thoracic spine, which is the most frequent location. Erosive sclerotic changes involve the vertebral endplates adjacent to the disc space. **B:** AP radiograph of area of spondylodiscitis in lower thoracic spine, again showing erosive sclerotic changes at the level of the disc space.

FIG. 13. A: Lateral radiograph of thoracolumbar spine showing typical shear fracture of ankylosing spondylitis involving L1 vertebra without deformity. **B:** Lateral radiograph 6 weeks later showing increasing deformity with 20° of kyphosis at fracture site. **C:** Lateral radiograph 4 months following injury showing progression of deformity with fracture kyphosis measuring 30°. Patient had intractable pain, and difficulty standing without support. The fracture-deformity is typical of that seen in ankylosing spondylitis, but this patient had a previous history of malignant melanoma. **D:** Bone scan showing changes consistent with fracture of L1, without evidence of neoplastic disease elsewhere. **E:** Lateral view of the same 51-year-old patient. In view of the history of malignancy, biopsy of L1 was performed revealing secondary malignant melanoma. **F:** Lateral radiograph showing immediate preoperative alignment with fracture kyphosis measuring 42°. At operation the vertebral bodies of L1–L3 were involved with malignant melanoma, "color coded" with black pigment. The three vertebral bodies were resected with reconstruction using fresh frozen femoral allograft supplemented with autogenous rib graft. **G:** Lateral radiograph 6.5 months postoperatively showing allograft in position with correction of deformity. **H:** Lateral postoperative view of patient. The patient's spinal pain was relieved, but he later developed metastasis elsewhere. When there is a suspicion of malignancy, it should be considered in the diagnosis and appropriate investigation carried out.

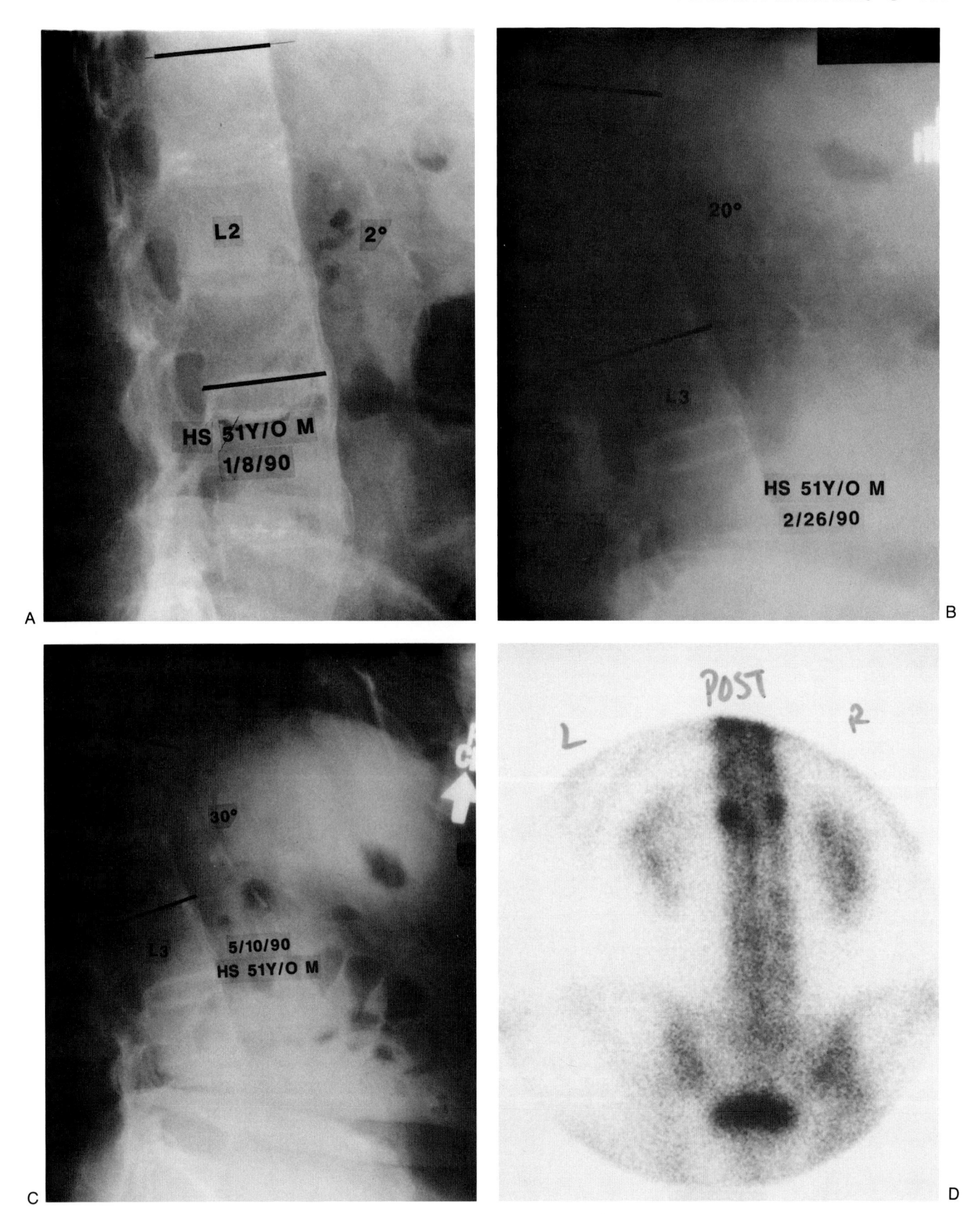

SPINE FRACTURES IN ANKYLOSING SPONDYLITIS ● 403

Figure continues

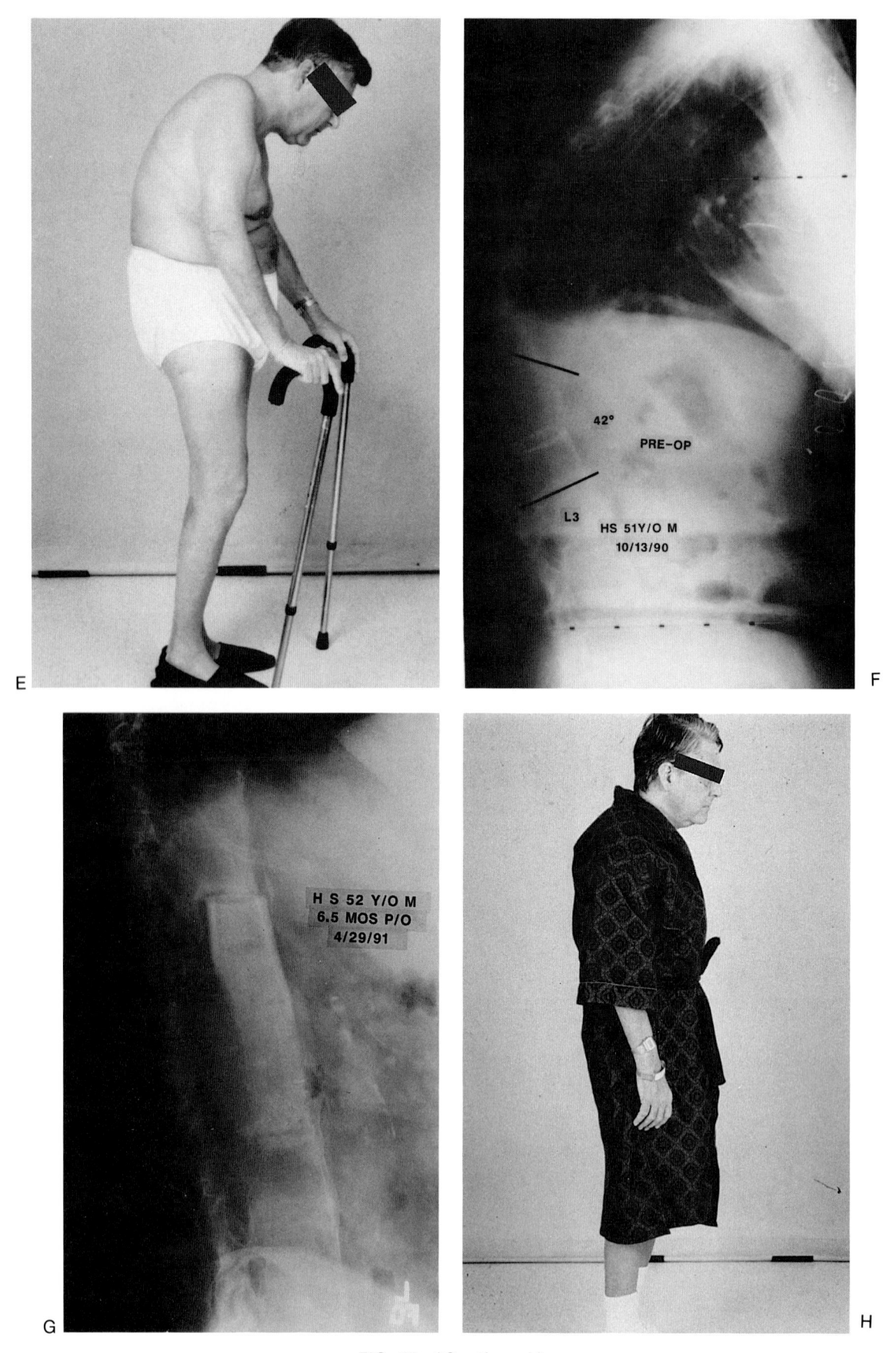

FIG. 13. *(Continued.)*

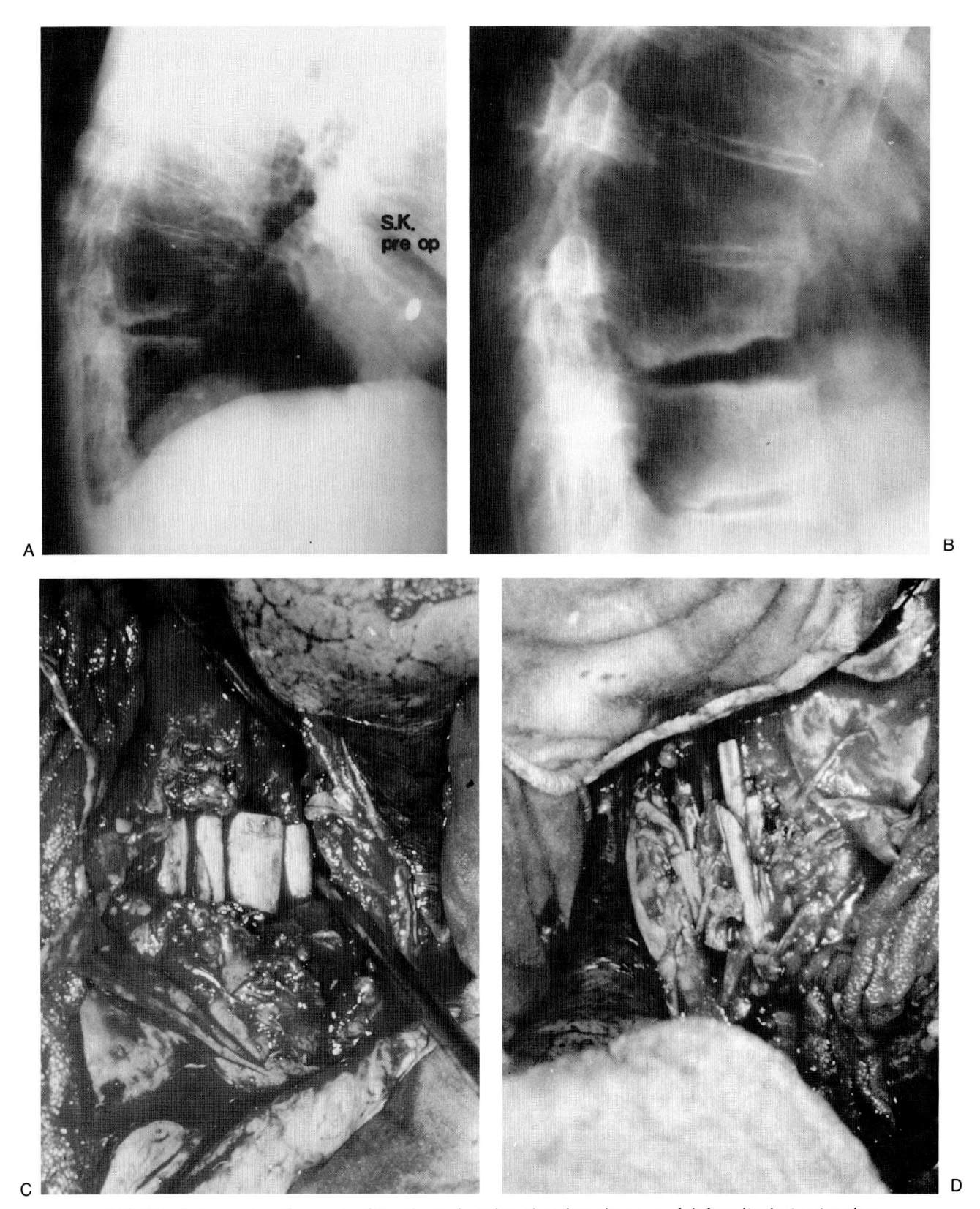

FIG. 14. A: Lateral radiograph of the thoracic spine showing absence of deformity, but extensive destructive change of spondylodiscitis at T9–T10. The patient suffered immediate severe pain following total hip arthroplasty due to lack of bony support anteriorly. **B:** Close-up lateral view showing extent of endplate destruction and absorption at disc space. **C:** Anterior exposure of spine showing excision of the area of spondylodiscitis with multiple fibular strut grafts. **D:** Final operative view showing addition of further onlay cortical and cancellous bone grafts.

Figure continues

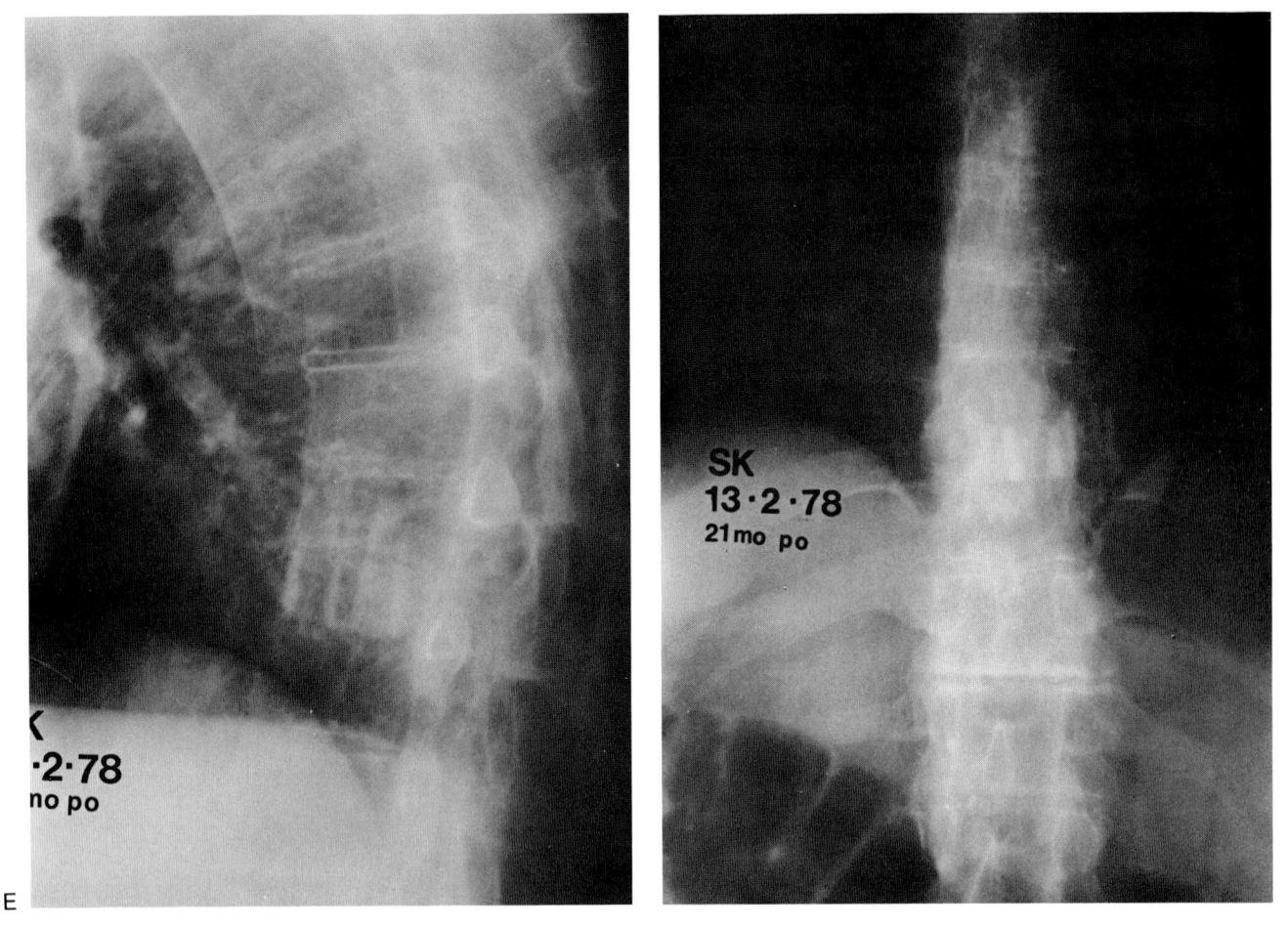

FIG. 14. (*Continued.*) **E:** Lateral radiograph 21 months postoperatively showing successful grafting and normal spinal alignment. **F:** Postoperative AP radiograph showing fusion 21 months postoperatively. The patient's pain was relieved by stabilization of the spine with anterior strut graft fusion.

Twenty-four of the 26 patients had surgical correction of their main deformity. The aim was to correct the kyphotic deformity completely, shifting the weight-bearing line of the upper body posteriorly to produce a balanced spine. When the spondylodiscitis was in the area of the deformity and contributed to it, correction of the deformity resulted in fusion at the site of the spondylodiscitis. Fusion occurred when the axis of the involved disc space was shifted from a vertical to a more transverse position, replacing any shear force by vertical compression with healing of the lesion. There were two cases that required multiple thoracic anterior strut grafting and posterior Harrington compression rod instrumentation for severe angular thoracic kyphotic deformities associated with destructive spondylodiscitis (46–48). Another patient required anterior fibular strut grafting for pain at the site of gross destructive spondylodiscitis that was not associated with deformity (Fig. 14).

The majority of patients with spondylodiscitis are asymptomatic; the lesion is noted on routine radiologic examination. However, when the area of involvement is under stress, it may be painful and can contribute significantly to kyphotic deformity. In the treatment of severe cases with deformity, surgical correction produces a balanced spine and encourages fusion at the site of the spondylodiscitis (Fig. 11). Rarely, anterior grafting is indicated for gross, painful, destructive lesions without deformity (44,47,48).

It is important to recognize destructive lesions of the spine in patients with ankylosing spondylitis. The lesions should be evaluated carefully, considering the differential diagnosis and the patient's symptoms. Bone scans can be helpful in diagnosing and following these lesions (11,36). The role of surgery depends on spinal alignment, severity of symptoms, and necessity for biopsy.

SUMMARY

1. Due to ossification and osteoporosis, the spine in ankylosing spondylitis is extremely susceptible to fracture.

2. The typical injury is a shear fracture through the fused elements due to a rigid column of bone above and below and may result from minor trauma. The most common site of injury is at the cervicothoracic junction.
3. The ankylosing spondylitis patient with neck pain following even trivial trauma should be considered to have a fracture until proved otherwise.
4. The best diagnostic aid in diagnosing the fracture is a lateral tomogram, along with cervical radiographs.
5. Fractures of the spine in ankylosing spondylitis patients are very unstable, with significant risk for displacement.
6. The patient with a cervical fracture should be immobilized with halo cervical traction and gradual correction to at least the preinjury position, followed by immobilization in a halo cast for 4 months.
7. Spondylodiscitis is often confused with fracture pseudarthrosis. Spondylodiscitis is an erosive lesion that occurs at the disc space and involves the surrounding endplates, while fracture pseudarthrosis results from a shear crack through the weaker vertebral body.
8. The majority of patients with spondylodiscitis are asymptomatic. When the lesion is under shear stress with fracture disruption of the posterior elements, surgical intervention may be required.
9. All physicians dealing with emergency care or the treatment of patients with arthritic disease should be aware of the potential for subtle presentation and disastrous complications of unrecognized fracture of the spine in ankylosing spondylitis.

REFERENCES

1. Andersson JA. Rontgenbilden vid spondyloarthritis ankylopoetica. *Nord Med* 1937;14:2000.
2. Amamilo SC. Fractures of the cervical spine in patients with ankylosing spondylitis. *Orthop Rev* 1989;18(3):33944.
3. Ball J. Articular pathology of ankylosing spondylitis. *Clin Orthop* 1979;143:30–37.
4. Bechterew VM. The classic-stiffening of the spine in flexion, a special form of disease. *Clin Orthop* 1979;143:4–7.
5. Bergmann EW. Fractures of the ankylosed spine. *J Bone Joint Surg* 1949;31A(3):669–671.
6. Bohlman HH. Acute fractures and dislocation of the cervical spine. An analysis of three hundred hospitalized patients and review of the literature. *J Bone Joint Surg* 1979;61A(8):1119–1142.
7. Broom MJ, Raycroft JF. Complications of fractures of the cervical spine in ankylosing spondylitis. *Spine* 1988;13(7):763–766.
8. Calin A. Ankylosing spondylitis. *Clin Rheum Dis* 1985;11(1):41–60.
9. Cawley MID, Chalmers TM, Kellgren JH, Ball J. Destructive lesions of vertebral bodies in ankylosing spondylitis. *Ann Rheum Dis* 1972;31:345.
10. Detwiler KN, Loftus CM, Godersky JC, Menezes AH. Management of cervical spine injuries in patients with ankylosing spondylitis. *J Neurosurg* 1990;72(2):210–215.
11. Dilorio G, Sundaram M. Radiologic case study. Fracture with pseudarthrosis in ankylosing spondylitis. *Orthopaedics* 1990;13(1):118, 120–123.
12. Fang D, Leong JC, Ho EK, Chan FL, Chow SP. Spinal pseudarthrosis in ankylosing spondylitis. Clinicopathological correlation and the results of anterior spinal fusion. *J Bone Joint Surg* 1988;70B(3):443–447.
13. Fardon DF. Odontoid fracture complicating ankylosing hyperostosis of the spine. *Spine* 1978;3(2):108–112.
14. Farhat SM, Schneider RJM. Traumatic spinal extradural hematoma associated with cervical fractures in rheumatoid spondylitis. *J Trauma* 1973;13:591–599.
15. Fast A, Parikh S, Marin EL. Spine fractures in ankylosing spondylitis. *Arch Phys Med Rehabil* 1986;67(9):595–597.
16. Fazl M, Bilbao JM, Hudson AR. Laceration of the aorta complicating spinal fracture in ankylosing spondylitis. *Neurosurgery* 1981;8(6):732–734.
17. Foo D, Sarkarati M, Marcelino V. Cervical spinal cord injury complicating ankylosing spondylitis. *Paraplegia* 1985;23:358–363.
18. Gold RH, Bassett LW, Seeger LL. The other arthritides. Roentgenologic features of osteoarthritis, erosive osteoarthritis, ankylosing spondylitis, psoriatic arthritis, Reiter's disease, multicentric reticulohistiocytosis, and progressive systemic sclerosis. *Radiol Clin North Am* 1988;26(6):1195–1212.
19. Graham B, Van Peteghem PK. Fractures of the spine in ankylosing spondylitis. Diagnosis, treatment and complications. *Spine* 1989;14(8):803–807.
20. Grisolia A, Bell RL, Peitier LF. Fractures and dislocations of the spine complicating ankylosing spondylitis. A report of six cases. *J Bone Joint Surg* 1967;49A(2):339–344.
21. Guttmann L. Traumatic paraplegia and tetraplegia in ankylosing spondylitis. *Paraplegia* 1967;5:188–203.
22. Hart FD. The stiff aching back. The differential diagnosis of ankylosing spondylitis. *Lancet* 1968;1(545):740–742.
23. Hershmann EB, Bercik RJ, Allen SC, Fielding JW. Correction of chin-on-chest deformity in ankylosing spondylitis through a fracture site—a case report. *Clin Orthop* 1985;201:201–204.
24. Hunter T, Dubo H. The spinal complications of ankylosing spondylitis. *Semin Arthritis Rheum* 1989;19(3):172–182.
25. Hunter T, Dubo H. Spinal fractures complicating ankylosing spondylitis. *Ann Intern Med* 1978;88(4):546–549.
26. Hunter T, Dubo HI. Spinal fractures complicating ankylosing spondylitis. A long-term follow-up study. *Arthritis Rheum* 1983;26(6):751–759.
27. Juric S, Coumas JM, Giansiracuse DF, Irwin RS. Hemothorax—an unusual presentation of spinal fracture in ankylosing spondylitis. *J Rheumatol* 1990;17(2):263–266.
28. Kanefield DG, Mullins BP, Freehafer AA, Furey JS, Horenstein S, Chamberlin WB. Destructive lesions of the spine in rheumatoid ankylosing spondylitis. *J Bone Joint Surg* 1969;51A(7):1369–1375.
29. Kewalramani LS, Taylor TG, Albrand OW. Cervical spine injury in patients with ankylosing spondylitis. *J Trauma* 1975;15(10):931–934.
30. Kiwerski J, Wieclawek H, Garwacka I. Fractures of the cervical spine in ankylosing spondylitis. *Int Orthop* 1985;8:243–246.
31. Masi AT, Medsger TA Jr. A new look at the epidemiology of ankylosing spondylitis and related syndromes. *Clin Orthop* 1979;143:15–29.
32. Murray SC, Persellin RH. Cervical fracture complicating ankylosing spondylitis: a report of eight cases and review of the literature. *Am J Med* 1981;70(5):1033–1041.
33. Osgood CP, Abbasy M, Mathews T. Multiple spine fractures in ankylosing spondylitis. *J Trauma* 1975;15(2):163–166.
34. Osgood C, Martin LG, Ackerman E. Fracture-dislocation of the cervical spine with ankylosing spondylitis. Report of two cases. *J. Neurosurg* 1973;39(6):764–769.
35. Podolsky SM, Hoffmann JR, Pietrafesa CA. Neurologic complications following immobilization of cervical spine fracture in a patient with ankylosing spondylitis. *Ann Emerg Med* 1983;12(9):578–580.
36. Resnick D, Williamson S, Alazraki N. Focal spinal abnormalities on bone scans in ankylosing spondylitis: a clue to the presence of fracture or pseudarthrosis. *Clin Nucl Med* 1981;6(5):213–217.

37. Salathiem M, Jiohr M. Unsuspected cervical fractures: a common problem in ankylosing spondylitis. *Anesthesiology* 1989; 70(5):869–870.
38. Sharma RR, Mathad NV. Traumatic spinal fracture in ankylosing spondylitis (a case report). *J Postgrad Med* 1988;34(3):193–195.
39. Simmons EH. Surgery of the spine in rheumatoid arthritis and ankylosing spondylitis. In: Cruess RL, Mitchell NS, eds. *Surgery of rheumatoid arthritis*. Philadelphia: Lippincott, 1971; 93–110.
40. Simmons EH. The surgical correction of flexion deformity of the cervical spine in ankylosing spondylitis. *Clin Orthop* 1972; 86:132.
41. Simmons EH. Kyphotic deformity of the spine in ankylosing spondylitis. *Clin Orthop* 1977;128:65.
42. Simmons EH. Surgery of the spine in rheumatoid arthritis and ankylosing spondylitis. In: Evarts CM, ed. *Surgery of the musculoskeletal system*, vol 2, Sec 4. Edinburgh: Churchill Livingstone, 1983;85–153.
43. Simmons EH. Surgery of the spine in ankylosing spondylitis and rheumatoid arthritis. In: *Operative orthopaedics*, vol 3. Philadelphia: Lippincott, 1988;2077–2114.
44. Simmons EH. The surgical correction of flexion deformity of the cervical spine in ankylosing spondylitis. In: *The cervical spine*, 2nd ed. Philadelphia: Lippincott, 1989;505–528.
45. Simmons EH. Ankylosing spondylitis and rheumatoid arthritis. In: Laurin CA, Riley LH Jr, Roy-Camille R, eds. *Atlas of orthopaedic surgery*, vol 1. Paris: Masson, 1989;505–528.
46. Simmons EH. Surgical treatment of ankylosing spondylitis in the spine. In: Evarts CM, ed. *Surgery of the musculoskeletal system*. New York: Churchill Livingstone, 1990;2331–2393.
47. Simmons EH. Surgical treatment of ankylosing spondylitis. *Bull Hosp Jt Dis Orthop Inst* 1989;49(2):111–130.
48. Simmons EH, Duncan CP. Fracture of the cervical spine in ankylosing spondylitis—an analysis of its influence on severe deformity presenting for spinal osteotomy. *Clin Orthop* 1978;133: 277.
49. Simmons EH, Goodwin CB. Spondylodiscitis: a manifestation of ankylosing spondylitis. *Orthop Trans* 1984;8(1):165.
50. Trent S, Armstrong GW, O'Neil J. Thoracolumbar fractures in ankylosing spondylitis. High-risk injuries. *Clin Orthop* 1988;227: 61–66.
51. Weinstein PR, Karpman RR, Gall EP, Pitt M. Spinal cord injury, spinal fracture, and spinal stenosis in ankylosing spondylitis. *J Neurosurg* 1982;57(5):609–616.
52. Woodruff FP, Dewing SB. Fracture of the cervical spine in patients with ankylosing spondylitis. *Radiology* 1983;80:17–21.
53. Young JS, Chesire DJE, Pierce JA. Cervical ankylosis with acute spinal cord injury. *Paraplegia* 1977–78;15:133–146.

28

Systemic Complications of Spinal Cord Injuries

Avital Fast

Spinal cord injury (SCI), especially at high thoracic levels, has far reaching effects on all the body systems and may lead to numerous systemic complications. In the very high thoracic lesions, these complications may be similar or identical to those found in quadriplegic patients, may lead to significant morbidity, and may shorten the life expectancy of the affected individual. In the early decades of this century, SCI led to devastating complications and early mortality. In the 1950s, 35% of quadriplegic patients died within the first 3 months following SCI (34).

Improved understanding of the pathophysiological changes that occur in SCI and early aggressive management have improved the quality of life and led to near normal life expectancy in many individuals. In the late 1970s the mortality rate within the first 3 months following injury was 6.8% for complete quadriplegics and 1.4% for incomplete cervical SCI patients (34).

In the following discussion, systemic complications and the current prevailing therapeutic approaches are presented. A short discussion of anatomy and physiology is included when necessary.

RESPIRATORY COMPLICATIONS

Pulmonary complications are very common in patients with SCI and account for significant morbidity and mortality. In the early acute stages of SCI, mostly in the first 3 months, pulmonary complications may be responsible for the very high mortality rate—up to 40% (4,49). An extensive epidemiological study of 5131 patients has shown that the leading cause of death in quadriplegics was pneumonia (16).

Spinal lesions below the C5 segment spare the diaphragm, thus allowing the patient to inhale. In high thoracic levels most of the expiratory muscles are paralyzed. As a result, the patient is unable to actively exhale. This leads to marked reduction in the vital capacity (up to 65%), decreased or absent expiratory reserve volume, and reduced respiratory force (27).

During normal respiration, inhalation produces negative pleural pressure, which is produced by the descent of the diaphragm and, to a lesser extent, by chest expansion (59). In the acute stages of SCI, when the patient is still in spinal shock, all the muscles are completely paralyzed and flaccid. As a result, paradoxical movements of the rib cage may occur, thus compromising the patient's breathing. At this stage, as the diaphragm moves down, the rib cage is sucked in, producing a paradoxical movement. A similar phenomenon may be seen in patients sustaining a low paraplegia. In these patients, a moderate decrease in the expiratory reserve volume is produced as the flaccid pelvic floor bulges out during expiration (25,27). Many SCI patients demonstrate improvement in pulmonary function tests several months postinjury even in the absence of actual neurological recovery. This may occur due to spasticity of the intercostal and abdominal muscles, which may improve the diaphragmatic function by decreasing or abolishing the paradoxical movements (43,52). It has been shown that by the third to fifth week after injury, the forced vital capacity is rapidly improving. This change in pulmonary function could be attributed to reflex contractions of the intercostal muscles (43).

A recent review (59) of pulmonary complications in patients with SCI revealed that they were very common. The following complications were enumerated: pneumonia—57%, atelectasis—35%, respiratory failure—18%, and pulmonary emboli—10%. The same complications were observed in the chronic stages of SCI as well.

A. Fast: Department of Rehabilitation Medicine, St. Vincent's Hospital & Medical Center of New York, New York, NY 10011; and Department of Rehabilitation Medicine, New York Medical College, New York, NY.

The most prevalent complications in the first month following injury were respiratory failure and atelectasis (59). Even patients with lesions sparing the innervation to the diaphragm can go into respiratory difficulties due to accumulation of secretions and the formation of mucus plugs. Inadequate expiratory airflow compromises secretion clearing and may lead to atelectasis and infections.

These complications can cause acute hypoxemia with arterial Po_2 levels dropping below 60 mmHg. This occurs most likely due to ventilation perfusion imbalance. Inability to take a deep breath and inefficient mucociliary clearance lead to microatelectasis, which in turn causes ventilation perfusion imbalance (43). Most patients with this complication will respond to oxygen enrichment of the inspired air. If oxygen supplementation fails to improve the blood gases, ventilatory support is required. Early aggressive management including endotracheal intubation and tracheostomy may be necessary. These procedures account for the improved survival rates in the early stages of SCI (56). The most suitable location for SCI patients at these early stages is the intensive care unit. Around the clock monitoring by experienced staff combined with frequent chest radiographs and routine blood gases may reduce morbidity. (See Chapter 12.)

A few weeks following injury most quadriplegic patients will improve their forced vital capacity and will be expected to maintain reasonable blood gases without assistance. Patients with high lesions such as C8/T1 or T1/T2 may be unable to maintain acceptable gas exchange while sitting and require an abdominal binder to improve their pulmonary functions (43).

At the early stage, pulmonary function tests should frequently be performed and the physician should be prepared to provide those patients with progressively deteriorating pulmonary functions respiratory assistance. In cases where mucus plugs lead to pulmonary function compromise, aggressive management including chest percussions, turning the patient in bed from the supine to the prone position, deep-breathing exercises, intermittent positive pressure breathing, or bronchoscopy to remove mucus plugs and clear airway secretions may be utilized (49,59). Subsequently, the inspiratory muscles can be exercised with the goal of increasing their strength and endurance. This can be accomplished by periodic breathing against resistance. In this fashion the auxiliary respiratory muscles as well as the diaphragm may favorably respond to the increased load.

CARDIOVASCULAR COMPLICATIONS

The two components of the autonomic nervous system, the parasympathetic and sympathetic divisions, modulate the cardiovascular system. The preganglionic parasympathetic cells are located in the brain stem and the sacral spinal cord (S2–S4). Whereas the cranial outflow is involved with the cardiovascular system, the sacral outflow is involved with pelvic organs and does not influence the cardiovascular system. The main target organ of the cranial outflow is the heart. The fibers reach the heart via the vagi nerves, which are located outside the spinal cord and remain intact during SCI.

The preganglionic cells of the sympathetic system are located in the intermediolateral horn of the spinal cord. They can be found in the thoracic portion of the spinal cord (T1–L1). Preganglionic fibers coming out of the cells travel to the paravertebral and prevertebral ganglia. Postganglionic fibers emanate from these ganglia and course to their target organs. The most important target organs are the heart, arteries, and veins. Sympathetic activation leads to vasoconstriction and tachycardia, resulting in elevation of the blood pressure.

In high thoracic cord lesions, the sympathetic nervous system remains active and functioning. The spinal injury, however, disrupts fibers traveling from high centers through the cord, leading to isolation of the sympathetic system from supraspinal excitatory and inhibitory influence. As a result, the isolated sympathetic system may respond to peripheral stimuli without supraspinal control. This may result in significant disruption of the cardiovascular system and in the case of severe unchecked facilitation may lead to serious and life-threatening complications.

The segmental organization of the sympathetic system within the spinal cord is of importance. The heart and the big vessels are located above the diaphragm and are supplied by sympathetic cells originating within T1 to T7. The splanchnic vessels receive their sympathetic innervation from cells located at T5 and below. This organization has clinical relevance, as is discussed later.

In the initial stages of SCI, during the spinal shock phase, all the activities within the transected cord temporarily cease. This period usually lasts from a few minutes to several hours. Occasionally, it lasts for about 2 to 3 weeks. In cases with high thoracic lesions, preganglionic sympathetic cells are inactivated due to the spinal shock. As a result, the sympathetically mediated regulatory reflexes are temporarily abolished. The plasma epinephrine and norepinephrine levels drop precipitously and peripheral vasodilatation predominates (48). Due to the persistent vasodilatation, the blood pressure tends to be lower than normal.

The impaired ability to achieve vasoconstriction and loss of autonomic responses compromise the patient's response to hypovolemia, which commonly occurs in patients with trauma and leads to severe hypotension. Due to unopposed parasympathetic activity, the patient may develop sinus arrest or severe bradycardia during manipulation of the upper respiratory airways (i.e., suction or endotracheal intubation), thus further compromising the cardiovascular system (24).

Diffuse widespread paralysis leads to blood pooling in the peripheral veins and decreases venous return. If the patient attempts to sit up or is brought to the upright position, via a tilt table, postural hypotension develops. If the upright position is maintained, the patient may lose consciousness.

Unlike the response of able-bodied individuals, quadriplegic patients do not show an increase in the level of catecholamines in response to tilting to the upright position (47). This may occur also in high thoracic cord injury patients. They develop lightheadedness and sweating above the lesion and may go into syncope if the upright position is maintained.

As the spinal cord gets out of the spinal shock phase, the autonomic system can be conditioned and "taught" to properly respond to postural changes, thus maintaining the blood pressure in the upright position. Reconditioning can be accomplished through gradual exposure of the patient to the upright posture. This is accomplished in the clinical setting by the use of a tilt table or by gradually elevating a reclining wheel chair. Applying ace bandages over the lower extremities combined with an abdominal binder may decrease the amount of blood pooled in the lower extremities and thus reduce the tendency toward hypotension.

In the rare patient who is unresponsive to the above regime, a trial of fludrocortisone and ergotamine products is warranted. The steroid preparation helps retain fluids, thus increasing the plasma volume. Ergotamine works as a vasoconstrictor by inhibiting receptor reuptake of norepinephrine at sympathetic nerve endings (33,37). The combination of these drugs may be helpful in rare cases where postural hypotension persists beyond the early stages of spinal shock. Postural hypotension is more common in complete high thoracic SCI and is less of a problem in patients with lower lesions or patients with incomplete SCI.

AUTONOMIC DYSREFLEXIA

Autonomic dysreflexia (AD) tends to occur in patients with complete high thoracic and cervical lesions. AD will not occur in patients with lesions below T6 to T8. AD usually does not appear in the first 4 weeks following injury.

Since unchecked facilitation of the isolated spinal sympathetic system is the underlying pathophysiological mechanism, AD does not appear while the patient is in spinal shock. It tends to appear in the first 8 weeks following injury. In most cases, AD may be well established by 6 months following injury.

Patients suffering from AD complain of excruciating headache. They appear ill and anxious. Physical examination may detect increased spasticity, profuse sweating (usually above the level of the lesion), piloerection, flushing of the face, extreme hypertension, and bradycardia. Lack of immediate therapeutic intervention may risk the patient's life. The patient may develop convulsions and cerebral bleeding and die.

Pathophysiologically, the hallmark of AD is unchecked sympathetic overactivity in the spinal cord below the level of the lesion. This occurs in response to persistent peripheral stimulation, most likely emanating from the bladder or the rectum. In response to a blocked catheter leading to an overdistended bladder or in the presence of fecal impaction, a surge of continuous afferent impulses reaches the spinal cord below the level of the lesion. Because of the spinal lesion, the afferent stimuli cannot reach the brain and the patient remains unaware of the impending catastrophy. At a certain point of time, in response to the peripheral stimuli, the "isolated" spinal cord responds to the afferent stimuli with unchecked facilitation. Sympathetic overactivity leads to extreme vasoconstriction and hypertension. The baroreceptors, in an effort to lower the blood pressure, slow the heart rhythm. The patient may have increased spasticity, which results from overactivity of the anterior horn cells. Autonomic dysreflexia is seen in patients with SCI at T6 or at higher levels. It is rarely seen in patients with lesion below the T8 level (44).

Since the splanchnic blood vessels receive their sympathetic innervation through neural segments below T6, spinal cord injuries at higher levels can lead to severe, sustained splanchnic vasoconstriction during AD. This leads to sudden shunting of large amounts of blood from the splanchnic area into the circulation, thus raising the blood pressure. In patients with lesions below T8, the splanchnic vessels remain under central control and do not participate in the autonomic dysreflexic process. Blood shunted from vessels that participate in the autonomic crisis (the lower extremities vasculature) can easily be accommodated in the splanchnic vessels, thus preventing hypertension (40).

The causes of AD include catheter occlusion with bladder overdistension, fecal impaction, overgrown toenails, decubiti, infections, and unidentified abdominal catastrophies. Upon identification of the dysreflexic syndrome, the physician should immediately check the urinary outflow and the patency of the catheter. If no urinary obstruction is observed the physician should perform a rectal examination to rule out fecal impaction. Commonly, the physician will find that the catheter has been blocked, leading to an overdistended bladder. Following careful and gradual urinary drainage, the blood pressure will normalize and the AD syndrome may disappear. Occasionally, no immediate apparent cause can be found and the AD syndrome persists. Since this is a medical emergency with potential fatal complications, the blood pressure should be forced down by intravenous or fast-acting oral medications: vasodilators (hydralazine), calcium channel blockers (nifedipine), ganglion blockers (guanethidine), and alpha blockers (phenoxybenzamine) are among the drugs being used (45). In patients who are prone to develop AD, local anesthetics should be used before manipulations of the urinary tract; that is, local anesthetics may be injected into the urethra before a catheter is being placed. In these patients, preventive oral administration of calcium channel blockers (i.e., nifedipine) may be helpful in ameliorating the autonomic response, and thus lowering the risk of acute hypertension (45). In the absence of an apparent cause for AD, following blood pressure control the physician should carefully examine the patient. Since patients with complete SCI have no sensation below the level of the lesion, an abdominal emergency should always be considered. In the presence of increased spasticity or vague abdominal complaints, the physician should resort to ancillary tests to rule out catastrophies such as a perforated viscus. In the case of a pregnant paraplegic or quadriplegic patient, the gynecologist as well as the anesthesiologist should be familiarized with AD. Uterine contractions may be the source of strong spinal sympathetic response and should be considered if natural delivery is allowed to occur.

THROMBOEMBOLIC COMPLICATIONS

Thromboembolic complications are very common in patients with SCI and cause significant morbidity and mortality. The prevalence of deep venous thrombosis (DVT) in patients with SCI is high. Estimates may vary and depend on the diagnostic procedures being performed. Diagnosis based only on clinical examination may be unreliable and overlook DVT in a significant number of patients—up to 50% (9). DVT and pulmonary emboli (PE) tend to be more common in the early stages of SCI. In the first 3 months following injury the risk of DVT is at its peak (68).

If prophylactic anticoagulation is not administered, thromboembolic complications may be clinically apparent in up to 40% of the patients (67). Utilization of specific diagnostic studies such as ^{125}I-labeled fibrinogen, impedance plethysmography, and venography increases the diagnostic yield. These diagnostic techniques may detect DVT in up to 100% of acute SCI patients (66). It is clear then that clinical examination is not sensitive enough and may overlook a significant number of patients who develop DVT in the early stages postinjury. The patient's age, weight, level of injury, and preceding surgery have no predictive value as to who might develop DVT (53).

In patients with complete lesions, there is complete muscular paralysis below the level of the lesion. As a result, the ankle pump mechanism of lower extremity musculature does not work. Peripheral venous pooling, stagnating, sluggish circulation, and hypercoagulability increase the tendency to develop DVT (66). Myllynen et al. (53) compared the incidence of DVT in two groups of patients. One group sustained spinal fractures with cord injury. The second group consisted of patients who sustained spinal fractures without neurological compromise. All the paralyzed patients developed DVT. Nine percent of them had PE. Patients who were immobilized because of the spinal fracture, but were neurologically intact, did not develop DVT or PE (57). This study clearly demonstrates that it is the cord injury and not immobilization per se that is responsible for the high rate of thromboembolic complications.

Since clinical examination is not a reliable indicator as to which patient might develop DVT, and since most if not all SCI patients do develop DVT, all patients should be anticoagulated in the early stages following injury. In addition, calf compression boots and ace bandages should be applied.

Heparin is the drug of choice in the early postinjury phase. It can be administered intravenously or subcutaneously. The therapeutic dosage may vary between 10,000 and 30,000 units per day. It has been shown that in low-dose levels a significant number of patients may still develop DVT, whereas in the higher doses the risk of bleeding is substantial (31). The newly manufactured low molecular weight heparin is more effective, has a lower rate of side effects, and thus should be the initial drug of choice (30). For protracted anticoagulation Coumadin is recommended.

Anticoagulation should be administered for the first 3 months. With the appearance of spasticity, and when the patient's level of activity increases, the administration of Coumadin may be discontinued.

Some patients develop thromboembolic complications much later in the course of SCI. In cases at high risk (immobile, repeated urinary tract infections with urosepsis, evidence of intravascular coagulation, previous DVT), anticoagulation should be administered on an individualized basis, for longer periods of time—up to 6 months (20,57). In patients with recurrent pulmonary emboli, a year or two of anticoagulation should be considered. If emboli persist despite adequate Coumadin dosage, the introduction of a Greenfield filter into the inferior vena cava should be considered. The filter (umbrella) will prevent the thrombi from reaching the lungs.

HETEROTOPIC OSSIFICATION

Up to 20% of SCI patients may become impaired due to heterotopic ossification (28). Heterotopic ossification (HO) tends to develop in spastic patients. The process usually appears surrounding major joints—hips and knees in the case of paraplegic patients. At times, huge masses of abnormal bone can be detected (Fig. 1).

Several weeks following injury, and usually within 3 months, the patient develops swelling, warmth, and sometimes erythema in the vicinity of the joint. These may occasionally be combined with systemic fever. In addition to the above observations, the clinician may notice limitation in the passive range of the involved joint. In many patients the clinical presentation of HO resembles that of DVT. A duplex scan is then indicated to rule out or confirm the presence of DVT.

In the early stages of HO, radiological studies of the involved joint will not demonstrate any abnormality. Laboratory examination may detect an elevated alkaline phosphatase. Although this test is nonspecific, it is the most convenient and earliest indication that the patient develops HO (28). Bone scan can confirm the diagnosis at a later stage.

Once the diagnosis is established, efforts to normalize the range of motion of the involved joint should cease. Etidronate disodium (disodium ethane-1-hydroxy-1,1-diphosphonate or EHDP) should be started. This medication has been demonstrated to inhibit calcium phosphate precipitation and blocks its transformation to hydroxyapatite. Etidronate should be given for about 6 months in a dosage of 20 mg/kg/day (28). Upon maturation and completion of HO formation, when the alkaline phosphatase returns to normal levels or when the bone scan becomes less intense, surgical intervention may be contemplated. It should be performed about 12 months following the detection of HO. It is believed that at such a late period the stimulus causing HO has weakened or does not persist.

The indications for surgical intervention are limited range of motion that interferes with the activity of daily living, vascular compromise due to pressure exerted by the mass of abnormally formed bone, and an increased risk of abnormal pressure on the skin that may increase the risk of decubiti (65).

Infections, fractures due to excessive osteoporosis, bleeding, and recurring HO are among the most common postoperative complications.

URINARY COMPLICATIONS

Care of the genitourinary system is of paramount importance in preventing serious morbidity and mortal-

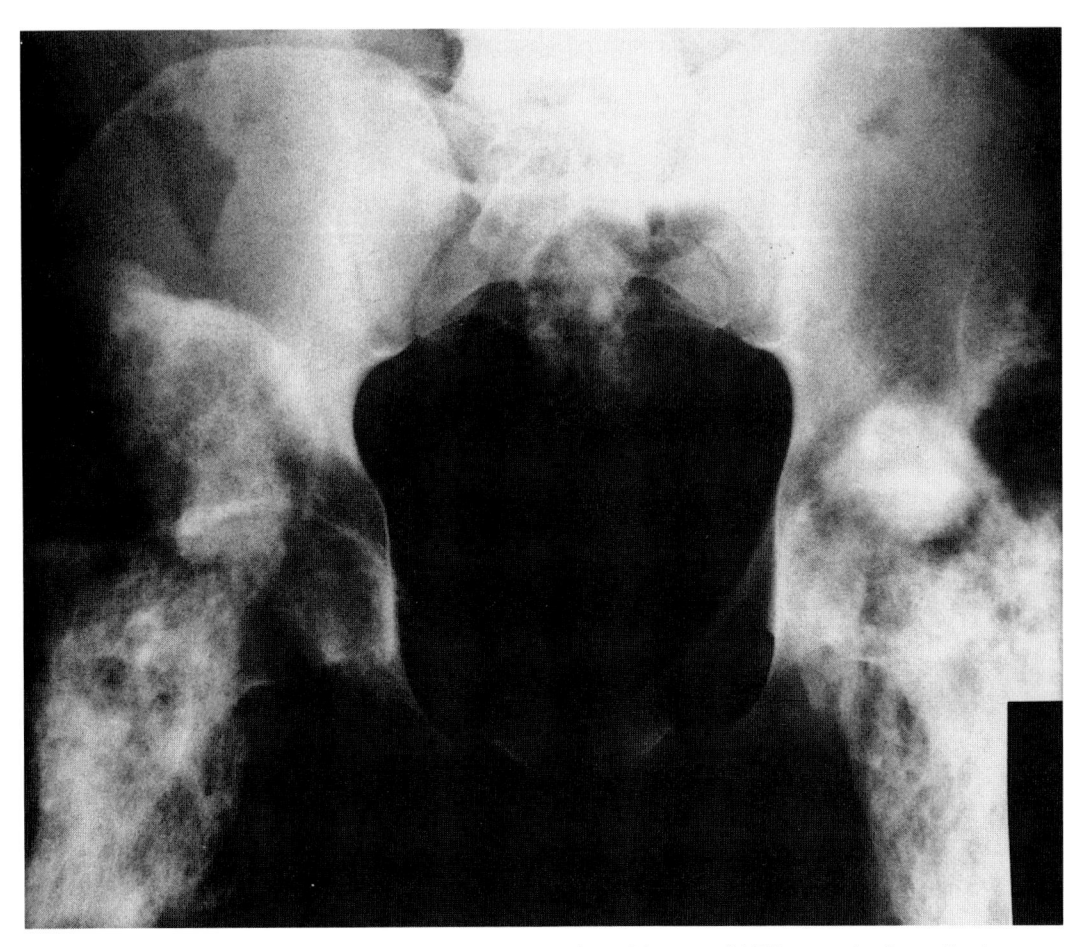

FIG. 1. Extensive heterotopic ossification in a 36-year-old T6 paraplegic patient.

ity in SCI patients. In the mid-1950s, dysfunction of the genitourinary system was the most common cause of death in the early stages post-SCI (60). Prior to World War II, most SCI victims died within a year postinjury. In most cases ascending urinary infection, urosepsis, and decubiti were the leading causes of death (1). The lower urinary tract is discussed first.

Innerveration of the Bladder

The parasympathetic center for micturition is located at the S2–S4 cord segments and is connected to the bladder via the pelvic nerves. The pudendal nerves, conveying somatic fibers, originate at the same levels and innervate the external urinary sphincter. The sympathetic system's contribution to micturition is still debatable. According to some researchers, this system plays an important role in bladder filling and urine storage. This is accomplished via inhibitory influences on the parasympathetic system and increased outlet resistance. The latter effect is accomplished by smooth muscle activity at the bladder base and the proximal urethra, functioning as a sphincter (8,55). The efferent sympathetic fibers originate at the T11–L2 spinal cord segments and reach the bladder and urethra via the hypogastric nerves. The hypogastric and pelvic nerves consist primarily of efferent fibers but have been shown to include afferent fibers as well (69).

The urinary bladder, with the help of its sphincters, has two main functions. It serves as a reservoir and thus is responsible for urinary continence. At this stage, the bladder wall is relaxed and accommodates the inflowing urine. The internal and external urinary sphincters remain tightly closed at this stage, thus allowing continence even when the intra-abdominal pressure is rising (i.e., during laughing, sneezing). The second function of the bladder is to allow complete volitional emptying. At this stage the bladder wall is contracting while the sphincters are simultaneously relaxing. Under normal physiological condition, there is complete emptying of the bladder without residual volume.

The act of micturition is very complex and requires coordination between the forces of expulsion and retention. In spinal cord injuries the delicate balance between these forces is affected, resulting in urinary dysfunction. In the early phases of SCI, during the spinal shock phase, the urinary bladder is completely flaccid. At this stage urine is continuously accumulating in the bladder but no bladder contractions can be observed.

If early drainage is not secured, the bladder will be filled to capacity and bladder wall overstretching will occur. Bladder overdistension may damage the nerve fibers located in the bladder wall, adversely affecting bladder function at later stages. Once the bladder has filled to maximal capacity, overflow incontinence will occur (28).

The insertion of an indwelling catheter will allow complete bladder emptying and avoid overdistension. The problem with an indwelling catheter, however, is that it serves as a source of infection and will, sooner or later, lead to urinary tract infections, urosepsis, and significant morbidity.

A much better approach, one that simulates normal physiological conditions, is to catheterize the bladder intermittently. This technique requires around-the-clock well-trained staff who are familiar with the pathophysiological changes that occur in SCI.

Upon arrival in the SCI unit, the goal and methodology of intermittent catheterization are explained and the patient is required to regulate the amount and the time of fluid intake. Catheterization is then performed intermittently with a straight catheter and the amount of urine is recorded. Patients who retain functional upper extremities can be taught to catheterize themselves in an aseptic technique and record the amount of urine that is drained each time.

The spinal center of micturition, located at the S2–S4 segments, is usually the first to recover from spinal shock. As the spinal cord below the level of the lesion recovers, bladder tone returns and bladder contractions become possible. In patients with low SCI that affect the sacral segments, the bladder remains atonic and areflexic at all times. Bladder emptying in these patients can be achieved by straining (i.e., during the Valsalva maneuver) or by Credé's maneuver. In the latter instance the patient compresses the lower abdomen while sitting on the toilet. This elevates the intra-abdominal pressure and increases the forces of expulsion, thus forcing the urine out. If the residual volume remains high despite adequate trials of bladder emptying, the patients may be managed continuously by intermittent catheterization. Although a very high percentage of these patients may have bacteruria in the acute stage (32), long-term follow-up shows that they may have relatively infrequent positive urine cultures and rare febrile urinary tract infections, while their kidney function remains stable (50).

As the spinal cord recovers from spinal shock, the bladder tone returns and bladder contractions may be observed. Initially, these contractions may not be strong enough and may fail to open the bladder neck region. Urine may spurt out but complete bladder emptying may not occur and the postvoiding residual urine remains high (above 100 cc).

When bladder contractions improve, the clinician should try to obtain reflex bladder contractions in response to peripheral stimuli. Tapping of the abdominal wall, pulling the pubic hair, and sometimes anal stimulation may provoke bladder contraction and urination.

Clinical experience demonstrates that patients

whose bladders were appropriately managed during the early stages following SCI will develop moderate amounts of spasticity. On the other hand, patients who are poorly managed during the early stages and sustain repeated urinary tract infections and sepsis will develop severe spasticity with severe autonomic disturbances.

In many patients, simultaneous contractions of the bladder and the external urinary sphincter are observed. As the bladder contracts the sphincter tightens, thus creating bladder–sphincter dyssynergia (50).

The bladder may become hypertrophic and develop trabeculation, and urinary reflux, due to vesicoureteral dysfunction, occurs (22). Occasionally, as the bladder contracts, the patient may develop autonomic dysreflexia. If vesicoureteral dysfunction is not identified early, it will lead to urinary reflux with significant morbidity. Pyelonephritis, renal calculi, and ultimately renal failure will occur (15).

The frequency of kidney stones in SCI patients ranges from 7% to 32% and is significantly more common in patients with reflux (35). Renal stones are most likely to develop within 3 months postinjury and are more common in male patients with complete SCI (17). Continuous drainage with Foley catheter does not prevent reflux formation. It increases the risk of infection and therefore does not protect the kidney from further damage.

The prevalence of urinary stones is surprisingly higher in patients managed with continuous drainage (i.e., Foley catheter) as opposed to those managed with intermittent catheterization (18,41). In many patients renal calculi are associated with pyelonephritis. These patients may eventually develop recurrent sepsis and die.

Early identification of these complications mandates an immediate, aggressive therapeutic approach. It should be noted, however, that urinary tract infection in an asymptomatic patient who has an indwelling catheter does not mandate antibiotic therapy. Blood cultures should be obtained and the patient should be monitored closely. If the patient becomes symptomatic, a 10-day course of antibiotics should be prescribed (46,64). All efforts should be made to get rid of the indwelling catheter.

In patients with vesicoureteral dysfunction due to a spastic sphincter, the physician should try to reduce the spasticity by antispastic medications (i.e., baclofen), so that the external urinary sphincter will allow adequate bladder emptying.

In a patient with a small-capacity hypertonic bladder, anticholinergic medications may be administered in order to reduce the bladder tone and allow retention of more urine in the bladder, thus reducing the tendency toward reflux. If satisfactory emptying does not occur (less than 100 cc of residual volume), the patient should be taught to perform intermittent self-catheterizations. In selected male patients who fail to respond to an adequate conservative management, sphincterotomy combined with external condom catheter may be indicated. Occasionally, posterior rhizotomy combined with an implantable anterior sacral root stimulator should be contemplated (46).

Although less common today, end-stage renal disease is a well-known complication of long-standing SCI. It usually results from reflux, stasis, kidney infections, calculi, and secondary amyloidosis. The availability of hemodialysis has significantly prolonged life in these patients. Spinal cord injury dialysis patients, however, do not fare as well as nonparalyzed dialysis patients. Sepsis and amyloidosis lead to earlier deaths than in the nonparalyzed group. Septicemia usually originates from the urinary tract or from pressure sores and is the leading cause of mortality in up to 76% of the patients (2,62).

Amyloidosis can be found in a very high percentage of SCI patients and may be responsible for significant morbidity as well (3).

GASTROINTESTINAL COMPLICATIONS

In the early stages postinjury, upper gastrointestinal bleeding secondary to stress ulcers may be encountered. Up to 20% of the patients may bleed, most of them from the stomach due to stress-induced gastritis and erosions (21). This complication is not unique to the cord-injured patient. It may appear in most cases admitted to an intensive care unit following any major trauma. The recently introduced protocol of extremely high steroid doses can also contribute to and increase the risk of bleeding. The physician taking care of the SCI patient has to anticipate this potential complication and try to avoid it by frequent administration of antacids or H_2 antagonists.

Within 72 hr of SCI, about half of the patients may develop ileus accompanied by gastric dilatation. In low thoracolumbar lesions the ileus appears immediately. In higher lesions its appearance may be delayed. Stress ulcers and pancreatitis may appear within the first month. These usually resolve as the patients come out of the spinal shock.

The most troublesome gastrointestinal problems, which start early and become chronic, are concerned with gastrointestinal motility: delayed gastric emptying, gastric dilatation, and ileus and colonic distention leading to constipation (61,63). It has been demonstrated that patients with SCI have a prolongation of the colonic transit time (51). In some patients, gastroesophageal reflux, hiatus hernia, and diverticulosis may appear in high frequency (29). At these early stages, upper gastrointestinal bleeding and perforated ulcers occur in up to 3.5% of the patients, especially in complete cervical SCI patients (29). Berlly and Wilmot (6) retrospectively evaluated 945 charts of acute SCI patients. Almost 5% of the patients developed abdominal pathology within the first 4 weeks postinjury. At greater risk were patients with complete lesions above T5. Upper gastrointestinal bleeding and pancreatitis appeared as early as 3 days postinjury. Decadron was found to be a risk factor for pancreatitis but not for peptic disease (6).

In later stages, the most common complaint, especially in chronic SCI patients, is fecal impaction.

A prospective study of 127 chronic SCI patients documented symptomatic gastrointestinal problems in 27% of the patients. Patients with more complete injuries were more likely to have symptoms (63). Most of these patients had postprandial distension and difficulty with evacuation. A significant number of them had symptoms related to gastroesophageal reflux. Hemorrhoids were symptomatic in most of the patients. Patients with lesions above T5 tended to have a higher prevalence of difficulties with evacuation, requiring occasional disimpaction. Only two patients had fecal incontinence requiring a colostomy. Vague abdominal pain relieved by passing gas or bowel care was found in most patients. Autonomic dysreflexia, although clearly more commonly associated with genitourinary problems, was also seen in relation to gastrointestinal dysfunction. Twenty-three percent of the patients required at least one hospitalization related to evaluation or management of a gastrointestinal problem (63). Of all the gastrointestinal complications of SCI, the patients are mostly disturbed by loss of voluntary control of defecation and distressed by fecal incontinence.

The orthopaedic surgeon taking care of SCI patients should bear in mind the importance and difficulty of diagnosing acute abdominal emergencies in patients with complete lesions. Up to 10% of the fatality rate of SCI patients may occur due to abdominal emergencies. Due to severe neurological impairment, early and timely detection of these emergencies may be difficult. Thorough understanding of the pathophysiological processes taking place in SCI may be required in order to establish the diagnosis and reduce the morbidity and mortality associated with these emergencies.

During the spinal shock phase, abolition of cord activity including the autonomic responses may compromise the diagnostic acumen of the unwary physician. At this stage most or all of the signs found in acute abdomen are abolished. In high thoracic injuries, the abdominal wall may remain soft even in the presence of peritonitis and the patient may remain asymptomatic without pain. Even the blood count may not be entirely helpful since many patients develop urinary infections and or pneumonia at early stages, which affect the blood picture.

Radiological studies will detect air-filled dilated intestines or air under the diaphragm if perforation has occurred. Abolition of autonomic responses may lead to hypotension and bradycardia, which may further confuse the inexperienced clinician.

Maintaining a high level of suspicion combined with close monitoring, repeated laboratory testing (i.e., repeated hematocrits and white blood counts), and peritoneal lavage may guide the physician toward the correct diagnosis (6,51).

In the more chronic stages of SCI, especially in high complete lesions, the patients tend to become severely spastic. In these patients, the abdominal wall may feel rigid at all times and may not yield the information obtained during physical examination of nonparalyzed patients. Increased spasticity may interfere with the abdominal examination and may mask an acute abdomen. During an abdominal emergency, the spinal patient may perceive dull, poorly localized pain that should not be ignored. He/she may not feel well and will tend to lose his/her appetite. Increasing levels of spasticity, reflex sweating, sudden progressive abdominal distension, and a full blown or partial autonomic dysreflexia may appear (23,38). Patients with low cord lesions may present without autonomic phenomena. These patients, however, may localize the abdominal pain, thus making diagnosis relatively easy. Patients with incomplete cord lesions have more accurate sensations and should be diagnosed early.

In a review of 42 SCI patients that were operated on for acute abdominal emergencies, the most common findings were bowel obstruction (16 patients), perforated viscus (11 patients), and acute appendicitis (10 patients). Three patients had a perforated bladder, one suffered from ruptured spleen, and one patient had acute cholecystitis (38). Of 10 patients with appendicitis, eight had the cord lesion above the splanchnic outflow (T8). All these patients had, at the time of operation, perforation of the appendix with a periappendiceal abscess. Two patients with lower cord lesions were diagnosed early and operated on. In these patients, perforation of the appendix was not found.

These cases clearly demonstrate the difficulties encountered in diagnosing abdominal emergencies and the complications emanating from late interventions (38).

METABOLIC–ENDOCRINE COMPLICATIONS OF SCI

Prolonged bed rest and immobilization, which in high cord lesions involves most of the skeletal muscles, lead to an increased skeletal atrophy accompanied by substantial calcium loss.

It has been shown that short-term bed rest, in nonparalyzed patients, decreases the bone mineral content of lumbar vertebrae at a rate of about 1% per week (26). Negative calcium balance is one of the most consistent early metabolic changes occurring in SCI.

As early as 1 day postinjury, SCI patients start to lose excessive amounts of calcium in the urine. The hypercalciuria of SCI is greater than that observed during recumbency without cord damage (11). Patients with complete lesions lose more calcium and magnesium than patients with incomplete lesions. In the first 2 weeks postinjury, there is also increased urinary excretion of phosphate. After 2 weeks the urine phosphate levels return to normal. Since hydroxyproline is the main amino acid found in collagen, a major component of bone matrix, it is also found in increasing amounts in the urine of SCI patients and serves as a reliable indicator of collagen breakdown due to bone resorption. Skeletal collagen secretion is of longer duration and greater magnitude in quadriplegic patients. In these patients, there is also breakdown of skin collagen. The pathogenesis leading to skin collagen breakdown is still unclear. Skeletal collagen loss may prevent recalcification, prolong the hypercalciuria, and eventually end up in osteoporosis (13,54).

In most SCI patients, the serum calcium levels remain within normal limits, even when hypercalciuria is at its peak. In a small percentage of quadriplegic patients, especially in young males, serum hypercalcemia may be observed. Changes in body fluid distribution, renal vasodilatation due to sympathetic paralysis, and hormonal modulation, specifically higher calcitonin levels, may contribute to the development of hypercalcemia (12). Prompt identification of this complication and an aggressive therapeutic intervention may prevent the complications associated with hypercalcemia.

In immobilized healthy subjects hypercalciuria peaks at 4 weeks. In patients with SCI, however, hypercalciuria peaks at approximately 2.5 months postinjury and remains higher than normal for several months (5). Early rehabilitation intervention incorporating exercises may shorten the hypercalciuric period.

In patients with long-standing cord injury, the bone mineral content of the paralyzed extremities is significantly reduced. Dual photon absorptiometry studies, which were performed 2 to 25 years following injury, have revealed significant osteoporosis in the long bones. The femoral shaft has demonstrated a decrease of 25% in bone density and the proximal tibia had lost up to 50% of its mineral content. Of interest was the finding that brace usage did not change the mineral content of the paralyzed extremities. The lumbar spine, due to its weight-bearing state, continued to preserve its mineral content. SCI patients who sustain lower extremity fractures had the lowest bone mineral content (7).

Osteoporosis leads to lower limb fractures in up to 6% of SCI patients. Lower extremity fractures are more common in paraplegic patients since they retain more mobility than quadriplegic patients. Mild trauma, which may not inflict significant injury in healthy individuals, may be of sufficient force to break the osteoporotic bone. In the presence of a complete lesion, the patient may not be aware of the trauma that caused the fracture and does not feel pain. This may interfere with early diagnosis of the fracture.

Management of these fractures should take into account the anesthetic skin and the fact that these patients do not use their lower extremities for weightbearing. For simple fractures, especially fractures below the midfemur, well padded splints may suffice. These splints may be used in the treatment of ankle, tibia, and femoral shaft fractures. Frequent skin inspections are recommended. When skeletal traction is considered, the increased risk of infection and the fact that the bone stock is poor should be kept in mind. The atrophied flaccid musculature combined with poor vascular tone increases the likelihood of hematoma formation, which may get infected. In the presence of urosepsis or decubiti, the hematoma may get infected even in closed fractures (19).

Patients with femoral neck fractures should be operated on. In these patients an adequate prophylactic antibiotic coverage should be instituted. All efforts should be made to keep the patient mobile and out of bed so that pressure sores will be prevented. The general condition of the patient is more important than fracture alignment. Even with poor alignment and partial immobilization, long bone fractures will heal in paraplegic patients, sometimes with extensive callous formation.

In the early stages postinjury, all SCI patients go through a period of negative nitrogen balance. Life support equipment interferes with their oral intake. The patients lose their appetite due to depression. These factors combined with the catabolic state, accompanying the spinal injury, result in significant weight loss, especially in quadriplegic patients. I recently saw a patient with a complete C2 injury who developed anasarca within a few weeks of injury despite the fact that he was in an intensive surgical unit throughout the entire period!

Patients with high lesions lose more weight and their serum albumin levels are lower than those observed in paraplegic patients. In the acute stage following injury, these patients lose nitrogen in amounts equivalent up to 181 g of protein or 900 g of muscle mass (14). Laven et al. (42) studied the nutritional status of 51 SCI patients. The patients were assessed at 2, 4, and 8 weeks postinjury. One hundred percent of the patients had decreased albumin levels, 62% had decreased carotene, 37% transferrin, 25% ascorbate, 24% thiamine,

20% folate, and in 11% of the patients the copper levels were low. The source of weight loss in the SCI patients appeared to be the muscles rather than the fatty tissues. They documented statistically significant reduction in upper as well as lower extremity muscle circumferences in quadriplegic patients between 2 and 4 weeks postinjury. Of interest was the fact that despite the participation of professionals familiar with SCI and dietary requirements, the caloric intake and dietary supply did not meet the demand in these patients (42).

Pressure sores also contribute to negative nitrogen balance. Big decubiti can lead to a significant protein loss, which in turn may interfere with their healing, thus creating a vicious cycle that may endanger the patient. It has been shown that patients with low albumin levels do not heal their decubiti as early and quickly as those with adequate albumin levels (39). Furthermore, malnutrition may contribute to depressed immune function, leading to increased susceptibility to infections (10). It is clear then that aggressive nutritional support supervised by physicians familiar with this subject is of extreme importance, especially in the early stages of SCI. With adequate nutritional support the patient's catabolic response may be reduced and the secondary complications of malnutrition avoided.

Anemia is one of the most commonly observed complications in patients with multiple trauma. It has been documented in the acute stages of high spinal lesions even in the absence of detectable blood loss.

In a prospective study of 28 acute cervical cord injuries, low erythrocyte counts, hemoglobin, hematocrit, and red cell mass were documented in more than 70% of the patients. Seventy percent of these patients had normochromic, normocytic anemia. Most patients, however, may have normal erythropoietin levels with normal reticulocyte counts (36).

The exact causes and pathophysiological mechanisms leading to anemia are still not conclusively clear. Stress-induced changes, nutritional deficiencies such as decreased folic acid, endocrine changes, and altered bone marrow maturation may be important contributing factors (36,58). Anemia may also be observed in the chronic stages of SCI. In late stages following injury, anemia is much more common in patients with decubiti ulcers, specifically the deep ones. However, many chronic SCI patients may have slightly decreased blood volume, plasma volume, and red cell mass even in late stages following injury. Although anemia of SCI is usually mild and rarely requires transfusion, its presence combined with other nutritional and metabolic changes may interfere in the rehabilitation process (36).

As has been demonstrated, SCI affects most if not all the systems of the body. The short-term and long-term effects of SCI affect the quality of life and may, if not adequately managed, shorten the life span of the SCI victim.

REFERENCES

1. Abramson AS. Modern concepts of management of the patient with spinal cord injury. *Arch Phys Med Rehabil* 1967;48:113–121.
2. Barton CH, Vaziri ND, Gordon S, Filles S. Renal pathology in endstage renal disease associated with paraplegia. *Paraplegia* 1984;22:31–41.
3. Barton CH, Vaziri ND, Gordon S, Eltorai L. Endocrine pathology in spinal cord injured patients on maintenance dialysis. *Paraplegia* 1984;22:7–16.
4. Bellamy R, Pitts FW, Stauffer ES. Respiratory complications in traumatic quadriplegia. *J Neurosurg* 1973;39:596–600.
5. Bergmann P, Heilporn A, Schonterns A, Paternot J, Tricot A. Longitudinal study of calcium and bone metabolism in paraplegic patients. *Paraplegia* 1977–78;15:147–159.
6. Berlly MH, Wilmot CB. Acute abdominal emergencies during the first four weeks after spinal cord injury. *Arch Phys Med Rehabil* 1984;65:687–690.
7. Biering-Sorensen JB, Schaadt O. Bone mineral content of the lumbar spine and lower extremities years after spinal cord lesion. *Paraplegia* 1988;26:293–301.
8. Blaivas JG. The neurophysiology of micturition: a clinical study of 550 patients. *J Urol* 1982;127:958–963.
9. Chu DA, Ahn JH, Ragnarsson KT, Helt J, Folcarelli P. Deep venous thrombosis: diagnosis in spinal cord injured patients. *Arch Phys Med Rehabil* 1985;66:365–368.
10. Claus-Walker J, Halstead LS. Metabolic and endocrine changes in spinal cord injury. IV. Compounded neurologic dysfunctions. *Arch Phys Med Rehabil* 1982;63:632–638.
11. Claus-Walker J, Campos RJ, Carter RT, Valbone C, Lipscomb HS. Calcium excretion in quadriplegia. *Arch Phys Med Rehabil* 1972;53:14–20.
12. Claus-Walker J, Carter RE, Campos RJ, Spencer WA. Hypercalcemia in early traumatic quadriplegia. *J Chron Dis* 1975;28:81–90.
13. Claus-Walker J, Sign J, Leach CS, Hattoin DV, Hubert CW, DiFerrante N. The urinary excretion of collagen degradation products by quadriplegic patients and during weightlessness. *J Bone Joint Surg* 1977;59A:209–212.
14. Cloninger MC. Nutritional management of patients with spinal injury: paraplegia vs. quadriplegia. *Arch Phys Med Rehabil* 1980;61:489.
15. Damanski M. Vesico-ureteric reflux in paraplegia. *Br J Surg* 1965;49:1761–1766.
16. Devivo MJ, Kartus PL, Stover SL, Rutt RD, Fine PR. Cause of death for patients with spinal cord injuries. *Arch Intern Med* 1989;49:1761–1766.
17. DeVivo MJ, Fine PR, Cutter GR, Maetz HM. The risk of renal calculi in spinal cord injury patients. *J Urol* 1984;131:857–860.
18. Editorial comment. *J Urol* 1989;141:859–860.
19. Eicherrholtz SN. Management of long bone fractures in paraplegic patients. *J Bone Joint Surg* 1963;45A:299–310.
20. El Masri WS, Silver JR. Prophylactic anticoagulant therapy in patients with spinal cord injury. *Paraplegia* 1981;19:334–342.
21. Epstein N, Hood DC, Ransohoff J. Gastrointestinal bleeding in patients with acute spinal cord trauma: effects of steroids, cimetidine and mini dose heparin. *J Neurosurg* 1981;54:16–20.
22. Fam B, Yalla SV. Vesicoureteral dysfunction in spinal cord injury and its management. *Semin Neurol* 1988;8:150–155.
23. Fast A. Reflex sweating in patients with spinal cord injury. A review. *Arch Phys Med Rehabil* 1977;58:435–437.
24. Fikoff G, Marcelino V. Peripheral vascular disorders in spinal cord injured patient. *Phys Med Rehabil State of Art Rev* 1987;1:443–457.
25. Forner JV. Lung volumes and mechanics of breathing in tetraplegics. *Paraplegia* 1980;18:258–266.

26. Frolner V, Toft B. Vertebral bone loss: an unheeded side effect of therapeutic bed rest. *Clin Sci* 1983;64:537–540.
27. Fugl-Meyer AR. Effects of respiratory muscle paralysis in tetraplegic and paraplegic patients. *Scand J Rehabil Med* 1971;3:141–150.
28. Garland DE. A clinical perspective on common forms of acquired heterotopic ossification. *Clin Orthop* 1991;263:13–29.
29. Gore RM, Mintzer RA, Calenoff L. Gastrointestinal complications of spinal cord injury. *Spine* 1987;6:538–544.
30. Green D, Lee MY, Lim AC, et al. Prevention of thromboembolism after spinal cord injury using low-molecular-weight heparin. *Ann Intern Med* 1990;113:571–574.
31. Green D, Lee MY, Ito VY. Fixed-vs-adjusted–dose heparin in the prophylaxis of thromboembolism in spinal cord injury. *JAMA* 1988;260:1258.
32. Gribble MJ, McCallum NM, Schecter MT. Evaluation of diagnostic criteria for bacteremia in acutely spinal cord injured patients undergoing intermittent catheterization. *Diagn Microbiol Infect Dis* 1988;9:197–206.
33. Groomes TE, Huang CT. Orthostatic hypotension after spinal cord injury: treatment with fludrocortisone and ergotamine. *Arch Phys Med Rehabil* 1991;72:56–58.
34. Hachen HJ. Idealized care of the acutely injured spinal cord in Switzerland. *J Trauma* 1977;17:931–936.
35. Hall MK, Hackler RH, Zampieri TA, Zampieri JB. Renal calculi in spinal cord injured patient: association with reflux, bladder stones, and foley catheter drainage. *Urology* 1989;34:126–128.
36. Huang CT, DeVivo MJ, Stover SL. Anemia in acute phase of spinal cord injury. *Arch Phys Med Rehabil* 1990;71:3–7.
37. Jennings G, Esler M, Holmes R. Treatment of orthostatic hypotension with dihydroergotamine. *Br Med J* 1979;2:307.
38. Jules GL, Eltorai M. The acute abdomen in spinal cord injury patients. *Paraplegia* 1985;23:118–123.
39. Kermani SR, Siddiqui M, Zain S, Kazi ZK. Biochemical studies on pressure sore healing in paraplegics. *Paraplegia* 1970;8:36–41.
40. Kewalramani LS. Autonomic dysreflexia in traumatic myelopathy. *Am J Phys Med* 1980;59:1–21.
41. Lamid S. Long term follow-up of spinal cord injury patients with vesicoureteral reflux. *Paraplegia* 1988;26:27–34.
42. Laven GT, Huan CT, DeVivo MJ, Stover SL, Kuhlemeier KV, Fine PR. Nutritional status during the acute stage of spinal cord injury. *Arch Phys Med Rehabil* 1989;70:277–282.
43. Ledsome JR, Sharp JM. Pulmonary function in acute cervical cord injury. *Am Rev Respir Dis* 1981;124:41–44.
44. Linden R, Joiner E, Freehafer AA, Hazel C. Incidence and clinical features of autonomic dysreflexia in patients with spinal cord injury. *Paraplegia* 1980;18:292–293.
45. Linden R, Leffler EJ, Kedia KR. A comparison of the efficacy of an alpha-1-adrenergic blocker and the slow calcium channel blocker in the control of autonomic dysreflexia. *Paraplegia* 1985;23:34–38.
46. Madersbecher H. The various types of neurogenic bladder dysfunction: an update of current therapeutic concepts. *Paraplegia* 1990;28:117–229.
47. Mathias CJ, Christensen NJ, Corbett JL, Frenkel HL, Goodwin TJ, Peart WS. Plasma catecholamines, plasma renin activity and plasma aldosterone in tetraplegic man, horizontal and tilted. *Clin Sci Mol Med* 1975;49:291–299.
48. Mathias CJ, Christensen NJ, Frankel HL, Spalding JMK. Cardiovascular control in recently injured tetraplegics in spinal shock. *Q J Med* 1979;48:273–287.
49. McMichan JC, Michel L, Westbrook PR. Pulmonary dysfunction following traumatic quadriplegia: recognition, prevention, and treatment. *JAMA* 1980;243:528–531.
50. McGuire EJ, Brady S. Detrusor-sphincter dyssynergia. *J Urol* 1979;121:774–777.
51. Menadro G, Bausano G, Corrazziari RE. Large bowel transit in paraplegic patients. *Dis Colon Rectum* 1987;30:924–928.
52. Morgan MDL, Gourlay AR, Silver JR. Contribution of the rib cage to breathing in tetraplegia. *Thorax* 1985;40:613–617.
53. Myllynen P, Kammonen M, Rakkanen P, Bostman O, Lalla M, Laasonen E. Deep venous thrombosis and pulmonary embolism in patients with acute spinal cord injury: a comparison with nonparalyzed patients immobilized due to spinal fractures. *J Trauma* 1985;25:541–543.
54. Naftchi NE, Viau AT, Sell GH, Lowman EW. Mineral metabolism in spinal cord injury. *Arch Phys Med Rehabil* 1980;61:139–142.
55. Norlen L, Sundin T. Influence of the sympathetic nervous system on the lower urinary tract and its clinical implication. *Int Rehabil* 1982;4:37–43.
56. O'Donohue WJ, Baker JP, Bell GM. Respiratory failure in neuromuscular disease. Management in a respiratory intensive care unit. *JAMA* 1976;235:733–735.
57. Perkash A, Prakash V, Perkash I. Experience with the management of thromboembolism in patients with spinal cord injury. *Paraplegia* 1978;16:322–331.
58. Perkash A, Brown M. Anemia in patients with traumatic spinal cord injury. *Paraplegia* 1982;20:235–236.
59. Polatty CR, McElaney MA, Marcelino V. Pulmonary complications in the spinal cord injury patient. *Phys Med Rehabil State of Art Rev* 1987;1:353–373.
60. Posniak AO, Weiss A, Tobis JS. Management of the neurogenic bladder. *Arch Phys Med Rehabil* 1956;37:755–759.
61. Price N, Schubert ML, Vijay MR. Gastrointestinal disease in the spinal cord injury patient. *Phys Med Rehabil State of Art Rev* 1987;1:475–488.
62. Stacey WR, Midha M. The kidney in the spinal cord injury patient. *Phys Med Rehabil State of Art Rev* 1987;1:415–423.
63. Stone JM, Nino-Murcia M, Wolfe VA, Perkash I. Chronic gastrointestinal problems in spinal cord injury patients: a prospective analysis. *Am J Gastroenterol* 1990;85:1114–1119.
64. Stover SL, Lloyd LK, Waites KB, Jackson AB. Urinary tract infection in spinal cord injury. *Arch Phys Med Rehabil* 1989;70:47–54.
65. Stover SL, Niemann KMW, Tulloss JR. Experience with surgical resection of heterotopic bone in spinal cord injury patients. *Clin Orthop* 1991;263:71–77.
66. Todd JW, Frisbie JH, Rossier AB, et al. Deep venous thrombosis in acute spinal cord injury: a comparison of ^{125}I fibrinogen leg scanning, impedance plethysmography and venography. *Paraplegia* 1976;14:50–57.
67. Van Hove E. Prevention of thrombophlebitis in spinal cord injury patients. *Paraplegia* 1978–79;16:332–335.
68. Walsh JJ, Tribe CR. Phlebo-thrombosis and pulmonary embolism in paraplegia. *Int J Paraplegia* 1965;3:209–213.
69. Wein AJ. Lower urinary tract function and pharmacologic management of lower urinary tract dysfunction. *Urol Clin North Am* 1987;14:273–296.

29

Post-Traumatic Syringomyelia

A General Review

Jafar J. Jafar, Ramesh Babu, Bernard Sigel, and Junju Machi

Post-traumatic syringomyelia is a chronic, progressive disorder of the spinal cord characterized pathologically by cavitation within the substance of the spinal cord and clinically by delayed onset of progressive neurological deficits corresponding to spinal cord segments distant from the level of original injury. In 1827, Charles Olliver d'Angre first used the term "syringomyelia." Hallopeau (10) described the necropsy appearance of unconnected cystic lesions in the spinal cord in 1871. Harvey Cushing in 1898 reported post-traumatic syringomyelic syndrome following a gunshot wound to the cervical spinal cord (3). Gordon Holmes (11) in 1915 drew attention to the cavitary lesions in the neighborhood of primary traumatic cord lesions, which explained the delayed progression of the neurological deficits corresponding to the spinal cord segments away from the level of initial traumatic lesions (24). Strong (29) in 1919 described the syrinx (post-traumatic cyst) of the cervical spinal cord.

EPIDEMIOLOGY

The improvement in the survival of patients with spinal cord injury and increasingly sophisticated diagnostic techniques have increased the incidence of post-traumatic cysts. In 1985, in a review of the world literature, Rossier found 181 cases (27); however, there were 330 cases published by 1984. Of course, the figures in 1991, though not staggering, are still very high. Barnett and Jousse (1) reported an incidence of 1.2% over a period of 26 years and Vernon et al. (32) found a 1.6% incidence over a 10-year period among spinal cord injured patients. In 1985, Rossier et al. (27) reported an incidence of 3.2%. It has also been found that post-traumatic syringomyelia is more common in complete lesions with quadriplegia (7.9%) compared to incomplete lesions producing quadriparesis (2.6%). The incidence of syringomyelia in complete versus incomplete paraplegic patients is not significantly different (1.4% versus 2.4%) (27). Overall, in the population with traumatic paraplegia, the incidence ranges from 0.9% to 7.9% (1,27). Barnett and Jousse (1) stated an incidence of 1.8% in paraplegics compared to 0.2% in tetraplegic patients. This is contrary to the data of Rossier and co-workers, who found that post-traumatic syringomyelia was more common in quadriplegics than in paraplegics. The site of the syrinx also varies depending on the series. Shannon et al. (28), Vernon et al. (32), and Watson (34) observed that post-traumatic syringomyelia is more common in thoracic and thoracolumbar spinal cord injuries. Accordingly the thoracic cord was involved in 67.5%. Post-traumatic syringomyelia does not occur commonly in the cervical cord; the reported incidence ranges from 5.8% to 15% (1,32). This is presumably due to the high mortality associated with cervical spinal cord injuries.

Post-traumatic syringomyelia can initially manifest itself up to 30 years following the initial injury, with an average presentation between 4 and 9 years. It is often difficult to pinpoint the exact date of onset of cyst formation, because the patients are not routinely sub-

---

J. J. Jafar and R. Babu: Department of Neurosurgery, New York University Medical Center, New York, NY 10016.
B. Sigel and J. Machi: Surgical Research Division, Department of Surgery, Medical College of Pennsylvania, Philadelphia, PA 19129.

jected to neuroimaging studies unless they are symptomatic. Generally, patients remain asymptomatic with relatively small cysts. Occasionally, a post-traumatic syrinx is acute, related to coughing or straining, and can occur as early as 2 months after injury (32). Lyons et al. (17) observed that the mean period between the initial injury and the onset of new symptoms was 101 months for incomplete lesions and 39 months for complete lesions. The time from trauma to the onset of symptoms was longer in patients with thoracolumbar injuries than in those with cervical cord injuries (13.5 years versus 8.6 years) (27). It is not known whether the severity of injury has anything to do with this "incubation" period (25,27,28).

The initial injury can vary from minor to severe. In minor trauma, the formation of syringomyelia can explain the major neurological signs that develop.

Post-traumatic syringomyelia has been described in blunt injuries, stab wounds, thoracic disc protrusions, following spinal anesthesia, and in gunshot wounds (32). Usually it occurs as a late sequel to minor or moderate spinal cord injuries with or without post-traumatic adhesive arachnoiditis (27). Straining maneuvers like coughing and sneezing act as precipitating factors in increasing the size of the syrinx and the extent of cord dissection.

PATHOGENESIS

In 1915, Gordon Holmes (11) presented the first systematic pathological study of a series of cases. He showed central areas of degeneration within the spinal cord at sites adjacent to gunshot wounds extending over several segments, depicting the possible future syrinx. Holmes believed that the cavities he observed not long after injury were created by transuded fluid and degeneration products under pressure, tracking away from the site of injury along the pathway of least resistance. Cystic cavities have been found above and below the initial injury. Cysts develop in areas of previous liquefactive necrosis. However, more subtle cord injuries, including petechial hemorrhages or microinfarcts, lead to softening of the cord and later formation of cysts. Barnett et al. (2) found that local trauma inflicted on the spinal cord may result in local cystic lesions replacing the necrotic hemorrhagic tissue. The exact pathogenesis of the disease is not only multifactorial but also controversial.

Various mechanisms have been described for the development of syringomyelia. Initially, there is crush necrosis at the site of injury associated with hematomyelia. This is followed by liquefaction of the intracordal hematoma and later lysosomal autodigestion and absorption of blood and necrotic tissue, followed by cavitation. Kao and Chang (14) explain the autolysis of neural tissue by the lysosomal enzymes transported to the site of injury along traumatized axons. Foo et al. (7) feel that the post-traumatic syringomyelia is the result of cystic degeneration of the damaged cord tissue near the site of original injury.

The second step in cyst formation is the enlargement and extension of the syrinx. Secretion of the cyst fluid by the lining, passage of cerebrospinal fluid (CSF) via enlarged perivascular spaces, or direct communication with the subarachnoid space have all been suggested as means whereby the size of the cyst is enhanced by increasing its fluid volume.

Enlargement of the cysts occurs following activities that increase the intrathoracic or intra-abdominal pressure—coughing, sneezing, or exercise—activities that effectively distend the epidural veins and result in an increase in the transmission of CSF through the cord. The normal movements of the cord become limited by any adhesive arachnoiditis at the site of the injury, which produces an added dimension to the enlargement of intramedullary cavities under stressful conditions. Hemorrhage into the syrinx is a rare cause of acute syrinx extension (2).

PATHOLOGY

Wozniecicz et al. (37), in their autopsy series of 120 patients who died in a rehabilitation center following spinal cord injury, described both total and partial disorganization of the spinal cord. The total disorganization of the cord may be associated with a central core of necrosis extending up and down from the level of injury, whereas the partial disorganization and necrosis were mainly confined to the "watershed" area between the anterior and posterior spinal artery territories. The watershed area, which is anatomically at the junction of the posterior columns and the posterior horns (11,31), is the area where early or limited syrinx formation is generally seen. The tissue in the gray matter between the posterior horns and the posterior columns is also inherently fragile and is easily broken down. The necrosis that occurs at the site of primary injury is generally due to crush injury, and extension above and below is thought to be due to adjacent local ischemia.

Ultrastructurally, a syrinx is lined largely by cell processes of astrocytes; the caudal end of a syrinx is lined by flattened ependymal cells and these are thought to represent the central canal. Whether the central canal gives rise to, or is partially incorporated into, the cavity is speculative (26). The cysts rarely, if ever, communicate with the fourth ventricle, with the central canal, or with the subarachnoid space at the level of the original injury (2,13,16,21). Barnett et al. (2), Peerless and Durward (23), Durward et al. (5), and Quencer et al. (25) noted that the fluid in the syrinx was similar to CSF but was of a higher protein content. The increased protein content is thought to result from active secretions of fluid from the glial cyst lining. Also, the cyst is thought to have arisen from a previous area of necrosis and hemorrhage, which would contribute to the higher protein content (27). Rossier compared the syrinx fluid to the lumbar CSF, which by virtue of relative stagnation (sluggish circulation) has a higher content of protein compared to the rest of the CSF spaces (27).

SYMPTOMS AND SIGNS

A small syrinx can stay asymptomatic and is only detected at autopsy, or the onset of symptoms, when they occur, may be sudden, indicating acute increase in the size of the cavity caused by sudden coughing and sneezing.

The most common presenting symptom is pain (62.5%). Sensory loss above the level of the lesion occurs in 25% of the patients, followed by increased motor weakness (5%) and increased spasticity (27,32). Other noteworthy symptoms such as excessive sweating, decreasing reflexes, and arthropathy are often missed during routine follow-up.

Pain is rarely below the level of the original injury. The pain is usually localized to the spinous processes at the site of the original injury in 50%. The pain often radiates along the arms or trunk. The nature of the pain varies from a dull aching to a constant or an intermittent shocklike pain. An ascending sensory level with a dissociated sensory loss and depressed reflexes corresponding to the level of the syrinx are also common features. A new onset of motor weakness or worsening function of the joints due to muscle weakness is the next commonly detected finding. Some observers found deteriorating sensory or motor function below the original injury site (1,28); others (27) found approximately 50% had worsening sensory function below the original injury level and only 16% had changes in motor function below that site. The sensory and motor deficits may be unilateral (1,32) or bilateral (27). Horner's syndrome is not a constant feature. Patients may have facial hypesthesia, dysphonia, atrophy of the tongue, or progressive dysphagia, indicating the extension of the syrinx into the brain stem.

Secondary changes in joints are also a common occurrence. The early symptoms and signs may ascend and pain may eventually be replaced by hypalgesia. In evaluating spinal cord injured patients with new neurological complaints months or years after blunt trauma, one should suspect the presence of syringomyelia, especially in the presence of a mixed upper and lower motor neuron deficit, a dissociated sensory loss, or a neurogenic bladder.

RADIOLOGY

For many years myelography with oil- or water-soluble contrast media was the investigation of choice, replacing air myelography. Endomyelography (15) was also used for a few years and in fact has been responsible for the conception of drainage procedures as a treatment for the syrinx. Recently, myelography with CT/myelography has become the most commonly used neuroimaging procedure. Delayed computed tomography (CT) scans of the spine, done 6 to 24 hr after the injection of metrizamide in the subarachnoid space, has avoided some of the false-negative results previously encountered in these cases. The optimal delay for the dye to penetrate the spinal cord after a subarachnoid injection is approximately 3 to 8 hr (12,27,36). However, the need for hospitalization and the difficulty in evaluating the cervical and cervicomedullary areas have made this investigation less popular, particularly with the advent of magnetic resonance imaging (MRI).

MRI has been very useful and dependable in diagnosing these lesions (9). The loculi and septa in syringomyelic cavities can be reliably visualized (Figs. 1 and 2).

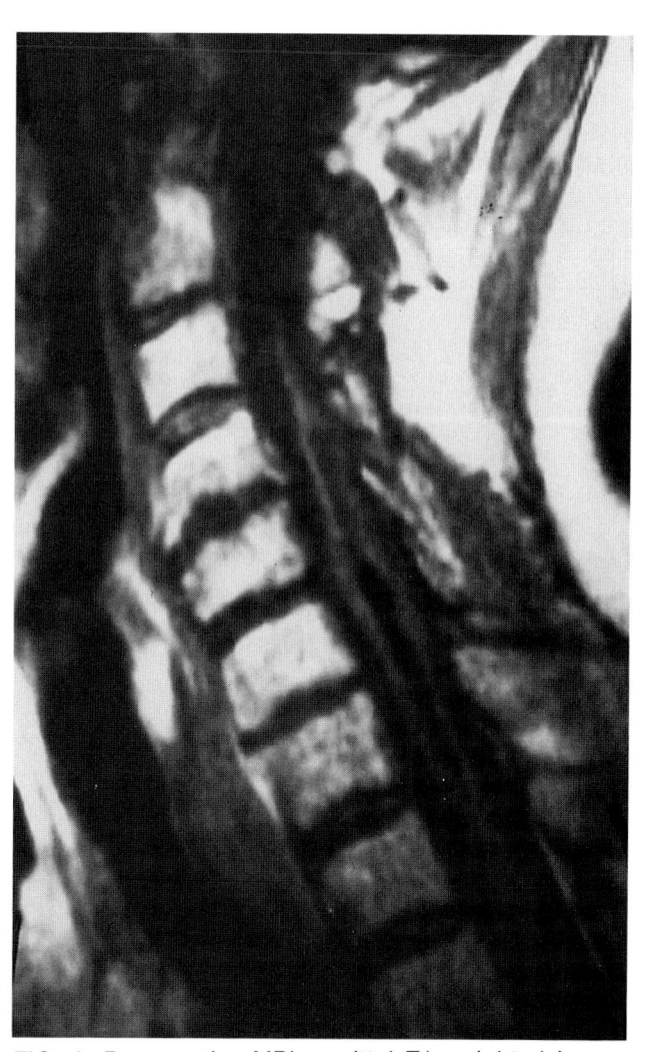

FIG. 1. Preoperative MRI: sagittal T1 weighted image. Midline slice demonstrates a CSF intensity cyst within the spinal cord extending from C5 to T1. Atrophy of the cord is seen above and below the cyst.

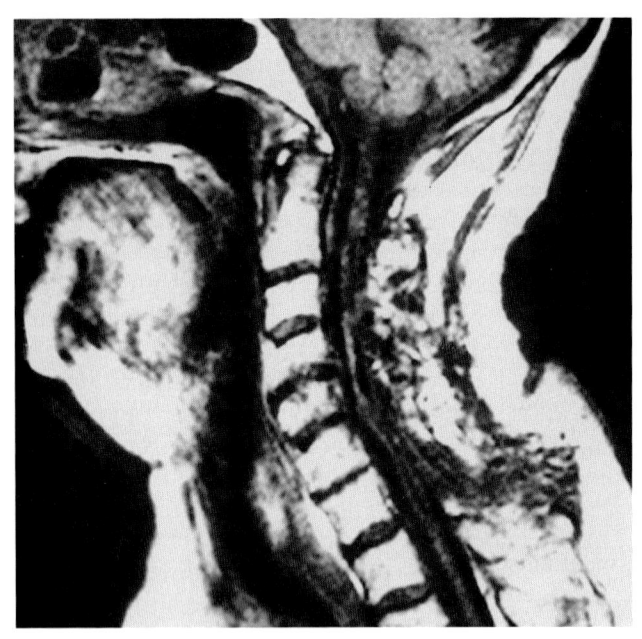

FIG. 2. Postoperative MRI: sagittal T1 weighted image. Midline slice demonstrates decrease in size of the cyst at the lower cervical area with postoperative changes.

MRI has also been helpful in delineating "remote post-traumatic syringomyelia" away from the original injury site. It also gives insight into the contents of the syrinx, whether clear or bloody, and can delineate the size of the cord and associated soft tissue anomalies such as disc protrusions. Though the ferromagnetic devices used in stabilization procedures in traumatic fractures and dislocations of vertebrae produce imaging artifacts, the development of MRI-compatible metallic devices should eliminate that.

ELECTROPHYSIOLOGICAL STUDIES

The characteristic finding in electrophysiological studies is a subjective sensory loss with an intact sensory electrical response (6). In electromyography, synchronous firing of involved muscles and prolonged "F" wave latencies were seen in syringomyelia (4). The prolongation of "F" wave latency reflects anterior horn cell dysfunction, perhaps as a consequence of acute interstitial edema occurring after sudden increases in the size of the syrinx. Electrical studies are also useful in the follow-up period after surgery as the normalization of "f" wave latency indicates the reversal of this anterior horn cell dysfunction. In post-traumatic syringomyelia there are no specific somatosensory evoked potentials reported.

ULTRASONOGRAPHY

Ultrasonography has been useful intraoperatively as well as postoperatively (22). During surgery, it helps to identify the syrinx and the septa. Ultrasonography may identify the lesion at surgery even though the preoperative CT/myelography is negative. MRI has avoided these false-negative results. Ultrasonography also reveals the dimensions of the syrinx including its caudal and rostral extensions. This enables the surgeon to make the minimal necessary myelotomy with the exact placement of the drainage catheter. Using a frequency of 7.5 MHz, a high-resolution image of the spinal cord, its contents, and its coverings can be obtained. The central canal is best imaged in sagittal slices; in axial planes the dural sac and subarachnoid space can best be seen.

In the postoperative period, the position of the catheter in the syrinx may be seen with percutaneous ultrasonography, which can detect the slippage of the catheter, an increase in the size of the syrinx, or good shunt function with collapse of the syrinx.

SURGICAL MANAGEMENT

Though the natural history of post-traumatic syringomyelia is not very well established, some patients with the disorder definitely get progressively worse. Previously quadriplegic patients may become bedridden or ventilator dependent and may also develop unrelenting pain. Some patients also develop arthropathy secondary to muscular weakness. Surgery may stop the progression of the deficits and help bring about neurological recovery. Since we are unclear as to the natural history of this disorder, it is rather difficult to definitely conclude that surgical intervention stops the progression or changes the pace of the disease in the long term. Though the incidence of post-traumatic syringomyelia is low, it is worthwhile to follow these spinal injured patients with frequent MRI scans in order to detect cysts in the early stages. Surgery is suggested for intractable pain, progressive muscle weakness, neuropathic joints (1), and progressive neurological deterioration (30). Drainage of the cyst is the chief aim of surgery for syringomyelia. It is doubtful whether drainage of small syrinxes is of any help to patients (27). It is clear, however, that small cysts may become larger, may coalesce, and then become symptomatic. Rossier et al. (27) and Peerless and Durward (23) do not advocate surgery for patients who have mild symptoms and are stable with small cysts.

In 1959 Freeman (8) first performed a syringotomy in a patient. McLean et al. (18) communicated the syrinx with the subarachnoid space by performing a cordectomy at the level of the syrinx. Since post-traumatic syringomyelia, unlike hydromyelia, does not communicate with the fourth ventricle, plugging the obex is not indicated (20,27).

Multiple surgical procedures have been advocated for the treatment of post-traumatic syringomyelia. Included among these are myelotomy, syringosubdural shunt, syringocisternal shunt, syringoperitoneal shunt, syringopleural shunt, laminectomy, and cordectomy (17).

The operation performed depends on the level of the cord injury as well as the neurological deficits. Cordectomy and placement of a shunt into the syrinx may be indicated in complete lesions of the thoracic and lumbar areas (1). If the lesion is incomplete, insertion of the tube into the syrinx at or just above the original injury site is advocated (1). Making extra holes in the shunt tubes often increases the efficiency of the tube in terms of drainage (23). Shannon et al. (28) and Quencer et al. (25) recommend placement of two shunts if the syrinx is large or multiloculated; however, placement of the catheter in the larger part of the cyst (30) or in the lowermost extent of the syrinx (23) also has been suggested. Cordectomy and placement of the catheter in the proximal stump of the resected cord have less chances of shunt malfunction. In cases where a myelotomy is performed and a syringostomy catheter placed, effective drainage may be impeded by the collapse of the syrinx around the tube. Syringosubdural shunting is mentioned only to be condemned as it is associated with a high failure rate. Myelotomy and placement of a shunt catheter are occasionally hazardous in partial paraplegics with small syrinxes or in patients with syrinxes at the cervical and lumbar enlargements; hence in this group of patients, a laminectomy and keeping the dura open or a duroplasty producing an artificial meningocele has been advocated by some (35).

SURGICAL TECHNIQUE

In our institute, syringopleural shunting is the most commonly performed operation for the treatment of post-traumatic syringomyelia. Over the years, we have found that the failure rate with syringosubarachnoid shunts has been higher than with syringopleural shunts. We have also had favorable results with syringoperitoneal shunts.

As for any neurosurgical operation, positioning is very important. The prone position is ideal for the exposure of the spine while allowing good access to the lateral thorax for placement of the pleural catheter. The operation is always performed with somatosensory evoked potential monitoring.

The patient is positioned on the operating table on two chest rolls. A suitable radiolucent frame is also used for intraoperative radiographic localization especially in the high thoracic areas. Prior to draping the patient, the site of the proposed laminectomy is identified with a radiograph. A second radiograph is often needed after the skin incision and muscle dissection have exposed the posterior elements of the vertebrae.

A single-level, total, or hemi-laminectomy is performed at the area of maximum diameter of the syrinx. In patients where the syrinx is of moderate size and not multiloculated, we do a hemi-laminectomy. Once the laminectomy is performed, the exact site, size, and configuration of the syrinx is confirmed by ultrasonography (Figs. 3 and 4). The rest of the operation is performed with a microscope. While performing a syringopleural shunt, one does not need to open the dura widely away from the syrinx, but in cases of syringosubarachnoid shunting, the dura must be opened away from the syrinx area in order to get to the healthy arachnoid. This is important since subarachnoid shunts become less efficient when placed in the vicinity of the injured site due to adhesions and scarring.

Once the dura is opened, it is tied down to the paraspinal muscles with 4-0 Neurolon sutures. The arachnoid is carefully opened and tacked up to the inner surface of the dura with hemostatic clips. We prefer to perform a midline myelotomy for the insertion of the tube. The myelotomy may be performed at the thinnest part of the cord, which corresponds to the largest diameter of the syrinx, or at the dorsal root entry zone. We have found the Edwards–Barbaro shunt tube (Heyer-Shulte, manufactured by American V. Mueller, Chicago, IL) to be the most optimal shunt system for this operation. The proximal T-tube arms are trimmed to the desired length and inserted into the syrinx. The vertical limb of the T-tube is anchored to the dura. The arachnoid is closed with 6-0 Tevdek and the dura is

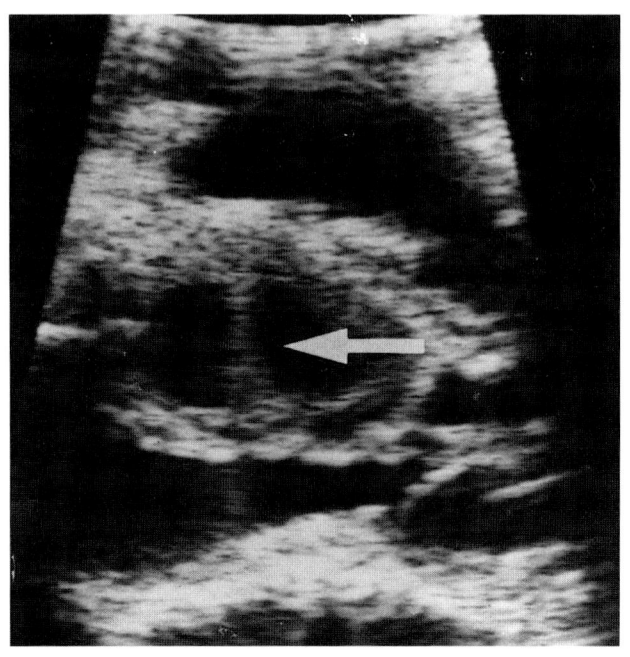

FIG. 3. Sonogram showing a longitudinal view of the syrinx with a clear septation between the two compartments (*arrow*). The transducer is slightly oblique to the long axis of the cord.

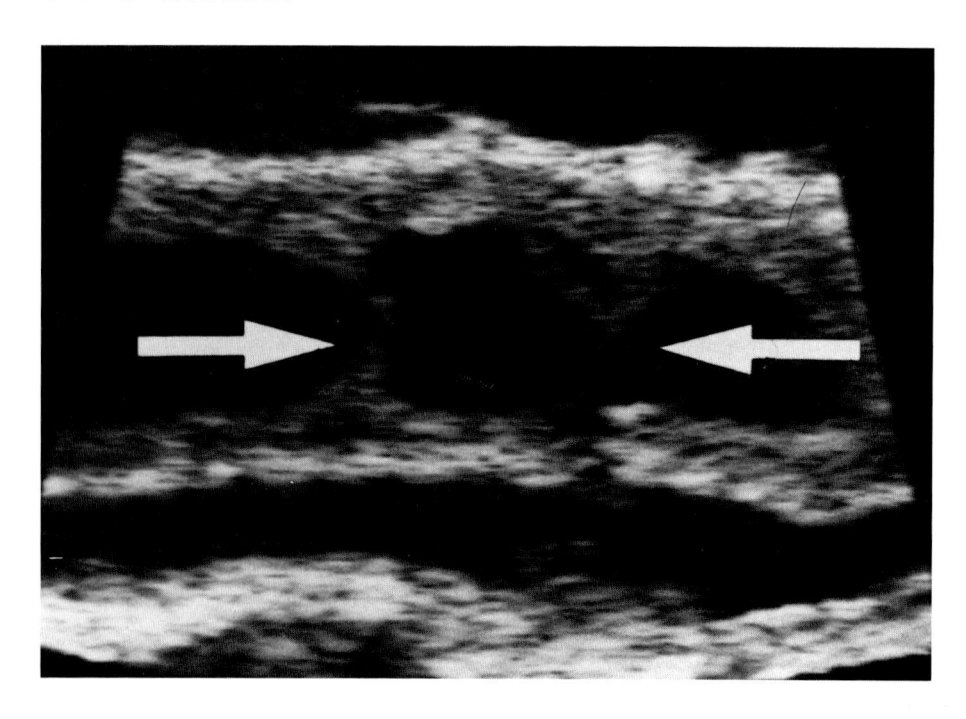

FIG. 4. Sonogram of a spinal cord showing syringomyelia with two septa (*arrows*) dividing the syrinx into at least three compartments.

closed watertight with 4-0 Neurolon. The vertical limb is connected to a distal tubing. An antisiphon device can be placed between the T-tube and the distal tube.

A 5-cm thoracotomy incision is made in the posterior axillary line in the eighth intercostal space. Alternatively, in cases where the inferior border of the scapula comes in the way of the incision, one may resort to an incision in the sixth intercostal space at the midaxillary line. The latissimus dorsi muscle is split along its muscle fibers and the intercostal muscles are detached from the upper part of the lower rib, thus avoiding injury to the neurovascular bundle, which lies on the lower surface of the upper rib. Deep cerebellar retractors are applied to the adjoining ribs, exposing the pleura. The distal end of the shunt tube is tunneled subcutaneously. At this stage, the anesthesiologist is asked not to ventilate the patient for a few seconds, during which the pleura is punctured either with a pair of bayonet forceps or a #15 blade. The distal end of the shunt tube is introduced into the pleural cavity swiftly. If inadvertently a large opening is made in the pleura, a purse string suture with 5-0 Tevdek is placed, otherwise closure of the pleura is not necessary. The wound is irrigated with normal saline and at the same time the anesthesiologist is asked to perform a Valsalva maneuver in order to expel any air trapped in the pleural cavity during the introduction of the distal catheter. Later, both the wounds are closed in a routine manner.

SURGICAL RESULTS

Patients who have the operation often show some deterioration immediately after the surgery due to the surgical manipulation. These patients ultimately improve. Late postoperative deterioration of these patients is explained by adhesive arachnoiditis and shunt malfunction. An attempt to decrease the complication can be made by using Silastic tubing, which is less irritating.

Surgical results are better with large cysts (25,30). The surgical results are improved if the duration of the presenting symptoms are shorter (23,30). Quencer et al. (25), however, noted no such correlation. Rossier et al. (27) found that patients with pain from 4 to 6 years had a good improvement.

After surgery, pain is decreased in the majority of the patients. Motor improvement is more frequent than sensory (28,33). This phenomenon is due to the presence of syrinx in the gray matter between the posterior horn and the posterior columns. The pyramidal tracts, by virtue of their position, are affected at a later stage and therefore have a better recovery. In one report (7), sensory improvement was better than the motor. Shannon et al. (28) found that incomplete cord lesions do better than complete cord lesions. However, Rossier et al. (27) do not concur with this. Vernon et al. (33) in their series report that 56% of the patients had less pain; sensory improvement was noted in only 33.3%, and in 56% the progression of the disease was arrested.

In order to alleviate pain Nashold and Bullitt (19) suggested performing a dorsal root entry zone lesion either at the time of the syringostomy or in the event of recurrence of pain.

As mentioned earlier, immediately after surgery one might notice transient neurological deterioration, which is due to the surgical manipulation. Delayed neurological deterioration may be due to placement of the tube in the subdural space instead of the subarachnoid space, slippage of the tube, blockage of the tube due to collapse of the syrinx, or adhesive arachnoiditis (1,23,30).

CONSERVATIVE TREATMENT

Since the benefits of surgery outweigh conservative management, few patients were electively treated conservatively. Of the six patients who were treated conservatively by Barnett and Jousse (1), only two patients improved and the rest deteriorated. Vernon et al. (32) observed a worsening neurological state in all their patients who were followed conservatively. Watson (34) observed that while numbness, sensory loss, and reflex loss remain unchanged, motor weakness can improve. None of the patients of Rossier have improved while conservatively managed, and only 6 out of the 29 remained stable. He also observed further deterioration the longer the patients were followed.

It is conceivable that if all patients are followed for a longer period of time, eventual deterioration will become evident. Untreated cases have progressed slowly or rapidly to severe disability. There are no objective criteria to predict the outcome of patients who are going to worsen and, if so, how fast or how slow. Remissions in sensory deficits and replacement of pain by hypalgesia after many years may occur (32). Although surgical treatment has been shown to be beneficial in the arrest of progression, deterioration in the condition of patients following surgery has been noted. Due to the low risk of surgery, we advocate surgical intervention in patients harboring a post-traumatic syrinx.

REFERENCES

1. Barnett HJM, Jousse AT. Syringomyelia as a late sequel to traumatic paraplegia and quadriplegia—clinical features. In: Barnett HJM, Foster JB, Hudgson P, eds. *Syringomyelia*. London: Saunders, 1973;129–153.
2. Barnett HJM, Jousse AT, Ball MJ. Pathology and pathogenesis of progressive cystic myelopathy as a late sequel to spinal cord injury. In: Barnett HJM, Foster JB, Hudgson P, eds. *Syringomyelia*. Philadelphia: Saunders, 1973;174–219.
3. Brierley JB. The penetration of particulate matter from the cerebrospinal fluid into the spinal ganglia, peripheral nerves, and perivascular spaces of the central nervous system. *J Neurol Neurosurg Psychiatry* 1950;13:203–215.
4. Di Benedetto M, Rossier AB. Electrodiagnosis in post-traumatic syringomyelia. *Paraplegia* 1977;14:286–295.
5. Durward QJ, Rice GP, Ball MJ, Gilbert JJ, Kaufman JCE. Selective spinal cordectomy—clinicopathological correlation. *J Neurosurg* 1982;56:359–367.
6. Fincham RW, Cape CA. Sensory nerve conduction in syringomyelia. *Neurology (Minneapolis)* 1968;18:200–201.
7. Foo D, Bignami A, Rossier AB. A case of post-traumatic syringomyelia. Neuropathological findings after 1 year of cystic drainage. *Paraplegia* 1989;27:63–69.
8. Freeman LW. Ascending spinal paralysis: case presentation. *J Neurosurg* 1959;16:120–122.
9. Gabriel KR, Crawford AH. Identification of acute post-traumatic spinal cord cyst by magnetic resonance imaging: a case report and review of the literature. *J Pediatr Orthop* 1988;8:710–714.
10. Hallopeau FM. Sur une faîte de sclérose diffuse de la substance grise et strophie musculaire. *Gazzy Med (Paris)* 1871;25:183.
11. Holmes G. The Goulstonian Lectures on spinal injuries of warfare. *Br Med J* 1915;2:769–774.
12. Isherwood I, Fawcitt RA, Forbes W St C, Nettle JRL, Pullan BR. Computed tomography of the spinal canal using metrizamide. *Acta Radiol Suppl (Stockh)* 1971;355:299–305.
13. Jensen F, Reske-Nielsen E. Post-traumatic syringomyelia. A review of the literature and two new autopsy cases. *Scand J Rehabil Med* 1977;9:35–53.
14. Kao CC, Chang LW. The mechanism of spinal cord cavitation following spinal cord transection. Part I—A correlated histochemical study. *J Neurosurg* 1977;46:197–209.
15. Kendall B, Symon L. Cyst puncture and endomyelography in cystic tumors of the spinal cord. *Br J Radiol* 1973;46:198–204.
16. Klawans HJ Jr. Delayed traumatic syringomyelia. *Dis Nerv Syst* 1968;29:525–528.
17. Lyons BM, Brown DJ, Calvert JM, Woodward JM, Wriedt CHR. The diagnosis and management of post-traumatic syringomyelia. *Paraplegia* 1987;25:340–350.
18. McLean DR, Miller JDR, Allen PBR, Ezzeddin SA. Post-traumatic syringomyelia. *J Neurosurg* 1973;39:485–492.
19. Nashold BS Jr, Bullitt E. Dorsal root entry zone lesions to control central pain in paraplegics. *J Neurosurg* 1981;55:414–419.
20. Nurick S, Russell JA, Deck MDF. Cystic degeneration of the spinal cord following spinal cord injury. *Brain* 1970;93:211–222.
21. Oakley JC, Ojemann GA, Alvord EC Jr. Post-traumatic syringomyelia. *J Neurosurg* 1981;55:276–281.
22. Pasto ME, Rifkin MD, Rubenstein JB, Northrup BE, Cotler JM, Goldberg BB. Realtime ultrasonography of the spinal cord: intraoperative and post operative imaging. *Neuroradiology* 1984;26:183–187.
23. Peerless SJ, Durward QJ. Management of syringomyelia—a pathophysiological approach. *Clin Neurosurg* 1983;30:531–576.
24. Piatt JH Jr. Post-traumatic syringomyelia. In: Wilkins RH, Rengachary SS, eds. *Neurosurgery Update II*. New York: McGraw, 1991;1761–1763.
25. Quencer RM, Green BA, Eismont FJ. Post-traumatic spinal cord cysts: clinical features and characterization with metrizamide computed tomography. *Radiology* 1983;146:415–423.
26. Reddy KKV, Del Bigio MR, Sutherland GR. Ultrastructure of the human post-traumatic syrinx. *J Neurosurg* 1989;71:239–243.
27. Rossier AB, Foo D, Shillito J, Dyro FM. Post-traumatic syringomyelia. Incidence, clinical presentation, electrophysiological studies, syrinx protein and results of conservative and operative management. *Brain* 1985;108:439–461.
28. Shannon N, Symon L, Logue V, Cull D, Kang J, Kendall B. Clinical features, investigation and treatment of post-traumatic syringomyelia. *J Neurol Neurosurg Psychiatry* 1981;44:35–42.
29. Strong OS. A case of spinal cord injury and a subsequent unilateral syringomyelia. *Neurol Bull* 1919;2:277.
30. Tator CH, Meguro K, Rowed DW. Favorable results with syringosubarachnoid shunts for the treatment of syringomyelia. *J Neurosurg* 1982;56:517–523.
31. Turnball IM, Brieg A, Hassler O. Blood supply of the cervical spinal cord in man—a microangiographic cadaver study. *J Neurosurg* 1966;24:951–965.
32. Vernon JD, Silver JR, Ohry A. Post-traumatic syringomyelia. *Paraplegia* 1980;20:339–364.
33. Vernon JD, Silver JR, Symon L. Post-traumatic syringomyelia, the results of surgery. *Paraplegia* 1983;21:37–46.
34. Watson N. Ascending cystic degeneration of the cord after spinal cord injury. *Paraplegia* 1981;19:89–95.
35. Williams B. Post-traumatic syringomyelia, an update. *Paraplegia* 1990;28(5):296–313.
36. Winkler SS, Sackett JF. Explanation of metrizamide brain penetration. A review. *J Comput Assist Tomogr* 1980;4:191–193.
37. Wozniecicz B, Filipowicz K, Swiderska SK, Deraka K. Pathophysiological mechanism of traumatic cavitation of the spinal cord. *Paraplegia* 1983;21(5):312–317.

30

Post-Traumatic Syringomyelia

Surgical Management and Case Reports

Bernard Williams

Syringomyelia is an important but uncommon entity that does not deserve the dignity of being called a disease. A disorder with many causes, it is relevant to start this chapter by pointing out that the most common cause of syringomyelia is disordered cerebrospinal fluid (CSF) dynamics; the commonest grouping of these cases is associated with abnormalities at the foramen magnum (7,29,31). These cases may be grouped as hindbrain-related syringomyelia, and it is important to realize that they are different from the post-traumatic cases. The hindbrain-related varieties of syringomyelia are often associated with other causative conditions, such as hindbrain herniation, hydrocephalus, spina bifida, bony abnormalities at the base of the skull, or tumors. When syringomyelia complicates thoracolumbar fractures, the central nervous system was normal before the injury, and the two varieties of the condition should not be confused. This chapter is concerned with syringomyelia in association with fractures. Other causes of syringomyelia in orthopaedic practice are not covered.

The diagnosis of syringomyelia is not always easy and, when discovered, the causes are sometimes obscure. When scoliosis complicates the picture, the problems of elucidation become complicated because deformities may also produce cord damage, local arachnoiditis, and obstruction of the CSF pathways. Under these circumstances, determining causes is often difficult, and some cases must be regarded as idiopathic. In the post-traumatic cases the central nervous system, including the anatomy and physiology of the CSF pathways, almost always was normal before the trauma. The cause of the problem is therefore the spinal injury.

Minor cystic changes in the spinal cord after complete or incomplete spinal injury are common; sizeable cavities that track along the cord and cause neurologic deficits are less common. The nomenclature is unclear: some authors prefer the term "cystic myelopathy" rather than syringomyelia. (It may be that cystic myelopathy should be reserved for the smaller type of cyst.) Greenfield preferred to reserve the term syringomyelia for cavities that extended over several segments.

Post-traumatic syringomyelia is one of the serious late complications of spinal injury, appreciation of which only recently has become widespread. As a complication of paraplegia, it is of overwhelming importance to those who suffer from it. The results of the disease process may contribute greatly to an end disability, even for those who, for a time, seem to have made an apparently complete recovery from spinal injuries (12,18,19,21).

INCIDENCE

The incidence of syringomyelia after paraplegia is unclear. Clamant syringomyelia, which demands treatment, is probably less than 3%. Watson (27) suggested 1.1% in 1972. Barnett and Jousse (5) gave 2.3% for their complete paraplegics in 1976 and suggested that the condition was more common in partial paraplegics. Rossier et al. (19) in 1985 gave 3.2%. This increasing

---

B. Williams: Midland Centre for Neurosurgery and Neurology, Warley, Birmingham B67 7JX, United Kingdom.

incidence may be due to greater awareness of the condition over the past two decades as well as to the use of magnetic resonance imaging (MRI) scans.

Small cysts opposite the fracture are common, but the question of whether they should be drained is difficult to answer (2). Individual cases require individual decisions, and a policy of observation with repeated MRI scans often may be chosen when the level does not ascend for more than a few centimeters above the site of injury (Figs. 1 and 2).

The morphology of the cystic enlargement is variable. A simple cyst, which may be of any size, may be seen opposite the fracture, as in Case 1. Sometimes there is a cyst that appears to be separate from an upward or downward prolongation and may be separate from both, as shown in Fig. 3. The region also may be marked by only one septum at the site of fracture, as in Cases 2 and 3, where the spinal cord findings are strikingly different below the paraplegia from those above. This may be accompanied by a zone of stenosis, as shown in Fig. 4. Sometimes the cord is wide open opposite the site of injury, with wide connection both upward and downward, as shown in Fig. 5. This type of communication is usual in those patients who have a wide canal. Thus it is seen most frequently in the postarachnoiditic cases.

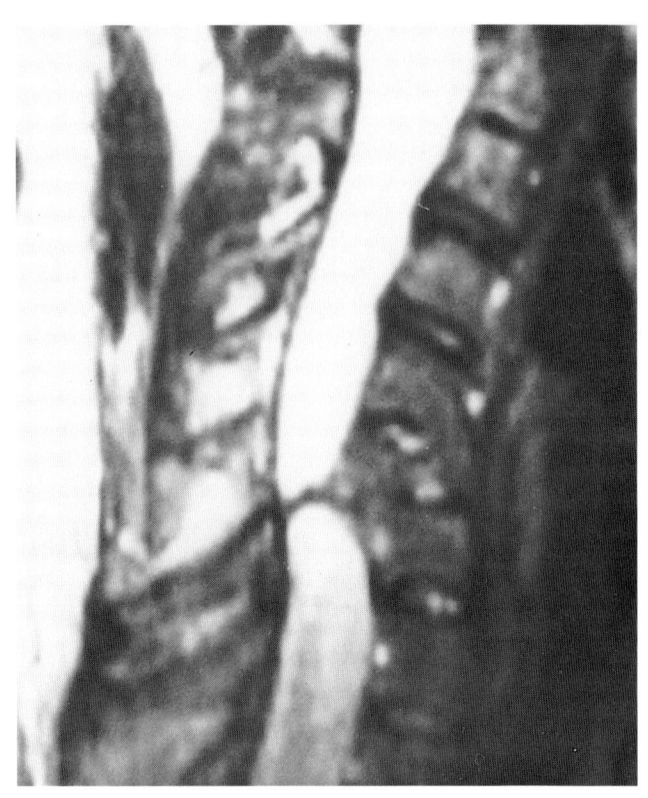

FIG. 2. A T2-weighted MRI image will often show a zone of arachnoiditis more clearly than the T1 image. Contrast this with Fig. 1, which is of the same case.

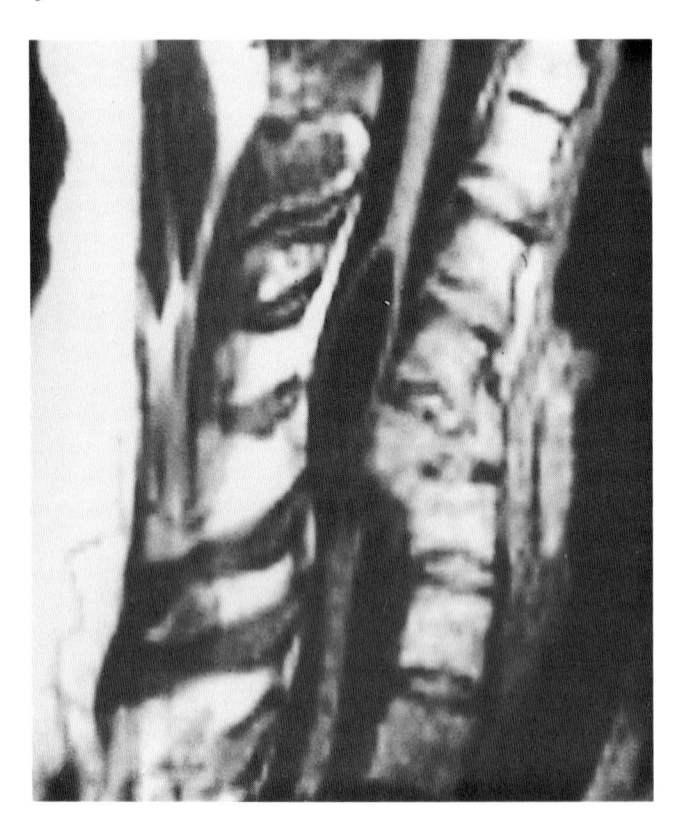

FIG. 1. A tense primary cyst opposite a C6 fracture. A cyst with this configuration is likely to be under raised pressure and to be contributing to the deterioration in arm function that had taken place over the previous few months. Drainage was not helpful to this patient.

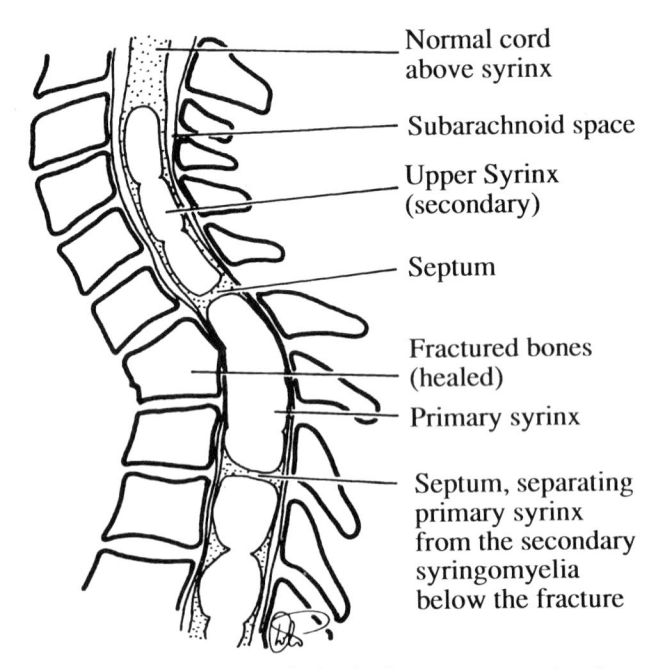

FIG. 3. A common morphological appearance after fracture. A primary syrinx opposite the fracture site suggests that hematoma might have caused an initiatory cavity. Septa may be intact, as shown here, in relation to a primary syrinx but may also be intact at more distant situations.

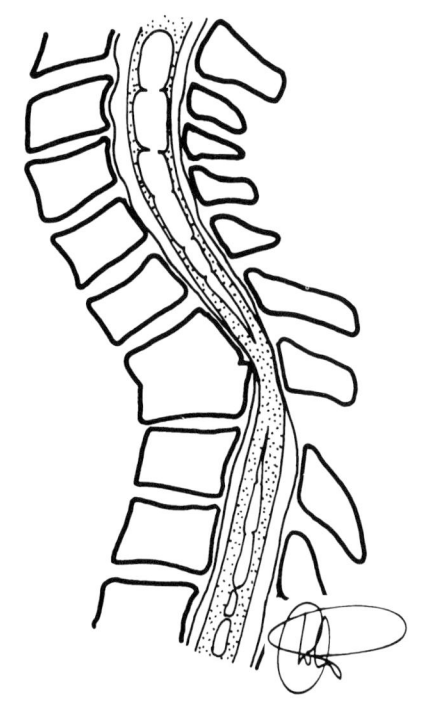

FIG. 4. Stenosis at the site of fracture is sometimes accompanied by syringomyelia either above or below the site of maximum damage with no primary syrinx visible on investigation or determinable at operation. A syrinx above and below is not so common as only one syrinx.

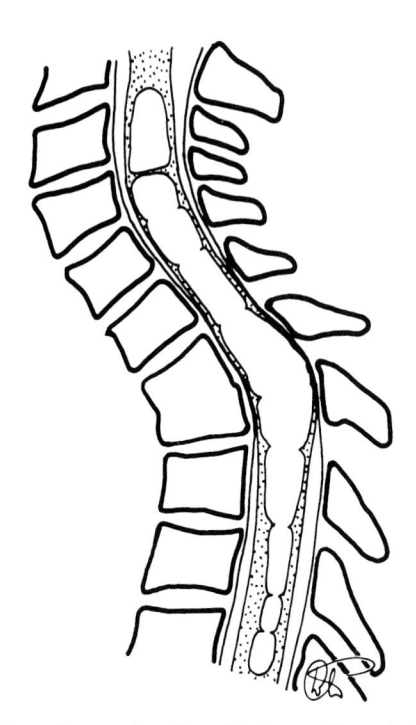

FIG. 5. Dilatation at the site of injury with no intact septation close to the site of damage is a common finding. In postarachnoiditic cases where there is no fracture, the cord may appear to be pulled open by adhesive arachnoiditis.

TIME OF ONSET

The time of onset of the cystic degeneration is not known in sufficient detail to justify conclusions. Large medical centers with adequate MRI facilities are accumulating data, and more information will be forthcoming.

The clinical onset or the time of diagnosis varies from a few months to over 30 years after injury. There may be a bimodal distribution, suggesting two separate etiological factors, but this requires elucidation (30).

MECHANISMS OF ONSET

The most obvious mechanism that may be suggested as initiating a cavity in the cord opposite the site of injury is the formation of an acute cavity due to liquefied cord contents, edema, and blood effusion. The acute accumulation of fluid after injury is well known (8).

The presence of a primary cyst, as in Figs. 1 and 3, might suggest this mechanism. The soft, gray matter allows tracking of the fluid core upward, often for two segments or so, as well as transient ascent of the clinical lesion for one or two segments. This is followed by descent of the clinical dermatomal level again after some weeks and is not uncommon.

HEMATOMYELIA

Greenfield pointed out that overt bleeding within the spinal cord after injury is uncommon. The same findings were stressed by Kakoulas (10), with the observation that ascending epidural hematomas and ascending spinal artery thrombosis are likewise rare. Kakoulas wrote that the central traumatic hemorrhagic necrosis of the cord is not a space-taking lesion. Liquefaction and the formation of a cavity are usual. Such cavities may be multicompartmental and crossed by astrocytic webs of residual tissue and vascular structures. This may explain cases wherein the protein is high or varies in differing loculi of the syrinx.

ENLARGEMENT OF CYSTIC SPACES

The spinal canal is subject to continuous pressure swings that are mediated by the venous channels. There are large veins that partly occupy the epidural space and are in free, valveless communication with the plexuses of veins around the vertebral bodies. These in turn freely transmit volumes of blood that produce concomitant pressure swings from the azygos, hemiazygos, and other abdominothoracic veins. The intraspinal compartments, particularly the intradural

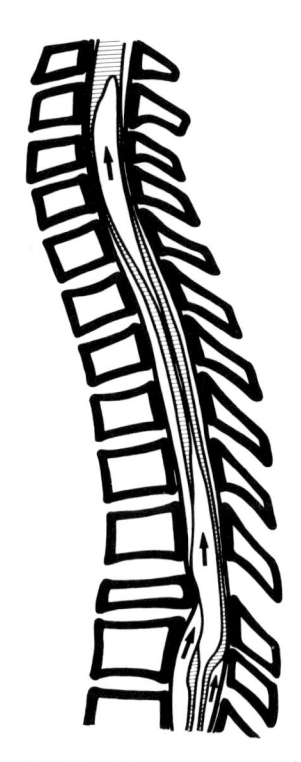

FIG. 6. Proposed method for pressure differentials forcing fluid into the syrinx. This would be perhaps more convincing if there were either a visible communication or if the cord changed in dimensions in the way shown. There are difficulties in understanding the place of septation when considering a diagram of this kind.

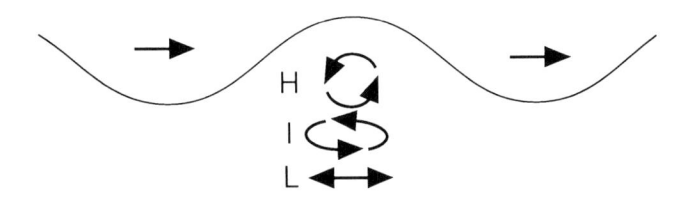

FIG. 8. The energy transmission of waves in a tank is accompanied by circular movement of particles close to the surface as shown on the left of this figure. Particles next to a flat bottom can only move in a linear direction; intermediate particles as shown on the right side of the figure move in an elliptical manner.

fluids, are therefore subject to relatively violent pressure swings in response to such stresses as lifting, coughing, sneezing, and shouting. In the normal human, the result of transient high pressure in the spine, such as produced by a cough, is movement of the cerebrospinal fluid up the subarachnoid spaces into the head, followed by return of the fluid to the resting distribution. The head end of the neuraxis provides a relatively compliant closure at the top of the spinal canal. It might be thought that the elevation of venous pressure would also produce venous engorgement in the head simultaneously with the spine. However, the venous capacity, especially in the neck, provides a reservoir for the venous blood, and backing up of blood in the veins all over the body is available to accommodate the volume.

Conversely, the cerebrospinal fluid, when compressed in the spine, has no where else to go in the short term, and it therefore moves with almost ballistic speed up and down the neuraxis. A volume of about 12 ml passes into the head with a cough; this upward movement is over in about one-tenth of a second. The pressures involved in a cough often exceed 100 mmHg, and the total energy provides a potentially destructive force (24,29–33).

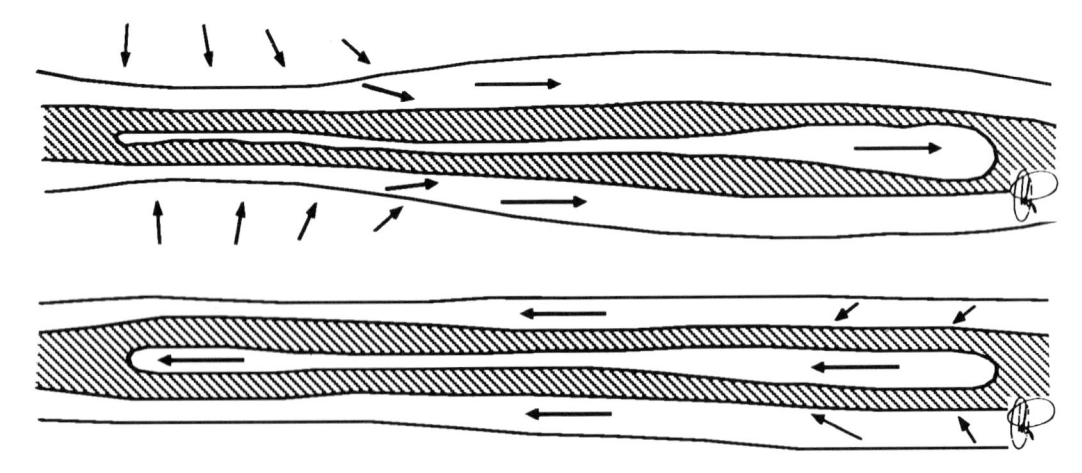

FIG. 7. Simplified idea of the slosh mechanism applicable to all types of syringomyelia. When compression is applied to the outside of the dura by distending epidural veins, cerebrospinal fluid moves upward in the subarachnoid space. This will compress the spinal cord and then after the episode of straining there will be a rebound as shown in the lower figure. Obviously the existence of septa confounds this idea of a long wavelength as shown in this figure and Fig. 6.

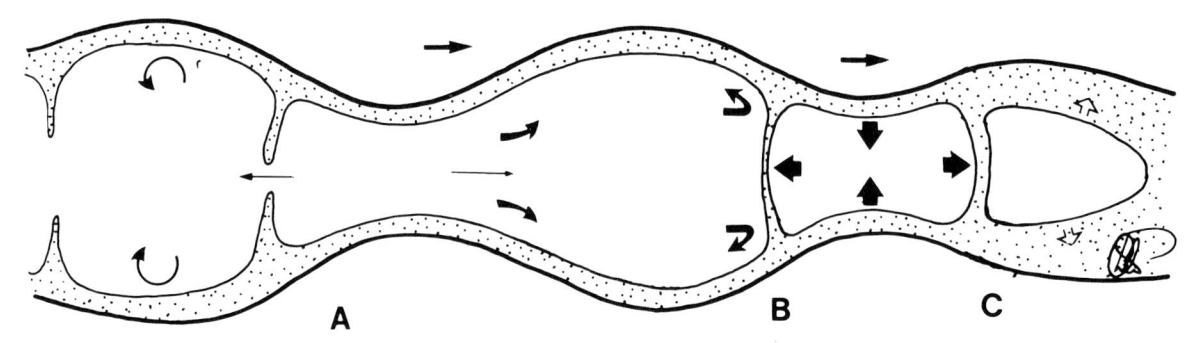

FIG. 9. The spinal cord may have waves similar to Fig. 8 but folded around to form an annulus. Particles in the middle of the cord may move upward and downward in a manner analogous to particles on the floor of a tank. There may be small zones of movement close to the surface. If the distance between the septa at A and B were one wavelength, then there would be no need for fluid to be transmitted up and down through the septations, which could remain intact. If the septations were to move, however, as shown between B and C, then wave energy might be transmitted along the cord by a change in the shape of the cells produced by septation without the septa transmitting pulses of fluid. It might be that the energy in the walls of the cord might lead to development of a separate cavity beyond an intact septum as shown by the clear arrows to the right of C.

It seems likely that the energy of the pulsation sets up pressure gradients across the walls, either on the lines suggested in Fig. 6 or through the walls during the propagation of waves, as suggested by Figs. 7 to 10. It seems probable that the fracture site is the site of entry of CSF into the syrinx, perhaps augmented by exchange of fluid through the walls of the syrinx after it has developed (Fig. 10).

The walls of the spinal cord are not waterproof. There are potential spaces along the vessels of the cord; these were described by Virchow and Robin. Whether or not the histologists are correct in condemning them as postfixation artifacts, it seems they have the capacity to transmit fluid. They are sites of weakness, and fluid may seep through them in either direction.

On inspection, the walls of the cord in the region of damage are so thin that they may visibly weep CSF, which may allow flattening of the syrinx cavity during the preparation of the operative site.

It is unreasonable to regard the impulse forces that act on any intracord collection of fluid as the only mechanism. Some cases of syringomyelia are due to spinal adhesive arachnoiditis without trauma. The commonest causes are meningitis, particularly tuberculous, and epidural abscess. Arachnoiditis may occur in response to Myodil (Iophendylate, Pantopaque), and some cases are idiopathic. In a center treating syringomyelia of all types, the ratio in primarily spinal syringomyelia, excluding tumors, is about four post-traumatic for each nontraumatic case. If the acute liquefactive changes plus a variable amount of hemorrhage are discounted, the mechanisms of syringomyelia are probably similar in both the post-traumatic and the postinflammatory types. The important similarities include the blockage of the CSF pathways around the cord, the

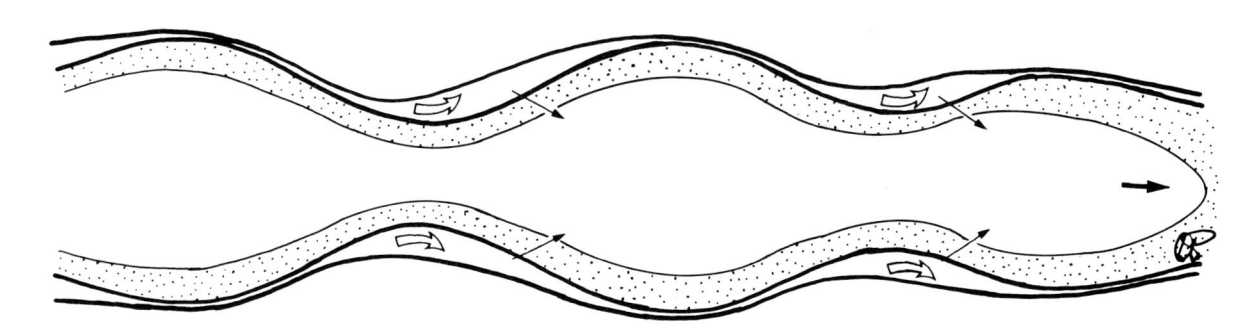

FIG. 10. All forms of syringomyelia seem to be able to fill or to maintain themselves to a limited extent even after the filling mechanism has partially been disabled by surgery. The free movement of contrast medium across the walls, for example, suggests that there is easy fluid exchange. When considering wave motion such as shown in Fig. 9, it may be reasonable to suppose that zones of pressure difference between the subarachnoid space and the intrasyrinx cavity might drive fluid directly across the walls under certain circumstances.

tendency to upward extension of the syrinx cavities, particularly in association with straining, and the tendency to progress, sometimes many years after the causative lesions. The main clinical difference between types seems to be that, in some of the post-traumatic cases, the condition becomes evident early, only a few months after the initial cord involvement. This may result from a hematoma at the site of injury.

CLINICAL PRESENTATION

The clinical presentation is variable, and the condition is often not diagnosed for many years after the symptoms have become egregious (4,5,11–13,16,23, 25,30,33). The symptoms may be grouped into those of pain, motor, sensory, structural, and autonomic features, although an anatomic classification such as neurological involvement contiguous with the level, ascending problems, arm symptoms appearing above the paraplegic level leaving a gap, bulbar features, and features below the neurological level might also be useful. It may be accompanied by deterioration below the fracture in partial paraplegics. Such deterioration may be due to arachnoiditis or gliosis as well as cavitation. The most common combination is both motor and sensory symptoms with pain as shown in a Venn-Euler diagram (Fig. 11).

Pain is common in post-traumatic syringomyelia. A paraplegic in a pain clinic has syringomyelia until otherwise proved. There are many causes of pain in a paraplegic. Local nerve damage and disordered function of the damaged cord tissues may be at fault. Local arachnoiditis or the formation of cystic loculi around the damaged cord may play a part in distorting the cord and contribute to the production of abnormal impulses that travel up the pain pathways. Such pain may be referred to the level of injury or any level below it; when localized to the abdomen, pain often gives rise to severe diagnostic difficulties. In addition to pain arising from the cord, the arms and necks of paraplegics take more strain than the arms of walkers, and cervical spondylotic myelopathy and radiculopathy may be more common than in the population at large. The arms may be damaged by crutches, especially around the elbow, leading to nerve damage; and the median nerves may similarly be damaged by direct trauma from crutches or sticks. When syringomyelia is present, it is probably responsible for pain arising from central structures, notably the area of the posterior root entry zone and the substantia gelatinosa. There is experimental evidence as well as observation of hindbrain-related syringomyelia to suggest that this mechanism is important.

The pain may be felt around the level of the neurological damage, below the level, or anywhere above the sensory loss of the paraplegia. As with other manifestations of syringomyelia, the symptoms are often strikingly unilateral. There is a frequent association with straining of the sort discussed under pathogenesis. The association of the pain with straining seems more common than in the hindbrain-related cases. The pain that accompanies coughing may be described as a tearing or ripping pain. It is often confined to a small zone of the body, usually unilateral. This pain is often not a complaint of the patient in the paraplegia clinic because often it has lasted for a few days or even only for a few impulse-related events. Its replacement by a variety of numbness or dysesthetic sensory loss may be rapid. The patients will often remember the pain with clarity because of its severity but may need to be questioned.

Not all pain in the region of the fracture or above will abate after successful operation; it may be replaced by dysesthesia. Some patients may have pain that is troublesome throughout the illness and difficult to eradicate by treatment (7). Pain around the trunk or the abdomen in the region of the fracture is difficult to analyze, and unsuccessful abdominal investigations are often initiated. Headaches are common, although the explanation seems obscure.

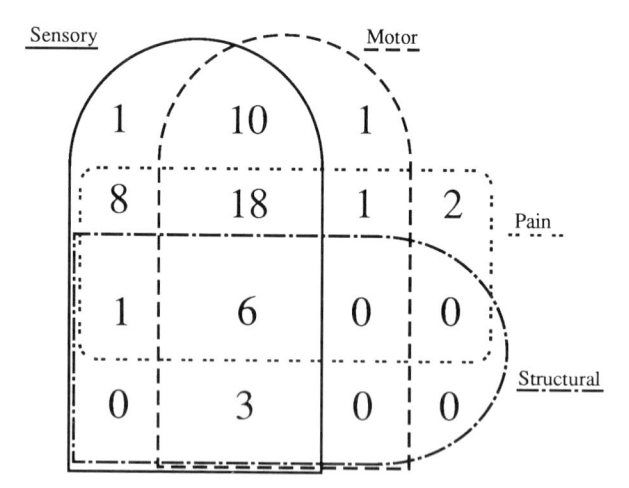

FIG. 11. Venn–Euler diagram of the symptom groupings in 51 cases of primarily spinal syringomyelia. These cases all have spinal arachnoiditis, but not all of them were traumatic. The numbers indicate the intersections of the symptom groupings. For example, only one patient had sensory abnormality without pain, one had motor abnormality without any other features, two had pain alone, and none of them had only structural changes. The largest group is when sensory, motor, and pain are involved, which is over one-third of the cases.

SENSORY LOSS

The classical loss of the gross syringomyelic is not often seen nor, for that matter, is it seen often in hindbrain-related cases in a modern practice (7,31). Most patients should be diagnosed before they develop neuropathic joints or have gross trophic changes, such as the thickened fingers of Marfan's syndrome, or scarring from painless burns. The dissociated nature of the loss, that is, the loss of pain and temperature sensation without the loss of light touch or joint movement sense, is the description of the classical neurological texts but, again, is not the commonest finding (7). Patients are often vague about their loss and do not find it easy to describe levels when tested for dermatomal involvement.

The area of involvement of the classical hindbrain-related case is often seen. It is unilateral and goes up to the side of the neck, involving the whole of the upper limb. This area tends to be involved early, and the advance of the sensory loss is more by increase in the severity of the loss rather than by extension of the involved area. Examiners on different days may obtain dissimilar maps. The losses are often both incomplete and fluctuant; the description that the hand feels as if it has a glove on, or is tingly or clumsy, is more common than the description of protopathic or spinothalamic loss when the patients describe loss of ability to discriminate temperature, sometimes even reversing the sensation and feeling cold for hot.

MOTOR LOSS

As with the sensory loss, the motor deficits are often vague, with variable severity from one day to another. Many patients feel strong until taking physical exercise when the arms, or more usually one arm, suddenly weaken. This has been reported by basketball players, weight lifters, a canoeist, and other athletes. As with the sensory loss, there may be sudden motor loss at any time. Sudden deterioration is again likely to be associated with a sudden strain, such as a fall from a wheelchair or a traffic accident (12) (see Case 4). Such sudden deteriorations are likely to leave a residual permanent deficit.

What might be described as the classical syringomyelic motor features are those of the involvement of the cervical enlargement by the cavity. Thus they often start with the small muscles of the hand. Wasting of the first dorsal interosseous is often an early sign and fasciculation is also most commonly seen at this site. Any muscle group may be affected first, triceps and scapular muscles. In the more fully developed case, the small muscles of the hand become so affected that there is a claw deformity followed by progressive loss of the forearm and upper arm musculature. As with the sensory losses, a dermatomal level is often not definable and generalized thinning of the upper limb musculature and nonspecific weakness with loss of the ability to transfer may be all the patient's motor complaints.

TENDON REFLEXES

Loss of the tendon reflexes in the arms may be due to damage to the reflex arc, the lower motor neuron, or the sensory relays in the dorsal horn of the gray matter. Sometimes the tendon reflexes are unexpectedly spared. Nevertheless, the careful scrutiny of the arm reflexes may be almost diagnostic in the early stages of the disease. Hoffmann's reflex and the long finger tendon flexors can also be sought, sometimes with clearly abnormal results. The triceps jerks, in particular, are easy to test in the majority of patients with upper limb pain or weakness due to peripheral nerve disease. There may only be an asymmetry, but all the tendon reflexes should be noted and the examination should be extensive.

STRUCTURAL CHANGES

Advancing structural changes are less common in the post-traumatic syringomyelia patients than in those who have hindbrain-related disease. Kyphoscoliosis is related to the fracture and has usually been corrected by the team looking after the original injury. Charcot joints do occur and may be severe because of the excessive use of the arms. Burns on the hands, which are painless, and trophic changes in the forms of contractures and thickening of the fingers are uncommon.

AUTONOMIC DYSFUNCTION

There may be more autonomic disturbances in the post-traumatic group of patients with syringomyelia than in the hindbrain-related cases. It might be thought that the general instability of the isolated cord was responsible, as in the tendency for paraplegic patients to suffer autonomic dysreflexia. Interesting features come from the cord above the injury.

Horner's syndrome (Bernard's syndrome) is more common in the post-traumatic cases than in hindbrain-related. The manifestations are often incomplete; anisocoria may be present without ptosis or sweating disturbance. The presumed affected site is the lateral gray matter, which contains sympathetic neurons. The relevant outflow is probably at T1. This is above the majority of thoracolumbar fractures and the exact explanation remains obscure. Horner's syndrome, which changes side with the patient's change of position, has also been seen, but no reports of this have been found in hindbrain-related syringomyelia.

The sweating disturbances found in post-traumatic syringomyelia are often gross (7,22). There may be hyperhidrosis or the skin may be dry. The lower body may be affected and the disturbance is likely to be symmetrical. Upper limb manifestations are often asymmetrical and may be associated with differences in skin color. Hyperhidrosis may be followed in a proportion of cases by dryness of the skin, which may extend upward to involve the face.

Asymmetry of vascular reactions on one side are not uncommon; blushing or anger may affect one side only, and the erythematous reaction to sunburn may affect one side more than the other.

CHANGES BELOW THE LEVEL OF INJURY

It is probable in the majority of cases with syringomyelia below the level of injury and not extending above that the diagnosis is not made. Only one such case has been seen in this clinic. The results in a partial paraplegic are more important than in a complete paraplegic. In the latter some of the changes may be beneficial; for instance, the reflex spasms that may have been troublesome may be lessened by the syrinx. In general, however, the changes are disadvantageous and include sweating disturbances and deteriorating bladder function with impairment of reflex emptying. In one illustrative patient, Case 2, the bowel dysfunction was so severe that a colostomy was necessary. It is not possible to be sure that the syringomyelia was responsible. Improved bladder function after treatment may be reported.

Reliable clinical evidence of a descending syrinx is loss of tendon reflexes. As with the reflexes in the arms, the pattern may reflect more destruction in the lumbar enlargement than in the intervening zone, and the ankle jerks may disappear while one or both knee jerks are preserved.

RADIOLOGY

The radiology of the acute injury may be of interest. Past thoracic damage may affect the choice of side for syringopleural shunting. Hemothorax is of significance. There is no correlation with the type of bony injury, whether the bony canal is large or small, or whether there is a reduced subluxation or not. Radiologic confirmation may be by myelography, endomyelography, postmyelography computed tomography (CT) examinations, and more recently by MRI examination.

MYELOGRAPHY

This is presently performed with water-soluble, nonionic contrast media. Myodil (Pantopaque, Iophendylate) is no longer used, although cases are still being seen in whom the arachnoiditis produced by injury may be complicated by effects of contrast medium.

Myelography will show localized arachnoiditis at the site of injury. Injections in the cervical spine are probably more informative than injections after lumbar puncture, but lumbar puncture is painless in the complete paraplegic. The cisternal route is safe; hindbrain herniation is unlikely. There may be septa and dilated, pouchlike structures formed by thin membranes in the subarachnoid space that are not well seen on MRI scan. The usual result is that some contrast will pass the obstruction. Sometimes there appears to be a complete block. The diameters of the cord above or below the fracture may be enlarged. The patients may have an enlarged cord with no symptoms, or they may have egregious symptoms with normal cord diameters. The radiologic confirmation of a syrinx is better done by demonstration of the cavity than by looking at the external diameter.

Contrast may sometimes enter the cavity of the syringomyelia immediately. This is uncommon, and when it occurs it usually does so from the injection of contrast into the lumbar sac, below the site of injury. There are a few cases in which a communication has been recorded (13,20).

Entry of contrast into the syrinx cavity is shown on postmyelographic CT scans. This will also demonstrate, almost always, that the contrast has gone past the site of obstruction in the subarachnoid space (21). A scheme of postmyelographic imaging is to view the region of the filling mechanism—in the post-traumatic cases this is the fracture site—in detail at about 1 hr. Sometimes positive contrast is in the syrinx at this stage, but it is uncommon and suggests a relatively free communication as mentioned above. If the myelogram is done in the morning, then it is often convenient for the scan to be repeated at the end of the working day, about 4 to 6 hr after the first scan (29,31). At this time careful axial cuts should be done from the site of the cord damage to the areas of clinical suspicion, usually up to the medulla and down to the conus. Tiny cavities may be picked up in this way when an MRI scan may be unsuccessful (Fig. 12).

In a proportion of cases the situation in respect to intracord cavities will be unclear at 6 hr and repeat scans on the morning after myelography, at about 22 to 24 hr, may show a cavity clearly compared with the subarachnoid space, which will largely be free of contrast at that time.

The timing of the filling of the cavities and the relative density of the opacification do not shed any light on the filling mechanism. The cavity in a tumor case, where there is an intrinsic cord tumor producing a proteinaceous fluid and where the filling of the syrinx is almost certainly due to the secretion of the fluid from the tissue of the tumor, may be as striking as that seen in cases where the fluid is presumably forced in by anatomic variations at the site of the injury.

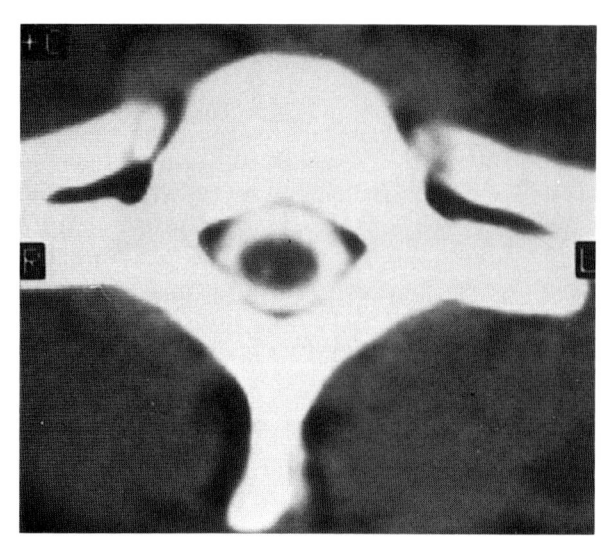

FIG. 12. Postmyelography CT scan is useful for picking up tiny cavities, and its resolution may exceed that of the MRI scanner depending on equipment quality. In this case, a tiny cavity can be seen on the right to correlate with clinical symptoms and confirm the diagnosis.

ENDOMYELOGRAPHY

Endomyelography may be carried out by injection of contrast medium into the syrinx cavity by direct cord puncture. Lateral cervical puncture for post-traumatic syringomyelia has been described (21). The results are not vital for the surgeon; the pictures are much the same as each other. Once a tightly filling syrinx is established, the treatment is clear and the extent or the width of the syrinx is irrelevant. A surgeon about to operate for post-traumatic syringomyelia would like to know the anatomy of the region close to the fracture. Does the upper cavity communicate with the lower one? Does the patient have a primary cyst that is separated by a septum from the upper syrinx? Are there other septa close to the site of proposed insertion of the drain? These things are useful to know, but in my practice endomyelography is seldom used.

There is a limited value in extensive radiological studies. A careful exploration yields more information about the nature of the local arachnoiditis, which is difficult to assess radiologically. Perioperative ultrasound is of value for finding cysts and sepation (15).

MAGNETIC RESONANCE IMAGING

MRI scanning provides the quickest and most complete images of the syringomyelia cavities and shows the tension in the cyst as well as the presence and number of the septa (1,14,15,21). The disadvantages include the poor quality of scanners available, the use of surface coils leaving the edges of the picture dark, and difficulty in imaging all parts of the syrinx on one pic-

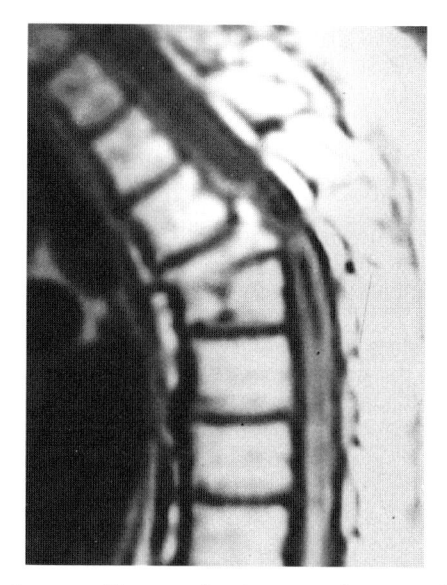

FIG. 13. A case with a small primary syrinx exactly opposite the fracture. There is an almost equally small, insignificant looking syringomyelia below this, stretching for just over three vertebrae, which would not justify surgery. The syrinx above the fracture is tightly full and has multiple septations in it. The axial cuts showed a perfectly round tense cavity that went up as high as C2. The patient was beginning to suffer motor deficit, and surgery in a case of this kind should be regarded as urgent.

ture when scoliosis or other causes of malalignment are present in relation to the fracture (Case 3) (Figs. 13 and 14). Although septa may be seen, and may be imaged on axial cuts, it is not possible to be sure whether they are intact or perforated because the septa neither

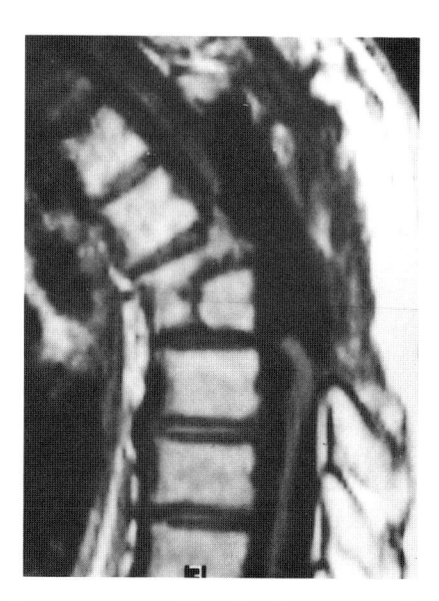

FIG. 14. Same case as Fig. 13 after transection of the cord and syringopleural shunt. The upper cavity has almost completely disappeared. The cord below has folded over slightly. Note the sizeable artificial meningocele that is probably more responsible for the success of this operation than the drain.

keep still, nor are they flat. The septations almost certainly move in time with even minor pulsations.

Images weighted to show CSF, as in Fig. 2, may show the CSF pathways clearly but sometimes it is difficult to be sure whether the signal is intrasyrinx or subarachnoid. Development of MRI will bring improvements in syringomyelia management. Techniques for straightening out the spine so that all of the syrinx appears on one image and methods of carrying out cine MRI, perhaps combined with stress testing of the CSF pathways, must contribute more, not only to understanding the pathogenesis but also to surgical management of these cases. Flow void is easily seen in T2-weighted images and cine MRI techniques are being developed to illustrate flow. MRI has often been omitted in the preoperative assessment of my cases but has proved invaluable in outpatient surveillance.

TREATMENT

Rossier made the statement that there was no benefit in operating on a patient with a small syrinx (19). All large syrinxes were small at some stage and it seems likely that if they were competently treated then, they would not become large. A counsel of perfection would be to treat when it was demonstrated that cavities were enlarging but before they become symptomatic. There is no possibility, however, of any large series having no postoperative complication rate, and if small syrinxes could be shown to resolve or to remain asymptomatic frequently, then a waiting policy might be justifiable with small syrinxes that were silent or giving only minimal problems.

The state of the remaining cord function below the injury is obviously important in deciding the timing of operation. A partial paraplegic with adequate bladder and sexual function who can walk well enough to get around at work is only likely to be interested in an operation with no complication rate.

INDICATION FOR OPERATION

A tensely full syrinx extending for several segments upward to involve the cervical enlargement demands operation. It does not matter what the symptoms are or even if the patient is asymptomatic. Such lesions are dangerous and neurologic deficits are likely to progress suddenly and not to be reversible.

A modest sized cavity in a cord opposite a fracture and not extending for more than one vertebra does not demand operation. If symptoms are not attributable to it and especially if there is only a partial paraplegia, then the probability is that it should not be operated on.

In between these two extremes there lies a difficult set of decisions. The difficulty comes in interpreting whether or not a cyst is "tense" and what is the significance of the extent of the cavities. Additionally, the severity and type of symptoms have to be taken into account when the radiologic indications are unclear. Total as opposed to incomplete paraplegia may swing a decision toward early operation. Ascent of the level of loss is unacceptable in either the cervical or the lumbar enlargements and since the level of functioning tissue is sometimes difficult to ascertain, laminectomy may best be avoided in some patients.

WHEN TO TREAT

The onset of symptoms may be sudden and involve loss of function that never returns. The complication rate of laminectomy and production of an artificial meningocele must be low, and it seems likely that this will suffice for small syrinxes in partial paraplegics or patients with injuries of the cervical or lumbar enlargements where drainage via a myelotomy might be hazardous. Early treatment has a good deal to commend it.

PRINCIPLES OF TREATMENT

Drainage, by whatever route, may be insufficient. Preferable is removal of the cause rather than the drainage of the resulting abnormality. The cause of the syrinx, that is, the place where the greater part of the fluid gets into the cavity, is almost certainly at the site of the fracture. If the cavity is drained, it will go flat, and parts of the wall may adhere internally. Flattening the cavity will almost certainly block the draining catheter. Healing of the cavity does not prevent another cavity from developing alongside it or at a different level (2). If there is a filling mechanism still acting, or even if there is a sizeable residual syrinx in another part of the cord, then a new syrinx may readily form alongside the flattened syrinx. In illustrative Cases 1 and 5, recurrence was affecting another part of the cord. Sometimes the syrinx changes sides. Treatment should therefore be directed at the cause, or specifically to the disablement, of the filling mechanism.

The creation of a free access of the fluid to traverse the site of the injury in an upward or downward direction is therefore the most logical step to take in the management of this disorder. The prevention of a postoperative arachnoiditis is part of this aim.

The next most desirable feature is to prevent the cord from being held open at the site of the arachnoiditis, making it easy for fluid to pass into the site of the primary cavity. The drainage of the syrinx is subsidiary to the above aims; the maneuver is worth doing because it helps to open up the subarachnoid spaces and encourages the syrinx cavity to heal. The contention that the widest part of the syrinx should be drained (2) is open to criticism if the filling mechanism remains intact.

STANDARD OPERATION

The standard operation that I have evolved in my own practice is illustrated between Figs. 15 and 17.

The incision is made over at least three laminae and preferably five. The soft tissue, epidural fat, and ligamentum flavum are removed from the inside of the laminae before the dura is flapped up. The aim is to gain a smooth access for the CSF from the subarachnoid space to the artificial meningocele. As the dura is opened, a small piece may be taken out to use as a graft. The dura is sutured backward along the sides of the wound; the ends of the dura are not left as a slit but are converted into a V-shaped flap as shown in Fig. 15. If left as a slit, then suturing the dura backward tends

FIG. 15. Standard operation as described in the text. Note the long laminectomy. The dura is sutured upward and downward with a flap at the ends of the incision. A small patch is taken from the dura to seal off the myelotomy. Arachnoid is opened and carefully sutured back.

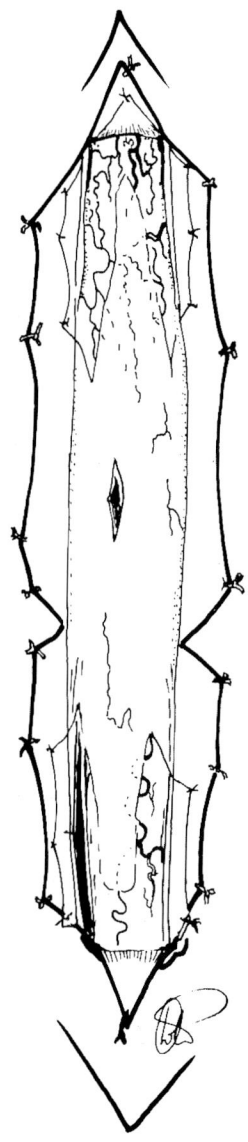

FIG. 16. After opening up the subarachnoid spaces at the top and the bottom a myelotomy is made. If a probe passed upward encounters a septum, a separate myelotomy may be necessary at a higher site. If a septum is encountered just beyond the top of the laminectomy, then it is probable that draining the accessible part of the syrinx and opening the subarachnoid spaces will provide a cure. The decision is facilitated by making a large laminectomy.

to produce a narrowing. The arachnoid is difficult to handle; it is often loosely adherent at the ends of the exposure to the middle of the spinal cord. It may therefore be divided laterally more easily than close to the midline as shown in Fig. 17. It adheres to the pia at the site of the fracture and should be undissected. The arachnoid may be sutured upward after the dura is in position. Sometimes part of the dentate ligament may be divided and sutured up with it. If it is divided close to the cord, the dentate ligament will take a suture more readily than the filmy arachnoid. The use of a micro-

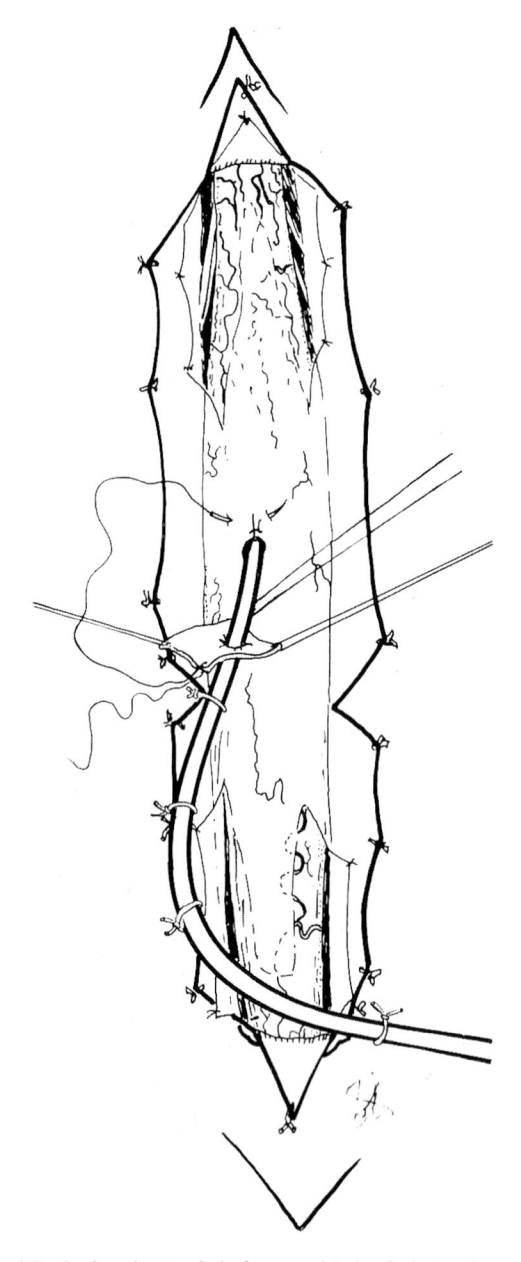

FIG. 17. A simple straightforward tube is introduced and the cord sutured to narrow the myelotomy. Big sutures should be avoided in a partial paraplegic, and Tisseel may be preferred to fasten the patch in position. Note that the drainage tube must be securely sutured to surrounding structures.

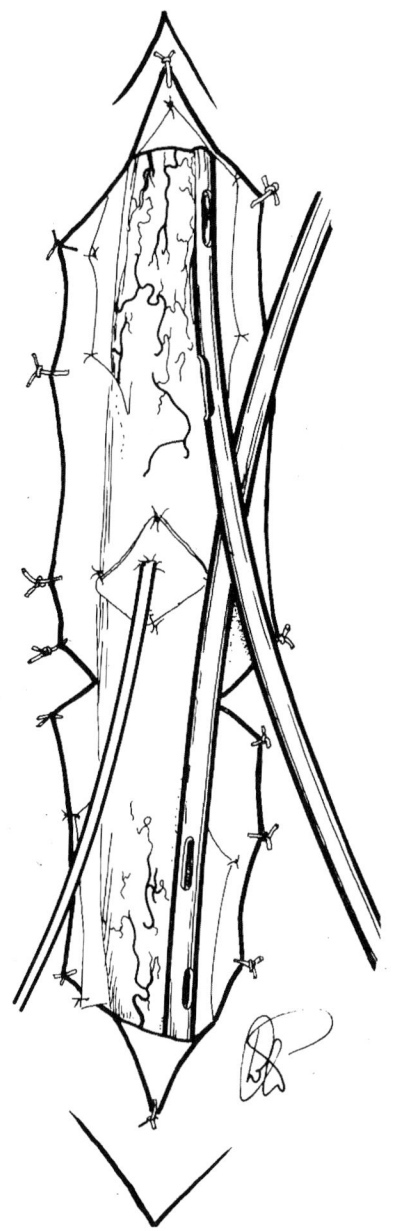

FIG. 18. The subarachnoid space may be held open by the use of stents. In this case two pediatric chest drainage tubes of 12 French gauge have been used to hold open the subarachnoid space and maintain its continuity with the artificial meningocele. They can be removed after 2 or 3 days. If the syrinx is drained externally it may be removed at the same time.

scope is helpful for this part of the procedure. Good clearance of the arachnoid above and below is probably the most essential part of the procedure. Nerve roots passing the site of maximum cord drainage may be functional and should be respected (Figs. 15–17).

The myelotomy site can be chosen anywhere that is convenient in the total paraplegic but in the partial paraplegic the myelotomy site needs to be chosen with care. The midline and the posterior root entry zone are the usual sites.

If the drainage tube is to be inserted into a low-pressure extrathecal area such as the pleura or peritoneum, care must be taken to prevent fluid from entering the myelotomy site. A dural patch as shown in Figs. 17 and 18 may be sutured or fastened with Tisseel (immunofibrin glue).

DECOMPRESSION

The place of pulsation in the etiology and the maintenance of the syrinx is discussed above. The creation of a free access of the fluid to traverse the site of the injury in an upward or downward direction is therefore desirable in the management of this disorder.

The abolition of the pressure differences and the opening up of the constriction associated with the arachnoiditis or the backward gibbus of damaged bones seem important. Even in a patient with partial preservation of cord function, as in Case 1, leaving the dura open may be associated with improvement.

Closure of the dura may be likened to closing the breech of a gun. It reconstitutes the barrel formed by the dura and enables the fluid, which finds its way into the cord, to be violently propelled upward under the influence of violent pressure changes, such as coughing, and to excavate new cavities or keep the existing cavities under tension. Nonclosure of the dura may be the most important surgical prophylaxis against this group of disorders.

Grafts provoke fibrosis. A Silastic graft will cause dense fibrosis on the back and on the front surface. Fascia lata grafts seek a blood supply. If they lie against cord and roots, the grafts will often adhere, giving a more severe arachnoiditis than previously.

When closing a laminectomy, some blood inevitably runs down and coats the back of the cord and blocks the subarachnoid spaces. To keep the passageway open between the subarachnoid spaces above and below and the artificial meningocele stents may be left as shown in Fig. 18 and removed through the skin after 2 or 3 days.

SYRINGOSUBARACHNOID SHUNTING

The use of syrinx to subarachnoid shunting, although it is frequently successful as reported by Barnett and co-workers (4,5), McLean et al. (13), and others (24,33), may be criticized. There may be some residual elasticity in the cord that allows a myelotomy to deflate a syrinx. Such a hole in the cord may allow a cavity to fill as well as to empty. Any drainage tube or "wick" left to keep a myelotomy open may provoke further fibrosis.

DRAINAGE TO PLEURA OR PERITONEUM

If the cavity is to be effectively drained, it should probably not be by a variety of myelotomy but by a shunt to a low-pressure area such as the pleura or the peritoneum (3,11,13,29,31,32). Drainage of the cord to the pleura, or externally, has the advantage that the space-occupying qualities of the enlarged cord are lessened and the subarachnoid spaces are opened up after the collapse of the swollen syrinx.

I presently favor a simple drainage tube with multiple perforations. Metal junction pieces interfere with imaging and silicone Y-, K-, or T-shaped tubes all require big myelotomies.

It is not always easy to find the cavity. Perioperative ultrasound may help. The important thing is to put the tube in so that it *must* work. It must go right into the syrinx cavity, not alongside it, for 2 in. at least. The bottom end must go into the pleura.

Care must be taken to keep the lung pressure high and not to damage the lung. Air in the pleural cavity may cause the syrinx to inflate with air, in time with the respirator. This provides proof of patency of the drain but is not a pretty sight.

VALVES OR NOT?

The purpose of valves such as Holter, Hakim, or Pudenz valves as used in ventriculoatrial or ventriculoperitoneal shunting of CSF from the ventricles in the treatment of hydrocephalus is not only to prevent reflux but, more importantly, to prevent overshunting with resultant collapse of the ventricular system and the production of serious complications such as acute subdural hematomas.

They have the advantage that they can sometimes be palpably pumped, and sometimes CSF can be aspirated to establish the patency of differing parts of the system.

None of these factors apply to valves when draining the inside of a syrinx. The point of a hydrocephalus shunt is to lower the pressure to normal. In the majority of post-traumatic syringomyelia patients, the overall CSF pressure is normal because the absorptive mechanism in the head is intact. The intention is to flatten the cavity; the cavity is abnormal, unlike the cerebral ventricles, which are normal and should not be flattened. There is no likelihood that the syrinx will fill up so rapidly that the shunt needs to run for a while. The probability is that the flow through the drain is minuscule (2) and soon stops.

If a hydrocephalus shunt is put in the drainage system, it complicates the system and if it keeps the pressure up in the normal range the valve may stop it from working. Therefore, do not put in a valve.

AVOIDANCE OF DRAINS

I do not use drains in the treatment of midbrain-related syringomyelia. If the primary treatment to negate the filling mechanisms is successful, the drain only provides unwelcome complications. Particularly in partial paraplegics, the myelotomy or the increase in local irritation produced by having a drainage tube may be adverse features. It is therefore reasonable to abjure the use of syrinx drains altogether. I am having success using this method.

DIVISION OF THE CORD

The most effective disablement of the filling mechanism is excision of the area of damaged cord as shown in Fig. 19. This recommendation was also made by Durward, et al. (6). The thinned cord, through which the CSF almost certainly enters, and the zone of arachnoiditis are thereby removed, the funnel-shaped lower end of the upper syrinx is closed, and the drainage tube is conveniently placed. Maximal access to the subarachnoid space of surging fluid is thereby attained. Of my personal cases with cord transection in this series, none has deteriorated after operation. This technique is limited to complete lesions (29–33).

The removal of the damaged area of cord may also be indicated for the removal of dysfunctional tissue, which may be thought responsible for pain (6).

ILLUSTRATIVE CASES

CASE 1. This man was born normally and was well until his road traffic accident at the age of 21. He was strapped in a car and sustained fractures of L3 and T9. The patient had an almost complete paraplegia at T9 with a little preservation of perineal and bladder sensation. At the age of 25, while competing in the Stoke Mandeville games, he noted a severe pain across the top of his shoulder brought on by a cough. Subsequent coughing caused exacerbation. He then had "a sort of cramping feeling" in the left hand. He then noted that hot objects in the left hand felt cold and vice versa. This inversion passed after months and became replaced by a more dense loss of sensation, which spread into the face and up to the vertex of the head. He had a period of marked hyperhidrosis in the legs, which was symmetrical but which lessened over several months.

Investigations showed an expanded cord immediately above and below the T9 fracture. Since he had no pain and no motor losses, he was reluctant to have

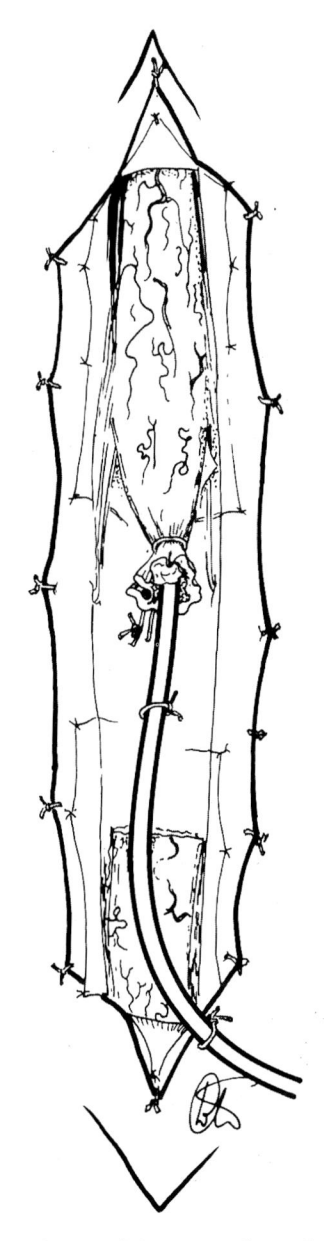

FIG. 19. The most complete correction of syringomyelia when paraplegia is total is to transect the area of damage and to close off the bottom end with a drain. The cord should be sutured to the posterior longitudinal ligament to prevent it migrating upward.

surgery. After some months during which he did not improve, he agreed to have this done.

A syringopleural shunt was done at around T3 or T4 and the drainage tube passed upward to C5 or C6; the cord was enlarged.

Postoperatively there was a slight increase in sensation on the left side but little improvement in the trigeminal loss. Three and a half years later, at the age of 32, he had a sudden relapse with sensory loss on the right side although his previous symptoms had been on the left. There was aggravation of pain in the neck and some weakness of both arms; the patient was alarmed

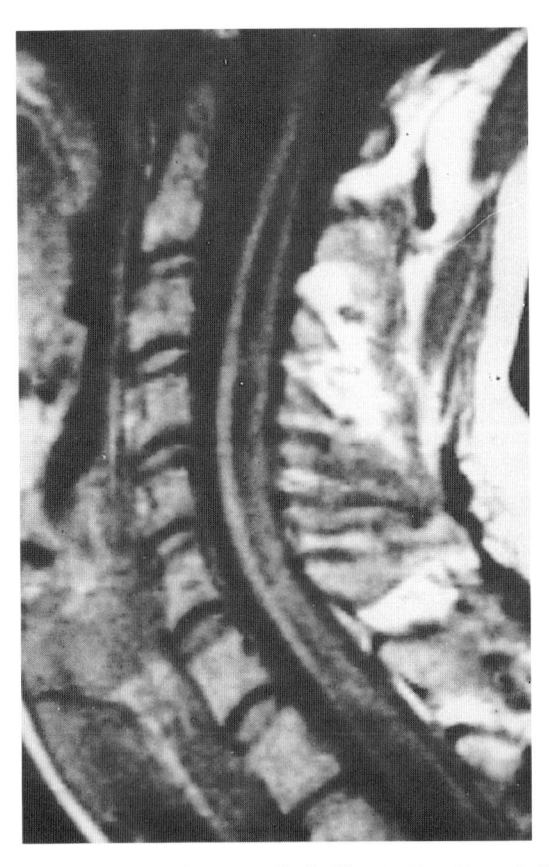

FIG. 20. Cervical syringomyelia in illustrative Case 2. This syrinx is not tense but it is big enough to threaten arm function and to be associated with extensive sensory loss.

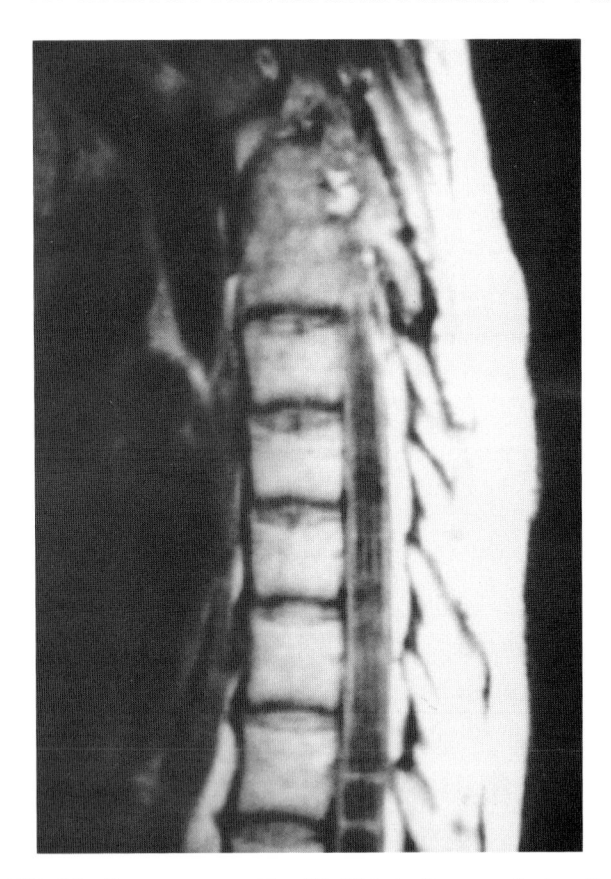

FIG. 21. Same case as Fig. 20. This is the area below the fracture. It can be seen that the syrinx is extremely tense; there are two well-formed septations at the bottom of the scan. Vertical lines can be seen as the white matter columns standing out against the distending syrinx. This patient had severe bladder and bowel problems, which may well have been contributed to by the syrinx.

at the change of side although the left-sided symptoms had not worsened. Postmyelography CT scans showed a small syrinx. He was advised to have the cord transected or ligated above the site of maximum arachnoiditis but the patient then declined.

Five years later MRI scan showed a tapered thin-walled syrinx going up for 2½ vertebrae above the fracture. There were microcystic changes in the cord of the neck, particularly opposite C5–C6.

Myelography failed to confirm the suspicion of cervical compression from discs. It seems probable that the problems of this man were not properly addressed because the site of damage was not operated on. T3 was chosen because it would drain the cervical enlargement without a myelotomy at that site.

CASE 2. This girl was 15 at the time of a motorcycle accident, which left her a total paraplegic from a T5–T6 fracture. At the time of her examination 2 years later for insurance purposes, she had a dissociated sensory loss in the right forequarter. She was reassured by the neurologist that cysts within the cord that did not progress to motor loss did not require treatment. After some years she sought further advice about this persisting problem.

On examination at the age of 25, she had no motor loss and no gross autonomic features although she had excessive "goosebumps" and sometimes excessive sweating. Colostomy had been done for bowel problems.

MRI showed the syrinx to extend from C1 to the conus. Although the upper syrinx was not tight, the lower part of the cord was tightly filled with some septations present (Figs. 20 and 21). Operation was advised and a section of cord about 1.5 cm long was removed including the most damaged part. A complete septum was discovered at surgery about 1 cm above the site of cord transection. A drain was used to the right pleural cavity. It was inserted in the manner shown in Fig. 19, but no attempt was made to drain the lower syrinx. There was immediate improvement in the sensory loss and the left side, which she had previously thought of as normal, felt a deep and unpleasant itching. She developed an intermittent and variable left

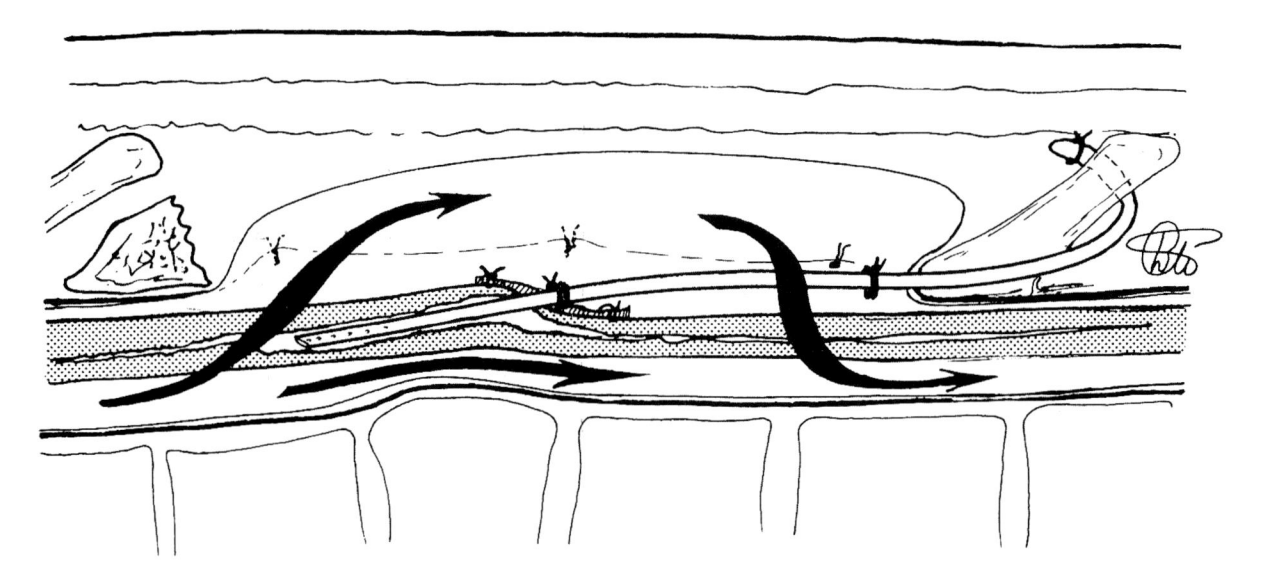

FIG. 22. In a partial paraplegic where the cord is not to be divided, the ideal operative result is suggested here. The ventral pathway may not be opened up as suggested by the *arrow*, but, provided a free access is available from the subarachnoid space to the artificial meningocele, pressure differences are minimized and an adequate depulsation is provided.

pupillary dilatation without ptosis (Fig. 22). She suffered a marked change in the autonomic responses of the skin so that the left side flushed more strongly than the right in response to anger or embarrassment. Reddening due to sunburn was symmetrical.

Three weeks after discharge from hospital she developed severe headache, which came on overnight. This was eased slightly by lying down. At the time of her readmission there had been slight improvement but the pain was still exaggerated by either sitting up or lying with the right side down. There were no signs of infection. The MRI scans showed an excellent result (Figs. 23 and 24). The CSF pressure was unrecordably low. It seemed the drainage tube had become dislodged, and that low CSF pressure due to overshunting was the cause of her problem. The cord had not been sutured to the posterior ligament as in Fig. 19. The shunt was removed without reopening the laminectomy. The recovery of the headache was immediate. A repeat MRI scan 1 year after the shunt removal showed unchanged appearances with the upper and lower syrinx greatly collapsed, although the septations were still visible. Power remained full. The sensation had improved with the only residual sensory loss being along the inner border of the right forearm and palm. There was no change in her other signs; she thought her hands were more nimble and precise than before operation. Her intermittent anisocoria, presumably due to a partial right Horner's syndrome, remained.

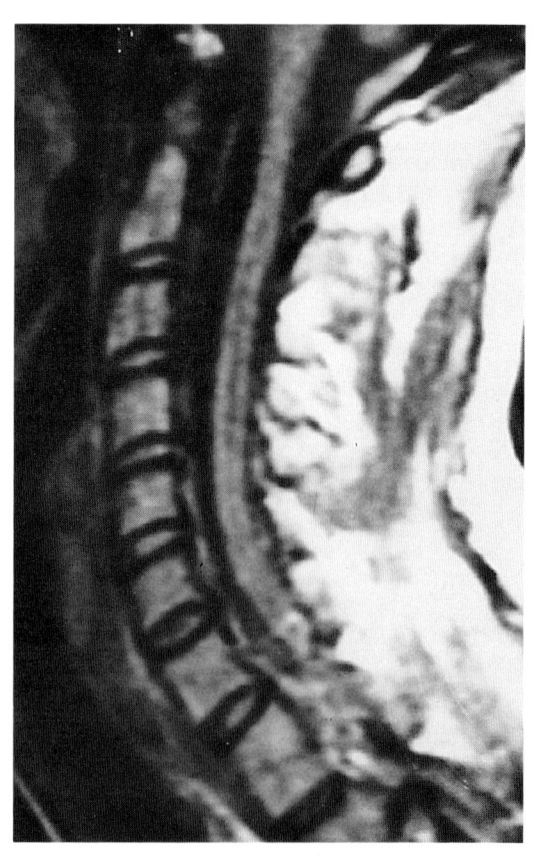

FIG. 23. Case 2 postoperative. Note the improvement in filling of the upper syrinx cavity when compared with Fig. 21. There was marked clinical improvement.

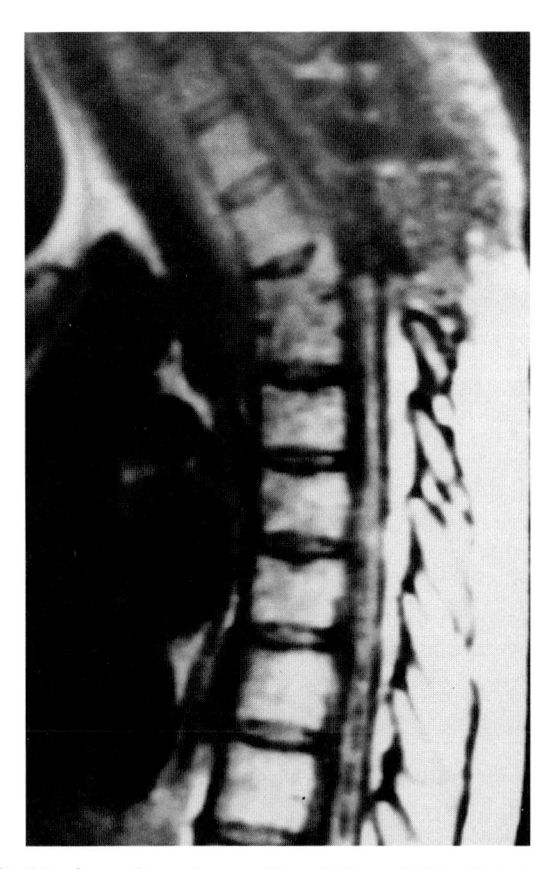

FIG. 24. Case 2 postoperative. It is notable that, in this case, the drain was only put into the upper syrinx but the transection and the artificial meningocele have produced a striking improvement in the appearance of the lower syrinx, which was not drained. This is common and suggests that the drainage is not so important as the concept of disabling the filling mechanism.

CASE 3. This man was thrown off a city wall and sustained an immediate complete paraplegia from a T6–T7 fracture. There was a bilateral hemothorax and hemomediastinum. A left-sided syringomyelia syndrome developed gradually and was diagnosed within 2 years of the assault. There was no impulse-related feature. The sensory features were of "a painful tingly numbness" with dissociated loss and an interscapular pain. There was no weakness, the power was full, the left triceps jerk was depressed, and the biceps and supinator jerks absent. He had noted increased sweating of the right leg and had had bladder difficulties treated by sphincterotomy.

MRI scanning (see Figs. 13 and 14) showed a tight, multiseptated syrinx from C1 to the upper dorsal region. At operation the cord was divided above what seemed to be a complete septum, and a neat, almost complete septum with a small round hole in the center was identified above the level of transection. A drain was inserted upward, and the cord was sutured around it, to the posterior longitudinal ligament to prevent ascent.

Postoperatively, the patient reported immediate sensory improvement, which continued to improve for many weeks. There was also some bladder improvement. Postoperative MRI scans confirm the flattening of the syrinx (Fig. 14).

CASE 4. A 21-year-old woman was involved in a traffic accident in 1970 with a crush fracture of T5 and complete paraplegia. Just over 2 years later she noted numbness of the left side of the face going down to the level of the paraplegic sensory loss. The tendon reflexes were depressed in the left arm. There were no motor features and it was thought justifiable to leave the condition unoperated and uninvestigated. She followed advice to curtail physical activity but remained able to transfer, drive, dress herself, and perform her own toilet functions until a second road traffic accident in 1985. In this injury she was severely jolted but sustained no fractures and no head injury. Immediately after this she had severe neck pain and marked increase in the leg spasms. She lost the ability to transfer and had to give up her job. She thought that she was unable to transfer because of the spasms rather than because of weakness. There was loss of dexterity, general "stiffening up" of the hand, and the arm generally was clinically assessed as slightly weakened. Sensory loss was bilateral at this stage but still left more than right. MRI examination confirmed a tense syrinx from the medulla to T7 with a constriction at T5.

At the age of 38 she consented to operation, although she was worried about the bladder getting worse because she had a partially automatic bladder which she thought might be giving some sensation. She agreed that transection should be left to the surgeon's judgment. Dorsal laminectomy was done, as were resection and ligation of a severely damaged part of the cord that did not seem possibly to be functional, with a syringopleural drain from the upper syrinx to the right pleural cavity.

There was some immediate improvement. She could make a fist, for instance, on the day after operation; previously she could not. Six weeks later the arms were stronger and the hands more nimble. Sensation improved on both sides but was not back to normal, with left remaining worse than right. The pain disappeared from the neck and arms. Spasms in the legs seemed immediately worse but improved about 3 or 4 months after the operation. The bladder function was unchanged. She was able to get back to work for the first time since her second accident.

MRI scan postop showed marked diminution in syrinx size. The result in this case could almost certainly have been improved if operation had been undertaken at the time of diagnosis.

CASE 5. This man fell off rocks at the age of 22, sustaining a fracture of L1 with a severe conus lesion. It was difficult to be sure if this was complete or not. He had good dorsiflexion of the feet but no useful calf muscle power; the buttock area and posterior perineum were partly numb but the bladder, bowel, and sexual functions seemed almost normal.

Syringomyelia features started 2 years after injury with a burning sensation in the left side of the abdomen, which ascended slowly over a further year to affect the thorax and the arm. His bladder control worsened so that he was occasionally incontinent. On examination at the age of 25 the motor power of the arms was normal. Tendon reflexes were depressed in the arms and the left knee; abdominal reflexes were absent on the left together with the left gluteal reflex. Sensation showed the most intense loss on the ulnar border of the left arm. There was generalized depression of sensitivity over the left side up to the face with sparing of the front of the left thigh. Endomyelography was unsuccessfully attempted together with attempted removal of Myodil (Iopamidol), which had been put in elsewhere. Myelography showed a complete blockage of the subarachnoid space; the cord was not discernibly enlarged. Operation was projected but because of the good function in the conus and the severe increase in deficit that might be expected if the neurological level were to ascend even one level, the laminectomy and the dissection of the conus were approached in a cautious manner. At laminectomy there was no enlargement of the conus; the damaged area was not fully exposed because of the fear of damaging the cord above the neurological level. Four attempts to obtain fluid by needling were unsuccessful. A terminal ventriculostomy was done, partly because it was hoped that the laminectomy itself might have been effective through altering the pulsatile dynamics of the situation and partly because Gardner has claimed that the central canal down to the filum may be successful in draining all syrinxes.

The initial result was successful with improvement of the sensation in the left hand and also the backs of both legs. He needed to intermittently catheterize for 5 days but then improved to his normal standard. The tendon jerks returned, although less briskly than on the right. He thought that the legs were stronger, but this was difficult to verify objectively. He stabilized over several months with improved thermal sensation over part of the left arm and the fingertips.

Three months after operation he noticed a stabbing back pain followed by the ascent of numbness from the iliac crest to the sternum on the left side only, with no further involvement of the leg. This was similar to the sensations accompanying the initial involvement and slowly spread again to reinvolve the arm. During a bout of influenza in which he had a cough, the symptoms spread to involve the previous area and hot and cold again became indistinguishable over the entire left arm. The sensory loss spread into the back of the scalp. Hyperhidrosis developed over the entire left side. The left arm became mildly weak. The condition slowly progressed and 9 months after the operation he became incontinent of urine.

The examination findings were that the tendon reflexes had again disappeared. Three years after the initial operation it was clear that all the benefits of that procedure had been erased and that his condition was worse than preoperative. He observed that if he sneezed while standing up it made him feel ill for a long period, but that if he laid down sneezing was not troublesome.

Reoperation was considered. Myelography with follow-on CT scan confirmed a cavity from the medulla down to T5; the cavity was not visible below this level.

A low cervical laminectomy was therefore done with a syrinx to pleural shunt. The improvement once again affected all modalities of cord function. Although the legs had not seemed to be much affected, the improvement in sensation was greater than after the first operation. The improvements persisted without relapse for 2 years. Symptoms then started in the right upper limb.

He was readmitted for investigations at the age of 30. The residual signs in the left arm were much as before: there were no motor, reflex, or gross sensory signs in the right arm. There was still a complete block at L1. Follow-on CT scans showed there to be apparently three separate syrinx cavities in the cord just above the fracture, which dwindled in the upper thoracic cord, and two small syrinxes, on each side in the cervical region. It seemed likely that these five cavities were communicating with each other to some extent but they might have been completely separate.

None of these seemed big enough to drain and the question of reoperating at the original site was discussed with the risks to the lumbar enlargement function being observed. It was again decided to await events.

Five years later at the age of 36 it was clear that the situation was deteriorating unrelentingly. The left hand was developing weakness with wasting and with claw deformity, the sensory picture was worsening such that the risks to the lumbar enlargement of the cord would have to be faced in view of the necessity to act to save his arms. MRI at this time showed one big syrinx. The cervical syringopleural shunt was plainly not working.

Reexploration of the lumbar enlargement was carried out with a marked upward extension of the laminectomy. The area of the Silastic graft showed severe fibrosis all around the graft on both the back of the cord and behind the graft. The syrinx was entirely above the zone of dense fibrosis. This was partly cut away and the arachnoid dissected upward beyond the zone of arachnoiditis. A midline myelotomy was made and a drain inserted. It was brought through the skin and drained into a bile bag. Two temporary stents were used to open the arachnoid spaces into the artificial cisterna magna. They were brought out through the skin and all the drains were removed after a few days. The improvements were again striking but varied greatly from day to day in the immediate postoperative period. The long-term results are awaited but MRI examinations at 18 months and clinical results at 2 years are excellent. The message from this case is that boldness is necessary and also that drainage away from the filling mechanism is ineffective.

RESULTS

Short-term results in the surgical management of post-traumatic syringomyelia are excellent for the production of improvement in the cord signs. In partial paraplegics the results are relatively worse than in complete paraplegics. Myelotomy often produces a deficit and part of the problem in such cases is commonly due to progressive gliosis and collagenosis from arachnoid adhesions as well as disordered CSF pulsation.

Barbaro (2) has recently tried to analyze published work and has indicated widespread disarray in publications dealing with results (3,12,18,19,21,26,32,33).

Some authors do not distinguish between types of syringomyelia or between complete and incomplete paraplegics and most authors, such as myself, have operated by varying techniques as their experience increased. They are always beset by the problem that the most recent variation in their operative technique seems to be yielding the best results precisely because they are the most recent and the short-term results are best.

There is not much value in analyzing whether it is pain, motor, sensory, or autonomic features which do best. All the symptoms are likely to improve. The important observations are that it is the cases who are operated on early that do best (3), that if the cases are untreated then a significant proportion will worsen (5,19), sometimes suddenly (Case 4), and that MRI surveillance plus reintervention when necessary is likely to provide the best long-term management.

Specific complications deserve a mention. Displacement of drainage tubes is an obvious complication and this may produce overshuntage of the CSF pathways with headaches (Case 2) or even subdural hematomas. Sepsis or wound breakdown are no commoner than in the rest of neurosurgery; in my own cases I have had no sepsis and only one wound that required resuturing.

FUTURE WORK

Further analysis of surgical material, particularly the correlation of morphological variants such as the type of local cyst, the existence of septations, and the odd occurrence of a completely blocked zone at the site of injury with separate cysts below and above needs to be done. The morphology may be correlated with the possibly bimodal distribution of the time of onset of the syrinx after the trauma in the post-traumatic cases.

It is a matter of some urgency to see how many paraplegic cases get small syrinxes, at what age they arise, and how many of them enlarge or become symptomatic. Prognostic features may be identified from the morphology. Early syrinxes may heal. Serial MRI scans from a sizeable population at an early stage may identify what proportion of cases have an early hematoma and what fraction of these then become a clear fluid-containing cavity. How many of these then develop a syrinx? In how many cases will a syrinx form without any seminal cavity?

Routine MRI scans after both conservatively managed paraplegia and those managed with the aid of cord exploration and myelotomy may well yield information in favor of either system. It seems likely that evacuation of a hematoma followed by leaving the dura open will minimize the chances of a syrinx developing. The likelihood of syringomyelia, occurring in less than 5% of paraplegics, of course would not constitute a sole or sufficient indication for cord exploration in the acute stage, and the need for stabilization of the bones of the spine is a dominating requirement at the time of injury.

Perhaps the most immediate chance for improving the management of these patients lies in the refinement of MRI techniques to analyze the filling mechanisms in small cyst cases. The passive, low-pressure cyst that merely occupies the space formerly occupied by cord, which has now gone necrotic, may well look different from the tense cyst burgeoning with jets of cerebrospinal fluid, which is about to spread upward into new regions of the cord.

CONCLUSIONS

Post-traumatic syringomyelia is an uncommon but important late complication of all spinal features above L2 whether or not paraplegia persists.

The clinical presentation is variable and includes pain and sweating disturbances as well as the more obvious and frequently expected sensory and motor disturbances. Frequent MRI examinations of post-trauma patients may be the most effective method of monitoring for its occurrence. Large steel prostheses impede all varieties of imaging and should be avoided if possible or removed if doubt persists. Titanium or carbon fiber prostheses may be preferable because of their lack of magnetic properties. Loops should be avoided, if possible, because of the effects of electrical circuits becoming established within these loops.

If cystic dilatation of the cord is present, consideration should be given to surgery. Specialist centers with particular expertise are better placed to give advice than individual surgeons without comprehensive experience.

Long, tense syrinxes affecting the cervical enlargement pose a threat to arm function and strongly indicate surgery. A cyst of less than one or two segments above the site of cord damage and a slack appearance favor conservative management. Intermediate cases demand care in decision-making. Surgery is easy and safe if the patients have complete paraplegia. Partial paraplegics are at risk of deterioration at the time of surgery, whatever procedure is done.

Operations may be recommended differently by experienced surgeons. I advise operation at the site of injury, wide decompression, and nonclosure and nongrafting of the dura with myelotomy and temporary or no damage. Other techniques may eventually prove to be superior, but I presently believe that the principle underlying success is the disablement of the filling mechanism by the provision of a wide, depulsating decompression of the site of injury combined with drainage to an extrathecal site. I presently favor the pleura when using internal drainage but both temporary external syrinx drains and no drainage at all have appeal and seem to be as helpful.

Transection of the cord with closure of the bottom of the syrinx affords the most complete protection for the total paraplegic. There are convincing arguments to be made against the use of drainage for the widest part of the syrinx while leaving the site of the paraplegia untouched.

REFERENCES

1. Aichner F, Poewe W, Rogalsky W, et al. Magnetic resonance imaging in the diagnosis of spinal cord. *J Neurol Neurosurg Psychiatry* 1985;48:1220–1229.
2. Barbaro NM. Surgery for primarily spinal syringomyelia. In: Batzdorf U, ed. *Syringomyelia: concepts in diagnosis and treatment*. Baltimore: Williams & Wilkins, 1991;183–198.
3. Barbaro NM, Wilson CB, Gutin PH, et al. Surgical treatment of syringomyelia: favourable results with syringoperitoneal shunting. *J Neurosurg* 1984;61:531–538.
4. Barnett HJM, Botterell EH, Jousse AT, Wynn-Jones M. Progressive myelopathy as a sequel to traumatic paraplegia. *Brain* 1966;89:159–173.
5. Barnett HJM, Jousse AT. Post-traumatic syringomyelia (cystic myelopathy). In: Vinken PJ, Bruyn GW, eds. *Handbook of clinical neurology*, vol 6. Amsterdam: North-Holland, 1976;113–157.
6. Durward QJ, Rice GP, Ball MJK, Gilbert JJ, Kauffman JCE. Selective spinal cordectomy: clinicopathological correlation. *J Neurosurg* 1982;56:359–367.
7. Foster JB. Neurology of syringomyelia. In: Batzdorf U, ed. *Syringomyelia: current concepts in diagnosis and treatment*. Baltimore: Williams & Wilkins, 1991.
8. Frankel HL. Ascending cord lesion in the early stages following spinal injury. *Paraplegia* 1969;6:111–118.
9. Jefferson AA. Cordectomy for intractable pain in paraplegia. In: Lipton S, Miles JB, eds. *Persistent pain*, vol IV. London: Academic Press, 1983;115–132.
10. Kakoulas B. Pathology of spinal injuries. *Central Nerv Syst Trauma* 1984;1:117–129.
11. Lacert P, Trottier S, Durand J, Pannier S, Grossiord A. Syndromes syringomyéliques tardifs chez la paraplégiques. *Rev Neurol (Paris)* 1977;133(5):325–338.
12. La Haye PA, Batzdorf U. Post-traumatic syringomyelia. *West J Med* 1988;148:657–666.
13. McLean DR, Miller JDR, Allen PBR, Ezzedin SA. Post-traumatic syringomyelia. *J Neurosurg* 1973;39:485–492.
14. Peerless SJ, Durward QJ. Management of syringomyelia: a pathophysiological approach. *Clin Neurosurg* 1983;30:531–576.
15. Quencer RM. The injured spinal cord: evaluation with magnetic resonance and intraoperative sonography. *Radiol Clin North Am* 1988;26:1025–1045.
16. Quencer RM, Green BA, Eismont FJ. Post-traumatic spinal cord cysts: clinical features and characterization with metrizamide computed tomography. *Radiology* 1983;146:415–423.
17. Rafael M, Malpica A, Ruiz C, et al. Paraplejia traumática crónica: diagnóstico y tratamiento. *Mundo Médico* 1991;18:11–19.
18. Rossier AB, Werner A, Wildie, Berney J. Contribution to the study of late cervical syringomyelia syndromes after dorsal or lumbar traumatic paraplegia. *J Neurol Neurosurg Psychiatry* 1968;31:99–105.
19. Rossier AB, Foo D, Shillito J, Dyro FM. Posttraumatic cervical syringomyelia. *Brain* 1985;108:439–461.
20. Savoiardo M. Syringomyelia associated with post-meningitis spinal arachnoiditis. Filling of the syrinx through a communication with the subarachnoid space. *Neurology* 1976;26:551–554.
21. Shannon N, Symon L, Logue V, Cull D, Kang J, Kendall BE. Clinical features, investigation and treatment of post-traumatic syringomyelia. *J Neurol Neurosurg Psychiatry* 1981;44:35–42.
22. Stanworth P. The significance of hyperhidrosis in patients with post-traumatic syringomyelia. *Paraplegia* 1982;20:282–287.
23. Suzuki M, Davis C, Symon L, Gentili F. Syringoperitoneal shunt for treatment of cord cavitation. *J Neurol Neurosurg Psychiatry* 1985;48:620–627.
24. Tator CH, Meguro K, Rowed DW. Favourable results with syringosubarachnoid shunts for treatment of syringomyelia. *J Neurosurg* 1982;56:517–523.
25. Umbach I, Heilporn A. Post-spinal cord injury syringomyelia. *Paraplegia* 1991;29:219–221.
26. Vernon JD, Silver JR, Symon L. Post-traumatic syringomyelia, the results of surgery. *Paraplegia* 1983;21:37–46.
27. Watson N. Personal communication, 1972; quoted by Barnett and Jousse, ref. 5.
28. Williams B. On the pathogenesis of syringomyelia: a review. *J R Soc Med* 1980;73:798–806.
29. Williams B. Progress in syringomyelia. *Neurol Res* 1986;8:130–145.
30. Williams B. Post-traumatic syringomyelia, an update. *Paraplegia* 1990;28:296–313.
31. Williams B. Malformations. In: Swash M, Oxbury J, eds. *Clinical neurology*, vol 2. New York: Churchill Livingstone, 1991;1533–1575.
32. Williams B, Page N. Surgical treatment of syringomyelia with syringopleural shunting. *Br J Neurosurg* 1987;1:63–80.
33. Williams B, Terry AH, Jones HWF, McSweeney T. Syringomyelia as a sequel to traumatic paraplegia. *Paraplegia* 1981;19:67–80.

31

Late Deformities

Steven D. Glassman and Jean-Pierre C. Farcy

Late deformity following thoracolumbar fracture is a consequence of acute or chronic spinal instability. As early as 1949 Nicoll classified thoracolumbar injuries as stable or unstable based on the integrity of the interspinous ligaments. Although the issue of post-traumatic deformity was considered, Nicoll concluded that "the best results were obtained when the affected vertebral bodies fused spontaneously in the deformed position" (44). Forty years later, newer techniques including computed tomography (CT) scan and magnetic resonance imaging (MRI) have added specificity to diagnosis and classification. Treatment options have expanded to include anterior or posterior instrumentation for correction and fusion. Despite these advances, the development of deformity following thoracolumbar fracture remains a significant cause of morbidity. The definition and diagnosis of spine stability, although discussed extensively, continues to be a controversial concept.

In 1963 Holdsworth (28) presented a classification of thoracolumbar injuries and introduced the concept of a burst fracture. He described the mechanism of the burst fracture thus: "the nucleus of the disc is forced into the vertebral body which explodes." He also stated that because of the intact ligaments, a burst fracture was a stable injury (29).

In 1970, Roberts and Curtiss (48) evaluated a series of patients with traumatic paraplegia and assessed the prognosis for stability. Although spontaneous fusion was documented in only 62% of cases, thoracolumbar burst fractures were noted to be more stable than rotational fracture dislocations. On this basis, a 6-week period of bed rest was recommended with the expectation that progressive deformity would not occur. In 1977 Whitesides (54) raised the issue of progressive kyphosis following thoracolumbar burst fractures. This evaluation was based on a two-column model of the spine; the anterior column resisted compression and the posterior column resisted tension. In the case of a burst fracture, the inability of the anterior column to resist axial compression was identified as the differentiating factor between a stable and an unstable injury. Whitesides also stressed the fact that "unstable fractures cannot be expected to spontaneously become stable by bone union" (54).

Until that time, thoracolumbar fractures were classified by radiographic criteria, which were consistent with a two-column model of the spine (47,54,55). In 1983, Denis (13) proposed a three-column model of the spine (Fig. 1). This advance in conceptualization was paralleled by increased capacity of the CT scan to visualize these fractures in terms of three columns. The three-column classification identifies a "middle column" composed of the posterior one-third of the vertebral body, posterior annulus fibrosis, and posterior longitudinal ligament (12). In particular, the burst fracture is differentiated from the wedge compression fracture by the presence of middle-column disruption in the burst fracture.

Treatment algorithms can roughly be divided on the basis of the neurologic status at the time of injury. Operative intervention is well accepted in cases of incomplete neurologic deficit, since decompression is required to promote neurologic recovery. In cases of intact neurologic status, treatment decisions involve an evaluation of deformity and stability and are far more controversial.

Patients may present with late deformity and neurologic deficit following thoracolumbar fractures as the result of no treatment, unsuccessful brace treatment,

---

S. D. Glassman: Department of Orthopaedic Surgery, University of Louisville, School of Medicine, Louisville, KY 40292.
J.-P. C. Farcy: Department of Orthopaedic Surgery, Columbia University College of Physicians and Surgeons; and Columbia–Presbyterian Medical Center, New York, NY 10032.

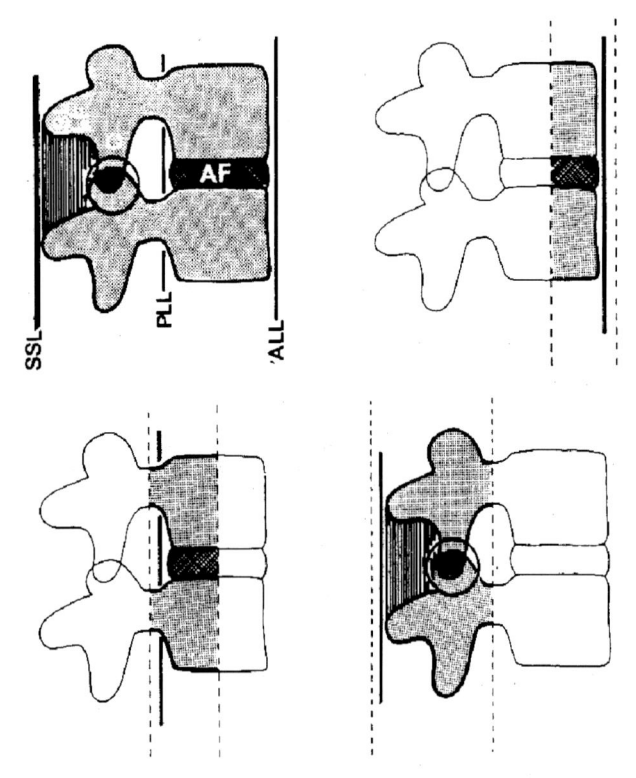

FIG. 1. The three-column model of the spine describes a middle column. Injury to the middle column is characteristic of a burst fracture. From ref. 13.

inappropriate operative treatment, or despite seemingly appropriate operative treatment. In general, late deformity can be considered in terms of either a stable or an unstable deformity. This division is significant for understanding the risk and rate of progression, as well as the characteristics of the deformity and associated neurologic symptoms. Since 1949, there has been significant evolution in the understanding of thoracolumbar fractures in terms of etiology, biomechanics, diagnosis, treatment, and outcome. Recent efforts have been directed toward identifying, at the time of injury, those patients at increased risk for progressive deformity.

DEFINING STABILITY

Classification schemes for thoracolumbar injuries have frequently been based on the mechanism of injury. In conjunction with his original description of the burst type fracture, Holdsworth (29) categorized five "types of violence" to which the spine is subjected. These included pure flexion, flexion and rotation, extension, and direct shear, as well as the vertical compression mechanism responsible for the "burst" fracture. According to Holdsworth's scheme, these injuries were further divided into stable or unstable types. This determination of stability was not clearly quantified but was assessed in relation to physical examination of the back, radiographic characteristics, and neurologic findings. Burst fractures were considered to be uniformly stable injuries.

Whitesides introduced the concept that a burst fracture might be either stable or unstable, based on the integrity of two columns. Stable fractures are those in which the spine can withstand axial compression forces anteriorly, tension forces posteriorly, and rotational stresses in torsion (54). An unstable fracture, therefore, cannot meet these criteria without progression of deformity or compromise of neural elements. This approach to classification reflected Whitesides' observation of progressive kyphosis among a subset of thoracolumbar fractures that should have been stable according to Holdsworth's classification system (33,54,55).

In 1983, Denis (13) presented a three-column model of the spine and a correlated classification system for thoracolumbar injuries. He divided major spine injuries into four categories: compression fractures, burst fractures, seat belt type fractures, and fracture dislocations. Seat belt type injuries are characterized by failure of both the posterior and middle columns in tension. These injuries then are subdivided both on the basis of one versus two levels of injury, and bony versus ligamentous disruption. Fracture dislocations are characterized in the Denis classification as a failure of all three columns resulting from compression, tension, rotation, or shear. Subtypes of fracture dislocations include: type A, flexion rotation; type B, shear; and type C, flexion distraction. Burst fractures are characterized by disruption of the posterior vertebral body wall or "middle column." Burst fractures were subdivided further by specific radiographic findings and mechanism of injury into five subtypes, "A" through "E" (Fig. 2). While this three-column model of spine stability has been widely accepted, the application of this classification system has been hindered by its complexity.

Ferguson and Allen (23) proposed a mechanistic classification of thoracolumbar fractures that differentiates between compressive flexion and vertical compression injuries. Although the concept of middle-element disruption is similar to Denis' middle-column fracture, the Ferguson–Allen classification separates middle-column disruption into tension versus compression. A middle-column compressive injury, classified as "vertical compression," is considered significantly more stable than the analogous middle-column "compressive flexion" injury. Radiographically, vertical compression injuries were identified by shortening of the posterior vertebral body wall when compared to the compressive flexion injuries.

How does one define spinal stability? In Holdsworth's original description, the burst fracture

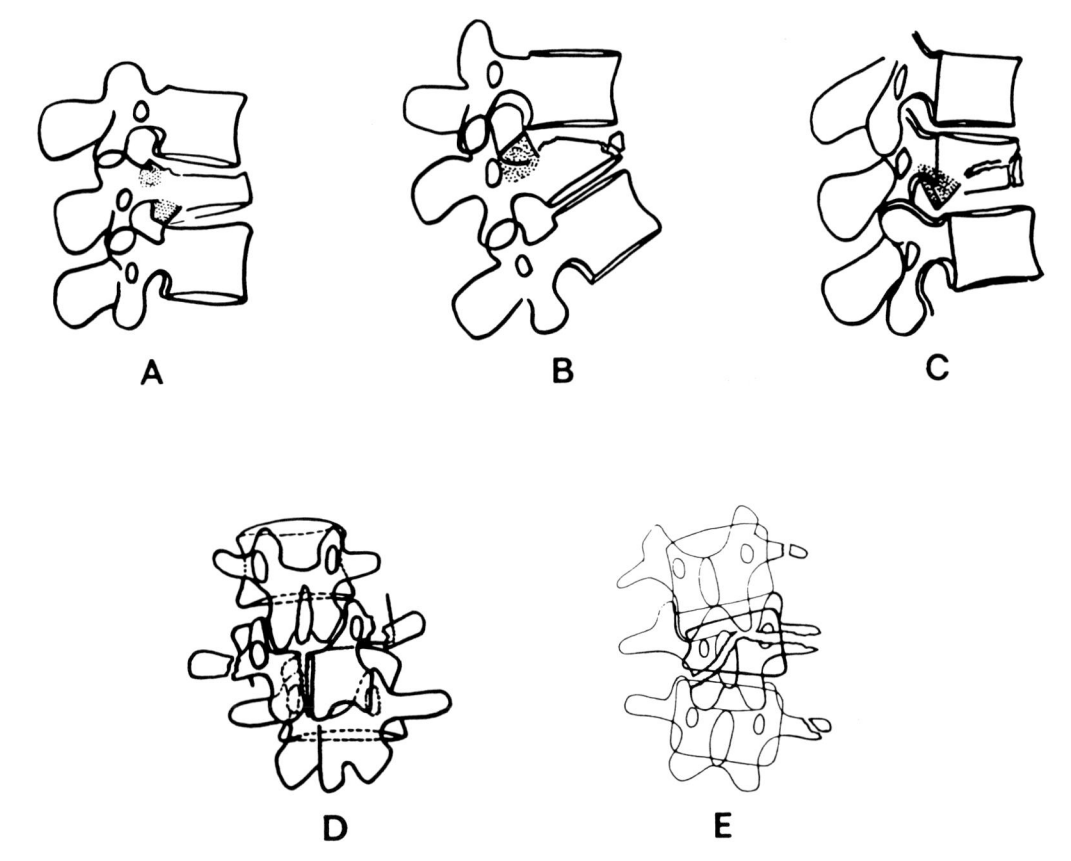

FIG. 2. Subdivision of burst fractures into five types, "A" through "E." Application of this classification has been hindered by its complexity. (From ref. 13.)

was classified as a stable injury (28). Subsequently, authors have differentiated between stable and unstable burst fractures on the basis of posterior-element disruption, degree of kyphotic deformity, severity of spinal canal compromise, and presence or absence of neurologic deficit (6,13,14,40,53). Most classification schemes define stability in relation to both biomechanical factors and neurologic findings. The rationale for considering the patient's neurologic status in an evaluation of biomechanical stability, as outlined by White and Panjabi (53), is that, in most cases, the neurologic deficit is indicative of the severity of trauma. This also reflects the difficulty in evaluating ligamentous and soft tissue injury in a more quantitative fashion. Although inclusion of the neurologic status can be justified as the ultimate indicator of instability, a combined radiographic and clinical classification has not readily provided prognostic information.

The advent of MRI technology has improved our ability to assess soft tissue injury in association with thoracolumbar fractures. A modification of the Denis model considers both a bony and ligamentous component in each of the three columns of the spine (20). The anterior column is composed of the anterior longitudinal ligament and the anterior two-thirds of the disc and vertebral body. The middle column is the posterior longitudinal ligament and the posterior one-third of the disc and vertebral body. The posterior column consists of the posterior bony elements, joint capsules, and interspinous ligaments (Fig. 3). One unit of stability is accorded for either bony or ligamentous disruption in any of the three columns. Instability is suspected with disruption of three or more of the six total elements. In a study of thoracolumbar burst fractures, this stability index, in conjunction with an evaluation of sagittal deformity, was predictive of progressive kyphosis (21).

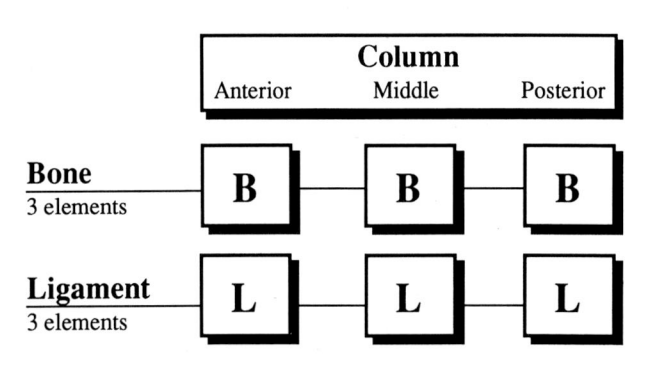

FIG. 3. A modified three-column model of the spine that considers the ligamentous components in each column.

In summary, evaluation of stability involves an assessment of the characteristics and severity of the deformity, in conjunction with an assessment of the remaining stabilizing elements. A deformity that is progressive is, by definition, unstable in some fashion. The concept of progression is crucial because it is the treatment indicator for both imaging and clinical findings. Late instability may be insidious and extremely difficult to document. Only repeated, careful, clinical evaluation can appreciate the development of symptoms and loss of function. Correlation of clinical and radiographic progression is important as a guide to optimal treatment decisions.

PRESENTATION OF LATE DEFORMITY

Late deformity is a description that encompasses a broad range in terms of timing and severity. The division between early and late treatment may be considered by chronologic progression, advancement through a series of treatment modalities, or physiologic progression of fracture healing. Classification by time alone, for example, greater than 6 months following injury, has the advantage of simplicity and reproducibility but, unfortunately, elapsed time is not an effective predictor of outcome. It is the presence of a healed fracture, a malunion, or an established pseudarthrosis that will ultimately determine the course of a late deformity.

A critical factor in the management of late deformity is the division between stable and unstable late deformity. Stable late deformity is essentially a malunion and carries the risks of spinal stenosis. Unstable late deformity is more analogous to a pseudarthrosis with the attendant risks of acute instability. In general, stable late deformity would be more likely subsequent to a burst fracture, whereas unstable late deformity would be associated with a Chance fracture or fracture dislocation (9). An understanding of stable and unstable late deformity can provide an indication of whether a late deformity is likely to become a progressive deformity.

The clinical presentation following thoracolumbar injury may be as pain, deformity, mechanical instability, or neurologic deficit. All these symptoms can be explained as a consequence of acute or chronic instability. Back pain was the most frequent presenting complaint in several series, being noted in 70% to 90% of cases (40,41,52). Two distinct patterns of back pain were commonly reported. Pain may occur at the apex of the deformity and be exacerbated by upright activities and relieved by bed rest. When accompanied by crepitus on flexion and extension, apical back pain may be indicative of gross instability (40). Low back pain, radicular or nonradicular, is also a frequent sequela of thoracolumbar fracture. Low back pain may be the result of either stenosis at the level of the fracture or compensatory hyperlordosis secondary to the thoracolumbar kyphosis. Pain related to compensatory hyperlordosis may be particularly confusing in older patients with underlying lumbar degenerative disease.

The pattern of back pain provides an indication of the mechanics and stability of the deformity. In cases of chronic, slowly progressive instability, pain characteristic of spinal stenosis is more likely to develop. Gross instability, often associated with a pseudarthrosis or ligamentous injury, would likely yield symptoms of mechanical instability.

Although pain in some cases is clearly a reflection of neural compression, neurologic function is generally evaluated in terms of motor, sensory, or bowel and bladder function. Motor function is measured either by Frankel grade or Motor Index Score (MIS) (24,39). A careful neurologic examination is the most important component in the clinical evaluation of late deformity following thoracolumbar injury. Malcolm et al. (41) reported a history of progressive neurologic deficit in five of 27 thoracolumbar fractures with post-traumatic kyphosis. In addition to direct neural compression, other potentially complicating factors such as local vascular insufficiency of the cord, extradural and intradural fibrosis, and arachnoiditis were cited. Occult disc rupture in association with spine fracture has also been reported (45). Neurodiagnostic evaluation using electromyogram (EMG), nerve conduction studies, or somatosensory evoked potentials may assist in the quantification of neurologic deficit (8). In the future, motor evoked potentials may provide a similar analysis over a more complete range of spinal cord function (17).

Thoracolumbar injuries often involve the conus medullaris, resulting in bowel or bladder dysfunction that may occur even in the absence of other neurologic signs or symptoms. Cystometrics or urodynamics provide a useful adjunct in the evaluation of acute or chronic injury at the thoracolumbar level. Recently, cortical evoked potentials have been shown to be more sensitive than cystometrograms in detecting bladder dysfunction in a canine model of cauda equina compression (11). In a study of 48 thoracolumbar injuries treated by anterior decompression, McAfee et al. (42) reported a preoperative conus medullaris lesion in 32 cases. Similarly, Transfeldt et al. (52) found that a high percentage of patients requiring delayed decompression had associated bladder dysfunction.

Although radiographic progression of kyphotic deformity is pathognomonic of the syndrome of late deformity, less than 50% of the patients in Malcolm's series were subjectively aware of this progression (41). The perception of instability may be correlated to the degree of motion on flexion and extension lateral radiographs. This provides quantitative evidence for the differentiation between stable and unstable late deformity. The radiographic evaluation of late deformity begins with posteroanterior (PA) and lateral plain radiographs. Deformity can occur in both frontal and sagittal planes, but segmental kyphosis remains the most classic deformity.

The kyphotic deformity may be quantified by measurement of the Sagittal Index. Sagittal Index is defined as the measurement of segmental kyphosis at the level of a given mobile segment (i.e., one vertebra and one disc) adjusted for the baseline sagittal contour at that level (21). Associated deformities may include scoliosis, lateral translation, spondylolisthesis, or rotational malalignment. Each of these deformities may be indicative of the nature and extent of the original injury. For example, a scoliosis may be secondary to an element of lateral compression. Rotational malalignment or lateral translation is more suggestive of an unstable deformity. Despite the availability of sophisticated imaging techniques, plain radiographs are still the mainstay of evaluation, and their importance should not be minimized.

Subsequent radiologic evaluation may include CT scan, MRI scan, tomograms, myelography, and discography. In each case, the appropriate study should be chosen to address specific questions in conjunction with the clinical examination. A streamlined, problem-directed radiologic evaluation is most likely to provide clinically useful information.

CT scan and tomograms may aid assessment of the stability or instability of a given deformity by identifying a pseudarthrosis at the level of the fracture. Flexion and extension radiographs or MRI scan may provide additional information as to the degree of ligamentous involvement. CT scan or lateral tomography also may be helpful in quantifying the adequacy of anterior bone stock, since insufficient bony support can result in later collapse despite initial healing. It is essential that all radiographic findings be correlated with the clinical examination.

Evaluation of canal compromise and neural compression is accomplished by CT and/or MRI scans. Whereas CT scan is accurate in imaging the bony anatomy, the MRI scan better visualizes the soft tissue components, such as ligament or disc material. Although the accumulation of experience with the MRI scan has refined its diagnostic accuracy, myelogram is still the gold standard for evaluation of neural compression. This is particularly important in patients with low back pain following thoracolumbar fracture. Pain related to thoracolumbar deformity and primary lumbar degenerative disease may exist simultaneously and must be differentiated. Discography may have a role in evaluating low back pain associated with thoracolumbar deformity. Particularly in the older patient with lumbar degenerative changes, lumbar discography or differential lumbar and thoracolumbar injections may delineate the source of pain. Finally, the documentation of neural compromise must be assessed in conjunction with clinical findings in order to optimize treatment outcome.

RISKS FOR PROGRESSIVE DEFORMITY

Risk factors for late progression of deformity following thoracolumbar injury have been categorized according to various characteristics. Malcolm (40) proposed a division based on factors being either intrinsic or extrinsic to the spinal column. An alternative division is to categorize risk factors as being primarily patient related, fracture related, or treatment related.

Patient-specific risk factors are indicative of healing potential and include age, bone quality, chronic medical illness, and associated injuries. Trauma victims are predisposed to malnutrition on the basis of their multiple injuries. Nutritional deficiency presents an immediate risk in terms of impaired healing and may potentiate the risk of pseudarthrosis and unstable late deformity. Chronic malnutrition may lead to osteoporosis, compounding the loss of structural integrity in an anterior column already compromised by fracture and kyphotic deformity. Fracture secondary to metabolic bone disease or tumor often will be complicated by delayed healing. Although thoracolumbar trauma is unusual in the elderly, this situation presents a difficult clinical management problem as the result of impaired healing and, therefore, progression to late deformity.

Neurologic injury, whether central cord level, or peripheral, may influence the course of an associated spine deformity. This spectrum ranges from peripheral nerve injury to complete paraplegia. Maintenance of spinal alignment and stabilization of deformity are crucial in patients with paraplegia. When stabilization is achieved, rapid rehabilitation is facilitated, thus optimizing remaining function.

The anatomic characteristics of the thoracolumbar fracture or dislocation are obviously a pivotal predictor of progressive deformity. Progression of kyphotic deformity is influenced both by the magnitude of the initial deformity and the degree of instability. Goutallier and Louis (25) have demonstrated that the degree of local kyphotic deformity correlates to the destruction of the bony substance of the involved vertebral body after fracture. Controversy exists as to whether a thoracolumbar injury, if intrinsically unstable, can obtain long-term stability as the result of bony healing (36,48,55). Jacobs et al. (30) reported that vertebral body fracture, because it is through cancellous bone, would heal rapidly following reduction by distraction. In contrast, Benson (2) states that even fractures which are initially stable may later collapse into kyphosis because of insufficient anterior bone stock.

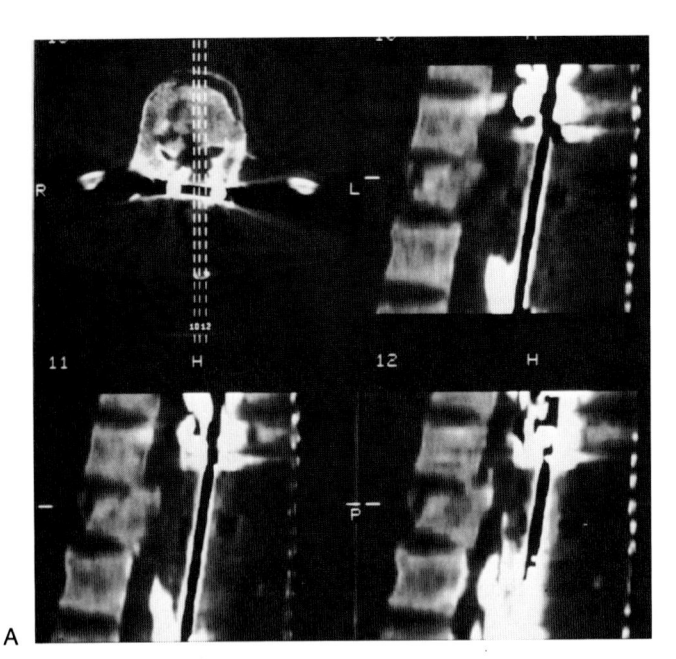

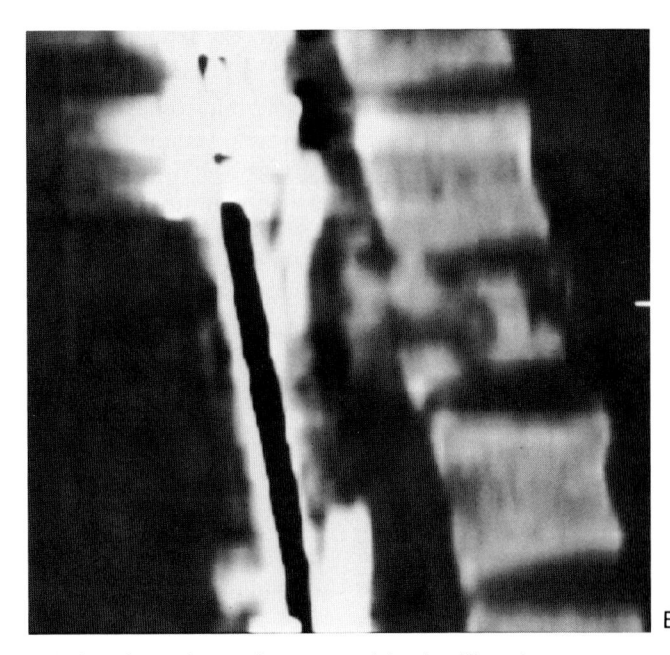

FIG. 4. A: A CT scan following posterior instrumentation for a burst fracture with significant kyphotic deformity. Despite restoration of the cortical outline, the structural integrity of the vertebral body is severely compromised. **B:** Reconstruction of anterior column following vertebrectomy and iliac crest strut graft is indicated.

Our experience has been that, in the presence of significant loss of osseous stock, bony healing will not occur even though the preinjury vertebral height was restored by reduction and stabilization. Instead, the gap will be filled by fibrous tissue that cannot restore the structural integrity of the vertebral body (21) (Fig. 4). The point at which anterior column bony destruction will require anterior stabilization to avoid progressive deformity can be correlated to the Sagittal Index.

Restoration of sagittal contour by reduction is an important factor in the treatment of thoracolumbar injuries. Stabilization without reduction and, in particular, without reconstruction of sagittal contour, has been questioned (14,21,41). Malcolm et al. (41) reported that, if reduction was not performed prior to instrumentation and fusion, solid arthrodesis was not obtained and results were poor. Adequate reduction led to solid fusion even if correction was incomplete or partial loss of reduction occurred postoperatively (41,51). In our experience, nothing short of anatomic restoration of frontal and sagittal plane contours represents a valid treatment goal.

Ligamentous instability is often difficult to document clearly unless there is significant posterior distraction or lateral translation on plain radiographs. The MRI scan provides an improved visualization of soft tissue injury and may ultimately allow quantification of ligamentous damage. When healing does occur, fibrous scar, which is more bulky, offers less strength, and has poor elastic qualities, replaces the original ligamentous tissue. Krompinger et al. (36) postulate that kyphosis greater than 30° over one mobile segment may be a marker for occult facet subluxation and posterior column injury. Disc disruption is particularly destabilizing because of the critical role of the strong annular fibers (49). Also, when disrupted, the disc tends not to heal; rather, it degenerates. Transection studies in monkeys indicate that disc disruption alone may result in greater kyphosis than vertebral body injury since both of the surrounding levels are compromised (1).

The risk of progressive deformity following thoracolumbar injury is obviously affected by initial treatment decisions. Late deformity may occur following either brace or surgical treatment. The role of brace treatment has been reviewed extensively and both good and bad results have been reported (24,27,30,36,46). In terms of surgical intervention, isolated laminectomy has clearly been identified as a source of iatrogenic deformity (3,6,43,48). Nonetheless, late deformity may develop despite seemingly adequate instrumentation and fusion if biomechanical stability is not reestablished (21,41,51).

TREATMENT OPTIONS

Instability of the Thoracolumbar Junction

Treatment of late deformity following thoracolumbar injury is difficult, and excellent results are unusual. Treatment options include conservative therapy, stabilization in situ, and reduction of deformity. In each case, associated neural decompression may or may not be indicated. Regardless of treatment modality, realistic expectations in terms of risk for persistent pain or neurologic deficit, incomplete correction of deformity, and the complexity of any procedure must be maintained.

Conservative therapy must be considered as a reasonable option, since surgical outcomes are frequently suboptimal. Nonoperative therapy may be applicable to a late deformity with gradual onset of pain. Patients may benefit from intermittent bracing, physical therapy, or anti-inflammatory medications. Chronic use of narcotics should be aggressively avoided. Epidural blocks may be either an efficacious treatment or an effective temporizing measure for post-traumatic spinal stenosis in this group of patients. Long-term bracing is often disadvantageous, resulting in subsequent muscle weakness, which exacerbates the underlying problem. Finally, pain clinic referral may be a useful adjunct to nonoperative treatment if a quality pain clinic is available.

Surgical treatment of late deformity and associated symptoms is determined by the severity, duration, and specific characteristics of the injury. Surgical intervention can broadly be categorized as either a stabilization in situ or reduction of deformity. These goals may be achieved via anterior, posterior, or combined surgical approaches. In either case, a satisfactory outcome is possible only if solid arthrodesis and satisfactory decompression are obtained. On the surface, stabilization in situ may appear simpler and safer than reduction but several authors have pointed to a decreased fusion rate in cases treated without reduction (41,51). It is therefore important to stress that long-term safety (i.e., preservation of neurologic function) is enhanced only if stabilization in situ is successful. On this basis, stabilization in situ might be an appropriate choice for an injury with significant instability but mild deformity.

Reduction of late deformity is a complex problem and anatomic reduction is rarely achieved. An unstable deformity may be mobile enough that reduction via a single approach, either anterior or posterior, is feasible. Traditionally, anterior grafting was accompanied by posterior instrumentation for stabilization, but recent technical improvements have made single-stage anterior instrumentation and fusion a viable alternative (32,34,35). Experimental studies in the calf spine have demonstrated that instrumentation with Cotrel–Dubousset (C-D) rods, Steffee plates, or the Kaneda device in combination with anterior bone grafting afforded significantly greater immediate stability than bone grafting alone (26).

More commonly, late deformities are rigid and require some combination of anterior and posterior osteotomies for reduction. In the simplest form, anterior discectomies are followed by posterior instrumentation with or without osteotomy. The margin of safety is maximized if care is taken to avoid any lengthening of the neural elements. This approach will often yield only a modest reduction of deformity but improvement in the arthrodesis rate has been independent of the degree of correction (21,41,51).

A more anatomic reduction can be obtained if the clinical situation warrants an expanded procedure. However, the risks of the procedure are obviously expanded as well. Technical expertise, experience, and comprehensive spinal cord monitoring are all critical to a successful outcome. Anterior release can be extended to include resection of the posterior longitudinal ligament or to vertebrectomy. In conjunction with posterior osteotomies, spinal shortening may allow significant reduction without neural compromise.

An alternative approach involves a three-stage procedure consisting of posterior osteotomies and anterior bone grafting followed by posterior instrumentation. The advantage is that the reduction may be achieved at the time of anterior bone grafting. No loosening of the graft will occur, as opposed to an attempted posterior reduction following anterior grafting. If anterior reduction were undertaken first, the neural elements would be stretched over a posterior fulcrum, the fixed posterior column. The preceding osteotomies preserve the basic concept of spinal shortening to facilitate reduction (38). The extent of this procedure is justified only in selected cases.

Another option is the "eggshell vertebrectomy," a transpedicular approach that allows anterior release via a posterior exposure. Potential indications for the eggshell vertebrectomy include a contraindication to thoracotomy or the necessity for a multilevel anterior release. The procedure is technically difficult and is not considered a "smaller" procedure, although only one exposure is required. In general, the anterior release obtained via transpedicular vertebrectomy is less effective than vertebrectomy via the thoracoabdominal approach.

Whether or not reduction is attempted, combined anterior and posterior surgery may be considered to enhance fusion rate. Malcolm and co-workers (40,41) recommended circumferential fusion on the basis of a 50% failure rate following anterior fusion alone. A potential disadvantage of the combined fusion is that posterior instrumentation often involves a longer segment fusion. Alternative solutions include the addition of anterior instrumentation (16,35) or short segment posterior instrumentation with pedicle screws. Posterior instrumentation without fusion for reduction and stabilization requires hardware removal following anterior graft healing and is more appropriate in the acute setting (21).

The second significant treatment decision involves the need for neural decompression. With rare exceptions, compression is anterior and requires some form of anterior decompression. Possible approaches include the posterolateral (37) or thoracoabdominal routes (7,41,55). The efficacy of late decompression following thoracolumbar fracture has been questioned because, although the potential for neurologic improvement has been documented, the recovery of useful function is less common (3,4,21,31,52). Transfeldt et al. (52) point out that the benefits of delayed decompression must be evaluated separately regarding the effects on motor function, bowel and bladder function, and pain.

Motor function is usually assessed either by Frankel grade or Motor Index Score (24,39). While the Motor Index Score offers a more quantified evaluation, postoperative improvement may represent strengthening as the result of physical therapy rather than return of neurologic function (52). Even with actual recovery of function, small changes in neurologic function at the thoracolumbar level may not translate into improvement with activities of daily living. An exception is in deficits of bowel or bladder function. Several studies suggest that recovery of bladder function is more likely to follow late decompression (52,56). This potential for recovery has been attributed to the presence of injury to the conus medullaris rather than to the cord.

Pain associated with late deformity may be secondary to instability, neural compromise, or a combination of factors. For this reason, pain relief after delayed decompression is difficult to attribute to any single element of the surgical procedure. Nonetheless, pain relief does appear to be more reliable than motor recovery following delayed decompression. Transfeldt et al. (52) differentiated between mechanical pain, central dysesthetic pain, and pain secondary to spasticity. Spasticity was not improved by decompression, and relief of mechanical pain was attributed to stabilization. Central dysesthetic pain, however, was improved in 83% of patients undergoing delayed anterior decompression (52).

Instability of the Thoracic and Lumbar Spines

Although less frequent than thoracolumbar injuries, thoracic and lumbar injuries display unique characteristics that should be noted. In the thoracic spine, the ribs provide an element of stability against rotation, so that instability takes place in the sagittal rather than the transverse plane. When the anterior column, composed of discs and bodies, is disrupted, deformity develops in kyphosis. A subsequent subluxation of the facet joints will facilitate an increase of the normal physiologic kyphosis, creating more rapid development of sagittal deformity.

Malunion most likely results from multilevel injuries or burst fractures that were treated conservatively as compression fractures. When the kyphotic deformity increases, the overall spinal canal diameter will decrease at the level where the anterior column buckled. The cord is stretched over the bone, and the patient may present with pain, weakness, and signs of long tract irritation. The overriding issue is the compromised spinal cord.

Ideally, these patients are treated by correction of the angular kyphosis (5). Following anterior decompression, a tricortical iliac crest strut graft, fixed by a lateral A-O type plate, is one effective method of stabilization. Patients who have already undergone posterior decompressive laminectomies, or who require laminectomies to treat a post-traumatic syrinx, will require circumferential fusion. The posterior instrumentation will always be placed in compression, with rods contoured to match the normal thoracic kyphosis. This will provide enough stability to avoid any type of postoperative orthosis, since the mechanical efficiency of orthoses with regard to protection of the thoracic spine is questionable.

Many authors have stressed the issue of scarce blood supply to the thoracic cord (10,15,18–22,35,50). It is often difficult to determine whether neurologic loss following thoracic spine injury or anterior thoracic surgery is due to medullary ischemia. Kostuik denied any major vascular problems suggestive of medullary ischemia in 350 anterior approaches for which ligature of the segmental vessels above and below the lesion was usually performed.

In our experience, thoracic decompression is extremely dangerous in cases of late deformity. MRI scan evaluation is crucial because patients with spinal cord atrophy are at high risk for deterioration after surgery. In these cases, arteriogram is indicated to assess the actual blood supply to the thoracic cord; if doubt remains, we prefer to perform stabilization in situ, without decompression. Even if the blood supply appears adequate, preservation of the segmental vessels at the level of the division in the foramen must be kept in mind by performing ligature and division as far anteriorly as possible.

Lumbar instability will result in a cauda equina or root level compression. It is important to determine how much of the pain described could be related to a different origin, such as arachnoiditis or post-traumatic arthritis. The principle of treatment still is to correct the sagittal deformity, but an anterior approach may not be required; a posterior osteotomy extended laterally to the pedicles and posterior instrumentation in compression are usually adequate. Reduction must be accompanied by thorough posterior decompression. Post-traumatic arachnoiditis must be recognized because it is unlikely to improve with surgery, and comprehensive conservative treatment must be contemplated.

CLINICAL OUTCOME

Since 1985, 54 patients have been treated for late deformity and neurologic compromise. At the time of injury, these patients would have met our criteria for surgery but they either refused surgery, were treated conservatively, or had suboptimal surgical treatment. Surgical failures were the result of deficiencies such as approximate correction, incomplete decompression, laminectomy without fixation, or inadequate fixation. The various treatments that we now call suboptimal may have been state of the art when they were performed. In retrospect, these treatments failed to accomplish complete decompression, anatomic correction of the deformity, and successful, stable arthrodesis.

We have undertaken revision surgery in these 54 patients with late deformities and late neural compression. Our approach in the first 31 cases consisted of staged procedures to obtain anterior release, posterior osteotomies, circumferential bone grafts, and internal fixation in the anatomic position. The patients' deformities were corrected and solid anterior and posterior arthrodeses developed, bridging the vertebrae in both the front and back. The patients showed improvement in level of pain and function. Those patients who had neurologic improvement following revision surgery were cases in which complete decompression, restoration of frontal and sagittal alignment, and solid fusion were achieved.

The surgical techniques are demanding and require planning and trained teams working together. Significant complications were encountered in the first 31 patients who underwent surgery. They were: one CSF leak, one deep infection, one pulmonary embolus, one paraplegia, and two hardware failures. Nonetheless, the surgical successes far outnumbered the failures in this difficult group of patients.

In analyzing our complications in the first 31 cases, deep infection and pulmonary embolus were felt to be the most difficult complications to deter. Complications related to technical difficulties were recognized: they decreased with successive cases. Other potential problems such as length of the procedure, blood loss, and instability between procedures that prevented proper nursing care were identified. To minimize some of the technical problems of staged procedures, a combined simultaneous approach was developed. Its advantages are (a) elimination of instability between procedures, (b) protection against dislodgment of the anterior strut graft, (c) osteotomies and reduction under anterior and posterior visual control, and (d) application of posterior fixation with direct control of the anterior graft to maintain the optimal reduction.

OUR PREFERRED TECHNIQUE

Our preferred technique for treatment of thoracolumbar malunion or pseudarthrosis involves simultaneous anterior and posterior decompression, correction of deformity, and fusion with fixation (Fig. 5). The technique is appropriate for severe kyphotic deformity as indicated by a Sagittal Index greater than 25°. The simultaneous technique requires two teams with appropriate experience in spine surgery as well as comprehensive spinal cord monitoring. The principles and the philosophy of the technique are described.

Many instrumentation systems are available, and all have "pros and cons." Certainly, it is personal training and experience that make a surgeon select a given instrumentation. Our preferred instrumentation is a combination of hooks, screws, and rods from the C-D instrumentation. There are difficulties inherent to the C-D system, but when the difficulties are overcome, it definitely provides a very versatile system that allows us to "play with" distraction and compression as necessary. It also allows the desired correction and provides an extremely rigid construct that guarantees a solid fixation. Obviously, if the same philosophy and approach are respected, other anterior and/or posterior instrumentation systems will be able to achieve the same goals.

The patient is placed securely in the lateral position so that the table can be safely tilted in either direction (Fig. 6). The patient is draped circumferentially to facilitate access to the back, flank, chest, and abdomen. Surgical adjuncts such as somatosensory evoked potentials, access for radiographs, and operating table manipulation are all verified prior to incision.

Via the posterior approach, previous instrumentation, if any, is removed. Following hardware removal, the uppermost level of fixation is selected, generally two levels above the deformity. Hook sites are prepared bilaterally, using closed thoracic laminar hooks to form a "claw" encompassing two vertebral levels. Hooks with a small foot may be used to minimize the potential for canal obstruction.

Simultaneously, a large thoracoabdominal approach

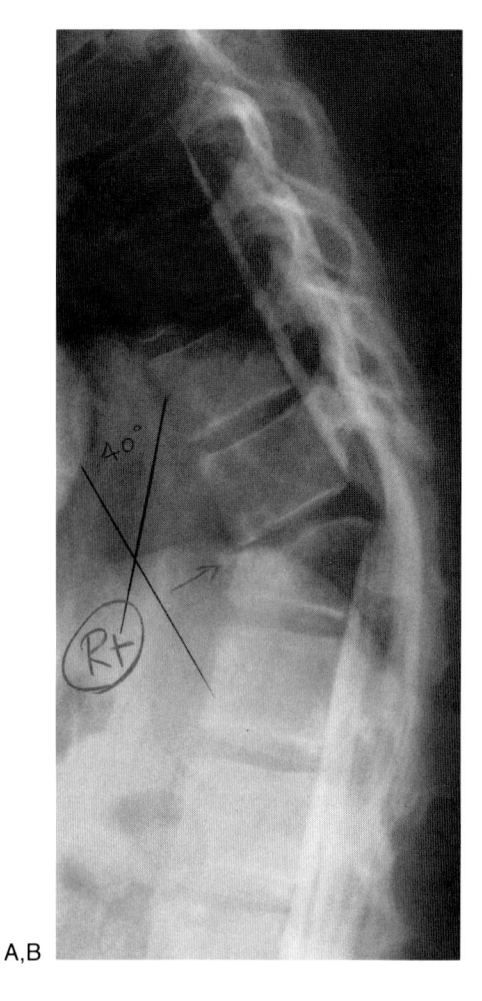

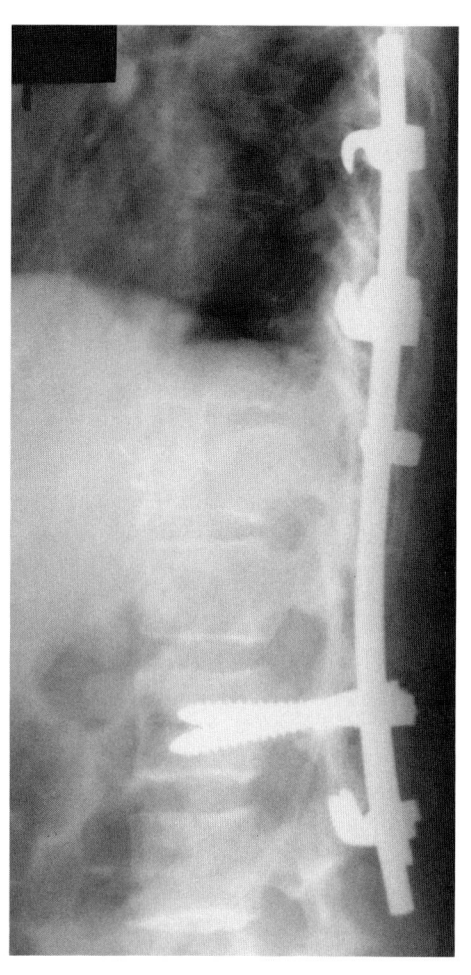

FIG. 5. Patient is a 39-year-old woman who suffered a T12 fracture with significant posterior ligamentous injury 1 year prior to her procedure. **A:** Preoperative radiograph reveals a 40° kyphosis at the T11–T12 level. **B:** Postoperative radiograph demonstrates anatomic reduction and ideal graft placement.

is developed via a tenth rib resection. The diaphragm is divided, leaving a 1-in. cuff attached to the chest wall to facilitate reconstruction. After ligature of the segmental vessels, the arcuate ligament is divided and the vertebral column is exposed. When both anterior and posterior aspects of the spine have been exposed, the osteotomies are planned and performed. Simultaneous direct visualization of the deformity has been helpful in selecting the most efficient site for correction. A posterior "chevron" osteotomy is made with a Leksell rongeur and Capener gouges (Fig. 7A,B). A Kerrison rongeur and cottonoids protect the dura for completion of the osteotomy. It is critical that adequate osteotomy precede any anterior reduction so that the neural elements are not stretched over an elongated posterior column.

After the "chevron" osteotomy has been performed and extended anteriorly, it is always possible, even in cases of large deformities, to find the remnant of a disc space anteriorly. This space is enlarged, an osteotome

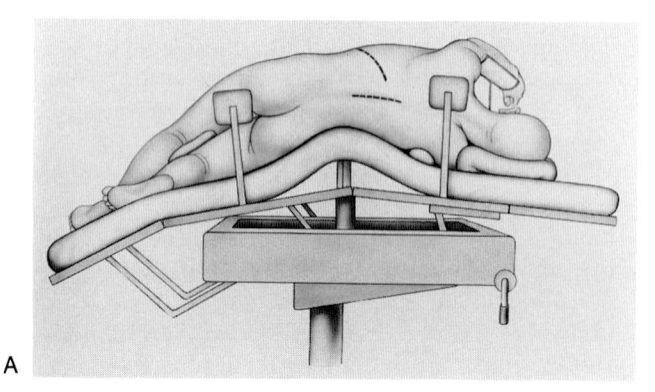

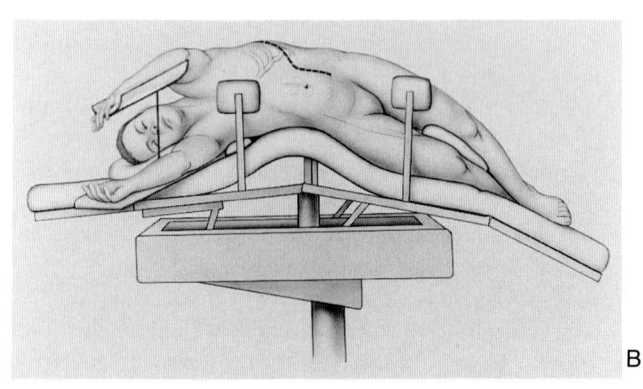

FIG. 6. A,B: Patient is placed in the lateral position. Bolsters allow access to the back, flank, chest, and abdomen and permit the table to be safely tilted in either direction.

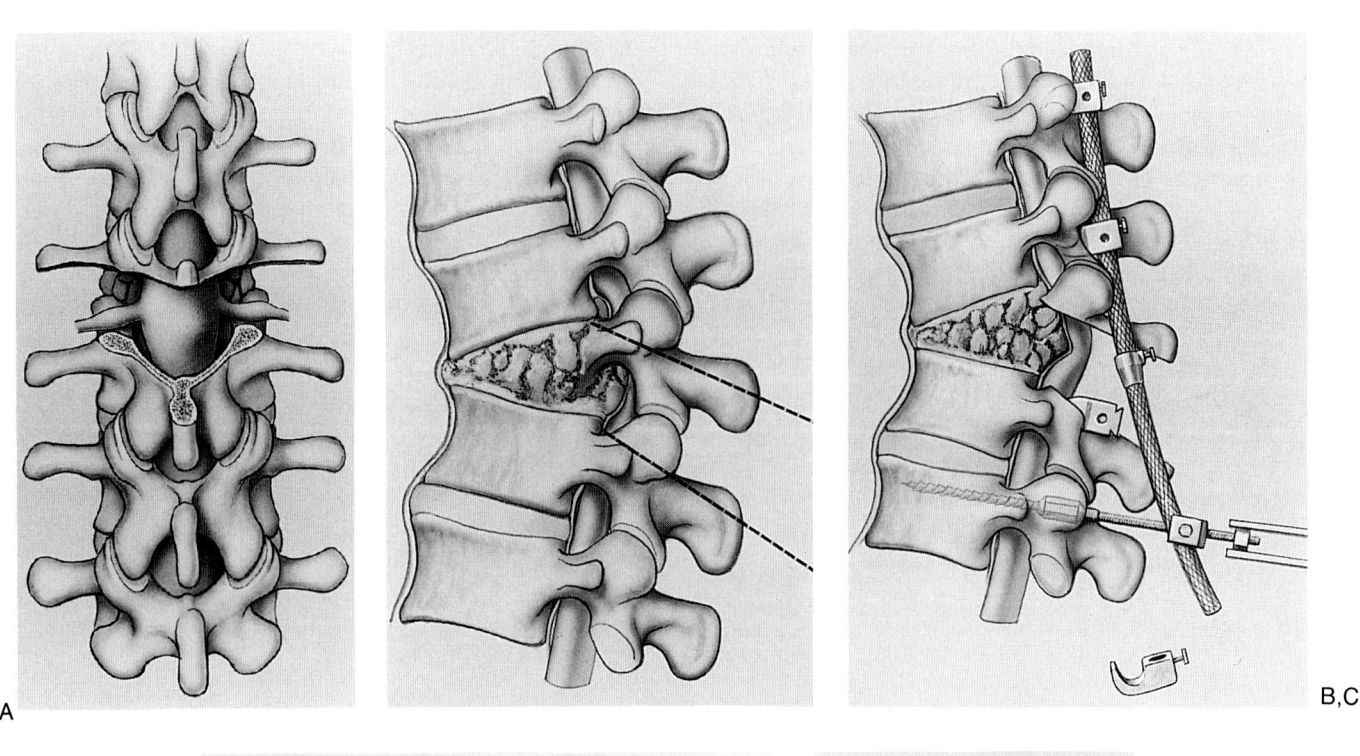

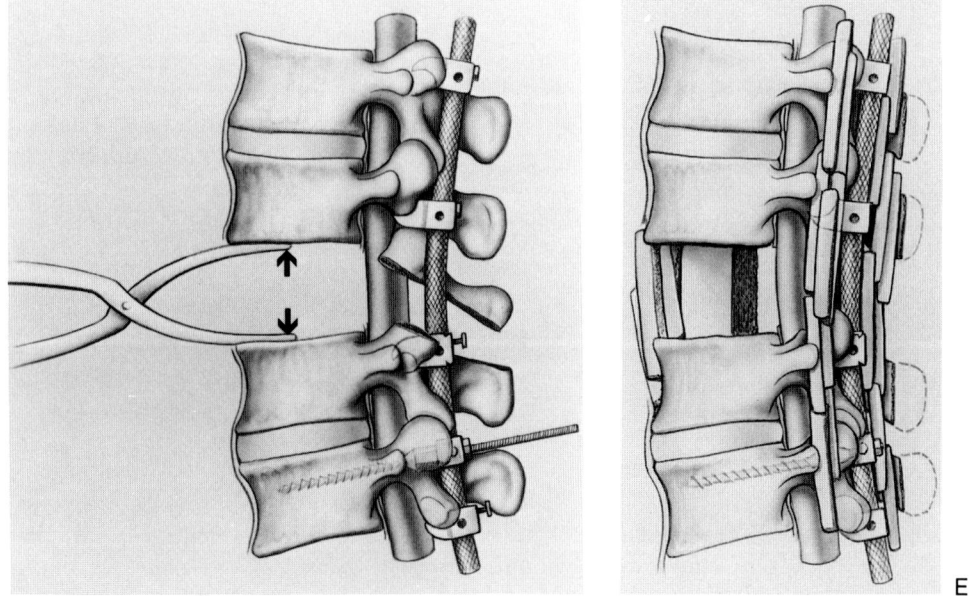

FIG. 7. AP **(A)** and lateral **(B)** views of posterior chevron osteotomy. **C:** Posterior instrumentation is placed and secured proximally. The distal aspect of the instrumentation is not firmly fixed. **D:** Under direct anterior and posterior control, the strut graft is placed and posterior instrumentation is secured. **E:** Following compression of the posterior construct, cross-link and posterior bone graft are placed.

is introduced, and a gentle lever arm applied. After release of the anterior column, a complete resection of the body with the old fracture can be performed, with dissection carried out to the canal. The posterior longitudinal ligament is often adherent to the retropulsed bone, and epidural veins are likely to be encountered. If bleeding makes complete decompression difficult, bipolar coagulation, or packing with Avetine and/or thrombin-soaked Gelfoam provides hemostasis.

After adequate anterior decompression and posterior osteotomy, correction of the deformity is initiated. Posterior instrumentation may be placed and affixed to the two cephalad claws, with compression applied to produce a solid anchorage. The rods are contoured to provide an appropriate reduction, based on the measured Sagittal Index. At this point, the distal aspect of the instrumentation is not firmly fixed (Fig. 7C). Anterior reduction is obtained using a laminar spreader for placement of an anterior bone graft. The strut graft may be bicortical or tricortical iliac crest, or allograft bone. Rib strut graft is rarely used. Autologous cancellous bone is then packed anteriorly to the strut graft. Compression of the posterior instrumentation is then undertaken with direct control of the anterior strut to ensure forceful impaction of the graft (Fig. 7D).

A double-threaded pedicle screw is inserted into each of the two pedicles of the vertebral body two levels below the osteotomy. Torque applied to the nut of the double threaded screw will drive the C-D rod toward the spine; this maneuver allows the posterior osteotomy to close. Two upgoing offset hooks are inserted beneath the laminae of the vertebra into which the screws were inserted, in order to obtain a second set of "claws" distally. When adequate compression across the anterior strut graft has been obtained, the instrumentation is firmly fixed. A cross-link is applied to the posterior instrumentation and the resected rib is cut into matchsticks for posterior bone graft (Fig. 7E).

As demonstrated in Figure 8, complete decompression has been achieved, and re-expansion of the dural sac has set the stage for potential neurological improvement.

Success of this simultaneous technique is dependent on the entire operative team and ancillary assistance. The management of hemodynamics is crucial and can be aided by careful attention to blood conservation techniques. Predonation of three to four units of autologous blood is recommended if the patient is a suitable candidate. Preoperative hemodilution of two additional units of blood is also recommended. During the procedure, a Cellsaver (Haemonetics, Braintree, MA) technique is used for salvage of shed blood, usually resulting in two to three units of RBCs (red blood cells). It is important to monitor the administration of Cellsaver blood, as these washed RBCs are devoid of other blood components. If a significant volume of Cellsaver blood is used, associated factors such as FFP and platelets must also be replaced. Postoperatively, the Solcotrans (Richards Medical, Memphis, TN) drainage system is utilized for recovery of RBCs from wound drainage. This frequently provides an additional unit of RBCs in the early postoperative period. Overall, this regimen has improved the margin of safety surrounding this major surgical intervention.

Postoperatively, the stability that has been achieved allows almost immediate mobilization and early physical therapy. Among the 23 patients treated with this simultaneous technique, the average blood loss and operating time have both decreased significantly. The Motor Index Score has increased an average of 18 points, and the Sagittal Index has been corrected to an average of 5°. Complications have been minimal: one superficial infection and two CSF leaks. Overall, this technique has given us the opportunity to save time

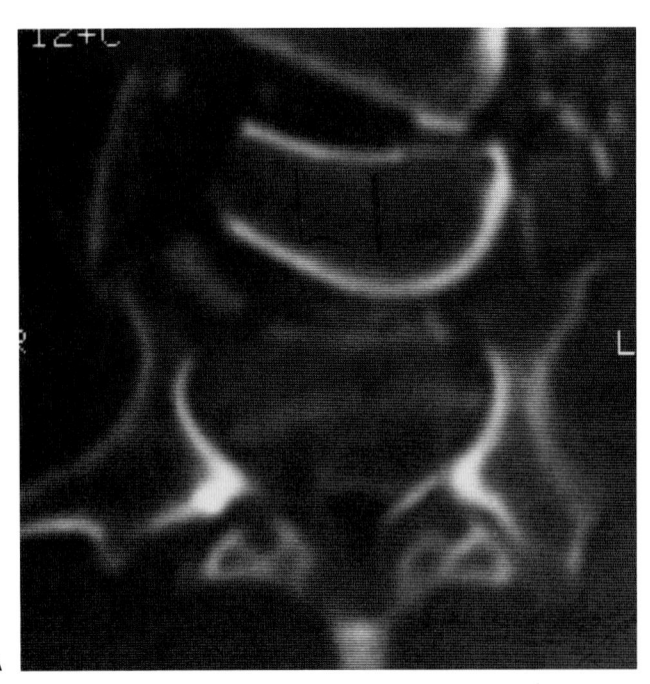

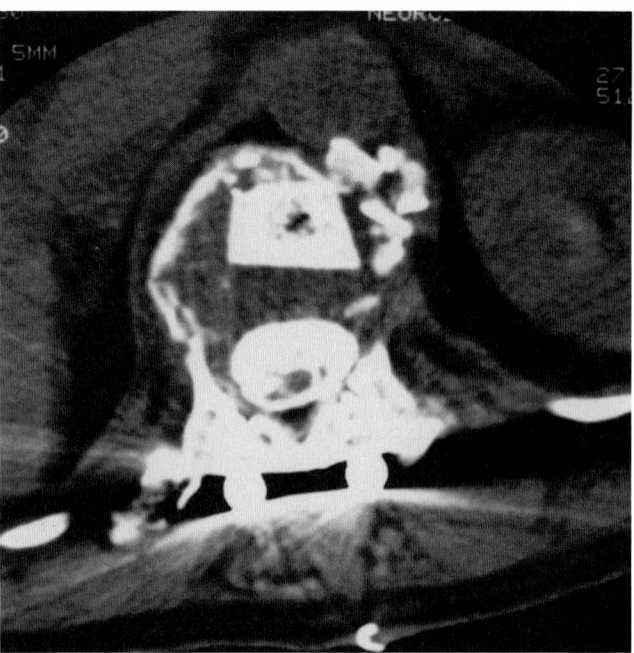

FIG. 8. A: CT scan of a patient who underwent an anterior attempt to decompress the canal after a burst fracture. The canal is occupied 100%, and there is a total block visible on CT/myelogram. **B:** A CT/myelogram of the same patient after simultaneous anterior and posterior procedures shows the anterior strut allograft and the posterior rod fixation.

and blood. In most cases, the surgery is performed with autologous transfusion only.

In general, the results of surgery for late deformity, neurologic deficit, and pain following thoracolumbar fracture are less satisfactory than for analogous procedures in the acute setting. Reduction of deformity is difficult to achieve (21), and significant improvement in neurologic function is unusual (52). Pain may be addressed via stabilization or decompression, but relief is frequently incomplete. As is true for much of spine deformity, late deformity following thoracolumbar injury is easier to prevent than it is to treat.

REFERENCES

1. Argenson C, Dintimille H. Lesions traumatiques experimentales durachis chez le singe. *Rev Chir Orthop* 1977;63:430–431.
2. Benson DR. Unstable thoracolumbar fractures, with emphasis on the burst fracture. *CORR* 1988;230:14.
3. Bohlman HH, Eismont FJ. Surgical techniques of anterior decompression and fusion for spinal cord injuries. *Clin Orthop* 1981;154:57.
4. Bohlman HH, Freehafer A, DeJak J. Late anterior decompression of spinal cord injuries. *J Bone Joint Surg* 1975;57A:1025.
5. Bradford DS. Deformities of the thoracic and lumbar spine secondary to spinal injury. Bradford DS, Lonstein JE, Moe JH, Ogilvie JW, Winter RB, eds. *Moe's textbook of scoliosis*, 2nd ed. Philadelphia: Saunders, 1987;435–463.
6. Bradford DS. Spinal instability: orthopedic perspective and prevention. *Clin Neurosurg* 1980;27:591.
7. Bradford DS, Winter RB, Lonstein JE, Moe JH. Techniques of anterior spinal surgery for the management of kyphosis. *CORR* 1977;128:129–139.
8. Celesia GG. American Electroencephalographic Society Guidelines for intraoperative monitoring of sensory evoked potentials. *J Clin Neurophysiol* 1987;4(4):397–416.
9. Chance GQ. Note on a type of flexion fracture of the spine. *Br J Radiol* 1948;21:452–453.
10. Crock HV, Yoshizawa H. *The blood supply of the vertebral column & spinal cord in man*. New York: Springer-Verlag, 1977.
11. Delamarter RB, Bohlman HH, Bodner D, Biro C. Urologic function after experimental cauda equina compression: cystometrograms versus cortical-evoked potentials. *Spine* 1990;15:864.
12. Denis F. Spinal instability as defined by the three column concept in acute spinal trauma. *Clin Orthop* 1984;189:65–67.
13. Denis F. The three column spine and its significance in the classification of acute thoracolumbar spinal injuries. *Spine* 1983;8:817.
14. DeWald RL. Burst fractures of the thoracic and lumbar spine. *Clin Orthop* 1984;189:150.
15. Dommisse GF. The blood supply of the spinal cord. *J Bone Joint Surg* 1974;56B(2):225–235.
16. Dunn HK. Anterior stabilization of thoracolumbar injuries. *Clin Orthop* 1984;189:117.
17. Edmonds HL, Paloheimo MPJ, Backman MH, Johnson JR, Holt RT, Shields CB. Transcranial magnetic motor evoked potentials (tcMMEP) for functional monitoring of motor pathways during scoliosis surgery. *Spine* 1989;14:683.
18. Farcy JPC, Roye DP, Weidenbaum M. Cotrel–Dubousset instrumentation technique for revision of failed lumbosacral fusion. *Bull Hosp Jt Dis Orthop Inst* 1987;47:1–12.
19. Farcy JPC, Weidenbaum M. Pitfalls in fracture fixation with Cotrel–Dubousset instrumentation. In: *Proceedings of the 5th International Congress on Cotrel–Dubousset instrumentation*. Montpellier: Sauramps Medical, 1989;103–110.
20. Farcy JPC, Weidenbaum M. A preliminary review of the use of Cotrel–Dubousset instrumentation for spinal injuries. *Bull Hosp Jt Dis Orthop Inst* 1988;48(1):44.
21. Farcy JPC, Weidenbaum M, Glassman SD. The Sagittal Index in the management of thoracolumbar burst fractures. *Spine* 1990;15:958.
22. Farcy JPC, Weidenbaum M, Sola C. Surgical management of severe cervical kyphosis following extensive laminectomies. *Spine* 1990;15(1):41–45.
23. Ferguson RL, Allen BL. A mechanistic classification of thoracolumbar spine fractures. *Clin Orthop* 1983;189:77.
24. Frankel HL, Hancock DO, Hyslop G, et al. The value of postural reduction in the initial management of closed injuries of the spine with paraplegia and tetraplegia. Part I. *Paraplegia* 1969;7:179–192.
25. Goutallier D, Louis R. Indications theraputiques dans les fractures instables du rachis. *Rev Chir Orthop* 1977;63:475–481.
26. Gurr KR, McAfee PC, Shih CM. Biomechanical analysis of anterior and posterior instrumentation systems after corpectomy. *J Bone Joint Surg* 1988;70A:1182–1191.
27. Guttman L. Spinal deformity in traumatic paraplegics and tetraplegics following surgical procedures. *Paraplegia* 1969;7:38–49.
28. Holdsworth FW. Fractures, dislocations, and fracture-dislocations of the spine. *J Bone Joint Surg* 1963;45B:6.
29. Holdsworth F. Fractures, dislocations, and fracture-dislocations of the spine. *J Bone Joint Surg* 1970;52A:1534.
30. Jacobs RR, Asher MA, Snider RK. Thoracolumbar spine injuries: a comparative study of recumbent and operative treatment in one hundred patients. *Spine* 1980;5:463–477.
31. Johnson JR, Leatherman KD, Holt RT. Anterior decompression of the spinal cord for neurologic deficit. *Spine* 1983;8:396.
32. Kaneda K, Kuniyoshi A, Masanori F. Burst fractures with neurologic deficits of the thoracolumbar–lumbar spine. *Spine* 1984;9:788–795.
33. Kelly RP, Whitesides TE. Treatment of lumbodorsal fracture-dislocations. *Ann Surg* 1968;167:705.
34. Kostuik JP. Anterior fixation for fractures of the thoracic and lumbar spine with or without neurologic involvement. *Clin Orthop* 1984;189:103–115.
35. Kostuik JP, Matsusaki H. Anterior stabilization instrumentation and decompression for post-traumatic kyphosis. *Spine* 1989;14(4):379–396.
36. Krompinger WJ, Frederickson BE, Mino DE, Yuan HA. Conservative treatment of fractures of the thoracic and lumbar spine. *Orthop Clin North Am* 1986;17:161.
37. Larson SJ. Lateral extracavitary approach to traumatic lesions of the thoracic and lumbar spine. *J Neurosurg* 1976;45:628–637.
38. Leatherman KD, Dickson RA. Two-stage corrective surgery for congenital deformities of the spine. *J Bone Joint Surg* 1979;61B:324–328.
39. Lucas JT, Ducker TB. Motor classification of spinal cord injuries with mobility, morbidity and recovery indices. *Am Surg* 1979;45:151–158.
40. Malcolm BW. Spinal deformity secondary to spinal injury. *Orthop Clin North Am* 1979;10(4):917.
41. Malcolm BW, Bradford DS, Winter RB, Chou SN. Post-traumatic kyphosis. *J Bone Joint Surg* 1981;63A:891.
42. McAfee PC, Bohlman HH, Yuan HA. Anterior decompression of traumatic thoracolumbar fractures with incomplete neurological deficit using a retroperitoneal approach. *J Bone Joint Surg* 1985;67A:89.
43. Morgan TH, Wharton GW, Austin GN. The results of laminectomy inpatients with incomplete spinal cord injuries. *Paraplegia* 1971;9:14.
44. Nicoll EA. Fracture of the dorso-lumbar spine. *J Bone Joint Surg* 1949;31B:376.
45. Pratt ES, Green DA, Spengler DM. Herniated intervertebral discs associated with unstable spinal injuries. *Spine* 1990;15(7):662–666.
46. Reid DC, Hu R, Davis LA, Saboe LA. The nonoperative treatment of burst fractures of the thoracolumbar junction. *J Trauma* 1988;18:1188.
47. Roaf R. A study of the mechanics of spinal injuries. *J Bone Joint Surg* 1960;42B:810.
48. Roberts JB, Curtiss PH. Stability of the thoracic and lumbar

spine in traumatic paraplegia following fracture or fracture/dislocation. *J Bone Joint Surg* 1970;52A:1115.
49. Roberts S, Manage J, Urban JPG. Biochemical and structural properties of the cartilage end plate and its relation to the intervertebral disc. *Spine* 1989;14:166–174.
50. Robertson JM, Whitesides TE. Surgical reconstruction of late posttraumatic thoracolumbar kyphosis. *Spine* 1985;10:307–312.
51. Streitz W, Brown JC, Bonnett CA. Anterior fibular strut grafting in the treatment of kyphosis. *CORR* 1977;128:140.
52. Transfeldt EE, White D, Bradford DS, Roche B. Delayed anterior decompression in patients with spinal cord and cauda equina injuries of the thoracolumbar spine. *Spine* 1990;15:953.
53. White AA, Panjabi MM. *Clinical biomechanics of the spine*, 2nd ed. Philadelphia: Lippincott, 1990.
54. Whitesides TE. Traumatic kyphosis of the thoracolumbar spine. *Clin Orthop* 1977;128:78.
55. Whitesides TE, Shah SG. On the management of unstable fractures of the thoracolumbar spine: rationale for use of anterior decompression and fusion and posterior stabilization. *Spine* 1976;1:99.
56. Young R, Brooks WH, Tibbs PA. Anterior decompression and fusion for thoracolumbar fractures with neurological deficits. *Acta Neurochir* 1981;57:287.

32

Rehabilitation Principles in the Management of Thoracolumbar Spine Fractures

Kristjan T. Ragnarsson

Every person who sustains a fracture of the spine is likely to require some form of rehabilitation treatment, regardless of whether the fracture results in a neurological deficit or not, or if the fracture is considered stable or unstable. Clearly, however, the individual whose spinal fracture is accompanied by a neurological deficit will be in greater need for rehabilitation services than the person who is neurologically intact. All fractures of the spine, even those that are considered stable, are associated with acute pain, which will require a certain degree of spinal immobilization. Later consequences of the fracture and of the necessary immobilization are likely to include some degree of chronic pain and physical deconditioning. The range of rehabilitation services that are required will vary depending on the specific symptoms and the extent of the physical disability. At a minimum, these services may consist of providing the patient with simple activity instructions or a soft spinal orthosis, whereas the patient with major neurologic deficits would require spinal immobilization by means of surgery and/or by application of extensive rigid spinal orthosis, involvement in a comprehensive inpatient rehabilitation program, and lifelong follow-up services. Optimal care of the patient with a spinal fracture will thus require good collaboration between the orthopaedic or neurological surgeon and the physiatrist, that is, the medical specialist in physical medicine and rehabilitation.

PRINCIPLES OF PHYSICAL MEDICINE AND REHABILITATION

The field of physical medicine and rehabilitation overlaps with many other medical and surgical specialties. Physical medicine is perhaps one of the oldest of the therapeutic approaches of traditional medicine along with the treatment by chemicals and surgery. *Physical medicine* may be defined as that branch of medicine that uses different physical agents in the management of disease and disability, for example, heat, cold, light, water, electromagnetic forces, and a variety of mechanical agents such as massage, exercise, traction, manipulation, and mechanical apparatus (25). *Rehabilitation medicine* is defined as the maximum restoration of physical, psychological, vocational, recreational, and economic function within the restrictions of the physical disability by multidisciplinary team intervention (42). The medical specialty of physical medicine and rehabilitation is often referred to as physiatry and its practitioners as physiatrists.

The patient with a major fracture of the thoracolumbar spine, regardless of the presence or absence of neurological deficits or the extent of such deficits, should be seen in consultation by the physiatrist within 48 hr of injury. The rehabilitation interventions that are initiated at this stage will depend on the stability of the spine and the general medical condition, as well as on

---

K. T. Ragnarsson: Department of Rehabilitation Medicine, Mount Sinai School of Medicine, New York, NY 10029.

the physical findings, but in general these interventions tend to be mostly preventive in nature, that is, gentle mobilization of extremity joints, joint splinting, breathing exercises, and so on. A more intensive rehabilitation program may be initiated when the spine has been judged stable and medical and surgical complications have been dealt with.

THE SPINAL INJURY REHABILITATION TEAM

At the heart of successful rehabilitation for any individual with a severe physical disability, such as spinal cord injury, is the multidisciplinary rehabilitation team (Table 1), which consists of many different health professionals. Under the direction of the physiatrist, members of the multidisciplinary rehabilitation team become involved as judged appropriate by the patient's medical and surgical condition. The members of the team meet regularly to discuss the patient's medical, neurological, functional, psychological, vocational, and social status, as well as the functional potential. At these meetings, specific rehabilitation goals are set, needs for equipment, home modifications, and personal assistance are projected, and discharge date, whether from the inpatient or outpatient program, is predicted. The physiatrist meets with the patient and the family after each meeting to review the recommendation of the team, explain to them the components of the rehabilitation program and its goals, and address all their questions and concerns. Each member of the rehabilitation team plays an important and specific role in the patient's rehabilitation. In order to expedite the rehabilitation process, it is important that the team members work simultaneously toward the final goals. Communication between the patient, the physiatrist, and the rehabilitation team members is of enormous importance to ensure that all concerns are expressed and addressed in a timely manner.

TABLE 1. *Multidisciplinary spinal cord injury rehabilitation team*

Physician (physiatrist, consultants)
Rehabilitation nurse
Physical therapist
Occupational therapist
Psychologist
Social worker
Vocational counselor
Recreational therapist
Orthotist
Driver educator
Home economist
Equipment coordinator/vendor
Educator
Patient and family

FUNCTIONAL ASSESSMENT

Measurable benefits must result from any accepted medical and surgical treatment. In contrast to other medical fields, the outcome of rehabilitation interventions cannot be measured by eradication of symptoms or survival rate, since there is usually a lasting disability that does not affect life expectancy. The effectiveness of rehabilitation interventions is assessed by how independent the patient becomes in the different aspects of self-care, mobility, and communication as a result of this treatment. The terms impairment, disability, and handicap have been carefully defined by the World Health Organization in order to express in functional terms the impact of a physical deficit on a person (50). *Impairment* is "a loss or abnormality of psychological, physical or anatomical structure of function," for example, paraplegia. *Disability* is "any restriction or lack (resulting from an impairment) of an ability to perform an activity in a manner within the range considered normal for a human being," for example, paraplegia resulting in an inability to walk. *Handicap* is "a disadvantage for a given individual resulting from an impairment or disability that limits or prevents the fulfillment of a role that is normal (depending on age, sex and social and cultural factors) for that individual," for example, the individual is paraplegic and unable to ambulate and therefore not able to meet the demands of the job and thus unable to return to work.

The functional performance in the different activities of self-care, mobility (Table 2), and communication must be regularly and numerically assessed during the rehabilitation treatment for the purpose of documentation and monitoring of changes in function. Several grades of independence/dependence may be defined for this purpose, for example, completely independent, independent with devices, requires personal assistance of varying degree (i.e., reminding, supervision, "spotting," or physical help), or is completely dependent. Accurate functional assessment requires collection of

TABLE 2. *Skills for self-care and mobility*

Eating and drinking
Dressing and undressing
Bathing and grooming
Toileting
Managing bladder and bowel functions
Manipulating small objects
Caring for health and fitness
Moving in bed
Changing position
Walking on level surface
Climbing stairs
General wheelchair skills
Using a manual wheelchair
Using a powered wheelchair

diverse data, which are gathered by several means, for example, physical examination, observation, review of records and reports, and verbal accounts from nurses, therapists, as well as from the patient and the family. Several functional assessment scales exist; some are simple and easy to use but provide inadequate information, whereas others are detailed and time consuming. Computer technology has facilitated collection analysis and plotting of data and has enabled clinicians to record the patient's progress numerically both during inpatient and outpatient rehabilitation. The scale that has gained the greatest acceptance by rehabilitation professionals is the Functional Independence Measure (FIM) (Fig. 1) (18).

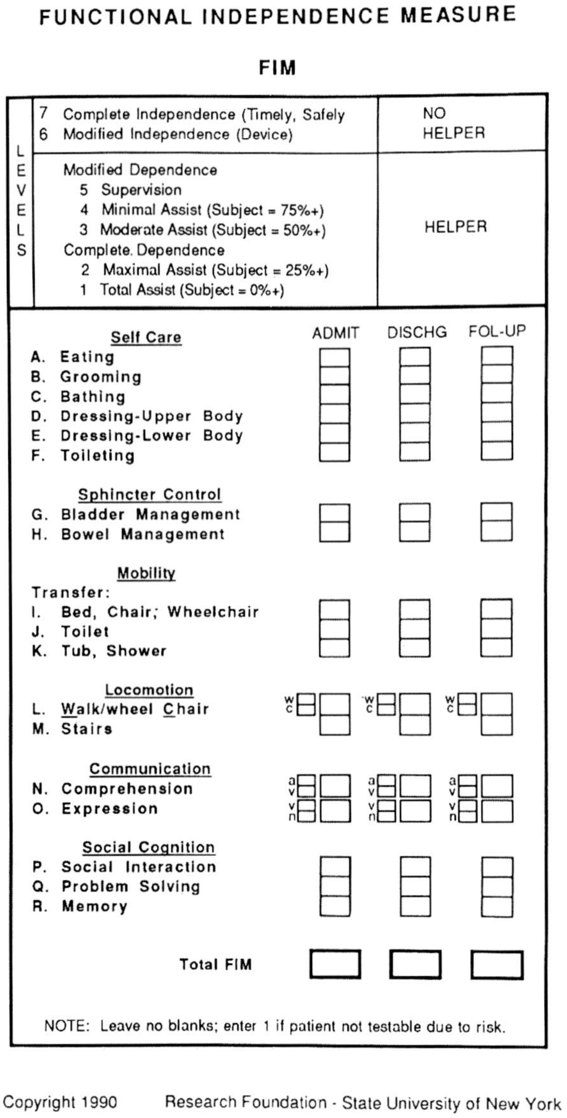

FUNCTIONAL INDEPENDENCE MEASURE

FIM

LEVELS	7 Complete Independence (Timely, Safely) 6 Modified Independence (Device)	NO HELPER

	Modified Dependence
	  5 Supervision
	  4 Minimal Assist (Subject = 75%+)
	  3 Moderate Assist (Subject = 50%+)
	Complete Dependence
	  2 Maximal Assist (Subject = 25%+)
	  1 Total Assist (Subject = 0%+)
		HELPER

	ADMIT	DISCHG	FOL-UP
Self Care A. Eating B. Grooming C. Bathing D. Dressing-Upper Body E. Dressing-Lower Body F. Toileting			
Sphincter Control G. Bladder Management H. Bowel Management			
Mobility Transfer: I. Bed, Chair; Wheelchair J. Toilet K. Tub, Shower			
Locomotion L. Walk/wheel Chair M. Stairs			
Communication N. Comprehension O. Expression			
Social Cognition P. Social Interaction Q. Problem Solving R. Memory			
Total FIM			

NOTE: Leave no blanks; enter 1 if patient not testable due to risk.

Copyright 1990   Research Foundation - State University of New York

FIG. 1. Functional Independence Measure (FIM). A scale to assess and monitor function of persons with disabilities. (From ref. 18).

ORTHOTIC MANAGEMENT OF THE FRACTURED SPINE

The spine has three major functions. It provides support and mobility for the body and a protective shield for the spinal cord. The anatomy of the spine has been described in detail in Part I of this book. With respect to orthotic management of the fractured thoracolumbar spine, the reader must know the anatomical structure and relationships of the vertebrae, the intervertebral discs, ligamentous connections, vascular supply, spinal cord, and nerve roots. The intervertebral discs serve as the main cushioning mechanism against vertical compression forces, but in addition, the three basic physiologic curves of the spine in the anterior–posterior plane (i.e., cervical lordosis, thoracic kyphosis, and lumbar lordosis) serve to diminish the effects of compressive forces and to adjust the body to the upright position. Multiple factors influence the posture of the spine, but the pelvic or lumbosacral angle is of particular importance since the entire spine balances on the sacrum as its foundation. The lumbosacral angle in turn is affected by position of the main lower limb joints. Additionally, the posture of the spine is affected by heredity, habit, structural abnormalities, distribution of body fat, and physical conditioning.

Three-dimensionally the spine has three main planes of motions: flexion/extension, lateral bending, and rotation. Additionally, some longitudinal or axial motion in the form of distraction/compression occurs. The mean motions of the different segments of the spine are shown in Table 3, although it should be noted that investigators differ in their opinions with regard to the exact degree of motion at different levels. The ligaments of the spine have several different functions, but in essence they are elastic elements that resist tensile forces but buckle with compression. They thus allow physiological segmented motion with minimum muscle energy cost, while providing spinal stability along with muscles and protecting the spinal cord by restriction of motion (49). Without muscles the spinal column is not stable and buckles with even minimal compression

TABLE 3. *Mean motion of the spine (in degrees)*

Movement	Cervical	Thoracic	Lumbar
Flexion	60	15	40
Extension	78	15	25
Total flexion–extension	138	30	65
Lateral flexion, right	44	15	20
Lateral flexion, left	44	15	20
Total lateral flexion	88	30	40
Rotation, right	78	40	5
Rotation, left	78	40	5
Total rotation	156	80	10

Adapted from ref. 37.

forces. Only with combined intrinsic and extrinsic support is the spine able to withstand the great forces that it is subjected to during daily life and work. During motion the spinal canal changes in dimension while its contents (i.e., the spinal cord and its associated structures) do not slide up and down but deform in a fashion similar to an accordion because of their elastic nature (6). This elasticity, however, may be lost with injury. Clinical stability of the spine is a critical, although an elusive, concept subject to many different definitions. Clinical instability may be defined as the loss of the ability of the spine under physiological loads to maintain its pattern of displacement so that there is no initial or additional neurologic deficit, no major deformity, and no incapacitating pain (49). Physiologic loads in turn are defined as those incurred during normal activities. Spinal instability is also frequently defined simply as loss of two of the three structural columns of the spine (10,19).

A spinal orthosis is prescribed following a fracture, primarily in order to protect or immobilize the painful or unstable vertebral column and to allow effective healing. When an orthosis is prescribed to allow healing of a spinal fracture or of a surgical spinal fusion, it usually must be worn for at least 10 to 12 weeks. The efficacy of the attempted protection and immobilization is often hard to judge given the difficulty in clinically examining the deep-seated joints of the spine and assessing their motions. The orthotic prescription, however, must be based on as accurate identification of the biomechanical deficits as possible.

Two basic methods of control are employed when correcting or stabilizing spinal deformities: (a) longitudinal traction or distraction and (b) counteractive horizontal forces [i.e., the three-point pressure system (8)]. The size of the body area over which the corrective forces can be applied and the tolerance of the underlying tissues are important factors to be considered when the exact design of the orthosis is determined.

Numerous designs of spinal orthoses are available, although the biomechanical effects of most tend to be similar. The exact orthotic design selected frequently depends more on local customs and availability rather than on specific indications. The Spinal Technical Analysis form may be helpful to the clinician to document the major spinal impairment, assess the biomechanics, identify treatment objectives, and recommend the proper orthosis (29). The prescribing physician should make it clear to the patient that the spinal orthosis is only a temporary intervention that is applied to allow proper healing during the postinjury or postoperative period. If clinically possible, the patient should be instructed to perform certain trunk exercises and practice good protective body mechanisms in order to reduce deconditioning effects on the trunk muscles and to avoid emotional dependency on the orthosis.

In order to discourage the confusing use of eponyms and to improve communication, a systemic nomenclature for orthotic devices was developed in 1973 by a national task force and this nomenclature has since become standard. Here spinal orthoses are classified according to the spinal segments involved: cervical orthoses (CO), head–cervical orthoses (HCO), thoracolumbosacral orthoses (TLSO), lumbosacral orthoses (LSO), and cervicothoracolumbosacral orthoses (CTLSO). Spinal orthoses may be further classified as rigid, semirigid, or flexible, and depending on the prescription indication, as corrective or supportive.

Unless life-saving interventions are needed, the individual with acute spinal cord injury must immediately have the entire spine immobilized on a spinal stabilization traction board in order to prevent any secondary spinal disruption, which could cause further injury. This immobilization must include both ends of the spine (i.e., the head and the pelvis), since position and movement of these parts may influence spinal alignment.

Effective immobilization of the lumbosacral regions is quite difficult to achieve by orthotic means although frequently attempted. A molded rigid pelvic girdle or a hip spica, carefully padded, is generally required for maximum external stabilization. On the other hand, the thoracic spine, particularly its upper half, tends to be relatively stable given the support of an intact rib cage, which minimizes displacement after fracture and/or dislocation. As noted in Table 3, the thoracic spine allows considerably greater rotation than flexion/extension and lateral bending, while the reverse is true for the lumbar spine. This is mainly due to the anatomical differences in articular facet orientation.

Lumbosacral orthoses (LSO) and thoracolumbosacral orthoses (TLSO) may be prescribed for numerous common clinical conditions and symptoms besides fractures. These orthoses are primarily used to diminish pain, to provide body support, to control spine motion and alignment, to compensate for muscle weakness, and to correct deformities. Different materials may be used for fabrication and numerous designs are available. The materials used in the fabrication of spinal orthoses are usually combinations of cloth, leather, plaster, metal, plastic, and rubber. The different designs provide different degrees of spinal support and accordingly may be referred to as belts, corsets, braces, or jackets. Optimal trunk support is obtained by applying pressure over the entire abdominal wall, thereby raising the intra-abdominal pressure, and by simultaneously applying the three-point pressure system. When the intra-abdominal pressure is raised by supporting weak abdominal muscles with a rigid orthotic support, the stress on the spine is decreased by generating a semirigid hydropneumatic cylinder anteriorly and laterally. This cylinder distributes the vertical

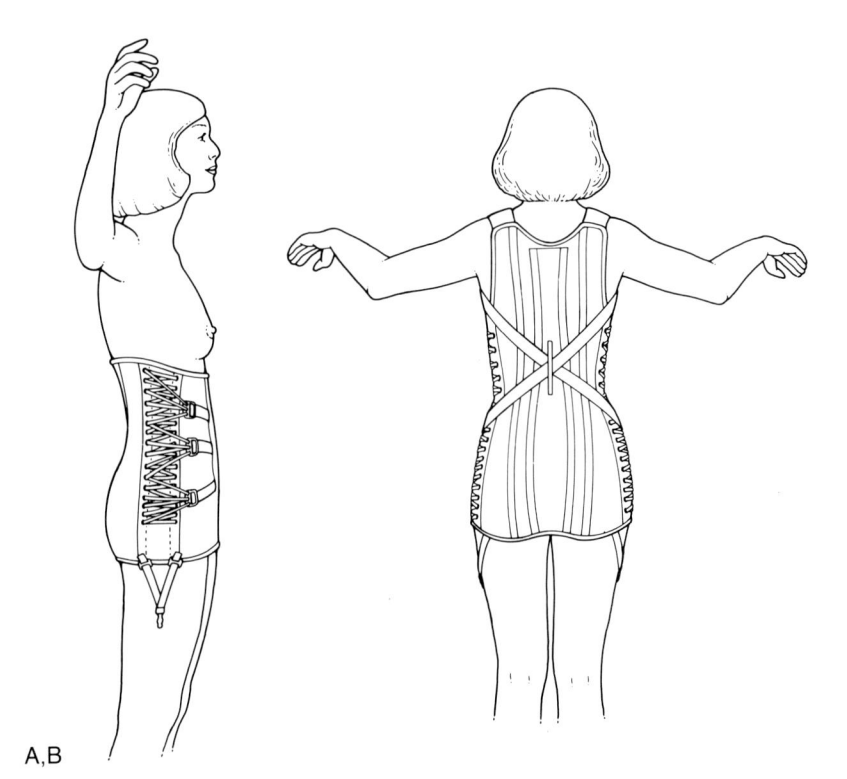

FIG. 2. A: Flexible lumbosacral orthosis (LSO, corset), lateral view. **B:** Flexible thoracolumbosacral orthosis (TLSO, corset) with shoulder straps and posterior metal stays (posterior view).

force and reduces the lumbar lordosis. It has been shown that elevation of the intra-abdominal pressure by this means may reduce the load on the intervertebral discs by 30% in the lumbar spine and 50% in the thoracic spine (32). Control of spinal motions and maintenance of realignment are better provided by applying the three-point pressure system than by abdominal wall support. The effectiveness of this system is quite variable depending on orthotic design. As with all orthotic devices, sensory feedback is an additional effective influence in inhibiting motion and correcting trunk position.

Corsets, either a flexible LSO or a TLSO (Fig. 2), are made of different fabrics with adjustable sets of braces or straps, which are tightened to provide support for the abdominal muscles and thus the trunk. They are usually reinforced with rigid paraspinal metal stays. Corsets are relatively ineffective in mechanically restricting motion, but rather act as a reminder to limit motion. They are comfortable and generally effective in reducing pain and are thus prescribed for various painful back disorders, including stable compression fractures of the lumbar and lower thoracic spine.

When greater restriction of spinal motion is required, a more rigid orthosis is prescribed. The old "Chairback" LSO (Fig. 3) consists of a metal pelvic band inferiorly that extends posteriorly across the pelvis between the greater trochanter on each side just below the iliac crest. Superiorly, there is a thoracic band transversely located 1 in. below the scapulae.

These bands are connected by two paraspinal metal uprights. The Knight LSO additionally has two lateral metal uprights. Both orthoses have an anterior apron, which is usually made of fabric. The Knight–Taylor

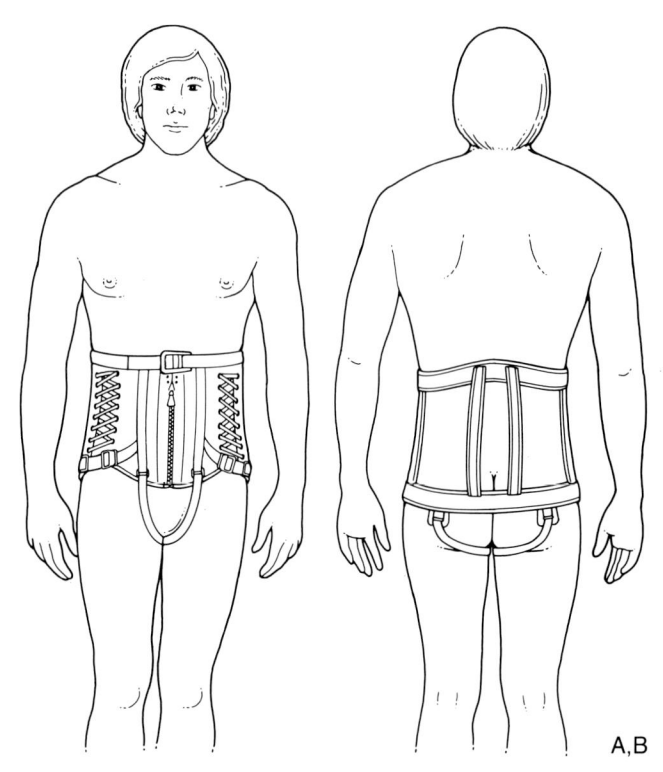

FIG. 3. Lumbosacral orthosis (LSO, Knight spinal brace). **A:** Anterior view. **B:** Posterior view.

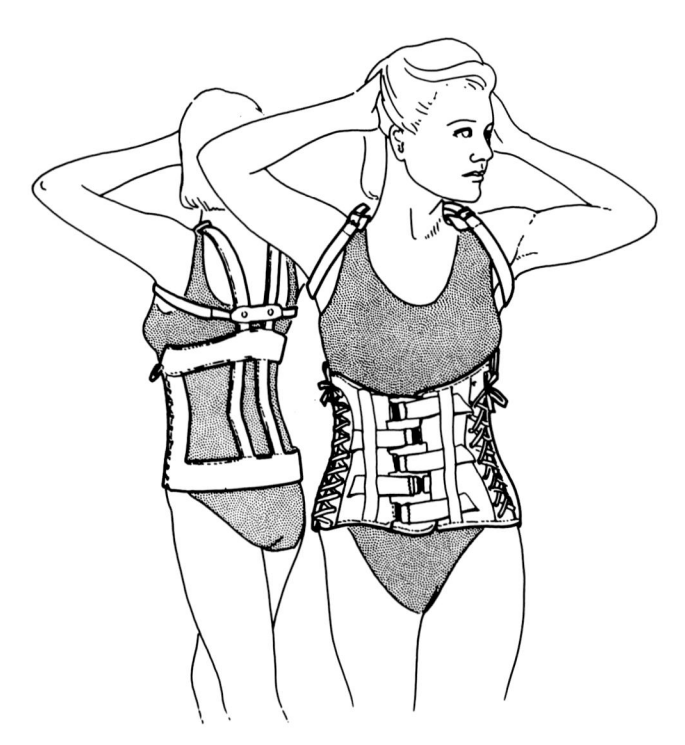

FIG. 4. Thoracolumbosacral orthosis (TLSO, Knight–Taylor spinal brace). (From ref. 39.)

TLSO (Fig. 4) is a modification of the Knight LSO, where the two rigid posterior paraspinal uprights are extended upward along the extent of the thoracic spine and the thoracic band is extended anteriorly and superiorly to the pectoral region to prevent rotation, lateral bending, and flexion of the spine. Axillary straps attached to this orthosis have little effect on the spine but may be placed to retract the shoulders. Perineal straps may also be placed to prevent sliding of the orthosis up and down. A cervical extension may be added to this orthosis if needed. These orthoses are relatively comfortable and easily adjusted and are frequently used for relatively stable fractures of the thoracolumbar spine, or after surgical stabilization of any unstable fracture. They reduce gross motion and provide trunk support but are inadequate for treatment of unstable fractures as they do not produce complete three-dimensional control.

Different designs of spinal hyperextension TLSO are available, for example, the Jewett, CASH, and Baker orthoses. These orthoses use the three-point pressure system by applying pressure anteriorly on the pelvis or pubis below and the sternum above by means of pads attached to a firm metal frame. Posteriorly, pressure is applied over the lower thoracic and upper lumbar spine by a pad that is attached to the anterior metal frame by adjustable straps. These orthoses provide no abdominal muscle support and limit motion in only one plane, that is, flexion. Although they are lightweight, they may be uncomfortable since the corrective forces are distributed over a relatively small area. The Jewett orthosis (Fig. 5) is probably most commonly used of these, especially for anteriorly wedged compression fractures of the lower thoracic and upper lumbar spine or after surgical stabilization of fractures in this region. Adequate breast and axillary relief may sometimes be difficult to obtain while maintaining spinal control with the Jewett orthosis. Many patients have found the cruciform anterior spinal hyperextension (CASH) orthosis (Fig. 6) more comfortable, which may account for its increasing popularity.

Custom-molded spinal jacket or total contact TLSO (Fig. 7) is the most rigid design. It is prescribed for maximum restriction of motion in the three dimensions and for trunk support. This orthosis may be made of plaster of Paris or plastic materials. The orthosis is usually bivalved and the anterior and posterior halves are connected by Velcro straps. The jacket is firmly molded around the pelvis below. Above it may extend to the manubrium of the sternum anteriorly in order to control both rotation and flexion. Posteriorly it extends to the midportion of the scapula. When needed, a cervical extension may be added to this orthosis. When it is important to restrict motion across the lumbosacral region, a hip spica orthosis may have to be applied. Here a rigid thigh socket extends to the supracondylar region of the thigh in one limb and to the level of the hip joint on the opposite side. An external drop lock may be placed at the hip in order to inhibit motion

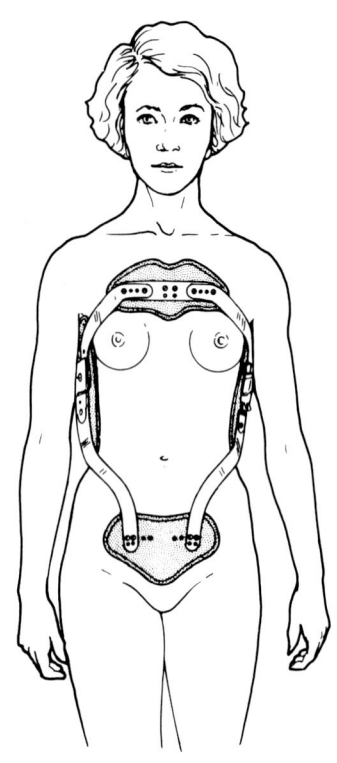

FIG. 5. Jewett hyperextension (TLSO) orthosis. (From ref. 37.)

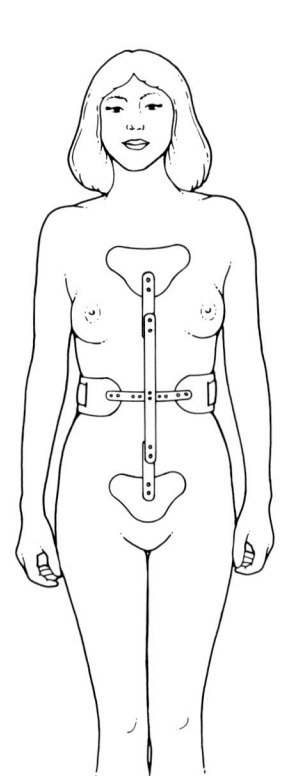

FIG. 6. Cruciform anterior spinal hyperextension (CASH) orthosis (TLSO).

while the patient is standing, ambulating, or sitting and to allow motion when resting in the supine position. The rigid TLSO body jacket is prescribed for unstable fractures of the spine that may not be surgically stabilized or when the adequacy of the surgical stabilization is in question. Additionally, these are frequently used for certain spinal metastases. Even when well fitted, the TLSO jacket tends to be warm and somewhat uncomfortable. Comfort may be increased by placement of holes in the jacket to improve skin breathing. Large cutout pieces from the orthosis should be avoided as these may reduce its mechanical functions. As noted above, any form of appropriate orthotic support, which is used to allow better healing of a fractured or surgically fused spine, usually needs to be continued for at least 10 to 12 weeks. During this time static exercises of the trunk muscles should be performed in order to reduce muscle atrophy and to facilitate the eventual weaning of the orthosis.

ELECTRODIAGNOSTIC STUDIES

Electrodiagnostic studies are usually performed and interpreted by physiatrists or neurologists. When expertly done, these studies may be useful as additions to the clinical examination, often confirming a pathological process, its localization, main characteristics, and severity. The referring physician needs to understand the basic principles involved in these studies in order to be able to critically judge the objective findings and the examiner's interpretation of these. These studies consist of electromyography (EMG), nerve conduction measurement studies (NCS), and elicitation and recording of evoked cerebral potentials. Electrodiagnostic studies are essentially risk-free but may be uncomfortable to the awake patient. A pleasant and clinically skillful examiner can do much to make this test more comfortable for the patient.

Electromyography

Electromyography is the detection and recording of electrical activity from muscles, usually by inserting a small coaxial needle electrode. This electrode detects tiny intramuscular electrical potentials that are amplified and may either be acoustically or visually displayed and recorded. The variations of the electrical potentials in number and configuration provide the information that is of diagnostic value. Unfortunately, EMG findings are hardly ever pathognomonic for a given disease and must be interpreted in light of the clinical findings.

A normal muscle is electrically silent at rest. Upon insertion or with any movement of the needle electrode, there is a brief burst of electrical activity referred to as *insertional activity*. Usually this activity averages less than 300 milliseconds (msec) in duration. This is seen on the oscilloscope as a series of sharp spikes followed by a flat line. Increased insertional activity is a nonspecific pathological finding that indi-

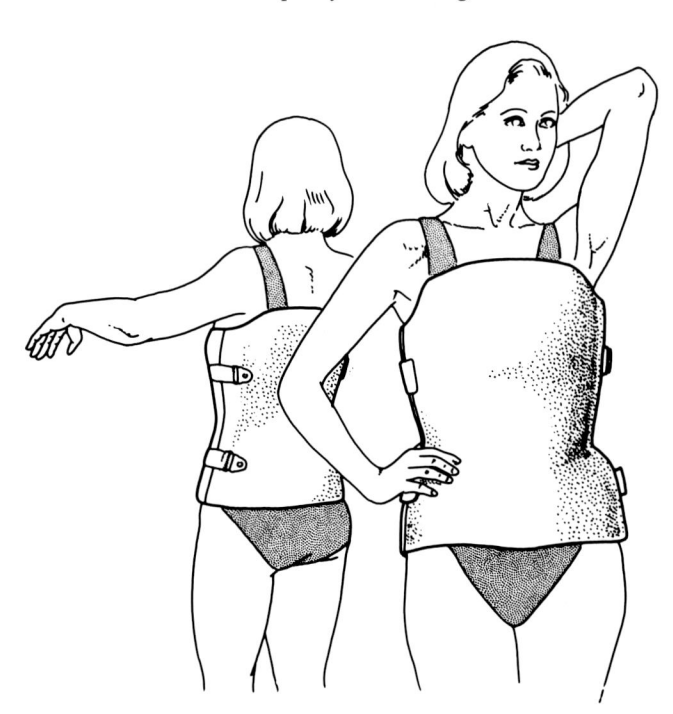

FIG. 7. Total contact TLSO or custom-molded spinal jacket. (From ref. 39.)

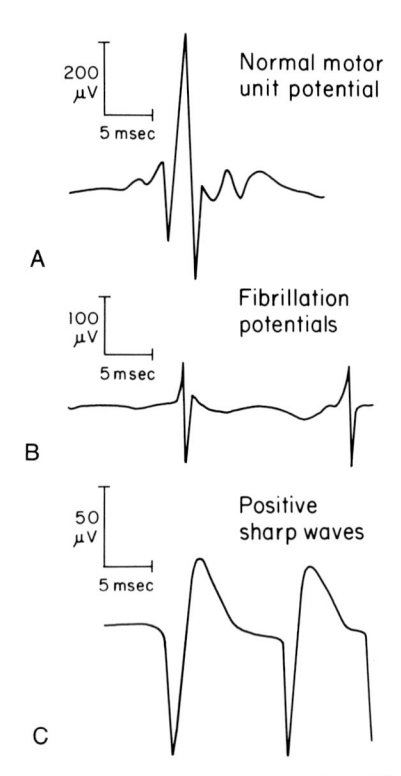

FIG. 8. A: Normal motor unit potential. **B:** Fibrillation potentials. **C:** Positive sharp waves.

cates muscle hyperactivity for both myopathic and neuropathic reasons. A single *motor unit potential* (Fig. 8A) is the smallest electrical activity that can be generated by voluntary effort. It reflects electrical firing of one motor neuron through its axon and simultaneous and synchronous contraction of all muscle fibers innervated by that axon. The motor unit potential is usually biphasic or triphasic and measures 4 to 12 msec in duration. Depending on the number of contracting muscle fibers and their proximity to the needle, the amplitude may vary between 300 microvolts (μV) and 5 millivolts (mV). A motor unit potential, much larger in amplitude (10–20 mV) may be seen in anterior horn cell disease and other conditions that result in collateral sprouting of the axon to denervated muscle fibers.

After degeneration of a nerve fiber, the efferent stimulus may fail to reach all the muscle fibers of the motor unit simultaneously. The resulting motor unit action potential may then have a greater number of spikes, be lower than normal in amplitude, and be of longer duration. These potentials are referred to as *polyphasic potentials*. They are of clinical significance, if they have more than seven to eight spikes and repeat themselves consistently (i.e., constitute more than 10% of all the recorded motor units). Polyphasic potentials of low amplitude and short duration are typically seen in myopathic disease, whereas in neuropathic disease these tend to be of higher amplitude and longer duration.

During a normal vigorous muscle contraction, the oscilloscope screen will fill with countless motor unit potentials and disappearance of the baseline. This appearance is referred to as a complete *interference pattern*. In neurogenic disease the interference pattern may be incomplete (i.e., an interrupted baseline is present), while demonstrating relatively high amplitude, whereas in myopathy the interference pattern is typically complete, even upon a clinically weak muscle contraction, but the amplitude is low.

Besides causing prolonged insertional activity and generating polyphasic potentials, damage to the motor neuron and its axon usually results in spontaneous appearance of very small but distinctly pathological electrical potentials while the muscle is at rest. These are referred to as *fibrillations* (Fig. 8B). They are usually biphasic, or rarely triphasic, in shape and measure less than 2 msec in duration and 50 to 100 μV in amplitude. They are often accompanied by monophasic *positive sharp waves* (Fig. 8C) of variable amplitude and duration, usually 50 to 100 μV and 5 to 10 msec, respectively. Fibrillations and positive sharp waves appear approximately 2 weeks after nerve injury but usually disappear after complete reinnervation and within 3 to 10 years if no reinnervation occurs. While these potentials are typical for lower motor neuron disease, they may also be seen, although more rarely, in myopathy and upper motor neuron disease.

Nerve Conduction Measurement Studies

Nerve conduction velocity may be measured objectively and accurately in a relatively easy fashion. After a ground electrode is connected, a recording electrode is placed on the skin over a given muscle. The corresponding nerve is next stimulated at two different points, one proximally and the other distally (Fig. 9). A supramaximal stimulus is used to ensure that all motor nerve fibers are stimulated. The speed of the conducted stimulus along the nerve is calculated by measuring the distance between the proximal and distal stimulation sites in centimeters, and dividing this number by the difference in latency, that is, the conduction time from the two stimulation sites to the pick-up electrode. The time is expressed in milliseconds and the results in meters per second (m/sec). Nerve conduction velocity is affected by many factors including the diameter of the nerve and its myelin sheath thickness, environmental temperature, and the patient's age, but average velocity is normally 50 to 70 m/sec in the upper extremities and 45 to 55 m/sec in the lower extremities. Conduction time of sensory nerve fibers may be measured in a similar fashion by evoking and recording their electrical

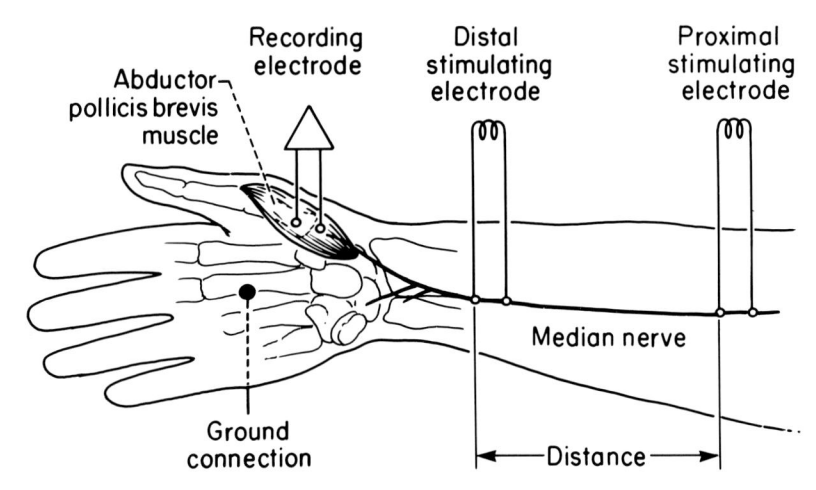

FIG. 9. Nerve conduction velocity measurement of the median nerve. Proximal stimulating electrode is placed at the elbow and a distal stimulating electrode at the wrist. Recording electrode is placed over the abductor pollicis brevis. The ground electrode is placed on the back of the hand. The difference in conduction time from the two stimulation sites to the recording electrode will indicate the nerve conduction velocity.

potentials either in "antidromic" or "orthodromic" fashion. Nerve conduction velocity is clinically slowed along the entire nerve in neuropathic disease and segmentally in entrapment conditions.

EMG and NCS are of some clinical value in assessing the patient with spinal fracture. It is important for the clinician to recognize that even in the presence of neurological damage, no EMG abnormalities will appear for at least 2 weeks after the injury. Any EMG abnormalities detected during those first 2 weeks can be interpreted as being due to preexisting conditions. Neurological impairment due to spinal fracture may be due to injury to the spinal cord, the nerve roots, or both. Injury to the nerve roots, including the cauda equina, will result in EMG evidence of denervation approximately 2 weeks after injury; that is, an appearance of fibrillations and positive sharp waves, prolonged insertional activity, and, if some voluntary motion is present, incomplete interference pattern and polyphasic motor unit action potentials. When the spinal cord is injured, similar findings may be detected in muscles innervated by neurological segments and roots at the level of the lesion, since injury to the cord results in segmental loss of anterior horn cells and is usually associated with some injury to the nerve roots as well. Thus a cervical spinal cord injury causing quadriplegia is usually associated with spasticity and relative paucity of EMG findings in the trunk and lower extremities, but results in clinical signs of lower motor neuron damage in the upper extremities with widespread EMG abnormalities. A fracture at the thoracolumbar junction or in the lumbar spine, which injures the conus of the cord and the cauda equina, will be associated with extensive EMG changes in the lower extremities.

Nerve conduction studies are usually normal following spinal fractures since it is rare that all neurons, both motor and sensory, as well as the nerve roots, which make up a major nerve, are complete destroyed. Extensive damage of these elements, however, may reduce the size of the action potential upon stimulation.

Evaluation of different peripheral reflexes by recording EMG responses following electrical stimulation of a mixed peripheral nerve or tapping of a tendon may be useful in order to assess the integrity of the peripheral nerve system at different levels and the excitability of the spinal cord, for example, the Hoffman reflex (H-reflex), the F-wave, the tendon tap reflex (T-reflex), and the tonic vibration reflex (23).

Evoked Potentials

Electrical activity was first recorded from the brain more than a century ago (5) and for more than half a century it has been known that alpha waves may be blocked by eye opening. In 1947 Dawson (9) first reported the use of photographic averaging of the electroencephalogram (EEG) by superposition, which he found to improve his technical ability to resolve synchronized responses to a specific event. This enabled him to demonstrate large somatosensory evoked potentials (SEP) on the EEG in certain forms of myoclonus and subsequent elicitation of such cerebral electrical responses by stimulation of a peripheral nerve. Since that time advances in electronics and computer technology have made the recording of various cerebral evoked potentials (EP) easier for the evaluation of a number of clinical conditions affecting the nervous system.

NORMAL

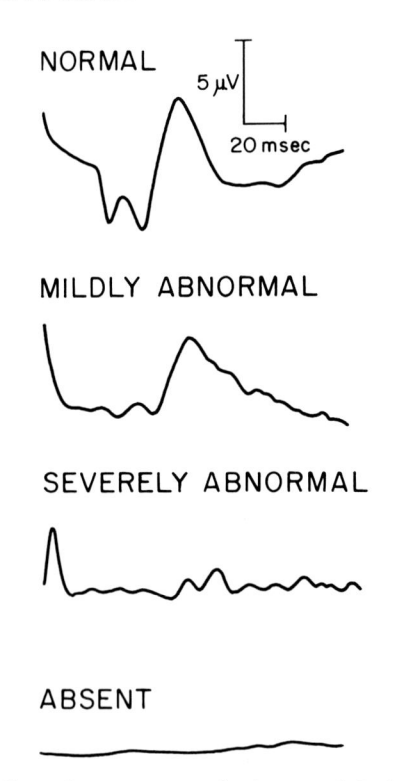

MILDLY ABNORMAL

SEVERELY ABNORMAL

ABSENT

FIG. 10. Somatosensory evoked potentials (SEPs).

Complete evaluation of the patient with thoracolumbar spine fracture should include recording of SEPs (Fig. 10). Additionally, during major spinal surgery on the neurologically spared and anesthetized patient, many clinicians choose to monitor SEPs continuously intraoperatively. The technique usually employed during a recording and monitoring of SEPs involves repetitive electrical stimulation of a mixed peripheral nerve or a pure sensory nerve, usually the median nerve at the wrist and the posterior tibial nerve at the ankle. Stimulation activates the large myelinated and fast conducting sensory fibers within the nerve, which carry the stimulus proximally through the corresponding plexus and dorsal nerve roots to the spinal cord. Within the spinal cord the impulse is carried in the ipsilateral dorsal columns to the contralateral sensory regions in the cerebral cortex. Scalp electrodes are carefully placed over specific cortical sites for picking up the action potential. The cerebral EP is very small but with proper amplification and signal averaging it is clearly identified and recorded. The SEP latency, amplitude, and configuration provide valuable but not absolute information on neurological function along the route of the stimulus.

While recording of SEPs is often included in the initial evaluation of the patient with new spinal fracture, its value is somewhat limited as a diagnostic and prognostic tool for spinal cord function. Since this test only provides information on the conduction in the posterior columns of the cord, false-positive results are common. Monitoring of SEPs has found its greatest usefulness during major surgical procedures on the spine (33), when altered wave forms and longer latencies compared with preoperative results may indicate a new impingement of the spinal cord tissue or diminished blood flow. These findings may alert the surgeon to stop or change the surgical maneuvers. This technique may spare the surgeon the need to do a "wake-up test" during the procedure, which not only is disrupting but has also been reported to result in accidental extubation and dislodgement of implanted rods (33). Unfortunately, increased neurological deficits may occasionally occur without intraoperative recording of SEP changes. Alteration of SEPs may also occur due to factors other than neurological deficits, for example, different anesthetic agents and drugs (e.g., halogenated agents, Fentanyl in a bolus form, diazepam), body temperature lower than 35°C, electrolyte changes, increased Pco_2, hypotension, and excessive stimulation rate (33).

In order to increase the usefulness of EP testing, different techniques are under evaluation or have been tested clinically. These techniques include spinal–spinal evoked responses, that is, stimulating and recording directly on the cord above and below the lesion during an open surgical operation and recording motor evoked responses that are elicited by stimulating the groin through a scalp electrode placed over the motor cortex of the brain, either with electricity or in a less painful fashion with localized magnetic field, and recording EMG signals from the distally appropriate muscles. Evaluation of the motor responses provides information on conduction velocity within the descending pathways of the cord, activation mechanisms of the alpha motor neurons, and distribution of the impulse to different muscles. Unfortunately, motor responses have little or no prognostic value since their elicitation has only been reported in muscles that the patient was able to contract voluntarily.

REHABILITATION MANAGEMENT OF THE NEUROLOGICALLY INTACT PATIENT WITH THORACOLUMBAR SPINE FRACTURE

In general, it appears that surgical stabilization of the fractured spine is done more often than previously. Regardless of the presence or absence of neurological deficits, several basic indications exist, both for performing internal surgical stabilization of the fractured thoracolumbar spine and for choosing nonsurgical management. These indications should be clear to the rehabilitation clinician as well as to the surgeon. The main surgical indications would be (a) gross spinal instability as defined in the orthopaedic literature (10,14,21), (b) gross misalignment of the spine, (c) incomplete neurological deficits, especially if these are progressive, and (d) irreducible fracture-dislocation. The relative indications for a nonsurgical management approach (31) include the presence of anterior compression fracture of the vertebral body resulting in less than 3.5-mm displacement, multiple spinal fractures, especially if these are not adjacent to each other, and spinal fracture of more than 3 weeks duration. Additionally, fractures of the upper thoracic spine (i.e., between T1 and T10) that are not associated with any neurological deficits are best treated nonsurgically since this part of the spine is inherently stable (31). Surgical stabilization of a fracture in this part of the thoracic spine in the neurologically intact patient is associated with high risk of surgically induced neurological trauma, perhaps related to the small size of the spinal canal and the delicate vascular supply to the cord. However, if surgery is undertaken, careful intraoperative monitoring of SEPs is necessary. Fractures of the thoracic spine above T6 should preferably be treated initially with skeletal traction and subsequently by placing the patient in CTLSO. For fractures below T6, a TLSO (e.g., plastic laminated body jacket, Knight–Taylor or Jewett orthosis) should be applied and worn at all times, even during periods of bed rest, for up to 3 months or during the time that any degree of spinal instability is suspected. Stable fractures (e.g., anterior wedge compression fractures) may require a brief period of bed rest while pain is most severe. The extent of orthotic support that is required for these fractures will depend on the severity of the patients complaints, clinical findings, and the radiological appearance of the fracture.

Fractures between T11 and L2 are frequently unstable, especially when caused by a major injury, and may thus warrant surgical stabilization. When the patient is neurologically intact, initial management should be nonsurgical, but undertaken with great care. The patient should be placed in the horizontal position, prone or supine, on a Stryker frame, standard hospital bed, or a special hospital bed (e.g., the Roto-Rest bed). Depending on the exact type of the fracture and dislocation, pillows may be placed in key areas to maintain proper alignment of the spine. When surgical stabilization of these fractures is completed, orthotic immobilization with a TLSO is needed for 10 to 12 weeks. If surgical stabilization is not done for some reason, 4 to 6 weeks of strict bed rest may be required. This is followed by prolonged immobilization with a spinal orthosis. During the period of bed rest, the patient will require careful observation, excellent nursing care, and appropriate physical therapy in order to prevent medical complications (e.g., urinary tract infections, pressure sores, deep venous thrombophlebitis).

Fractures of the lumbar and the sacral spine may result in varying degrees of neurological deficits or none at all. Below the L2 vertebral level the neurological deficits are caused by damage to the cauda equina and/or the nerve roots but not to the spinal cord, which in the adult ends at the L2 vertebra. These deficits may vary greatly in extent. Both the fracture and minor neurological deficits may initially be easily missed, especially when the patient has sustained multiple other injuries, and a careful clinical examination therefore needs to be done.

While most fractures of the spine heal well and with acceptable alignment in approximately 3 months, the patient may continue to complain of pain for a much longer period of time, even when no neurological deficits can be found. These patients require a careful evaluation, assurances, and a long-term outpatient rehabilitation program that may include physical therapy with different modalities, as well as psychological and vocational counseling similar to that recommended for other patients with chronic low back pain.

REHABILITATION OF THE PATIENT WITH SPINAL CORD INJURY

The incidence of traumatic spinal cord injury (SCI) in the United States is estimated to be approximately 30 new injuries per million inhabitants each year. Thus approximately 8000 new injuries to the spinal cord occur annually. Due to improved life expectancy after SCI, there are now between 180,000 and 250,000 people alive in the United States, who have sustained SCI (12,20). Motor vehicle accidents cause almost half of these injuries, but approximately 15% are due to falls, sports injuries, and gunshot wounds each (44). At the time of the injury, two-thirds of all SCI victims are between 15 and 30 years of age, and 80% are male. A slight maturity of persons with spinal cord injury has quadriplegia or quadriparesis due to injuries to the cervical spine in contrast to less than 50% who have paraplegia or paraparesis due to injuries to the thoracolumbar spine. With improving emergency care and acute interventions, neurologically incomplete injuries have now become more common than complete injuries.

Acute Care

The rehabilitation outcome is affected by all events that occur from the time of injury. Everything that is done, or for that matter not done, from the time of injury will affect the outcome for the patient. This includes extraction of the patient from the site of injury, immobilization of the spine, and transportation by the emergency medical technicians. Subsequently, the outcome depends on the specific medical and surgical interventions, that is, administration of medications (e.g., high-dose methylprednisolone) (3), surgical stabilization of the spinal column, and decompression of the spinal cord as well as on the general acute medical care.

The rehabilitation interventions should start even during the early acute phase or as soon as the presence of SCI has been verified. The level of injury and the neurological deficit need to be established (11) in order to predict functional outcome and plan properly the rehabilitation program. The neurological level of injury has been defined as the lowest (most caudal) neurological segment with both normal motor and sensory function. It is well recognized that the zone of partial preservation (ZPP), which is also known as the zone of injury, may span up to three consecutive neurological segments caudal to the point of damage to the spinal cord. In this zone there is frequently some preservation of motor and sensory function. Neurologically complete injuries have no preservation of any motor and sensory function below the ZPP, whereas the incomplete injury demonstrates some motor and/or sensory function below the ZPP. The incomplete injuries can be anatomically classified according to the distribution of spared, abnormal, or absent function in different major tracts of the spinal cord as was discussed previously in Part III of this book. The incomplete injuries may vary with respect to neurological sparing from only sacral sensory sparing to virtually complete recovery. In this respect, Frankel's classification of incomplete injuries has been found to be very useful (11,15), both for clinical assessment and collection of research data: (A) complete absence of motor and sensory function below ZPP, (B) preserved sensation only, (C) preserved motor (nonfunctional), (D) preserved motor (functional, key muscle grade greater than $3/5$), and (E) complete recovery except for perhaps abnormal reflexes.

Assessment of voluntary muscle strength relies on the manual muscle test system, where strength is graded from 0 and 5: grade 0, absent–total paralysis; grade 1, trace–palpable or visible contraction; grade 2, poor–active movement through full range of motion of the joint with gravity eliminated; grade 3, fair–active movement through full range of motion of the joint against gravity; grade 4, good–active movement through full range of motion of the joint against resistance; grade 5, normal or full strength for age, body size, and so on. During the muscle strength assessment, the patient should be lying down and the key muscles should be tested both with gravity eliminated and against gravity (11). In order to document numerically changes in motor function over time, the Motor Index Score is most helpful (11). Here each of the key muscle groups for the 10 key neurological segments of the spinal cord is tested on both sides of the body and given a numerical score of 0 to 5, that is, for C5 the elbow flexors, for C6 the wrist extensors, for C7 the elbow extensors, for C8 the finger flexors, for T1 the hand intrinsic muscles, for L2 the hip flexors, for L3 the knee extensors, for L4 the ankle dorsiflexors, for L5 the big toe extensors, and for S1 the ankle plantar flexors. Thus a minimum score of 0 is possible and a maximum score of 100. In neurologically complete lesions, that is, Frankel class A or B, it is not uncommon to observe the neurological level drop by one or even two neurological segments over many months after inquiry while the paralysis usually remains complete below the zone of partial preservation. Those who have incomplete cord lesions, that is, Frankel class C or D, and even occasionally Frankel class B, may experience neurological improvement, the extent of which is difficult to predict accurately, especially early after the injury. In general, however, the earlier that this recovery starts and the faster that it proceeds, the more substantial it usually will be.

The early care of the SCI patient is geared toward preventing further cord damage, whether related to spinal instability, ischemia, or other pathological events, as well as to prevent life-threatening complications such as hypotension, aspiration pneumonia, and ventilatory failure. The unstable spine initially needs to be stabilized by external means (i.e., skeletal traction, appropriate orthoses, proper bed) or by surgical internal fixation. Respiratory complications such as aspiration pneumonia, atelectasis, hemothorax, bruised lungs, and fractured ribs frequently occur in patients with fractures of the thoracic spine. Preexisting pulmonary conditions, smoker's lungs, and obesity may further make respiratory care difficult. Cardiovascular complications such as cardiac dysrhythmia and hypotension, which are frequently seen in quadriplegics, may also be present in patients with high paraplegia who have lost supraspinal sympathetic control. Deep venous thrombosis occurs frequently and may result in pulmonary embolism and death and therefore needs to be actively prevented by proper anticoagulation and by other means (48). Various gastrointestinal complications are frequently seen during the acute phase including paralytic ileus, peptic ulcer, and pancreatitis (2,34) besides the irregular and uncontrolled bowel evacuation. Voluntary control over bowel evacuation is lost and results in stool incontinence. As soon as bowel activity restarts following the period of paralytic ileus, bowel evacuation management should be started. Bladder control is also lost. During the acute stage of SCI there is a flaccid paralysis of the detrusor muscle of the bladder, which requires insertion of a Foley catheter. The catheter is kept in place until a program of intermittent catheterization can be started (43,51). Increased metabolic demands and inadequate nutritional management may result in marked weight loss and malnutrition. Pressure sores frequently develop during the acute phase, particularly on the sacrum and on the heels, since the patient is frequently kept for lengthy periods of time in the supine position on a relatively firm surface. The SCI physicians and nurses may pay greater attention to establishing the diagnosis and initiating life-saving measures than providing preventive skin care and as a result pressure sores may develop unnoticed. Proper positioning of the patient and use of special mattresses and beds as well as regular turning will help to prevent the development of pressure sores as well as to aid in the prevention of joint contractures.

In order to ensure the optimal care of the individual with SCI from the onset of injury and throughout life, it is best that the patient be referred immediately after the injury to one of the SCI model systems of care. Here expert management is provided from the onset to prevent complications, to facilitate both the acute and the rehabilitative care, and to provide lifelong follow-up. The SCI model systems of care have had a huge impact on survival, quality of care, length of institutional stay, and functional outcome (44). The acute care of individuals with SCI is usually provided by surgeons from the orthopaedic, neurosurgical, and trauma services, with a heavy input from physiatrists, anesthesiologists, and internists who all work together in a multidisciplinary fashion to manage and prevent the different complications that may occur during the acute phase. While certain rehabilitation interventions are started as early as 24 hr after the injury, these tend to be limited in scope and mostly preventive while the patient is still in the intensive care unit or on the acute service.

Subsequent Management and Rehabilitation

The SCI patient is ready for more comprehensive rehabilitation, when medical complications have been brought under control and the spine has been stabilized. The fractured spine may be stabilized either by application of orthotic devices or by surgical instrumentation with bony fusion.

No individual with SCI should receive comprehensive rehabilitation in isolation from other similarly disabled individuals. A minimum number of acute SCI admissions to the rehabilitation center must be at least 30 per year for the program to be adequate with respect to staff training and development of SCI-specific components of the program. Clearly, the staff/patient ratio and the physical facilities are also important.

Patients with SCI should optimally receive inpatient rehabilitation in a hospital-based rehabilitation unit, with an in-house resident physician coverage and medical and surgical consultation services available on a 24-hr basis. When serious medical complications arise during the rehabilitation course, which interfere with the patients ability to attend therapy for more than three consecutive days, the patient should be transferred to the appropriate medical or surgical service for definitive care.

Upon admission to the inpatient rehabilitation service, the admitting physiatrist must undertake a comprehensive evaluation in order to plan and appropriately implement the comprehensive rehabilitation

TABLE 4. *Functional goals for different key SCI levels*

Skills	C4	C5	C6	C7	C8–T1	T2–T12	L1–L3	L4–S1
Self-care skills								
Feeds	O	P	P	I	I	I	I	I
Dresses	O	D	D	P/I	I	I	I	I
Grooms	O	D/P	P	P/I	I	I	I	I
Cares for bladder/bowel	O	D	D/P	I	I	I	I	I
Bathes	O	D	P	P	I	I	I	I
Wheelchair skills								
Operates powered wheelchair	I	I	I	I	I	I	I	I
Propels manual wheelchair	O	P	P/I	I	I	I	I	I
Transfers to and from wheelchair	O	D	P	I	I	I	I	I
Bed Mobility	O	D	P	I	I	I	I	I
Communication skills								
Uses telephone	P	P	I	I	I	I	I	I
Writes	O	D/P	P	P	I	I	I	I
Types	P	P	P	P	I	I	I	I
Ambulation skills	O	O	O	O	O	D	P	P
Orthotic devices needed	ECU	UEO	UEO	UEO		KAFO	KAFO	KAFO
Transportation skills								
Drives with hand controls	O	D/P	P	I	I	I	I	I
Uses train/plane	O	D	D	P/I	I	I	I	I
Uses bus without lift	O	O	O	O	O	O	O	P

Abbreviations: I, completely independent; P, partly or completely independent with special equipment; D, dependent but can assist; O, not possible; ECU, environmental control unit; UEO, upper extremity orthosis; KAFO, knee–ankle–foot orthosis; AFO, ankle–foot orthosis.

program. The physiatrist must first address two basic questions: (a) What is the neurological level of cord injury and the extent of the neurological deficit? (b) What are the clinical problems and current complications that are present or can be anticipated and how are these best prevented or managed? The neurological assessment and the different syndromes of SCI are addressed elsewhere in this book. Once the level and the neurological deficit have been established, functional goals for self-care and mobility can be predicted with a good degree of accuracy for most patients (Table 4). The physiatrist establishes the rehabilitation goals for the patient and prescribes a specific and detailed evaluation and intervention program for the various members of the multidisciplinary team to follow. These instructions include nursing orders, administration of medications, and specific diagnostic tests, such as a urologic evaluation, pulmonary function tests, appropriate radiologic and electrodiagnostic studies, and blood and urine tests. The physiatrist also prescribes the specific exercises and training methods to be given by the physical and occupational therapists, as well as interventions provided by psychologists and vocational counselors.

On the inpatient rehabilitation unit the prescribed rehabilitation program is immediately implemented. During the first week the actual participation of the patient may be disrupted by the patient's medical condition or by special evaluations and tests. Thereafter, the patient usually spends 4 to 6 hr daily in an active therapy program in addition to participation in bladder and bowel training, practice time in self-care activities, and involvement in educational and recreational programs. Team conferences are held within 1 week of admission where the patient's medical, neurological, functional, psychological, social, and vocational condition, as well as his/her potential and prognosis are presented and discussed. The major and specific rehabilitation goals are set (Table 5), equipment needs are assessed, and a discharge date is predicted. The physiatrist and the social worker meet with the patient and

Table 5. *SCI: goals of inpatient rehabilitation*

1. Maximum function as allowed by the neurological level and other limitations
2. Balanced bladder emptying
3. Bowel routine established
4. Health maintenance education obtained
5. Psychological adjustment progressing
6. Accessible community housing available
7. Appropriate adaptive equipment obtained
8. Transportation arranged
9. Vocational plans and referrals made
10. Community resources referrals made (physicians, VNS, support groups, OVR, vendors, insurance, information networks, etc.)

TABLE 6. *Conditions and complications associated with spinal cord dysfunction*

1. Paralysis
2. Sensory loss
3. Neurogenic bladder
4. Neurogenic bowel
5. Sexual dysfunction
6. Autonomic hyperreflexia
7. Pain
8. Spasticity
9. Joint contractures
10. Heterotopic ossification
11. Metabolic disturbances
12. Circulatory disorders
13. Respiratory insufficiency
14. Pressure sores
15. Psychological, social, and vocational problems

the family shortly after this conference to discuss these issues and to answer any questions that they may have regarding the patient's medical condition and the rehabilitation program. Reevaluation conferences are held every 2 weeks to discuss the patient's progress. After each conference the physiatrist again meets with the patient and the family for further discussions and planning. Communication between rehabilitation team members is facilitated through frequent meetings during which the medical, psychological, and social issues related to the patient are clarified and specific concerns that any member of the team may have about any patient are shared and discussed.

A number of clinical conditions and complications are associated with SCI (Table 6). Each of these conditions must be anticipated, addressed, prevented, or properly managed. Several of these conditions are briefly discussed as they relate to the paraplegic individual in the following paragraphs.

Paralysis and Sensory Loss

Functional Restoration

When the neurological level has been established, it is possible to predict with reasonable certainty which functional goals the patient may realistically reach and which assistive devices he/she will require (Table 4). It is clear that the lower the level of injury and the more incomplete the neurological loss is, the more muscles there are under voluntary control, the higher is the Motor Index Score, and the greater is the functional potential. Paraplegics should as a rule become totally self-sufficient in the various activities of daily living and independently mobile in a wheelchair unless they are impaired by a secondary disability or complication, for example, obesity, advanced age, failure of a major organ system, or severe spasticity. In order to reach this level of independence, an appropriate exercise and training program has to be initiated. Joint range of motion exercises for the paralyzed limbs, which were initiated during the acute phase, are continued, but greater emphasis is placed on strengthening exercises for all the normally and partly innervated musculature using a variety of weights, pulleys, and ergometers. These are the muscles that the patient will have to rely on in order to make up for the strength lost in the paralyzed muscles. Specific muscle reeducation exercises are initiated for muscles weakened, but not totally paralyzed, by the spinal cord damage. When preparing for self-sufficiency, particular attention is directed to strengthening the trapezius, deltoid, triceps, latissimus dorsi, and wrist extensor muscles, which are the key muscles for transfers to and from a bed or wheelchair as well as for crutch walking. As endurance, body balance, and strength in these key muscles increase, patients begin exercise classes on mattresses where they are taught to turn from side to side, come to a sitting position, move about in the sitting position, and transfer with a sliding board to the wheelchair. The goal of these exercises is to increase mobility in order to achieve as much functional independence as possible in such activities as bed mobility, wheelchair transfers, and dressing.

Wheelchairs

Most paraplegics will require a wheelchair for locomotion, both indoors and outdoors. When prescribing an appropriate wheelchair the physiatrist must take into account the user's disability, prognosis, physical characteristics, functional skills, and personal preferences (46). The general and specific aspects of the wheelchair to be prescribed must be well known to the prescribing physician. Preferably, the paraplegic individual should personally test different wheelchair designs and consider different options before obtaining the new wheelchair, given the importance of this device, both with respect to the patient's mobility and self-image. Wheelchair training must be provided not only to ensure proper operation of the wheelchair on level surfaces and inclines, but also for maneuvering on curbs and steps, transferring into and out of the chair, falling safely, getting back into the chair from the ground, and pulling the chair into an automobile after transfer. Proper maintenance techniques, handling, and storage of the wheelchair should also be taught.

Ambulation

In theory, all paraplegic patients can learn to ambulate with crutches and lower limb orthoses given adequate motivation, upper extremity strength, and training. The type of orthoses described seems to make little difference. Unfortunately, very few paraplegic individuals continue to use the orthoses following discharge from the rehabilitation program since the metabolic cost of such ambulation is so great and the speed of walking is so slow that few ever become ambulatory in the community. As a general rule, only paraplegics who have pelvic control and adequate quadriceps strength to provide knee stability, at least on one side, are able to ambulate functionally in the community (22), that is, they require one ankle–foot orthosis (AFO) and one knee–ankle–foot orthosis (KAFO) besides the crutches (47). Nonetheless, it may be indicated to prescribe lower extremity orthoses for those with complete thoracic paraplegia for several reasons. The cultural pressures to ambulate by any possible means are strong and the psychological benefits from such ambulation may be considerable. There are several recognized physiological benefits related to the upright position and the physical exercise that occurs with ambulation with orthoses. Some paraplegic individuals succeed, despite the odds, in using the orthoses functionally for standing transfers and even for limited functional locomotion within the household or in the community.

Functional Electrical Stimulation

In recent years, a great deal of interest has been generated by the use of computer controlled functional electrical stimulation (FES) on multiple lower limb muscle groups (28). If such electrical stimulation is given in proper sequence, ambulation indeed can be accomplished, although still at a relatively slow pace and at increased energy cost. Although FES technology has advanced rapidly during the last two decades, no FES system for ambulation meets adequately all the clinical requirements of safety, reliability, function, energy expenditure, ease of use, cosmesis, and cost. Experimentally, hundreds of individuals with paraplegia, both in the United States and abroad, have learned to ambulate by this means, and currently at least one such system is being marketed (Fig. 11). FES systems for ambulation may differ in several ways with respect to the components used, but the main design features are usually similar. The *electrodes* may either be placed on the surface of the skin or percutaneously at the motor point of the muscle. Percutaneously placed electrodes are generally preferred by most investigators as they generate better muscle selectivity, more consistent muscle response, and less skin irritation, despite a considerable failure rate and the occurrence of occasional burns and infections (28). *Muscle control* may be obtained either by an open or a closed loop

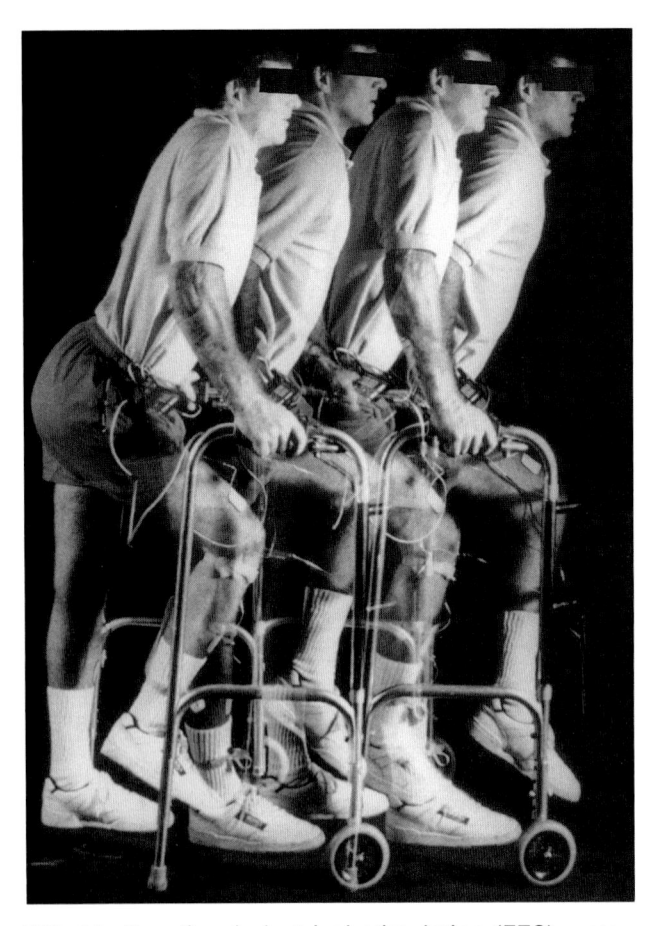

FIG. 11. Functional electrical stimulation (FES) system for ambulation. ("Parastep" produced by Sigmedics, Inc. Northfield, IL 60093. Reproduced with permission.)

system. In an open loop control system programmed patterns of electrical stimulation are created for specific muscles in a specific individual in order to accomplish a specific motor task but there is no automatic correction for changes in muscle contraction, or in circumstances. In a closed loop system the computer receives feedback information from peripherally placed sensors about a given movement and institutes corrective action or gives a warning signal when aberrations occur. The number of stimulation *channels* may vary between 4 and 48, but in current clinical experimental programs either 4 or 8 channels are most commonly used. The number of programmed physical activities depends on the FES system's capability and skill of the user. Some systems allow only a single activity (e.g., standing), whereas the most advanced systems can be programmed for as many as 24 different activities (e.g., standing, walking, climbing, or descending stairs, or performing different physical exercises). *Sensory feedback* may be provided simply by instructing the patient to use the residual sensory functions (i.e., visual, auditory, vestibular, proprioception), but in the more sophisticated systems sensory feedback is provided by attaching sensory devices on the stimulated limbs, which can provide the computer with information regarding joint positions and which allows the velocity and acceleration of movement to be calculated by the microprocessor that controls the stimulator (36). *Orthoses* of different designs are currently used by most FES systems to provide joint stability in order to prevent injuries, to decrease energy cost, to increase limb control, and to reduce the number of electrodes required. *Canes, crutches, and walkers* are used to improve standing and ambulation balance, thus making ambulation safer and more effective.

Paraplegic individuals ambulating with FES systems have been reported to ambulate at the average speed of 12 to 18 meters per minute (m/min) (24) with a maximum speed of 50 to 60 m/min for the best performers. Endurance on level surfaces usually is 100 to 200 m with maximum distance traveled of 400 m (28). Oxygen consumption during standing and walking with FES is similar to that measured for paraplegic ambulation with KAFOs, but similar to orthotic gait, it is two to three times higher than during walking for nondisabled people (27). However, it appears that energy cost of ambulation may not increase significantly as the speed of FES-generated ambulation increases in contrast to the rising energy consumption that occurs with accelerated ambulation using KAFOs and crutches (27). Daily care and the application of an FES ambulation system may take between 30 and 60 min daily. Although *cosmesis* has improved with miniaturizing of system components, these are still conspicuous and there location and size may interfere with their performance of certain activities.

The ideal candidates for FES ambulation are individuals with thoracic spastic paraplegia, that is, a cord lesion and upper motor neuron involvement between T4 and T11. Those with higher level paraplegia, or with quadriplegia, in general have impaired supraspinal control over the sympathetic nervous system, a condition that significantly decreases their exercise capacity. Paraplegic individuals with cord lesions at T12 or below usually have significant lower motor neuron damage, which prevents effective muscle contraction upon stimulation. Since the electrical stimulus is normally painful, the subject's sensation at the stimulated sites must be impaired. Joint movements in the lower limbs must not be limited by excessive spasticity or the presence of joint contractures and quite obviously the subject must be generally healthy and emotionally stable. Intensive training for 1 to 2 months is needed for most candidates in order for them to discover if this mode of ambulation is possible and practical.

During the experimental application of FES systems for ambulation, it became clear that a lengthy preparatory period was required where stimulation of the targeted muscles was needed to increase their strength

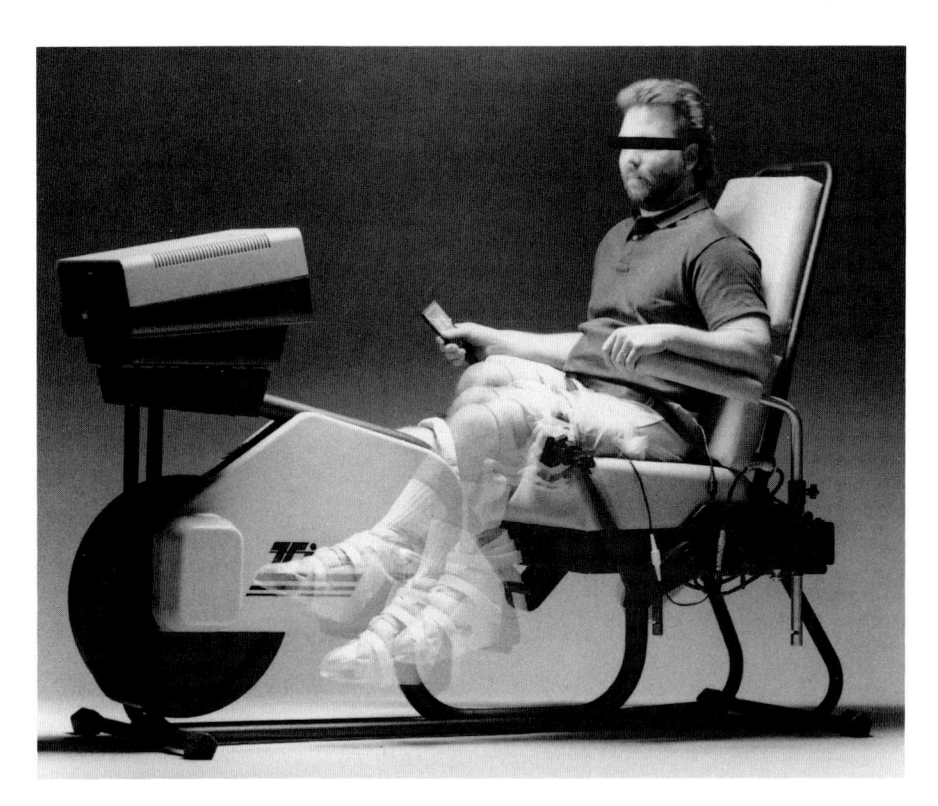

FIG. 12. Functional electrical stimulation (FES) ergometer. ("ERGYS" produced by Therapeutic Technologies, Inc. Tampa, FL 33634. Reproduced with permission.)

and endurance. Many participating subjects observed that while the ambulation by means of FES was not what they expected, the physical training proved to be very beneficial. Subsequently, the development and marketing of a computerized FES ergometer (exercise cycle) (Fig. 12) for exercising paralyzed muscles and improving fitness has enabled hundreds, if not thousands, of individuals with SCI to participate regularly in such therapy. While such regular active exercise of the paralyzed muscles has been shown to have several documented therapeutic benefits (e.g., increased bulk and strength of the paralyzed muscles, improved cardiovascular endurance and circulation, sustained elevation of endorphins), other theoretical health and functional benefits remain unproven (38,40).

Bladder and Bowel Dysfunction

Most paraplegic individuals experience sphincter disturbances, which may be evident as retention or incontinence of stools and urine. While the *neurogenic bladder* is initially best managed with an indwelling Foley catheter, this catheter should be removed at the earliest possible time and a program of intermittent catheterization initiated (43,52). If the bladder resumes reflex functioning, male patients are fitted with an external condomlike collecting device that is connected to a urinary leg bag. If spontaneous voiding does not occur, intermittent catheterization needs to be done at least every 4 to 6 hr, striving to maintain the bladder volume at less than 500 cc at all times. Urodynamic studies need to be performed periodically to ensure that intrinsic bladder pressure does not rise excessively. When the catheterized urine specimen measures more than 500 cc, a more frequent catheterization is required, and if the intrinsic bladder pressure rises excessively, administration of anticholinergic medications may additionally be indicated. If voiding occurs, whether spontaneous or voluntary, intermittent catheterization can be reduced in frequency and halted altogether when postvoiding residual urine volumes are less than 50 to 100 cc, the intrinsic bladder pressure is acceptable, and the urinary tract is free of complications. Since no external collecting devices for paraplegic female patients are effective, intermittent catheterization for bladder emptying is usually continued indefinitely and anticholinergic agents are used to reduce bladder detrusor muscle contractions and ensure continence between catheterizations. All paraplegic patients, male or female, should be taught intermittent self-catheterization as early as possible, preferably using a disposable kit. Regular surveillance of the urinary tract needs to be done for the rest of the patient's life, assessing in particular the condition of the upper urinary tract with respect to dilatation, stone formation, renal function, and the intrinsic pressure of the bladder.

The *neurogenic bowel* is optimally managed by establishing a routine of bowel evacuation that should occur at predictable times, at hours similar to what the patient had prior to the SCI. Tendency for constipation may be counteracted by administration of stool softeners, high fiber bulk increasing laxatives, and adequate fluid intake. Peristalsis of the entire bowel may be enhanced by daily administration of stool softeners (i.e., docusate sodium, Colace) or laxatives, such as Senekot tablets or granules, which are taken 6 to 8 hr before the anticipated bowel evacuation. The actual bowel evacuation may be triggered by inserting into the rectum a suppository that stimulates the defecation reflex by its bulk, gaseous distention of the rectum or chemical irritation of the mucosa. Stimulation of the rectum digitally to initiate this reflex is a time honored method that many paraplegics quickly adapt for this purpose.

Other Dysfunctions

Sexual dysfunction associated with paraplegia needs to be addressed (7). Sexual counseling is provided by different members of the rehabilitation team on an individual basis and by organizing seminars on human sexuality and adjustment. Genital sensation and erectile capability may be lost to a different degree depending on the level and extent of the neurological deficit and for the male ejaculation is usually not possible. Sexual rehabilitation emphasizes that paraplegia does not cause loss of sexuality since sexuality is a part of the whole person. Sexual drive is not lost although function is impaired. The anatomy and physiology of sexual function are explained to the patients and their spouses and general guidelines for success are given. Communication and strengthening of relationships between partners are emphasized and the physical aspects of sexual performance are clarified in order to make expectations compatible with performance capability. For most paraplegics deficient neurological function should not interfere with establishing a solid personal relationship with one's partner, being sensitive to the partner's desires, or reducing the ability to please and enjoy. Sexual rehabilitation stresses that, if sexual comfort is taught, sexual competence may result. Fertility is usually addressed in these sessions; women are advised that their fertility is not affected by the SCI and that contraception is required if they do not desire to become pregnant, while male fertility is adversely affected by the SCI primarily due to the patient's inability to ejaculate. Educational material is provided regarding electroejaculation for collection of semen and subsequent artificial insemination, which has dramatically altered the fertility of paraplegic males in recent years (1).

Autonomic hyperreflexia may occur in all quadriplegics and also in those paraplegics who have neurological level at T5 or above (13). This is usually characterized by the clinical complaints of headaches and sweating, and the findings of elevated blood pressure and bradycardia. It is usually caused by an obstructed bladder or bowel or other form of irritation in the sacral dermatomes. Immediate intervention is required in order to prevent disastrous consequences (i.e., cerebral hemorrhage from severe hypertension). Catheterization of the bladder or evacuation of the bowel usually results in dramatic disappearance of symptoms but occasionally administration of nerve blocking agents may be required.

Pain is a common complaint among paraplegics. Pain in the shoulder and upper limbs is usually related to the hard work that is required during rehabilitation and performance of the activities of daily living. Radicular pain or hyperesthesia at the level of the lesion and dysesthetic pain below are all common complaints that are difficult to manage successfully. Different neuroactive medications may be tried and assurances given. In the most difficult cases of dysesthetic pain, neurosurgical procedures such as dorsal root entry zone (DREZ) surgery have been advocated (17).

Spasticity of varying degree is frequently seen in patients with thoracic level of paraplegia. While mild or moderate spasticity is in no way harmful, more severe spasticity needs to be treated (30). Fundamental for the patient is to perform thorough stretching of all joints in the paralyzed limbs each morning and to prevent irritation from a variety of sources on the paralyzed parts of the body. Oral baclofen in different doses is frequently very effective in reducing spasticity with minimum side effects and for intractable spasticity intrathecal administration of this medication has given excellent results (35). Selective nerve blocks and different neurosurgical procedures may be indicated in rare instances.

Joint contractures may occur in the paraplegic individual for different causes, that is, severe spasticity, muscle imbalance, and inadequate stretching or range of motion exercise program. Development of heterotopic ossifications may also result in severe ankylosis if not aggressively treated (26,45).

Metabolic disturbances with negative calcium and nitrogen balance occur primarily during the acute phase of SCI, but its consequences (i.e., osteoporosis and muscle atrophy) continue thereafter. The osteoporosis, which clinically appears to be more severe in individuals with flaccid type of paraplegia than spastic, may result in fractures of the long bones in the paralyzed limbs with trivial injury. Surgical interventions of these fractures is best avoided since healing with abundant callus formation is usually the rule and exact realignment of the fracture is not of paramount importance for the nonambulatory individual (16,41).

Circulatory disturbances of different types are common. Orthostatic hypotension is usually only experienced in the paraplegic individual following any lengthy period of bed rest. Edema of the paralyzed lower limbs may be seen during both the acute and chronic phases. When it occurs during the acute phase, deep vein thrombophlebitis (DVT) must be suspected, particularly if the edema is unilateral. Prophylactic anticoagulation with low dose subcutaneous heparin for the first 3 months after SCI is usually recommended. If the diagnosis of DVT is established, full anticoagulation must be initiated and continued for at least a period of 3 months. DVT during the chronic phase of paraplegia is much less common than during the acute phase but must be considered and appropriately treated. Chronic and symmetrical edema of the lower limbs is usually related to leg dependency and reduced muscle contractions. Compressive stockings may be of some help but are a nuisance for the patient to put on and diuretics are generally not indicated. Elevation of the legs is usually adequate treatment for minor degrees of leg edemas.

Respiratory problems are frequently present during the acute phase of thoracic paraplegia because of associated rib fractures and lung contusions. The intercostal respiratory muscles may also be paralyzed to an extent that is determined by the level of the injury. This may result in diminished respiratory function with clinically reduced cough strength. Respiratory infections should be aggressively treated with early administration of antibiotics and other respiratory care as needed.

The *psychological, social, and vocational implications* of SCI are profound. While proper counseling and intervention are started during the acute rehabilitation phase, these must be continued aggressively following discharge. The *psychologist* assists the patient and the family in coping with their reactive depression and grief through individual counseling, as well as by assisting the rehabilitation team members in managing the patient. Although psychological counseling is both needed and helpful and psychiatric intervention may occasionally be required, most paraplegic individuals respond best to the general emotional support from their family members and the entire rehabilitation staff, as well as to the opportunity to be able to work physically at reducing their disability (4). Eventually, most patients learn to cope with their disabilities through the process of intellectualization and the passage of time.

A rehabilitation *social worker* is assigned to each patient. The social worker assists the patient and the family in securing economic resources, such as health insurance, social security, and compensation, obtaining authorization and payment for prescribed devices, arranging for transportation, nursing and attendant care, home modification, and another appropriate posthospital care. When all these issues are addressed in a timely manner, proper planning for discharge is accomplished and a smooth transition will likely occur from the hospital to community living. During the rehabilitation course the social worker frequently acts as a liaison between the patient, the family, and the different members of the rehabilitation team.

The *vocational counselor* plays an important role on the rehabilitation team since few criteria for rehabilitation success are as significant as return of the patient to work. Unless the paraplegic patient is capable of returning to his/her previous job, there are multiple steps on the route to vocational success. The vocational counselor facilitates the paraplegic individual's entry into the labor market through multifaceted services. The patient is interviewed and evaluated with respect to education and aptitude. Counseling, guidance, and planning are provided at a pace that is sensitive to the patient's readiness to become involved in the vocational process. Given the profound impact of paraplegia on the patient's personal life, very few consider return to work in a different capacity a high priority during the acute phase of SCI, whereas during the chronic phase this becomes a major issue. At the appropriate time the vocational counselor provides the necessary interventions, for example, remediation, education, career exploration, job trials, job site analysis, job seeking skills training, job development, specialized placement, and follow-up services.

Outpatient Rehabilitation and Follow-up Care

The rehabilitation of the paraplegic individual is far from over at discharge from the inpatient rehabilitation service, even if the patient has become maximally independent in the activities of daily living and mobility. Inpatient length of stay at most rehabilitation centers has been diminishing rapidly over the last two decades and thus there has been less time to allow the patient to adjust emotionally to the disability and to anticipate what may await in the community with respect to social, vocational, and recreational issues. Proper outpatient rehabilitation has therefore become more important and needs to be carefully coordinated and provided in an effective manner. After discharge from the inpatient service, further rehabilitation and community reintegration certainly cannot be left only to the patient and the family. The goals of rehabilitation do not change much upon discharge (Table 5), but if the patient has become maximally self-sufficient and mobility independent, the outpatient program traditionally will focus primarily on the psychologically, socially, vocationally, and recreationally oriented goals rather than on further physical exercise. It may be debated how many outpatient rehabilitation interventions should be prescribed for the paraplegic individual and for how long these should be continued after discharge. A program that consists only of psychological, social, and vocational counseling is frequently not acceptable to the patient whose thoughts are centered on the physical disability and functional loss. In order to ensure compliance and participation in the outpatient program, it may be feasible to prescribe physical and occupational therapy in order to improve physical fitness and functional skills through a variety of means, that is, ambulation with orthoses and crutches, FES for ambulation or fitness training, biofeedback training, high level wheelchair activities, and so on. Continuation of this program may then depend on the patient's active participation in the community reintegration oriented activities, such as, counseling sessions, educational classes, and meeting of support groups.

A carefully organized lifelong follow-up plan is crucial for ultimate success. The recommended frequency of outpatient visits to the physician for the uncomplicated patient with paraplegia is as follows. The first visit should occur within 4 to 6 weeks of discharge, and the subsequent visits should be scheduled at least every 3 months for the next 1 year, every six months for the following 2 or 3 years, and annually thereafter. More frequent visits obviously are needed when medical problems arise or are unsolved. While loss of function in self-care and mobility will predictably occur with aging, premature functional loss may have multiple other causes, including neurological, musculoskeletal, psychological, and social, and therefore such loss requires a complete and careful assessment.

Prognosis

The life expectancy of SCI persons has increased dramatically during the last few decades, although it is still less than that for able-bodied individuals. Accurate figures are difficult to come by, but it is generally believed by clinicians and actuaries that the mean life expectancy for paraplegic individuals who survive the acute phase and receive optimal care and social support is only slightly less than normal. Paraplegic individuals with incomplete neurological lesions tend to survive longer than those with complete lesions. Renal complications are no longer among the most common causes of death (44). Currently, respiratory complications, cardiovascular disorders, and violence, including suicides, are all more common causes of death than renal disorders. Psychological and social success is difficult to assess, but in general the majority of SCI persons appear to make a successful adaptation and between one-third and one-half of all paraplegics eventually become competitively employed. For others there exists a vocational disincentive as many people have to risk giving up financial benefits and the security of health care insurance when returning to work. While the functional prognosis for mobility and self-care for a paraplegic individual can be predicted with reasonable accuracy depending on the level of the neurological lesion, individual variations are common with some individuals falling short of the anticipated goals, while others by sheer motivation and practice accomplish what may have been thought impossible by the clinicians.

REFERENCES

1. Bennett CJ, Seager SW, Fasher EA, et al. Sexual dysfunction and electroejaculation in men with spinal cord injury. review. *J Urol* 1987;139:453–457.
2. Berlly MH, Wilmot CB. Acute abdominal emergencies during the first four weeks after spinal cord injury. *Arch Phys Med Rehabil* 1984;65:687–690.
3. Bracken MB, Shepard MJ, Collings WF, et al. A randomized controlled trial of methylprednisolone or naloxone in the treatment of acute spinal cord injury. *N Engl J Med* 1990;322:1405–1411.
4. Brackett TO, Condon N, Kindelan KM, Bassett L. The emotional care of a person with spinal cord injury. *JAMA* 1984;252:793–795.
5. Brazier MAB. *A history of the electrical activity of the brain: the first half century.* London: Pittman Medical, 1961.
6. Breig A. *Biomechanics of the central nervous system: some basic and normal and patholoic phenomena.* Stockholm: Almquist and Wiksell, 1960.
7. Comfort A, ed. *Sexual consequences of disability.* Philadelphia: George F Stickley Company, 1978.
8. Cotch MT. Biomechanics of the thoracic spine. In: American Academy of Orthopaedic Surgeons. *Atlas of orthotics, biomechanical principles and application.* St Louis: CV Mosby, 1975.
9. Dawson GD. Cerebral responses to electrical stimulation of peripheral nerve in man. *J Neurol Neurosurg Psychiatry* 1947;10:134–140.
10. Denis F. The three column spine and its significance in the classification of acute thoracolumbar spinal injuries. *Spine* 1983;8:817–831.
11. Donovan WH, Maynard FM, McCluer S, Menter RR, Ragnarsson KT, Weingarden S, Wilmot CB. *Standards for neurological classification of spinal injury patients.* Chicago: American Spinal Injury Association, 1990.
12. Ergas Z. Spinal cord injury in the United States: a statistical update. *Cent Nerv Syst Trauma* 1985;2:19–30.
13. Erickson RP: Autonomic hyperreflexia: pathophysiology and medical management. *Arch Phys Med Rehabil* 1980;61:431–440.
14. Ferguson RL, Allen BL. A mechanical classification of thoracolumbar spine fractures. *Clin Orthop* 1984;189:77.
15. Frankel H, Hancock D, Hyslop G, et al. The value of postural reduction in the initial management of closed injuries to the spine with paraplegia or tetraplegia. *Paraplegia* 1969;7:179–192.
16. Freehafer AA, Hazel CN, Becker CL. Lower extremity fractures in patients with spinal cord injury. *Paraplegia* 1981;19:367–372.
17. Friedman AH, Nashold BS. DREZ lesions for relief of pain related to spinal cord injury. *J Neurosurg* 1986;65:465–469.
18. *Guide for the use of the uniform data set for medical rehabilitation.* State University of New York at Buffalo, 82 Farber Hall, SUNY Main Street, Buffalo, NY 14214; 1990.
19. Haher TR, Tozzi JM, Lospinuso MF, et al. The contribution of the three columns of the spine to spinal stability: a biomechanical model. *Paraplegia* 1989;27:432–439.
20. Harvey C, Rothschild BB, Asmann AJ, Stripling T. New estimates of traumatic SCI prevalence: a survey-based approach. *Paraplegia* 1990;28:537–544.
21. Holdsworth FW. Fractures, dislocations and fracture-dislocations of the spine. *J Bone Joint Surg* 1979;52A:1534–1551.
22. Hussey RW, Stauffer ES. Spinal cord injury: requirements for ambulation. *Arch Phys Med Rehabil* 1973;54:544–547.
23. Kimura J. *Electrodiagnosis in diseases of nerve and muscle, principles and practice.* Philadelphia: FA Davis, 1983;353–398.

24. Kralj A, Bajd T, Turk R. Enhancement of gait restoration in spinal injured patients by functional electrical stimulation. *Clin Orthop* 1988;233:34–43.
25. Krusen FA. *Physical medicine*. Philadelphia: Saunders, 1941.
26. Lall S, Hamilton BB, Heinemann A, Betts HB. Risk factors for heterotopic ossification in spinal cord injury. *Arch Phys Med Rehabil* 1989;70:387–390.
27. Marsolais EB, Edwards BG. Energy costs of walking and standing with functional neuromuscular stimulation and long leg braces. *Arch Phys Med Rehabil* 1988;69:243–249.
28. Marsolais EB, Kobetic R. Development of practical electrical stimulation system for restoring gait in the paralyzed patient. *Clin Orthop* 1988;233:64–74.
29. McCollough NC. Biomechanical analysis of the spine. In: American Academy of Orthopaedic Surgeons. *Atlas of orthotics, biomechanical principles and application*. St Louis: CV Mosby, 1975.
30. Merritt JL. Management of spasticity in spinal cord injury. *Mayo Clin Proc* 1981;56:614–622.
31. Meyer PR. Fractures of the thoracic spine: T1–T10. In: Meyer PR, ed. *Surgery of the spine trauma*. New York: Churchill Livingstone, 1989;525–571.
32. Morris JM, Lucas DB, Bresler B. Role of the trunk in the stability of the spine. *J Bone Joint Surg* 1961;43A:337–351.
33. Nainzadeh NK. Somatosensory evoked potentials: assessment and management in lumbar spine surgery. In: Camins M, O'Leary P, eds. *The lumbar spine*. New York: Raven Press, 1987.
34. Neumayer LA, Bull DA, Mohr JD, Putnam CW. The acutely affected abdomen in paraplegic spinal cord injury patients. *Ann Surg* 1990;212:561–566.
35. Penn RD, Savoy SM, Corcos D, Latash M, Gottlieb G, Parke B, Kroin JS. Intrathecal baclofen for severe spinal spasticity. *N Engl J Med* 1989;320:1517–1521.
36. Petrofsky JS, Phillips CA, Stafford DE. Closed loop control for restoration of movement in paralyzed muscle. *Orthopaedics* 1984;7:1289–1302.
37. Ragnarsson KT. Orthotics and shoes. In: DeLisa JA, ed. *Rehabilitation medicine: principles and practice*. Philadelphia: Lippincott, 1988;chap 16.
38. Ragnarsson KT. Physiological effect of functional electrical stimulation-induced exercises in spinal cord injured individuals. *Clin Orthop* 1988;233:53–63.
39. Ragnarsson, KT. Rehabilitation of patients with physical disabilities caused by tumors of the musculoskeletal system. In: Lewis MM, ed. *Musculoskeletal oncology—a multidisciplinary approach*. Philadelphia: Saunders, 1992;chap 23.
40. Ragnarsson KT, Pollack SF, Twist D. Lower limb endurance exercise after spinal cord injury: implications for health and functional ambulation. *J Neurol Rehabil* (*in press*).
41. Ragnarsson KT, Sell GH. Lower extremity fractures after spinal cord injury: a retrospective study. *Arch Phys Med Rehabil* 1981;62:418–423.
42. Rusk HA. *Rehabilitation medicine*. St Louis: CV Mosby, 1977.
43. Sperling KB. Intermittent catheterization to obtain catheter free bladder function in spinal cord injury. *Arch Phys Med Rehabil* 1978;59:4–8.
44. Stover SL, Fine PR, eds. *Spinal cord injury: the facts and figures*. Birmingham: The University of Alabama, 1986.
45. Stover SL, Hataway CJ, Zeiger HE. Heterotopic ossification in spinal cord injured patients. *Arch Phys Med Rehabil* 1975;56:199–204.
46. Todd SP. Choosing a wheelchair system. *J Rehabil Res Dev Clin Supp* 1990. 2:1–118.
47. Waters RL, Yakura JS, Adkins R, Barnes G. Determinants of gait performance following spinal cord injury. *Arch Phys Med Rehabil* 1989;70:811–818.
48. Weingarden SI, Weingarden DS, Belen J. Fever and thromboembolic disease in acute spinal cord injury. *Paraplegia* 1988;26:35–42.
49. White AA, Panjabi MM. *Clinical biomechanics of the spine*, 2nd ed. Philadelphia: Lippincott, 1990.
50. *World Health Organization international classification of impairment, disabilities and handicaps: a manual or classification relating to consequences of disease*. Geneva: World Health Organization, 1980.
51. Wyndaele JJ, DeSy WA, Claessens H. Evaluation of different methods of bladder drainage used in the early care of spinal cord injury patients. *Paraplegia* 1985;23:18–26.
52. Guttman L, Frankel H. The value of intermittent catheterization in the early management of traumatic paraplegia and tetraplegia. *Paraplegia* 1966;4:63–84.

Index

A

ABCS (Alignment, Bone, Cartilage, Soft tissue) approach, to radiography of thoracolumbar fractures, 73, 80, 81–84
Abdominal emergencies, in spinal cord injury, 416
Absorptiometry, for bone mass measurement
  dual photon, 350, 351
  dual x-ray, 350
  single photon, 350, 350–351
Abuse, child, and spinal cord injury without radiographic abnormalities (SCIWORA), 320
Action potential
  compound muscle, 110. *See also* M-wave studies
  motor unit, 113, 115, 470
  sensory nerve, 111
Acute abdominal emergencies, in spinal cord injury, 416
AD. *See* Autonomic dysreflexia
Adhesive arachnoiditis, syringomyelia caused by, 433, 436
AFO. *See* Ankle-foot orthosis
Age
  bone loss related to, 344
  nerve conduction velocity affected by, 110
Alar fractures. *See also* Sacrum
  sacral, 245, 246
  treatment of, 246, 247
Alkaline phosphatase levels, in heterotopic ossification, 413
Alpha blockers, for hypertension in autonomic dysreflexia, 170, 412
Ambulation, for paraplegic patients, 477
  functional electrical stimulation systems for, 477–478
Amyloidosis, in spinal cord injury, 415
Anal sphincter, external, electromyography of, 115–116
Analgesics, in acute management of osteoporotic vertebral fractures, 353
Anemia, in spinal cord injury, 418

Aneurysmal bone cyst, of spine, 374
Angiography, in spinal tumors, 365
Ankle-foot orthosis, for ambulation of paraplegic patients, 477
Ankylosing spondylitis
  rheumatoid arthritis differentiated from, 385
  spinal fractures in, 385–408
    differentiation of fracture pseudarthrosis from spondylodiscitis and, 397–406
    flexion deformity of neck and, 388–395, 396
    mechanism of, 385–387
    spinal cord injury and, 391–393
Annulus fibrosus, 16, 46
  resistance of to rotation, 236
Antacids, for prophylaxis of GI bleeding in spinal cord injury, 415
Anterior approach
  for low lumbar burst fractures, 230–232
    indications for, 232–233
  for spinal tumors, 367–368, 369–370, 371
  for thoracolumbar fractures, 255–263, 267, 268, 273
    for fracture debridement and canal decompression, 261–263
    historical review of, 252
    retroperitoneal, 260–261
    thoracoabdominal, 258–260
    transthoracic, 256–258
    versus posterior approach, 274, 275–277
Anterior cord syndrome, 42, 163
Anterior fixation devices, 252–254, 267–278
  biomechanical evaluation of, 270–271
  clinical results with, 272, 273
  history of, 267–269, 270
  for late deformity, 456
  for spinal tumors, 369–370, 371
Anterior longitudinal ligament, 16

degree of elongation of prior to failure, 48
facet capsule stability and, 235
Anterior ring epiphysis avulsion, in children, extension/distraction injury causing, 317
Anterior techniques of decompression and fixation, 251–266, 267–278
  anterior approach and, 255–263
    canal decompression and, 261–263
    fracture debridement and, 261–263
    historical review of, 252
    retroperitoneal, 260–261
    thoracoabdominal, 258–260
    transthoracic, 256–258
  anterior fixation devices and, 252–254
  biomechanical evaluation of, 270–271
  for burst fractures, 267–278
    indications for, 271
    rationale for decompression and, 272
    versus posterior surgery, 274, 275–277
  future developments in, 264
  historical review of, 251–254, 267, 268, 270
  results of, 263–264, 272, 273
  for secondary spinal deformities in children, 337
  and thoracolumbar fracture treatment, 254–255
    historical review of, 251–252
Anticholinergic agents, for hypertonic bladder, 415
Anticlinal phenomenon, 14
Anticoagulation, for thromboembolism prevention in spinal cord injury, 171, 174, 412
Antidiuretic hormone, syndrome of inappropriate secretion of, in spinal cord injury, 171
Antispasmodic agents, in acute management of osteoporotic vertebral fractures, 353

485

A-O Fixateur Interne, 287, 288. *See also* Dick's device
    for posterior fixation and fracture reduction in thoracic spine, 251
    results of, 263
A-O plates
    for anterior fixation and fracture reduction in thoracic burst fractures, 269, 270
    biomechanical evaluation of, 291
    clinical results of, 272
A-O screws, biomechanical evaluation of, 290
Arachnoid, spinal, 36
Arachnoiditis, adhesive, syringomyelia caused by, 433, 436
Arcus vertebrae. *See* Vertebral arch
Armstrong plate, for anterior fixation and fracture reduction in thoracic spine, 252
    for burst fractures, 269, 270
Arteria spinalis anterior. *See* Spinal arteries, anterior
Arterial blood gas analysis, spinal cord oxygenation monitored by, 168
Arthrodesis
    for fracture/dislocations in children, 324
    for seat belt fracture in children, 324
Articular processes
    superior and inferior, 11
    torsion affecting, 49
Atelectasis, in spinal cord injury, 170, 409, 410
Atropine, for bradycardia in spinal cord injury, 169
Automobile accidents, spine injuries caused by, 61–62
    flexion injuries, 73–74
Autonomic dysreflexia (autonomic hyperreflexia), after spinal cord injury, 47, 170, 411–412, 416, 435
    rehabilitation and, 480
Autonomic evaluation, 116. *See also* Sympathetic skin response
Autonomic hyperreflexia. *See* Autonomic dysreflexia
Autonomic nervous dysfunction
    in spinal cord injury, 169–170, 411–412, 416, 480
    in syringomyelia, 435–436
Axial compression loads
    accommodation of spinal components to, 46–48
    facet joints affected by, 236
Axillary nerve, neurographic testing of, 110
Axonotmesis, neurography in, 109

B
Back pain
    following conservative treatment for burst fractures, 217–218
    in late deformities, 452
        after surgery, 456
    in osteoporotic vertebral fracture, 345, 353–354
    in post-traumatic syringomyelia, 423, 434
        surgery for relief of, 426
    in spinal cord injury, rehabilitation and, 480
    in spine tumors
        anatomic considerations and, 360
        treatment decisions and, 361
Baclofen, for spasticity in spinal cord injury, 480
Baker orthosis, 468
Basic multicellular unit, bone remodeling and, 341
Battered child/battered baby syndromes, and spinal cord injury without radiographic abnormalities (SCIWORA), 320
Bed rest
    in conservative management of burst fractures, 217–218
    for spinal cord injury, metabolic and endocrine complications and, 416–417
Bekhterev's disease (ankylosing spondylitis)
    rheumatoid arthritis differentiated from, 385
    spinal fractures in, 385–408
        differentiation of fracture pseudarthrosis from spondylodiscitis and, 397–406
        flexion deformity of neck and, 388–395, 396
        mechanism of, 385–387
        spinal cord injury and, 391–393
Bending loads, thoracolumbar spine affected by, 49
    failure and, 53–54
Bernard's syndrome (Horner's syndrome), in syringomyelia, 423, 435
Biconcave fractures, osteoporotic, radiology of, 347
Bizarre high-frequency discharges (complex repetitive discharges), in electromyography, 114, 115
Bladder
    catheterization of in spinal cord injury, 171, 414–415
        early management and, 174, 474
    distension of, autonomic dysreflexia caused by, 411
    dysfunction of
        in late deformities, 452

in spinal cord injuries, 171, 174, 414–415, 474
    rehabilitation and, 479–480
    innervation of, spinal cord injury and, 414–415
    neurogenic. *See also* Bladder, dysfunction of
        rehabilitation and, 479
Blood-brain barrier, and acute spinal cord injury, 40
Blood flow, spinal cord, in acute injury, 40, 168
Blood gas analysis, spinal cord oxygenation monitored by, 168
BMU. *See* Basic multicellular unit
Body fixator, intervertebral, for anterior fixation and fracture reduction in thoracic burst fractures, clinical results of, 272
Body temperature
    nerve conduction velocity affected by, 110
    somatosensory evoked potentials affected by, 105
Boehler classification, of thoracolumbar fractures, 131
Boehler method, for conservative management of thoracolumbar fractures, 179
    for burst fractures, 189
    for compression fractures, 188, 291
        results of, 191–192
    for thoracic vertebral fractures, 199
Bone cement, for stabilization in spinal tumors, 365–367
Bone cyst, aneurysmal, of spine, 374
Bone fragments, intracanal, unreduced, fate of, 127, 143, 184, 218–219, 220, 254, 261, 267, 293. *See also* Burst fractures
Bone grafts, for stabilization in spinal tumors, 271, 365–367, 370
Bone loss
    age-related, 344
    factors causing, 341
Bone mass
    factors controlling, 340
    measurement of, 350–353
        techniques for, 350
    reduction of in osteoporosis, 339, 340–341
Bone mineral content, in spinal cord injury, 417
Bone remodeling, 365–367, 370
    menopause affecting, 342–344
    and osteoporotic fractures, 341–342
Bone resorption, in bone remodeling, 341
Bone scans, in spinal tumors, 364
Bone tumors, spinal, 359–382. *See also specific type and* Spinal tumors

giant cell, 375
  incidence of, 359
  malignant, 375–379
  primary, 372
    benign, 267–278
    incidence of, 359
Bony lesions, in traumatic spine and spinal cord injuries in children, evolution of, 329–330
Bowel, neurogenic, 479–480. *See also* Bowel dysfunction
Bowel dysfunction
  in late deformities, 452
  in spinal cord injury, 474
    rehabilitation and, 479–480
Bowel regimen, in early spinal cord injury management, 174, 474
Brachial plexus, neurographic testing of nerves derived from, 109, 110
Bracing
  in conservative management of burst fractures, 217–218
  and preservation of sagittal profile in low lumbar burst fractures, 224
  for secondary spinal deformities, at level of injury, 331–333
Bradycardia, in spinal cord injury, 169, 411
Breast cancer, spinal metastasis in, 380
Browne-Séquard syndrome, 162
  in children, 319
Burst fractures, 74, 134, 135, 137, 143–145
  anterior decompression and instrumentation for, 267–278
    biomechanical evaluation of, 270–271
    clinical results of, 272, 273
    indications for, 271
    rationale for decompression and, 272
    versus posterior surgery, 274, 275–277
  bed rest for, 217–218
  bracing for, 217–218
  in children, 314, 315
    spinal stability after, 323
    treatment of, 324
  classification of, late deformities and, 450–451
  conservative management of, 215–222, 293–294
    clinical outcome and, 219–220
    complications related to, 218
    controversial aspects of, 215
    radiographic changes over time following, 218
    and unreduced intracanal bony fragments, 218–219, 220
  CT scan of, 85, 86, 87

facet injury and, 238
fixation for, 203, 204, 205, 267–278
and high-energy blunt trauma producing unstable injuries with or without neurologic deficit, 217
Holdsworth classification and, 132
instability and, 55, 140, 143–147
of L2 vertebrae, 164, 165
and low-energy trauma producing stable injuries without neurologic deficit, 216–217
low lumbar (L3-L4-L5 fractures), 164, 165, 223–234
  anterior approach to, 230–232
    indications for, 232–233
  neural decompression and, 224–230
    anterior approach for, 232
    retroperitoneal flank approach to, 230–231
    retroperitoneal paramedial approach to, 231–232
  sagittal profile and, 223–224
    anterior approach and, 232
  with subluxation, 224, 225
  transperitoneal anterior approach to, 232
lumbar, 147–148, 223–234
  fixation of, 210
mechanism of, 195–196
without nerve compromise, treatment of, 189
  conservative, 216–217, 217–218
with neurologic compromise
  conservative management of, 217–218
  surgery for, 180, 181–184, 185–188
posterior fixation for, 294–302
radiography of, 74, 75, 81, 82
sacral, 248
  treatment of, 249
stability and, 55, 140, 143–147, 215–216
  radiographic criteria of, 216
treatment, 189
ultrasonography of, 127

C
C-D instrumentation. *See* Cotrel-Dubousset instrumentation
Calcitonin, in management of osteoporotic vertebral fractures
  acute, 353
  chronic, 354
Calcium
  acute spinal cord injury affecting extracellular concentration of, 41, 168
  in chronic management of osteoporotic vertebral fractures, 354

loss of in spinal cord injury, 416–417, 480
Calcium channel blockers
  in cord resuscitation, 168
  for hypertension in autonomic dysreflexia, 412
Canal decompression. *See* Decompression surgery
Canal stenosis, after treatment of thoracolumbar fracture, 191
Canalis neurentericus. *See* Neurocentral canal (neurenteric canal)
Cardiovascular dysfunction, in spinal cord injury, 169–170, 410–411, 474
  rehabilitation and, 480–481
Cartilaginous lesions, in traumatic spine and spinal cord injuries in children, evolution of, 329–330
CASH orthosis, 468, 469
Casting, and preservation of sagittal profile in low lumbar burst fractures, 224
Catheterization, urinary bladder, in spinal cord injury, 171, 414–415
  early management and, 174, 474
Cauda equina, 19
Cauda equina nerve roots, injury to, 164, 165
Central cord syndrome, 162–163
  in children, 319
Central motor latency, of motor evoked potential, 108
Central sacral canal fractures, 245, 248–249
  treatment of, 249
Cerebrospinal fluid, blockage of flow of, myelography for demonstration of, 97
Cervical fractures
  in ankylosing spondylitis, 388–395, 396
  epidemiology of, 60
Cervical lordosis, 17
Cervical orthoses, 466
Cervicothoracic junction, MRI for evaluation of, 71
Cervicothoracolumbosacral orthoses, 466
"Chairback" lumbosacral orthosis, 467
Chance fracture, 54, 74, 138, 140, 150, 189, 196
  in children, spinal stability after, 323
  conventional radiography of, 74, 75
  CT scan of, 90
  facet subluxation and, 240
  posterior fixation for, 291
Chance-like fracture, in children, 315
"Chevron" osteotomy, for reduction in late deformity, 458

Child abuse, and spinal cord injury without radiographic abnormalities (SCIWORA), 320
Children
  spinal deformities in, after traumatic spine and spinal cord injuries, 327–337
    at level of lesion, 329–333
    at levels below lesion, 333–337
    and normal growth of spine, 327–329
    prevention of, 335–336
  thoracic and lumbar spine injuries in, 307–325
    anterior ring epiphysis avulsion, 317
    burst fractures, 314, 315
      treatment of, 324
    classification of, 311–319
    clinical diagnosis of, 319–320
    compression fractures, 311–315
      treatment of, 323–324
    computed tomography of, 321
    cord injuries, 308–309
      without radiographic abnormalities (SCIWORA), 309, 320–321
    epidemiology of, 308–309
    fracture/dislocations, 316
      treatment of, 324
    fractures, 308–309
    imaging of, 321
    literature review of, 307–308
    magnetic resonance imaging of, 321
    myelography of, 321
    neurocentral cartilage separation, 318, 319
    pars interarticularis fractures, 319
    pathoanatomy and, 311
    posterior avulsion of ring margin epiphysis (rim fracture), 317–319
    radiography of, 321
    seat belt injuries, 315–316
      treatment of, 324
    spine stability after, 321–323
    tomography of, 321
    treatment of, 323–324
    vertebral growth and, 309–310
Chondrification centers, formation of, 3
Chondrosarcomas, of spine, 378, 379
  incidence of, 359
Chordomas, 379
  incidence of, 359
Circulatory disturbances. See Cardiovascular dysfunction
CMAP. See Compound muscle action potential
CMG. See Cystometrography

CO. See Cervical orthoses
Collagen breakdown, in spinal cord injury, 417
Colles' fractures, osteoporotic, 339, 340
Colloids, for volume loading in spinal cord injury, 169
Colon transit time, prolonged, in spinal cord injury, 415
Colonic distention, in spinal cord injury, 415
Columna vertebralis. See Vertebral column
Complete cord lesions, 163–165
  at T11-T12 vertebral level, 163–164
  at T12-L1 vertebral level, 164
  timing of surgery for, 180–181
Complex repetitive discharges, in electromyography, 114, 115
Compound muscle action potential, 110. See also M-wave studies
Compression fractures, 134, 135, 136, 141–143
  in children, 311–315
    spinal stability and, 321–322
    treatment of, 323–324
  facet injury and, 238
  indications for surgery in, 188–189
  mechanism of, 195
  of thoracic spine, 195
  treatment of, 188–189
    in children, 323–324
  wedge, 140
Compression instrumentation, for bilateral facet dislocation, 237
Compression loads
  facet joints affected by, 236
  thoracolumbar spine affected by, 46–48
    failure and, 51–53
Computerized tomography
  in children's spinal injuries, 321
  in late deformities, 453
  in low lumbar burst fractures, 224
  postmyelography, in post-traumatic syringomyelia, 436, 437
  in post-traumatic syringomyelia, 423
  quantitative, in bone mass measurement, 350
  in sacral fractures, 245
  in spinal tumors, 365
  in thoracic and lumbar vertebral fractures, 84–90
    and clinical decisions about conservative therapy, 216
    pitfalls of, 89–90
Constipation, in spinal cord injury, 415
Conus medullaris, injury to, 164
Conventional radiography
  in children's spinal injuries, 321
  in osteoporotic vertebral fractures, 346–347

  in sacral fractures, 245
  in spinal tumors, 364–365
  in thoracic and lumbar vertebral fractures, 69–84
    ABCS approach in evaluation of, 73, 80, 81–84
    and assessment of post-traumatic vertebral stability, 84
    diagnostic considerations in, 73–81
    pitfalls of, 84
    technical considerations in, 69–73
Cord division, for syringomyelia, 442
Cord edema, MRI demonstrating, 96
Cord resuscitation, 167–168
Cord transection, MRI of, 93
Cord trauma. See Spinal cord injury
Cordectomy, for post-traumatic syringomyelia, 425
Corpus vertebrae. See Vertebral body
Cortex, trabecularization of, 344
Cortical latency, of motor evoked potential, 107, 108
Corticosteroids, for acute spinal cord injury, 41, 168, 175
Costotransversectomy, for anterior approach to spinal tumors, 370
Cotrel-Dubousset instrumentation, 284, 285, 288
  biomechanical evaluation of, 270, 290, 291
  for burst fractures, 301, 302
  for flexion injuries, 291
  for flexion/distraction injuries, 291
  for fracture/dislocations, 292
  for late deformity, 457
  for lumbar fractures, 209–212
  for preservation of sagittal profile in low lumbar burst fractures, 224
  for secondary spinal deformity in children, 337
  for thoracic fractures, 199–201
  for thoracolumbar fractures, 201–203
Cotrel-Dubousset pedicle screws, 288
  biomechanical evaluation of, 290, 291
Coumadin, for thromboembolism prevention in spinal cord injury, 412
Credé's maneuver, for bladder emptying in spinal cord injury, 414
Cruciform anterior spinal hyperextension (CASH) orthosis, 468, 469
Crush fractures
  in osteomalacia, 348
  osteoporotic, 345, 347
    radiology of, 347
  in Paget's disease, 348

in primary hyperparathyroidism, 348–350
in renal osteodystrophy, 348
Crystalloids, for volume loading in spinal cord injury, 169
CT. *See* Computerized tomography
CT-myelography
 for post-traumatic syringomyelia, 423
 for spinal tumors, 365
CTLSO. *See* Cervicothoracolumbo-sacral orthoses
Curvatures of spine, 17–19, 49
 development of, 8–9
Custom-molded spinal jacket, 468–469
Cutting cone, in bone remodeling, 341
Cystic myelopathy. *See also* Syringomyelia
 intraoperative ultrasonography of, 128–130
Cystometrography, in central sacral canal fractures, 249
Cytochrome oxidase activity, acute spinal cord injury affecting, 41

D

Debridement, fracture, with anterior approach, 261–263
Decompression surgery
 anatomic rudiments of, 24
 anterior techniques of, 251–266
  anterior approach and, 255–263
   canal decompression and, 261–263
   historical review of, 252
   retroperitoneal, 260–261
   thoracoabdominal, 258–260
   transthoracic, 256–258
  for burst fractures, 267–278
   rationale for, 272
   results of, 263–264, 272, 273
  and thoracolumbar fracture treatment, 254–255
   historical review of, 251–252, 267
  versus posterior surgery, 274, 275–277
 for bilateral facet dislocation, 237
 for burst fractures, in children, 324
 in early spinal cord injury management, 175–178
 with intraoperative ultrasonography, 127–128
 for late deformity, 456, 457
 for low lumbar burst fractures, 224–230
  anterior approach for, 232
 in neurologic deterioration following recumbent management, 218
 for post-traumatic syringomyelia, 441

results of, 191–193
 for sacral fractures, 249
 for spinal deformities
  in children, after traumatic spine and spinal cord injuries, 330
  secondary, at level of injury, 330
 for spinal tumors, neural function preservation and, 367–368
 for thoracic vertebral fractures, 199.
 for thoracolumbar fractures, 180–184, 185–188
  anterior techniques for, 254–255, 267–278
  historical review of, 251–252
  with neurologic compromise, 180, 181–184, 185–188
Decoulx-Rieunau classification, of thoracolumbar fractures, 132
Decubiti, pressure (pressure sores), in spinal cord injury, 418, 474–475
 prevention of, 174
Deep tendon reflexes, in thoracic spine fracture
 in apparently neurologically intact person, 159
 in paraplegic, 160
 diagnosing level of, 162
Deep vein thrombosis, in spinal cord injury, 412
 heterotopic ossification differentiated from, 413
 prevention of, 171, 412
  intermittent pneumatic compression stockings for, 174
Dejerine arcuate tract, 37
Delayed gastric emptying, in spinal cord injury, 415
Denis classification, of thoracolumbar fractures, 133–140
 in children, 311–319
 integration of with other classifications, 141–156
Denis type I fractures, 141–143. *See also* Compression fractures
Denis type II fractures, 143–145. *See also* Burst fractures
Denis type III fractures, 148–149. *See also* Seat belt fractures
Denis type IV fractures, 149–154, 155. *See also* Fracture/dislocations
Diastematomyelia, 7
Diazepam, in acute management of osteoporotic vertebral fractures, 353
Dick device, 287–288
 for anterior fixation and fracture reduction in thoracic spine, 199
 biomechanical evaluation of, 270–271, 289, 291

Diltiazem, in cord resuscitation, 168
Dimethyl sulfoxide, in cord resuscitation, 168
Disability, definition of, 464
Disc. *See* Intervertebral disc
Disc herniation
 fracture and, CT scan of, 85
 MRI of, 93, 94
Discectomy, prophylactic, for bilateral facet dislocation, 237
Discus intervertebralis. *See* Intervertebral disc
Dislocations, 134, 135, 139. *See also* Fracture/dislocations
 in children, 316
 facet
  complete bilateral thoracolumbar, 236–237
  unilateral, 237
 fixation for, 203
 flexion injuries and, 76, 77
 instability and, 55
 posterior fixation for, 292–293
Disodium ethane-1-hydroxy-1, 1-diphosphonate. *See* Etidronate disodium
Distal motor latency, 111
Distraction
 for thoracolumbar fractures with neurologic compromise, 181
 thoracolumbar spine affected by failure continuum and, 53–54
 flexion injuries causing, 74–76
Diverticulosis, in spinal cord injury, 415
Diving, spinal accidents caused by, 62
DML. *See* Distal motor latency
Dopamine, for hemodynamic insult in spinal cord injury, 170
Dorsal horn, 36
Dorsal root entry zone surgery, for pain in spinal cord injury, 480
Double body sign, in complete bilateral thoracolumbar facet dislocation, 236
"Dowager's hump," 345
DPA. *See* Dual photon absorptiometry
Drains, for syringomyelia, 442
DREZ surgery. *See* Dorsal root entry zone surgery
"Droit devant" ("straight ahead") technique, 26–28
Drummond instrumentation, biomechanical evaluation of, 289
Dual photon absorptiometry, for bone mass measurement, 350, 351
Dual x-ray absorptiometry (DXA), for bone mass measurement, 350, 351

Dunn device
  for anterior fixation and fracture reduction in thoracic spine, 252, 253
    for burst fractures, 267, 270
  biomechanical testing of, 289
  results of, 264
Dura mater, spinal, 36
Dural tears
  in lumbar fractures, repair of, 206, 207, 224, 226
  myelography demonstrating, 96, 97
  and surgery for spinal cord injury, 176
DVT. See Deep vein thrombosis
Dwyer device, for anterior spinal fixation, 267
DXA. See Dual x-ray absorptiometry
Dysreflexia, autonomic, after spinal cord injury, 170, 411–412, 416
  rehabilitation and, 480
Dysrhythmias, in spinal cord injury, 169

E
ECG abnormalities, in spinal cord injury, 169
Edwards sleeves, 283
  biomechanical testing of, 289
  for posterior fixation and fracture reduction in thoracic spine, 251–252
Edwards-Barbaro shunt tube, for post-traumatic syringomyelia, 425
"Eggshell vertebrectomy," for late deformity, 455
EHDP. See Etidronate disodium
Electrodiagnostic studies. See Electrophysiology of spine
Electrogenic pump, acute spinal cord injury affecting, 40–41, 174–175
Electrolyte disorders, in spinal cord injury, 171
Electromyography, 112–116, 469–470
  case study of, 118
  and commonly tested muscles and their segmental innervation, 113
  discharge pattern and, 115
  of external anal sphincter, 115–116
  motor unit recruitment and, 113, 115
  neural structures evaluated by, 99
  in post-traumatic syringomyelia, 424
  recording technique for, 113
  in rehabilitation of spine fractures, 469–470
  single motor unit action potential analysis and, 113, 115
  spontaneous activity and, 113–114, 115
Electrophysiology of spine (electrodiagnostic testing of spine), 99–121
  autonomic techniques and, 116
  case study of, 116–118
  electromyography, 112–116
    in rehabilitation, 469–470
  evoked potentials
    motor, 105–108, 109
    in rehabilitation, 471–472
    somatosensory, 100–105
  nerve conduction studies, 110–112
    in rehabilitation, 470–471
  neurography, 109–112
  in post-traumatic syringomyelia, 424
  prognosis of spinal cord trauma and, 116, 482
  in rehabilitation, 469–472
Embryonic mesoblast, 3
Emergency procedures, in spinal cord injury, 173–174
EMG. See Electromyography
Empty facet sign, in complete bilateral thoracolumbar facet dislocation, 236
End-stage renal disease, in spinal cord injury, 415
Endocrine complications, in spinal cord injury, 416–418
Endomyelography, for post-traumatic syringomyelia, 423, 437
Endotracheal intubation, for respiratory failure in spinal cord injury, 170, 410
Endplate, compression loads affecting, 16–17
  rupture and, 51–52
Eosinophilic granuloma, spine affected in, 375
  spinal tumor differential diagnosis and, 363
EP. See Evoked potentials
Ephedrine, for hemodynamic insult in spinal cord injury, 169
Epidural abscess, syringomyelia caused by, 433
Erb's point, somatosensory evoked potential at, 101, 102, 103
Ergometer, FES, 479
Ergotamine, for postural hypotension in spinal cord injury, 411
Estrogen, in chronic management of osteoporotic vertebral fractures, 354
Etidronate disodium
  in chronic management of osteoporotic vertebral fractures, 355
  for heterotopic ossification, 413
Euler's formula, 49
Evoked potentials, 471–472
  motor, 105–108, 109, 472
    case study of, 117
    nerves stimulated by and muscles recorded from for level diagnosis, 100
    neural structures evaluated by, 99
    normal values of, 108, 109
    in rehabilitation of spinal fractures, 472
    root stimulation for, 107–108
    safety issues and, 106
    stimulation and recording techniques for, 106–108
    transcranial stimulation for, 107
  rehabilitation of spinal fractures and, 471–472
  somatosensory, 100–105, 472
    body temperature affecting, 105
    case study of, 117
    median nerve, 102
    nerves stimulated by and muscles recorded from for level diagnosis, 100
    neural structures evaluated by, 99
    nomenclature of, 102–105
    normal values of, 102–105
    peripheral neuropathies affecting, 105
    peroneal nerve, 104, 105
    rehabilitation of spinal fractures and, 472
    stimulation and recording techniques for, 100–102
    sural nerve, 104, 105
    tibial nerve, 103–104
    waveforms of, 102–105
Ewing's sarcoma, of spine, 379
Exercise, in chronic management of osteoporotic vertebral fractures, 354
Extension injuries
  mechanism of, 81
  radiography of, 80, 81
External anal sphincter, electromyography of, 115–116
External fixator (Magerl), 287
  biomechanical evaluation of, 289, 290
Extrapleural approach, for spinal tumors, 369–370

F
F-wave, 112
F-wave studies, 112
  for motor evoked potential interpretation, 108
  neural structures evaluated by, 99
  in post-traumatic syringomyelia, 424

Facet joints
  anatomy of, 235–236
  biomechanics of, 235–236
  injury of
    bilateral dislocation, 236–237
    burst versus compression
      fractures and, 238
    clinical considerations and,
      237–242
    compression loads and, 53, 236
    CT scan of, 87
    failure to recognize, 237–238
    isolated dislocation, 237
    management of, 235–243
    unilateral dislocation, 237
  lumbar, 236
  range of motion of, 235–236
  subluxation of, 238–242
  thoracolumbar, complete bilateral
    dislocation of, 236–237
  torsion affecting, 49
  widening of, in ABCS approach to
    plain film interpretation, 82
Failure continuum
  with anterior column under
    compression, 51–53
  with posterior elements under
    distraction, 53–54
  with rotation combined with various
    loads, 54, 55
"Far-out syndrome," 248
Fasciculation potentials, in
  electromyography, 114
Fecal impaction, in spinal cord injury,
  416
Femoral neck fractures, in spinal cord
  injury, 417
Femoral nerve, neurographic testing
  of, 109, 110
Ferguson method, for radiography of
  sacral fractures, 245
FES. See Functional electrical
  stimulation
FES ergometer, 479
Fibrillation potentials, in
  electromyography, 114, 115,
  470
FIM. See Functional Independence
  measure
Final common pathway, 37
Fingerprints approach, to radiography
  of thoracolumbar fractures, 73
  in extension injuries, 80, 81
  in flexion injuries, 77
  in rotary injuries, 77–78
  in shearing injuries, 78, 79
Fixation
  of alar fractures with pelvic
    instability, 246
  anterior techniques of, 251–266
    anterior approach and, 255–263

historical review of, 252
retroperitoneal, 260–261
thoracoabdominal, 258–260
transthoracic, 256–258
for burst fractures, 267–278
fixation devices and, 252–254
results of, 263–264
in thoracolumbar fracture
  treatment, 254–255
  historical review of, 251–252
indications for, 472–473
for late deformity, 457
for lumbar fractures, 208, 209–212
posterior instrumentation for,
  279–306
  biomechanical testing of, 288–291
  devices available for, 279–288
  versus anterior approach, 274,
    275–277
and preservation of sagittal profile
  in low lumbar burst fractures,
  224
for secondary spinal deformities, at
  level of injury, 331
for spinal tumors, 365–367, 368–369
  anterior techniques for, 369–370,
    371
for thoracic vertebral fractures,
  199–201
for thoracolumbar fractures,
  201–203, 204, 205
  anterior techniques for, 254–255,
    267–278
  historical review of, 251–252
for unilateral facet dislocation, 237
Flank approach, retroperitoneal, for
  low lumbar burst fractures,
  230–231
"Flatback syndrome," 281
Flaval ligament. See Ligamentum
  flavum
Flexeril, in acute management of
  osteoporotic vertebral
  fractures, 353
Flexion injuries
  in ankylosing spondylitis, 386, 387
  of neck, 388–395, 396
  mechanisms of, 73–74
  posterior fixation for, 291
  radiography of, 73–77
Flexion/distraction injuries, 140,
  148–149, 150. See also Seat
  belt fractures
  in children, 316
  mechanism of, 195–196, 197
  posterior fixation for, 291, 292
  treatment of, 189
Fludrocortisone, for postural
  hypotension in spinal cord
  injury, 411

Foraminal fractures, sacral, 245,
  246–248
  treatment of, 247–248
Foraminotomy
  for sacral fracture/dislocation, 249
  for sacral fractures causing sciatica,
    247
Fracture/dislocations, 134, 135, 139,
  149–154, 155
  in children, 316
    spinal stability after, 323
    treatment of, 324
  facet, unilateral, 237
  and failure continuum with rotation,
    54, 55
  instability and, 55
  mechanism of, 196, 197
  MRI for evaluation of, 71
  posterior fixation for, 292, 293
  sacral, 248
    treatment of, 249
  treatment of, 190
    in ankylosing spondylitis, 393
Fracture patterns, in pathologic
  fractures, 363–364
Frankel classification, of spinal cord
  injury, 42, 159
Functional electrical stimulation, for
  ambulation of paraplegic
  patients, 477–479
Functional Independence measure,
  465
"Functional treatment," of
  thoracolumbar fractures, 179
Fusion. See also Fixation
  for late deformity, 455–456, 457
  for secondary spinal deformities, at
    level of injury, 331

G
Ganglion blockers, for hypertension in
  autonomic dysreflexia, 170, 412
Gangliosides, for acute spinal cord
  injury, 41, 168, 175
Gastric atony, in spinal cord injury,
  171
Gastric dilatation, in spinal cord
  injury, 415
Gastric emptying, delayed, in spinal
  cord injury, 415
Gastritis, stress-induced, and
  gastrointestinal bleeding in
  spinal cord injury, 415
Gastroesophageal reflux, in spinal
  cord injury, 415, 416
Gastrointestinal bleeding, in spinal
  cord injury, 171, 415–416
Gastrointestinal dysfunction, in spinal
  cord injury, 171, 415–416, 474
Gaucher's disease, spine affected in,
  375

Gaucher's disease (*contd.*)
  spinal tumor differential diagnosis and, 362, 363
Genitourinary dysfunction, in spinal cord injury, 171, 413–415
Giant cell tumor of bone, spinal, 375
  incidence of, 359
Glucocorticoids (glucocorticosteroids), for acute spinal cord injury, 41, 168, 175
GM$_1$ gangliosides, for acute spinal cord injury, 41, 168, 175
Goll and Burdack tract, 37
Gray matter, spinal, 36
Greenfield filter, for thromboembolism prevention in spinal cord injury, 171, 174, 412
Grinding injuries. *See* Rotary injuries
Growth plates, and spine injury in children, 309
Guanethidine, for hypertension in autonomic dysreflexia, 412

H

H$_2$ blockers, for prophylaxis of GI bleeding in spinal cord injury, 171, 415
H-reflex, 112
H-reflex studies, 112
  neural structures evaluated by, 99
Hakim valve, for draining a syrinx, 441
Halo vest, for cervical fractures in ankylosing spondylitis, 393, 395
Handicap, definition of, 464
Hansen's node (primitive node), 1
Harms "cage"
  for anterior fixation and fracture reduction in thoracic burst fractures, 270
  for vertebral bone tumors, 377, 378
Harms-Zielke instrumentation, for anterior fixation and fracture reduction in thoracic burst fractures, 270
"Harri-Luque" system, 282, 283
  biomechanical evaluation of, 289
Harrington instrumentation, 280, 281–282
  biomechanical evaluation of, 270, 289, 290, 291
  for burst fractures, 294, 295, 296
  for decompression of spinal canal with intraoperative ultrasonography, 127–128
  for flexion injuries, 291
  for flexion/distraction injuries, 291, 292
  for fracture/dislocations, 292, 293
  and preservation of sagittal profile in low lumbar burst fractures, 224
  for thoracic fractures, 199
  for thoracolumbar fractures, 251, 252, 280, 281–282
    results of, 263
HCO. *See* Head-cervical orthoses
Head-cervical orthoses, 466
Headache, in autonomic dysreflexia, 411
Hemangioma, spinal, 372–373
Hematomyelia, 431
Hemivertebra, 8
Hemodialysis, for end-stage renal disease, 415
Hemomediastinum, thoracic vertebral fractures and, 196–197
Hemopneumomediastinum, thoracic vertebral fractures and, 198
Hemorrhoids, in spinal cord injury, 416
Hemothorax, thoracic vertebral fractures and, 197–198
Heparin, for thromboembolism prevention in spinal cord injury, 171, 174, 412
Hernia, hiatus, in spinal cord injury, 415
Herniation, intervertebral disk fracture and, CT scan of, 85
  MRI of, 93, 94
Heterotopic ossification, in spinal cord injury, 412–413
  deep vein thrombosis differentiated from, 413
  rehabilitation and, 480
Hiatus hernia, in spinal cord injury, 415
Hip fractures, osteoporotic, epidemiology of, 339
Histiocytosis X, spine affected in, 375
HO. *See* Heterotopic ossification
Hoffmann's reflex, in post-traumatic syringomyelia, 435
Holdsworth's classification, of thoracolumbar fractures, 131–132
Holter valve, for draining a syrinx, 441
Hooks
  for fixation in lumbar fractures, 209–210
  for fixation in thoracic fractures, 199–201
  for fixation in thoracolumbar fractures, 201–203
  for preservation of sagittal profile in low lumbar burst fractures, 224
Horner's syndrome, in syringomyelia, 423, 435
Howship's lacuna, in bone remodeling, 341
Hydralazine, for hypertension in autonomic dysreflexia, 412
Hydroxyproline levels, in spinal cord injury, 417
Hyperbaric oxygen therapy, in cord resuscitation, 168
Hypercalcemia, in spinal cord injury, 417
Hypercalciuria, in spinal cord injury, 417
Hyperextension fractures, in children, treatment of, 324
Hyperhidrosis, in post-traumatic syringomyelia, 436
Hyperparathyroidism
  primary, crush fractures in, 348–350
  secondary, in renal osteodystrophy, crush fractures and, 348
Hyperreflexia, autonomic. *See* Autonomic dysreflexia
Hypertension, in autonomic dysreflexia, 411
Hypokalemia, in spinal cord injury, 171
Hyponatremia, in spinal cord injury, 171
Hypotension, in spinal cord injury, 169, 410–411
  postural (orthostatic), 411
  rehabilitation and, 480–481
Hypothermia therapy, in cord resuscitation, 168

I

I-plate, Syracuse
  for anterior fixation and fracture reduction in thoracic spine, 252, 253
  for burst fractures, 269
  biomechanical evaluation of, 270–271
  clinical results of, 272
Ileus, in spinal cord injury, 171, 415
Iliac strut graft, for anterior fixation and fracture reduction in thoracic burst fractures, biomechanical evaluation of, 270
Immobilization
  in conservative treatment of thoracolumbar fractures, 179
    results of, 191–192
  for spinal cord injury, metabolic and endocrine complications and, 416–417
Impairment, definition of, 464
Inferior vena cava filters, for thromboembolism prevention in spinal cord injury, 171, 412
Insertional activity, 469

Instability, 141. *See also* Stability
  Louis' quantification of, 132, 133
  Nicoll classification and, 131, 141
  spinal tumors and, 365
  of thoracolumbar fractures, 54–56
  Watson-Jones classification and, 131
"Instrument long, fuse short" strategy, for fracture management, 282
Instrumentation. *See* Fixation
Intensive care unit, spinal cord injury management in, 167–172
  cardiovascular management and, 169–170
  electrolyte disorders and, 171
  gastrointestinal management and, 171
  genitourinary management and, 171
  indications for admission and, 167
  nutrition and, 171
  respiratory management and, 170–171
  spinal cord resuscitation and, 167–168
  thromboembolism prevention and, 171
Interbody devices, for anterior fixation and fracture reduction in thoracic burst fractures, 270
Interference pattern, in electromyography, 470
Intermediate zone, 36
Intermittent pneumatic compression stockings, for deep vein thrombosis prevention, 174
Internal fixation
  of alar fractures with pelvic instability, 246
  anterior techniques of, 251–266
    anterior approach and, 255–263
    historical review of, 252
    retroperitoneal, 260–261
    thoracoabdominal, 258–260
    transthoracic, 256–258
  for burst fractures, 267–278
  fixation devices and, 252–254
  results of, 263–264
  in thoracolumbar fracture treatment, 254–255
    historical review of, 251–252
  indications for, 472–473
  for late deformity, 457
  for lumbar fractures, 208, 209–212
  posterior instrumentation for, 279–306
    biomechanical testing of, 288–291
    devices available for, 279–288
    versus anterior approach, 274, 275–277

and preservation of sagittal profile in low lumbar burst fractures, 224
  for secondary spinal deformities, at level of injury, 331
  for spinal tumors, 365–367, 368–369
    anterior techniques for, 369–370, 371
  for thoracic fractures, 199–201
  for thoracolumbar fractures, 201–203, 204, 205
    anterior techniques for, 254–255
    historical review of, 251–252
  for unilateral facet dislocation, 237
Interspinous ligament, 16
  degree of elongation of prior to failure, 48
  torsion affecting, 49
Intertransverse ligament, 16
Intervertebral body fixator, for anterior fixation and fracture reduction in thoracic burst fractures, clinical results of, 272
Intervertebral disc, 16
  bending loads affecting, 49
  compression loads affecting, 46, 47
  failure and, 51–53
  herniation of
    fracture and, CT scan of, 85
    MRI of, 93, 94
  shear forces affecting, 48
  tension forces affecting, 48
  torsional stresses affecting, 48–49
Intervertebral disc space, widening or narrowing of, in ABCS approach to plain film interpretation, 82
Intervertebral joint, disruption of, 56
Intracanal bony fragments, unreduced, fate of, 218–219, 220
Intraoperative ultrasonography, 123–130
  basic physics underlying, 123
  for cord trauma evaluation, 130
  in cystic myelopathy, 128–130
  decompression of spinal canal and, 127–128
  normal anatomy and, 124, 125–126
  technique for, 123–125
Intrapleural approach, for spinal tumors, 369–370
Intubation
  endotracheal, for respiratory failure in spinal cord injury, 170, 410
  nasogastric, for gastrointestinal dysfunction in spinal cord injury, 171
Iophendylate. *See* Myodil

Isthmic spondylolysis, microtraumatic injuries causing, 319
IVBF. *See* Intervertebral body fixator

J
Jacobs rod, 284
  biomechanical evaluation of, 289, 290
Jewett orthosis, 468
Joint contractures, in spinal cord injury, rehabilitation and, 480
Joint dysfunction, in post-traumatic syringomyelia, 423
"Jumped facet," 237
Junctura intercorporealis, 15
Juncturae columnae vertebralis. *See* Vertebral joints
Juncturae zygapophyseales. *See* Posterior joints
Juvenile kyphosis (Scheuermann's disease)
  osteoporosis differentiated from, 349, 350
  and spinal cord injury without radiologic abnormalities (SCIWORA), 320–321

K
KAFO. *See* Knee-ankle-foot orthosis
Kaneda device
  for anterior fixation and fracture reduction in thoracic spine, 252, 253
    for burst fractures, 267, 268, 270
  biomechanical evaluation of, 270, 289
  results of, 264
Kidney cancer, spinal metastasis in, 381, 382
Kidney stones, in spinal cord injury, 415
Knee-ankle-foot orthosis, for ambulation of paraplegic patients, 477
Knight lumbosacral orthosis, 467
Knight-Taylor spinal brace, 467–468
Kostuik-Harrington device
  for anterior fixation and fracture reduction in thoracic spine, 252, 253
    for burst fractures, 267–269, 270
  biomechanical evaluation of, 270–271
  results of, 263, 272, 273
Kyphoscoliosis, in post-traumatic syringomyelia, 435
Kyphosis
  evaluation of instability and, 154, 155

Kyphosis (*contd.*)
  following nonoperative management of thoracolumbar fractures, 218
  as late deformity, 452–453
  thoracic, 17, 49
  after thoracolumbar fracture, 56

L

L1, injuries at level of, 164
L2
  burst fractures of, 164, 165
  growth of, 310
  spinal cord ending at, 19
L3-L4-L5 fractures, 164, 165, 223–234
  anterior approach to, 230–232
    indications for, 232–233
  neural decompression and, 224–230
    anterior approach for, 232
  retroperitoneal flank approach to, 230–231
  retroperitoneal paramedial approach to, 231–232
  sagittal profile and, 223–224
    anterior approach and, 232
  transperitoneal anterior approach to, 232
Lamina
  injuries of, CT scan of, 87
  neuralis, development of, 2
  prechordalis. *See* Prechordal lamina
  of vertebral arch, 11–12
    structure of, 12
Laminectomy
  for burst fractures, 294
  for lumbar fractures, 206, 207
  for post-traumatic syringomyelia, 425
    surgical technique for, 425
  for sacral fracture/dislocation, 249
  and spinal deformities in children after traumatic spine and spinal cord injuries, 329–330
  and spinal stability after spinal injury in children, 323
  for spinal tumors, neural function preservation and, 367–368
  for thoracic fractures, 199
Lap-type seat belts, flexion injuries and, 74. *See also* Seat belt fractures
Late deformities, 449–461
  definition of stability and, 450–452
  presentation of, 452–453
  risks for progression of, 453–454
  stable, 452
  treatment of, 455–457
    clinical outcome and, 457
    conservative, 455
    preferred technique for, 457–460
  unstable, 452

Lateral femoral cutaneous nerve, neurographic testing of, 110
Lateral recess, 22
Lateral translation, as late deformity, 453
Lazaroides, in cord resuscitation, 168
Ligamentotaxis, for burst fractures, 294, 296
Ligamentous lesions, in traumatic spine and spinal cord injuries in children, evolution of, 329–330
Ligamentum denticulum, 36
Ligamentum flavum, 16–17
  and anteroposterior diameter evaluation of vertebral canal, 22
  degree of elongation of prior to failure, 48
Ligamentum interspinale. *See* Interspinous ligament
Ligamentum intertransversarium. *See* Intertransverse ligament
Ligamentum longitudinale anterius. *See* Longitudinal ligaments, anterior
Ligamentum longitudinale posterium. *See* Longitudinal ligaments, posterior
Ligamentum supraspinale. *See* Supraspinous ligament
Limb fractures, osteoporotic, in spinal cord injury, 417
Linea primitiva. *See* Primitive line
Lipid peroxides, in acute spinal cord injury, 41
Load
  accommodation of spinal components to, 46–49
  facet joints affected by, 236
Locking hook spinal rod system, 284
Longitudinal ligaments
  anterior, 16
    degree of elongation of prior to failure, 48
    facet capsule stability and, 235
  posterior, 16
    degree of elongation of prior to failure, 48
    facet capsule stability and, 235
    integrity of, and stability of burst fractures, 145–146
Looser's zone fractures, 348
Lordosis
  cervical, 17
  lumbar, 17, 49
    and low lumbar burst fractures, 223–224
Louis
  quantification of instability by, 132, 133
  three-column concept of, 133

LSO. *See* Lumbosacral orthoses
Lumbar fractures, 206–212
  burst, 147–148, 223–234
  fixation for, 208, 209–212
  low (L3-L4-L5 fractures), 164, 165, 223–234
    anterior approach to, 230–232
      indications for, 232–233
    neural decompression and, 224–230
      anterior approach for, 232
    retroperitoneal flank approach to, 230–231
    retroperitoneal paramedial approach to, 231–232
    sagittal profile and, 223–224
      anterior approach and, 232
    transperitoneal anterior approach to, 232
  treatment of, 206–212
  types of, 206
Lumbar lordosis, 17, 49
  and low lumbar burst fractures, 223–224
Lumbar nerve roots, in injuries at T12-L1 level, 164
Lumbar potential, 101
Lumbar spinal cord. *See also* Lumbar spine; Lumbar vertebrae
  arteries of, 19–21
  venous drainage of, 21
Lumbar spine. *See also* Lumbar spinal cord; Lumbar vertebrae; Spine
  anatomy of, 159, 206
  instability of, as late deformity, 456–457
    treatment of, 456–457
  organogenesis of, 1–10
  physiology of, 206
  radiography of, 72, 73
Lumbar vertebrae. *See also* Lumbar spine
  characteristics of, 12–13
  nerve connections in, 19
  targeting for pedicular screw insertion, 26–28
Lumbosacral facet dislocation, unilateral, 237
Lumbosacral junction, 17
Lumbosacral orthoses, 466, 467
Lung cancer, spinal metastasis in, 379–380
Luque instrumentation, 283
  biomechanical evaluation of, 270, 289, 290, 291
  inappropriateness of for burst fractures, 294
  for thoracic vertebral fractures, 199
Lymphoma
  spinal, 375–377
  spinal canal invasion by, 360

M

M-wave studies
  for motor evoked potential interpretation, 108
  normal values of, 109
McAfee classification, of thoracolumbar fractures, 140
Magerl external fixator, 287
  biomechanical evaluation of, 289, 290
Magnesium, loss of in spinal cord injury, 417
Magnetic resonance imaging
  in children's spinal injuries, 321
  in late deformities, 453
  in post-traumatic syringomyelia, 423–424, 437–438
  in sacral fractures, 245
  in spinal tumors, 364
  in thoracic and lumbar vertebral fractures, 90–97
Magnetoelectric stimulation, for motor evoked potentials, 105–108
  root, 107–108
  safety issues and, 106
  stimulation sites and recording techniques for, 106–108
  transcranial, 107
Mannitol, in cord resuscitation, 168
Marginal rim, 6
Marginal ring, development of, 310
Marie-Strümpell disease (ankylosing spondylitis)
  rheumatoid arthritis differentiated from, 385
  spinal fractures in, 385–408
    differentiation of fracture pseudarthrosis from spondylodiscitis and, 397–406
    flexion injuries of neck and, 388–395, 396
    mechanism of, 385–387
    spinal cord injury and, 391–393
Mechanical ventilation, for respiratory failure in spinal cord injury, 170, 410
Median nerve
  neurographic testing of, 109, 110
  somatosensory evoked potentials from, 102
Mediastinal effusion, thoracic vertebral fractures and, 196–197, 198
Medulla spinalis. See Spinal cord
Medullar vascularization, 19–21
Medullary infarction, in children, 319
Medullary lesions, in spinal cord injury without radiologic abnormalities (SCIWORA), pathophysiology of, 320–321

Meninges, spinal cord, 35–36
Meningitis, syringomyelia caused by, 433
Meningocele, 7
Menopause
  bone mass loss and, 340, 342–344
  and osteoporotic thoracolumbar fractures, 339
  role of in osteoporotic fractures, 342–344
MEPs. See Motor evoked potentials
Mesoderma embryonicum. See Embryonic mesoblast
Metabolic disturbances, in spinal cord injury, 416–418
  rehabilitation and, 480
Metastatic disease of spine, 379–382
  incidence of, 359–360
  vertebral fractures in, 348
"Method of Boehler." See Boehler method
Methylprednisolone, for acute spinal cord injury, 41, 168, 175
Metrizamide, for CT scans of post-traumatic syringomyelia, 423
Meurig-Williams spinous process plates, 280–281
Microatelectasis, in spinal cord injury, 410
Micturition, spinal center of, 414
Milkman's fractures, 348
Milwaukee brace, for secondary spinal deformities, at level of injury, 333
MIS. See Motor index score
Morscher plate, for anterior fixation of cervical spine, 264
Motility, gastrointestinal in spinal cord injury, 415–416
Motor deficits, in post-traumatic syringomyelia, 435
Motor evoked potentials, 105–108, 109, 472
  case study of, 117
  nerves stimulated by and muscles recorded from for level diagnosis, 100
  neural structures evaluated by, 99
  normal values of, 108, 109
  in rehabilitation of spinal fractures, 472
  root stimulation for, 107–108
  safety issues and, 106
  stimulation and recording techniques for, 106–108
  transcranial stimulation for, 107
Motor examination, in thoracic spine fracture
  in apparently neurologically intact person, 159
  in complete paraplegia, 160
  diagnosing level of, 162

Motor function, in late deformities, 452
  postoperative, 456
Motor index score
  for assessing late deformities, 452
  postoperative, 456
  for assessing spinal cord injury, 42
Motor nerve conduction, 111
  case study of, 117
Motor root stimulation, magnetoelectric, for motor evoked potentials, 107
Motor unit action potentials, 113, 115, 470
Motor unit recruitment, 113, 115
Motor vehicle accidents
  flexion injuries caused by, 73–74
  spine injuries caused by, 61–62
Motor weakness, in post-traumatic syringomyelia, 423
Motorcycle accidents, flexion injuries caused by, 73–74
MRI. See Magnetic resonance imaging
MUAPs. See Motor unit action potentials
Multiple myeloma, spinal, 375
Muscle strength assessment, 474
Musculocutaneous nerve, neurographic testing of, 110
Myelocele, 7
Myelography
  in children's spinal injuries, 321
  in post-traumatic syringomyelia, 423, 436, 437
  in sacral fractures, 245
  in spine tumors, 365
  in thoracic and lumbar vertebral fractures, 96, 97
Myeloma, spinal, 375
Myelomeningocele, 7
Myelopathy
  cystic. See also Syringomyelia
  intraoperative ultrasonography of, 128–130
  injury causing, spinal cord injury without radiographic abnormalities (SCIWORA) and, 320
Myelotomy, for post-traumatic syringomyelia, 425, 440
  surgical technique for, 425, 440
Myodil, arachnoiditis caused by, syringomyelia and, 433, 436

N

"Naked facets," in ABCS approach to plain film interpretation, 82, 83
Naloxone, in cord resuscitation, 168

Nasogastric intubation, for gastrointestinal dysfunction in spinal cord injury, 171
NCS. *See* Nerve conduction studies
Neck, flexion injuries of, in ankylosing spondylitis, 388–395, 396
Negative nitrogen balance, in spinal cord injury, 417–418
  rehabilitation and, 480
Nerve conduction studies, 110–112
  age affecting, 110
  F-wave, 112
  H-reflex, 112
  motor, 111
  in rehabilitation in spinal fractures, 470–471
  safety issues in, 110–111
  sensory, 111–112
  temperature affecting, 110
Nerve conduction velocity, 470
  age affecting, 110
Nerve root lesions, in traumatic spine and spinal cord injuries in children, evolution of, 330
Nerve roots, in thoracic spine, 21–22
Nervi spinales. *See* Spinal nerves
Neural decompression. *See* Decompression surgery
Neural elements. *See also* Spinal cord
  physiology and pathophysiology of, 35–44
Neural tube
  development of, 2–3
  nonclosure of, combined neurologic and bone anomalies associated with, 7
Neurapraxia, neurography in, 109
Neurenteric canal (neurocentral canal), 1, 2
Neurocentral cartilage separation, in children, 319
  treatment of, 324
Neurogenic bladder. *See also* Bladder, dysfunction of
  rehabilitation and, 479
Neurogenic bowel. *See also* Bowel dysfunction
  rehabilitation and, 479–480
Neurogenic shock, 41
Neurography, 109–112
  in axonotmesis, 109
  and commonly tested nerves and their segmental innervation, 109–110
  F-wave studies and, 112
  H-reflex studies and, 112
  motor nerve conduction and, 111
  nerve conduction studies, 110–112
  neural structures evaluated by, 99
  in neurapraxia, 109

in neurotmesis, 109
safety issues and, 110–111
sensory nerve conduction and, 111–112
Neurologic deficit (neurologic injuries). *See also* Paraplegia
  with complete cord lesions, 163–165
  with incomplete thoracic lesions, 162–163
  with L2 burst fractures, 165
  with L3-L4-L5 fractures, 165
  with sacral fractures, 165
  spinal anatomy and, 157–159
  in spinal cord injury
    assessment of, 41–42
    complete, 41
    incomplete, 41–42
  in spinal fracture in ankylosing spondylitis, 385
  in spinal tumors, 363–364
    anatomic considerations and, 360
    location and, 363
    rate of development of, 363
    treatment decisions and, 361
    surgery for, 180–184, 185–188
    results of, 191–193
    timing of, 180–181
  with T1-T10 vertebral fractures, 159–162
  with T11-T12 vertebral fractures, 163–164
  with T12-L1 vertebral fractures, 164
Neuromeningeal dynamics, 37–38
Neurophysiologic evaluation of spine (electrodiagnostic testing), 99–121
  autonomic techniques and, 116
  case study of, 116–118
  electromyography, 112–116
    in rehabilitation, 469–470
  evoked potentials
    motor, 105–108, 109
    in rehabilitation, 471–472
    somatosensory, 100–105
  nerve conduction studies, 110–112
    in rehabilitation, 470–471
  neurography, 109–112
  in post-traumatic syringomyelia, 424
  prognosis of spinal cord trauma and, 116, 482
  in rehabilitation, 469–472
Neuroporus caudalis, nonclosure of, combined neurologic and bone anomalies associated with, 7
Neurotmesis
  in injuries at T12-L1 level, 164
  neurography in, 109
Nicoll classification, of thoracolumbar fractures, 131
Nifedipine
  in cord resuscitation, 168

for hypertension in autonomic dysreflexia, 412
Nitrogen balance, negative, in spinal cord injury, 417–418
  rehabilitation and, 480
Nodus primitivus. *See* Primitive node
Nonsteroidal antiinflammatory drugs, for pain from osteoporotic vertebral fractures, 353
Norepinephrine, for hemodynamic insult in spinal cord injury, 170
Notochord, development of, 1, 2
Notochordal process, formation of, 1–2
Nucleus pulposus, 16
Nutrition, in spinal cord injury, 171, 417–418

O

Obturator nerve, neurographic testing of, 110
Olerud device, for posterior fixation and fracture reduction in thoracic spine, 251
"Open book" pelvic injuries, foraminal fractures and, 248
Organogenetic defects, 7–9
Orthoses. *See also specific type*
  for ambulation of paraplegic patients, 477
  with functional electrical stimulation system, 478
  for secondary spinal deformities, at level of injury, 333
  for spinal fractures, 465–469
Orthostatic (postural) hypotension, in spinal cord injury, 411
  rehabilitation and, 480–481
Ossification, heterotopic, in spinal cord injury, 412–413
  deep vein thrombosis differentiated from, 413
  rehabilitation and, 480
Ossification centers, development of, 4–6
Osteoarthrosis, after "instrument long, fuse short" fracture management, 282
Osteoblastomas, of spine, 373–374
  incidence of, 359
Osteoblasts, in bone remodeling, 341, 342
  age affecting, 344
Osteochondromas, of spine, 373
  incidence of, 359
Osteoclasts, in bone remodeling, 341
Osteocytes, in bone remodeling, 341
Osteodystrophy, renal, vertebral crush fractures in, 348
Osteogenesis imperfecta, vertebral fractures in, 350

Osteoid osteomas, of spine, 373
  incidence of, 359
Osteomalacia, vertebral crush
    fractures caused by, 348
Osteomas, osteoid, of spine, 373
  incidence of, 359
Osteomyelitis, in spinal tumor
    differential diagnosis, 363
Osteoporosis
  Colles' fractures in, 339, 340
  hip fractures in, 339
  limb fractures in, spinal cord injury
      and, 417
  in paraplegia, rehabilitation and,
      480
  pull-out strength of pedicle screws
      affected by, 290
  in spinal cord injury, 417
  thoracolumbar fractures in, 339–358
    acute management of, 353–354
    age-related bone loss and, 344
    bone mass measurement and,
        350–353
    bone remodeling and, 341–342
    calcium and, 354
    chronic treatment of, 354
    clinical features of, 344–346
    differential diagnosis of, 348–350
    epidemiology of, 339–340
    exercise and, 354
    interrelationships among fractures
        and, 340
    menopause and, 342–344
    pain and, 345, 353–354
    pathophysiology of, 340–344
    pharmacologic therapy and,
        354–355
    radiologic appearance of, 346–347
    spinal tumor differential diagnosis
        and, 363
    treatment of, 353–355
Osteosarcomas, of spine, 379
  incidence of, 359
Osteotomy, "chevron," for reduction
    in late deformity, 458
Ovarian function, loss of, bone mass
    loss and, 343
Oximetry, pulse, spinal cord
    oxygenation monitored by, 168
Oxygen therapy, hyperbaric, in cord
    resuscitation, 168

P
Paget's disease
  and spinal osteosarcomas, 379
  vertebral crush fractures in, 348
Pain
  in late deformities, 452
    after surgery, 456
  in osteoporotic vertebral fracture,
      345, 353–354
  in post-traumatic syringomyelia,
      423, 434
    surgery for relief of, 426
  in spinal cord injury, rehabilitation
      and, 480
  in spine tumors
    anatomic considerations and, 360
    treatment decisions and, 361
Pancreatitis, in spinal cord injury,
    415, 416
Pantopaque. *See* Myodil
Paralysis
  in spinal cord injury, rehabilitation
      and, 476–481
  from spinal tumors
    anatomic considerations and, 360
    treatment decisions and, 361
  vertebral growth affected by, 328
Paralytic ileus, in spinal cord injury,
    171, 415
Paramedian approach, retroperitoneal,
    for low lumbar burst fractures,
    231–232
Paraplegia/paraparesis, 62
  complete, 160–162
    diagnosis of level of, 162
  with complete cord lesions, 163–165
    diagnosis of level of, 162
  with incomplete thoracic lesions,
      162–163
  with L2 burst fractures, 165
  with L3-L4-L5 fractures, 165
  and paralysis below level of injury,
      333–334
  physical examination in, 160–162
  with sacral fractures, 165
  spinal anatomy and, 157–159
  syringomyelia after. *See* Post-
      traumatic syringomyelia
  with T1-T10 vertebral fractures,
      159–162
  with T11-T12 vertebral fractures,
      163–164
  with T12-L1 vertebral fractures, 164
Paraspinal soft tissue mass, in ABCS
    approach to plain film
    interpretation, 82, 83
Parathyroid hormone, and bone mass
    loss after menopause, 343
Paraxial mesoblast, 3
Parenteral alimentation, in early
    spinal cord injury management,
    174
Pars interarticularis, 11
  fractures of
    in children, 319
    clinical considerations and,
        237–242
Partial volume averaging effect, in CT
    scans, 89

Passive range of motion exercises, in
    early management of spinal
    cord injury, 174
Pathologic fractures, of thoracolumbar
    spine, neoplastic infiltration
    causing, 363–364
Pedicle, 11
  structure of, 12, 24–26
Pedicle fixation, 285–288. *See also
    specific type*
  biomechanical evaluation of, 270
  for preservation of sagittal profile in
      low lumbar burst fractures, 224
  results of, 263
  for unilateral facet dislocation, 237
Pedicle screws, 285–287
  biomechanical evaluation of, 290,
      291
  for burst fractures, 294–302
  for fixation in lumbar fractures, 209
  insertion of
    anatomic rudiments of, 24–32
    hazards related to, 32
    along pedicular axis, 28–29
    "straight ahead" ("droit
        devant") technique for,
        26–28
    targeting lumbar vertebrae for, 28
    targeting thoracic vertebrae for,
        26–28
  for late deformity, 456, 460
Pelvic injuries, sacral fractures
    accompanying, 245
Pelvic instability, with alar fracture,
    treatment of, 246, 247
Perfusion pressure, spinal cord,
    monitoring, 168
Pericardial effusion, thoracic vertebral
    fractures and, 198
Peripheral neuropathy, somatosensory
    evoked potentials affected by,
    105
Peroneal nerves
  neurographic testing of, 109, 110
  somatosensory evoked potentials
      from, 104, 105
Phenoxybenzamine, for hypertension
    in autonomic dysreflexia, 412
Phenylephrine, for hemodynamic
    insult in spinal cord injury, 170
Phosphate, loss of in spinal cord
    injury, 417
Phrenic nerve, neurographic testing
    of, 110
Physical medicine. *See also*
    Rehabilitation
  definition of, 463
  principles of, 463–464
Pia mater, spinal, 36

Plain film radiography
  in children's spinal injuries, 321
  in osteoporotic vertebral fractures, 346–347
  in sacral fractures, 245
  in spinal tumors, 364–365
  in thoracic and lumbar vertebral fractures, 69–84
    ABCS approach in evaluation of, 73, 80, 81–84
    and assessment of post-traumatic vertebral stability, 84
    diagnostic considerations in, 73–81
    pitfalls of, 84
    technical considerations in, 69–73
Plasmacytoma, solitary, of spine, 375, 376
Plate systems, for anterior fixation and fracture reduction in thoracic spine, 253
Pluridirectional tomography, for thoracic and lumbar vertebral fractures, 90, 91, 92
Pneumatic compression stockings, intermittent, for deep vein thrombosis prevention, 174
Pneumonia, in spinal cord injury, 409
Polyphasic potentials, 470
Positive sharp waves, in electromyography, 114, 115, 470
Post-traumatic syringomyelia, 421–427, 429–448
  autonomic dysfunction and, 435–436
  case studies of, 442–447
  and changes below the level of injury, 436
  in children, 330
  clinical presentation of, 423, 434
  conservative treatment of, 427
  cord division for, 442
  decompression surgery for, 199, 200, 441
  drainage of, 424–425, 438
    to pleura or peritoneum, 441
  drains in management of, 442
  electrophysiological studies of, 424
  endomyelography of, 423, 437
  enlargement of cystic spaces and, 431–434
  epidemiology of, 421–422
  hematomyelia and, 431
  incidence of, 421, 429–430
  magnetic resonance imaging of, 423–424, 437–438
  mechanisms of onset of, 431
  morphology of, 430, 431
  motor loss and, 435
  myelography of, 423, 436, 437
  pathogenesis of, 422
  pathology of, 422–423
  radiology of, 423–424, 436
  sensory loss and, 434–435
  structural changes and, 435
  surgical management of, 424–427
    future work in, 447
    indications for, 438
    principles of, 438–439
    results of, 426–427, 447
    standard operation for, 439–441
    technique for, 425–426
    timing of, 438
  symptoms and signs of, 423, 434
  syringosubarachnoid shunting for, 441
  tendon reflexes affected in, 435
  time of onset of, 431
  treatment of, 438
  ultrasonography of, 424
  ultrastructural appearance of, 422–423
  valves in management of, 441
Posterior avulsion of ring margin epiphysis, 317–319
Posterior fixation devices, 279–288. *See also specific type*
  biomechanical testing of, 288–291
Posterior instrumentation
  for burst fractures, 294–302
  for late deformity, 456
  for secondary spinal deformities in children, 337
  for spinal tumors, 372
  for thoracolumbar fractures, 279–306
    biomechanical testing of, 288–291
    devices available for, 279–288
    versus anterior approach, 274, 275–277
Posterior joints, vertebral, 16–17
Posterior longitudinal ligament, 16
  degree of elongation of prior to failure, 48
  facet capsule stability and, 235
  integrity of, and stability of burst fractures, 145–146
Postural hypotension (orthostatic hypotension), in spinal cord injury, 411
  rehabilitation and, 480–481
Potassium
  acute spinal cord injury affecting extracellular concentration of, 40–41
  imbalances of in spinal cord injury, 171
Potential
  action
    compound muscle, 110. *See also* M-wave studies
    motor unit, 113, 115, 470
    sensory nerve, 111
    single motor unit, 113, 115
  fasciculation, 114
  fibrillation, 114, 115
  lumbar, 101
  motor evoked, 105–108, 109
    case study of, 117
    nerves stimulated by and muscles recorded from for level diagnosis, 100
    neural structures evaluated by, 99
    normal values of, 108, 109
    root stimulation for, 107–108
    safety issues and, 106
    stimulation and recording techniques for, 106–108
    transcranial stimulation for, 107
  somatosensory evoked, 100–105
    body temperature affecting, 105
    case study of, 117
    median nerve, 102
    nerves stimulated by and muscles recorded from for level diagnosis, 100
    neural structures evaluated by, 99
    nomenclature of, 102–105
    normal values of, 102–105
    peripheral neuropathies affecting, 105
    peroneal nerve, 104, 105
    stimulation and recording techniques for, 100–102
    sural nerve, 104, 105
    tibial nerve, 103–104
    waveforms of, 102–105
Pre-osteoclasts, in bone remodeling, 341
Prechordal lamina, 2
Pressure decubiti (pressure sores), in spinal cord injury, 418, 474–475
  prevention of, 174
Primary ossification centers, of vertebra, 4
Primitive line, 1
Primitive node (Hansen's node), 1
Processus articularis superior and inferior. *See* Articular processes, superior and inferior
Processus notochordalis. *See* Notochordal process
Processus spinosus. *See* Spinous process
Processus transversus. *See* Transverse process
Prostate cancer, spinal metastasis in, 380
Pseudarthrosis
  after Cotrel-Dubousset instrumentation for lumbar fixation, 211

late deformities and, 453
spondylodiscitis differentiated from, 387, 397–406
and thoracolumbar fractures in ankylosing spondylitis, 387
Pseudomyotonia (complex repetitive discharges), in electromyography, 114, 115
Psoas stripe, loss of, in ABCS approach to plain film interpretation, 82, 83
Psychologic problems, after spinal cord injury, rehabilitation and, 481
PTH. See Parathyroid hormone
Pudendal nerve, neurographic testing of, 110
Pudenz valve, for draining a syrinx, 441
Pulmonary dysfunction, in spinal cord injury, 170–171, 409–410, 474
rehabilitation and, 481
Pulmonary emboli, in spinal cord injury, 409
Pulmonary function tests, in spinal cord injury, 170, 410
Pulse oximetry, spinal cord oxygenation monitored by, 168

Q
Quadriplegia (quadriparesis), from spinal cord injury, 62
Quantitative computed tomography, for bone mass measurement, 350

R
Radial nerve, neurographic testing of, 109, 110
Radiation therapy, for spinal tumors, neural function preservation and, 367–368
Radices spinales. See Nerve roots
Radiculopathy, in children, 319–320
Radiography, conventional
in children's spinal injuries, 321
in osteoporotic vertebral fractures, 346–347
in sacral fractures, 245
in spinal tumors, 364–365
in thoracic and lumbar vertebral fractures, 69–84
ABCS approach in evaluation of, 73, 80, 81–84
and assessment of post-traumatic vertebral stability, 84
diagnostic considerations in, 73–81
pitfalls of, 84
technical considerations in, 69–73

Range of motion exercises, passive, in early management of spinal cord injury, 174
Recessus lateralis. See Lateral recess
Rectal exam, in thoracic spine fracture
in apparently neurologically intact person, 159
in paraplegic, 160–162
diagnosing level and, 162
Reduction
of alar fractures with pelvic instability, 246
of bilateral facet dislocation, 237
in conservative treatment of thoracolumbar fractures, 179
results of, 191–192
of late deformity, 455
operative, dangers of in ankylosing spondylitis, 391–393
of thoracic vertebral fractures, 199
of unilateral facet dislocation, 237
Reflexes
tendon, in post-traumatic syringomyelia, 435
in thoracic spine fracture
in apparently neurologically intact person, 159
in paraplegic, 160
diagnosing level and, 162
Rehabilitation, 463–483
ambulation and, 477
bladder dysfunction and, 479–480
bowel dysfunction and, 479–480
electrodiagnostic studies and, 469–472
electromyography and, 469–470
evoked potentials and, 471–472
functional assessment and, 464–465
functional electrical stimulation and, 477–479
functional goals and, 475
functional restoration and, 476–477
nerve conduction measurement studies and, 470–471
for neurologically intact patient with thoracolumbar fracture, 472–473
orthotic management of fractured spine and, 465–469
paralysis and, 476–481
for patient with spinal cord injury, 473–482
acute, 473–475
follow-up-care, 481–482
inpatient, 475–481
outpatient, 481–482
prognosis and, 482
principles of, 463–464
sensory loss and, 476–481

systemic problems and, 480–481
team for, 464
wheelchairs and, 477
Rehabilitation medicine. See also Rehabilitation
definition of, 463
Remodeling, bone
menopause affecting, 342–344
and osteoporotic fractures, 341–342
Renal cancer, spinal metastasis in, 381, 382
Renal failure, in spinal cord injury, 415
Renal osteodystrophy, vertebral crush fractures in, 348
Renal stones, in spinal cord injury, 415
Respiratory dysfunction, in spinal cord injury, 170–171, 409–410, 474
rehabilitation and, 481
Respiratory failure, in spinal cord injury, 409, 410
Resuscitation, spinal cord, 167–168
Retroperitoneal approach
for anterior techniques of decompression and fixation, 260–261
flank, for low lumbar burst fractures, 230–231
paramedian, for low lumbar burst fractures, 231–232
for spinal tumors, 370
Reversal phase, of bone remodeling, 342
Rezaian device, for anterior fixation and fracture reduction in thoracic burst fractures, 270
Rheumatoid arthritis, ankylosing spondylitis differentiated from, 385
"Rheumatoid" spondylitis. See Ankylosing spondylitis
Rhizotomy, for hypertonic bladder, 415
Rim fracture, 317–319
treatment of, 324
Ring margin, posterior avulsion of, 317–319
Risser-Cotrel frame
for reduction of thoracic fractures, 199
for reduction of thoracolumbar fractures, 179
Rod sleeves (Edwards), 283
biomechanical testing of, 289
Rods. See also specific type
for anterior fixation and fracture reduction in thoracic burst fractures, 269, 270
for fixation in lumbar fractures, 209

Root escape, in injuries at T12-L1 level, 164
Root stimulation, magnetoelectric, for motor evoked potentials, 107
Rotary injuries, 54, 55
  CT scan of, 87, 88
  mechanism of, 77
  MRI of, 95
  radiography of, 77–78
Rotational malalignment, as late deformity, 453
Rotational movements. *See also* Rotary injuries
  thoracolumbar spine affected by, 48–49
  fracture/dislocation and, 54, 55
Roy-Camille plates and screws, 288
  biomechanical evaluation of, 289, 290, 291
  for thoracic vertebral fractures, 199
"Rugger jersey" spine, 348

S

S1, characteristics of, 14–15
S2, characteristics of, 15
Sacral burst fractures, 248
  treatment of, 249
Sacral canal, 15
Sacral fractures, 165, 245–249
  classification of, 245–249
  diagnosis and management of, 245–249
  roentgenographic findings of, 245
  zone I (alar zone), 246
  zone II (foraminal zone), 246–248
  zone III (central sacral canal), 248–249
Sacral sciatica, foraminal fractures and, 246–248
Sacral screws
  for fixation in lumbar fractures, 208, 209
  insertion of, anatomic rudiments of, 29–32
Sacral spine. *See also* Spine
  anatomy of, implant insertion and, 11–33
  organogenesis of, 1–10
Sacral vertebrae, first two, 14–15
Sacrotuberous ligament avulsion, in alar fracture with pelvic instability, 247
Sacrum (ala), 14–15
  organogenesis and ossification of, 6, 7
Sagittal index, 155
  in late deformities, 453
Sagittal profile, and low lumbar burst fractures, 223–224
  anterior approach for surgery of, 232, 233

Salmon calcitonin, in acute management of osteoporotic vertebral fractures, 353
Saphenous nerve, neurographic testing of, 109
Sarcoma, Ewing's, of spine, 379
SCBF. *See* Spinal cord blood flow
Schantz screws, in Dick internal fixator, 287
Scheuermann's disease
  osteoporosis differentiated from, 349, 350
  and spinal cord injury without radiographic abnormalities (SCIWORA), 320–321
Schmorl's nodes, in osteoporosis, 347
SCI. *See* Spinal cord injury
Sciatica, sacral, foraminal fractures and, 246–248
SCIWORA (spinal cord injury without radiographic abnormalities), in children
  incidence of, 309, 320–321
  pathophysiology of medullary lesions in, 320–321
  treatment of, 324
Sclerotome, migration of, 2, 3–6, 7
  chondrification stage of, 3, 4
  ossification stage of, 4–6, 7
  precartilaginous stage of, 3, 4
Scoliosis
  hemivertebra and, 8
  as late deformity, 453
  after spinal injury in children, 323
Seat belt fractures, 54, 74, 75, 134, 135, 138, 148–149, 150. *See also* Flexion/distraction injuries
  in children, 315–316
    spinal stability after, 323
    treatment of, 324
  fixation for, 203
  mechanism of, 195–196, 197
  treatment of, 189
    in children, 324
Senegas plate, for anterior fixation and fracture reduction in thoracic burst fractures, 269, 270
Sensibility, in thoracic spine fracture
  in apparently neurologically intact person, 159
  in paraplegic, 160
    diagnosing level and, 162
Sensory loss
  in post-traumatic syringomyelia, 434–435
  spinal cord injury rehabilitation and, 476–481
Sensory nerve action potential, 111
Sensory nerve conduction, 111–112
  case study of, 117

SEPs. *See* Somatosensory evoked potentials
Septicemia, in spinal cord injury dialysis patients, 415
Sexual dysfunction, in spinal cord injury rehabilitation, 480
Shear forces. *See also* Shearing injuries
  thoracolumbar spine affected by, 48
Shearing injuries
  in ankylosing spondylitis, 387
  mechanism of, 78, 79
  radiography of, 78, 79
SIADH. *See* Syndrome of inappropriate antidiuretic hormone secretion
Single motor unit action potentials, in electromyography, 113, 115
Single photon absorptiometry, for bone mass measurement, 350, 350–351
Sinus arrest, in spinal cord injury, 411
Slot device, for anterior fixation and fracture reduction in thoracic spine burst fractures, 267, 270
SNAP. *See* Sensory nerve action potential
Social worker, rehabilitation, 481
Sodium, acute spinal cord injury affecting extracellular concentration of, 40–41
Sodium fluoride, in chronic management of osteoporotic vertebral fractures, 355
Soft tissue damage, MRI of, 95
Soft tissue mass, paraspinal, in ABCS approach to plain film interpretation, 82, 83
Solitary plasmacytoma, spinal, 375, 376
Somatic reflexes, spinal centers for, 36
Somatosensory evoked potentials, 100–105, 472
  body temperature affecting, 105
  case study of, 117
  median nerve, 102
  nerves stimulated by and muscles recorded from for level diagnosis, 100
  neural structures evaluated by, 99
  nomenclature of, 102–105
  normal values of, 102–105
  peripheral neuropathies affecting, 105
  peroneal nerve, 104, 105
  in rehabilitation of spinal fractures, 472
  stimulation and recording techniques for, 100–102
  sural nerve, 104, 105

tibial nerve, 103–104
waveforms of, 102–105
Somite, development of, 2, 3
Somitus. *See* Somite
Sonography. *See* Ultrasonography
SPA. *See* Single photon absorptiometry
Spasticity, in spinal cord injury, rehabilitation and, 480
Spatial summation, and motor evoked potentials, 107
Sphincterotomy, for hypertonic bladder, 415
Spina bifida, 7
Spina bifida occulta, 7
Spinal adhesive arachnoiditis, syringomyelia caused by, 433, 436
Spinal arteries, 19–21, 37
  anterior, 19, 37
  posterior, 37
Spinal canal, decompression of, with intraoperative ultrasonography, 127–128. *See also* Decompression surgery
Spinal cerebellar tract
  anterior ventral, 37
  posterior, 37
Spinal column. *See* Vertebral column
Spinal cord. *See also* Spine
  cysts of. *See also* Syringomyelia
    intraoperative ultrasonography of, 128–130
  edema of, MRI demonstrating, 96
  embryology of, 35
  funicles of, 19
  growth patterns of, 2, 3
  injury of. *See* Spinal cord injury
  lesions of
    complete, 163–165
      at T11-T12 vertebral level, 163–164
      at T12-L1 vertebral level, 164
      timing of surgery for, 180–181
    in traumatic spine and spinal cord injuries in children, evolution of, 330
  meninges of, 35–36
  morphology of, 36–37
  neuromeningeal dynamics and, 37–38
  vascularization of, 19–21, 37
Spinal cord blood flow, in acute injury, 40
Spinal cord injury. *See also* Spine trauma; Vertebral column, injuries of
  acute, 38–40
  age and, 59, 61, 67
  in ankylosing spondylitis, 391–393
  autonomic dysfunction in, 169–170, 170, 411–412, 416
    rehabilitation and, 480
  biochemical derangement and, 40–41, 174–175
  bladder dysfunction in, 171, 174, 414–415, 474
    rehabilitation and, 479–480
  bladder innervation affected in, 414–415
  bowel dysfunction in, rehabilitation and, 479–480
  cardiovascular complications in, 169–170, 410–411
    rehabilitation and, 480–481
  causes of, 61–62
  in children
    epidemiology of, 308–309
    without radiographic abnormalities (SCIWORA)
      incidence of, 309, 320–321
      pathophysiology of medullary lesions in, 320–321
      treatment of, 324
    spinal deformities secondary to, 327–337
  complications of, 409–419, 476. *See also specific type*
  electrolyte disorders and, 171
  emergency management of, 173–174
  endocrine complications and, 416–418
  epidemiology of, 59–63, 65–68
  ethnicity and, 66–67
  functional impairment and, 62
  gastrointestinal complications and, 171, 415–416
  genitourinary complications and, 171, 413–415
  hemodynamic changes and, 40
  heterotopic ossification and, 412–413
  incidence of, 59–60, 66–67
  intensive care of patient with, 167–172
    indications for admission and, 167
  intraoperative ultrasonography in evaluation of, 130
  joint contractures in, rehabilitation and, 480
  male to female ratio of, 60, 61, 66–67
  management of
    early, 173–178, 473–475
    in intensive care unit, 167–172
    medical, 174–175
    principles of, 173–174
    surgical, 175–178, 180–184, 185–188
    results of, 191–193
  mechanical insult in, 38–40
  metabolic disturbances in, 416–418
    rehabilitation and, 480
  MRI demonstrating, 93, 96–97
  neurologic assessment of, 41–42
  nutrition and, 171
  pain and, rehabilitation and, 480
  paralysis and, rehabilitation program for, 476–481
  prognosis and, 116, 482
  psychological implications of, rehabilitation and, 481
  without radiographic abnormalities (SCIWORA), in children
    incidence of, 309, 320–321
    pathophysiology of medullary lesions in, 320–321
    treatment of, 324
  rehabilitation in, 473–482
    acute care and, 473–475
    ambulation and, 477
    follow-up care, 481–482
    functional electrical stimulation in, 477–479
    functional goals for, 475
    functional restoration and, 476–477
    inpatient, 475–481
      goals of, 476
    outpatient, 481–482
    prognosis and, 482
    team for, 464
    wheelchairs in, 477
  respiratory complications in, 170–171, 409–410
    rehabilitation and, 481
  seasonality affecting incidence of, 61
  sensory loss and, rehabilitation program for, 476–481
  sexual dysfunction in, rehabilitation and, 480
  social implications of, rehabilitation and, 481
  spasticity in, rehabilitation and, 480
  spinal cord resuscitation and, 167–168
  sports- and recreation-related, 62
  thromboembolic complications and, 412
    prevention of, 171, 412
  urinary complications and, 171, 413–415
  vocational implications of, rehabilitation and, 481
Spinal cord resuscitation, 167–168
Spinal curvature, 17–19, 49
  development of, 8–9
Spinal deformities
  late, 449–462
    definition of stability and, 450–452

Spinal deformities, late (contd.)
   presentation of, 452–453
   risks for progression of, 453–454
   stable, 452
   treatment of, 455–457
     clinical outcome and, 457
     conservative, 455
     preferred technique for, 457–460
   unstable, 452
  progressive, risks for, 453–454
  after traumatic spine and spinal cord injuries in children, 327–337
   and evolution of bony/cartilaginous/and ligamentous lesions, 329–330
   and evolution of spinal cord and nervous system lesions, 330
   at level of lesion, 329–333
   at levels below lesion, 333–337
   normal growth of spine and, 327–329
   pathophysiology of, 329–330, 333–335
   prevention of, 335–336
   treatment of, 330–333, 335–337
Spinal fractures. See also Thoracolumbar fractures; Vertebral fractures
  in ankylosing spondylitis, 385–408
   and differentiation of fracture pseudarthrosis from spondylodiscitis, 397–406
   flexion injuries of neck and, 388–395, 396
   mechanism of, 385–387
   spinal cord injury and, 391–393
  orthotic management of, 465–469
Spinal injury rehabilitation team, 464
Spinal instrumentation. See Fixation
Spinal jacket, custom-molded, 468–469
Spinal ligaments, 16
  tension forces affecting, 48
  disruption and, 54
Spinal nerves, in three month embryo, 2
Spinal orthoses, 465–469. See also specific type
Spinal roots, 21–22
Spinal shock, 41, 410–411
  bradycardia in, 169, 411
  in children, 319
  hypotension in, 169, 410–411
  management of, 169–170
Spinal tumors. See also specific type
  anatomical considerations and, 360–361
  differential diagnosis of, 363
  imaging studies of, 364–365
  incidence of, 359–360
  location of, 363
  metastatic, 379–382
  neurologic deficits from, 363–364
   treatment decisions and, 361
  pain caused by, treatment decisions and, 361
  pathological fractures and, 363–364
  presentation of, 361–363
  primary, 372, 375–379
   benign, 372–375
   incidence of, 359
   malignant, 375–379
  surgical management of, 359–384
   anterior approaches and instrumentation in, 369–370, 371
   approaches for, 369–372
   combined approaches for, 372
   goals of, 365–369
   indications for, 363
   posterior approaches and instrumentation in, 372
  treatment decisions and, 361–363
Spine. See also Spinal cord; Vertebral column
  in ankylosing spondylitis, 385
  biopsy of, 361–362
  bone-related anomalies of, 8–9
  combined neurologic and bone anomalies of, 7
  curvature of. See Spinal curvature
  electrophysiology of (electrodiagnostic testing of), 99–121
   autonomic techniques and, 116
   case study of, 116–118
   electromyography, 112–116
    in rehabilitation, 469–470
   evoked potentials
    motor, 105–108, 109
    in rehabilitation, 471–472
    somatosensory, 100–105
   nerve conduction studies, 110–112
    in rehabilitation, 470–471
   neurography, 109–112
   in post-traumatic syringomyelia, 424
   prognosis of spinal cord trauma and, 116, 482
   in rehabilitation, 469–472
  external support of, 50
  growth of, 9, 327–329
   patterns of, 2, 3
  organization of, 49–50
  organogenesis of, 1–7
  organogenetic defects of, 7–9
  ossification of, 1–3, 4–6, 7
  overview of, 17–19
  sagittal curvatures of, 49
  trauma to. See Spine trauma
  tumor-like lesions affecting, 375
  tumors of. See Spinal tumors
Spine trauma (spine injuries). See also specific type and Spinal cord injury
  calculated angles in, 18, 19
  causes of, 61
  in children, 307–325
   anterior ring epiphysis avulsion, 317
   burst fractures, 314, 315
    treatment of, 324
   classification of, 311–319
   clinical diagnosis of, 319–320
   compression fractures, 311–315
    treatment of, 323–324
   computed tomography of, 321
   epidemiology of, 308–309
   fracture/dislocations, 316
    treatment of, 324
   fractures, 308–309
   imaging in, 321
   magnetic resonance imaging of, 321
   myelography of, 321
   neurocentral cartilage separation, 318, 319
   pars interarticularis fractures, 319
   pathoanatomy and, 311
   posterior avulsion of ring margin epiphysis (rim fracture), 317–319
   radiography of, 321
   seat belt injuries, 315–316
    treatment of, 324
   spinal deformities secondary to, 327–337
   spine stability after, 321–323
   tomography of, 321
   treatment of, 323–324
   vertebral growth and, 309–310
  intraoperative ultrasonography in, 123–130
   basic physics underlying, 123
   cord trauma evaluation and, 130
   cystic myelopathy and, 128–130
   decompression of spinal canal and, 127–128
   normal anatomy and, 124, 125–126
   technique for, 123–125
Spinotectalis tract, 37
Spinous process
  development of, 3
  structure of, 12
Spinous process plates, 280–281
Splanchnic vasoconstriction, in autonomic dysreflexia, 411
Spondylitis, ankylosing
  rheumatoid arthritis differentiated from, 385

spinal fractures in, 385–408
  and differentiation of fracture
    pseudarthrosis from
    spondylodiscitis, 397–406
  flexion injuries of neck and,
    388–395, 396
  mechanism of, 385–387
  spinal cord injuries and, 391–393
Spondylodiscitis, pseudarthrosis
  differentiated from, 387,
  397–406
Spondylolisthesis
  as late deformity, 453
  MRI of, 93
Spondylolysis, isthmic,
  microtraumatic injuries
  causing, 319
Spontaneous activity, in
  electromyography, 113–114,
  115
Sports injuries, spinal, 62
SSR. See Sympathetic skin response
Stability
  of burst fractures, 215–216
    radiographic criteria for, 216
  spinal, 51. See also Instability
    late deformities and, 450–452
    post-traumatic
      assessment of, 84
      in children, 321–323
    and surgery for spinal tumors,
      365–367
Stabilization surgery. See also
  Fixation
  for bilateral facet dislocation, 237
  in early spinal cord injury
    management, 175–178
  for secondary spinal deformities, at
    level of injury, 331
  for spinal tumors, 365–367, 368–369
Stable injuries, 55
Steffee pedicular screw-plate system,
  288
Steffee plates
  biomechanical evaluation of, 270,
    289, 291
  for posterior fixation and fracture
    reduction in thoracic spine,
    251–252
Steffee screws, biomechanical
  evaluation of, 290
Steroids, for acute spinal cord injury,
  41, 168, 175
  gastrointestinal bleeding and, 415
"Straight ahead" ("droit devant")
  technique, 26–28
Stress ulcers, and gastrointestinal
  bleeding in spinal cord injury,
  415–416
Subluxation
  facet, 238–242

with low lumbar burst fracture, 224,
  225
Sucralfate, for prophylaxis of GI
  bleeding in spinal cord injury,
  171
Superoxide dismutase, in acute spinal
  cord injury, 41
Suprascapular nerve, neurographic
  testing of, 110
Supraspinous ligament, 16
  degree of elongation of prior to
    failure, 48
Sural nerve
  neurographic testing of, 109, 110
  somatosensory evoked potentials
    from, 104, 105
Surgery
  for bilateral facet dislocation, 237
  decompression. See also
    Decompression surgery
    anatomic rudiments of, 24
    anterior techniques of, 251–266
    with intraoperative
      ultrasonography, 127–128
    in early spinal cord injury
      management, 175–178
    for fixation. See also Fixation
      anterior techniques of, 251–266
    for lumbar fractures, 206–212
    orthopaedic principles of, 179–194
    for post-traumatic syringomyelia,
      424–427
      results of, 426–427
      technique for, 425–426
    for spinal cord injury, dural tears
      and, 176
    for spinal tumors, 359–384
      anterior approaches and
        instrumentation in, 369–370,
        371
      approaches for, 369–372
      combined approaches for, 372
      goals of, 365–369
      indications for, 363
      posterior approaches and
        instrumentation in, 372
    for thoracolumbar fractures
      anterior techniques of, 251–266
      without nerve compromise,
        188–190
      with neurologic compromise,
        180–184, 185–188
      technique for, 181–184,
        185–188
      timing of, 180–181
      results of, 191–193
Sweating disturbances, in post-
  traumatic syringomyelia,
  435–436
Sympathetic overactivity, in
  autonomic dysreflexia, 411

Sympathetic skin response, 100, 116
  neural structures evaluated by, 99
Sympathomimetics, for hemodynamic
  insult in spinal cord injury, 169
Syndrome of inappropriate
  antidiuretic hormone secretion,
  in spinal cord injury, 171
Syracuse I-plate
  for anterior fixation and fracture
    reduction in thoracic spine,
    252, 253
  for burst fractures, 269
    biomechanical evaluation of,
      270–271
    clinical results of, 272
Syringocisternal shunts, for post-
  traumatic syringomyelia, 425
Syringomyelia
  epidural abscess causing, 433
  meningitis causing, 433
  post-traumatic, 421–427, 429–448
    autonomic dysfunction and,
      435–436
    case studies of, 442–447
    and changes below the level of
      injury, 436
    in children, 330
    clinical presentation of, 423, 434
    conservative treatment of, 427
    cord division for, 442
    decompression surgery and, 199,
      200, 441
    drainage of, 424–425, 438
      to pleura or peritoneum, 441
    drains in management of, 442
    electrophysiological studies of,
      424
    endomyelography of, 423, 437
    enlargement of cystic spaces and,
      431–434
    epidemiology of, 421–422
    hematomyelia and, 431
    incidence of, 421, 429–430
    magnetic resonance imaging of,
      423–424, 437–438
    mechanisms of onset of, 431
    morphology of, 430, 431
    motor loss and, 435
    myelography of, 423, 436, 437
    pathogenesis of, 422
    pathology of, 422–423
    radiology of, 423–424, 436
    sensory loss and, 434–435
    structural changes and, 435
    surgical management of, 424–427
      future work in, 447
      indications for, 438
      principles of, 438–439
      results of, 426–427, 447
      standard operation for, 439–441
      technique for, 425–426
      timing of, 438

Syringomyelia, post-traumatic (*contd.*)
symptoms and signs of, 423, 434
syringosubarachnoid shunting for, 441
tendon reflexes affected in, 435
time of onset of, 431
treatment of, 438
ultrasonography of, 424
ultrastructural appearance of, 422–423
valves in management of, 441
spinal adhesive arachnoiditis causing, 433, 436
Syringoperitoneal shunts, for post-traumatic syringomyelia, 425, 441
Syringopleural shunts, for post-traumatic syringomyelia, 425, 441
surgical technique for, 425–426
Syringostomy, for post-traumatic syringomyelia, 424
Syringosubarachnoid shunting, for post-traumatic syringomyelia, 441
Syringosubdural shunts, for post-traumatic syringomyelia, 425

T

T1 to T10 vertebral fracture, 159–162
management of, 195–210
T1 to T11 incomplete thoracic lesions, 162–163
T7, growth of, 310
T11-T12 vertebral injuries, 163–164
T12
injuries at, 163–164
thoracolumbar transition at, 13–14
^{99m}Tc bone scan, in spinal tumors, 364
Teardrop fractures, 54
stability of, 56
Temperature
nerve conduction velocity affected by, 110
somatosensory evoked potentials affected by, 105
Temporal summation, and motor evoked potentials, 107
Tendon reflexes, in post-traumatic syringomyelia, 435
Tension forces, thoracolumbar spine affected by, 46–48
failure and, 53–54
Tethered chain concept, 320
Tetraplegia
and paralysis below level of injury, 333–334
vertebral growth affected by, 328
Texas Scottish Rite Hospital instrumentation, 285, 286

for preservation of sagittal profile in low lumbar burst fractures, 224
Thoracic cage, injury of, 195–201
associated lesions and, 197–198
description of, 195–196
internal fixation and, 199–201
mechanism of, 195
neurologic status after, 198
treatment of, 199–201
neurosurgical, 199, 200
Thoracic facet joints, anatomy and biomechanics of, 235–236
unilateral dislocation of, 237
Thoracic kyphosis, 17, 49
Thoracic spinal cord. *See also* Thoracic spine; Thoracic vertebrae
arteries of, 19–21
venous drainage of, 21
Thoracic spine. *See also* Spine; Thoracic spinal cord
anatomy of, 157
incomplete lesions of, 162–163
instability of, as late deformity, treatment of, 456–457
MRI for evaluation of, 71
neurologic injuries associated with fracture of, 159–164
normal radiographic appearance of, 70
organogenesis of, 1–10
tumors of. *See also* Spinal tumors
metastatic, incidence of, 360
neurologic deficits and, 360, 361
Thoracic vertebrae. *See also* Thoracic spine
characteristics of, 12, 13
fractures of, 185–201. *See also* Thoracolumbar fractures
associated lesions and, 197–198
description of, 195–196
internal fixation for, 199–201
mechanism of, 195
neurologic status after, 198
treatment of, 199
neurosurgical, 199, 200
nerve connections in, 19
radiography of, pitfalls of, 71
targeting for pedicular screw insertion, 26–28
Thoracoabdominal approach, for anterior techniques of decompression and fixation, 258–260
Thoracolumbar facet dislocation, complete bilateral, 236–237
Thoracolumbar fractures, 201–203, 204, 205. *See also specific type and* Spine trauma; Spinal fractures; Vertebral fractures
anatomic and physiologic considerations in, 201

in ankylosing spondylitis, 387
anterior techniques in management of, 251–266, 267–278
anterior surgical approaches for, 255–263
biomechanical evaluation of devices for, 270–271
historical review of, 251–254
indications for, 271
rationale for decompression and, 272
results of, 263–264, 272, 273
role of, 254–255
versus posterior surgery, 274, 275–277
burst. *See* Burst fractures
classification of, 131–156
historic perspective of, 131–141
instability and, 141, 450–451
late deformities and, 450–451
decompression surgery for, 180–184, 185–188
anterior techniques for, 251–266
deformity after, consequences of, 56
disruption of spinal components in, 51
and failure continuum with anterior column under compression, 51–53
and failure continuum with posterior elements under distraction, 53–54
and failure continuum with rotation combined with various loads, 54, 55
fixation for, 201–203, 204, 205
imaging of, 69–98
algorithm for, 97
applications of, 94–97
and assessment of post-traumatic vertebral stability, 84
in children, 321
computed tomography, 84–90
pitfalls of, 89–90
conventional radiography, 69–84
ABCS approach to, 73, 80, 81–84
and assessment of post-traumatic vertebral stability, 84
diagnostic considerations in, 73–81
pitfalls of, 84
technical considerations in, 69–73
magnetic resonance imaging, 90–97
myelography, 97
pluridirectional tomography, 90, 91, 92

Thoracolumbar fractures (contd.)
  late deformities following, 449–462
  management of
    conservative, 179–180, 215–222
      clinical outcome of, 219–220
      complications related to, 218
      controversial aspects of, 215
      and fate of unreduced
        intracanal bony fragments,
        218–219, 220
      indications for, 473
      radiographic changes over time
        following, 218
      results of, 191–192
    historical review of, 251–252
    rehabilitation principles in,
      463–483
    surgical
      anterior techniques for,
        251–266
      indications for, 472–473
      orthopaedic principles of,
        179–194
      results of, 191–193
  mechanical failure associated with,
    51–56
  without nerve compromise, surgery
    for, 188–190
  with neurologic compromise,
    surgery for, 180–184, 185–188
  osteoporotic, 339–358
    in spinal tumor differential
      diagnosis, 363
  pathologic
    metastatic disease causing, 348
    neoplastic infiltration causing,
      363–364
  posterior instrumentation for,
    279–306
    biomechanical testing of, 288–291
    devices available for, 279–288
    versus anterior approach, 274,
      275–277
  potential instability of, 54–56
  progressive deformity after, risks
    for, 453–454
  stability of, 54–56, 215–216
  types of, 201
Thoracolumbar junction, 17
  anatomy of, 157–159
  facet dislocations at, 236
  injuries at level of, 201. See also
    Thoracolumbar fractures
  instability of, as late deformity,
    treatment of, 455–456
Thoracolumbar spine. See also Spine
  accommodation of to load, 46–49
  anatomy of, 157–159
    implant insertion and, 11–33
  bending loads affecting, 49
  biomechanics of, 45–57

bony stability of, 158
compression loads affecting, 46–47
fractures of. See Thoracolumbar
  fractures
neurologic compromise caused by,
  361
organization of, 49–50
post-traumatic deformity of,
  consequences of, 56
potential vulnerability of, 45–46
protection of from mechanical
  failure, biomechanics of, 46
shear forces affecting, 48
stability of, 51
tension forces affecting, 48
torsional stresses affecting, 48–49
tumors of. See also specific type
    and Spinal tumors
  anatomical considerations and,
    360–361
  differential diagnosis of, 363
  imaging studies of, 364–365
  incidence of, 359–360
  location of, 363
  metastatic, incidence of, 360
  neurologic deficits from, 363–364
    treatment decisions and, 361
  pain caused by, treatment
    decisions and, 361
  pathological fractures and,
    363–364
  presentation of, 361–363
  surgical management of, 359–384
    anterior approaches and
      instrumentation in, 369–370,
      371
    approaches for, 369–372
    combined approaches for, 372
    goals of, 365–369
    indications for, 363
    posterior approaches and
      instrumentation in, 372
    treatment decisions and, 361–363
Thoracolumbar transitional vertebrae
  characteristics of, 13–14
  potential vulnerability of, 45–46
Thoracolumbosacral orthoses
  for secondary spinal deformities, at
    level of injury, 333
  for spinal fractures, 466, 467–469
Three-column concept of spine
  Denis', 133
  late deformities and, 449, 450
  Louis', 133
Three-dimensional computerized
  tomography, 88, 89
Three-zone classification of sacral
  fractures, 245–249
Thromboembolism, in spinal cord
  injury, 412
  heterotopic ossification
    differentiated from, 413

prevention of, 171, 412
  intermittent pneumatic
    compression stockings for,
    174
  pulmonary, 409
Thyrotropin-releasing hormone, in
  cord resuscitation, 168
Tibial nerve
  neurographic testing of, 109, 110
  somatosensory evoked potentials
    from, 103–104
TLSO. See Thoracolumbosacral
  orthoses
Tomography
  for children's spine injuries, 321
  computerized. See Computerized
    tomography
  pluridirectional, for thoracic and
    lumbar vertebral fractures, 90,
    91, 92
  for sacral fractures, 245
Torsion, thoracolumbar spine affected
  by, 48–49
  fracture/dislocation and, 54
  posterior fixation for, 293
Total contact TLSO, 468–469
Trabecular architecture, changes in in
  menopause, bone remodeling
  affected by, 343–344
Tracheostomy, for respiratory failure
  in spinal cord injury, 410
Traction, for alar fractures with pelvic
  instability, 246
Transcranial stimulation,
  magnetoelectric, for motor
  evoked potentials, 107
Translational injuries, 140
Transperitoneal anterior approach
  for low lumbar burst fractures, 232
  for spinal tumors, 370
Transthoracic approach, for anterior
  techniques of decompression
  and fixation, 256–258
Transverse process, 11
  development of, 3
  structure of, 12
Traumatic spinal cord injury. See
  Spinal cord injury
Triceps jerk, in post-traumatic
  syringomyelia, 435
Trilaminar embryonic disc, formation
  of, 1
TSRH. See Texas Scottish Rite
  Hospital instrumentation
Tuberculosis, in spinal tumor
  differential diagnosis, 363
Tuberculous meningitis, syringomyelia
  caused by, 433
Tubus neuralis. See Neural tube
Turner's syndrome, bone mass loss
  and, 343

U

Ulcers, stress, and gastrointestinal bleeding in spinal cord injury, 415–416
Ulnar nerve, neurographic testing of, 109, 110
Ultrasonography
  intraoperative, 123–130
    basic physics underlying, 123
    for cord trauma evaluation, 130
    in cystic myelopathy, 128–130
    decompression of spinal canal and, 127–128
    normal anatomy and, 124, 125–126
    for post-traumatic syringomyelia, 424
    technique for, 123–125
  postoperative, for post-traumatic syringomyelia, 424
Unstable injuries, 55
Urinary bladder
  catheterization of in spinal cord injury, 171, 414–415
    early management and, 174, 474
  distension of, autonomic dysreflexia caused by, 411
  dysfunction of
    in late deformities, 452
    in spinal cord injuries, 171, 174, 414–415, 474
      rehabilitation and, 479–480
  innervation of, spinal cord injury and, 414–415
  neurogenic. *See also* Bladder, dysfunction of
    rehabilitation and, 479
Urodynamics, in diagnosing level of paraplegia, 162
Uterine contractions, autonomic dysreflexia and, 412

V

Valves, for draining a syrinx, 441
Vasodilatation, in spinal shock, 410
Vasodilators, for hypertension in autonomic dysreflexia, 412
Ventilation, mechanical, for respiratory failure in spinal cord injury, 170
Ventral horn, 36
Vermont fixator, biomechanical evaluation of, 289, 290
Vertebra plana, in tumor-like lesions affecting spine, 375
Vertebrae, 11–12
  external configuration of, 11–12
  fractures of. *See* Vertebral fractures
  growth of, 309–310, 327–328
  lumbar
    characteristics of, 12–13
    nerve connections in, 19
    targeting for pedicular screw insertion, 26–28
  ossification of, 4–6, 7
  pile arrangement of, 50
  sacral, first two, 14–15
  spine growth at level of, 327–328
  structure of, 12
  thoracic, characteristics of, 12, 13
  thoracolumbar transitional, characteristics of, 13–14
Vertebral arch, 11–12
Vertebral body, 11
  bending loads affecting, 49
  compression loads affecting, 47–48
  fractures of, 53. *See also* Vertebral fractures
    epidemiology of, 60–61
  structure of, 12
  tension forces affecting, 48
Vertebral body plates, biomechanical evaluation of, 289
Vertebral canal, encroachment of in spinal injury, CT scan of, 87
Vertebral column. *See also* Spine
  alignment and anatomy
    abnormalities of, 81–82
    MRI of, 93
  angles of, 18–19
  bony integrity abnormalities of, 82
  cartilage or joint space abnormalities of, 82, 83
  injuries of. *See also* Spinal cord injury
    epidemiology of, 60–62
  overview of, 17–19
  pile arrangement of, 50
  post-traumatic stability of, assessment of, 84
  radiography of in trauma, 73
  soft tissue abnormalities of, 82–84
Vertebral deformities, in osteoporosis, radiologic evaluation of, 346–347
Vertebral foramina, sagittal and transverse diameters of, 22
Vertebral fractures. *See also* Spinal fractures; Spine trauma
  asymptomatic, osteoporotic fractures differentiated from, 348
  in children, epidemiology of, 308–309
  debridement of with anterior approach, 261–263
  epidemiology of, 60–62
  imaging of, 69–98
    algorithm for, 97
    applications of, 94–97
    and assessment of post-traumatic vertebral stability, 84
    in children, 321
    computerized tomography, 84–90
      pitfalls of, 89–90
    conventional radiography, 69–84
      ABCS approach to, 73, 80, 81–84
      and assessment of post-traumatic vertebral stability, 84
      diagnostic considerations in, 73–81
      pitfalls of, 84
      technical considerations in, 69–73
    magnetic resonance imaging, 90–97
    myelography, 97
    osteoporosis and, 346–347
    pluridirectional tomography, 90, 91, 92
  metastatic disease causing, 348
  in osteogenesis imperfecta, 350
  in osteomalacia, 348
  osteoporotic, 339–358
    age-related bone loss and, 344
    bone mass measurement and, 350–353
    bone remodeling and, 341–342
    calcium in management of, 354
    clinical features of, 344–346
    differential diagnosis of, 348–350
    epidemiology of, 339–340
    exercise in management of, 354
    incidence of, 340
    interrelationships among fractures and, 340
    menopause and, 342–344
    pain and, 345, 353–354
    pathophysiology of, 340–344
    pharmacologic therapy in management of, 354–355
    radiology of, 346–347
    in spinal tumor differential diagnosis, 363
    treatment of, 353–355
      acute, 353–354
      chronic, 354
  in Paget's disease, 348
  paraplegia associated with, 159–165
  pathologic
    metastatic disease causing, 348
    neoplastic infiltration causing, 363–364
  in primary hyperparathyroidism, 348–350
  in renal osteodystrophy, 348
  in Scheuermann's disease, 349, 350
  treatment of, in ankylosing spondylitis, 393

Vertebral isthmus, 11
Vertebral joints, 15–17. *See also specific type*
　intervertebral disc, 16
　junctura incorporealis, 15
　ligaments of, 16
　posterior, 16–17
Vertebrectomy, "eggshell," for late deformity, 455
Vesicoureteral dysfunction, in spinal cord injury, 415
Vitamin D deficiency, in osteomalacia, vertebral crush fractures and, 348
Vitamin E, for acute spinal cord injury, 41
Vocational counselor, rehabilitation and, 481

Volume loading, for hypotension in spinal cord injury, 169

W

Watson-Jones classification, of thoracolumbar fractures, 131
Weaning, from mechanical ventilation, 170–171
Wedge fractures, 140
　instability of, 55
　osteoporotic, 340
　　radiology of, 347
Weight loss, in spinal cord injury, 417–418
Weiss springs, 282–283
　biomechanical evaluation of, 289
Wheelchairs, 477

White matter, spinal, 36, 37
"Winking owl" sign, 360

Y

Yuan plate, for anterior fixation and fracture reduction in thoracic burst fractures, 269, 270
　clinical results of, 272

Z

Zielke device
　for anterior fixation and fracture reduction in thoracic burst fractures, 267, 270
　biomechanical evaluation of, 291
Zone of partial pressure, 474